The SAGE Handbook of

Social Studies in Health and Medicine

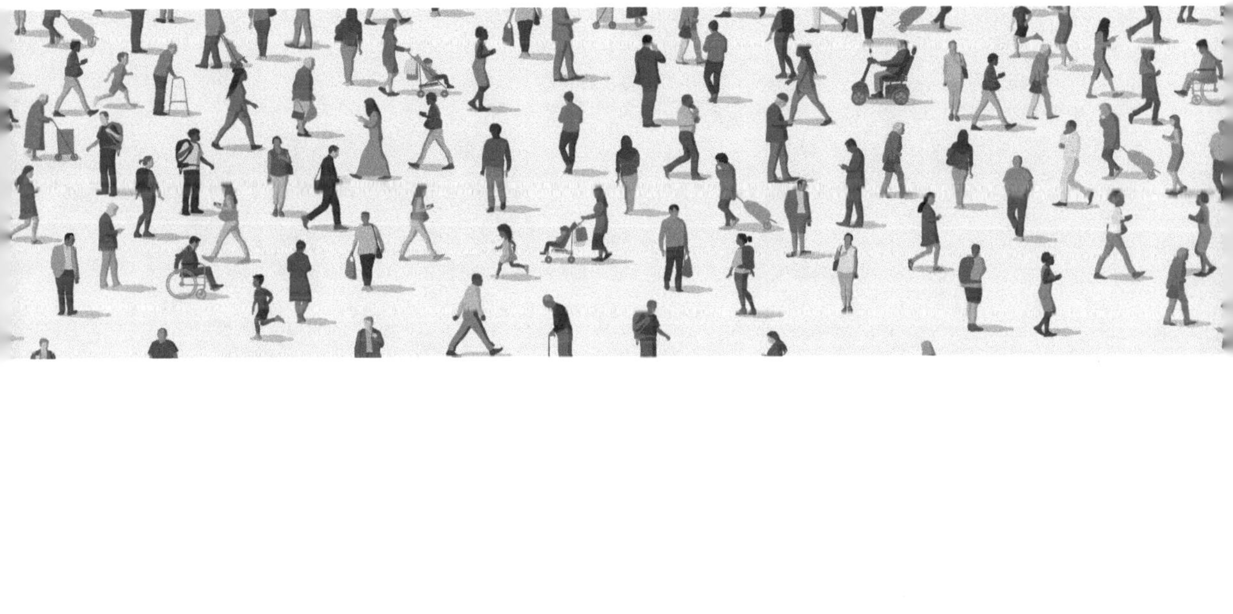

The SAGE Handbook of

Social Studies in Health and Medicine

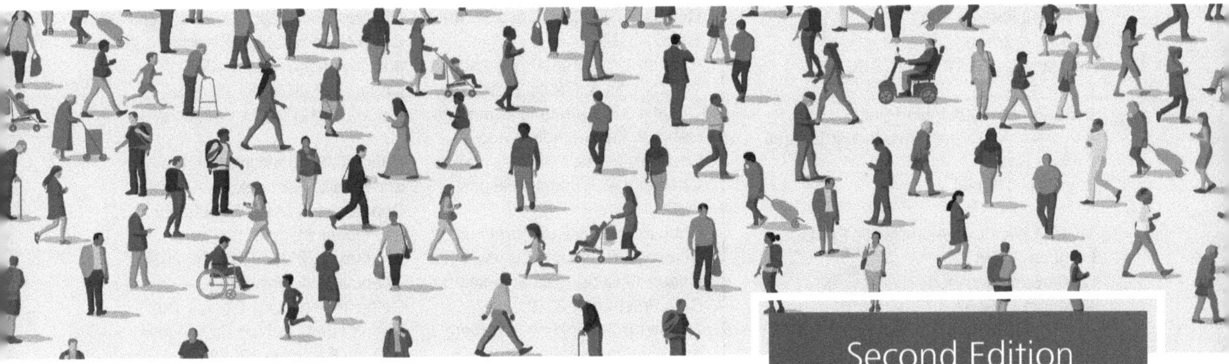

Second Edition

Edited by

Susan C. Scrimshaw

Sandra D. Lane

Robert A. Rubinstein

and Julian Fisher

SAGE reference

Los Angeles | London | New Delhi | Singapore | Washington DC | Melbourne

SAGE

Los Angeles | London | New Delhi
Singapore | Washington DC | Melbourne

SAGE Publications Ltd
1 Oliver's Yard
55 City Road
London EC1Y 1SP

SAGE Publications Inc.
2455 Teller Road
Thousand Oaks, California 91320

SAGE Publications India Pvt Ltd
B 1/I 1 Mohan Cooperative Industrial Area
Mathura Road
New Delhi 110 044

SAGE Publications Asia-Pacific Pte Ltd
3 Church Street
#10-04 Samsung Hub
Singapore 049483

Editor: Natalie Aguilera
Assistant Editor: Eve Williams
Production Editor: Prachi Arora
Copyeditor: Sarah Bury
Proofreader: Derek Markham
Indexer: Cathryn Pritchard
Marketing Manager: Chazelle Keeton
Cover Design: Naomi Robinson
Typeset by Cenveo Publisher Services
Printed and bound by CPI Group (UK) Ltd, Croydon, CR0 4YY

MIX
Paper from responsible sources
FSC www.fsc.org FSC® C013604

Library of Congress Control Number: 2021948537

British Library Cataloguing in Publication data

A catalogue record for this book is available from the British Library

978-1-5264-4066-2

Contents

List of Figures

List of Tables

List of Boxes

Notes on the Editors and Contributors

THE EDITORS

Susan C. Scrimshaw, PhD, was an editor and author for the first edition of this Handbook. She is a medical anthropologist who grew up in Guatemala and has worked globally, particularly in Latin America and with Latino and African American populations in the US. She was Dean of the University of Illinois at Chicago School of Public Health, and President of Russell Sage College. She was elected to the National Academy of Medicine in 1993, and is a Fellow of the American Anthropological Association, the Society for Applied Anthropology and the American Association for the Advancement of Science. Her awards include the Margaret Mead Award, the Adam Yarmolinsky Medal, and a Hero of Public Health Gold Medal presented by former President Vicente Fox of Mexico. Her research includes community participatory research methods, combining qualitative and quantitative research, health disparities, pregnancy outcomes, health communication, and culturally appropriate delivery of health care.

Sandra D. Lane is Laura J. and L. Douglas Meredith Professor of teaching excellence in Public Health and Anthropology at Syracuse University and a Research Professor in the Department of Obstetrics and Gynecology at Upstate Medical University. She received her PhD in medical anthropology from the joint program at the University of California at San Francisco and Berkeley, and an MPH in epidemiology from the University of California at Berkeley. Her research focuses on the impact of racial, ethnic and gender disadvantage on maternal, child, and family health in urban areas of the United States and the Middle East. She is the recipient of the 2019 George Foster Practicing Medical Anthropology Award from the Society for Medical Anthropology.

Robert A. Rubinstein, PhD, MsPH is a distinguished Professor of Anthropology and Professor of International Relations at the Maxwell School of Syracuse University. His medical anthropology work is on infectious eye disease, psychosocial epidemiology, health inequalities, and on integrating epidemiological and anthropological methods. His political anthropology research focuses on cross-cultural aspects of conflict and dispute resolution. He is an originator of the field of the anthropology of peacekeeping, in which he has conducted empirical research and policy studies. Rubinstein has collaborated with the International Peace Academy, the United Nations Departments of Peacekeeping Operations and Internal Oversight Services, and the United States Army Peacekeeping Institute. He is the author or editor of nine books and more than 100 journal articles and book chapters. He received the 2016 Victor Sidel and Barry Levy Award for Peace from the American Public Health Association, and the 2010 Robert B. Textor and Family Prize for Anticipatory Anthropology from the American Anthropological Association.

Julian Fisher is a policy advisor and analyst with focused expertise in lifelong learning, health workforce education, social and environmental determinants of health, and health in all policy approaches. Julian holds adjunct teaching positions: Research Assistant Professor, Department of Public Health and Preventive Medicine (SUNY Upstate Medical University, New York, USA), and School of Health Sciences and Public Health (University of Georgia, Tbilisi, Georgia). He is on the Board of Directors of the World Accelerated Medically Trained Clinicians Network. His work experience covers a diverse range of professional domains, including international public health policy and advocacy (consultancies for UN agencies including WHO, UNESCO and UNEP), health profession (federation) management, health workforce undergraduate and postgraduate education, both classroom and web-based. His work has been based in geographical locations, including Europe, Africa (Tanzania, South Africa), Saudi Arabia, Falkland Islands and Antarctica within various sectors and organizations. Julian Fisher earned his BDS (Dentistry) from Birmingham University in 1985, a MSc (HIV/AIDS) from Stellenbosch University, South Africa in 2002, and a MIH (International Health) from Charité University, Berlin in 2006.

THE CONTRIBUTORS

Corinne Yawę'nęhà·wi' Abrams, MPH, her name means "She Carries the Day." She is an enrolled member of the Tuscarora Nation, within the state of New York. She follows the traditional ways and teachings of the Longhouse. She received her Master of Public Health in Environmental Health and Epidemiology from the University at Buffalo. In addition, her research interests include food sovereignty, and health disparities for Native American populations.

Vinya Ariyaratne, MD, MPH, MSc is a physician by training and a Board Certified Specialist in Community Medicine. He is a past President of the College of Community Physicians of Sri Lanka (CCPSL). Dr Vinya Ariyaratne is the President of the Sarvodaya Shramadana Movement, which is Sri Lanka's largest non-governmental grassroots development organization. Dr Ariyaratne also serves as the Director General of the newly established Sarvodaya Institute of Higher Learning (SIHL) and as a board member of Sarvodaya Development Finance (SDF), the economic empowerment arm of the Sarvodaya Movement.

Nesrine Benyahia has a PhD in Health Law from Descartes University at Paris. After several years in the medical device industry, she joined a law firm by creating the e-health and data protection department. In 2018, Nesrine founded Dr Data, a company dedicated to health data protection and valorization, which is her main professional activity as CEO. She is an associate member of the Law & Health Institute at Paris (Inserm), and the President of the digital department at the French Health Digital Society. Nesrine is also certified from MIT Business School in Blockchain technologies, and ISO27001 Lead implementer for health information system security.

Dessa Bergen-Cico, PhD, is a Professor of Public Health and Coordinator of the Addiction Studies Program, and Neuroscience faculty at Syracuse University, USA. Dessa is an Affiliated Research Investigator at the Veterans Administration Center for Integrative Healthcare, a Fellow of the American Academy of Health Care Providers in the Addictive Disorders. Dessa has earned two Fulbright Research awards and has conducted site-based research on substance use and recovery in the Republic of Georgia and Thailand. Dr Bergen-Cico is the author of more than 50 scholarly publications, including the book *War and Drugs: The Role of Military Conflict in the Development of Substance Abuse* (2012, 2015, Routledge).

Christopher Boudreaux is an associate professor of economics at Florida Atlantic University and a research fellow for the Phil Smith Center for Free Enterprise. His research interests include entrepreneurship, innovation, and the economic analysis of public policy. He received his PhD and MS from Florida State University and his BS from Nicholls State University.

Martina Breuning, Dr. phil., is a psychologist and researcher at the University Clinic Freiburg, Germany. Since 2008 she has been conducting qualitative research and teaching qualitative methods. Her current research interests include the gains and challenges of multifaceted applications of patient experiences in the health sector and new ways of participation. She is a member of the international collaboration, DIPEx international, which is engaged in the collection, analysis and application of patients' narratives worldwide.

Annette Burns is a psychologist researching loneliness at Ulster University and the Institute of Public Health in Ireland since 2018. She has a background in Psychology (BA) and Applied Social Research (MSc) and completed a structured PhD in Population Health and Health Services Research exploring smoking in those with mental health difficulties in 2018. She is Chair of the Psychological Society of Ireland's Science and Public Policy Committee. Her research interest include loneliness, health inequalities, mental health, interventions and mixed methods research. She has led on and contributed to loneliness publications related to health care use, video call interventions, physical activity as well as consensus building on definitions, measurement and ongoing knowledge gaps in relation to loneliness in older adults.

Courtney Butler is a staff advisor within the College of Computer, Math and Natural Sciences at the University of Maryland, College Park, and a research associate with the Consortium of Race, Gender and Ethnicity. She formerly served as a healthcare administrator at Johns Hopkins University School of Medicine in the departments of Dermatology and Neurosurgery. Her research interests look to interrogate race/ethnicity, class, and gender as overlapping systems of inequality and their subsequent impacts on health. She received the 2019–2020 Provost's Professional Academic Advisor of the Year award.

Michael Calnan is a Professor of Medical Sociology who is involved with teaching and research in the Sociology of Health and Health Policy. His research has involved a mixture of theoretical, policy, and empirical analysis which has used both quantitative and qualitative methods. His recent funded research has included projects which have focused on trust in different health systems, dignity in health care for people in later life and the social influences on decision-making by the National Institute for Health and Care Excellence (NICE) in relation to technological appraisals. He has published extensively in journals and books about a range of health-related topics. His most recent book is entitled: *Health Policy, Power and Politics: Sociological Insights* (2020, Emerald).

Lorraine M. Conroy, ScD, CIH, is Professor and Division Director of Environmental and Occupational Health Sciences at the University of Illinois at Chicago (UIC), School of Public Health. She serves as the Director for the UIC Center for Health Work, a NIOSH-funded Center of Excellence in Total Worker Health®. The focus of the UIC Center is precarious work, understanding the scope of and working conditions associated with precarious work and developing multi-level intervention strategies to turn unhealthy work into healthy work. She is also the co-Director of the Occupational Safety Program and Director of the Pilot Projects Research Training Program in the Illinois Occupational Safety and Health Education and

Research Center. Dr Conroy is certified in the comprehensive practice of industrial hygiene by the American Board of Industrial Hygiene. She earned her undergraduate degree in Chemical Engineering from the University of Massachusetts, Amherst, and a master and doctoral degree in Environmental Science and Physiology, with a focus in industrial hygiene from Harvard University, School of Public Health.

Ian Couper is Director of the Ukwanda Centre for Rural Health and Professor of Rural Health in the Department of Global Health, Faculty of Medicine and Health Sciences, Stellenbosch University, since 2016. This follows more than 13 years at the University of the Witwatersrand (Wits), where he established the Wits Centre for Rural Health. He still holds an appointment as visiting professor in the Wits Department of Family Medicine and Primary Care. While at Wits, he also served in the North West Provincial Department of Health, leading the development of family and rural medicine, as part of 26 years of service in the public health system. He is an executive member and past chair of the World Organization of Family Doctors (WONCA) Working Party on Rural Practice. He is the African section editor of *Rural and Remote Health*, and an associate editor of *BMC Medical Education*. He has been involved in educational support in a number of African universities. He has held visiting appointments at Monash and Flinders Universities in Australia and the University of Washington in the USA.

Patricia Cuff, MS, MPH, is a Senior Program Officer for the Board on Global Health within the division of Health and Medicine where she directs the Global Forum on Innovation in Health Professional Education – a position she has held since 2012. Patricia is also working on a special COVID-related project with select academies in Africa. Patricia worked for 11 years on the African Science Academy Development Initiative where she was the Country Liaison to the Uganda National Academy of Sciences. She has directed and co-directed multiple studies at the National Academies including Clinical Trials During the 2014–2015 Ebola Outbreak, Options for Overseas Placement of US Health Professionals, and Enhancing the Behavioral and Social Science Content of Medical School Curricula. Patricia joined the Academies staff to work on the report, *Emerging Microbial Threats to Health in the 21st Century*. Before coming to Washington, DC, Patricia worked at St Luke's-Roosevelt Hospital Center in New York City in the field of HIV-nutrition as a counselor, researcher, and lecturer on topics of adult and pediatric HIV. She received a MS in Nutrition and a MPH in Population and Family Health from Columbia University, and performed her undergraduate studies at the University of Connecticut.

Miguel Cuj is a Guatemalan-K'iche Maya Anthropology Doctoral student at Vanderbilt University. He has a Nutrition degree from San Carlos University in Guatemala, which was supported by the Guatemalan Maya Educational Foundation scholarship program. He has worked on several projects in rural Guatemala with the Maya population. Miguel has a Master of Arts in Latin American Studies, a Masters in Anthropology, and a certificate in Global Health. His research interests are anthropology of food and nutrition, structural violence, global health, foodways, K'iche' Maya food, bio-communicability, and cultural models.

Robbie Davis-Floyd, PhD, Adjunct Professor, Department of Anthropology, Rice University, Houston and Fellow of the Society for Applied Anthropology, is a well-known medical anthropologist, international speaker and researcher in transformational models in childbirth, midwifery, obstetrics, and reproduction. She is author of over 80 journal articles and 24 encyclopedia articles, and of *Birth as an American Rite of Passage* (1992, 2003, University of California Press) and of its 3rd, revised and updated edition (2022, Routledge); she is also author of *Ways of Knowing about Birth: Mothers, Midwives, Medicine, and Birth Activism* (2018, Waveland Press). She is co-author of *From Doctor to Healer: The Transformative Journey* (1998, Rutgers University Press) and *The Power of Ritual* (2016); and lead or co-editor of 16 collections, including the award-winning *Cyborg Babies: From Techno-Sex to Techno-Tots* (1998, Routledge) and *Childbirth and Authoritative Knowledge: Cross-Cultural Perspectives: (1997, University of California Press; The "seminal" Birth Models That Work* (2009, University of California Press); *Birth in Eight Cultures* (2019, Waveland Press); *Birthing Models on the Human Rights Frontier: Speaking Truth to Power* (2021, Routledge); *Sustainable Birth in Disruptive Times* (2021, Springer Nature); and the solo-edited *Birthing Techno-Sapiens: Human-Technology Co-Evolution and the Future of Reproduction* (2021, Routledge). She has also lead-edited a Special Issue of *Frontiers in Sociology* on "The Global Impact of COVID-19 on Maternity Care Practices." In process is a 3-volume series on *The Anthropology of Obstetrics and Obstetricians: The Practice, Maintenance, and Reproduction of a Biomedical Profession* (Routledge). She currently serves as Lead Editor for a Routledge series called "Social Science Perspectives on Childbirth and Reproduction." Most of her published articles are freely available on her website: www.davis-floyd.com.

Tom Douglass, PhD, is a medical sociologist. He currently works as a Research Associate at Ulster University on the National Institute for Health Research-funded "Real Complaints" project working within the qualitative arm. He holds degrees in Sociology and Social Policy (BA Hons), winning the prize for highest graduating average, and Social Research Methods (MA) both from Russell Group institutions. Subsequently he achieved a PhD in Sociology (concentrated within Medical Sociology) from the University of Kent. His past research has been concerned with the exploration of the pharmaceuticalization of society. He has also published on the dynamics of pharmaceutical regulation, vaccines, and trust within health care settings.

Pamela I. Erickson, Dr PH, PhD, is a medical anthropologist at the University of Connecticut, Storrs Campus in the Department of Anthropology. She is also affiliated with the Institute for Collaboration on Health, Intervention, and Policy (Storrs Campus) and the Department of Community Health in the School of Medicine (Farmington Campus). Her research interests include human reproduction, sexual decision-making, and risk reduction among adolescents and emerging adults, global health, the impact of global climate change on health, health and human rights, qualitative research methods, ethnomedicine, and the causes and implications of Waorani raiding in Amazonian Ecuador. She has conducted research in East Los Angeles CA, Hartford CT, Ecuador, India, Mexico, Nepal, Panama, and the Philippines.

Linda Forst, MD, MPH a Professor of Environmental and Occupational health Health Sciences at the University of Illinois at Chicago (UIC), School of Public Health. She is the director of the Great Lakes Center for Occupational and Environmental Safety and Health, a World Health Organization Collaborating Center. Her research is in occupational health surveillance and interventions that protect the health of disadvantaged working populations, including migrant labor and workers hired through temporary staffing companies. She teaches toxicology and occupational and environmentally disease, both locally and globally. Her research focus is on occupational health surveillance, and preventing exposure to heavy metals and pesticides. She maintains an Occupational Medicine practice in Chicago.

Cynthia A. Frank, PhD, RN, is a medical anthropologist who is affiliated with the Yale University School of Medicine as a clinical researcher and the University of Connecticut where she is an adjunct professor in the Department of Anthropology. She has extensive experience in clinical care and infectious disease research, primarily HIV infection. Her research interests include disease-related stigma, biomedicine and its health care providers, infectious diseases, and substance use disorders.

Suzanne M. Gaulocher, PhD, MPH, is Assistant Professor in Public Health and is the Director of the Center for Healthy Communities at Plymouth State University. She holds a PhD from the University of Wisconsin at Madison where she was a part of the Center for Sustainability and the Global Environment, focusing on the intersection of human and environmental health. Her research and teaching center around the intersection between human health and the environment with focus on community engagement, social justice and health equity.

Nicolas Giraudeau is a dental surgeon, an Associate Professor and a Hospital Practitioner at the University of Montpellier and at the University-Hospital of Montpellier. He is deputy head of the dental education and research center, responsible for the first-consultation and telemedicine team. Following his diploma as a dental surgeon (2009), Dr Giraudeau studied health law at the Faculty of Law and Political Science of the University of Montpellier and obtained a Master degree. Then he continued with a PhD entitled "The medical act challenged by the oral telemedicine" (2014). He is now a member of a political science research team working on the use of digital technology within health policies. He is in charge of the e-DENT program: an oral telemedicine project, enabling remote oral consultation. He is in charge of Telemedicine for the French Digital Health Society. He is also a digital health expert with the WHO, a member of the Experts Committee in charge of the creation and writing of the handbook for the WHO mOralHealth program. He is the president of the Montpellier University Foundation.

Elizabeth A. Goldblatt, PhD (UCLA), MHA/PA (Portland State University), is an educational consultant on inter-professional education and collaborative practice for the complementary and integrative health professions. She was a founding member and Acting Executive Director of the Academic Collaborative for Integrative Health (ACIH; formerly ACCAHC) and later served as Chair of the ACIH board. She represents ACIH on the National Academy of Medicine's Global Forum for Global Innovations in Health Professional Education. She was on the leadership team of the University of Arizona's National Center for Integrative Primary Healthcare. She teaches integrative health and medicine systems at several colleges. She was president and vice-president of the Council of Colleges of Acupuncture/OM and co-chaired the Education Committee of the North American Acupuncture/OM Council. She served on the Board of Trustees for Pacific University and was president of the Oregon College of Oriental Medicine (1988–2003), and Provost, Vice President of Academic Affairs and Director of Institutional Assessment at ACTCM (2004–2012).

Stacy Gomes, EdD, MAEd, is Vice President of Academic Affairs at Pacific College of Health and Science where she has worked since 1997. She received her master's degree in education technology, instructional design at San Diego State University in 1997 and her doctorate in educational leadership at the University of La Verne in 2006. Her expertise is in higher education accreditation, assessment and program evaluation. She writes, consults, and trains on accreditation, assessment, curriculum design, faculty development, program evaluation, research design, student learning, and integrative medicine. She serves on the Boards of the Academic Collaborative for Integrative Health, the Council of Colleges of Acupuncture & Oriental Medicine, and the UCSD Center for Integrative Medicine, among others.

Lionel Green-Thompson currently serves as the Dean: Faculty of Health Sciences at the University of Cape Town, South Africa. He served previously as the Dean at Sefako Makgatho Health Sciences University (2018–2020) after working as the Assistant Dean: Teaching, Learning and Undergraduate Affairs (2014–2018) at Wits University. He served as a co-author panellist for the ASSAf Consensus Report: Reconceptualising health professions education in South Africa. This report released in 2018, represented a national response to the Lancet Commission of 2010. Lionel has also served on the education workstream, which contributed to the 2030 Human Resources for Health Strategy: Investing in the Health Workforce for Universal Health Coverage for the South African government. He is a specialist anaesthesiologist by training and completed a PhD in 2014 entitled "The nature of social accountability in South African medical education and practice." Lionel has an interest in the assessment of learning in both clinical and cognitive domains. He currently represents the SA Committee of Medical Deans (SACOMD) in engagements with the Colleges of Medicine of SA with a view to the development of workplace-based assessments for specialist education. He currently serves on the board of the Rural Health Advocacy Project (RHAP) and Towards Unity for Health (TUFH). He is a member of AMEE and serves on the AMEE Research Committee, co-chairing a Network for Medical Education in Resource Constrained Environments (MERCS).

Christine Holmberg, Dr. phil., M.P.H., is professor of Social Medicine and Epidemiology at the Brandenburg Medical School Theodor Fontane. She is an anthropologist and epidemiologist by training whose research aims to understand epidemiological knowledge production and knowledge transfer. She is particularly interested in the effects of such knowledge on medical practice, communities, and patients' experiences. Her most recent work is concerned with a more nuanced conceptualizing of social health to engage with and ameliorate people-centered health care structures. She has recently co-edited the volume *Narratives in Practice: Potentials and Challenges of Using Narratives in Health-related Context* (2018, Oxford University Press). Professor Holmberg is a member of DIPEx international and DIPEx Germany (www.krankheitserfahrungen.de), a project that aims to improve understanding of personal health experiences for the benefit of communities, researchers and the health sector, including health care professionals and policy makers.

Alex Hryhorczuk, JD, MPP, is the Chief Data Officer at sr4-Data Information Systems (DIS) in Evanston, Illinois. His work involves developing information systems to make data more useful for building community resilience to public health threats. He received his BA from Georgetown University, his JD from the University of Illinois, and his MPP from the University of Chicago Harris School of Public Policy, with certificates in international development and global conflict studies. Prior to joining sr4-DIS, he interned at the Chicago Council on Global Affairs and was in private law practice.

Daniel Hryhorczuk, MD, MPH, FACMT, is a Professor Emeritus of Environmental and Occupational Health Sciences and Epidemiology at the University of Illinois School of Public Health. He received his BA from Northwestern University and MD and MPH degrees from the University of Illinois. He is board-certified in Occupational and Environmental Medicine and in Medical Toxicology. He is a fellow of Collegium Ramazzini. He is the past Director of the

Great Lakes Centers for Occupational and Environmental Health (a World Health Organization Collaborating Centre) and of Chicago's Toxikon Consortium. He has served on the National Advisory Committee for Occupational Safety and Health, the Children's Health Protection Advisory Committee, and the Board of Scientific Counselors for the National Center for Environmental Health. His research has focused on the effects of environmental stressors on human health, especially in countries of the former Soviet Union.

Lois Jircitano, PhD, JD, MA, Deyi:Hwagenhahs, means "She Argues for her People." Dr Jircitano is an enrolled member of the Kanienkehaka/Mohawk from Six Nations Grand River, Oshweken, Ontario, Canada. She received her Doctorate in Educational Leadership, Administration and Policy in 2001, a Juris Doctor in 1982, and a Master of Arts in American Studies 1990 from the State University of New York at Buffalo. Her current research interest includes examination of American education law/policy and cultural trauma of Indian children.

Jok Madut Jok is a Professor of Anthropology at the Maxwell School of Citizenship and Public Affairs at Syracuse University. His areas of specialization include security, governance, democracy, and development in South Sudan and Sudan. He has also written extensively about gender, sexuality and reproductive health, humanitarian aid, ethnography of political violence, gender-based violence, and war and slavery and the politics of identity in South Sudan and Sudan. He is the author of *Breaking Sudan: The Search for Peace* (2017, Oneworld Publications), *Sudan: Race, Religion and Violen*ce (2007, One World Publication), *War and Slavery in Sudan* (2001, University of Pennsylvania Press), and *Militarization, Gender and Reproductive Health in South Sudan* (1998, Edwin Mellen Press). He is co-editor with J. Ryle, J. Willis, and S. Baldo of *The Sudan Handbook* (2011, James Currey). Before joining Maxwell he was visiting professor of anthropology, University of Oxford, and Fellow of Linacre College. He had also served in the government of South Sudan as undersecretary in the Ministry of Culture and Heritage (2010–2013). He is the founding director of the Sudd Institute, a public policy research center. He earned his PhD in Anthropology from the University of California, Los Angeles, his MA in Medical Anthropology from the American University in Cairo, and his BA in the Faculty of Arts & Humanities from the University of Alexandria, Egypt.

Irma Kirtadze, MD, PhD, is an Assistant Professor of the Addiction Studies, Arts and Science faculty at Ilia State University, Georgia. Irma is an Affiliated Senior Researcher at the Addiction Research Center Alternative Georgia. Dr Kirtadze has earned NIDA Distinguished International Scientist Collaboration Award (DISCA) in 2014 and has conducted site-based research fellowship on substance use and recovery at the Horizon clinic at Chapple Hill (NC, USA). Irma is the author of more than 30 scholarly publications, including the chapter "Changing Patterns of Drug Use in Georgia: A Case Vignette" in N. el-Guebaly, G. Carrà and M. Galanter (eds.), *Textbook of Addiction Treatment: International Perspectives* (2015, Springer).

Ambika Krishnakumar, PhD, is a Professor in the Department of Human Development and Family Science at Syracuse University. Her research and publications are interdisciplinary and involve studies of cross-cultural comparisons in the areas of family and youth dynamics, including the use of health and social services. Dr Krishnakumar's international research includes work conducted in Trinidad and Tobago, Guyana, China, Ukraine, and Thailand. Her current work involves the examination of youth sexual behaviors and identification of background and situational predictors of intimate partner violence in the United States and the Caribbean.

Jean-Paul L'Huillier is currently assistant Professor of economics at Brandeis University, and previously was at the Einaudi Institute for Economics and Finance and a visiting Faculty member at Yale University. An expert on the study of business cycles, his recent research concentrates on how to perform suitable monetary policies in environments of chronic liquidity traps, and on understanding medium-term macroeconomic boom-bust cycles. He has published more than 10 academic articles in refereed journals including the American Economic Review, the Journal of Monetary Economics, American Economic Journal: Macroeconomics, the Journal of Money, Credit, and Banking, and the Journal of Economic Dynamics and Control.

Gerard Leavey is the Director of the Bamford Centre at Ulster University. Prior to this, he was the Director of Research for Barnet, Enfield & Haringey Mental Health NHS Trust in London and a researcher in the Department of Mental Health Sciences, University College London. As a social worker he spent several years with Jewish Care, working with Holocaust survivors. His research career has focused mainly on mental health services. He has published widely on service pathways and access by minority ethnic, migrant and disadvantaged populations. His work ranges from epidemiological studies on ethnic elders and refugee children to qualitative investigations of community-level agencies such as schools and faith-based organizations, and their role in the recognition and management of mental illness. He is the lead on an EU-funded project on the use of intergenerational exchange to combat social exclusion in rural and isolated regions of Europe.

Ibu Robin Lim CPM, is a Filipino-American midwife, mother, grandmother, and founder of Yayasan Bumi Sehat, a non-profit organization in Indonesia. Lim also serves on the board of Bumi-Wadah Philippines, where she is known as "Lola Robin." Her Passion is Human Rights in Childbirth. She believes that each individual is an essential "Piece of Peace"; therefore, by protecting the mothers in childbirth and the newborns (our smallest citizens of Earth) we may build peace, one Baby, one Mother, one Family at a time.

Douglas A. Luke is the Irving Louis Horowitz Professor in Social Policy and Director of the Center for Public Health Systems Science at the Brown School at Washington University in St Louis. Dr Luke is a leading researcher in the areas of public health policy, implementation science, and systems science. His research focuses on the evaluation, dissemination, and implementation of evidence-based public health policies. During the past decade, Dr Luke has worked on applying systems science methods to important public health problems, especially social network analysis. He has published two systems science review papers in the *Annual Review of Public Health*, and the first study to employ new statistical network modeling techniques on public health data was published in the *American Journal of Public Health* in 2010. Dr Luke received his PhD in clinical and community psychology in 1990 from the University of Illinois at Urbana-Champaign.

Deborah Lupton is SHARP Professor in the Faculty of Arts & Social Sciences, University of New South Wales, Sydney, Australia. She is located in the Centre for Social Research in Health and the Social Policy Research Centre and leads the Vitalities Lab and the UNSW Node of the ARC Centre for Automated Decision-Making + Society. She is the author/co-author of 19 books, including *Digital Sociology* (2015, Routledge), *The Quantified Self* (2016, Polity Press), *Digital Health* (2017, Routledge), *Fat* (2018, 2nd edition, Routledge) and *Data Selves* (2019, Polity Press). She is a Fellow of the Academy of the Social Sciences in Australia and holds an Honorary Doctor of Social Science degree awarded by the University of Copenhagen.

Bianca N. Manago is an Assistant Professor of Sociology at Vanderbilt University. She received her PhD in sociology and MS in applied statistics from Indiana University. Broadly, her research examines the factors that shape two related forms of inequality: stigma, a measure of social exclusion, and status, the extent to which one is perceived as respected and competent. Her current projects investigate topics such as the effect of mental illness labels on stigma, the relationship between status, social contexts, and physiological stress responses, and how inequality can be reduced in small group interactions. These questions require a variety of methodological approaches, including experiments (laboratory and survey-based), in-depth qualitative interviews, and nationally representative survey data.

Mary Corey March lives in San Francisco with her husband and daughter. Her education has alternated between art and academics (one undergraduate degree in each, one Masters in each, including an MFA from the San Francisco Art Institute). She is an avid traveler who pursues an extensive array of interests and studies which inform and feed her artwork. Her first publicly displayed commission was done at the age of 16 and her work has been shown throughout the US and internationally. In May 2017 she became disabled with CFS/ME. After an adjustment period she has continued her artwork with the help of assistants.

Manu Raj Mathur, PhD, MPH, is a Dental Surgeon with a PhD in Epidemiology and Population Health from University College London and a Masters in Public Health from the University of Glasgow (UK). He is currently Senior Research Scientist and Associate Professor at Public Health Foundation of India (PHFI), New Delhi. He was a 2010–2011 Fogarty International Clinical Research Scholar, and won a Wellcome Trust scholarship for his doctoral studies, and a Wellcome Trust Mid-Career Fellowship to undertake work on psychosocial determinants inequalities in oral health in India. His areas of expertise are in operations and health systems research and health promotion. He has worked on many projects funded by the Government of India, WHO, BMGF, USAID and NIH, and is currently leading large-scale projects from MRC UK, the Global Bridges Consortium, the Government of India and the Rockefeller Foundation. He is author of many peer-reviewed journal articles and of multiple global health book chapters. He currently serves as the Group Programme Chair for the Global Oral Health Inequalities Research Network of International Association for Dental Research.

Humayra Mayat is a medical student at SUNY Upstate pursuing Internal Medicine. Humayra is invested in pursuing a career in public health with an emphasis on health disparities. As a medical student, Humayra has served as a service learning leader at the Rahma Free Clinic and helped plan her school's first Health Justice Conference. Humayra aspires to continue to foster her passion for advocacy and programming to better serve her future patients and surrounding community.

Julia McDaniel is a Cultural Anthropology PhD Candidate at the Maxwell School of Citizenship and Public Affairs at Syracuse University. Her research focuses on Congolese and Somali refugee maternal health experiences in displacement and resettlement contexts. She is interested in transnationalism, political economy, maternal health, conflict, power, policy, and the applications of technology to aid marginalized and underserved populations. Julia has worked domestically and internationally on issues of gender, public policy, leadership, social justice, and human rights with the US Peace Corps, USAID, NYU, DFID, and community organizations that serve local populations. She earned her MPA in International Public Policy from New York University and her BA in International Relations and French Language and Literature from the State University of New York College at Geneseo.

Thierry Moulin graduated from the University of Lyon, France, in 1981 and obtained a PhD degree in medicine and another PhD degree in human biology from the University of Franche-Comté, France, in 1998. His principal fields of expertise in neurology include cerebrovascular diseases, emergency neurology, and neuroimaging. In 2001, he founded the Réseau des Urgences Neurologiques, Franche-Comté, to develop the use of telemedicine tools to manage the remote treatment of stroke patients within the region. Since 1990, he has been involved in various studies to develop new stroke treatments. He is a cofounder of the Société Française de Neuro-Vasculaire and is a long-standing member of numerous other medical societies, including the American Academy of Neurology, European Neurological Society, the European Stroke Council, and European Stroke Organisation. He is a reviewer for several medical journals, including the *Revue Neurologique*, *European Neurology*, the *Journal of Neurology, Neurosurgery and Psychiatry*, *Cerebrovascular Diseases*, and *Stroke*. He is joint-editor-in-chief of *Digital Health*. He has worked at the University Hospital of Besançon since 1984, held a Research Fellowship in cerebrovascular diseases at the University Hospital of Lausanne in Switzerland (1990–1992), and has occupied the position of a Professor of Neurology at the University Hospital of Besançon since 2001 and the head of the Department of Neurology since 2013. In 2006, he was elected the Vice President of the Scientific Council of the University of Franche-Comté. He has been the dean of the Medicine Faculty since 2017. In 2011, he was elected President of the French Stroke Society (SFNV) and in 2013, President elected French Telemedicine Society (SFT) and Past-President in 2019. He is the author or co-author of more than 200 articles published in peer-reviewed journals and has contributed to more than 50 books.

Deepti Nagrath, Dr. Nagrath is a Dental Surgeon with a Master's of Science in Clinical Research and is currently perusing PhD in Epidemiology. She has multiple years of experience as a public health researcher and is currently working as a Senior Research Assistant at Public Health Foundation of India (PHFI), New Delhi. Currently she is involved in a multi country randomized controlled clinical trial, she has also previously worked on projects funded by the Government of India, MRC, WHO and CDC.

Lutchmie Narine, PhD, is Professor and Chair of the Department of Public Health at Syracuse University. His research interests are in the areas of health policy and management, focusing on various aspects of the access and use of health services. Dr Narine has implemented international health projects and conducted research in a variety of countries, including Canada, Hungary, Saudi Arabia, Thailand, Trinidad and Tobago, and Ukraine. His current research involves data collection from three Southern Caribbean countries to understand the factors that influence risk-taking behaviors among emerging youth and ultimately their use of health and other services.

Roger O'Sullivan is the Director of the Ageing Research and Development Division within the Institute of Public Health in Ireland and visiting Professor at Ulster University. He was Director of The Centre for Ageing Research and Development in Ireland (2007–2015). Professor O'Sullivan has written, edited, and published on issues relating to social policy, substantially in the area of ageing and older people. In 2018 he co-established the International Loneliness and Social Isolation Research Network, and in 2019 established the Gerontological Society of America interest group on loneliness and isolation with Professors Prohaska and Lubben. In 2020 he led the global "Coping with Loneliness, Isolation and Covid-19" study. Professor O'Sullivan was awarded membership through distinction of the Faculty of Public Health–UK in 2017 and in 2020 he was made Fellow of the Gerontological Society of America.

David Otiashvili, MD, PhD, is a Director of the Addiction Research Centre Alternative Georgia and Associate Professor of Healthcare at the School of Natural Sciences and Medicine, Ilia State University, Tbilisi, Georgia. He spent 10 years in clinical work, treating patients with substance use disorders. As a NIDA Hubert Humphrey Fellow, he studied substance abuse research at Johns Hopkins University, Baltimore, USA. For the last decade his major focus has been substance use-related research, including policy research, and education programs in addiction science. David has been involved with harm reduction and drug policy advocacy at a national and regional level. He is an official lobbyist for drug policy and drug legislation in the Georgian Parliament. He serves as representative of the civil society sector in the Georgian Interagency Drug Policy Coordinating Council.

Jay Jeong Hyun Park earned her BA degree in Sociology graduating with honors cum laude at Syracuse University, USA. Jay JH is currently a graduate student of Sociology with a focus in criminological sociology at Korea University, Seoul.

Deborah Parra-Medina, PhD, MPH, is Professor of Mexican American and Latina/o Studies and Director of the Latino Research Institute at The University of Texas at Austin. Dr Parra-Medina has substantial experience in health promotion, public health epidemiology, health disparities in chronic disease, and community-based interventions among under-served and minority populations. Over the past 20 years, she has served as Principal Investigator for 17 grants funded for over $19 million, published over 65 scientific articles, presented at many national and international conferences, and received awards for research, teaching, and service. Dr Parra-Medina was named Fellow of the American Academy of Health Behavior in 2016. She received the American Public Health Association Mayhew Derryberry Award in 2013 for outstanding contributions to research in the behavioral sciences.

Bernice A. Pescosolido is Distinguished Professor of Sociology and Director of the Indiana Consortium for Mental Health Services Research at Indiana University. Trained as a medical sociologist at Yale University, her work focuses on the social and cultural aspects of health and health care. In particular, she has developed theoretical models focusing on the power of human connectedness to influence individuals' response to the onset of illness in the Network Episode Model, to suicide in the network translation of Durkheim's theory, and to the stigma of mental illness and addictions in the FINIS Model. Her focus on social networks has guided her empirical projects in these areas, including the Indiana Network Mental Health Study and the US National Stigma Studies. She was elected to the National Academy of Medicine in 2016.

Klaus von Pressentin is a family physician and head of the Division of Family Medicine in the School of Public Health and Family Medicine at the University of Cape Town, South Africa. As a clinician-scientist and -educator, he has a sustained record of primary care research, teaching and practice. Prior to joining the University of Cape Town in 2020, he worked mainly in the rural areas of the public health system over the previous two decades. He completed his PhD in 2017, which evaluated the impact of family physicians within the district health system of South Africa. His research focuses on health service strengthening, health systems (especially human resources for health), as well as educational aspects in family medicine and health professions education. His current voluntary activities include serving as the Editor-in-Chief of the *South African Family Practice Journal* (the official journal of the South African Academy of Family Physicians), as well as serving on the Council of the College of Family Physicians, Colleges of Medicine of South Africa.

Thomas Prohaska is an Emeritus Professor and Dean (retired) at George Mason University College of Health and Human Services. He is also an Emeritus Professor in the School of Public Health at the University of Illinois Chicago. He is currently a Trustee for RRF Foundation for Aging. His research background is in Public Health and ageing, including physical activity, chronic disease management, and dissemination and diffusion of community-based intervention programs to promote health and well-being among older adults. He has been on numerous national and international advisory committees, including the National Advisory Committee for the Robert Wood Johnson Foundation, the Pan American Health Organization (PAHO), and the CDC Healthy Aging Research Network. Awards include the national UCLA Distinguished Professor Gerontology/Geriatrics Award, Fellow Gerontological Society of America, and the Philip Weiler Award for Leadership in Aging and Public Health, American Public Health Association.

Beth Prusaczyk is an Instructor at the Institute for Informatics and in General Medical Sciences at Washington University School of Medicine in St Louis. Dr Prusaczyk is an implementation scientist who specializes in improving health care for vulnerable older adults, such as those living in rural areas or with dementia, by understanding how to better implement existing research findings into practice and policy. Her work focuses on how systems science, existing health care data, and health information technology can both inform and speed up this implementation process. Dr Prusaczyk received her PhD and MSW from the Brown School at Washington University in St Louis, and completed her postdoctoral training at Vanderbilt University Medical Center. She also served as a Health and Aging Policy Fellow and American Political Science Association Congressional Fellow (2018–2019).

Tumisang Ramarea is currently a graduate student studying Decision and Risk Analysis in the Department of Management Science and Engineering at Stanford. He believes he is in this world to love and to be loved. One of the ways he hopes to love is through catalyzing the impact of initiatives and projects aimed at ending economic poverty. He plans to do this primarily by applying his engineering education to support rational and intelligent decision-making within high-impact organizations. Born and raised in Botswana, Ramarea has a bias towards organizations that work in or on Emerging Markets. He also hopes to help end economic poverty by investing in youth-owned businesses in Botswana and providing mentorship to academically gifted students from marginalized backgrounds.

Stephan Rist is emeritus Professor of human geography at the Institute of Geography of the University of Bern. He is holder of the UNESCO Chair "Natural and Cultural Heritage of Sustainable Mountain Development." He also works at the Centre for Development and Environment (CDE) of the University of Bern, working in the Cluster on Sustainability Governance of Land and Natural Resources. His geographic focus is on Latin America and Africa. He is involved in several international research projects dealing with critical sustainability assessments, political ecology, agroecology, sovereignty and sustainability in food systems, food democracy and local knowledge, social movements, and transdisciplinary approaches of research aiming at the enhancement of societal transformation in view of environmental justice.

Mariel Rivera is a PhD candidate at Syracuse University in the Department of Anthropology. Her research interests are within medical anthropology with a specific focus on reproductive health. She is interested in how race and gender influence reproductive and maternal health experiences. For her doctoral research, she is focusing on the use of community-based doulas in Syracuse, New York, who specifically work with Black women and other women of color.

Gary Rodziewicz, MD, is a board-certified neurosurgeon, now retired from being an Associate Professor of Neurosurgery at SUNY Upstate Medical Center in Syracuse, NY. He has an interest in innovative treatments for PTSD and other disorders.

Jesús Gómez Rossi (Spain/Argentina) is a DMD and health economist from the London School of Economics and Political Science working at the Charité- Universitätsmedizin. His research focuses on developing new forms of health service provision for high-need populations in different income settings through digital health solutions such as AI or biosensors for diagnostics. His projects demand developing forward-thinking strategies that push for greater digitalization, with the final aim of increasing access to higher quality health care for everyone.

Aparna Roy is Lead, Climate Change and Energy, at the Centre for New Economic Diplomacy (CNED) Climate Change and Energy, Centre for New Economic Diplomacy, and an Associate Fellow, Observer Research Foundation, New Delhi, India. Aparna's research interests include the politics of climate change, resilience building, and environmental governance. Aparna contributes regularly to public scholarship via platforms such as the *Times of India*, *Hindustan Times*, and *The Hindu*. She holds a Bachelor's degree in Political Science (Honours), and Masters degrees in Sociology and International Development. She was a Commonwealth scholar at the University of Bristol.

Barbara Rylko-Bauer, PhD, is adjunct Associate Professor in the Department of Anthropology at Michigan State University. Her work has focused on applied anthropology, health care delivery, structural violence and health inequities, political violence and war, narrative analysis, and prisoner-doctors in the Holocaust. She has published on these topics in numerous book chapters and peer-reviewed articles. Her most recent books are *Global Health in Times of Violence* (2009, School for Advanced Research Press) and *A Polish Doctor in the Nazi Camps: My Mother's Memories of Imprisonment, Immigration, and a Life Remade* (2014, University of Oklahoma Press), which received several awards, including being recognized as a Michigan Notable Book. She is also a recipient of the Rudolph Virchow Prize.

Norah A. Schwartz is a senior research professor at the Colegio de la Frontera Norte in Tijuana, Mexico, and an adjunct faculty member at San Diego State University. She received a Masters degree in Public Affairs from the Lyndon B. Johnson School of Public Affairs, University of Texas at Austin, and a doctoral degree in medical anthropology from the Joint Medical Anthropology Program at the University of California, San Francisco and Berkeley. Dr Schwartz's research interests revolve around child health and the prevention of chronic illness and disability on the US–Mexico border. Schwartz is an adaptive athlete and member of an adaptive rock climbing team in southern California. She began her professional career as a residential supervisor in group homes and as an advocate for disability rights.

Falk Schwendicke (Germany) is a Full Professor at the Charité-Universitätsmedizin, DMD, and specialist in public health. His work focused on public health, health economics, epidemiology and the development, evaluation and implementation of digital health solutions, especially those involving artificial intelligence. He has authored over 300 articles, edited various books and provided over 20 book chapters on a range of issues. Falk was awarded a range of prestigious awards, among them the Basil Bibby and Lion Award of the International Association for Dental Research (IADR), numerous awards of the German Society of Conservative Dentistry as well as the David Sackett Award of the German Network for Evidence-based Medicine.

Andrea V. Shaw is a physician at SUNY Upstate University, where she is an Assistant Professor of Internal Medicine and Pediatrics. She directs Upstate's Refugee medicine primary care program and works closely with community partners supporting a diverse population of refugees in their years after resettlement. Andrea also leads a clinical education partnership in East Africa through the Institute for Global Health and Translational Science at Upstate. Over the years, she has had various experiences in research, education, and clinical service working in East Africa. She completed her undergraduate BS at Cornell University, her MD at SUNY Upstate Medical University, and her combined Internal Medicine and Pediatric residency training at Duke University Medical Center.

Johannes Siegrist is Senior Professor of Medical Sociology at the Heinrich-Heine- University Düsseldorf, Germany. He received his PhD in sociology in 1969 (University of Freiburg) and held professorships for medical sociology at the Universities of Marburg and Düsseldorf from 1973 to 2012. He was visiting professor at the Johns Hopkins University, Baltimore, USA (1981) and at Utrecht University (1994). Main topics of his extensive publication record are health-adverse psychosocial work environments (having developed the effort–reward imbalance model of stressful work) and social inequalities in health. He edited international books in these fields and is currently co-editor of a new handbook series in occupational health sciences. In addition to his collaboration in distinct European research networks, he chaired several national and international academic societies and served as a consultant to the World Health Organization. Among other distinctions, he is a member of Academia Europaea (London) and a corresponding member of the Heidelberg Academy of Sciences.

Merrill Singer, PhD, is Emeritus Professor of Anthropology and Senior Research Scientist at the Center for Health, Intervention and Prevention, at the University of Connecticut. Dr Singer's work has focused on infectious disease and environmental health and includes research on HIV/AIDS, STIs, hepatitis, Ebola, tick-borne diseases, and arbovirus diseases. He is the author of 34 books, and over 200 peer-reviewed articles. Social justice, the social determinants of health, syndemics, and critical medical anthropology have been enduring themes of his research and applied work. His most recent books include *A Companion to the Anthropology of Environmental Health* (2016, Wiley-Blackwell), *Social Justice and Medical Practice: Life History of a Physician of Social Medicine* (2017, Routledge), and *Climate Change and Social Inequality: The Health and Social Costs of Global Warming* (2018, Routledge). His research has been supported through grants from NIH, CDC, and the US Department of Health and Human Services. Dr Singer has been awarded the Society for Medical Anthropology's Career Achievement Award, the Solon T. Kimball Award for Public and Applied Anthropology from the American Anthropological Association, the Society for the Anthropology of North America's Distinguished Achievement in the Critical Study of North America, and the Rudolph Virchow Prize.

Roger Strasser is Professor of Rural Health, University of Waikato, New Zealand, Professor of Rural Health and Founding Dean Emeritus of the Northern Ontario School of Medicine

(NOSM), Canada. Between 2002 and 2019, Professor Roger Strasser was NOSM Founding Dean and CEO. He is a leader in the global reform of rural health professional education and research. Recognizing the importance of context and community in medical education and research, Professor Strasser has become one of the world's foremost authorities on rural, socially accountable medical education, and a sought-after speaker and advisor. Prior to 2002, Roger Strasser was Professor of Rural Health and Head of the Monash University School of Rural Health in Australia and had an international role with the World Organization of Family Doctors (WONCA) as Chair of the Working Party on Rural Practice (1992–2004).

Theresa Tribaldos is a geographer and political scientist by training and leads one of the research groups at the Centre for Development and Environment and at the Institute of Geography at the University of Bern. Her research focuses on sustainability and justice questions in food systems and interventions to make these systems more sustainable, transdisciplinary research approaches for sustainable development, and the contributions science can make to sustainability transformations. She has worked in different research and implementation projects in the global North and South. She also has experience as a consultant in the sustainability of the Swiss food system, Swiss agricultural policy, or projects for supporting regional development in Swiss Alpine regions. Innovative and transdisciplinary methodologies and the collaboration with different types of actors are among her core interests.

Bryan S. Turner is Emeritus Professor of Sociology at the Graduate Center CUNY and Professor of Sociology at the Australian Catholic University. His early research was in the sociology of religion with special reference to Islam. He published *Weber and Islam* (1974, Routledge and Kegan Paul) 1974. Later he worked on medical sociology, publishing *The Body and Society* (1984: Basil Backwell) and *Medical Power and Social Knowledge* (1987: Sage). He is the founding editor of the journal *Citizenship Studies* and the *Journal of Classical Sociology*.

He was awarded the LittD from Cambridge University in 2009 and received the Max Planck award in 2015, creating the Centre for Citizenship, Social Pluralism and Religious Diversity at Potsdam University Germany, where he has an Honorary Professorship. His recent research has centred on vulnerability, happiness, and well-being. In 2019 he published (with Contreras-Vejar and Tice) *Regimes of Happiness* (2019: Anthem). With Aristotle's concept of Eudaimonia, he combines this interest in happiness with questions about the success or failure of whole societies. Professor Turner is an Honorary Fellow of The Edward Cadbury Centre for the Study of Public Understanding of Religion University of Birmingham, UK.

Cecilia Vindrola-Padros is a medical anthropologist interested in applied health research and the development of rapid approaches to research. She has written extensively on the use of rapid qualitative research and currently co-directs the Rapid Research, Evaluation and Appraisal Lab (RREAL) with Dr Ginger Johnson. Cecilia works across five interdisciplinary teams, applying anthropological theories and methods to study and improve healthcare delivery in the UK and abroad. She is a researcher on the NIHR-funded Rapid Service Evaluation Team (RSET), a collaboration between UCL and the Nuffield Trust. She is the past Director of the Qualitative Health Research Network (QHRN) and a fellow of the Society for Applied Anthropology (SfAA). Cecilia works as a Senior Research Fellow in the Department of Targeted Intervention, UCL and Social Scientist at the NIAA Health Services Research Centre (HSRC), Royal College of Anaesthetists (RCoA).

Margaret Voss is an Associate Professor in the Department of Nutrition and Food Studies and a faculty affiliate in the Interdisciplinary Program in Neuroscience at Syracuse University. She teaches courses in nutritional biochemistry, nutritional genomics, and metabolism. She is interested in how humans change the environment and the consequent health repercussions for both human and non-human vertebrates. Her current research projects all examine the link between environmental influences (e.g., anthropogenic disturbance, photoperiod, food availability, dietary components, and substrate availability) and genotypic expression, specifically changes in metabolism, reproductive physiology, and the timing of embryonic development.

Bhavneet Walia is an Assistant Professor of Public Health in Falk College at Syracuse University and a Faculty Affiliate in the Syracuse University's Aging Studies Institute and Lerner Center for Public Health Promotion. Dr Walia uses econometric modeling to understand issues of mortality, mental wellness, and physical wellness among populations that feature unique and, in some respects, elevated risk exposures (e.g., refugee populations, agricultural migrant workers, and contact sport participants). Her chief areas of research include health and labor econometrics. Her current research examines the mental and physical wellness effects of community gardening programs for refugees, social media and health, the economic and social effects of the H-2A Work Visa program (for agricultural laborers), and the mortality risk factors associated with participation in contact sports. Dr Walia teaches undergraduate and graduate Public Health in health data analysis. Her research has appeared in journals, including the *Journal of Organizational Behavior*, *Economics Letters (2)*, *Journal of Public Economic Theory*, *American Journal of Economics & Sociology*, *Journal of Economic Education*, *Journal of Sports Economics*, and *Southern Economic Journal*. Her work has been cited in national media outlets, including *Pacific Standard Magazine* and WalletHub.com. She is Editor of the *Journal of Development Innovations* and Associate Editor of the *Academy of Economics & Finance Journal*.

N. Ewen Wang, MD, is associate Director of Pediatric Emergency medicine and Professor in the Department of Emergency Medicine and Pediatrics at Stanford University Medical School. She has a strong interest and dedication to community health, medical education, and researching disparities in pediatric emergency care, both internationally and in California. Her research focuses on identifying and decreasing disparities in regionalized specialty care for children in California. Her current endeavors are focusing on trauma care and mental health access for children.

Deena White, Ph.D, is Professor of Political Sociology at the Université de Montréal, whose research focuses on whose research focuses on policy implementation involving community and citizen participation, partnerships, and network governance. From 2011 to 2021, she was director of ARIMA, a research partnership focused on local social service and action networks. Since then, she has been facilitating a Living Lab on Immigration-Inclusion-Participation, working with professionals and immigrants to mobilize social innovation. She has published *inter alia* on participation as a policy instrument, the organization of civil society, and the coordination of community-based and institutional services.

Linda M. Whiteford PhD, MPH, is Professor Emerita of Anthropology at the University of South Florida where she was Associate Vice President for Global Strategies, Associate Vice President for Academic Affairs and Strategic Initiatives, and Vice Provost. Dr. Whiteford was also the Founding Co-Director of the WHO Collaborating Center for Social Marketing and Social Justice at USF. She is Past President of the Society for Applied Anthropology, and the 2018 recipient of the Sol Tax Award for contributions to Applied Anthropology. Her research focuses on translating anthropological research into global health policies and practices, particularly concerning infectious and contagious water-related diseases. Dr. Whiteford's research has been funded by the National Science Foundation, and she consults for the World Bank, and The US Agency for International Development. Significant publications include: Primary Health Care in Cuba: The Other Revolution; Anthropological Ethics for Research and Practice; Globalization, Water and Health: Resources in Times of Scarcity; and Global Health in Times of Violence.

Lina Williatte-Pellitteri holds a PhD in law, is authorized to supervise research (HDR), and is Professor at the Law Faculty of the Catholic University of Lille. She is co-holder of the Law and Ethics Chair in digital health at the Faculty of Law and Medicine of the Catholic University of Lille. She is the director of a research center that studies the relationships between risk and the law. Her research has enabled her to integrate national think tanks around digital health. As such, she is vice-president of the French Digital Health Society in charge of the human and social sciences component and sits on ministerial working committees. Lina Williatte-Pellitteri is also a lawyer at the Lille Bar, partner of her firm, where she mainly deals with questions around the implementation of digital health projects.

Ruth Enid Zambrana is a Distinguished University Professor in the Harriet Tubman Department of Women, Gender and Sexuality Studies, Director of the Consortium on Race, Gender and Ethnicity and affiliate Professor of Family Medicine at the University of Maryland, Baltimore, School of Medicine. Her scholarship applies a critical intersectional lens to structural inequality and racial, Hispanic ethnicity, gender and economic disparities in population health and higher education trajectories. She has published widely on health inequity in women's health, maternal and child health, socioeconomic health disparities and life course impacts on health and mental well-being of traditionally and historically underrepresented minorities. Major awards include the 2013 American Public Health Association Latino Caucus, Founding Member Award for Vision and Leadership, 2013 University of Maryland Outstanding Woman of Color Award for her lifetime achievements, and the 2011 Julian Samora Distinguished Career Award by the American Sociological Association, Sociology of Latinos/as Section.

Wencheng Zhang is currently a doctoral student in the Department of Sociology at Syracuse University. Her research interests lie primarily in two areas: intergenerational relationships in ageing families and social determinants of health across the life course. Recently, she has been investigating how intergenerational ties influence the well-being of older adults and how early life conditions, adulthood exposures, and social context interact with one another to shape the health outcomes in adulthood.

Acknowledgements

We would like to thank the contributors from around the world who participated in the creation of this volume, patiently handled multiple edits and queries, and responded to our requests for innovative updates and new chapters.

We greatly appreciate our Advisory Board Members, who helped shape the vision for this edition of the Handbook in the planning stages, and who responded generously to requests to review chapters. Afaf Meleis, Allan Stern and Ruth Zambrana in particular were instrumental in providing feedback to authors along with Lutchmie Narine and Joan Ablon. Special thanks to Allan Stern who edited multiple chapters, and helped ensure readability across disciplines. In addition to the participation of Advisory Board Members, Monica Schoch-Spana, Clementine Fujimura, David Larsen and CorriZoli provided helpful reviews and Jean-Paul L'Huillier provided valuable comments on several chapters.

With sadness, we remember Professor Evan Weissman of Syracuse University, who was in the process of writing the chapter on food when he died suddenly at the age of 42 on April 9, 2020. Because of Evan's leadership on this topic, we chose a team to write the food chapter who share Evan's broad and nuanced perspective that integrates the analysis of food from farm to table, with a profound commitment to social justice.

We would like to thank our editor Colette Wilson, Reference Manager at SAGE Publishing, and our SAGE Publishing production editor, Prachi Arora for their suggestions, support, and encouragement.

Our thanks to each of our families who supported us as we worked through long Zoom calls and editing sessions. We enjoyed a remarkable team relationship as we guided this volume to completion, and our friendship deepened as we debated and learned from each other and from our authors.

This volume was completed during one of themost complex health and societal crisis in recent history, with the consequences likely to affect people's lives for many years to come. As events unfolded around the COVID-19 Pandemic and increased impacts of global warming, authors responded by including evidence and case studies to create both a valuable historical record and a work we believe is highly relevant for shaping the future of human and planetary health.

We dedicate this book to our planet and its peoples, and hope that it will inspire readers to learn with and from each other to tackle the immense challenges we confront.

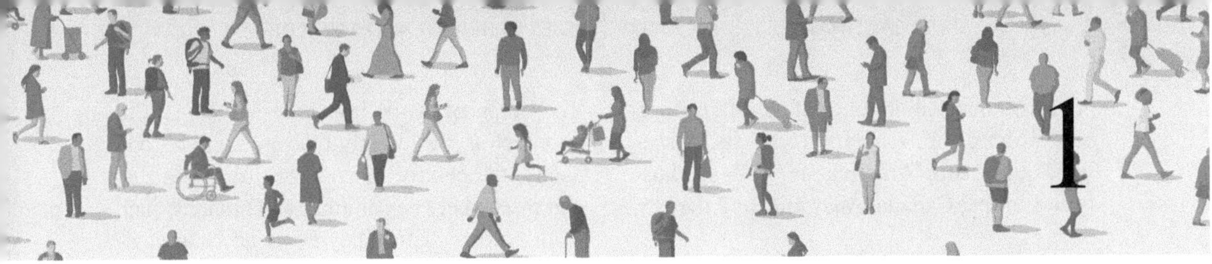

1 Introduction

Susan C. Scrimshaw, Sandra D. Lane, Robert A. Rubinstein, and Julian Fisher

HEALTH IN GLOBAL PERSPECTIVE

The first edition of *The Handbook of Social Studies in Health and Medicine* was published just over 20 years ago (Albrecht, Fitzpatrick, and Scrimshaw 2000), focusing on traditional social science disciplines as applied to health. This new edition incorporates the social, political and public health contexts of the 21st century. It goes beyond the social and behavioral sciences as they focus on individual behaviors and health systems to include broader health issues and a wider array of disciplines. In this *Handbook*, the social sciences are seen as interconnected with the health sciences, and with additional areas of science that influence the wider environmental issues that affect human and planetary health. Authors have been encouraged to analyze issues from multiple levels and perspectives, ranging from the individual, family, community, national and regional, through to the global. In addition to those multiple levels, a longitudinal perspective included in many chapters tackles the historical determinants of current health disparities, such as economic inequalities and unequal treatment of people, and how those determinants link to health systems and provide the context in which health systems, health behaviors and health injustices arise.

This edition adopts an inclusive approach to addressing health and related environmental issues across and within chapters, and to chapter authorship, which reflects the importance of a global view of local issues. We sought to include perspectives from local regions and communities, and the voices of members of those communities. Some of the chapters exemplify key issues through local or regional lenses, while others take on a global perspective. Seven of the original authors have updated their work, often adding co-authors to provide richer perspectives. Two original authors wrote entirely new chapters. Authors represent a wider range of countries, regions, and populations than in the first volume. Scholars from communities of indigenous peoples and refugees are represented along with scholars from Asia, Africa, India and Latin America as well as those from Europe, Canada, Australia, and the US.

HUMAN HEALTH IN THE CONTEXT OF PLANETARY HEALTH

Several important themes run through this volume. First, there is the theme of linking human health to environmental and planetary health. In this edition of the *Handbook of Social Studies in Health and Medicine*, we recognize that human health is inextricably bound to the effects of human activity on climate, water, land, bio and plant diversity and similar areas as they relate to the health of the planet. The chapters examine the effects of human use and abuse of the planet on health and societies through the lenses of food availability, water availability and quality, environmental hazards, occupational health, pandemics, economic stresses, refugee health, race, class and ethnicity and disasters. The chapter *Connecting Human Health to Nature Health: The Bridging Potential of Sustainable Food Systems* by Tribaldos and Rist (Chapter 29) explores the "One Health" concept: "Making the social sustainability outcomes explicit, allows linking the 'One Health' concept to biodiversity (in terms of genes, species and habitats of plants, microbes, and animals) and the bio-material world to the human side of health." The One Health concept states: "One Health is a collaborative, multi-sectoral, and trans-disciplinary approach – working at local, regional, national, and global levels – to achieve optimal health and well-being outcomes recognizing the interconnections between people, animals, plants and their shared environment" (One Health Commission 2021). World Health Organization One Health is an approach to designing and implementing programmes, policies, legislation and research in which multiple sectors work together to achieve better public health outcomes. The areas of work in which a One Health approach is particularly relevant include food safety, the control of zoonoses (diseases that can spread between animals and humans, such as flu, rabies, Rift Valley Fever and coronaviruses), and combatting antibiotic resistance (when bacteria change after being exposed to antibiotics and become more difficult to treat).

Several other chapters emphasize a more balanced and harmonious relationship between people and the planet through traditional and indigenous cultures. *Historical Trauma and Health Injustice in Indigenous Communities* (Chapter 12), *Cultural Variations in the Experience of Health and Illness* (Chapter 2), *Complementary and Integrative Health and Medicine Practices and Systems* (Chapter 23), and *Anthropological Approaches to Food and Nutrition* (Chapter 9) all discuss links between human and environmental health. The effects of humans on the environment have accelerated since the Industrial Revolution and we are witnessing the devastating consequences. As noted in the chapters on *The History of Changing Concepts of Health and Illness* (Chapter 5) and *The Social Causation of Health and Illness* (Chapter 4), people and societies have long organized themselves to induce and maintain wellness, with the understanding that this includes their environment (Clarkson, Morrissette, and Régallet 1992). The chapters reconnect important concepts of wellness and environment. Long-term neglect of these concepts now threatens the very survival of much of life on our planet. Many of the chapters explore the relationship between human health and planetary health, and discuss both problems and actions which need to take place going forward.

THE SOCIAL DETERMINANTS OF HEALTH

> "Yet the virus arrived on these shores, and it planted itself in the gaps of disparity. ... The virus exposed the vulnerabilities of all humans and the layers of hierarchy." (Wilkerson 2020, 356)

A second major theme revolves around the social determinants of health. The World Health Organization defines social determinants of health as "the conditions in which people are *born, grow, work, live, and age*, and the wider set of forces and systems shaping the conditions of daily life. These systemic forces include *economic policies and systems, development agendas, social norms, social policies and political systems*. … 50% of inequalities in major NCDs are *accounted for by social inequalities* in risk factors" (World Health Organization 2017, 1, original emphasis). We see health inequities as demonstrated by differences in rates and risk of disease and poor health, differences in severity of disease, and differences in disease outcomes between populations or groups. These in turn are intensified by disparate access to prevention and treatment services, differences in patterns of use of services, in health promotion and disease prevention behaviors, in behaviors in response to illness, in environmental and occupational risks, in community factors such as racism, stress, societal support, access to food, water, and other essential needs, community cohesion, and occasionally, by some degree of genetic risk. Each of these areas is discussed in one or more chapters in this *Handbook*, and together, they make up a large part of the social determinants of health (Bogard, Murray, and Alexander 2017).

Among the earliest work that led to the concept of social determinants of health was the Alameda Health Study in California, where longitudinal research on health habits documented a relationship with health outcomes. Behaviors related to factors such as healthy diet, increased physical activity and no tobacco use were associated with improved longevity (Bellock and Breslow 1972). Based on this work, Breslow argued in support of the then recently revised WHO definition of health, which included "physical, mental and social well-being, not merely the absence of disease or infirmity" and urged that medicine work to move people towards healthier behaviors (Breslow 1972, 1996). The results of the Alameda Health Study were transformational in moving medicine and public health from a disease model to a health promotion and health maintenance model.

Prior to the Alameda Health Study, Hans Selye published in 1956 a path-breaking work on stress and its impact on health. He proposed the concept of stress as an important influence on health and established the basis for studying the biological effects of stress on health. He proposed understanding the body's response to stress as an adaptation. He described some of the "diseases of adaptation" as heart disease, kidney disease, inflammatory diseases, cancer and mental health conditions, and argued for a more unified approach to biology and medicine (Selye 1956).

In parallel, the social and behavioral sciences, along with the medical sciences, were documenting social forces and individual and community behaviors that affect health. Medical anthropology, health psychology, medical sociology, health economics, social work and related disciplines contributed to understanding these social forces and added to the behavioral factors identified in the Alameda Health Study and in Selye's work on stress. For example, William Dressler documented the effects of racism and other forces creating increased stress for African American men and showed an association between stress, hypertension, and increased risk of heart disease (Dressler 1991, 1995). In 1992, Lobel et al. (1992) published data suggesting an association between pre-natal maternal stress and negative birth outcomes, including low birthweight even without premature delivery, as well as premature delivery. Data from the same study implicated stress and lack of social support in postpartum depression in addition to low birthweight, and implicated racism in producing increased stress for African American women (Collins et al. 1993; Engle et al. 1990).

Michael Marmot (2005) built on the body of work on the social determinants of health by reiterating the importance of social factors at the root of many inequalities in health and suggesting that the WHO adopt the term "social determinants of health" (SDH). His advocacy helped to launch the World Health Organization's independent Commission on Social Determinants of Health, which focused on turning public-health knowledge into political action, and which in 2008 published an ambitious agenda in *Closing the Gap in a Generation: Health Equity through Action on the Social Determinants of Health* (Commission on Social Determinants of Health 2008). The Commission drew on decades of study by social scientists on social-ecological issues in health (Anderson, Scrimshaw, et al. 2003; Evans et al. 2001) to recommend policies with the goal of improving health of the world's most vulnerable people. In 2008, the US National Academy of Medicine (then called the Institute of Medicine of the National Academies) held its annual meeting on the topic of *Is Biology Destiny?: The Social Determinants of Health*, a first for that organization. This was followed by a series of NAM and National Academy of Science consensus studies and workshops on multiple aspects of the topic. In the decade and a half since Marmot's publication, SDH have been mainstreaming into political discourse and health workforce education; a PubMed phrase-restricted search for articles using "social determinants of health" in their title, conducted on 14 February 2021, yielded 1,312 articles, with the bulk of those (913) being published in the five years 2015–2020. Researchers estimate that up to 90% of the factors that influence our health and survival arise from inadequate housing, poverty, exposure to violence, poor access to healthful foods, and similar conditions of disadvantage (Sederer 2016; Weber et al. 2018; Zambrana 1987).

Interest in SDH has also resulted in multiple conceptual models, or visual depictions with little consensus on a single version. One of the earliest was developed by the CDC Task Force on Community Preventative Services (Anderson, Fullilove, et al. 2003; Anderson, Scrimshaw, et al. 2003). More recent models that embrace many of the same elements include the WHO model (see *A Conceptual Framework for Action on the Social Determinants of Health* (Solar O 2010)), and the County Health Rankings Model (Fockele, Janeway, and Hsieh 2019). All three models describe the links between public policy and impacts on health outcomes and their consequences.

This *Handbook* envisions a holistic approach to social determinants of health, one that embraces the shared elements presented in many models, and expands the context to include planetary health, as discussed in the chapters in Part 4 on *Connecting Human Health to Nature Health: The Bridging Potential of Sustainable Food Systems* (Chapter 29) and *The Ecological Paradox: Health and Environment in the 21st Century* (Chapter 28). This expanded vision positions SDH within the UN 2030 Agenda for Sustainable Development and its 17 goals, and UN work across sectors through concepts such as One Health concept, which puts human health in the context of environmental health and emerging work on planetary health. Chapter 33, *Economic and Health Policy in the Context of the Sustainable Development Goals 2030 Agenda* discusses some of the issues raised by the 2030 Agenda. Ultimately, human health depends on people living within planetary boundaries. The case for this is made strongly in "Safeguarding human health in the Anthropocene epoch: report of The Rockefeller Foundation–*Lancet* Commission on Planetary Health" (Whitmee et al. 2015).

Stepping back to take a broad look at the areas encompassed in this book yields the model below that includes the concepts of planetary health and the social determinants of health, usually depicted separately. Planetary health is an emerging field but already speaks to many of the ideas put forward in the book. Thus, our model includes a wide range of areas. Topics such as climate, water, agricultural land, biodiversity, food sources, and environmental damage surround influences on the health of communities and individuals. Figure 1.1 draws on elements in multiple visualizations for the SDH, and in particular, the three mentioned above, but

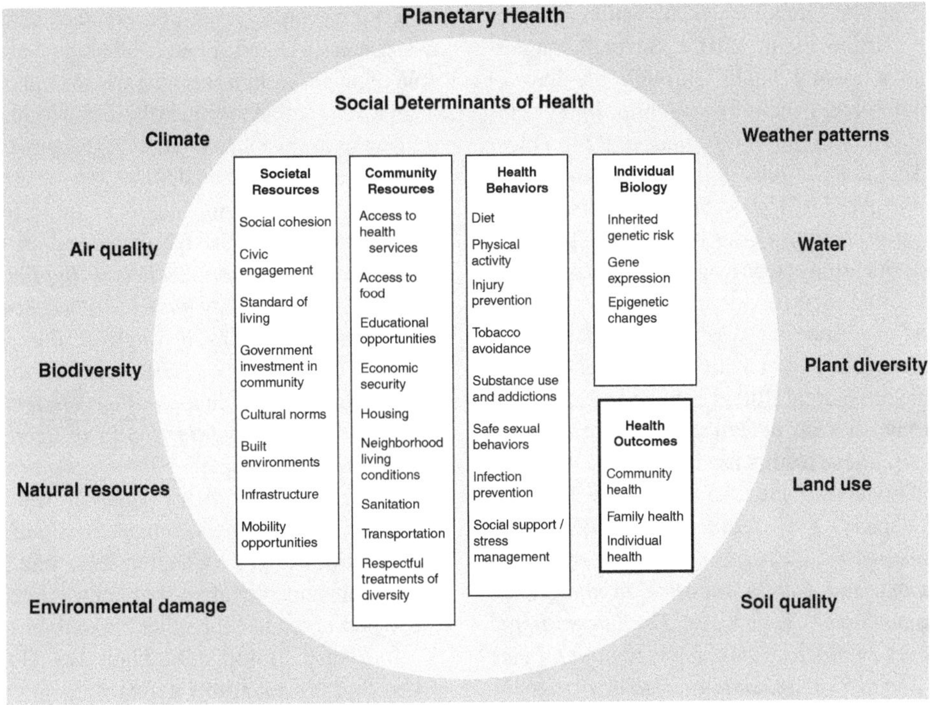

Figure 1.1 Social determinants of health in the context of planetary health

makes more explicit the elements of planetary health in order to picture a one-health model. In this view, the social determinants of health move from societal resources to community resources to health behaviors, and finally, to health outcomes at the community, family and individual levels. Our growing understanding of genetic risk, gene expression, and epigenetic changes is also reflected here, and is discussed in Chapter 11 on *Historical Trauma and Epigenetics*.

Initially, research on the social determinants of health focused on environmental and social risks that increased physical health problems, such as living in a food desert being associated with type 2 diabetes (Walker et al. 2014) or low birthweight (Lane et al. 2008). More recently, researchers focusing on depression, anxiety, and other mental health conditions began applying SDH concepts to psychological stressors that could increase emotional distress, using the framework "social determinants of mental health" (SDMH) (Alegría et al. 2018; National Academies of Sciences 2016). Subsequently, the SDMH approach has been applied to the study of how structural racism, and how exposure to interpersonal racism, is associated with poorer health and mental health (Paradies et al. 2015). Structural determinants of health such as institutional racism differentially impact disadvantaged communities, accentuating the vicious cycle of lower education and unstable employment, and unsafe housing. More directly related to psychological stress is increased allostatic load (the cumulative physiological consequences of chronic stress resulting from elevated levels of hormones released by the adrenal glands in response to racially-motivated treatment by others (McEwen 2005). Other authors have used the SDMH framework to examine and develop interventions for the adverse experiences civilians face in war situations, from which refugees flee (Bruno et al. 2019). Several chapters look at mental health through the lens of social forces, including *Mental Illness, the Global Landscape of Stigma, and the Power of Social Relationships* (Chapter 16) and *A Public Health Approach to Loneliness and Isolation among Older Adults* (Chapter 15). A major study from Kaiser Permanente in California identified that such adverse childhood experiences (ACEs) as loss of a parent or having a parent with substance addiction or severe mental illness can lead to increased chronic disease in adulthood (Gilgoff et al. 2020). These results are likely to be reflected in many communities around the world.

Chapters on *Historical Trauma and Epigenetics* (Chapter 11), *Historical Trauma and Health Injustice in Indigenous Communities* (Chapter 12), *The Intersectional Impact of Race, Class, Ethnicity, and Place on Social Determinants of Health across the Life Course* (Chapter 3), *Anthropological Approaches to Food and Nutrition* (Chapter 9), *Refugees, Life in Host Communities, and the Health Challenges* (Chapter 13), and in Part 4 chapters on *Syndemics and Structural Violence* (Chapter 30), The Social Determinants of Lifelong Learning (Chapter 34), and *Disasters and Health* (Chapter 31) also look at historical trauma as a continuum of multi-, inter-, and intra-generational harm. Emerging evidence in an evolving body of literature on epigenetics suggests that trauma may be inherited via the modulation of existing genes (Conching and Thayer 2019). Historical traumatic exposures potentially involving epigenetic changes include having ancestors who lived for generations under slavery, followed by Jim Crow laws and lynching; Native American children taken from their families and placed in brutal boarding schools; and severe famines, such as occurred in China and Ireland, and experiencing the direct effects and legacies of colonialism. The proceedings of a workshop on teaching the SDMH to health care students, hosted by the National Academy of Medicine, reviewed best-practice examples of how to help students to compassionately understand the various risks, stressors, and traumas affecting vulnerable populations in a way that the students can learn to take action to reduce those determinants in their future practice (National Academies of Sciences and Medicine 2020).

Finally, we cannot neglect the effects of racism on health. As discussed in the chapters on *The Intersectional Impact of Race, Class, Ethnicity, and Place on Social Determinants of Health across the Life Course* (Chapter 3), *Historical Trauma and Epigenetics* (Chapter 11), *Historical Trauma and Health Injustice in Indigenous Communities* (Chapter 12), *Occupational Health in the 21st Century* (Chapter 32), and *Refugees, Life in Host Communities, and the Health Challenges* (Chapter 13), unequal treatment and negative behavior towards those perceived as “the other” take their toll. Evolutionary biologist Stephen Jay Gould noted that “races aren’t definable, and even if definable, not very well defined. Racial variation is the original geographic variation of the species that spread, presumably from an African center, all over the world … when you measure the actual genetic differences among people, they’re astonishingly small” (Koch 1995, 14; Goodman 2000). Anthropologist Alan Goodman noted: “Because race and racism are sociopolitical realities, they affect individual biologies. Understanding this presents a new and radical biocultural agenda. The continuance of ‘race’ and ethnic differences in health calls for an explication of the biology of inequality and racism” (Goodman 2001, 31). Thus, the fact that race is not a valid concept for scientific measurement does not negate the fact that racism exists, and shapes how people are seen, defined and treated, which becomes part of the social determinants of health. This concept is further explored in detail in *Race: Are We So Different?* (Goodman, Moses, and Jones 2020). As discussed in multiple chapters in this *Handbook*, racism and its impacts are global, permeating virtually every nation.

METHODOLOGICAL AND EPISTEMOLOGICAL CONSIDERATIONS

Disease, illness, and conceptions of health are complex, interrelated phenomena. It follows that the simple explanations of these phenomena give only partial insights into them. Sometimes partial understandings can lead to inadequate and poorly fitting policies or interventions. The range of the chapters display some of the resulting diversity in methodologies and epistemological approaches in this area. Throughout the *Handbook*, the chapter authors describe ways in which this diversity affects our understanding. We highlight here four dimensions of this complexity: (1) methods, measurement, and research design; (2) multi-level investigations; (3) the importance of historical depth; and (4) different ways of knowing and constructing evidence.

Social science research in health and medicine includes many disciplines. Each has its own set of methodological guidelines that researchers use. Sometimes these rely on particular approaches to the collection of evidence, emphasizing, for example, quantitative techniques or qualitative approaches. In some circumstances, disciplinary methodological preferences form strong barriers between researchers, isolating them in disciplinary silos that reduce their knowledge of other fields.

Working within a quantitative paradigm, Campbell and Fiske showed that a more adequate understanding depends upon approaching the subject of study using multiple measures, each of which give a slightly different picture of that subject (Campbell and Fiske 1959). Similarly, qualitative researchers have developed the idea that fully understanding the subject of their work depends upon evaluating a social setting from multiple perspectives, and has led to the idea of triangulation (Atkinson et al. 2001). Triangulation in a qualitative context means finding different ways to assess what is being studied and looking at how these converge to inform the accuracy of the information obtained. It is a qualitative realization of a quantitatively demonstrated methodological advance.

In the first edition of this *Handbook*, Rubinstein, Scrimshaw, and Morrissey (Rubinstein, Scrimshaw, and Morrissey 2000) demonstrated the value of considering multiple levels of analysis, and recommended that health research follow "the rule of minimal inclusion" (Rubinstein, Laughlin, and McManus 1984), which stipulates that research designs include levels of organization, above and below the phenomenon being investigated. They argued that doing so provides a fuller picture than would be possible by looking at issues of health and illness only on the social level, or biological level, or psychological level. In essence, "the rule of minimal inclusion" is an application of the Campbell and Fiske insight and in a sense a suggestion for three-dimensional triangulation. Multilevel research has become a much more common approach (e.g., Cook et al. 2014).

Multilevel studies provide a much clearer picture of issues of health and illness and of the interaction among the cultural, social, psychological, and physical worlds in which issues of health are lived. With the development of newer fields of inquiry, like epigenetics and historical trauma affecting Indigenous peoples, contributors to this second edition of the *Handbook* show the importance of adding a fourth dimension to the understanding of health and illness. Such historical analyses demonstrate that the health status of contemporary populations is affected by the experiences of prior generations. These experiences may include various kinds of traumas which may lead to changes in the biological organisms that endure over time and also to the ways in which societies and cultures organize themselves and provide meaning about the health challenges they face (see Chapter 12 on *Historical Trauma and Health Injustice in Indigenous Communities* and Chapter 11 on *Historical Trauma and Epigenetics*).

Several of the chapters describe research methodologies that illuminate the recognition that experiences of health and illness rely as well on different ways of knowing. Studies that interpret meaning, rather than only categorizing and counting, provide essential information with which to craft interventions that fit better with the cultural understandings of the research participants. Social and political factors lead to the privileging of particular ways of understanding the world in what has been called "authoritative knowledge" – "the knowledge that is constructed and displayed by members of a community of practice as the basis for legitimate decision-making" (Jordan 1993, xii–xiii; and see Chapter 24 on *Childbirth, Midwifery and Obstetrics: Global Issues in Maternity Care*). The chapters use not only different methodological approaches derived from their disciplinary commitments, but also reflect other ways of knowing about the world, such as descriptions of the ways in which health phenomena are experienced. These descriptions may derive from introspection as in Chapter 8 on *Personal Experience of Illness and the Patient's Perspective Regarding Appropriate Healthcare* and Chapter 17 on *From Ableism to* Amplitude*: A Celebration of Dis/ability*; or from the collection of narratives of a community of affected individuals as in Chapter 10 on *Community Engaged Learning: Community Health and Learning through Service in Sri Lanka*, or from other kinds of knowledge-producing techniques as described in Chapter 7 on *Network Analysis: The Social Bridge to Health* and Chapter 22 on *Lay Participation in Healthcare Policy, Planning and Practice: To What End?*

It is important to recognize that these different ways of knowing provide information that can be useful for interpreting the world (Rubinstein, Laughlin, and McManus 1984). However, although it is important to engage seriously with a wide variety of information sources, it is also critical to understand that the information that each source provides support different kinds of claims about the world. For example, a double masked trial of an intervention provides information about the efficacy of that intervention, while an experiential account does not. At the same time, the experiential account provides information about what it may be like to experience the condition for which intervention is developed in a way that a double masked trial cannot. Both of these forms of information are important for engaging health and illness and disease but they do not substitute one for the other. We have sought to allow diverse voices to speak while also pointing out places where those voices provide appropriate support for the claims that they may be making. We have endeavored as well to be clear in the editing of this *Handbook* to point out instances in which claims from different ways of knowing about a health-related phenomenon may be in tension with one another and to show the extent and the limits of the support that each of the different ways of understanding provide for the claims being made in the chapters.

COMMUNICATION AND TECHNOLOGY

The vital importance of innovations in communication and technology also challenge our ability to address health concerns from the individual to the planetary levels. Two chapters in this volume focus specifically on these areas, Chapter 26 on *Digital Health: An Important Public Health Tool* and Chapter 27 on *Health Behaviors and Social Media*. Both areas are evolving rapidly. In health technology, wearable devices are transforming our ability to monitor and self-monitor health as well as to influence behaviors such as physical activity. Other devices, such as oximeters, allow for home measurement of blood oxygen levels, while smartphone and computer technology provide constant access to information. Technological innovations like these help individuals monitor their own physical and emotional state. Additionally, technological innovations available to institutions and organizations have enhanced the precision with which remote diagnosis and treatment can be conducted. The synergies created by technologies facilitate the conditions for information sharing among geographically and professionally diverse teams of professionals, providing insights and treatment opportunities not previously possible. Globally, there are wide disparities in the availability of these devices to individuals. Also, as discussed in Chapter 27 on *Health Behavior and Social Media*, there is wide variability in the reliability and accuracy of sources accessed by means of social media, which necessitates strategies for helping people distinguish the accurate from the misleading or inaccurate sources. This is complicated by health literacy.

Health literacy has been defined as "the degree to which individuals have the capacity to obtain, process, and understand basic health information and services needed to make appropriate health decisions" (Institute of Medicine 2004). Adults with limited health literacy have less knowledge of disease management and of health-promoting behaviors, report poorer health status, and are less likely to use preventive services (Institute of Medicine 2004; Levandowski et al. 2006). Health literacy is mediated by educational level, culture, language, the communication and assessment skills of people providing health care and information, and the ability of the media, the marketplace, and government agencies to provide health information in a manner appropriate to the audience (Lane et al. 2017). Health literacy is much more than reading levels, or even vocabulary, but must be understood and addressed in the context of culture and language. It is about communication and understanding, which are shaped by insider cultural world views and how language shapes understanding and meaning. For examples of this, see the chapters on *Anthropological Approaches to Food and Nutrition* (Chapter 9), *The Sociomaterial Nature of the Body and Medicine* (Chapter 6), and *Cultural Variation in the Experience of Health and Illness* (Chapter 2).

Health communication also involves the ability of health professionals and scientists to communicate clearly with each other across disciplinary boundaries, and then to communicate clearly with the wider lay communities (Scrimshaw 2019). In this edition of the *Handbook*, we have worked with the authors to encourage them to write their chapters in language accessible to those outside of their specific disciplines areas, in an effort to make it accessible to a wide range of basic, clinical, and social scientists working on health and environmental issues, as well as to policy makers and administrators.

HEALTH SYSTEMS AND HEALTH WORKFORCE

As described in Chapter 19 on *Comparative Health Systems: Paradigm Changes*, health systems around the world take many shapes and forms, and are constantly evolving. In addition to the Western biomedical systems, we have alternative health systems, as described in Chapter 23 on *Complementary and Integrative Health and Medicine Practices and Systems*, and ways of healing and maintaining health based on traditional cultural values and practices, as discussed in the chapters on *Cultural Variation in the Experience of Health and Illness* (Chapter 2), *Childbirth, Midwifery and Obstetrics: Global Issues in Maternity Care* (Chapter 24) and *The History of the Changing Concepts of Health and Illness* (Chapter 5). For individuals, there is a wide and sometimes conflicting array of services, with access to them limited by educational, economic, geographic, policy and cultural factors, as discussed earlier in the social determinants of health sections. As discussed in Chapter 22 on *Lay Participation in Healthcare Policy, Planning and Practice: To What End?*, and in Chapter 20 on *Health Service Utilization and Barriers to Health Care*, these services are often hierarchically separated from the people they intend to serve, and there is a failure to respect and respond to user and patient perspectives.

As noted in Chapter 8 on *Personal Experience of Illness and the Patient's Perspective Regarding Appropriate Healthcare*, and Chapter 6 on *The Sociomaterial Nature of the Body and Medicine*, people's lived experiences also influence health seeking and health maintenance behaviors. Part 2 in this *Handbook* deals with these lived experiences for health issues ranging from loneliness to mental illness to substance use to disability (*A Public Health Approach to Loneliness and Isolation among Older Adults, Mental Illness, the Global Landscape of Stigma, and the Power of Social Relationships, From Ableism to Amplitude: A Celebration of Dis/ability*, and *Social and Geopolitical Factors Influencing Trends in Substance Use*). This section also deals with the effects of historical traumas on health, such as war, famine and genocide (*Historical Trauma and Epigenetics, Historical Trauma and Health Injustice in Indigenous Communities, Refugees, Life in Host Communities, and the Health Challenges*). These are issues that many health systems and health practitioners struggle with, as they often don't fit neatly into disease categories for which there is a clinical solution, but instead, present complex problems which require complex and multifaceted solutions. Again, both these problems and solutions are tied to understanding and addressing the social determinants of health.

Another set of complex issues – longstanding cultural practices which endanger women, and the difficulty which health systems have in diagnosing and treating women and girls in some instances – is discussed in Chapter 14 on *Gender and Health* in Part 2, and in Chapter 6 on *The Sociomaterial Nature of the Body and Medicine*. The shifting definitions of gender and gender identity are also described, along with noting the need for more understanding and respectful treatment of transgender people. Even as there are cultural and sometimes religious struggles around these issues, the underlying health needs remain.

All of the challenges discussed in this Introduction place increasingly complex demands on health workers, and many of these are reflected in the chapters in Part 3: *Health Care Systems, Access and Use*, as in Chapter 19 on *Comparative Health Systems: Paradigm Changes* and Chapter 20 on *Health Service Utilization and Barriers to Health Care*. The issue of increasing medicalization of health is described for the pharmaceutical industry in Chapter 25 on *Medicalization and Pharmaceuticalization: A Conceptual Analysis*, as well as in Chapter 24 on *Childbirth, Midwifery and Obstetrics: Global Issues in Maternity Care* and in Chapter 5 on *The History of the Changing Concepts of Health and Illness* in Part 1. The difficulty of understanding health status and health-related quality of life is assessed in Chapter 21 on *Measuring Health and Health Related Quality of Life*.

In 2010, a *Lancet* commission on the health workforce published an analysis of three major health professions – medicine, nursing and public health – in terms of their evolution as a 21st century workforce (Frenk et al. 2010). The report on *Health Professions for a New Century* noted that the health professions have changed dramatically in the past 100 years and will continue to change in response to scientific and medical advances, population health needs, economic constraints, changing health policies, and much more. It also noted that practitioners in health include many more professions than the three featured in the report, and that future analyses will need to include these. In this *Handbook*, we have tried to include a wide variety of health practitioners, both as authors and as topics of discussion.

The 2010 *Lancet* report has stimulated discussions in institutions ranging from the US National Academy of Medicine to the World Health Organization. In 2016, the United Nations Secretary-General announced the appointment of a Commission on Health Employment and Economic Growth, which moved quickly to produce a report with recommendations on job creation, gender equity, education and competencies, certification, technology, data collection and management, health services organization and delivery, financing, dealing with humanitarian crises, international migration, and forming partnerships to ensure cooperation (Commission on Health Employment and Economic Growth 2016).

In 2016, the US National Academy of Medicine's Board on Global Health published a report on *A Framework for Educating Health Professionals to Address the Social Determinants of Health* (National Academies of Sciences 2016). The chapter on *Futures of Health Professions Education* builds on this and the World Health Organization's work. It reflects ongoing efforts to encourage those involved in health and social care, ranging from physicians to community health workers, to respond to the rapidly changing environment in which health and illness must be considered. Education, continuing education, credentialing, licensing and interprofessional collaboration are all in urgent need of updating.

CONCLUSIONS: THE NEED FOR INTERDISCIPLINARY AND GLOBAL UNDERSTANDING, RESPECT, AND PRACTICE

This introduction was written in early 2021, in the midst of the COVID-19 pandemic. Human society is facing immense challenges with the current pandemic, testing health care and public health institutions, lifestyles and livelihoods, conventional ways of working, access to food and other necessary resources, and social relationships in ways not experienced since the last two great world wars.

While it may be comforting to imagine a swift return to a 'new normal', scientific evidence suggests that this may be more of a dress rehearsal for more extreme and unpredictable challenges emerging from Climate Change and antimicrobial resistance, for example. The COVID-19 pandemic yet again emphasizes the need to shift from seeing problems to be solved in an insular way to accepting that these are complex and evolving challenges. This will require solutions to be agile and part of an ongoing process requiring high levels of trust and cooperation as a global effort. The UN 2030 Agenda for Sustainable Development and its 17 Sustainable Development Goals provide the basis for global dialogue and action, but these will be ineffective if they remain disconnected from the everyday lives of people. This edition of the *Handbook* covers many issues from individual and community health to the environment, social determinants of health and health equity, occupational health, global warming, stressed food and water systems, refugees, disasters and pandemics. All highlight the interdependency and intersection of challenges and the complexity of both problems and solutions.

This edition highlights the need for respect, understanding, and cooperation, and we identify three key areas.

First, interdisciplinary cooperation is essential to solve the problems at hand. We encourage readers of this *Handbook* to explore beyond their comfort zone and seek to understand a wide range of disciplinary and substantive areas. Improving the health of our planet and of our populations is dependent on multi- and interdisciplinary solutions. This also means cultivating respect for all disciplinary areas, and respecting the multiple methodologies that can be used to inform decision-making. There is tension between the sciences which inform human and planetary health and development. Understanding and working to dissipate this tension is essential for success in developing effective strategies and solutions.

A second area requiring respect, understanding, and cooperation is the need to work together across dimensions of geographic space, national boundaries, and populations.

The era of scientific and policy dominance from economically advantaged nations is under pressure to give way to a more global understanding, but this trend needs to accelerate in order to address common problems. This edition includes the voices from the field, and from practice, education, research and policy from scientists and policy makers from all the world's regions, and from populations deeply affected by historic inequities. We encourage our readers to continue to expand the range of those providing input on science and policy. The refrain "don't reinvent the wheel" is a positive and practical note to close this edition. We can learn from traditional and indigenous cultures not only in terms of solutions but, more importantly, how to relate to our surroundings and the planet.

This *Handbook* focuses on balance and interdependency as we seek to understand and solve challenges to our very survival. Our authors and our advisory board members have helped us to understand this interdependency through their work and their advice. We are grateful for the time and effort they have contributed.

We are pleased to have introduced readers to ideas that we hope will help them move beyond a traditional behavioral sciences focus on individual behaviors and health systems to include broader health issues and a wider array of disciplines, including those associated with the social determinants of health and links between human health and planetary health. Many of the themes presented in this edition of the *Handbook* are brought into stark relief by the COVID-19 pandemic, during which the chapters were written. This work points towards the measures necessary to solve the problems identified here. Finally, it shows the value of actualizing a predominant characteristic of humanity, that, *in extremis*, working together is essential for the good of society as a whole, and for the survival of the complex interdependent web of life on this planet.

REFERENCES

Albrecht, Gary L., Ray Fitzpatrick, and Susan C. Scrimshaw, eds. 2000. *The Handbook of Social Studies in Health and Medicine*. London, UK: Sage Publications.

Alegría, M., A. NeMoyer, F.I. Bagué, Y. Wang, and K. Alvarez. 2018. "The social determinants of mental health: where we are and where we need to go." *Current Psychiatry Reports* 20 (95): 1–13. doi: 10.1007/s11920-018-0969-9.

Anderson, Laurie M., Mindy C. Fullilove, Susan C. Scrimshaw, and Jonathan E. Fielding. 2003. "The *Guide to Community Preventive Services*: interventions in the social environment to improve community health: a systematic review." *American Journal of Preventive Medicine* 24 (3S): 1–82.

Anderson, Laurie M., Susan C. Scrimshaw, Mindy C. Fullilove, Jonathan E. Fielding, and Task Force on Community Preventive Services. 2003. "The *Community Guide*'s model for linking the social environment to health." *American Journal of Preventive Medicine* 24 (3S): 12–20.

Atkinson, Paul, Amanda Coffey, Sara Delamont, John Lofland, and Lyn Lofland, eds. 2001. *Handbook of Ethnography*. London, UK: Sage Publications.

Bellock, Nedra B., and Lester Breslow. 1972. "Relationship of physical health status and health practice." *Preventive Medicine* 1 (3): 409–421.

Bogard, Kimber, Velma McBride Murray, and Charlee Alexander, eds. 2017. *Perspectives on Health Equity and Social Determinants of Health*. Washington, DC: National Academy of Medicine.

Breslow, Lester. 1972. "A quantitative approach to the World Health Organization definition of health: physical, mental and social well-being." *International Journal of Epidemiology* 1 (4): 347–355.

Breslow, Lester. 1996. "Social ecological strategies for promoting healthy lifestyles." *American Journal of Health Promotion* 10 (4): 253–257.

Bruno, W., A. Kitamura, S. Najjar, A. Seita, and W.K. Al-Delaimy. 2019. "Assessment of mental health and psycho-social support pilot program's effect on intended stigmatizing behavior at the Saftawi Health Center, Gaza: a cross-sectional study." *Journal of Mental Health* 28 (4): 436–442. doi: 10.1080/09638237.2019.1608936.

Campbell, Donald T., and Fiske, Donald W. 1959. "Convergent and discriminant validation by the multitrait-multimethod matrix." *Psychological Bulletin* 56 (2): 81–105.

Clarkson, Linda, Vern Morrissette, and Gabriel Régallet. 1992. *Our Responsibility to the Seventh Generation: Indigenous Peoples and Sustainable Development*. Winnipeg, MB: International Institute for Sustainable Development.

Collins, Nancy L., Christine Dunkel-Schetter, Marci Lobel, and Susan C. Scrimshaw. 1993. "Social support in pregnancy: psychosocial correlates of birth outcomes and postpartum depression." *Journal of Personality and Social Psychology* 65 (6): 1243–1258.

Commission on Health Employment and Economic Growth. 2016. *Working for Health and Growth: Investing in the Health Workforce. Report of the High-Level Commission on Health Employment and Economic Growth*. Geneva: World Health Organization.

Commission on Social Determinants of Health. 2008. *Closing the Gap in a Generation: Health Equity through Action on the Social Determinants of Health – Final Report of the Commission Social Determinants of Health*. Geneva: World Health Organization.

Conching, A.K.S., and Z. Thayer. 2019. "Biological pathways for historical trauma to affect health: a conceptual model focusing on epigenetic modifications." *Social Science and Medicine* 230: 74–82. doi: 10.1016/j.socscimed.2019.04.001.

Cook, Jonathan E., Valerie Purdie-Vaughns, Illan H. Meyer, and Justin T.A. Busch. 2014. "Intervening within and across levels: a multilevel approach to stigma and public health." *Social Science and Medicine* 103: 101–109.

Dressler, William W. 1991. *Stress and Adaptation in the Context of Culture: Depression in a Southern Black Community*. Albany, NY: State University of New York Press.

Dressler, William W. 1995. "Modeling biocultural interactions: examples from studies of stress and cardiovascular disease." *American Journal of Physical Anthropology* 38 (S21): 27–56.

Engle, Patricia, Susan C. Scrimshaw, Ruth Enid Zambrana, and Christine Dunkel-Schetter. 1990. "Prenatal and postnatal anxiety in Mexican women giving birth in Los Angeles." *Health Psychology* 9 (3): 285–299.

Evans, Timothy, Margaret Whitehead, Finn Diderichsen, Abbas Bhuiya, and Meg Wirth, eds. 2001. *Challenging Inequities in Health: From Ethics to Action*. Oxford, UK: Oxford University Press.

Fockele, Callan, Hannah Janeway, and Dennis Hsieh. 2019. "Social determinants of health." In *Emergency Medicine Advocacy Handbook* (5th edition), edited by Nathaniel Schlicher and Alison Haddock, pp. 179–186. Irving, TX: Emergency Medicine Residents' Association.

Frenk, Julio, Lincoln Chen, Zulfiqqar A. Bhutta, Jordan Cohen, Nigel Crisp, Timothy Evans, Harvey Fieneberg, Patricia Garcia, Yang Ke, Patrick Kelley, Barry Kistnasamy, Afaf Meleis, David Naylor, Ariel Pablos-Mendez, Srinath Reddy, Susan C. Scrimshaw, Jaime Sepulveda, and David Serwadda. 2010. "Health professionals for a new century: transforming education to strengthen health systems in an interdependent world." *The Lancet* 376 (9756): 1923–1958.

Gilgoff, R., L. Singh, K. Koita, B. Gentile, and S.S. Marques. 2020. "Adverse childhood experiences, outcomes, and interventions." *Pediatric Clinics of North America* 67 (2): 259–273. doi:10.1016/j.pcl.2019.12.001.

Goodman, Alan H. 2000. "Why genes don't count (for racial differences in health)." *American Journal of Public Health* 90 (11): 1699–1702.

Goodman, Alan H. 2001. "Biological diversity and cultural diverstiy: from race to radical bioculturalism." In *Cultural Diversity in the United States: A Critical Reader*, edited by Ida Susser and Thomas C. Patterson, pp. 29–46. Malden, MA: Blackwell.

Goodman, Alan H., Yolanda T. Moses, and Joseph L. Jones. 2020. *Race: Are We so Different?* Malden, MA: Wiley-Blackwell.

Institute of Medicine. 2004. *Health Literacy: A Prescription to End Confusion*. Washington, DC: The National Academies Press.

Jordan, Bridgette 1993. *Birth in Four Cultures: A Crosscultural Investigation of Childbirth in Yucatan, Holland, Sweden, and the United States* (Fourth edition, revised and expanded by Robbie Davis-Floyd). Long Grove, IL: Waveland Press.

Koch, John. 1995. "Stephen Jay Gould you were called 'fossil face' as a boy, for being nuts about dinosaurs. Do you have a message for today's kids, who are often even more stigmatized for their scholarliness?" *The Boston Globe Magazine* 31 December: 14.

Lane, S.D., R.H. Keefe, R.A. Rubinstein, B.A. Levandowski, N. Webster, D.A. Cibula, A.K. Boahene, O. Dele-Michael, D. Carter, T. Jones, M. Wojtowycz, and J. Brill. 2008. "Structural violence, urban retail food markets, and low birth weight." *Health and Place* 14: 415–423. doi: 10.1016/j.healthplace.2007.08.008.

Lane, Sandra D., Sally J. Huntington, Lynn-Beth Satterly, Robert A. Rubinstein, Robert H. Keefe, and Amus Project Student Researchers. 2017. "Filling out the forms: health literacy among the uninsured." *Social Work in Health Care* 56 (8): 686–699.

Levandowski, Brooke A., P. Sharma, Sandra D. Lane, Noah Webster, Amanda Nestor, Donald A. Cibula, and Sally J. Huntington. 2006. "Parental literacy and infant health: an evidence-based Healthy Start intervention." *Health Promotion Practice* 7 (1): 95–102.

Lobel, Marci, Christine Dunkel-Schetter, and Susan C. Scrimshaw. 1992. "Prenatal maternal stress and prematurity: a prospective study of socioeconomically disadvantaged women." *Health Psychology* 11 (1): 32–40.

Marmot, Michael. 2005. "Social determinants of health inequalities." *Lancet* 365 (9464): 1099–1104. doi: 10.1016/S0140-6736(05)71146-6.

McEwen, Bruce S. 2005. "Stressed or stressed out: what is the difference?" *Journal of Psychiatry and Neuroscience* 30 (5): 315–318.

National Academies of Sciences, Engineering, and Medicine. 2016. *A Framework for Educating Health Professionals to Address the Social Determinants of Health*. Washington, DC: The National Academies Press.

National Academies of Sciences, Engineering, and Medicine. 2020. *Educating Health Professionals to Address the Social Determinants of Mental Health: Proceedings of a Workshop*. Edited by Patricia A. Cuff and Erin Hammers Forstag. Washington, DC: The National Academies Press.

One Health Commission. 2021. "One Health Commission." *One Health Commission*, www.onehealthcommission.org/: Accessed 16 February 2021.

Paradies, Y., J. Ben, N. Denson, A. Elias, N. Priest, A. Pieterse, A. Gupta, M. Kelaher, and G. Gee. 2015. "Racism as a determinant of health: a systematic review and meta-analysis." *PLoS One* 23 (9): e0138511. doi: 10.1371/journal.pone.0138511.

Rubinstein, Robert A., Charles D. Laughlin, Jr., and John McManus. 1984. *Science as Cognitive Process: Towards an Empirical Philosophy of Science*. Philadelphia, PA: University of Pennsylvania Press.

Rubinstein, Robert A., Susan C. Scrimshaw, and Suzanne E. Morrissey. 2000. "Classification and process in sociomedical understanding: towards a multilevel view of sociomedical methodology." In *The Handbook of Social Studies in Health and Medicine*, edited by Gary L. Albrecht, Ray Fitzpatrick and Susan C. Scrimshaw, pp. 36–49. London: Sage Publications.

Scrimshaw, Susan C. 2019. "Science, health, and cultural literacy in a rapidly changing communications landscape." *Proceedings of the National Academy of Sciences* 116 (16): 7650–7655.

Sederer, Lloyd I. 2016. "The social determinants of mental health." *Psychiatric Services* 67 (2): 234–235.

Selye, Hans. 1956. *The Stress of Life*. New York: McGraw-Hill.

Solar O, Irwin A. 2010. *A Conceptual Framework for Action on the Social Determinants of Health: Social Determinants of Health Discussion Paper 2 (Policy and Practice)*. Geneva: World Health Organization.

Walker, R.J., B.L. Smalls, J.A. Campbell, J.L.S. Williams, and L.E. Egede. 2014. "Impact of social determinants of health on outcomes for type 2 diabetes: a systematic review." *Endocrine* 47: 29–48. doi: 10.1007/s12020-014-0195-0.

Weber, Lynn, Ruth Enid Zambrana, M. Elizabeth Fore, and Deborah Parra-Medina. 2018. "Racial and ethnic health inequities: an intersectional approach." In *Handbook of the Sociology of Racial and Ethnic Relations, Second Edition*, edited by Hernan Vera and Joe R. Feagin, pp. 133–160. Cham, Switzerland: Springer.

Whitmee, Sarah, Andy Haines, Chris Beyrer, Frederick Boltz, Anthony G. Capon, Braulio Ferreira de Souza Dias, Alex Ezeh, Howard Frumkin, Peng Gong, Peter Head, Richard Horton, Georgina M. Mace, Robert Marten, Samuel S. Myers, Sahia Nishtar, Steven A. Osofsky, Subhrendu K. Pattanayak, Montira J. Pongsiri, Cristina Romanelli, Agnes Soucat, Jeanette Vega, and Derek Yach. 2015. "Safeguarding human health in the Anthropocene epoch: report of The Rockefeller Foundation–*Lancet* Commission on planetary health." *The Lancet* 386 (10007): 1976–2028.

Wilkerson, Isabel. 2020. *Caste: The Origins of our Discontents*. New York: Random House.

World Health Organization. 2017. *Social Determinants of Health Unit. Department of Public Health, Environmental and Social Determinants of Health*. Geneva: World Health Organization.

Zambrana, R.E. 1987. "A research agenda on issues affecting poor and minority women: a model for understanding their health needs." *Women & Health* 12 (3–4): 137–160.

PART 1

Culture, Society and Health

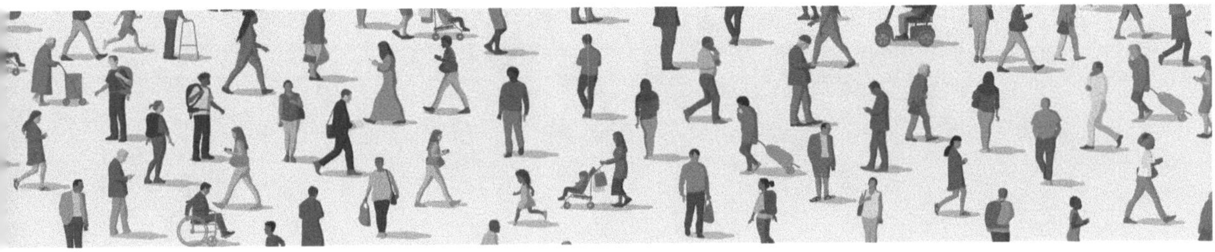

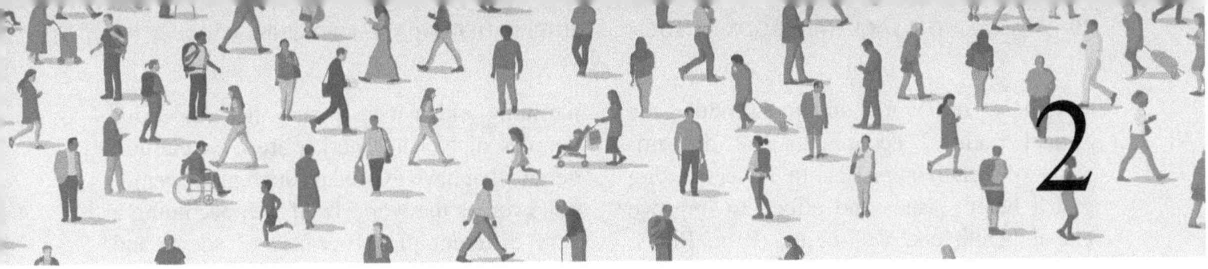

2

Cultural Variations in the Experience of Health and Illness

Pamela I. Erickson and Cynthia A. Frank

Every culture on our planet has developed a system for understanding the causes of illness and disease and devised ways both to prevent them and to help heal the bodies and minds of those afflicted. These ethnomedical systems are tremendously varied and each is an integral part of the culture in which it developed, currently exists, and evolves over time. Ethnomedical systems are cultural systems that reflect the dominant cultural themes of the societies in which they developed. For example, the primary ethnomedical system in the United States is biomedicine, which is based on a scientific, rationalistic approach to the world. It is also largely a for-profit (although there are some not-for-profit health insurance/maintenance companies – see https://achp.org/), hierarchical system that is oriented primarily toward the individual patient rather than to the broader social context of ill health (e.g., family, physical environment, poverty, sexism, racism, etc.) that Marmot (2005, 2006) has called the social determinants of health. Thus, biomedicine primarily reflects Americans' core cultural themes of independence, individualism, scientific positivism, and capitalism. Even though biomedicine developed in Europe and the United States, local cultural values of the different countries in Europe and in different areas of the United States affect how it is practiced *in situ*. For example, in the European Union and Canada, biomedical care is largely a nationalized, not-for-profit system funded by the government of each of the member nations and this reflects their more progressive, socially liberal value systems. Although biomedicine has become globalized, local cultures shape and reshape it to fit with their own cultural values. Ethnomedical systems other than biomedicine are also based on the core cultural themes of the cultures in which they developed and cannot be fully understood without some knowledge of the cultural values that guide the social, religious, economic, and political organization of the societies in which they are found.

We use a medical anthropological approach to examine the variety of ethnomedical systems in our world and to introduce the critical political economic/social determinants of health approach to understanding global health issues and efforts to improve global health and well-being (Birn, Pillay, and Holtz 2017; Singer and Erickson 2013). We begin with some key concepts from medical anthropology followed by an explanation of cultural views of health and illness based on the great ethnomedical systems in our world and how they relate to one another (Biomedicine, Ayurvedic medicine, Unani medicine, Traditional Chinese Medicine). We then address the smaller more local traditions (traditional healers, shamanism, sorcery, witchcraft) that are widespread in the world. Following this, we present a case study of a Hmong child's ethnomedical journey, the case of Lia Lee (Fadiman 1997), to illustrate the importance of understanding and learning the importance of accommodating different cultural beliefs about healing within biomedicine – what anthropologists call the emic or insider understanding and the etic or outsider understanding of health (Scrimshaw and Hurtado 1984). Finally, we describe some anthropological research methods that are useful for understanding culture and behavior and their implications for health.

CONCEPTS FROM MEDICAL ANTHROPOLOGY

Medical anthropology is the largest subfield within Cultural Anthropology, that branch of Anthropology devoted to understanding culture, which is a uniquely patterned set of beliefs and values that persist over time and distinguish one culture from another. Although medical anthropology also draws on other subfields, such as physical anthropology, linguistics, and archaeology, our primary concern in this chapter is to focus on the cultural understandings of medical systems. For example, the idea of karma and rebirth in India and the importance of harmony with nature among the indigenous peoples of North America are core cultural beliefs that have existed through many centuries even as the world itself was becoming a very different place because of social and economic changes (e.g., colonization and decolonization, the industrial revolution, globalization, global climate change). Anthropologists study the diversity of cultures in our world and seek to understand mechanisms of change and stability within them. We know culture changes, but we also know that core elements of culture (like karma and harmony) persist and provide a template for living in one's own culture.

Culture channels our natural biological urges (e.g., need for food, sex, elimination, and sleep) into culturally valued ways of expression and sets the limits for discouraged or prohibited ways of expression. It affects our social arrangements regarding kinship, gender roles, marriage, sex, reproduction and birthing, parenting, and death and dying. It also affects our food ways and what we think, what we do, what we believe, and how we express emotion. Important for the current chapter, culture shapes our understanding of health and illness: what causes illness/disease, when to seek care, and the appropriate healers to use for different health issues. Thus, culture plays a very important role in health, illness, and care-seeking, and this is why we often see conflict in cross-cultural interactions between patients and healers who themselves are not familiar with each other's health beliefs and behaviors. Indeed, this has been a major problem in global health efforts for decades. We are enculturated from birth into our own culture through our interactions with, observations of, and modeling of our own behavior on our parents, grandparents, siblings, relatives, friends, neighbors, teachers, and religious and community leaders. Culture provides us with a pattern for living our lives and gives us a sense of purpose, order, and meaning that feels natural and right – as though it were the only way to behave, feel, and think. This is why people often experience what anthropologists call "culture shock" (i.e., a sense of personal disorientation one may feel when experiencing an unfamiliar way of life) when we experience a different culture, especially one that is very different from our own. Cultures vary on the way they address the many issues of life primarily because there are many ways to solve the problems of life. Anthropologists embrace these cultural differences, and since the subfield began in the 1950s, medical anthropologists have often addressed issues of cross-cultural communication and miscommunication between patients and healers to help biomedical providers better interact with patients from a different culture to ensure a positive outcome for both (see Singer and Erickson 2011 for other examples).

Following Boas's advocacy for cultural relativism, medical anthropologists recognize the legitimacy of all medical systems and work to bring that understanding to biomedicine, which we regard as one of the many ethnomedicines in the world. Fortunately, in the last three decades, alternative medicine has become more widely accepted within the biomedical community and more practitioners have taken an interest in integrative medicine.[1] This is not surprising since healers from different medical traditions have a long history of borrowing remedies and procedures that work from one another because they are interested in healing their patients. For example, the Spanish conquistadors brought home the bark of the cinchona tree, a native to western Andean forests in South America, where it was widely and successfully used by local healers to treat malaria. From Spain, the bark spread across Europe and eventually to the whole world. Chloroquine (an anti-malarial drug) was synthesized from quinine, the active ingredient in cinchona bark that has long been one of the go-to global preventives and treatments for malaria.

Arthur Kleinman (1978, 1980) provided medical anthropology with a useful schematic for understanding health systems throughout the world. He identified three sectors of health care in every medical system: the popular sector, the folk sector, and the professional sector. The popular sector is nonprofessional and includes the individual and their social group (e.g., family, friends, neighbors, coworkers, religious communities, self-help groups, and people who have had special experience with a particular health problem). This is where health problems are first recognized and where the quest for treatment begins (e.g., home and/or herbal remedies, over-the-counter medicines, lifestyle change, spiritual guidance). It is estimated that 70 to 90 percent of all health care takes place in this sector (Helman 2007; Kleinman 1978). The folk sector includes many kinds of both secular and sacred healers who are not part of the professional sector but usually have some training under an older, more experienced mentor. Secular healers include folk healers, lay midwives, bone setters, and herbalists. Sacred healers include diviners, shamans, witches, and faith healers. All of these folk healers can be found in societies throughout the world and this sector has long been the traditional object of ethnomedical study for anthropologists. The professional sector includes the organized, legal healing professions in a society – for example, biomedicine and osteopathy in the United States, Traditional Chinese Medicine in much of Asia, and Ayurvedic and Unani medicine in India. Healers in this sector are recognized as physicians, dentists, nurses, pharmacists, physical therapists, chiropractors, and ancillary professions. This sector also includes licensed professionals from complementary and alternative medical systems (CAM) and the many indigenous healing systems labeled traditional medicine by the World Health Organization. The folk and professional sectors generally care for clients whose health problems are too serious for the popular sector, but that does not mean that the popular sector is ignored and people often seek help from different sectors at different times or simultaneously.

Kleinman also offered medical anthropology the important tool he called explanatory models (EMs). EMs contain explanations for the following issues: etiology, onset of symptoms, pathophysiology, course of sickness, and treatment and can be elicited from practitioners, patients, and family members for an illness episode (Kleinman 1978). These EMs are associated with the cultural health beliefs of those from whom they are elicited and can be very useful in understanding difference of belief among the practitioner, patient, and family. Further, Kleinman notes that EMs in the patient care group often conflict and can be examined and modified to further mutual understandings and agreements regarding care. Thus, elicitation of EMs can be very useful, especially when the practitioner and the patient are from different cultural groups. Reconciling differences in EMs can also be difficult as the practitioners tend to use disease models (technical information and treatment suggestions/plans) whereas patients and their families tend to use highly personal illness models that seek socially meaningful explanations as well as relief from the physical expression of the disease. Kleinman suggests that the reasons that folk healers endure despite biomedicine's success in disease treatment is because they treat the illness that patients experience as not only physical but also psychological, social, and often spiritual.

Following Kleinman's lead, medical anthropologists have come to regard *disease* as the objective pathology affecting the patient, *sickness* as the social manifestation of the disease or infirmity, and *illness* as the subjective experience of disease and sickness. Similarly, we use the words *curing* to refer to the removal or correction of organic pathology and *healing* to refer to the broader experience of the restoration of physical, mental, emotional, social, and spiritual health. Moreover, these linguistic differences represent the classic body/mind dualism that pervades Western medical notions of health. Many indigenous, traditional, and CAM therapies are theoretically attuned to the broader idea of health implied by the term *healing* and appeal to people who seek a more philosophical or cosmological answer to their afflictions (e.g., Why me, why now, what did I do to deserve this, how can I heal?).

Since the beginning of the subfield medical anthropologists have focused on understanding local medical systems and their perspective on illness and disease. For this reason, they became useful colleagues in the many international health and economic development programs that resulted after World War II and they remain useful to this day. They were especially useful for explaining local medical beliefs to biomedical personnel and helping local populations understand biomedicine better toward the goal of gaining buy-in from local communities for a variety of health initiatives such as vaccination campaigns, preventing and combatting infectious diseases, safe motherhood, and infant and child feeding programs. More recently, medical anthropologists have contributed to cultural understandings of HIV, Ebola, SARS, Zika, and currently COVID-19. Beginning in the 1980s and throughout the 1990s, many health workers and medical anthropologists realized and documented the tremendous negative impact neoliberal reforms and structural adjustment programs (SAPs) were having on local communities by destroying their economies and their medical, agricultural, and educational systems (Birn et al. 2017; Singer and Erickson 2013). This realization made understanding local interactions within the broader political, economic, and social framework very important for people's health and paved the way for the World Health Organization's interest in the social determinants of health.

In March 2005, the World Health Organization (WHO) established the Commission on the Social Determinants of Health (SDOH) to identify and address the particular social factors that lead to poor health (www.who.int/social_determinants/thecommission/en/). The Commission released its report in July 2008 and the evidence overwhelmingly supported the tremendous impact of social inequality on people's health and well-being in every country studied. Since its release and WHO's efforts to publicize the results widely, a global public health movement has developed to address social inequality and health in which medical anthropologists have been active, especially those who employ critical medical anthropology (CMA), a theoretical orientation that guides many anthropologists who work on global health issues (Singer and Baer 1995). Within this framework, medical anthropologists study the complex bio-socio-cultural interactions that impact health around the world, with particular attention to the social inequalities that produce health inequalities including unequal access to health care and resources and over-exposure to adverse living conditions (Singer and Erickson 2013). Health disparities and inequalities are more than the consequences of individual actions or decisions, they are heavily impacted by social inequality in many spheres of life, including lack of good education, safe housing, living-wage employment opportunities, access to health care, access to nutritious food and clean water, and the discrimination and stigma of institutionalized racism, sexism, and anti-LGBTQ sentiments. Today, accelerating global climate change further amplifies the negative health effects of social inequality among marginalized and poorer populations (Singer 2019). Thus, for critical medical anthropologists, the important issue is remedying social injustice and health inequities. The critical medical anthropological approach to global health marries well with the Social Determinants of Health model and adds to it an understanding of both local conditions, experiences, and perspectives of people afflicted and the social and structural factors that affect the health of individuals, families, and communities.

CULTURAL VIEWS OF HEALTH AND ILLNESS

Medical systems throughout the ages are a result of human behavior and subsistence strategies that shape and reshape the patterns of morbidity and mortality in a community (McElroy and Townsend 2015). They are embedded in the cultures in which they developed and they can and do evolve over time to adapt to changes in the ways people live and the kinds of illnesses that affect them. For example, modern biomedicine was based on the medical systems of early Western civilizations in Greece, the Roman Empire, and Persia that were all based on natural causes of disease. During the Dark Ages (500–1500 current era/CE) much of this knowledge was lost because the Catholic Church squashed it and maintained that disease was a test of faith, bringing back age-old ideas about supernatural causes of illness. During those dark years, the only repositories of the Western healing arts in Europe were monks, nuns, and folk healers who maintained knowledge of herbal medicine, surgery, wound treatment, and various physical manipulations (e.g., bone setters, midwives, etc.). During the Renaissance (1300–1650 CE) and Scientific Revolution (1450–1630), the ancient texts and healing practices from early Western civilizations were revived and once again became the basis for the development of biomedicine. Further cultural transformations during the Industrial Revolution (1750–1830) radically changed patterns of behavior and subsistence and brought new causes of disease and illness (e.g., coal- and smog-related diseases, malnutrition, health problems caused by substandard living and working conditions). Newer discoveries and developments in biomedicine, such as anesthesia, vaccines, antibiotics, pharmaceuticals, medical technological developments, and now the human genome, led to biomedicine becoming a global, hegemonic medical system (Magner 2005). Thus, it is that our medical systems change with changing cultural patterns of behavior and subsistence strategies, and hence our need to seek new forms of healing and curing.

Anthropologists George Foster and Robert Anderson (1978) introduced a typology of disease classification that can be used with any cultural system. They assert that human beings believe in four basic ideas about the cause of disease: (1) the patient or individual, (2) the natural world, (3) the social world, and (4) the supernatural world. Most ethnomedical systems emphasize either the first two, the individual and the natural world, or the last two, the social world and the supernatural, although there is some crossover in all ethnomedical systems. Ethnomedicines that emphasize the body and the natural world tend to favor naturalistic explanations of disease causation and those that emphasize the personal and the supernatural tend to favor personalistic explanations. As Erickson (2008) explained in *Ethnomedicine*, in naturalistic explanations the cause is impersonal and explained in systemic terms. The body is thrown into disequilibrium due to natural causes (e.g., malnutrition, infection, trauma, cancer, etc.) and it reacts to the threat from the natural world. In biomedicine and the humoral medical systems (e.g., Traditional Chinese Medicine, Ayurvedic medicine, and homeopathy) the goal of treatment is restoration of the body's normal equilibrium and the means to do so have long been medications, diet, exercise, rest, and attending to trauma. To these, biomedicine has added many new and powerful treatment avenues, including medical technologies, surgical procedures, pharmaceutical drugs, and the new and rapidly expanding possibility for genetic therapies. In personalistic systems, disease explanations involve the direct aggression of a human or supernatural being (e.g., witches, sorcerers, spirits, gods/God) against the victim that requires an individual narrative explanation for why the victim became ill. The cause of the illness is the disharmony between the people afflicted and their relationship to the social or supernatural world. Treatment entails restoring harmony by assuaging the supernatural agent or countermanding spells and hexes sent by witches and sorcerers. Both naturalistic and personalistic healing systems are internally consistent and attempt to heal the disease/illness to return the patient to good health.

Biomedicine is of course the extreme of naturalistic healing systems and Haitian Vodun (i.e., voodoo) is one of the more well-known examples of personalistic healing systems. Although these two systems are very different, their goal and that of all medical systems is to provide people with a culturally meaningful, coherent way to understand their illness, a plan to restore their health, and a means to reintegrate them back into their community after illness. It is important to remember that people when ill can and often do use other healing systems in conjunction with their primary system. Americans using the biomedical system often use other systems as well. Especially in cases of serious illness, they may seek religious or spiritual healers and use prayer to help them understand the ultimate reason for their suffering. In addition, other alternative healing strategies are often sought in conjunction with biomedicine; today many at the suggestion of their physicians seek alternative treatments such as reiki, meditation, massage, yoga, aroma therapy, etc. Similarly, Haitians using Vodun to regain harmony with the social or spiritual world may also seek out biomedicine when they believe it will help them (e.g., for cancer, surgery, broken bones, infectious diseases, etc.). As our world has become ever smaller, more connected, and more interdependent, patients are less wedded to their traditional healing systems and many are willing to try others. So it has been through the ages; healers have always traded information about healing strategies and have been open to new medicines and techniques when they saw good results from different practices in other healing systems. Patients as well, often seek out alternative ways to heal. This is not particularly surprising given that medical systems are always changing and people using those systems change along with them.

HISTORICAL MEDICAL TRADITIONS

There are three great classical medical traditions (so named by historians of biomedicine):

Ayurvedic medicine, Traditional Chinese Medicine (TCM), and Greek/Roman/Greco-Islamic (Unani) medicine. Each has an extensive written canon and they have all been influential in the old world for centuries, shaping many other local health systems over the ages in surrounding areas and countries. Today Ayurvedic medicine and TCM still stand as distinct medical traditions in India and China respectively and Greek medicine survives in the theory and practice of contemporary Unani medicine in Asia and the Middle East. Each of these traditions is briefly described below.

Ayurvedic medicine developed in India between 4500 BCE and 500 BCE (before current era). Its basic medical texts date from 1000–800 BCE (Magner 2005). Its goal was to prevent disease and maintain health rather than just treating disease after it appeared. Health was secured by maintaining balance in the three *doshas* or humors (wind, bile, and phlegm), which combined with blood to determine the body's vital functions. The body was made of five elements (earth, water, fire, wind, and ether). Health was achieved by sustaining harmony among the humors and body tissues (blood, muscle, fat, bone, nerves, semen, ova), normal digestion and elimination, and gratification of the senses, the mind, and the soul. One hundred and seven vital points in the body were named that referred to places where injuries could be serious or fatal. Imbalances of the humors led to illness and balance was restored through proper diet, behavior, exercise, fasting, purging, blood-letting, herbal remedies, Ayurvedic medicines, and surgery. In addition, religious ideas about *karma*, life cycle, yoga, diet, exercise, hygiene, meditation, and astrology had quasi-medical implications (Magner 2005) as did the idea of a life force/vital energy that animated the body (Lad 1995). The goal of these medical and religious factors was to maintain harmony in the body and in social and spiritual relationships. Moderation in living, compassion for others, and respect for the gods and spirits were important for a long and healthy life.

Traditional Chinese Medicine's basic foundations are found in the *I Ching* (The Book of Changes), believed to have been written in 3000 BCE, that outlines the Chinese philosophy of the dynamic balance of opposites and acceptance of the inevitability of change. The eight volume *Nei Ching* (The Yellow Emperor's Classic of Internal Medicine) dates to 300 BCE and describes the principles that have guided TCM for 2,500 years. These include the balance of yin and yang, the five phases or elements, and the daily factors that impinge on life (e.g., family, food, environment). TCM is guided by the idea that the world is a single, unbroken wholeness (*Tao*) that exists in every person and also that every person is a microcosm of the universe. Thus, TCM is embedded in nature, the body is viewed as an ecosystem, and medicine is based on nature metaphors (Beinfield and Korngold 1995).

Yin and yang are polar opposites that cannot exist without each other and whose balance fosters health and whose imbalance fosters illness. The five phases/elements include earth, metal, water, wood, and fire that are linked to each other by relationships of generation and destruction. The body contains qi (animating force/energy), moisture (body fluids), and blood (body tissues). The organs include five firm yin organs (heart, spleen, lungs, liver, kidneys) and five hollow yang organs (gall bladder, bladder, stomach, large intestines, small intestines) that are related to the five phases/elements. The organs are linked by a system of conduits through which qi flows.

In TCM, anatomy is thought about in terms of function rather than structure. Health is achieved by a maintaining balance of all contending forces (yin/yang, phases/elements) and the free flow of qi (i.e., the vital energy that animates the body internally). Illness results from blockage/depletion of qi or an imbalance of yin/yang or the five phases/elements. Diagnostic techniques include patient narrative and physical assessment by the physician (e.g., appearance, 50 pulses, tongue, temperature, joint flexibility, sensitivity of the 365 acupuncture points, and skin moisture) aimed at discovering the prevailing balance in the body. Prevention includes moderate lifestyle and attention to the balance of hot/cold and moist/dry. Treatment attempts to restore balance by use of acupuncture, readjusting qi, moxibustion (the burning of dried mugwort on particular acupuncture points on the body), medicines, diet, and exercise.

Greek medicine is the third great medical tradition that developed in ancient Greece and became the foundation for Western philosophy, science, and medicine. Although Greek medicine is believed to stem from the 8th century BCE, it is Hippocrates (460–361 BCE) who is remembered as the "Father of Medicine" (Magner 2005). The underlying principle of Greek medicine is that nature is a strong healing force and the physician's role is to help the body restore balance and heal itself. Hippocrates may have been the first to recognize that disease is a natural process that could be understood through rational study rather than the result of supernatural aggressions. He also emphasized that health can be affected by the environment and by social, religious, and political institutions, paving the way for the social determinants of health movement today.

To provide treatment, Greek physicians had to understand the temperament of their patients and how their way of living (i.e., food, drink, exercise) might affect health. They then applied the principle of humoral medicine (hot/cold balance) in treatment of the ultimate cause of disease, the imbalance of the four humors (yellow bile, blood, phlegm, and black bile), which were associated with the four elements (fire, air, water, earth) and four states (hot, cold, moist, dry). Thus, health was achieved by restoring the balance of the four humors. The patients' temperaments were associated with how much of each humor was present in their body. A choleric, hot-tempered temperament was associated with an abundance of yellow bile, the element fire, and with the hot-dry state; the sanguine, sturdy, cheerful temperament with an abundance of blood, the element air, and the hot-moist state; the phlegmatic, slow, dull temperament with and abundance of phlegm, the element water, and the moist-cold state; the melancholy, sad, depressed temperament with an abundance of black bile, the element earth, and the cold-dry state. The physician employed humoral theory to restore balance of the humors and help the body heal itself. Greek physicians used standard diagnostic techniques of observation, patient narrative, pulse, and urine examination and were adept at treating wounds, fractures, and other injuries with surgery.

Although Hippocrates is known as the father of modern medicine, it was Galen (130–200 CE) who advanced the idea that therapy must be based on understanding human anatomy and physiology, thus laying the foundation for modern, scientific medicine. Galen's writings dominated western European medical thought until the 16th century and were major medical sources for Persian physicians Al-Razi (Rhazes, 850–923 CE) and Ibn Sina (Avicenna, 980–1037 CE), whose writings preserved them during the Middle Ages. Their writings also contributed to the development of the Arab medical tradition known as Unani medicine, which is identical to Greek medicine in its theories and practices except for the use of surgery and wine in healing (Magner 2005). The other major medical tradition in Persia was Prophetic medicine that taught that faith was the way to deal with illness, much like the Catholic teachings during the European Dark Ages, and promoted traditional healing practices current during the Prophet Muhammad's (570–632 CE) lifetime (i.e., diet, medicines, bloodletting, and cautery). After the fall of the Roman Empire, the Greco-Roman medical traditions survived in the learning centers of Persia (500–1500) and Moorish Spain (711–1492). Today, Unani is an important medical system in India and Pakistan (Magner 2005).

In addition to these great medical traditions, there were and still are many other non-biomedical lay traditions both ancient and modern (Magner 2005). Midwifery, massage, bone setting, herbalism, faith healing, and spiritualism are all ancient forms of healing that seem to have existed throughout the world and still persist today. Some more modern (1800s–1900s) alternatives to biomedicine like osteopathy, chiropractic, naturopathy, and homeopathy have made it – after long struggles against biomedicine – into mainstream biomedical practice as respected, ancillary healing modes. Others, like nature cures and water cures have not been embraced by biomedicine but are not harmful. In addition, many non-Western healing modalities like meditation, yoga, reiki, and acupuncture are also accepted by biomedicine as ancillary healing modes. In the 1960s and 1970s, the Holistic Health and New Age movements emerged in reaction to a growing dissatisfaction with what was perceived as biomedicine's impersonal, reductionist, bureaucratic, costly, and dangerous practices. These movements, which included Green politics, environmental/ecological concerns, and a desire for a simpler more spiritual and natural way of life, advocated for natural foods and medicines, avoidance of processed food and pharmaceutical drugs, and less dependence on technology. Undoubtedly, the better nutritional practices of the holistic health movement can have a positive impact on overall health and the healthful impact of a healthy environment is noteworthy in these times of global warming and climate change.

The many indigenous medicines still extant in our world include a wide variety of peoples, places, and ideas about health and illness. They vary widely, being much attuned to specific environments and cultures, but one thing that seems common to most if not all of them is the idea that health is a result of harmony both within the individual and between the individual and the natural, social, and spiritual worlds (Cohen 1998; Parsons 1985; Reid 1983). In this they are much like the great medical traditions that saw balance as key to health, but they go beyond the body to include the balance of person with nature, with others, and with the spiritual realm. Indigenous groups have a long tradition of using herbal medicines as well as wound treatment, bone setting, midwifery, sorcery, shamanism, and witchcraft. All of these are still important theories of disease causation among indigenous peoples.

COMMON NON-BIOMEDICAL THEORIES OF DISEASE CAUSATION

As Mildred Blaxter notes, a pervasive belief about health in the postmodern world is "a lingering faith in a causal system outside science" (Blaxter 2004: 36). There are six domains that characterize these non-biomedical theories of disease causation: balance, body beliefs, the natural world, breach of conduct, malice, and the supernatural (Erickson 2008; Murdock 1980; Scrimshaw 2001, 2012; Scrimshaw and Lane 2020).

Body Balance

Body balance is basic to many healing systems (Magner 2005; Murdock 1980). Health results from an equilibrium of the body both internally and in relation to physical, social and supernatural environment. Illness results from an imbalance or blockage of the vital substance (e.g., humors) or force (e.g., energy) and/or a disharmony with the environment. Humoral systems counsel moderate lifestyles for health maintenance.

Hot-cold balance is another widespread theory found in many Asian, Mediterranean, and Latin American cultures in which disease is thought to be caused by an excess of hot or cold. The body is exposed to hot and cold in two ways – internally through consumption of food and drink and externally through physical activity, exposure to the elements, and interactions with other people. Balance is maintained by careful attention to eating a balance of hot and cold foods and avoiding excessive temperatures and heightened emotional states. Hot and cold are ascribed thermally or metaphorically to foods, objects, body states, emotions, diseases, and medicines and are locally determined classifications. Therapy involves restoring the hot/cold balance usually through dietary and herbal remedies guided by the theory of opposites (Foster 1953; Rubel and Hass 1996; Scrimshaw 2012; Weller 1983).

Energy balance is another common aspect of body balance theories in which blockage of some vital substance can cause disease (Beinfeld and Korngold 1995). One example from Chinese medicine is that the free flow of vital energy (i.e., qi) is essential to health. When qi is blocked, illness ensues. Acupuncture and acupressure are used to unblock qi and restore health. Another is the transfer of energy from one person or a group of people in Christian healing through laying on of hands or prayer.

Excessive emotions are thought to cause illness in many cultures as strong emotions can cause imbalance in the person (Murdock 1980; Scrimshaw 2001). Emotions such as anger, sorrow, fear, envy, love, hate, and jealousy are especially able to cause illness if not controlled.

Body Beliefs

Ethnomedical systems incorporate cultural beliefs about how the body should look, what the boundaries of the individual body are (e.g., how close is too close, who can touch whom), what the inner structure of the body is like, and how the body functions.

Beliefs about the organs and blood are often important in non-biomedical traditions. Many cultures associate illness with specific organs or body parts. Grief is often expressed as pain or heaviness in the heart (Good and Good 1981). Among the Hmong, the liver is associated with mental health, feelings, and personality. The womb is of concern worldwide as it is necessary for childbearing. In some cultures, blood is thought to be irreplaceable and any loss of blood is seen as dangerous. Some systems see an overabundance of blood, changes in its consistency, or its location in the body as a cause of disease. Menstrual blood has long been regarded as dangerous and polluting for men, especially in India and parts of Africa, where elaborate systems for separating women from the family during menstruation have removed the threat.

Pollution and contagion are also common themes in disease causation. Proximity to a corpse, for example, is often seen as dangerous. The Navajo avoid anything connected with death (e.g., body, dwelling, grave, archaeological sites) to prevent ghost sickness (Kluckhohn and Leighten 1962; Kunitz 1989). Hindus, too, find many things in daily life a source of ritual pollution (e.g., birth, death, food, sex) that require ritual purification. In the past, lower-caste individuals were also viewed as a source of pollution but this is rapidly disappearing.

Ingested substances are also problematic (Erickson 2008; Scrimshaw 2001). Food is often a source of illness according to the hot/cold theory discussed earlier, but also eating the wrong kind of food at the wrong time of day (e.g., heavy food before sleep) or eating spoiled, dirty, or raw food. Consumption of tabooed foods is also a common cause of illness. For example, eating certain foods during pregnancy or for ritual reasons under some conditions (e.g., before hunting or warring) are considered dangerous. In addition, many religions forbid certain foods altogether (e.g., pork in Judaism and Islam). Excessive use of alcohol, tobacco, and other drugs is almost universally considered dangerous and unhealthful.

Sex itself can also cause illness (e.g., sexually transmitted infections), but so can violation of sexual mores (Erickson 2008; Scrimshaw 2001). For example, parental adultery is thought to result in illness in a child in many parts of world and incest is thought to cause mental illness. Seemingly, anything outside of having sex in moderation with a culturally appropriate partner can result in illness to self or others.

Heredity and the Natural World

Most cultures recognize the health vulnerability of children and the elderly as well as the fact that some diseases are hereditary (e.g., hemophilia, depression, schizophrenia, sickle cell disease). In addition, the natural world (e.g., accidents, disasters) and its plants (e.g., poisoning, scratches) and animals (e.g., predation by large animals, reservoirs for diseases that affect humans, bites and stings of insects, microbial and fungal infections) can also cause illness.

Breach of Conduct

Bad behavior and breaches of taboo related to the core activities of human existence (e.g., sex, reproduction, sustenance, death) are widely thought to cause illness (Murdock 1980; Scrimshaw 2001). Birth is widely, perhaps universally, recognized as a dangerous time, as is death. Many cultures believe that improper respect of the dead and attention to proper burial can cause illness among the living. In many far eastern cultures where ancestors are revered (e.g., China, Korea), ancestors forgotten too soon or those who are angry can cause illness and/or misfortune among the living.

Malice

Malice and physical and psychological aggression against others are common sources of illness, injury, and death globally (Murdock 1980). Warfare, genocide, terrorism, torture, homicide, and battery are all too common in our world. These ills also lead to trauma, disease, death, epidemic diseases, starvation, and psychological suffering (Levy and Sidel 2000; World Health Organization 2002). As well, gossip, rumor, and slander are used globally to harm other people, sometimes at great cost to the accused (e.g., stoning of women accused of adultery in the circum-Caribbean and Muslim countries, ruining of reputations, ostracism).

Witchcraft and Shamanism

Witchcraft and shamanism are primary causes of harm and healing in many societies (Murdock 1980; Scrimshaw 2001). Witches and shamans are human beings thought to have supernatural powers. They can act on their own to harm/help another or their services can be enlisted by someone intending to do harm to another person. Witches rely on their own insights and inspiration to help or cause harm to others through magical means. Witches are more universally thought as causing harm and shamans more often thought to work for positive goals, although they can also cause harm. Unlike witches, shamans enter the spirit world (through drumming, chanting, alcohol, or drugs) to enlist help from their spirit helpers to heal or harm others. Witches and shamans, like other powerful healers, are both feared and revered and are frequently targets for murder attempts when practicing the dark side of their trade.

The Supernatural World

In all cultures, illness and misfortune have long been attributed to a variety of supernatural beings from one supreme being (e.g., God) to demons, devils, jinni, ghosts, and spirits that inhabit the natural environment (Murdock 1980). Supernatural beings may deliberately cause problems for humans or may do so only accidentally.

In the major world religions, illness is often seen as a punishment from God or the gods. In Christianity, Judaism, and Islam, for example, the will of God is an important cause of illness and misfortune and is often interpreted as a test of faith or a deserved punishment for sins. In Buddhism and Hinduism, misfortune is thought to be due to bad behavior in previous lives (i.e., bad karma).

For centuries, illness and misfortune have been attributed to fate, luck, and the stars (Magner 2005). Astrologers were important practitioners who could profile a person's life course, personality, and constitutional characteristics and weakness based on the alignment of the stars and planets at the time of birth. They could also determine auspicious times for important life events (e.g., weddings, making important decisions, building a house). China, India, Nepal, ancient Greece and Rome, Europe, and the Middle East all had some variation on fate and astrological influences on human life. Fortune tellers, too, have long been sought for advice and information about the future. Astrologers and fortunetellers have advised many people from kings and presidents to commoners.

Ghosts, devils, demons, jinni, and spirits are widely thought to cause harm to humans by intentional aggression (Erickson 2008; Murdock 1980; Scrimshaw 2001). In many cultures, spirits are thought to reside in certain places (e.g., sun, moon, stars, rivers, lakes, mountains, wind, etc.) and can cause harm to people who unwittingly cross their path or do not take care of their needs (e.g., proper respect, offerings). Another group of minor supernatural beings, such as fairies, gnomes, trolls, demons, and leprechauns, are thought to "play" with humans, sometimes causing misfortune. There are two main ways that such spirits cause harm to humans – by stealing their souls or possessing their body and mind. Soul loss is a common explanation for illness in western Asia and the Americas. From the Quechua in South America to the Inuit in Alaska, serious illness is thought to be caused by soul loss or theft. Soul loss can occur due to a fright that is more a matter of being in the wrong place at the wrong time than malice. Soul theft is deliberate aggression by a spirit at the bidding of a shaman and requires elaborate rituals to retrieve the soul, return it to the victim, and restore health. Spirit possession occurs when a spirit or supernatural being inhabits a person, replacing that person's being with their own. It can be used to heal or to harm.

Most ethnomedical systems do not maintain a single cause model of illness. Different illnesses are caused by different forces and can have several interacting causes. The goal of healers everywhere is to find the cause of illness, to cure the patient, and to help the patient find the meaning of their suffering. Biomedical health practitioners working with patients from different cultures need to pay attention to the explanatory models that their patients have about illness and to use that knowledge to make their own biomedical explanatory models mesh with the patient's. This may be difficult when the models are radically different, but it is important to understand and respect their beliefs rather than deny their importance. In the next section, we present a case study of clashing explanatory models of illness in the story of Lia Lee, a Hmong child being treated for epilepsy at a California hospital.

CASE STUDY: LIA LEE AND THE MEANING OF EPILEPSY

In her compelling book, *The Spirit Catches You and You Fall Down*, Anne Fadiman (1997), narrates the story of Lia Lee, born in 1982 to Hmong immigrants living in Merced, California, where they immigrated after fleeing Laos during the Viet Nam war era. The family had experienced extraordinary hardship and suffering before immigrating. Six of their children died during their dangerous journey from China to Laos and finally to Thailand, from which they were resettled as refugees in the United States. Lia was the Lee family's first child to be born in the United States and also the first born in a hospital. We have chosen Lia's case to illustrate the importance of understanding, learning, and accommodating different cultural beliefs about illness and healing within biomedicine.

When Lia was three months old she experienced the first of what would be many seizures that ultimately led to a biomedical diagnosis of epilepsy and a new journey navigating the American medical system. Her parents took her to the hospital for care, but Lia's symptoms (i.e., eyes rolled back, jerking of her arms, and fainting) were already familiar to the Lees. The Hmong have many beliefs about disease causation but the most common is soul loss. The soul, which is necessary for health, can be lost through strong emotions such as fear or anger. Lia's parents believed that the loud noise of a door being closed frightened Lia's soul out of her body (Fadiman 1997: 20–21). Further complicating things, what biomedical health care providers diagnosed as a seizure, Lia's family believed was *quag dab peg* (the spirit catches you and you fall down), a Hmong affliction. While they recognized that she had a serious medical condition, they interpreted her symptoms as a sign that she was being called to become a shaman, a traditional healer. This is particularly true for those who experience seizures because the seizures themselves are evidence of the person's ability to enter a trance and travel to the spirit world. This is a high honor among the Hmong.

Over the course of four years, Lia's seizures persisted and her parents continued to take her to the hospital because they understood the gravity of her medical condition. They did this despite the fact that they distrusted Western medicine, believing that the drugs prescribed for Lia were making her sick. They did not give her the medications as directed, not giving some and giving too much of others. Their ambivalence was evidenced by their ongoing use of traditional medical practices such as herbs and animal sacrifices, as well as relying on a shaman who was their traditional healer. The differences between shamans and biomedical providers would have been very clear to the Lees. Shamans make house calls, spend a long time with their patients, and make diagnoses without asking questions or touching the patient. They believe that the soul and spirits, particularly ancestral ones, can cause disease and illness. Biomedical care providers require the person who is ill to go to a facility to be seen where they generally spend a short time interviewing and examining the patient and order tests and procedures in order to make a diagnosis (Fadiman 1997: 33).

The physicians providing care for Lia became progressively frustrated with what they perceived as a lack of adherence to prescribed medical treatment and felt that her family was putting her at risk. Fadiman came to believe that the doctors didn't know if the Lees were ignoring their orders or just didn't understand what was expected of them. Visiting nurses were enlisted to help with medication adherence but ultimately one of Lia's pediatricians requested that Child Protective Services remove her from her parents' care and place her with a foster family. Lia remained in foster care for six months, at which point she suffered a prolonged seizure that the physicians were unable to stop for several hours. She was also found to be in septic shock, a life-threatening condition caused by a bacterial infection. Her physicians assumed that she would die from this systemic infection and allowed her to go home (Fadiman 1997: 177). Remarkably, Lia lived to the age of 30 without any further seizure activity (Fox 2012: A1). She had little brain activity and was unable to communicate, but was lovingly cared for by her family who continued to take her to see physicians and also treat her with traditional medical practices.

In the four years between her first seizure and the final one, Lia and her family experienced 15 admissions to the hospital (Fadiman 1997: 144) and 23 medication changes (Fadiman 1997: 46). The complexity of Lia's illness and her medication regimens would be difficult for any family, much less one that does not speak English or understand biomedical practices. Fadiman notes that the Hmong language does not have words that correlate with biomedical terms. She quotes Dan Murphy, the physician who diagnosed Lia with epilepsy, "The Hmong simply didn't have the same concepts that I did. For instance, you can't tell them that somebody is diabetic because their pancreas doesn't work. They don't have a word for pancreas. They don't have an *idea* for pancreas. Most of them had no concept that the organs they saw in animals were the same as in humans, because they didn't open people up when they died, they buried them intact" (Dan Murphy, MD, cited in Fadiman 1997: 69).

Ironically, a pediatric neurologist who provided medical care to Lia posited that the final seizure that resulted in brain damage was caused by the bacterial infection and subsequent septic shock. He did note that one of the anti-seizure medications that was prescribed for Lia can weaken the immune system and increase susceptibility to infections. He believed that her parents' non-compliance with her medication regimen did not cause the seizure and may have, in fact, prevented further compromise of her immune system (Fadiman 1997: 254–255).

There is much for biomedicine to learn from Lia's story in Fadiman's thorough and thoughtful account of the family's medical journey. Indeed, Kleinman's ideas about understanding the explanatory models of illness of both patients and their families and practitioners could have helped treatment options for Lia and her family by integrating biomedical perspectives with the patient's beliefs and allowing practitioners to understand belief obstacles and find culturally acceptable ways to work around them. Such culturally informed care could have eased the tensions that developed between the doctors and the family. But, Lia's biomedical practitioners did not attempt to understand how the Hmong, and specifically the Lees, understood and experienced Lia's illness.

One basic body belief among the Hmong is that each person has a finite amount of blood. Thus, the numerous laboratory tests ordered for diagnosis and treatment would have worried Lia's family. Neither did the team understand the significant role that spirituality plays in Hmong beliefs about health and disease. This is not surprising as spirituality is not generally considered important in biomedical care, although most hospital have religious leaders available for patients who want to consult them. Neither did the medical team know that Lia's family believed that she had *quag dab peg* and it was considered an honor. The gulf between Hmong and biomedical beliefs about illness and healing was enormous.

The medical team also knew that there was a language barrier, yet interpreters were not usually available when the family brought Lia to the hospital. The family would, at times, have their nephew, who speaks English, help with communication, but he was not always available when needed. Fadiman stresses the importance of having certified interpreters available as well as gender-specific health care providers who may be able to provide more relatable care. She also notes the value of allowing family to remain at the patient's bedside while hospitalized and to involve them in decision-making about health care. In this case, it would have been beneficial for the team to understand that Hmong community leaders must be involved in major decisions and that blood draws should be minimized. Allowing shamanic ceremonies in the hospital, when feasible, would have allowed the Lees to integrate their beliefs with those of biomedicine and provide Lia with "a little medicine and a little *neeb*" [shaman/traditional healer]. Ultimately, it is important for biomedical providers to understand the belief systems and linguistic needs of their patients when participating in their health care. But neither the biomedical health care providers nor the Lees tried to understand each other.

Speaking with Fadiman about Lia's case, Arthur Kleinman reflected on what is perhaps the most important lesson for biomedicine: insight into their own enculturation and how it shapes their view of the human body and their beliefs about health and disease. Practitioners are impacted by this enculturation just as much as their patients are shaped by the cultures in which they grew up. He asked, "If you can't see that your own culture has its own set of interests, emotions, and biases, how can you expect to deal successfully with someone else's culture?" (Kleinman, cited in Fadiman 1997: 261). Kleinman's explanatory models of illness can help health care providers gain insight into how people understand and experience illness, gaining the emic/insider perspective of the meaning of illness for an individual, perhaps leading to a much better outcome.

This poignant case study illustrates the importance and necessity for understanding and integrating cultural beliefs when dealing with disease and illness. This is of particular relevance to biomedicine, a medical system that views disease as universal and rarely, if ever, seeks to understand how individual patients think about and experience ill health. The experience of Lia Lee and her family, as they struggled to understand and cope with Lia's illness and her prescribed biomedical treatment, is often framed as a "clash" or "collision" between the Hmong and biomedical cultures. Yet it is more nuanced as it speaks to not only a lack of understanding about the belief systems of many involved in Lia's life and health care, but a lack of effort to gain insight and be empathetic. In the end, Lia's story highlights the critical importance of cross-cultural communication about explanatory models of illness held by providers, patients, and their families. Such discussions could help everyone to reach an understanding about the course of care and lead to better experiences for all involved.

ANTHROPOLOGICAL METHODS FOR UNDERSTANDING CULTURE, BEHAVIOR, AND HEALTH

Medical anthropologists use a wide number of research methods to understand the health and illness beliefs and behaviors of the people they study in other cultures and subcultures in their own countries. Here we discuss explanatory models, focus groups, interviews, and free list and pile sorting, all of which yield insights into health and illness beliefs and behaviors.

Explanatory Models

Earlier we introduced explanatory models (EMs) in the Concepts from Medical Anthropology section, where they were discussed as a tool for clinicians to understand what the patient believes about their illness episode regarding etiology, onset of symptoms, pathophysiology, the course of the sickness, and best treatment for the problem. Clinicians then communicate their own beliefs about the same issues and attempt to come to a reasonable course of action that makes sense to both patient and clinician. However, the elicitation of EMs by researchers regarding specific diseases/illnesses/health problems targeted in their study is an excellent way for researchers to quickly understand local ideas about the problem. A 20–30-minute interview with 20 to 30 local people can provide an understanding of the range of EMs in the community and could be undertaken using these five questions: What do you think causes X? What symptoms do people who have X present with and what do they do about them? What happens to the body when people have X? How long do people typically have X before they are cured? What are the best ways to treat X? This strategy is very like the open-ended interview discussed below, but targeted to understand EMs.

Focus Groups

Since the 1950s focus groups have been a mainstay of consumer research to understand how a small group of people (6–12 people) think about and react to different products. They require skilled moderators to lead the group discussion and another person to take notes and/or record the session that usually lasts one to two hours. For ethnographers, they can be an effective tool for probing group norms surrounding cultural issues of interest (e.g., how to plant a field, feed toddlers, where to hunt, attitudes toward abortion, etc.). For health care professionals, they can provide insider knowledge about how people view different things that can affect their health. For example, Erickson and colleagues used focus groups to understand why African American and Puerto Rican emerging adults (age 18–25) in Hartford who were in committed relationships had sex (i.e., cheated on partner) outside of the relationship. They asked focus group members (groups were comprised of same sex and ethnicity) why someone would cheat on their current partner and got a wide range of reasons that participants thought were acceptable or at least understandable (e.g., partner is in jail, to have a same-sex experience, revenge against a partner who cheated, to get money or drugs, excitement of new person, to get a particular kind of sex, unhappy in current relationship, access to housing and/or your children), and a few that were not acceptable (e.g., to emotionally hurt partner). These focus group responses revealed the complexity of cheating behavior and the impact it can have on health by sexual risk taking (Macauda et al. 2011).

Interviews

There are four kinds of interviews that anthropologists use: (1) informal, (2) unstructured, (3) semi-structured, and (4) structured (Bernard 2011). The difference among these interview types is the amount of control researchers have over the participants' responses, with informal interviews having the least control and structured interviewing the most control. Informal interviews are often used during initial periods of field work when researchers want to get a general idea of what people do and think about some area of interest (e.g., health care access, kinds of healers used, common health problems in the community, etc.). Unstructured interviews entail researchers having a plan in mind about the kinds of things they want to ask and then interviewing people when they see them in the community. This type of interview is often used when researchers are spending a long time in the community and have multiple opportunities to interview the same people several times to fill in topics not discussed and/or to ask about an unexpected new domain during the interviews that needs to be queried. Semi-structured interviews use an interview guide of topics to be covered in a particular order. They are often used for one-time interviews with a participant and the semi-structured nature of the interview allows querying each participant in the same way to produce reliable and comparable qualitative data. Structured interviews entail asking the same questions in the same order of all participants. Researchers may read the questions to the participant and record their answers or allow the participants to fill in the survey themselves (self-administered survey).

Semi-structured and structured interviews are probably the most useful types of interviews for health professionals as they are generally not seeking to learn about the whole culture and way of life of a group of people, but rather have more bounded interests in particular topics related to health (e.g., beliefs about disease X, how mental health issues are handled, knowledge of sexually transmitted infections). For example, Erickson and colleagues used semi-structured interviews to understand the "culture" of sexual and romantic behavior among African American and Puerto Rican emerging adults (18–25 years old) in Hartford. The interviews were 1–2-hour, open-ended interviews designed to allow participants to describe the natural history of their sexual and romantic relationships in the inner city. The interview guide consisted of open-ended questions that allowed interviewers to explore factors particular to each relationship that could help explain how decisions regarding sex and condom and contraceptive use were negotiated between partners. Their stories provided a general picture of the different ways young people begin their sexual lives, transition from one partner to the next, whether and with whom they used condoms and other contraceptives, and their feelings about their different relationships. A main finding was that having multiple partners (serial and concurrent) was normative for these young adults and condom use was normative only with new partners. Once a relationship became serious, condom use stopped, although multiple partners were still normative for a variety of reasons, elevating the risk of STI infection (Abraham et al. 2011; Macauda et al. 2011; Singer et al. 2006).

Free Lists and Pile Sorts

Free listing and pile sorting are simple but powerful methods for understanding cultural systems of classification that anthropologists call cultural domains. The domain can be either physical things (e.g., illness symptoms, causes of disease) or conceptual things (e.g., ideas about the safety and efficacy of vaccines, reasons for using different healing systems). In free listing, individual participants (20–30 people) are asked to write down all the things they think of that belong in a particular domain. The items are then analyzed to find the most salient 25–60 items (i.e., those mentioned by two or more participants) that can then be pile sorted by participants (20–30 people) to identify sub-domains of the larger domain. This is done by using a set of small cards with the name of the item and a code number on the back. Participants are asked to sort the cards into as many different piles as they want, based on how they think they belong together. The data are then analyzed using multidimensional scaling and Johnson's hierarchical clustering in order to define the different sub-domains of the broader domain of interest.

For example, Erickson and Frank (2017) asked 141 undergraduate and 27 graduate students in nine ethnomedicine classes between 2008 and 2017 to free list all of the causes of disease they could think of. The total number of items varied between 111 and 295 across classes but only about 50 were salient. The top ten causes of disease were consistent across the classes and included stress, viruses, environment, genetics, bacteria, pollution, animals, malnutrition, poor hygiene, and contaminated water. The students also pile sorted the top 50 items in order to identify sub-domains of causes of disease. The sub-domains included (1) Pathogens – small (e.g., virus, bacteria, parasites) and large (e.g., insects, animals, people), (2) Genetics (e.g., genes, mutations, heredity), (3) Environment – pollution (e.g., climate change, water issues) and toxins (e.g., radiation, chemicals), (4) Lifestyle Issues – behavior (e.g., exercise, hygiene, sleep, stress, sex, alcohol, tobacco, drugs) and food/diet issues (e.g., poor diet, obesity), (5) Natural Causes (e.g., age, accidents/injuries, disasters), and (6) Social Determinants of Health (e.g., poverty, living conditions, malnutrition). Overall, the students' knowledge and beliefs about what causes disease conformed to the biomedical model that emphasizes personal responsibility (behavior and lifestyle), accident and injury, genetics and heredity, germs, infections, contagions, acute and chronic illnesses, and environmental health hazards. Less likely to be mentioned by students were physical and emotional violence, war, and terrorist attacks, although this may change with their increasing frequency around the world.

ANTHROPOLOGY, HEALTH, AND ILLNESS

This chapter has aimed to provide accessible information about illness beliefs, theories of disease causation, complementary and alternative medicine (CAM), the importance of patients' health beliefs in the clinical encounter, and research methods medical anthropologists use to understand culture, health, and human behavior. The case study was chosen to highlight why, in our increasingly multicultural world, biomedicine needs to understand cultural differences in health beliefs and behaviors so they can achieve better outcomes for their multicultural patients. There is also a growing demand from students who are training for health care careers for more formal instruction about complementary and alternative medicines so they can become better practitioners when they graduate. Globalization has changed our world and the world of both biomedical and CAM healers. Anthropologists and others are researching and documenting this new world of illness and healing to understand the ways our culture and beliefs about illness and healing are changing and adapting to our multicultural world.

Note

1 "Integrative medicine, as defined by the American Board of Integrative Medicine® (ABOIM) and the Consortium of Academic Health Centers for Integrative Medicine, is the practice of medicine that reaffirms the importance of the relationship between practitioner and patient, focuses on the whole person, is informed by evidence, and makes use of all appropriate therapeutic approaches, healthcare professionals, and disciplines to achieve optimal health and healing." www.abpsus.org/integrative-medicine-defined, accessed 7-3-19.

REFERENCES

Abraham, Traci, Mark Macauda, Pamela Erickson, and Merrill Singer (2011). "And Let Me See Them Damn Papers!" The Role of STI/AIDS Screening among Urban African American and Puerto Rican Youth in the Transition to Sex without a Condom. *AIDS and Behavior* 15(7): 1359–1371.

Beinfield, Harriet and Efrem Korngold (1995). Chinese Traditional Medicine: An Introductory Overview. *Alternative Therapies* 1(1): 44–52.

Bernard, H. Russel (2011). *Research Methods in Anthropology. Qualitative and Quantitative Approaches*. 5th edition. Lanham, MD: AltaMira Press.

Birn, Anne-Emanuelle, Yogan Pillay, and Timothy H. Holtz (2017). *Textbook of Global Health*. 4th edition. Oxford, UK: Oxford University Press.

Blaxter, Mildred (2004). *Health*. Cambridge, UK: Polity Press.

Cohen, Ken ("Bear Hawk") (1998). Native American Medicine. *Alternative Therapies* 4(6): 45–56.

Erickson, Pamela I. (2008). *Ethnomedicine*. Long Grove, IL: Waveland Press.

Erickson, Pamela I. and Cynthia Frank (2017). *College Students' Changing and Stable Ideas about the Cause of Disease, 2008–2016*. Paper presented at the annual meetings of the Society for Applied Anthropology, Santa Fe, NM 3/29/17.

Fadiman, Anne (1997). *The Spirit Catches You and You Fall Down*. New York: Farrar, Strauss, and Giroux.

Fox, Margalit (2012). Lia Lee Dies: Life Went on around Her, Redefining Care by Bridging a Divide. *New York Times*, September 15, 2012, p. A1.

Foster, George M. (1953). Relations between Spanish and Spanish-American Folk Medicine. *Journal of American Folklore* 66: 201–217.

Foster, George M. and Barbara Gallatin Anderson (1978). *Medical Anthropology*. New York: John Wiley & Sons.

Good, Byron and Mary-Jo Delvecchio Good (1981). The Meaning of Symptoms: A Cultural Hermeneutic Model for Clinical Practice. In *The Relevance of Social Science for Medicine*. Leon Eisenberg and Arthur Kleinman (Eds.). Hingham, MA: D. Reidel, pp. 165–196.

Helman, Cecil G. (2007). *Culture, Health and Illness*. 5th edition. London: Hodder Arnold, an imprint of Hodder Education and a member of the Hodder Headline Group.

Kleinman, Arthur (1978). Concepts and a Model for the Comparison of Medical Systems as Cultural Systems. *Social Science and Medicine* 12: 85–93.

Kleinman, Arthur (1980). *Patients and Healers in the Context of Culture*. Berkeley: University of California Press.

Kluckhohn, Clyde and Dorothea Leighton (1962). *The Navajo: The American Museum of Natural History Library*. Revised edition. New York: Anchor Books, Doubleday.

Kunitz, Stephen J. (1989). *Disease Change and the Role of Medicine: The Navajo Experience*. Berkeley, CA: University of California Press.

Lad, Vasant (1995). An Introduction to Ayurveda. *Alternative Therapies* 1(3): 57–63.

Levy, Barry S. and Victor W. Sidel (Eds.) (2000). *War and Public Health*. Updated edition. Washington, DC: American Public Health Association.

Macauda, Mark M., Pamela I. Erickson, Merrill C. Singer, and Claudia C. Santelices (2011). A Cultural Model of Infidelity among African American and Puerto Rican Young Adults. *Anthropology & Medicine* 18(3): 351–364.

Magner, Lois N. (2005). *A History of Medicine*. 2nd edition. New York: Taylor & Francis.

Marmot, Michael (2005). The Social Determinants of Health Inequalities. *Lancet* 365(9464): 1099–1104.

Marmot, Michael (2006). Health in an Unequal World. *Lancet* 368: 2081–2094.

McElroy, Ann and Patricia K. Townsend (2015). *Medical Anthropology in Ecological Perspective*. Sixth edition. New York: Routledge.

Murdock, George Peter (1980). *Theories of Illness: A World Survey*. Pittsburg, PA: University of Pittsburgh Press.

Parsons, Claire D.F. (Ed.) (1985). *Healing Practices in the South Pacific*. Honolulu, HI: The Institute for Polynesian Studies/University of Hawaii Press.

Reid, Janice (1983). *Sorcerers, and Healing Spirits: Continuity and Change in an Aboriginal Medical System*. Canberra: Australian National University Press.

Rubel, Arthur J. and Michael R. Haas (1996). Ethnomedicine. In *Medical Anthropology: Contemporary Theory and Method*. Carolyn E. Sargent and Thomas M. Johnson (Eds.). Westport, CT: Praeger, pp. 113–130.

Scrimshaw, Susan C. (2001). Culture, Behavior, and Health. In *International Public Health: Diseases, Programs, Systems, and Policies*. Michael H. Merson, Robert E. Black, and Anne J. Mills (Eds.). Gaithersburg, MD: Aspen Publishers. pp. 53–78.

Scrimshaw, Susan C. (2012). Culture, Behavior, and Health. In *International Public Health: Diseases, Programs, Systems, and Policies*. 3rd edition. Michael H. Merson, Robert E. Black, and Anne J. Mills (Eds.). Burlington, MA: Jones & Bartlett, pp. 43–74.

Scrimshaw, Susan C. and Elena Hurtado (1984). Field Guide for the Study of Health-Seeking Behavior at the Household Level. *Food and Nutrition Bulletin* 6(2): 27–45.

Scrimshaw, Susan C. and Sandra D. Lane (2020). Culture, Behavior, and Health. In *Global Health: Diseases, Programs, Systems and Policies*. 4th edition. Michael H. Merson, Robert E. Black, and Anne J. Mills (Eds.). Burlington, MA: Jones & Bartlett, pp. 43–74.

Singer, Merrill (2019). *Climate Change and Social Inequality: The Health and Social Costs of Global Warming*. New York: Routledge.

Singer, Merrill and Hans Baer (1995). *Critical Medical Anthropology*. Amityville, NY: Baywood Publishing Co.

Singer, Merrill and Pamela I. Erickson (Eds.) (2011). *A Companion to Medical Anthropology*. Malden, MA: Wiley-Blackwell.

Singer, Merrill and Pamela I. Erickson (2013). *Global Health: An Anthropological Perspective*. Long Grove, IL: Waveland Press.

Singer, Merrill C., Pamela I. Erickson, Louise Badiane, Rosemary Diaz, Dugeidy Ortiz, Traci Abraham, and Anna Marie Nicolaysen (2006). Syndemics, Sex, and the City: Understanding Sexually Transmitted Diseases in Social and Cultural Context. *Social Science and Medicine* 63(8): 2010–2021.

Weller, Susan C. (1983). New Data on Intracultural Variability: The Hot-Cold Concept of Medicine and Illness. *Human Organization* 42: 249–257.

World Health Organization (WHO) (2002). *World Report on Violence and Health: Summary*. Geneva: World Health Organization.

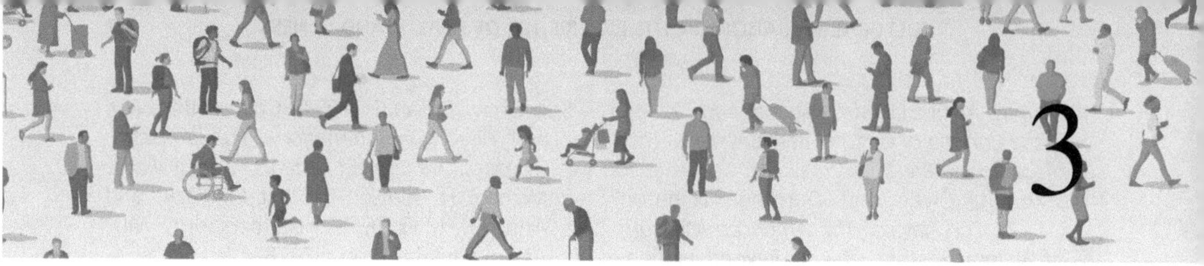

3

Social Determinants of Health: Intersectional Impacts of Race, Class, Ethnicity and Place

Ruth Enid Zambrana, Deborah Parra-Medina, and Courtney Butler

> "Health inequalities and the social determinants of health are not a footnote to the determinants of health. They are the main issue." (Marmot, 2018)

Health and well-being measures among the United States (US) population reflect persistent inequalities in morbidity, mortality, and life span, as well as inequities in access to quality health care services and public health interventions. A growing body of research has provided evidence and furthered understanding of the relationships between social determinants and health outcomes (American Medical Association [AMA], 2021; Braveman et al., 2017; Weber et al., 2018). Health equity, also referred to as "equity in health", reflects the ideal of a fair opportunity among all individuals to attain optimal health. The global goal of health equity is that all individuals have a fair opportunity to attain their full health potential and that no one should be disadvantaged from achieving this potential (World Health Organization [WHO], n.d.).

A key to decreasing health disparities, particularly among racial/ethnic groups, is the equitable distribution and availability of health care resources. The unique burden borne by African Americans and Latina/o groups in the US. is attributed to structural racism (Jones, 2018). Structural racism refers to the historical and contemporary policies, practices, and norms that create and maintain white supremacy through segregation of racial/ethnic communities and limited access to opportunity and upward mobility due to difficulties in securing quality education, jobs, housing, health care, and equal treatment in the criminal justice system (Urban Institute, 2020). Social determinants, ranging from class, race, ethnicity, neighborhood context, social and economic resources to structural racism in access to health and medical resources, contribute to observable, disparate effects on population health and equity (Williams et al., 2019).

Although race and ethnicity are associated with the maldistribution of health equity in the US, acknowledgement of the social determinants of health inequities is neither recent nor innovative. In his analysis of 1890 census data for Philadelphia, W. E. B. Du Bois noted that specific racial and ethnic disparities reflected "a vast set of problems having a common center [that] must be studied according to some general plan" (Du Bois, 1906). More than a century later, there is ongoing interest in further explicating the root causes of current differences and the associations between health inequities and race, ethnicity, gender, and socioeconomic status (White, 2011). In their interrogation of the meaning and contribution of socioeconomic status (SES) to health in the 20th century, Robert and House (2000) concluded that SES is among the many factors associated with poor health outcomes. According to Kindig and Stoddart (2003), population health "encompasses the examination of health outcomes, patterns of health determinants, and linked policies and interventions within a specific group" (p. 381). This definition of population health provides an aperture to clarify national discourses on the social determinants of health and associated health disparities and inequities with and among public health scholars, practitioners, and policy makers.

Reducing health disparities was the focus of the 2000 National Health Agenda of the Centers for Disease Control and Prevention (CDC, 1990). Although novel at the time, the public health response was an impediment rather than an engine of change because of the primary emphasis on understanding observed differences (health disparities) rather than focusing on the root causes of these disparities, social determinants. As a result, observed disparities served as the starting point of analysis and social determinants of health were mostly ignored. Notwithstanding these limitations, federal health agencies have continued to establish national health objectives aimed at improving the health of all Americans. Table 3.1 provides examples of these decennial Healthy People initiatives.

Despite the official identification of specific health indicators and support for collaborative, multi-sectorial efforts to address these high-priority health issues improvement in the 36 leading health objectives has been slow, and in some cases, undetectable. After two decades of defined health targets for specific race, ethnic, and socioeconomic status population groups, overall health disparities have remained resistant to significant change. Critics attribute this collective inability to make more significant progress on specific national goals towards the broader achievement of health equity to the dominant application of positivist biomedical frameworks; to the exclusion of more comprehensive intersectional, social determinants, and life course lenses; and to sampling frames not guided by demographic, geographic, and community factors (Bowleg, 2017; Parra-Medina & Fore, 2004; Pastor & Morello-Frosch, 2014; Weber & Parra-Medina, 2003). The persistence of these disparities and inequalities poses salient questions: Who is more vulnerable, or more "at risk?" What are the root causes of their vulnerability? Given the conceptual overlap between the constructs of risk and vulnerability, what is the rationale, or utility, of differentiating between them? Clearly, the current challenges of effectively addressing social determinants of health across intersectional population groups require increased clarity in terminology, acknowledgement of structural racism and precise descriptions of at-risk indicators (Braveman et al., 2017; Bowleg, 2021).

In this chapter, we examine health inequities associated with race, ethnicity, and socioeconomic status through an in-depth analysis of factors related to population health across the lifespan; assess three specific health conditions (Maternal and Child Health, HIV/AIDS)

Table 3.1 Healthy People 2000–2030 overarching goals

Healthy People 2000	• Increase the span of healthy life • Reduce health disparities • Provide access to preventive health services
Healthy People 2010	• Increase the span of healthy life • Eliminate health disparities across the categories of gender, race or ethnicity, education or income, disability, geographic location, and sexual orientation
Healthy People 2020	• Attain high-quality, longer lives free of preventable disease, disability, injury, and premature death • Achieve health equity, eliminate disparities, and improve the health of all groups • Create social and physical environments that promote good health for all • Promote quality of life, healthy development, and healthy behaviors across all life stages
Healthy People 2030	• Attain healthy, thriving lives and well-being, free of preventable disease, disability, injury and premature death • Eliminate health disparities, achieve health equity, and attain health literacy to improve the health and well-being of all • Create social, physical, and economic environments that promote attaining full potential for health and well-being for all • Promote healthy development, healthy behaviors and well-being across all life stages • Engage leadership, key constituents, and the public across multiple sectors to take action and design policies that improve the health and well-being of all

Sources:

Centers for Disease Control and Prevention (1990). *Healthy People 2000*. Available at: www.cdc.gov/nchs/healthy_people/hp2000.htm. Accessed on September 3, 2020.

Centers for Disease Control and Prevention (2010). *Healthy People 2010*. Available at: www.cdc.gov/nchs/data/hpdata2010/hp2010_final_review_overview.pdf. Accessed on September 3, 2020.

Office of Disease Prevention and Health Promotion (ODPHP) (2020). *Healthy People 2020*. Available at https://www.healthypeople.gov/2020/Leading-Health-Indicators. Accessed on June 29, 2021.

Office of Disease Prevention and Health Promotion (2021). Healthy People 2030. Available at https://www.healthypeople.gov/2020/About-Healthy-People/Development-Healthy-People-2030. Accessed on June 29, 2021.

that demonstrate the ways in which specific populations are at significantly higher risk than others throughout the life course; examine a recent example of COVID-19 and its impact on Latinos; and highlight policies and practices designed to assure equity with examples from three industrialized countries: Canada, Colombia, and Sweden.

POPULATION HEALTH ACROSS THE LIFE COURSE: INEQUITIES ASSOCIATED WITH RACE, ETHNICITY, AND SOCIOECONOMIC STATUS

The life course health approach takes into consideration an integrated continuum of exposures, experiences, and interactions from birth to old age, rather than a series of discrete steps or life stages (Braveman & Barclay, 2009). The accumulation of disadvantage over a lifetime reflects how social determinants impact health (García & Ailshire, 2019; Marmot, 2018). Central to the examination of social determinants of population health, equity is critical to assure the just allocation of financial, human, and health resources. Despite some doubts regarding the multiple causes of persistent health disparities, there is clear evidence that low SES and race/ethnicity are significantly associated with the equitable distribution of health care resources, including health insurance. The consequences of specific inequities (e.g., access to employment-linked health insurance), reflect social arrangements embedded in institutional systems that place specific populations at higher risk. Health research on poor and underserved groups often discounts existing structural and political considerations and underlying power relations that contribute to maintaining the status quo that advantages one group over another (Adepoju et al., 2015; Dill & Zambrana, 2009). The historic distribution of governmental resources, ranging from the provision of public health services to research funding, has concentrated more health resources in white, middle- and upper-income communities and prioritized research on diseases more prevalent in those groups (e.g., Parkinson's, Cystic Fibrosis, Crohn's). Application of an equity lens requires consideration of both population demographics and place to provide a meaningful interpretative context for population outcomes and to avoid individual attributions for illness. To provide purposeful contexts for improving health conditions, public health scholars have forged new multidisciplinary paradigms and created a trifocal approach to population health across the life course that includes an intersectional focus on socioeconomic status, race and place, and equitable access to health care services (Bowleg, 2021; Weber et al., 2018).

Over the past two decades, an increasing body of work in health outcomes research has centered the role of neighborhoods, including ethnic enclaves (Diez Roux, 2016; Pastor & Morell-Frosch, 2014; Robert & House, 2000; White, 2011). Measures of neighborhood structural characteristics include availability of resources, discrimination and perceived threats to self and property (Benjamins & Middleton, 2019; Lavizzo-Mourey et al., 2021). Clear evidence has accumulated showing that individuals living in socially and structurally disadvantaged neighborhoods report poorer health and dietary habits, and less physical activity relative to residents of advantaged neighborhoods (Arcaya et al., 2016; Sharkey, 2013; White & Borrell, 2006). Furthermore, lower socioeconomic groups tend to encounter other barriers and disadvantages where they live, work, and play – all of which impact health outcomes (Institute of Medicine [IOM], 2003; Amaro, 2014). Analytically rigorous population health research takes into consideration the cumulative health effects of resource-poor neighborhoods, including inadequate schools and deficient public health services, and its impact on the health and well-being of diverse racial/ethnic groups.

In summary, the application of a social determinant/social equity lens broadens the focus of examination to include diverse factors with impacts across the life course (these range from safe and adequate housing to protection from environmental toxins, provision of sufficient economic means to purchase nutritious food and over-the-counter medications, perceived and structural racism, access to quality health care, and availability to safe recreational spaces and other resources) (Braveman et al., 2011). In the subsequent sections, we examine two exemplars of population health inequality: maternal and child health and HIV/AIDS. Each exemplar illustrates how distinct intersections of race, class, gender, and sexuality contribute to disproportionately higher health risks across the life course.

Maternal and Child Health: A Life Course Perspective

There is a substantial body of literature on US maternal and child health indicators that unequivocally demonstrates adverse outcomes among disadvantaged, historically underrepresented minority women, including African Americans, Puerto Ricans, and American Indian/Alaskan Natives (Kamal et al., 2019). Although untoward birth outcomes (i.e., low birthweight and high infant mortality) have declined over the past 40 years, the reproductive health disparities among non-white racial/ethnic women highlight persistent inequality and unfair treatment (Ross et al., 2016; National Academies of Science, Engineering, and Medicine [NASEM], 2020; IOM, 2003). A robust body of recent maternal-child health research literature substantiates the cumulative impact of multiple, multi-layered social determinants including racism on the life course of racial/ethnic, low-income women (Center for Disease Control and Prevention [CDC], 2018; Gadson et al., 2017). Examples of these social determinants range from inadequate access to health insurance coverage and quality health and social services to food insecurity, low wages and/or high unemployment, and lack of available and affordable childcare (Butkus et al., 2020; Nagata et al., 2019; NASEM, 2020).

In the decade between 2005 and 2015, the national pregnancy-related mortality increased 11.7%, from 15.5 to 17.2 pregnancy-related deaths per 100,000 live births. Notably, Black women experienced the highest mortality ratio of 42.8 per 100,000, followed by American Indian/Alaskan Native women at 32.5 per 100,000 (CDC, 2019a). Comorbidities and risk factors for African American maternal/fetal morbidity include late entry into care, with only 66.6% of pregnant African American women initiating prenatal care in the first trimester 10.2% only receiving late or no care (Borrell et al., 2016; CDC, 2019b; Howell, 2018; Leonard et al., 2019). American Indian/Alaskan Native women are the most likely to initiate late or receive no prenatal care (12.6% and 19.6%), most likely to have pre-pregnancy diabetes (2.3% and 2%) and are most likely to be overweight or obese (66.6% and 73.6%) (CDC, 2019b). In contrast, some Hispanic women experience healthier birth outcomes regardless of socioeconomic background. US-born Hispanic women had higher rates of three adverse birth outcomes (preterm birth; low birth weight; small for gestational age) than did foreign-born Hispanic women. These higher rates persisted after adjusting for maternal characteristics, with Puerto Rican women consistently having the poorest birth outcomes. Adverse birth outcomes vary by country of birth among foreign-born Hispanic women. In one study, DeSisto and McDonald (2018) examined birth outcomes among a sample of foreign-born Hispanic women, two-thirds of whom were non-US-born Mexican women. They noted that any analyses of rates for foreign-born Hispanic women as a single group would have produced rates that were not representative of all Hispanic women, but rather masked differences by country of birth. Current data reveal that African American and Puerto Rican women are the most likely to rely on public health insurance (Medicaid 65.3% and 60.3%), have preterm births (14.13% and 10.87%), deliver by cesarean section (36.1% and 33.6%), and deliver infants with low birthweight (14.07% and 9.39%) (US Department of Health and Human Services, 2019).

The unequal provision of healthcare to low-income and racial and ethnic women is rooted in structural racism (e.g., low quality of care, implicit bias) (Colen et al., 2018; Black Women's Health Imperative, 1983; Sister Song Women of Color Reproductive Justice Collective, n.d.; Zambrana & Dill, 2006). Given that providers are more likely to stereotype low-income and racial and ethnic women (Zambrana et al., 1987)[1], it is not surprising that these women are less likely to develop trust and feel comfortable in communication with providers. There is evidence that providers' lack of socially appropriate communication contributes to increased risk for adverse birth outcomes among pregnant women with low health literacy and lack of trust (Attanasio & Kozhimannil, 2017; Colen et al., 2018) and to perceived experiences of disparity in quality of care (Profit et al., 2017). There is compelling evidence that racial/ethnic concordance in patient-provider dyads improves outcomes and patient satisfaction, knowledge of birthing options, agency in making birthing decisions, and trust between patient and provider (Ma et al., 2019; Mujica et al., 2020). Furthermore, patient-provider racial/ethnic concordance is associated with improved patient adherence to treatment recommendations and follow-up services (Nielsen et al., 2016; O'Malley et al., 2004), as well as increased bodily autonomy in the context of having birthing experiences congruent with personal values and choices (Lyerly, 2013; Mujica et al., 2020; Sheppard et al., 2004). Across both public and private health care institutions, health care professionals demonstrate implicit biases and their attitudes and actions contribute to unwelcoming climates (IOM, 2003). Broader institutional profit motives often promote rushed, ineffective interpersonal interactions and result in lower quality services.

Inequitable access to opportunities and resources perpetuates institutional racial hierarchies, creates and sustains racial inequities (Marmot, 2006; Williams et al., 2019), and contributes to a disproportionate burden on historically minoritized populations due to inadequate community-driven resources (NASEM, 2020; Sullivan, 2004). The following example further illustrates how institutional exclusionary practices and stereotypic representations of individual risk attributions result in access inequities among individuals with HIV/AIDS.

HIV/AIDS: Devastation, Care, and Containment

There is a robust body of HIV/AIDS scholarship in three areas: the trends in incidence and prevalence by race, ethnicity, class, and geographic location; transmission modalities, risk factors, and comorbidities of specific populations; and access to specific HIV-related services and barriers to quality health care (including testing and treatment). For many racial/ethnic members of the LGBTQ community, rates of HIV/AIDS have been increasing while access to quality care is not readily available and opportunities to contain the transmission of infections are low. By the end of 2018, an estimated 1.2 million people were living with AIDS in the US (CDC, 2018). However, among the HIV+ population, only 14.2%, or 1 in 7, were aware of their infection status. Almost 70% of newly diagnosed cases of HIV were attributed to male-to-male sexual contact, followed by heterosexual contact (24%) and injection drug use (7%). From 2010 to 2017, among gay and bisexual men, HIV diagnoses decreased 19% in Whites, remained stable in Blacks, and increased 17% in Latinos. HIV is largely an urban disease, unevenly situated across the nation, and varies geographically by race and ethnicity.[2] African Americans currently have the highest prevalence of new HIV diagnosis and people living with HIV, accounting for 42% of all new HIV diagnoses, of which 31% were men and 11% were women. Among those at increased risk, recent data showed a 42% increase in HIV among African American gay and bisexual men ages 25–34. Latinos make up 27% of all new HIV diagnoses (22% men and 4% women) and overall HIV prevalence among Latinos increased 6%. During the same period, among Latinas there was a 20% decrease in new HIV diagnoses due to heterosexual contact and a 25% decrease from injection drug use (CDC, 2020a).

Comorbidities complicate patient care outcomes because often HIV patients must manage multiple health conditions and maintain the recommended follow-up clinical visits for both primary and comorbid conditions. According to Zingmond et al. (2017), 83% of people living with HIV are aged 50 and older, and among those between 18 and 49 years, 63% had at least one comorbidity. Medical and psychiatric complications constitute the most common comorbidities among the HIV+ population. These include substance-use disorders, cardiovascular disease, mental illness (e.g., depression and suicidal ideation), and other viral complications such as viral hepatitis and tuberculosis. Smoking, substance use/dependence, homelessness, intimate partner violence, and risky sexual behavior are other health risks common among individuals at high risk of HIV transmission and those diagnosed with HIV (Eastwood et al., 2021; IOM, 2010; O'Malley et al., 2019). Although frequently present among the HIV population, these risk factors are not precursors of the disease. A growing priority is to provide HIV patients prompt and affordable access to screening and treatment for non-communicable diseases in low-resource settings with specific attention to African American and Latina/o populations. Examples of specific strategies aimed at more frequent testing and stigma reduction among at-risk groups include the implementation of a multi-disease chronic care model and bundling of HIV tests with screenings for other conditions (Currier & Havlir, 2017; Galvan et al., 2006; IOM, 2010).

In tandem with the more widespread societal acceptance of varying sexual and gender identities since the 1970's, there were increased corporate and pharmaceutical industry investments, which resulted in the development of drugs like AZT, that primarily targeted those who were insured and socially privileged (IOM, 2011). More recent pharmaceutical interventions, including new drugs and preventive medications such as PrEP, aim to reduce HIV/AIDS transmission rates. However, these more recent treatment options continue to be less available to low-income, Black/Latinos and transgender women, a reflection, in part, of the myriad social determinants that shape their lives, particularly poverty, limited knowledge of prevention measures, and lack of health insurance coverage (Garcia & Harris, 2017; Huang et al., 2018). The adverse impact of HIV/AIDS over the past four decades has fallen disproportionately on low-income racial and ethnic men and women. As illustrated in Figure 3.1, Black and Latino gay and bisexual men continue to experience the highest new infection rates compared to White men. Notably, HIV rates among African American heterosexual women are three to four times higher than new infections among people who inject drugs, data

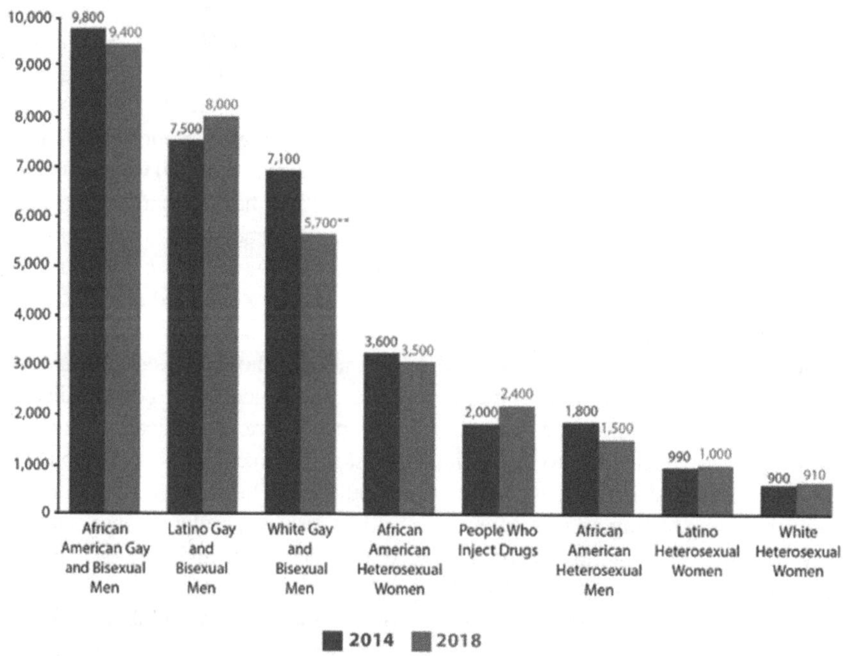

Figure 3.1 New HIV infections by race and transmission group, US 2014–2018

Source: CDC, Estimated HIV Incidence and Prevalence in the United States 2014–2018, 2020c

that challenge the stereotypic assumptions of race/ethnicity, drug use, and HIV/AIDS (CDC, 2020b).

A wide range of factors contribute to the continued disparity in rates of HIV infections and transmission among racial and ethnic minority groups. These social determinants include, but are not limited to, inadequate and unstable health insurance coverage, limited accessibility to preventive prescription measures such as PrEP, immunosuppression associated with comorbidities, repeated exposure to discrimination, low quality care, and high care costs, in addition to deficits related to other social determinants (e.g., nutrition, housing, education) (Phillips et al., 2021). These examples also demonstrate that the targeted national health goals to reduce disparities across major conditions have not been realized for all Americans.

COVID 19: Triple Pandemic of Race, Economics and Health

The Coronavirus Disease 2019 (COVID-19) epidemic in the US is a recent example of the practical impact of the social determinants of health among minority populations. Of note, Blacks and Latinos are represented disproportionately in essential work settings such as health care facilities, farms, factories, grocery stores, construction, and public transportation (US Bureau Labor Statistics, 2019; Schneider & Harknett, 2020). Workers in these settings had a higher potential for exposure to the coronavirus due to several factors. These included close contact with the public or other workers, inability to work from home, lack of access to personal protection equipment on the job, and not having access to paid sick days (Economic Policy Institute, 2020). Workers in these situations often cannot afford to miss work, even if they get sick, because they do not have enough money saved up for basic expenses and/or they are ineligible for benefits (Miller et al., 2020). Additionally, pandemic-related school closures contributed to increased food insecurity among children living in poverty who rely on school meal programs for nutritional support. Furthermore, employed women heads of household encountered the challenge of providing care for their children who were at home rather than in school; as a result, many women were not only unable to maintain their employment but were unable to provide for their family's essential needs.

Living conditions in low-income communities further increase risk for COVID-19 infection and/or transmission. Communities with higher racial and ethnic minority populations have higher housing density, more housing insecurity, scarcity of potable water, and more multigenerational households which makes it harder to follow prevention strategies (Branigin, 2020; Khunti et al., 2020; Taylor, 2019). COVID-19 is highly transmittable, and mitigation strategies include following healthy hygiene practices, staying at home when sick, practicing physical distancing to lower the risk of disease transmission, and use of a cloth face covering when physical distancing cannot be maintained. Uniform public health recommendations related to physical distancing or sheltering-in-place that did not consider local contexts and population characteristics may have been less effective (often for reasons beyond individual control). Social distancing was a privilege and the ability to isolate in a safe home, work remotely with full digital access, and sustain monthly income were components of this privilege (Benda et al., 2020; Yancy, 2020).

Nationally, Latinos and Blacks have contracted the virus at rates three times higher than Whites (Oppel et al., 2020). Mortality among Blacks is 3.6 times that of Whites and among Latinos is 2.5 times higher than Whites (Ford et al., 2020; Saenz, 2020). When nation-wide shut-downs were implemented to slow the spread of the infectious virus, it resulted in widespread loss of jobs and incomes, and health insurance, leaving millions of Americans without the means to meet their material and health needs (Berchick et al., 2019). According to the Pew Research Center (2020), although the pandemic affected almost everyone's work life, the impact was distributed unequally. Job loss and recovery were more challenging for specific racial/ethnic, gender, and nativity groups. Between February and June 2020, the lowest level of job loss was 7.5% among Whites, which reflected a loss of approximately one of every 13 jobs, compared to 12.3% loss among Latinos and 11.5% among Blacks (11.5%). During this period, Latinos lost about one of eight jobs and Blacks one of nine. Across all ethnic groups, men fared better than women, but the most elevated jobless rates occurred among women of color and immigrant Latinas (Saenz & Sparks, 2020).

Prior to the COVID-19 pandemic and associated economic fallout, poverty rates in the US were 22% among Blacks, 19% among Latinos, and 9% among Whites (The Henry J. Kaiser Family Foundation, 2018). Prior to the pandemic, the median wealth of white households across all income brackets was ten times the wealth of Black households and eight times that of Latino households (Kochhar & Cilluffo, 2017). As a result, individuals and families in these minority groups had less financial capacity to take necessary precautions amid the financial hardships that accompanied the pandemic. Beyond the health consequences of the pandemic, there will be significant financial implications stemming from inequalities related to joblessness and financial well-being. There will be consequences with potentially far-reaching effects for other aspects of life, potentially impacting both short-term and long-term health and well-being among already marginalized populations (CDC, 2019c).

A preponderance of clinical, epidemiologic, and social science evidence signals that other industrialized nations have implemented systemic approaches that optimize population health without increasing the burden of providing health care (Rostila, 2013). In the following sections, we broaden the focus to examine other approaches to the provision of health care.

INTERNATIONAL PATTERNS OF EFFECTIVE HEALTH CARE: PERSPECTIVES AND EXEMPLARS

Unique to the system of healthcare access in the US is an underlying value system that situates health as a privilege bestowed primarily based on access to private health insurance through an individual's (or an immediate family member's) stable full-time employment (Avgar et al., 2020). This framing of health care is a racialized institutional practice that excludes major segments of the US population, including domestic workers, farm workers, part-time employees, and small-business owners (IOM, 2003; Weber et al., 2018). Table 3.2 compares the basic value premises underlying the provision of health care in the US with those in other highly industrialized countries. Given these distinct value systems, it is not possible to compare the US health care system to those of most other countries (Marmot, 2018).

According to a Commonwealth Fund report that compared the health systems of 11 high-income countries, the US had the highest

Table 3.2 Health care as a privilege or right: polarized perspectives

United States	*Other Highly Industrialized Countries*
Health care is a privilege	Health care is a human right
Health care coverage is an individual responsibility	Health care coverage is a societal responsibility
Availability and affordability of health care is linked to an individual or family's employment status	Provision of health care is universal and afforded to all, regardless of employment type or status

health care expenditures as measured by percent of Gross National Product (i.e., 16.9%). Despite this high level of financial investment, the US ranked last overall and in three of five performance rankings: access, equity, and health care outcomes (Schneider et al., 2017). Three key health indicators clearly influenced the US ranking globally: newborn mortality, mortality amendable deaths, and morbidity amenable to health care. In 2018, the US ranked last in newborn mortality (i.e., newborn deaths per 1,000 live births), with the highest rates of newborn mortality occurring among specific subgroups: African American women, poor women, and Native American/American Indian women (Kamal et al., 2019). Similarly, the US ranked last in the number of mortality amenable deaths per 100,000 deaths, an indication of mortality among individuals who would not have died had they been insured or experienced quality health care. Additionally, the US ranked last in morbidity amenable to health care, a measure of access to, timeliness of, and continuity of health care to assure early diagnosis, treatment, and management of chronic conditions (Schneider et al., 2017). These data support the assertion that the US health sector is an illness-driven system rather than a wellness-driven system. Given that prevention drives the health care delivery systems in many other countries, there are challenges to making direct comparisons with the US. However, there is clear evidence that stark differences exist in equity, cost, values, and quality of care (Braveman et al., 2017; NASEM, 2017).

Despite vast and differing national histories, population demographics, political structures, and health care systems, there are numerous examples of effective, equity-driven health care delivery systems across the globe, which illustrate the variety of ways in which these systems either ameliorate or contribute to health inequities. In the following section, we examine equitable policies in three industrialized nations: Canada, Colombia, and Sweden. Each of these countries has instituted equitable policies that have contributed to the improvement of individual, community, and public health. The systemic approach in each of the exemplars demonstrates their governments' willingness to share responsibility in the health and well-being of its residents based on need rather than ability to pay. We begin with an overview of universal health care access in Canada, then examine employment-linked health benefits in Colombia, followed by a review of reproductive health services and gender rights in Sweden and Western Europe.

Universal Access to Health Care in Canada

Over the last two decades, health care in Canada has evolved from a delivery system that was primarily privately funded to a publicly available and financed system (Hutchinson et al., 2011; Pylypchuk & Sarpong, 2013). The federal government directly funds and/or delivers primary and supplementary services to specific population groups, including First Nations people living on reserves, Inuit, military personnel and eligible veterans, federal prison populations, and certain groups of refugee claimants. As a result of both the 1984 Canada Health Act and the 2004 Accord on Health Care Renewal, structural changes to the Canadian health care system were implemented to support access, quality, and long-term sustainability. Targeted areas of reform included: wait times management; Aboriginal health; home care; primary health care; a national pharmaceutical strategy; health care services in the North; medical equipment; prevention, promotion, and public health; and enhanced reporting on progress made on these reforms (Government of Canada, 2011; Martin et al., 2018). Most provincial and territorial governments offer and fund supplementary benefits for specific population groups (e.g., low-income residents and seniors) not covered under the Canada Health Act. These benefits include the cost of drugs prescribed outside hospitals, ambulance costs, and hearing, vision, and dental care.

Findings from a cross-national, population-based survey of both Americans and Canadians demonstrated absolute differences in health status, access, and utilization patterns (Lasser et al., 2006; Pylpchuk & Sarpong, 2013). The data indicated US residents were less healthy than Canadians, with higher rates of obesity (20.7% vs. 15.3%), physical inactivity (13.6% vs. 6.5%), diabetes (6.7% vs. 4.7%), hypertension (18.3% vs. 13.9%), arthritis (17.9% vs. 16%), and chronic obstructive pulmonary disease (1.9% vs. 1%). Furthermore, Americans were more likely to report unmet health care needs because of cost (7% vs. 0.8%) and less likely to have access to a regular medical doctor (79.6% vs. 84.9%). The Canadian approach to universal health care reflects a commitment to health equity, affordability, and access that has consistently produced better population health outcomes than the US health care approach.

Linkage of Employment and Health Insurance Structures in Colombia

The government of Colombia guarantees a state-mandated minimum living wage as well as government health insurance, disability benefits, and retirement. In 1993, the federal government approved Law 100, a universal health insurance program that guarantees a comprehensive health benefits package to all Colombian citizens irrespective of their ability to pay (Giedion & Uribe, 2009). Prior to the implementation of these reforms, only 24% of the population had health coverage; by 2016, 96% of the population had access to health insurance (Lamprea & García, 2016). As a result, Colombia is among the very few nations in the developing world with near-universal health insurance coverage (Pan American Health Organization [PAHO], 2017).

Colombia's universal health insurance system covers individuals under one of two regimes depending on income. The Contributory Regime (CR) covers workers and their families with monthly incomes above a minimum monthly amount (approximately US $170 per month). The Subsidized Regime (SR) covers individuals identified as economically poor in accordance with a proxy means test. SR eligibility is based on 14 indicators of household well-being, among which are access to public utilities, ownership of assets, rurality, educational attainment, and labor force participation. These poverty-targeting variables assess the ability to pay for health and social services and provide accessible and affordable coverage to those who need it the most (Gideon & Uribe, 2009). The elimination of financial barriers through the universal provision of no-cost preventative health care services promotes equity of access and reflects a position of health care as a basic social right (WHO, 2017). Colombia has one public health insurance plan, the Entidades Promotoras de Salud (EPS; Health Promotion Entities), in conjunction with multiple private health insurance plans organized into a broader system. The basic EPS policy serves as the foundation from which the individual can build a personalized policy. Purchase of a separate, private policy allows for certain expanded options (e.g., the freedom to choose your own doctor or specialist, quicker access, shorter wait times, enhanced concierge services). Of note, most preventative services in Colombia, including primary care, family medicine, and ambulatory obstetric/gynecologic visits, are free, regardless of insurance status.

In their study on the effectiveness, utilization, and risk protection of Colombia's insurance program, Miller et al. (2009) highlighted how subsidized regime (SR) coverage for poor populations was incentivized for local governments and families. Subsidies for local governments provided federal funding to increase health care insurance enrollment which resulted in families being less financially burdened with full, out-of-pocket costs. In a recent study, the National Demographic and Health Survey (ENDS), which was conducted in 2015, shows that in Colombia, 98% of women who had deliveries received antenatal care by trained personnel (doctors and nurses); 92% of these women received four or more prenatal check-ups during their last pregnancy, and 78% of the women received postnatal care at their last delivery. Although the government of Colombia has made a significant effort to prioritize the health of the nation, significant inequalities still exist.

Reproductive Health Services and Women's Rights in Sweden

Improving maternal and childbirth outcomes requires integrated delivery of services across a continuum of care. Within the Swedish health care system, prenatal care is available to all without cost, and almost all pregnant women participate (Stephansson et al., 2018). Preparation for the arrival of a child is supported across the continuum from antenatal to one-year postpartum care. This approach actively supports and enhances the mothering role and provides equitable and quality care via universal access to pre- and post-birth midwife providers and postpartum parental leave policies that promote positive parental bonding with the child.

Swedish antenatal care is organized into defined areas by geographic proximity to delivery hospitals, usually including all antenatal care units of the catchment area of a specified hospital. Each area has an antenatal care obstetrician and a midwife coordinator who are responsible for evaluating and improving the quality of care. The primary antenatal care providers are midwives linked to obstetricians through a referral system when needed (Stephansson et al., 2018). In 1974, the Swedish Parental Leave reform granted both parents 480 days (16 months) of combined, paid parental leave. Each parent has an exclusive right to 90 of those days and this leave time does not expire until the child is eight years old. This unprecedented parental leave fosters a longer postpartum recovery period, enhances parent/child bonding, and provides for more meaningful family time. In contrast, the Family and Medical Leave Act of 1993 (FMLA) requires US employers to grant 12 weeks of unpaid leave annually for parents of newborn or newly adopted children, given that the following requirements are met: parents must have worked for the employers for at least 12 months, for a total of at least 1,250 hours over the past 12 months, and at a location where the company employs 50 or more employees within 75 miles (US Department of Labor, 2020). Although many larger companies do include short-term disability in their standard employee benefits packages, many new mothers in the US must either forego spending quality time with their new child or risk not being paid a salary (Manuel & Zambrana, 2009).

Worldwide, maternity-related employment leave policies and the increased economic and social stressors to return to work can be major barriers to successful long-term breastfeeding (Jones et al., 2015; Robinson et al., 2019). Breastfeeding provides numerous health benefits for infants and mothers (Rollins et al., 2016; Sriraman & Kellams, 2016), and employer support for flexible work scheduling may help more women achieve their breastfeeding goals (Mirkovic et al., 2014). Of note, Sweden reported a 95.5% rate of breastfeeding initiation, one of the highest rates in the world. The majority (63%) of Swedish mothers breastfeed for at least six months, compared to 58% of American women who initiate breastfeeding and 51% breastfeed for at least six months (Lubold, 2019). Across these exemplars, the systemic approaches reflect a commitment by the government in each country to share responsibility for promoting the health and well-being of its residents, based on need rather than ability to pay.

PROMOTING POLICY DEVELOPMENT CONSISTENT WITH POPULATION HEALTH DATA

Between 2000 and 2010, there were no changes in 69% of the measured health indicators in the US (CDC, 2010). By 2020, 15.4% of the targeted health indicators had been met, with improvements shown among 38.5% of the indicators and no changes or worse outcomes among 40 of the indicators (Office of Disease Prevention and Health Promotion [ODPHP], 2020). Considering the inadequate progress in achieving national health benchmarks, three major policy initiatives – reproductive justice policy, universal healthcare, and the development of workforce diversity – would redirect national health care resources in an equitable direction. Achievement of national health goals requires policy actions that are driven by population health data embedded within a social determinant and life course equity perspective that fosters improvement in the health of the nation, not just the health of a few. Universal health care and the availability of quality health care across all segments of the population are key determinants of good health and longevity. We posit that successful achievement of the national Healthy People objectives requires access to universal health insurance coverage not linked to employment benefits, establishment of adequately resourced community-based health care systems, an improved continuum of maternal and child health care services, and competent health and medical workforce that is representative of the diverse racial and ethnic communities in the US, and particularly of the most disadvantaged communities.

The beginning of the life course, birth, is an important marker for the opportunity to initiate a healthy life course. Reproductive justice is an approach to assure a healthy beginning to life. It entails the provision of free or affordable healthcare, adequate and accessible maternal and child health services, including antenatal and postnatal services, and paid family leave. An underlying value of reproductive justice is to center each woman in the birthing experience, making it a normal biological, social, and cultural event during which she is able to exercise her bodily rights, select the provider of care, experience the birth in a community-co-located center or at home with dignity and respect, and engage in guided and mutual decision-making about medical interventions (Edmonds, 2014). In a recent report, NASEM (2020) proposed specific action strategies to improve both the quality of care and to reduce maternal and child mortality and morbidity. The report proffered three recommendations aimed at enhancing reproductive justice: (1) prioritize training and hiring of diverse, ethnically competent, and well-qualified maternal and child health care providers, particularly for primary care settings; (2) foster informed decision making in choice of maternal and childbirth settings, providers, risk, and specific care practices; and (3) improve and increase the educational pipeline opportunities within a diverse maternity care workforce that includes, for example, midwives, doulas (birth coaches), community-health workers, and nurse practitioners.

Quality of care is not only a function of the qualifications of the provider but also is related to the provider's ability to communicate with patients, administer the most appropriate health and medical treatment for the patient's specific health condition(s), and provide appropriate referrals and timely follow-up (IOM, 2003). Quality of care is central in reproductive justice and aligns with a health care workforce that is representative of disadvantaged and underserved communities. Medical and public health care providers drawn from their communities are critical to improving the population health of our racial/ethnic underserved communities (NASEM, 2020). Beyond informing the direct provision of care to individuals and families, reproductive justice focuses on integrated care across the lifespan and promotes optimal health for all. There are long-standing challenges to attaining equitable representation of racial and ethnic minorities within the US health care provider workforce (Sullivan, 2004). Among health care professionals, relative to their respective proportion among the general US population, African Americans and Hispanics (Mexican Americans and Puerto Ricans in particular) are underrepresented, and White and Asian professionals are disproportionately overrepresented (Association of American Medical Colleges, 2019). In the 1970s, there was a period of growth in the number of Latino and African American physicians, attributed to wider availability of financial assistance, increased availability of medical school admissions, and the implementation of programs focused on minority physician recruitment (Mader et al., 2016; Olivares-Urueta, 2012; Simpson & Aronoff, 1988). However, underrepresentation has continued to persist (Health Resources & Services Administration [HRSA], 2018). Increased diversity in the health care workforce is necessary to reduce national health disparities and improve patient outcomes. To increase representation of historic racial/ethnic groups, leaders in medical education must endorse the need for a more representative workforce, promote the value of socially, ethnically and class knowledge and competence among its workforce to promote appropriate care and ensure the ongoing development and implementation of pathways for increased and continued representation (Vick et al., 2018).

Further understanding of the wide range of social determinants and their relationships with population health is central to reversing patterns of adverse health outcomes among low-income racial/ethnic groups. The inclusion of specific population demographic descriptors at the intersections of race, class, gender and sexuality can provide direction to improve research rigor to identify effective preventive measures that promote increased health and well-being (Bowleg, 2021; Weber et al., 2018; Weber & Parra-Medina, 2003). Persistent, ongoing application of deficit models, at either the individual or population levels, contributes to the decontextualization of health conditions without regard to social determinants, such as poverty, discimination, and level of available resource levels. Addressing the structural racism that exists at the juncture of discrimination and quality of care is key in addressing health disparities and adverse outcomes (Benjamins & Middleton, 2019).

The COVID-19 pandemic provides a clear example of the interdependence of social determinants of health – e.g., race, ethnicity, socioeconomic status, and place – and demonstrates the urgent need for health care restructuring that ensures universal access to quality care for all Americans. At the US policy level, it is imperative that the essential value of health be recognized, both in terms of the implementation of our shared democratic ideals and to strengthen the economic and social well-being of the entire population.

Employing a public health equity lens is central to insightful and solution-driven research, effective interventions, to promoting new collaborations across medical, public health and sociomedical disciplines, and in forging a new tradition of comprehensive, interdisciplinary health perspectives. New perspectives can move the population health field forward to reflect and validate community-based knowledge and to serve an active role in the formulation of primary health care community-based programs and demonstrate respect and dignity for those they intend to serve. To achieve health equity, social justice must be placed at the center of all policy and actions, to ensure equal access to opportunities to achieve the highest possible level of well-being according to their economic needs and circumstances.

Notes

1 In the late 1980 s, an interdisciplinary group of investigators at UCLA were awarded a grant to launch a study on prenatal, medical and psychosocial risk factors associated with birth outcomes among Mexican-American, Mexican immigrant and African-American women. These pioneering groups of

studies identified multiple social determinants (stress, social supports, financial concerns, among others) as contributors to birth outcomes. Although conducted three decades ago, the findings are still very pertinent to the field of social determinants, disparities and inequities today (Zambrana et al., 1991; Lobel et al., 1992; Zambrana et al., 1996; Zambrana et al., 1997; Zambrana et al., 1999).

2 In 2018, the rate of new HIV diagnoses per 100,000 was 15.7 in the South, followed by 10.0 in the Northeast, 9.3 in the West, and 7.2 in the Midwest. African Americans make up the majority of new diagnoses in the South (53%), Midwest (48%) and Northeast (41%), and Latinos account for 40% of new diagnoses in the West and 98% in US dependent territories (including Puerto Rico). From 2010 to 2014, 84% of the total relative percent increase of new cases in Latinos was concentrated in six states (New York, Florida, Illinois, Texas, Arizona, and California) and Puerto Rico (CDC, 2020b).

REFERENCES

Adepoju, O. E., Preston, M. A., & Gonzales, G. (2015). Health care disparities in the post-Affordable Care Act Era. *American journal of public health, 105 Suppl 5*(Suppl 5), S665–S667. https://doi.org/10.2105/AJPH.2015.302611

Amaro, H. (2014). *The action is upstream: Place-based approaches for acheieving population health and health equity*,104 (6), 964. https://doi.org/10.2105/AJPH.2014.302032

American Medical Association. (2021). *Organizational strategic plan to embed racial justice and advance health equity, 2021–2023*. https://www.ama-assn.org/system/files/2021-05/ama-equity-strategic-plan.pdf

Arcaya, M. C., Tucker-Seeley, R. D., Kim, R., Schnake-Mahl, A., So, M., & Subramanian, S. V. (2016). Research on neighborhood effects on health in the United States: A systematic review of study characteristics. *Social science & medicine (1982), 168*, 16–29. https://doi.org/10.1016/j.socscimed.2016.08.047

Association of American Medical Colleges (2019). *Percentage of US medical school faculty by race/ethnicity, 2018*. Retrieved June 29, 2021, from www.aamc.org/data-reports/workforce/interactive-data/figure-15-percentage-full-time-us-medical-school-faculty-race/ethnicity-2018

Attanasio, L., & Kozhimannil, K. B. (2017). Health care engagement and follow-up after perceived discrimination in maternity Care. *Medical care, 55*(9), 830–833. https://doi.org/10.1097/MLR.0000000000000773

Avgar, A. C., Eaton, A. E., Givan, R. K., & Litwin, A. S. (2020). Paying the price for a broken healthcare system: Rethinking employment, labor, and work in a post-pandemic world. *Work and occupations, 47*(3), 267–279. https://doi.org/10.1177/0730888420923126

Benda, N. C., Veinot, T. C., Sieck, C. J., & Ancker, J. S. (2020). Broadband internet access is a social determinant of health!. *American journal of public health, 110*(8), 1123–1125. https://doi.org/10.2105/AJPH.2020.305784

Benjamins, M. R., & Middleton, M. (2019). Perceived discrimination in medical settings and perceived quality of care: A population-based study in Chicago. *PloS one, 14*(4), e0215976. https://doi.org/10.1371/journal.pone.0215976

Berchick, E. R., Barnett, J. C., & Upton, R. D. (2019). Current population reports, P60-267 (RV), health insurance coverage in the United States: 2018. *US Census Bur, 267*, 19. https://www.census.gov/content/dam/Census/library/publications/2019/demo/p60-267.pdf

Black Women's Health Imperative (1983). Retrieved September 3, 2020, from https://bwhi.org/

Borrell, L. N., Rodriguez-Alvarez, E., Savitz, D. A., & Baquero, M. C. (2016). Parental race/ethnicity and adverse birth outcomes in New York City: 2000-2010. *American journal of public health, 106*(8), 1491–1497. https://doi.org/10.2105/AJPH.2016.303242

Bowleg, L. (2017). Towards a critical health equity research stance: Why epistemology and methodology matter more than qualitative methods. *Health education & behavior: the official publication of the Society for Public Health Education, 44*(5), 677–684. https://doi.org/10.1177/1090198117728760

Bowleg, L. (2021). Evolving intersectionality within public health: From analysis to action. *American journal of public health, 111*(1), 88–90. https://doi.org/10.2105/AJPH.2020.306031

Branigin, A. (2020). Black communities are on the "frontline" of the COVID-19 pandemic. Here's why. *The Root*. Retrieved August 24, 2020, from www.theroot.com/black-communities-are-on-the-frontline-of-the-covid-19-1842404824

Braveman, P., Arkin, E., Orleans, T., Proctor, D., Acker, J., & Plough, A. (2017). What is health equity? *Behavioral Science & Policy, 4*(1), 1–14. https://www.rwjf.org/en/library/research/2017/05/what-is-health-equity-.html

Braveman, P., & Barclay, C. (2009). Health disparities beginning in childhood: a life-course perspective. *Pediatrics, 124 Suppl 3*, S163–S175. https://doi.org/10.1542/peds.2009-1100D

Braveman, P., Egerter, S., Williams, D. R. (2011). The social determinants of health: coming of age. *Ann rev public health*. 32: 381– 398. https://doi.org/10.1146/annurev-publhealth-031210-101218

Butkus, R., Rapp, K., Cooney, T. G., Engel, L. S., & Health and Public Policy Committee of the American College of Physicians (2020). Envisioning a better U.S. health care system for all: Reducing barriers to care and addressing social determinants of health. *Annals of internal medicine, 172*(2 Suppl), S50–S59. https://doi.org/10.7326/M19-2410

Centers for Disease Control and Prevention. (1990). *Healthy people 2000*. Retrieved September 3, 2020, from www.cdc.gov/nchs/healthy_people/hp2000.htm

Centers for Disease Control and Prevention. (2010). *Healthy people 2010*. Retrieved September 3, 2020, from www.cdc.gov/nchs/data/hpdata2010/hp2010_final_review_overview.pdf

Centers for Disease Control and Prevention. (2018). *National vital statistics report, Births: Final Data for 2017*. Retrieved May 2, 2020, from www.cdc.gov/nchs/data/nvsr/nvsr67/nvsr67_08_tables-508.pdf

Centers for Disease Control and Prevention. (2019a). *Pregnancy mortality surveillance system*. Retrieved June 29, 2021, from https://cdc.gov/reproductivehealth/maternal-infanthealth/pregnancy-mortality-surveillance-system.html

Centers for Disease Control and Prevention. (2019b). *National vital statistics report, births: Final data for 2018*. Retrieved May 2, 2020, from www.cdc.gov/nchs/data/nvsr/nvsr68/nvsr68_13-508.pdf

Centers for Disease Control and Prevention. (2019c). *Health equity considerations and racial and ethnic minority groups*. Retrieved August 23, 2020, from https://www.cdc.gov/coronavirus/2019-ncov/community/health-equity/race-ethnicity.html?CDC_AA_refVal=https%3A%2F%2Fwww.cdc.gov%2Fcoronavirus%2F2019-ncov%2Fneed-extra-precautions%2Fracial-ethnic-minorities.html

Centers for Disease Control and Prevention. (2020a). *HIV public health partners*. Retrieved May 3, 2020, from www.cdc.gov/hiv/group/index.html

Centers for Disease Control and Prevention. (2020b). *HIV surveillance report, 2018 (Updated)*, vol. 31. Retrieved June 29, 2021, from www.cdc.gov/hiv/library/reports/hiv-surveillance.html

Centers for Disease Control and Prevention. (2020c). *Estimated incidence and prevalence in the United States, 2014–2018*. Retrieved June 29, 2021, from https://www.cdc.gov/hiv/library/reports/hiv surveillance.html [see Figure 3.1.].

Colen, C. G., Ramey, D. M., Cooksey, E. C., & Williams, D. R. (2018). Racial disparities in health among nonpoor African Americans and Hispanics: The role of acute and chronic discrimination. *Social science & medicine (1982), 199*, 167–180. https://doi.org/10.1016/j.socscimed.2017.04.051

Currier, J. S., & Havlir, D. V. (2017). CROI 2017: Complications and comorbidities of HIV disease and its treatment. *Topics in antiviral medicine, 25*(2), 77–83. https://pubmed.ncbi.nlm.nih.gov/28598792/

DeSisto, C. L., & McDonald, J. A. (2018). Variation in birth outcomes by mother's country of birth among Hispanic women in the United States, 2013. *Public health reports (Washington, D.C.: 1974), 133*(3), 318–328. https://doi.org/10.1177/0033354918765444

Diez Roux A. V. (2016). Neighborhoods and health: what do we know? What should we do?. *American journal of public health, 106*(3), 430–431. https://doi.org/10.2105/AJPH.2016.303064

Dill, B. T., & Zambrana, R. E. (2009). Critical thinking about inequality: An emerging lens.

In B. Dill & R. Zambrana (Ed.), *Emerging Intersections* (pp. 1–21). Ithaca, NY: Rutgers University Press. https://doi.org/10.36019/9780813546513-003

Du Bois, W. E. B. (1906). *The Health and Physique of the Negro American*. Atlanta, GA: Atlanta University Press.

Eastwood, E. A., Nace, A. J., Hirshfield, S., & Birnbaum, J. M. (2021). Young transgender women of color: homelessness, poverty, childhood sexual abuse and implications for HIV care. *AIDS and Behavior*, *25*(1), 96–106. https://doi.org/10.1007/s10461-019-02753-9

Economic Policy Institute. (2020). *Black workers face two of the most lethal preexisting conditions for coronavirus—racism and economic inequality [online]*. Retrieved August 25, 2020, from www.epi.org/publication/black-workers-covid/

Edmonds, B. T. (2014). Shared decision-making and decision support: their role in obstetrics and gynecology. *Current Opinion in Obstetrics and Gynecology*, *26*(6), 523–530. https://doi.org/10.1097/GCO.9781473939523120

Ford, T., Reber, S., & Reeves, R. (2020). Race gaps in COVID-19 are even bigger than they appear. *Brookings*. Retrieved May 3, 2020, from www.brookings.edu/blog/up-front/2020/06/16/race-gaps-in-covid-19-deaths-are-even-bigger-than-they-appear/

Gadson, A., Akpovi, E., & Mehta, P. K. (2017). Exploring the social determinants of racial/ethnic disparities in prenatal care utilization and maternal outcome. *Seminars in perinatology*, *41*(5), 308–317. https://doi.org/10.1053/j.semperi.2017.04.008

Galvan, F. H., Bluthenthal, R. N., Ani, C., & Bing, E. G. (2006). Increasing HIV testing among latinos by bundling HIV testing with other tests. *Journal of urban health: bulletin of the New York Academy of Medicine*, *83*(5), 849–859. https://doi.org/10.1007/s11524-006-9072-3

García, C., & Ailshire, J. A. (2019). Biological risk profiles among Latino subgroups in the health and retirement study. *Innovation in aging*, *3*(2), igz017. https://doi.org/10.1093/geroni/igz017

García, M., & Harris, A. L. (2017). PrEP awareness and decision-making for Latino MSM in San Antonio, Texas. *PloS one*, *12*(9), e0184014. https://doi.org/10.1371/journal.pone.0184014

Giedion, U., & Uribe, M. V. (2009). Colombia's universal health insurance system. *Health affairs (Project Hope)*, *28*(3), 853–863. https://doi.org/10.1377/hlthaff.28.3.853

Government of Canada. (2011). *Canada's health care system*. Retrieved June 29, 2021, from www.canada.ca/en/health-canada/services/health-care-system/reports-publications/health-care-system/canada.html

Healthy People 2030. (2021). *Healthy people 2030: Building a healthier future for all*. Retrieved July 19, 2021, from https://health.gov/healthypeople

Health Resources & Services Administration Health Workforce. (2018). *The U.S. Health Workforce Chartbook – In Brief*. Retrieved August 10, 2020, from https://bhw.hrsa.gov/sites/default/files/bhw/health-workforce-analysis/research/hrsa-us-health-workforce-chartbook-in-brief.pdf

Henry J. Kaiser Family Foundation. (2018). *Poverty Rate by Race/Ethnicity*. Retrieved August 20, 2020, from www.kff.org/other/state-indicator/poverty-rate-by-raceethnicity/

Howell, E. A. (2018). Reducing disparities in severe maternal morbidity and mortality. *Clinical obstetrics and gynecology*, *61*(2), 387–399. https://doi.org/10.1097/GRF.9781473939523349

Huang, Y. A., Zhu, W., Smith, D. K., Harris, N., & Hoover, K. W. (2018). HIV preexposure prophylaxis, by race and ethnicity - United States, 2014–2016. *MMWR. Morbidity and mortality weekly report*, *67*(41), 1147–1150. https://doi.org/10.15585/mmwr.mm6741a3

Hutchison, B., Levesque, J. F., Strumpf, E., & Coyle, N. (2011). Primary health care in Canada: systems in motion. *The Milbank quarterly*, *89*(2), 256–288. https://doi.org/10.1111/j.1468-0009.2011.00628.x

Institute of Medicine (US) Committee on HIV Screening and Access to Care. (2010). *HIV screening and access to care: Exploring barriers and facilitators to expanded HIV testing*. National Academies Press (US). https://doi.org/10.17226/12932

Institute of Medicine (US) Committee on Lesbian, Gay, Bisexual, and Transgender Health Issues and Research Gaps and Opportunities. (2011). *The health of lesbian, gay, bisexual, and transgender people: Building a foundation for better understanding*. National Academies Press (US). https://doi.org/10.17226/13128

Institute of Medicine (US) Committee on Understanding and Eliminating Racial and Ethnic Disparities in Health Care, Smedley, B. D., Stith, A. Y., & Nelson, A. R. (Eds.). (2003). *Unequal treatment: Confronting racial and ethnic disparities in health care*. National Academies Press (US). https://doi.org/10.17226/12875

Jones, C. P. (2018). Toward the science and practice of anti-racism: Launching a national campaign against racism. *Ethnicity & disease, 28*(Suppl 1), 231–234. https://doi.org/10.18865/ed.28.S1.231

Jones, K. M., Power, M. L., Queenan, J. T., & Schulkin, J. (2015). Racial and ethnic disparities in breastfeeding. *Breastfeeding medicine: the official journal of the Academy of Breastfeeding Medicine, 10*(4), 186–196. https://doi.org/10.1089/bfm.2014.0152

Kamal, R., Hudman, J., & McDermott, D. (2019). *What do we know about infant mortality in the U.S. and comparable countries?* Retrieved May 3, 2020, from www.healthsystemtracker.org/chart-collection/infant-mortality-u-s-compare-countries/#item-start

Khunti, K., Singh, A. K., Pareek, M., & Hanif, W. (2020). Is ethnicity linked to incidence or outcomes of covid-19?. *BMJ (Clinical research ed.), 369*, m1548. https://doi.org/10.1136/bmj.m1548

Kindig, D., & Stoddart, G. (2003). What is population health?. *American journal of public health, 93*(3), 380–383. https://doi.org/10.2105/ajph.93.3.380

Kochhar, R., & Cilluffo, A. (2017). *How U.S. wealth inequality has changed since great recession*. Washington, DC: Pew Research Center. Retrieved August 25, 2020, from www.pewresearch.org/fact-tank/2017/11/01/how-wealth-inequality-has-changed-in-the-u-s-since-the-great-recession-by-race-ethnicity-and-income/

Lamprea, E., & García, J. (2016). Closing the gap between formal and material health care coverage in Colombia. *Health and human rights, 18*(2), 49–65. https://www.ncbi.nlm.nih.gov/pmc/articles/PMC5394995/

Lasser, K. E., Himmelstein, D. U., & Woolhandler, S. (2006). Access to care, health status, and health disparities in the United States and Canada: results of a cross-national population-based survey. *American journal of public health, 96*(7), 1300–1307. https://doi.org/10.2105/AJPH.2004.059402

Lavizzo-Mourey, R. J., Besser, R. E., & Williams, D. R. (2021). Understanding and mitigating health inequities - past, current, and future directions. *The New England journal of medicine, 384*(18), 1681–1684. https://doi.org/10.1056/NEJMp2008628

Leonard, S. A., Main, E. K., Scott, K. A., Profit, J., & Carmichael, S. L. (2019). Racial and ethnic disparities in severe maternal morbidity prevalence and trends. *Annals of Epidemiology, 33*, 30–36. https://doi.org/10.1016/j.annepidem.2019.02.007

Lobel, M., Dunkel-Schetter, C., & Scrimshaw, S. C. (1992). Prenatal maternal stress and prematurity: a prospective study of socioeconomically disadvantaged women. *Health psychology: Official journal of the Division of Health Psychology, American Psychological Association, 11*(1), 32–40. https://doi.org/10.1037//0278-6133.11.1.32

Lubold, A. M. (2019). Historical-qualitative analysis of breastfeeding trends in three OECD countries. *International breastfeeding journal, 14*, 36. https://doi.org/10.1186/s13006-019-0230-0

Lyerly, A. (2013). *A good birth: Finding the positive and profound in your childbirth experience*. New York: Penguin Random House.

Ma, A., Sanchez, A., & Ma, M. (2019). The impact of patient-provider race/ethnicity concordance on provider visits: Updated evidence from the medical expenditure panel survey. *Journal of racial and ethnic health disparities*, 6(5), 1011–1020. https://doi.org/10.1007/s40615-019-00602-y

Mader, E. M., Rodríguez, J. E., Campbell, K. M., Smilnak, T., Bazemore, A. W., Petterson, S., & Morley, C. P. (2016). *Status of underrepresented minority and female faculty at medical schools located within Historically Black Colleges and in Puerto Rico*. Medical education online, 21, 29535. https://doi.org/10.3402/meo.v21.29535

Manuel, T., & Zambrana, R. E. (2009). Exploring the intersections of race, ethnicity and class on maternity leave decisions: implications for public policy. In B. T. Dill & R. E. Zambrana (Eds.), *Emerging Intersections: Race, Class, and Gender in Theory, Policy and Practice* (pp. 123–149). New Brunswick, NJ: Rutgers University Press.

Marmot, M. G. (2006). Status syndrome: a challenge to medicine. *JAMA, 295*(11), 1304–1307. https://doi.org/10.1001/jama.295.11.1304

Marmot, M. G. (2018). *Addressing social determinants of health in primary care*. American Academy of Family Physicians. Retrieved June 29, 2021, from https://www.ctc-ri.org/sites/default/files/uploads/Addressing%20SDOH%20in%20PC.pdf

Martin, D., Miller, A. P., Quesnel-Vallée, A., Caron, N. R., Vissandjée, B., & Marchildon, G. P. (2018). Canada's universal health-care system: achieving its potential. *Lancet (London, England), 391*(10131), 1718–1735. https://doi.org/10.1016/S0140-6736(18)30181-8

Miller, C. C., Kliff, S., & Sanger-Katz, M. (2020). Avoiding coronavirus may be a luxury some workers can't afford. *The New York Times*, March 1. Retrieved August 23, 2020, from www.nytimes.com/2020/03/01/upshot/coronavirus-sick-days-service-workers.html

Miller, G., Pinto, D. M., & Vera-Hernández, M. (2009). *High-powered incentives in developing country health insurance: Evidence from Colombia's regimen subsidiado*. Cambridge: National Bureau of Economic Research. https://doi.org/10.3386/w15456

Mirkovic, K. R., Perrine, C. G., Scanlon, K. S., & Grummer-Strawn, L. M. (2014). Maternity leave duration and full-time/part-time work status are associated with US mothers' ability to meet breastfeeding intentions. *Journal of human lactation: official journal of International Lactation Consultant Association, 30*(4), 416–419. https://doi.org/10.1177/0890334414543522

Mujica, C., Alvarez, K., Tendulkar, S., Cruz-Gonzalez, M., & Alegría, M. (2020). Association between patient-provider racial and ethnic concordance and patient-centered communication in outpatient mental health clinics. *Journal of Psychotherapy Integration, 30*(3), 423–439. http://dx.doi.org/10.1037/int0000195

Nagata, J. M., Gomberg, S., Hagan, M. J., Heyman, M. B., & Wojcicki, J. M. (2019). Food insecurity is associated with maternal depression and child pervasive developmental symptoms in low-income Latino households. *Journal of hunger & environmental nutrition, 14*(4), 526–539. https://doi.org/10.1080/19320248.2018.1434101

National Academies of Sciences, Engineering, and Medicine, Health and Medicine Division, Board on Population Health and Public Health Practice, Committee on Community-Based Solutions to Promote Health Equity in the United States, Baciu, A., Negussie, Y., Geller, A., & Weinstein, J. N. (Eds.). (2017). *Communities in action: pathways to health equity*. National Academies Press (US). https://doi.org/10.17226/24624

National Academies of Sciences, Engineering, and Medicine; Health and Medicine Division; Division of Behavioral and Social Sciences and Education; Board on Children, Youth, and Families; Committee on Assessing Health Outcomes by Birth Settings, Backes, E. P., & Scrimshaw, S. C. (Eds.). (2020). *Birth settings in America: Outcomes, quality, access, and choice*. National Academies Press (US). https://doi.org/10.17226/25636

Nielsen, J. D., Wall, W., & Tucker, C. M. (2016). Testing of a model with Latino patients that explains the links among patient-perceived provider cultural sensitivity, language preference, and patient treatment adherence. *Journal of racial and ethnic health disparities, 3*(1), 63–73. https://doi.org/10.1007/s40615-015-0114-y

Office of Disease Prevention and Health Promotion (ODPHP) (2020). *Healthy People 2020*. Retrieved June 29, 2021, from https://www.healthypeople.gov/2020/Leading-Health-Indicators

Office of Disease Prevention and Health Promotion (2021). *Healthy People 2030*. Retrieved June 29, 2021, from https://www.healthypeople.gov/2020/About-Healthy-People/Development-Healthy-People-2030

Olivares-Urueta, M. (2012). The Latino/a health professions pipeline: An overview. *Hispanic Association of Colleges and Universities*. Retrieved June 29, 2021, from https://eric.ed.gov/?id=ED537729

O'Malley, A. S., Sheppard, V. B., Schwartz, M., & Mandelblatt, J. (2004). The role of trust in use of preventative screening services among low income African American women. *Preventive Medicine*, *38*, 777–785. https://doi.org/10.1016/j.ypmed.2004.01.018

O'Malley, T. L., Hawk, M. E., Egan, J. E., Krier, S. E., & Burke, J. G. (2019). Intimate partner violence and pre-exposure prophylaxis (PrEP): a rapid review of current evidence for women's HIV prevention. *AIDS and Behavior*, *24*(5), 1342–1357. https://doi.org/10.1016/j.ypmed.2004.01.018

Oppel Jr., R. A., Gebeloff, R., Rebecca Lai, K. K., Wright, W., & Smith, M. (2020). The fullest look yet at the racial inequity of coronavirus. *New York Times*, July 5. www.nytimes.com/interactive/2020/07/05/us/coronavirus-latinos-african-americans-cdc-data.html

Pan American Health Organization. (2017). *Social determinants of health in the region of the Americas [internet]*. https://www.paho.org/salud-en-las-americas-2017/uh-determinants.html

Parra-Medina, D., & Fore, E. (2004). *Behavioral studies*. In B. Beech & M. Goodman (Eds.), *Race and research: Perspectives on minority participation in health studies* (pp. 101–112) Washington, DC: American Public Health Association.

Pastor, M., & Morello-Frosch, R. (2014). Integrating public health and community development to tackle neighborhood distress and promote well-being. *Health affairs (Project Hope)*, *33*(11), 1890–1896. https://doi.org/10.1377/hlthaff.2014.0640

Pew Research Center. (2020). *Hispanic women, immigrants, young adults, those with less education hit hardest by COVID-19 job losses*. Retrieved August 2, 2020, from www.pewresearch.org/fact-tank/2020/06/09/hispanic-women-immigrants-young-adults-those-with-less-education-hit-,hardest-by-covid-19-job-losses/

Phillips, G., McCuskey, D., Ruprecht, M.M. Curry, C. W., & Felt, D. (2021) Structural interventions for HIV prevention and care among US men who have sex with men: A Systematic Review of Evidence, Gaps, and Future Priorities. *AIDS Behavior*. https://doi.org/10.1007/s10461-021-03167-2

Profit, J., Gould, J. B., Bennett, M., Goldstein, B. A., Draper, D., Phibbs, C. S., & Lee, H. C. (2017). Racial/ethnic disparity in NICU quality of care delivery. *Pediatrics*, *140*(3), e20170918. https://doi.org/10.1542/peds.2017-0918

Pylypchuk, Y., & Sarpong, E. M. (2013). Comparison of health care utilization: United States versus Canada. *Health services research*, *48*(2 Pt 1), 560–581. https://doi.org/10.1111/j.1475-6773.2012.01466.x

Robert, S. A., & House, J. S. (2000). Socioeconomic inequalities in health: Integrating individual-, community-, and societal-level theory and research. In G. L. Albrecht, R. Fitzpatrick, & S. C. Scrimshaw (Eds.), *The handbook of social studies in health and medicine* (pp. 115–135). Sage Publications Ltd. https://doi.org/10.4135/9781848608412.n9

Robinson, K., Fial, A., & Hanson, L. (2019). Racism, Bias, and Discrimination as Modifiable Barriers to Breastfeeding for African American Women: A Scoping Review of the Literature. *Journal of midwifery & women's health*, *64*(6), 734–742. https://doi.org/10.1111/jmwh.13058

Rollins, N. C., Bhandari, N., Hajeebhoy, N., Horton, S., Lutter, C. K., Martines, J. C., Piwoz, E. G., Richter, L. M., Victora, C. G., & Lancet Breastfeeding Series Group (2016). Why invest, and what it will take to improve breastfeeding practices? *Lancet (London, England)*, *387*(10017), 491–504. https://doi.org/10.1016/S0140-6736(15)01044-2

Ross, L., Gutiérrez, E., Gerber, M., & Silliman, J. (2016). *Undivided Rights: Women of Color Organizing for Reproductive Justice*. Chicago, IL: Haymarket Books.

Rostila, M. (2013). *Social capital and health inequality in European welfare states*. UK: Palgrave Macmillan.

Saenz, R. (2020). *COVID-19's surging impact on Latinos, a glimpse in August 2020*. Latino Decisions blog. Retrieved August 25, 2020, from https://latinodecisions.com/blog/covid-19s-surging-impact-on-latinos-a-glimpse-in-august-2020/

Saenz, R., & Sparks, C. (2020). *The inequities of job loss and recovery amid the COVID-19 Pandemic*. Retrieved August 25, 2020, from https://carsey.unh.edu/publication/inequities-job-loss-recovery-amid-COVID-pandemic

Schneider, D., & Harknett, K. (2020). *Essential and vulnerable: Service-sector workers and paid sick leave*. Berkeley, CA: The Shift Project. Retrieved August 25, 2020, from https://shift.hks.harvard.edu/files/2020/04/Essential_and_Vulnerable_Service_Sector_Workers_and_Paid_Sick_Leave.pdf

Schneider, E. C., Sarnak, D. O., Squires, D., & Shah, A. (2017). *Mirror, mirror 2017: International comparison reflects flaws and opportunities for better US health care*. The Commonwealth Fund. Retrieved September 3, 2020, from www.commonwealthfund.org/publications/journal-article/2017/jul/last-first-could-us-health-care-system-become-best-world?redirect_source=/publications/in-brief/2017/jul/last-to-first-could-us-health-system-become-best-in-world

Sharkey, P. (2013). *Stuck in place: Urban neighborhoods and the end of progress toward racial equality*. Chicago, IL: University of Chicago Press.

Sheppard, V. B., Zambrana, R. E., & O'Malley, A. S. (2004). Providing health care to low-income women: a matter of trust. *Family practice*, *21*(5), 484–491. https://doi.org/10.1093/fampra/cmh503

Simpson, C. E., Jr, & Aronoff, R. (1988). Factors affecting the supply of minority physicians in 2000. *Public health reports (Washington, D.C.: 1974)*, *103*(2), 178–184. https://www.ncbi.nlm.nih.gov/pmc/articles/PMC1477967/

Sister Song Women of Color Reproductive Justice Collective. (n.d.). *Reproductive Justice*. Retrieved May 2, 2020, from https://www.sistersong.net/reproductive-justice

Sriraman, N. K., & Kellams, A. (2016). Breastfeeding: What are the barriers? Why women struggle to achieve their goals. *Journal of women's health (2002)*, *25*(7), 714–722. https://doi.org/10.1089/jwh.2014.5059

Stephansson, O., Petersson, K., Björk, C., Conner, P., & Wikström, A. K. (2018). The Swedish pregnancy register - for quality of care improvement and research. *Acta obstetricia et gynecologica Scandinavica*, *97*(4), 466–476. https://doi.org/10.1111/aogs.13266

Sullivan, L. W. (2004). *Missing persons: Minorities in the health professions*. A Report of the Sullivan Commission on Diversity in the healthcare workforce. The Sullivan Commission. https://www.amsa.org/wp-content/uploads/2016/07/Sullivan_Commission.pdf

Taylor, J. (2019). *Racism, inequality, and health care for African Americans*. The Century Foundation. Retrieved August 24, 2020, from https://tcf.org/content/report/racism-inequality-health-care-african-americans/?agreed=1

Urban Institute. (2020). *Structural Racism in America*. Retrieved June 29, 2021, from www.urban.org/features/structural-racism-america

US Bureau of Labor Statistics. (2019). *Labor force characteristics by race and ethnicity, 2018*. Retrieved August 25, 2020, from www.bls.gov/opub/reports/race-and-ethnicity/2018/

US Department of Health and Human Services. (2019). *Infant mortality and Hispanic Americans*. Retrieved September 3, 2020, from https://minorityhealth.hhs.gov/omh/browse.aspx?lvl=4&lvlid=68

US Department of Labor. (2020). *Family and Leave Medical Leave (FMLA)*. Washington, DC: US Department of Labor. Available at: www.dol.gov/general/topic/benefits-leave/fmla. Missing date of retrieval.

Vick, A. D., Baugh, A., Lambert, J., Vanderbilt, A. A., Ingram, E., Garcia, R., & Baugh, R. F. (2018). Levers of change: a review of contemporary interventions to enhance diversity in medical schools in the USA. *Advances in medical education and practice*, *9*, 53–61. https://doi.org/10.2147/AMEP.S147950

Weber, L., & Parra-Medina, D. (2003). Intersectionality and women's health: charting a path to eliminating health disparities. *Advances in Gender Research*, *7*(3), 181–230. https://doi.org/10.1016/S1529-2126(03)07006-1

Weber, L., Zambrana, R. E., Fore, M. E., & Parra-Medina, D. (2018). Racial and ethnic health inequities: An intersectional approach. In: Batur P., Feagin J. (Eds.), *Handbook of the Sociology of Racial and Ethnic Relations*. Handbooks of Sociology and Social Research. Springer, Cham. https://doi.org/10.1007/978-3-319-76757-4_8

White, K. (2011). The sustaining relevance of W. E. B. Du Bois to health disparities research. *Du Bois Review: Social science research in race* *8*(1), 285–293. https://doi.org/10.1017/S1742058X11000233

White, K., & Borrell, L. N. (2006). Racial/ethnic neighborhood concentration and self-reported health in New York City. *Ethnicity & disease*, *16*(4), 900–908.

Williams, D. R., Lawrence, J. A., & Davis, B. A. (2019). Racism and Health: Evidence and Needed Research. *Annual review of public health*, *40*, 105–125. https://doi.org/10.1146/annurev-publhealth-040218-043750

World Health Organization. (n.d.). *Health Equity*. Retrieved September 17, 2020, from www.who.int/topics/health_equity/en/

World Health Organization & Alliance for Health Policy and Systems Research. (2017). *Primary health care systems (primasys): case study from Colombia: abridged version. Liscense: CC BY-NC-SA 3.0 IGO.* https://apps.who.int/iris/handle/10665/341065

Yancy, C. W. (2020). COVID-19 and African Americans. *JAMA*, *323*(19), 1891–1892. https://doi.org/10.1001/jama.2020.6548

Zambrana, R. E., & Dill, B. T. (2006). Disparities in Latina health: an intersectional analysis. In A. Schultz & L. Mullings (Eds.), *Gender, race, class, & health: Intersectional approaches* (pp. 192–227). San Francisco, CA: Jossey-Bass.

Zambrana, R. E., Dunkel-Schetter, C., Collins, N. L., & Scrimshaw, S. C. (1999). Mediators of ethnic-associated differences in infant birth weight. *Journal of urban health: bulletin of the New York Academy of Medicine*, *76*(1), 102–116. https://doi.org/10.1007/BF02344465

Zambrana, R. E., Dunkel-Schetter, C., & Scrimshaw, S. (1991). Factors which influence use of prenatal care in low-income racial-ethnic women in Los Angeles County. *Journal of community health*, *16*(5), 283–295. https://doi.org/10.1007/BF01320336

Zambrana, R. E., Mogel, W., & Scrimshaw, S. C. (1987). Gender and level of training differences in obstetricians' attitudes towards patients in childbirth. *Women & health*, *12*(1), 5–24. https://doi.org/10.1300/J013v12n01_02

Zambrana, R. E., Scrimshaw, S. C., Collins, N., & Dunkel-Schetter, C. (1997). Prenatal health behaviors and psychosocial risk factors in pregnant women of Mexican origin: the role of acculturation. *American journal of public health*, *87*(6), 1022–1026. https://doi.org/10.2105/ajph.87.6.1022

Zambrana, R. E., Scrimshaw, S. C., & Dunkel-Schetter, C. (1996). Prenatal care and medical risk in low-income primiparous, Mexican-origin and African-American women. *Families, Systems and Health*, *14*(3), 349–359. https://psycnet.apa.org/doi/10.1037/h0089920

Zingmond, D. S., Arfer, K. B., Gildner, J. L., & Leibowitz, A. A. (2017). The cost of comorbidities in treatment for HIV/AIDS in California. *PloS one*, *12*(12), e0189392. https://doi.org/10.1371/journal.pone.0189392

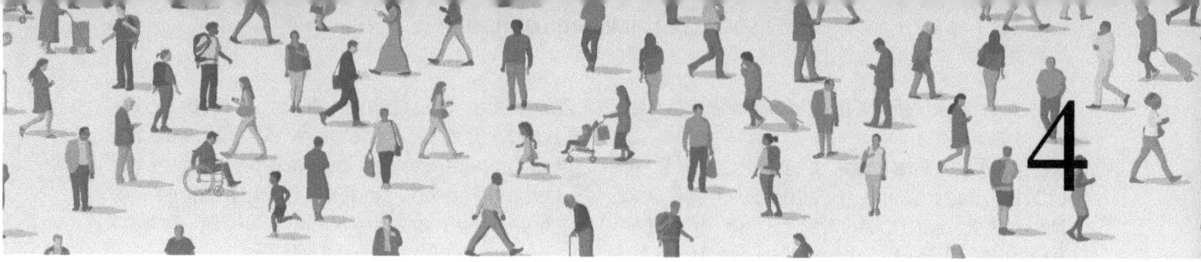

4

The Social Causation of Health and Illness

Johannes Siegrist

Box 4.1 Key Points

- The knowledge base on social causation of health and illness has been rapidly growing in the recent past, specifically by collaborative research between sociologists and epidemiologists.
- A large part of this knowledge was – and continues to be – devoted to the identification and explanation of social inequalities in health within and between societies.
- In a life course perspective, the period from early childhood to adolescence was shown to exert long-term effects on health, as analyzed by the three conceptual approaches of "critical period", "pathways", and "cumulative advantage/disadvantage".
- In addition, core social roles in midlife related to affiliation and productive activities are associated with differential health outcomes, depending on their material and psychosocial quality.
- A stress-theoretical framework proved to be useful in bridging social adversity in these roles with disease, applying sociological notions such as "social network", "social support", "control/autonomy", and "reward/recognition".
- Although additional research on the social determinants of health and disease is required, a body of available robust knowledge calls for implementation into models of good practice that aim at improving the health and well-being of populations.

INTRODUCTION

Sociology as a science is concerned with the description and explanation of societal phenomena and processes as they affect human populations and individuals. To a large extent, scientific progress in this field depends on input from specialized sub-disciplines that deal with particular areas of societal life in a systematic way. Health and illness, and the societal reactions towards them define the scope of one such sub-discipline, termed sociology of health or medical sociology (Cockerham 2010; Collier 2015; Mechanic 1978). The study of social factors that determine health and contribute to the development of ill health and disease defines an important area of research within this sub-discipline. A brief outline of its main historical achievements and its contribution to current debates on global challenges illustrates this importance (see below). However, as health and disease are also determined by factors that are not of a social nature, such as biological, psychological, or environmental conditions, research on social causation of health is an interdisciplinary task calling for integration of information from different scientific disciplines. Here, biomedical information is of primary importance, in particular as far as it results from studies of the distribution of health and disease across populations. This latter knowledge is produced by a distinct field of inquiry, epidemiology, and as far as the social distribution of health and disease across populations is the subject of this inquiry, the scientific contributions of social epidemiology (Berkman et al. 2014) and health-related or medical sociology are intrinsically intertwined. In this chapter, an attempt is made to demonstrate the strengths of combining sociological and epidemiological information in research on the social determinants of health and disease. Before reviewing major, yet selective evidence in a life course perspective, I address the rather basic question of what we understand by 'social causation'. Dealing with this question seems mandatory in view of the fact that different notions of causality are apparent from sociological studies of health and illness.

SOCIAL CAUSATION OF HEALTH: DIFFERENT NOTIONS

Sociology is a scientific discipline that is mainly based on observational studies, as the application of experimental research is limited, not least for ethical reasons. Whereas experimental study designs provide a convincing approach towards analyzing causal associations, observational studies use approximate methodological ways of demonstrating causal interference. Several basic requirements need to be met before causal inferences can be made. *First*, it is mandatory to distinguish between predicting and outcome variables, and to define these variables in an unambiguous way. In health-related sociology, there is no consensus on this latter criterion. For instance, the outcome variable 'health' has been defined in different ways, either in terms of absence of illness, absence of disease, or absence of sickness. Different from the normative notion of 'health' defined by the World Health Organization, these three terms reflect three different perspectives of the phenomenon: 'Illness' relates to the personal experience of states of unease, pain, or functional limitation reported by individual persons. 'Disease' is the professionally defined category of an abnormal state of physical or mental functioning, classified according to internationally established criteria of diagnoses. 'Sickness' denominates the burden of ill health for society, e.g., in terms of economic costs due to productivity losses.

Since 'disease' and 'illness' are defined on the basis of individual data, it is important to point to different notions of their social causation among medical sociologists. For instance, labelling theorists claimed that distinct mental disorders diagnosed by psychiatrists are in fact consequences of definitions of deviant behavior applied by significant others and legitimized thereafter by physicians as a means of social control (Scheff 1999). Social causation, in this perspective, means that the disorder is socially produced. A less radical position is found in social constructionism, where illness, the expression of symptoms, is shaped by powerful cultural and moral values, thus transforming bodily experience into socially approved behavior (Lorber 1997). Here, it seems difficult to apply the notion of social causation. Even if the outcome variable is defined in terms of diagnosed diseases, the notion of social causation can have different meanings. In their classical study on social class and mental illness, Hollingshead and Redlich (1958) observed a significant association between the prevalence and severity of certain types of treated mental disorders and social class membership, as defined by an index of relevant socioeconomic characteristics. An obvious interpretation of this association points to socially differentiated attribution of diagnoses by physicians. At a more subtle level, recent studies revealed that medical decision making is in part influenced by distinct patient characteristics, such as age, gender, or ethnic and sociocultural background (Lutfey et al. 2009). Clearly, if one intends to draw causal inference from some social characteristic to the occurrence of a disease, the two variables need to be defined in an unambiguous way at individual data level. This also holds true if the predicting variable is composed by aggregate- and individual-level data.

A *second* prerequisite of research on social causation concerns the temporal order where the predicting condition precedes the outcome event. To this end, prospective epidemiologic cohort studies define the gold standard of inquiry. Here, at baseline, where the exposure is assessed, the study population has to be free from the health outcome of interest. In this way, reverse causation can be excluded. For instance, it is widely assumed that the relationship between low income and ill health is explained by the fact that unhealthy people earn less money. Yet, if low income among initially healthy people increases the risk of developing ill health over time, this belief is considerably weakened (Cutler et al. 2008). For a long time, social epidemiologic cohort studies were restricted to one baseline assessment of the exposure and the analysis of relative risks of prospective health outcomes as a function of exposure level. More recently, changes of exposure over time were studied in addition to strengthen the evidence. To this end, different statistical approaches of analyzing within-person changes are available (Glymour and Kubzansky 2018).

Control of confounding is a *third* important prerequisite of causal inference in socio-medical research. If there is reason to interpret a statistical association within a prospective study design in terms of causality, there is still the problem that the association may be due to some underlying third variable. Therefore, the influence of relevant confounding factors in these associations needs to be controlled, e.g., by adjustment in multivariable regression analysis. Still, to strengthen evidence of a causal association supporting data explaining the pathways leading from exposure to disease are needed as a *fourth* requirement. For instance, if social isolation is prospectively related to an increased risk of cardiovascular disease, it is important to know if this association is due to an increase in unhealthy behaviors (e.g., smoking, lack of physical activity), or due to depressed mood and related stress-physiological responses (e.g., altered cortisol secretion or inflammatory activity) (Holt-Lunstad et al. 2015). Introducing and testing mediating constructs in research on social causation of health is a major challenge where the need of interdisciplinary collaboration is particularly evident.

In summary, the search for causation in observational research proves to be a demanding task. As obvious from the next sections of this chapter, many studies on social determinants of health still suffer from the fact that they do not meet all criteria required for demonstrating causal inference. Even worse, additional causality criteria were identified (Hill 1965), and new, rarely applied statistical tools are available to advance causal analysis, such as instrumental variables analysis, marginal structural models, as well as a systematic use of directed acyclic graphs (Glymour and Kubzansky 2018). Despite these limitations, we witness a substantial increase of knowledge on social determinants of health during the last two or three decades, where distinct theoretical models derived from sociology have enriched our understanding of how the social world affects human health and disease.

HISTORICAL DEVELOPMENTS AND GLOBAL CHALLENGES

Interestingly, the scientific study of social causes of health and illness originated from one of the most profound revolutions in the history of humankind, the double revolution of industrialization and democratic developments in the late 18th and early 19th centuries, especially in the United Kingdom, France, and somewhat later, Germany and the United States (Rosen 1979). Official statistics were established collecting administrative data on epidemics and their geographical and socioeconomic distribution; occupational medicine provided evidence on the pathogenic role of specific working conditions. For the first time, mental illness was studied in a socio-environmental perspective, and most researchers were directly involved in the health policy implications of their findings. Yet the scientific quality of this research was rather modest, as it was restricted to descriptive and correlational information, and as the underlying pathogenic models (e.g., the miasma theory of infectious diseases) were misconceived, as demonstrated by scientific breakthroughs in cellular pathology, virology, and related disciplines (Loomis and Wing 1990).

While the scientific discipline of sociology also originated from the industrial revolution, the two activities converged only a couple of decades later. In 1897, French sociologist Emile Durkheim published his landmark study on suicide (Durkheim 1951). This was the first investigation to test a set of sociological propositions dealing with an important cause of death that was unequally distributed across the French society. According to Durkheim, the risk of suicide was elevated among social groups characterized by a weakening or loss of social norms and values guiding interpersonal life. In consequence, egoistic or anomic tendencies precipitated socioemotional crises, distress and, ultimately, despair. Thus, suicide was interpreted as a socially caused event, not as an action based on individual motivation. It is important to mention that, in methodologic terms, Durkheim described suicidal episodes as *social facts* that were generated at a societal rather than at an individual level. Therefore, he studied the social patterning of health and disease using aggregate data as a distinct source of information.

Both seminal insights provided by Durkheim, the critical role of social anomie in explaining suicide, and the methodologic emphasis on social facts as a distinct category of analysis, were developed further by American sociologists during the first decades of the 20th century. For instance, Faris and Dunham (1939) demonstrated the use of ecological analysis in studies dealing with adverse effects of urban development, including mental illness. Hollingshead and Redlich (1958), as mentioned, reported a strong association between low social class membership and prevalence of certain types of mental illnesses. Perhaps even more important in theoretical terms, the concept of social anomia was elaborated in two landmark studies of mental illness, the Midtown Manhattan and the Stirling County Studies (Leighton et al. 1963; Srole et al. 1962). Srole et al. analyzed social anomia – a person's sense of normlessness, powerlessness, and helplessness – as result of Midtown's 'partial breakdown in the person-to-person private lines of communication' (Srole et al. 1962: 119). Its adverse effects on mental health became evident in the presence of critical life events and lack of group support that were more prevalent in lower socioeconomic groups (these core notions, not necessarily the appropriate terms, were already present in this interesting study!). Carrying further these ideas, Langner and Michael (1963) demonstrated the cumulative effects of deprived childhood and of stressful working and living conditions in adulthood on mental illness, thus pioneering, in an area that is currently of growing interest, the life course perspective of social epidemiology. In a similar approach, Leighton et al. (1963) advanced the idea of a pathogenic role of sociocultural disintegration in explaining the prevalence of psychiatric disturbance.

Whereas these studies still owed a lot to the Durkheimian paradigm of illness as a social rather than an individual fact, they increasingly referred to a concurrent sociological approach, the paradigm of '*social action*' developed most convincingly by Max Weber (Weber 1978). Social action theory claims that the ultimate unit of sociological analysis – the pattern of social interaction among persons – combines socio-structural (e.g., economic, historical) and individual (motivations, cognitions, emotions) information. In particular, different types of mismatch may arise between a society's structure of opportunities or constraints, and the socially patterned individual aspirations and needs (Merton 1938). In this sociological perspective, conflicts and pressures resulting from this mismatch were considered major causes of impaired health and well-being. Concepts such as social integration/disintegration, social support, social anomia, or social stress implicitly or explicitly refer to this paradigm.

During the early 1960s a number of socio-epidemiologic studies were undertaken with cardiovascular risk factors and coronary heart disease morbidity or mortality as outcome criteria. The two most important consequences of this shift from mental to physical disease were (1) the advancement of *stress-theoretical approaches* integrating sociological and biological information, and (2) the development of a *cross-cultural, comparative research* tradition within social epidemiology and medical sociology. This latter tradition provided us with a number of seminal insights into pathogenic effects on the cardiovascular system produced by rapid sociocultural change (Henry 1997; Henry and Cassel 1969; Scotch 1968; Tyroler and Cassel 1964), lack of stable sociocultural assets (Bruhn et al. 1966; Marmot and Syme 1976; Syme et al. 1964), poor social network and support (Berkman and Syme 1979), social status incongruence (Shekelle et al. 1969), and job loss (Kasl and Cobb 1970). Although at this stage of development the field suffered, to some extent, from conceptual inconsistency, the two decades ranging from the late 1950s to the late 1970s are now considered the founding period of a sociologically-driven epidemiology of chronic diseases. In 1977, Henry and Stephens published their book on *Stress, Health, and the Social Environment*. With this publication, for the first time, the crude links that existed between sociological constructs and disease endpoints were substantiated by physiological and pathophysiological evidence derived from social stress research in animals. Meanwhile, a growing number of investigations were performed that used biological markers of cardiovascular, hormonal and immune responses to stressful conditions to disentangle the processes mediating social exposures with the onset of bodily disease (Weiner 1992). This type of transdisciplinary research, conducted in a biopsychosocial perspective, has shaped major current developments of socio-medical research on social causation (see below).

The topic that attracted probably the highest attention of medical sociologists and social epidemiologists during the past few decades relates to the *socioeconomic inequalities in morbidity and mortality* of populations in modern societies. The traditional view maintained that excess morbidity and mortality were confined to socially deprived groups at the bottom of a society's hierarchy, whereas the large majority enjoyed fair or good health due to access to advanced health care, growing welfare, and health-promoting behaviors. However, starting with descriptive evidence from the United States in the late 1960s and early 1970s, robust evidence demonstrated so-called *social gradients* of morbidity and mortality: with each step one moves up on the social ladder, the better one's health. Thus, health inequalities are manifest across the whole of a society (Antonovsky 1967; Hinkle et al. 1968; Kitagawa and Hauser 1973). In the United Kingdom, Marmot et al. (1978) demonstrated a social gradient of morbidity and mortality due to cardiovascular disease and some other conditions of chronic disease according to occupational standing in the now famous Whitehall studies (Marmot et al. 1991). In Great Britain, this knowledge reached the broader public and the political scene with the publication of the *Black Report* on social inequalities in health (Department of Health and Social Security 1980). Numerous investigations on this topic emerged in other European countries, and several governments moved up this topic on their political agenda. While important scientific developments will be described below, the following paragraphs discuss the policy implications of research on social determinants of health in the frame of global challenges.

Global Challenges

As the disciplines of health-related sociology and social epidemiology were developed in the Global North, the problems they initially tackled were almost exclusively related to these societies. However, with the rise of *Low- and Middle-income countries*, with the expansion of economic globalization and world-wide spread of modern technologies, with growing transnational migration and urbanization, the study of social determinants of health was faced with new challenges. For instance, absolute poverty, starvation, and excessive levels of child mortality for a long time disappeared from the agenda of modern societies, but appeared as pressing problems in low-income countries. Here, the material dimension of social inequalities receives highest attention as substantial parts of urban populations still live in the disadvantaged conditions of slums, with lack of access to improved water supply, sanitation and health care, being exposed to poor nutrition, high morbidity and mortality (Baum 2018; World Health Organization 2008). For instance, in 2012, life expectancy at birth was 60 years among men in low-income countries, compared to 76 years in high-income countries, and among women, a respective difference of 19 years was even larger (Baum 2018: 256). These facts highlight the top of a huge number of serious threats to human health and well-being that are mainly due to socioeconomic deprivation in less developed countries. As an important response to these threats the *World Health Organization* set up a Commission on social determinants of health, under the lead of social epidemiologists, health sociologists and economists, to review scientific evidence on health inequalities in a global perspective, and to propose policy recommendations towards reducing these inequalities (WHO 2008). The report of the Commission concluded that "the poor health of the poor, the social gradient in health within countries, and the marked health inequities between countries are caused by the unequal distribution of power, income, goods, and services, … the consequent unfairness in the immediate, visible circumstances of people's lives … and their chances of leading a flourishing life" (WHO 2008: 1). Therefore, a detailed set of recommendations was elaborated, identifying actions on the social determinants of health at the level of international agencies, national governments, business, civil society, and local communities.

This is probably the first time that a core scientific matter of health-related sociology, the scientific evidence on social determinants of health, became the topic of an action plan at global level. Interestingly, a few years later, a second, similar report was initiated by the WHO's Regional Office for Europe (WHO 2014). This report focused on the large disparities of morbidity and mortality of populations in countries of Eastern vs. Western Europe. Again, this document consisted of a summary of robust scientific findings and the proposition of a set of specific *policy recommendations* derived from this knowledge, supplemented by case studies on models of good practice. Even at the national level, several governments set up commissions to produce national reports on social inequalities in health that could advise policy. So far, the British report *Fair Societies, Healthy Lives* is considered the most detailed and most influential one of these initiatives (Marmot 2010).

Taken together, these recent developments illustrate a growing awareness among scientific communities dealing with social determinants of health that their topic represents a challenge at a global level that requires engagement and collaboration with a variety of stakeholders committed to actions against health inequities. One can observe a similar process among scientists concerned with research on global climate change. In fact, there are strong reasons to recommend that these two movements should jointly operate towards strengthening a social and economic development that promotes health equity of a global population and the preservation of a sustainable ecological climate.

Despite these urgent needs, the scientific evidence base on social causation of health and illness is still debated to some extent, both within and outside of science, and there is an inherent tension as to how far this knowledge can serve as a convincing basis of far-reaching political decisions. Therefore, scientists should be aware of this tension and act in a self-critical, careful way. At the same time, efforts towards producing best available scientific knowledge should continue. In the following section, some significant recent extensions of the knowledge base on social determinants of health are reviewed and discussed.

SOCIAL CAUSATION OF HEALTH IN A LIFE COURSE PERSPECTIVE

In addition to the identification and description of social phenomena with relevance to health, sociology, as a science, aims at developing and testing theories that can explain observed associations. Theory development in the social sciences is a difficult task due to the variability, dynamics, and complexity of its object, the human society. For instance, it is widely accepted that there are different levels of sociological analysis: the macro-, the meso-, and the micro-sociological level. Research findings generated at each level are significant, but we hardly know how to link them within a comprehensive theoretical framework. Moreover, societal life at the same time is experienced as an objective (intersubjective) reality and as a subjectively defined, symbolically meaningful reality. Given these difficulties, it was proposed that sociological theories may be restricted to the so-called middle-range of analysis, whose scope of generalization is limited in time and space (Merton 1968). When using the term 'theory', we expect an analytical scheme or model that is able to produce new explanatory or predicting information and, by doing so, to exclude other, concurrent explanations. A powerful theory is characterized by independently confirmed explanations or predictions of poorly understood phenomena, or by unraveling connections between formerly unrelated features of the reality under study. It is based on valid measurement and aims at applying its parsimonious statements to a wide range of phenomena.

So far, a number of *middle-range theoretical models* were proposed and tested in health-related social sciences, but their diversity precludes any systematic classification or integration into a unifying framework. The theoretical concepts selected for this review mainly represent the *meso-sociological level* of analysis. This selection is justified by the fact that these models link socio-environmental conditions of everyday life to the actions, cognitions, and emotions and, hence, health outcomes of individuals (the Weberian paradigm). The emphasis of the meso-sociological level of analysis and its focus on core social roles through which people cope with the demands and opportunities of their proximate social environment does not exclude complementary macro-level analyses (the Durkheimian paradigm), where social determinants of health are explored with aggregate data. Examples of this latter approach are income distribution (Wilkinson and Pickett 2009), the structure of labor markets (Brenner 1997), or financial crises and socio-political upheavels (Stuckler et al. 2011). Yet, ultimately, these determinants need to be linked to biological and psychological information where the *embodiment of the social world* resulting in health or disease occurs. There is now a broad consensus that research on social determinants of health should adopt a *life course perspective* as a framework into which the different explanatory models need to fit. Two such stages, early life from pregnancy, early childhood to adolescence, and midlife, deserve special attention.

Childhood and Adolescence

The development of health starts with conception, based on the genetic imprint of parents and grandparents. During pregnancy, this development is highly vulnerable to influences mediated by mothers' behavior, emotions, and environmental exposures. A first theoretical model, '*critical period*', states that toxic influences during pregnancy have long-lasting adverse effects on elevated risks of morbidity and mortality in midlife. In other words, physiological dysregulation of the fetal organism in a distinct vulnerable phase of gestation produces irreversible damage that triggers long-term pathological development resulting in premature chronic disease. With the advent of epigenetic research, there is now convincing evidence of intergenerational transmission of social adversity and its effects on health. First evidence of this model came from Barkers' research on malnutrition during pregnancy, low birth weight, and increased cardiometabolic morbidity in midlife (Barker 1994). These early findings were replicated in several birth cohort studies, and, importantly, mothers' health-adverse behaviors that included smoking and alcohol abuse, were related to their deprived socioeconomic circumstances (Bartley 2017). Based on this evidence, the notion of 'social heritage' of health inequalities was proposed, pointing to the transgenerational transmission of socioeconomic disadvantage from parents to their children by critically disturbing normal embryonal development (Power and Kuh 2006). Determinants of these disturbances were not confined to adverse maternal health-related behaviors, but included environmental hazards, such as air pollution (Weck at al. 2008) as well as acute and chronic conditions of psychosocial stress. This latter association was studied more recently with emphasis on epigenetic processes related to biological aging and premature mortality. For instance, in a group of young adults whose mothers experienced a severely stressful life event during pregnancy, telomere length, a biomarker of cellular gaging, measured in white blood cells, was significantly shorter than in a control group of similar age (Entringer et al. 2011). Telomere length provides an estimate of expected cell divisions during one's remaining life time and, thus, a proxy indicator of estimated remaining life expectancy.

A wealth of research findings is available on the impact of *social disadvantage* during infancy and childhood on unequal adult health. Here, the notion of critical period relates to decisive stages of children's physical, emotional, cognitive, motivational, and moral development during the first decade of life. In these studies, social disadvantage was measured either by parental characteristics, such as socioeconomic position, housing and neighborhood quality, or by indicators of children's adverse immediate social environment, including experience of physical and emotional trauma (Davey Smith et al. 1998). In a recent review, childhood social adversity was associated with elevated risks of chronic disease and premature mortality in adulthood (Hughes et al. 2017).

While these associations provide an important extension of the traditional notion that adult socioeconomic position is a powerful determinant of later morbidity and mortality, it may not adequately capture the dynamics of social life. Therefore, a second conceptual approach was proposed, termed '*pathways model*' (Power and Kuh 2006). It assumes that social adversity experienced in early life exerts subtle, but significant effects on cognitive and physical development during childhood that result in less favorable educational and behavioral outcomes. These outcomes increase the probability that young people end up in lower socioeconomic positions in early adulthood. Being confined to a lower socioeconomic position in early adulthood goes along with exposure to new risks that contribute to increased illness and disease. Chains of risks as well as mediating effects are operating to result in social inequalities in health later on. Childhood cognitive ability is an example of this mediating effect. In a study by Osler et al. (2003), it was shown that poor parental socioeconomic conditions at birth are associated with reduced children's cognitive ability at school age. Moreover, low cognitive ability at school age was observed to increase the risk of premature adult mortality. Cognitive ability at school age mediated about a quarter of the effect of low childhood socioeconomic status on mortality (Osler et al. 2003).

With increasing availability of findings from birth cohort studies that started more than 50 years ago, thus demonstrating outcomes of longer-term life course trajectories, a third concept evolved, the model of '*cumulative advantage/disadvantage*' (Dannefer 2003). This model assumes a close link between the socio-structural disadvantage into which children are born, and the material and psychosocial resources or capabilities that are available for their further development. Both positive and negative effects can result from this interaction. Starting from a favorable socioeconomic background enables children to develop their capabilities to an optimal extent that in turn increase their career success in adult life. Conversely, given their poor material and psychosocial resources during childhood, young people's opportunities of escaping from their disadvantaged social background may be restricted, resulting in trajectories of cumulative relative social deprivation (Bartley 2017). The following *case study* offers convincing evidence on the negative consequences of these trajectories for people's health and survival.

CASE STUDY: LIFE COURSE CUMULATIVE SOCIOECONOMIC STATUS AND CARDIOVASCULAR MORTALITY

In their study of 7,846 men and women aged >50 years in England, Silvia Stringhini and co-authors (2018) analyzed cardiovascular disease (CVD) mortality during a mean 8.4-year follow-up period in relation to two complementary measures of cumulative socioeconomic status (SES). The first measure, an index of occupational trajectories, comprised four different combinations of paternal and own occupational status: 'stable high' (high paternal and own SES, based on three hierarchical categories); 'upward' (low or intermediate paternal SES, own high SES); 'downward' (high or intermediate paternal SES, own low SES); 'stable low' (low paternal and own SES). The second measure, a cumulative life course SES score, comprised four indicators: paternal and own occupational status (see above), educational degree (reflecting SES in early adulthood), and wealth in early old age. A sum score resulting in four quartiles indicated the amount of cumulative social disadvantage. Additionally, data on behavioral, psychosocial and physiological factors as potential mediators of these associations were collected. Associations of the two measures of social disadvantage with

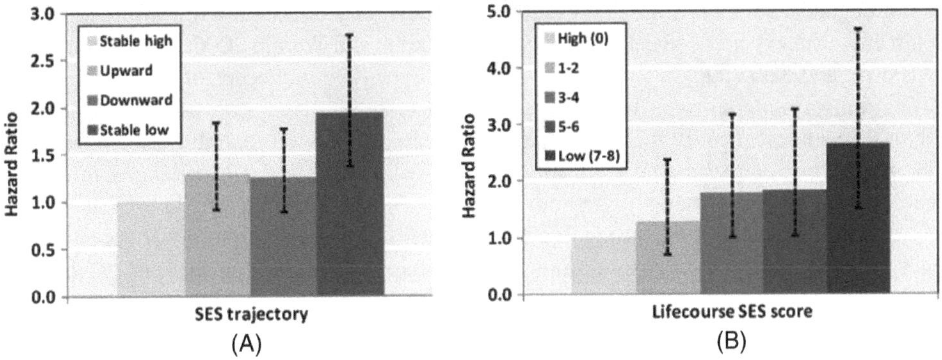

Figure 4.1 Association of life-course SES trajectory (A) and life-course cumulative SES score (B) with CVD mortality.*

Additional mediation analysis revealed that behavioral risk factors (smoking, alcohol, physical inactivity) and inflammatory markers (C-reactive protein, fibrinogen) provided the relatively largest contributions towards explaining these associations.

In conclusion, two complementary measures of cumulative socioeconomic disadvantage were associated with significantly elevated risks of cardiovascular mortality in this early-old population.

* Stringhini, S., Zaniotto, P., Kumari, M., Kivimäki, M., et al. (2018) 'Socio-economic trajectories and cardiovascular disease mortality in older people: The English Longitudinal Study of Ageing'. *International Journal of Epidemiology* 47: 42 (reproduced with permission from the Publisher)

CVD mortality were analyzed using multivariable logistic regression.

During the observation period, 438 participants died from CVD. Figure 4.1 demonstrates the results. A stable low life course SES trajectory (A) was associated with around double the risk of CVD mortality, compared to a stable high life course SES trajectory. Similarly, CVD mortality risk was significantly elevated in the highest quartile of a score reflecting life course cumulative social disadvantage (B).

Adolescence

The three models applied to the study of social determinants of health during childhood can also be applied to adolescence. This developmental phase is characterized by profound transformations at the biological level of puberty and growth, at the level of brain development, and at the psychosocial level of identity formation and extension of social relationships beyond primary groups. Therefore, all features of a 'critical period' can be identified. Critical life events and socioeconomic adversity experienced during adolescence have direct long-lasting negative effects on adult health (Viner et al. 2012). Moreover, these effects are modified by vulnerability factors acquired in early childhood. Low birth weight is one such example. Metabolic dysregulation during the years preceding puberty increases the risk of developing overweight (so-called 'adiposity rebound effect'). Overweight in adolescence in turn predisposes people to an elevated occurrence of cardio-metabolic disorders in adult life (Twig et al. 2016). Both conditions, low birth weight and overweight during adolescence, are socially graded, leaving girls and boys with a disadvantageous social background at higher risk. The social gradient of impaired lung function in adulthood, strongly related to respiratory disease, represents another example of a critical period effect modified by early childhood adversity. A low level of cognitive ability at school age explains a substantial part of the gradient of adult lung function, and low cognitive ability is more likely among adolescents who experienced early life adversity (Power and Kuh 2006).

The 'pathways model' is of particular significance in adolescence. In this view, a new track in the life course starts with adolescence, and this track is shaped by resources and capabilities acquired during earlier stages. *Health-related behaviors* define the most important track as adolescence is the period in life when young people experience, adopt, and eventually internalize these behaviors as part of an evolving *health lifestyle*. Numerous studies reported social gradients of health-adverse behaviors, such as smoking, alcohol and drug use, unhealthy diet, lack of physical exercise, and risky sexual behavior (Elgar et al. 2015; Jarvis and Wardle 2006; Richter 2010). How do these social gradients emerge? Several competing theoretical concepts were developed to explain the acquisition and maintenance or modification of health-related behaviors, among them the 'health belief model' (Becker 1974), the 'protection motivation theory' (Rogers 1983), and the 'transtheoretical model' (Prochaska et al. 2008). However, these concepts did not specifically address the social determinants of these behaviors. In this regard, Jessor and Jessor (1977) proposed to focus on latent functions of health-adverse behaviors. Adopting these behaviors is interpreted as a way of coping with situations that threaten adolescents' self-esteem, aiming at compensating failures of successful agency. There is reason to assume that the resources and capabilities required for successful agency were not well developed during childhood socialization of adolescents with a disadvantaged social background. These resources and capabilities are, among others, self-efficacy and self-confidence, goal orientation and achievement motivation, problem-solving competences, and optimism. With deficits in these resources, adolescents are more susceptible to adopting health-adverse behaviors, such as cigarette smoking, that regulate their mood, reduce their perceived stress, and offer some rewarding stimulation (Jarvis and Wardle 2006; Kristenson 2006).

Finally, the concept of 'cumulative advantage/disadvantage' can be applied to adolescence as well. Its central hypothesis states that a risk or advantage experienced in early life engenders consecutive risks or advantages at later stages of life. In terms of opportunities of future social advantage, the level of *educational attainment* during adolescence and young adulthood is of critical importance. Strong social gradients of educational attainment were repeatedly documented in economically advanced countries, with lower prevalence of tertiary education among those with lower parental socioeconomic status (OECD 2018). Young people from a disadvantaged social origin and with less educational skills are at high risk of experiencing unemployment or of being confined to dangerous or stressful jobs (Caspi et al. 1998). *Unemployment* in young adulthood and exposure to dangerous or stressful jobs in turn increase the risk of premature ill health and disease (Milner et al. 2013; Schnall et al. 2009). As another example, remaining in one's low social class of origin at the end of adolescence and in early adulthood was shown to be associated with a higher score, indicating accelerated epigenetic aging, compared to the score of those with the same origin, but social upward mobility at young age (Fiorito et al. 2017). A similar trend was observed in a British study with regard to differential risk of premature mortality (Davey Smith et al. 1997).

Taken together, three concepts of disentangling the complexities of developmental processes, critical period, pathways models, and cumulative advantage/disadvantage, proved to be useful in discussing the impact of social conditions on the health of children and adolescents.

Adulthood

Core social roles in midlife

The development and test of middle-range sociological theories on social causes of disease was particularly successful in the recent past. These theories are informed by basic sociological concepts of *social status* and *social role* (Merton 1968). Their fruitful application to human health is due to the fact that they bridge the social opportunity structure of positions ('statuses') and related access to social networks and to scarce resources with the material and psychosocial needs of individuals acting through their social roles. Hereby, the social roles related to affiliation and membership (partnership, family, close relationships, citizenship etc.) and those related to productivity (paid work, education, house and family work, volunteering etc.) are of primary importance. Obviously, some fundamental, widely prevalent human needs cannot be adequately met without a continued exchange of individuals with their proximal social environment. Beyond biological survival and reproduction, these fundamental needs include the recurrent experience of social ties and a related sense of belonging or self-integration (Bowlby 1969), the development of personal control or autonomy and related self-efficacy through goal-directed activities (Bandura 1997), and reinforced perceptions of social recognition by significant others and associated favorable self-esteem (Mead 2009). Accordingly, the social roles of partnership, parenthood, friendship or civic membership provide proximal social environments that enable individuals to experience trust, support, love, as well as emotional and material security. Their beneficial effects on health and well-being are briefly documented below. Yet, noxious effects on health that are attributable to lack or loss of social ties, serious conflicts, mistrust and betrayal have to be mentioned as well. Similarly, social roles offering or expecting productive activities, and specifically the work role, enable people to meet core material and psychosocial needs. These needs include the provision of regular income, the acquisition, maintenance and eventually improvement of social status and related benefits (social security and protection), the recurrent personal agency in terms of meeting goals, performing, exerting control and experiencing appreciation of one's achievements. Their beneficial effects on health and well-being essentially depend on the quality of work and employment. Conversely, poor quality of work and precarious employment threaten or prevent respective need satisfaction, with deleterious effects on health and well-being. Given their centrality in modern societies, *social roles related to affiliation and membership* and *social roles related to productive activities* have received major attention in health-related sociological and epidemiological research. Therefore, I briefly summarize relevant findings of this research.

Social ties and social support

Following the seminal work of Durkheim (1951) mentioned above, two concepts were developed that guided this line of research during the last few decades. '*Social network*' analyses examine the structural aspects of social relationships and ties, in terms of size, intensity, reciprocity, and duration, whereas '*social support*' identifies the functional aspects of these relationships, where one can distinguish the instrumental dimension from the emotional and the informational dimension. Moreover, it matters whether support is actually available if needed and whether it is perceived as appropriate (Berkman and Krishna 2014). A wide range of empirical studies explored the associations of these two concepts with indicators of health. The following *three hypotheses* were most often tested: (1) People with access to larger, more intense, proximate and enduring social networks enjoy better health and well-being than people with less well developed social networks or social isolation. (2) People who lack emotional and instrumental social support suffer from poorer health and well-being than those who benefit from appropriate available support. (3) Adverse effects of stressors on health are mitigated by the presence of strong social support (support as a moderator of this association).

Several systematic reviews and meta-analyses were performed in an attempt to summarize the findings on these hypotheses. Generally, these reviews were faced with the problems of heterogeneity of construct definitions and their measurements, of a wide range of health outcomes, and of a relative paucity of longitudinal studies. Despite these limitations, the main results can be summarized as follows. First, the evidence of an *association of social relationships with all-cause mortality* must be judged as very robust. A weak social network and/or social isolation goes along with an increase in mortality risk of about 50 percent, compared to the risk of a strong social network. Similarly, a low level of social support is associated with an increase in all-cause mortality risk of about 40 percent, compared to a high level of support (Holt-Lunstad et al. 2010; Holt-Lunstad et al. 2015). These associations were also observed, although in a lower number of reports, if the two measures of social relationships were related to mortality from cardiovascular disease (House et al. 1988). Second, in addition to mortality studies, incident *coronary heart disease* was found to be lower among people reporting strong social relationships (Berkman and Krishna 2014), and several studies observed strong associations of emotional and instrumental social support with mental health, and specifically *depression*. These findings were more pronounced in general populations than in populations with physical disability (Tough et al. 2017). Thus, the first two hypotheses are generally supported by empirical evidence, and findings confirm that they are valid across gender, age groups and ethnic background. However, third, the hypothesis of a buffering effect of social support was less often investigated. In this regard, the work of medical sociologist George W. Brown is of interest. Starting from the paradigm of life event research, Brown and Harris (1978) specified a model in which stressful life events adversely influence a person's affective health and well-being to the extent that a confident person or someone offering crisis support is absent. This vulnerability is intensified by poor self-esteem and self-blame of the person. This model found some support in a study of 353 mothers with a child under the age of 18 living at home. Onset of depression was best predicted by three variables: a lack of crisis support in the face of experienced life events or chronic difficulties, the person's self-blame, and her vulnerable psychosocial background (e.g., due to loss of a parent during childhood) (Brown et al. 1985). Brown's work on the social origins of affective disorder made a distinction to the field as it included *personal coping resources* in the analysis of relationships between social adversity and health. Moreover, it offered a detailed assessment method of the quality of stressful experience of threatening life events (Brown and Harris 1978).

Despite epidemiological evidence, the question of causality of relationships between social ties and morbidity or mortality is still debated. The *study of biomarkers* as pathways mediating the social with the biological reality offers one approach towards strengthening this link. More recently, investigations analyzed associations of social relationships with stress hormones, such as cortisol, immune markers, or leucocyte telomere length. As reviewed by Kim and Kawachi (2018), some support was found for the hypothesis that shorter telomere length is found in persons with poor social relationships (specifically lack of spousal support, living alone, low perceived support). Yet, few investigations demonstrated these associations in a prospective study design.

In summary, there is impressive evidence that *social roles* related to *affiliation and membership* can exert *beneficial effects on health* and well-being if they enable persons to experience the emotional and instrumental benefits of secure, trusting social ties, and of receiving the support needed in threatening situations. In the absence of these benefits, substantial negative effects on health and survival are documented.

Social productivity: control and reward

Among the social roles related to productivity, the *work role* is of central importance in modern societies, where employment conditions and the nature of work underwent significant changes. These changes are mainly due to technological advances and the impact of economic globalization. Participating in paid work can exert both beneficial and adverse effects on workers' health, depending on the quality and context of job tasks and work environments. To date, for many occupations, physical and chemical hazards are no longer the main threats to workers' health, but rather mental and emotional demands and threats, commonly labeled as *psychosocial work-related stressors*. To identify these stressors, the complexity and diversity of quality of work and employment needs to be tackled by applying a *theoretical model*. It is the aim of a theoretical model to reduce this complexity and to identify distinct critical dimensions at a level of generalization that allows for their use in a wide range of different occupations. Importantly, these critical dimensions should be based on stress-theoretical notions as the stress paradigm defines a common underlying frame of reference of research on psychosocial working conditions and health outcomes (Steptoe and Kivimäki 2012). While a variety of work-related stress models are available, two such models have been studied with particular intensity in recent past, both in the context of epidemiological cohort studies and of experimental stress research, the demand-control model and the effort-reward imbalance model.

The '*demand-control*' model posits that stressful experience at work results from a distinct job task profile defined by two dimensions, the psychological demands put on the working person and the degree of control available to the person to perform the required tasks (Karasek and Theorell 1990). This latter dimension is labelled 'decision latitude'. Jobs defined by high demands in combination with low control are stressful because they limit the individual's autonomy and sense of control while generating continued pressure ('high job strain'). Under these conditions, excessive arousal of the autonomic nervous system is expected to occur, activating the physiological system of the hypothalamic-pituitary-adrenocortical (HPA) stress axis with pronounced release of cortisol (Steptoe and Poole 2006). A third dimension, social support at work, was added to the original formulation. In this formulation, the highest level of strain would be expected in jobs that are characterized by high demand, low control and low social support at work or social isolation ('iso-strain jobs'). According to this model, it is the combined effect of high demand and low control that matters for health. 'Active jobs', offering a high degree of control and self-direction at work, are health-protective rather than health-damaging, even if associated with continued high demand.

A complementary model, '*effort-reward imbalance*', is concerned with stressful features of the work contract (Siegrist 1996). This model builds on the notion of social reciprocity, a fundamental principle of all types of costly transactions. Social reciprocity lies at the core of the work contract which defines distinct obligations or tasks to be performed in exchange with adequate rewards. These rewards include money, esteem and career opportunities (promotion, job security). Contractual reciprocity operates through norms of return expectancy, where effort spent by employees is reciprocated by equitable rewards from employers. The effort–reward imbalance model claims that lack of reciprocity occurs frequently under specific conditions. Failed reciprocity, in terms of high cost and low gain, elicits strong negative emotions and associated stress reactions with adverse long-term health consequences, by activating pain- and stress-related brain reward circuits (Schultz 2006). Distinct from the first model, this concept includes an intrinsic component in addition to the two extrinsic components, the personal pattern of coping with demanding work termed

Table 4.1 Conceptual differences: 'control' vs. 'reward'

	Control	*Reward*
Macro level	Access to occupational position offering challenge, responsibility, status	Access to occupational position offering security, continuity, promotion prospects
Meso level	Job task with autonomy, self-direction, skill development	Job enabling experience of fair pay, appreciation, support
Micro level (personal)	Self-efficacy	Self-esteem
Micro level (biological)	Low activation of SAM and HPA-axis	Low activation of pain- and stress-related brain-reward circuits

Abbreviations: SAM: Sympatho-adrenal medullary axis; HPA: Hypothalamus-pituitary-adrenocortical axis.

'over-commitment'. People characterized by over-commitment may strive towards continuously high achievement because of their underlying need for approval and esteem at work.

Although there is a slight overlap between 'demand' and 'effort' the two theoretical models complement each other by pointing to different dimensions of the psychosocial work environment. Table 4.1 delineates these differences with a focus on their *core-stress-theoretical notions*, *control* and *reward* respectively. At the macro-level of labor market arrangements, their focus is on those conditions of job acquisition that enable or threaten control vs. reward, while at the meso-level of organizations, the quality of work enabling or threatening autonomy and self-direction vs. fairness and recognition matters most. At the micro-level of personal experience, the models' focus is on strengthened or weakened self-efficacy vs. self-esteem, whereas at the level of biological response, the activation of stress responses due to stimulation or threat of control (SAM and HPA axis) differs somewhat from the activation due to stimulation or threat of reward (pain- and stress-related brain-reward circuits).

An extended description of these two stress-theoretical sociological models of a health-adverse psychosocial work environment and their underlying notions is justified by the fact that a large number of international studies investigated the health effects resulting from respective exposures. This extensive evidence is reviewed elsewhere (Kivimäki et al. 2018; Siegrist and Wahrendorf 2016) and only briefly summarized here. Two disorders with relevance to global public health were investigated with particular intensity: coronary heart disease and depression. More than 20 prospective cohort studies tested the job strain model, either in terms of a combination of demand and control, or in terms of single components, and several such studies analyzed the effort–reward imbalance model with regard to incident fatal or non-fatal coronary heart disease (CHD). Despite the heterogeneity of findings and despite the fact that in some studies expected effects were absent, the large majority confirmed that the *relative risk of CHD* following work stress exposure was *elevated by around 40 percent* (Dragano et al. 2017; Kivimäki et al. 2018). In these estimates, the influence of important cardiovascular risk factors was controlled by multivariable statistical adjustment. However, additional findings indicate that work stress is associated with some of these risk factors as well, such as high blood pressure, atherogenic blood lipids, and inflammatory markers (Eddy et al. 2017; Kivimäki et al. 2018). An equally large number of prospective investigations explored the effects of the two work stress models on *depression*. Overall, a *relative risk increase by 60 to 70 percent* was observed (Madsen et al. 2017; Rugulies et al. 2017). This risk was greatly increased if the effect of a co-manifestation of both models was analyzed (Juvani et al. 2018). Again, additional studies revealed associations of work stress with altered secretion of stress hormones, reduced immune competence, and increased inflammation, i.e., conditions relevant for the development of CHD and depression (Eddy et al. 2016).

From a sociological perspective, this evidence is of interest as it is based on studies from different cultures, from the Global North as well as from Low- and Middle-income countries. It should also be mentioned that work stress is more prevalent among lower socioeconomic status groups and in working populations characterized by precarious employment. Moreover, the effects of work stress on health are particularly pronounced among these latter vulnerable groups. Taken together, there is a robust body of knowledge available indicating that stressful psychosocial work environments experienced during midlife increase the risk of important mental and physical disorders. Therefore, efforts should be directed towards extending the provision of jobs and employment conditions with good quality that enable workers to recurrently experience control and reward.

According to the life course perspective, *transitions into old age* define the next stage where social determinants of health need to be analyzed, specifically so in view of rapidly aging societies. In line with the concept of cumulative advantage/disadvantage a wealth of research findings confirm that the conditions experienced during midlife exert powerful long-lasting effects on health and well-being in old age. In a series of coordinated longitudinal surveys of aging populations in several developed and developing countries, initiated by the Health and Retirement Study in the USA (Juster and Suzman 1995) and extended by the English Longitudinal Study of Ageing (Marmot et al. 2003), and the Survey of Health, Aging and Retirement in Europe (Börsch-Supan et al. 2011), this evidence is currently generated within a rapidly growing field of aging research. It is not possible to do justice to this rich new knowledge by a brief account within the restrictions of this chapter. Such an account would reveal that transitions into old age are not exclusively shaped by previous chains of advantage or disadvantage, but can also be characterized by disruptions and radical changes of life patterns. If disadvantageous, such disruptions may reflect the loss of close social ties, financial hardship, or accelerated frailty. If advantageous, these changes may reflect attempts towards healthy aging by selecting, optimizing and compensating one's personal and social resources (Baltes and Baltes 1990). Old age, therefore, offers new challenges to the study of social determinants of health and well-being.

CONCLUDING REMARKS

This chapter documents a rapid recent growth of sociological knowledge related to the determinants of health and disease. This growth of knowledge is evident even within the constraints of a selective account of research findings that focuses on social epidemiological studies with an attempt to identify causal inferences from socio-environmental conditions to elevated risks of morbidity and mortality. It goes unsaid that this selective approach fails to address complementary sociological research traditions, such as qualitative approaches. It also falls short of integrating the research findings conducted at the mesosocial level into multi-level analysis. There is still a considerable gap of knowledge on social determinants of health in developing countries, due to poorly developed research capacities in these countries, and the overarching focus on findings from modern Western societies may run the risk of bypassing relevant sociocultural and psychosocial dimensions that impact on health in other regions of the world. Moreover, this chapter has emphasized ill health and disease, i.e., the pathogenic perspective, at the expense of a salutogenic perspective, which focuses on social conditions that maintain and promote health. However, it is evident that the social conditions identified by theoretical models that explain elevated disease risks can act as health-protective factors if converted into their opposite (e.g., from low control and reward to high control and reward, from cumulative disadvantage to cumulative advantage).

This latter statement points to the need of strengthening research on interventions that evaluate the health effects of models of good practice. Although, admittedly, the conduction of intervention studies within social settings is a methodologically challenging task, such studies are urgently required. The theoretical models mentioned can inform the development and implementation of models of good practice. Educational arrangements in early childhood, pre-school and school environments, workplaces in organizations, and communities offer rich opportunities for intervention research. Even at the macro-level of national policies, beneficial effects on the health and well-being of populations due, for example, to improved social, labor market and tax policies, can be demonstrated by comparative cross-country studies. In conclusion, there is hope that scientific evidence generated by sociological and epidemiological research on social causation of health and disease will ultimately result in a sizeable reduction of social inequalities in health and in a further improvement of living conditions of populations around the globe.

REFERENCES

Antonovsky, A. (1967) 'Social class, life expectancy, and overall mortality'. *Milbank Memorial Fund Quarterly* 45: 31–73.

Baltes, P.B., and Baltes, M.M. (eds.) (1990) *Successful aging: Perspectives from the behavioral sciences*. New York: Cambridge University Press.

Bandura, A. (1997) *Self-efficacy: The exercise of control*. New York: Freeman.

Barker, D.J.P. (1994) *Mothers, babies and disease in later life*. London: British Medical Journal Group.

Bartley, M. (2017) *Health Inequality: An introduction to concepts, theories and methods* (2nd edition). Cambridge, UK: Polity Press.

Baum, F. (2018) *The new public health* (4th edition). Oxford: Oxford University Press.

Becker, M.H. (1974) 'The health belief model and sick role behavior'. *Health Education Monographs* 2: 409–19.

Berkman, L.F., Kawachi, I., and Glymour, M.M. (eds.) (2014) *Social epidemiology* (2nd edition). Oxford: Oxford University Press.

Berkman, L.F., and Krishna, A. (2014) 'Social network epidemiology', in L.F. Berkman, I. Kawachi, and M.M. Glymour (eds.), *Social epidemiology* (2nd edition). Oxford: Oxford University Press. pp. 234–89.

Berkman, L.F., and Syme, S.L. (1979) 'Social networks, host resistance, and mortality: A nine-year follow-up study of Alameda County residents'. *American Journal of Epidemiology* 109: 186–204.

Börsch-Supan, A., Brandt, M., Hank, K., and Schröder, M. (eds.) (2011) *The individual and the welfare state: Life histories in Europe*. Berlin: Springer.

Bowlby, J. (1969) *Attachment and loss. Vol.1: Attachment*. London: Hogarth Press.

Brenner, M.H. (1997) 'Heart disease mortality and economic changes, including unemployment, in Western Germany 1951–1989'. *Acta Physiologica Scandinavica. Supplementum*, 640: 149–52.

Brown, G.W., and Harris, T.O. (1978) *Social origins of depression*. London: Tavistock.

Brown, G.W., Craig, T.K.J., and Harris, T.O. (1985) 'Depression: Disease or distress? Some epidemiological considerations'. *British Journal of Psychiatry* 147: 612–22.

Bruhn, J.G., Chandler, B., Lynn, T.N., and Wolf, S. (1966) 'Social characteristics of patients with coronary heart disease'. *American Journal of Medical Sciences* 251: 629–37.

Caspi, A., Wright, B.R.E, Moffitt, T.T., and Silva, P.A. (1998) 'Early failure in the labor market: Childhood and adolescent predictors of unemployment in the transition to adulthood'. *American Sociological Review* 63: 424–51.

Cockerham, W.C. (2010) *Medical Sociology* (11th edition). Upper Saddle River, NJ: Pearson Prentice-Hall.

Collier, F. (ed.) (2015) *The Palgrave handbook of social theory in health, illness and medicine*. New York: Palgrave Macmillan.

Cutler, D.M., Lleras-Muney, A., and Vogl, T. (2008) *Socioeconomic status and health: Dimensions and mechanisms*. Washington, DC: National Bureau of Economic Research.

Dannefer, D. (2003) 'Cumulative advantage/disadvantage and the life course: Cross-fertilizing age and social science theory'. *Journals of Gerontology: Series B-Psychosocial Sciences and Social Sciences* 85: S327–S337.

Davey Smith, G., Hart, C., Blane, D., Gillis, C., et al. (1997) 'Lifetime socioeconomic position and mortality: Prospective observational study'. *British Medical Journal* 314: 547.

Davey Smith, G., Hart, C., Blane, D., and Hole, D. (1998) 'Adverse socioeconomic conditions in childhood and cause specific adult mortality: Prospective observational study'. *British Medical Journal* 316: 1631–5.

Department of Health and Social Security (1980) *Inequalities in health: Report of a working group chaired by Sir Douglas Black*. London: Department of Health Statistics and Surveys.

Dragano, N., Siegrist, J., Nyberg, S.T., Lunau, T., et al. (2017) 'Effort–reward imbalance at work and incident coronary heart disease: A multicohort study of 90,164 individuals'. *Epidemiology* 28: 619.

Durkheim, E. (1951) *The suicide*. New York: Free Press (original in French, 1897).

Eddy, P., Heckenheim, R., Wertheim, E.H., Kent, S., and Wright, B.J. (2016) 'A systematic review and meta-analysis of the effort-reward imbalance model of workplace stress with indicators of immune function'. *Journal of Psychosomatic Research* 9: 1–8.

Eddy, P., Wertheim E.H., Kingsley, M., and Wright, B.J. (2017) 'Associations between the effort–reward imbalance model of workplace stress and indices of cardiovascular health: A systematic review and meta-analysis'. *Neuroscience and Biobehavioral Reviews* 83: 252–266.

Elgar, F.J., Pförtner, T.K., Moor, I., De Clercq, B., et al. (2015) 'Socioeconomic inequalities in adolescent health 2002–2010: A time-series analysis of 34 countries participating in the Health Behaviour in School-aged Children study'. *The Lancet* 385: 2088–95.

Entringer, S., Epel, E. S., Kumsta, R., Lin, J., et al. (2011) 'Stress exposure in intrauterine life is associated with shorter telomere length in young adulthood'. *Proceedings of the National Academy of Sciences* 108: E513–E518.

Faris, R.E., and Dunham, H.W. (1939) *Mental disorders in urban areas: An ecological study of schizophrenia and other psychoses*. Chicago, IL: University of Chicago Press.

Fiorito, G., Polidoro, S., Dugué, P.A., Kivimaki, M., et al. (2017) 'Social adversity and epigenetic aging: A multi-cohort study on socioeconomic differences in peripheral blood DNA methylation'. *Scientific Reports* 7: 16266.

Glymour, M.M., and Kubzansky, L.D. (2018) 'Causal inference in psychosocial epidemiology', in M. Kivimäki, G.D. Batty, I. Kawachi, and A. Steptoe (eds.), *The Routledge international handbook of psychosocial epidemiology*. Abingdon, UK/New York: Routledge.

Henry, J.P. (1997) Cultural *change and high blood pressure*. Münster: Lit.

Henry, J.P., and Cassel, J.C. (1969) 'Psychosocial factors as risk factors in essential hypertension: Recent epidemiologic and animal experimental evidence'. *American Journal of Epidemiology* 90: 171–200.

Henry, J.P., and Stephens, P.M. (1977) *Stress, health, and the social environment*. New York: Springer.

Hill, A.B. (1965) 'The environment and disease: association or causation?' *Proceedings of the Royal Society of Medicine* 58: 295–300.

Hinkle, L.E. Jr., Whitney, L.H., Lehman, F.W., and Dunn, J. (1968) 'Occupation, education and coronary heart disease: Risk is influenced more by education and background than by occupational experiences, in the Bell system'. *Science* 161: 238–46.

Hollingshead, A.B., and Redlich, F.C. (1958) *Social class and mental illness: Community study*. New York: Wiley.

Holt-Lunstad, J., Smith, T.B., Baker, M., Harris, T., et al. (2015) 'Loneliness and social isolation as risk factors for mortality: A meta-analytic review'. *Perspectives on Psychological Science* 10: 227–37.

Holt-Lunstad, J., Smith, T.B., and Layton, J.B. (2010) 'Social relationships and mortality risk: A meta-analytic review'. *PLoS Medicine* 7: e1000316.

House, J.S., Landis, K.R., and Umberson, D. (1988) Social relationships and health. *Science* 241: 540–5.

Hughes, K., Bellis, A.M., Hardcastle, K.A., Sethi, D., et al. (2017) 'The effect of multiple adverse childhood experiences on health: A systematic review and meta-analysis'. *The Lancet Public Health* 2: e356–e366.

Jarvis, M.J., and Wardle, J. (2006) Social patterning of individual health behaviours: the case of cigarette smoking, in M. Marmot, and R.G. Wilkinson (eds.), *Social determinants of health* (2nd edition). Oxford: Oxford University Press. pp. 224–37.

Jessor, R., and Jessor, S.L. (1977) *Problem behavior and psychosocial development: Longitudinal Study of Youth*. New York: Academic Press.

Juster, F., and Suzman, R. (1995) 'An overview of the Health and Retirement Study'. *Journal of Human Resources* 30: 7–56.

Juvani, A., Oksanen, T., Virtanen, M., Salo, P., et al. (2018) 'Clustering of job strain, effort–reward imbalance, and organizational injustice and the risk of work disability: A cohort study'. *Scandinavian Journal of Work, Environment and Health* 44: 485–95.

Karasek, R., and Theorell, T. (1990) *Health work: Stress, productivity, and the reconstruction of working life*. New York: Basic Books.

Kasl, S.V., and Cobb, S. (1970) 'Blood pressure changes in men undergoing job loss: A preliminary report'. *Journal of Chronic Disease* 22: 259–78.

Kim, Y., and Kawachi, I. (2018) 'Social Networks', in M. Kivimäki, G.D. Batty, I. Kawachi, and A. Steptoe (eds.), *The Routledge international handbook of psychosocial epidemiology*. Abingdon, UK/New York: Routledge.

Kitagawa, E.M., and Hauser, P.M. (1973) *Differential mortality in the United States: A Study in socioeconomic epidemiology*. Cambridge, MA: Harvard University Press.

Kivimäki, M., Ferrie, J.E., and Kawachi, I. (2018) 'Workplace stressors', in M. Kivimäki, G.D. Batty, I. Kawachi, and A. Steptoe (eds.), *The Routledge international handbook of psychosocial epidemiology*. Abingdon, UK/New York: Routledge.

Kristenson, M. (2006) 'Socio-economic position and health: The role of coping', in J. Siegrist, and M. Marmot (eds.), *Social inequalities in health: New evidence and policy implications*. Oxford: Oxford University Press. pp. 127–51.

Langner, T.S., and Michael, S.T. (1963) *Life stress and mental health: The Midtown Manhattan Study*. New York: Free Press.

Leighton, D.C., Harding, J.S., Macklin, D.B., et al. (1963) *The character of danger: Psychiatric symptoms in selected communities*. New York: Basic Books.

Loomis, D., and Wing, S. (1990) 'Is molecular epidemiology a germ theory for the end of the twentieth century?' *International Journal of Epidemiology* 19: 1–3.

Lorber, J. (1997) *Gender and the social construction of illness*. London: Sage.

Lutfey, K.E., Link, C.L., Marceau, L.D., Grant, R.W., et al. (2009) 'Diagnostic certainty as a source of medical practice variation in coronary heart disease: Results from a cross-national experiment of clinical decision making'. *Medical Decision Making* 29: 606–18.

Madsen, I.E.H., Nyberg, S.T., Magnusson Hanson, L.L., Ferrie, J.E., et al. (2017) 'Job strain as a risk factor for clinical depression: Systematic review and meta-analysis with additional individual participant data'. *Psychological Medicine* 47: 1342–56.

Marmot, M.G. (2010) *Fair society, healthy lives*. The Marmot Review. London: Institute of Health Equity.

Marmot, M.G., Adelstein, A.M., Robinson, N., and Rose, G.A. (1978) 'Changing social-class distribution of heart disease'. *British Medical Journal* 2: 1109–12.

Marmot, M., Banks, J., Blundell, R., Lessof, C., and Nazroo, J. (eds.) (2003) *Health, wealth and lifestyles of the older population in England: The 2002 English Longitudinal Study of Ageing*. London: The Institute for Fiscal Studies.

Marmot, M.G., Davey Smith, G., and Stansfield, S. (1991) 'Inequalities in health twenty years on: The Whitehall II Study of British civil servants'. *The Lancet* 337: 1387–93.

Marmot, M.G., and Syme, S.L. (1976) 'Acculturation and coronary heart disease in Japanese Americans'. *American Journal of Epidemiology* 104: 225–47.

Mead, G.H. (2009) *Mind, self, and society: From the standpoint of a social behaviorist*. Chicago, IL: University of Chicago Press.

Mechanic, D. (1978) *Medical sociology*. New York: Free Press.

Merton, R.K. (1938) 'Social structure and anomie'. *American Sociological Review* 3: 672–82.

Merton, R.K. (1968) *Social theory and social structure*. New York: Free Press.

Milner, A., Page, A., and LaMontagne, A.D. (2013) 'Long-term unemployment and suicide: A systematic review and meta-analysis'. *PLoS One* 8: e51333.

OECD (2018) *Equity in education: Breaking down barriers to social mobility*. Paris: PISA, OECD Publishing.

Osler, M., Andersen, A.M., Due, P., Lund, R., et al. (2003) 'Socioeconomic position in early life, birth weight, childhood cognitive function, and adult mortality: A longitudinal study of Danish men born in 1953'. *Journal of Epidemiology and Community Health* 57: 681–6.

Power, C., and Kuh, D. (2006) 'Life course development of unequal health', in J. Siegrist and M. Marmot (eds.), *Social inequalities in health: New evidence and policy implications*. Oxford: Oxford University Press. pp. 27–53.

Prochaska, J.O., Coleen, A., Redding, C.A., and Evers, K.E. (2008) 'The transtheoretical model and stages of change', in K. Glanz, B.K. Rimer, and K. Viswanth (eds.), *Health behavior and health education*. San Francisco, CA: Jossey-Bass. pp. 97–122.

Richter, M. (2010) *Risk behaviour in adolescence: Patterns, determinants and consequences*. Wiesbaden: VS Verlag.

Rogers, R.W. (1983) 'Cognitive and physiological processes in fear appeals and attitude change: A revised theory of protection motivation', in J.R. Cacioppo and R.E. Petty (eds.), *Social psychology: A sourcebook*. New York: Guilford Press. pp. 153–76.

Rosen, G. (1979) 'The evolution of social medicine', in H.S. Freeman, S. Levine, and L. Reeder (eds.), *Handbook of medical sociology*. Englewood Cliffs, NJ: Prentice-Hall. pp. 23–45.

Rugulies, R., Aust, B., and Madsen, I.E.H. (2017) 'Effort–reward imbalance at work and risk of depressive disorders: A systematic review and meta-analysis of prospective cohort studies'. *Scandinavian Journal of Work, Environment and Health* 43: 294–306.

Scheff, T. (1999) *Being mentally ill* (3rd edition). Hawthorne, NY: Aldine de Gruyter.

Schnall, P., Dobson, M., and Rosskam, E. (eds.) (2009) *Unhealthy work: Causes, consequences, cures*. New York: Baywood.

Schultz, W. (2006) 'Behavioral theories and the neurophysiology of reward'. *Annual Review of Psychology* 57: 87–115.

Scotch, N.A. (1968) 'Sociocultural factors in the epidemiology of Zulu hypertension'. *American Journal of Public Health* 53: 1205–13.

Shekelle, R.B., Osterfeld, A.M., and Paul, O. (1969) 'Social status and incidence of coronary heart disease' *Journal of Chronic Diseases* 22: 381–94.

Siegrist, J. (1996) 'Adverse health effects of high-effort/low-reward conditions at work'. *Journal of Occupational Health Psychology* 1: 27–43.

Siegrist, J., and Wahrendorf, M. (eds.) (2016) *Work stress and health in a globalized economy: The model of effort–reward imbalance*. Cham, Switzerland: Springer International.

Srole, L., Langner, T.S., Michael, S.T., et al. (1962) *Mental health in the metropolis: The Midtown Manhattan Study* (Vol. 1). New York: McGraw-Hill.

Steptoe, A., and Kivimäki, M. (2012) 'Stress and cardiovascular disease'. *Nature* 9: 360–70.

Steptoe, A., and Poole, L. (2016) 'Control and stress', in G. Fink (ed.), *Stress: Concepts, cognition, emotion, and behavior*. Amsterdam: Elsevier. pp. 73–80.

Stringhini, S., Zaniotto, P., Kumari, M., Kivimäki, M., et al. (2018) 'Socio-economic trajectories and cardiovascular disease mortality in older people: The English Longitudinal Study of Ageing'. *International Journal of Epidemiology* 47: 36–46.

Stuckler, D., Basu, S., Suhrcke, M., Coutts, A., et al. (2011) 'Effects of the 2008 recession on health: A first look at European data'. *The Lancet* 378: 124–5.

Syme, S.L., Hyman, M.M., and Enterline, P.E. (1964) 'Cultural mobility and coronary heart disease in an urban area'. *American Journal of Epidemiology* 82: 334–46.

Tough, H., Siegrist, J., and Fekete, C. (2017) 'Social relationships, mental health and wellbeing in physical disability: A systematic review'. *BMJ Public Health* 17: 414.

Twig, G., Yaniv, G., Levine, H., Leiba, A., et al. (2016) 'Body-mass index in 2.3 million adolescents and cardiovascular death in adulthood'. *New England Journal of Medicine* 374: 2430–40.

Tyroler, H., and Cassel, J. (1964) 'Health consequences of cultural change – II: The effect of urbanization and coronary heart mortality in rural residents'. *Journal of Chronic Diseases* 17: 167–77.

Viner, R.M., Ozer, E.M., Denny, S., Marmot, et al. (2012) 'Adolescence and the social determinants of health'. *The Lancet* 379: 1641–52.

Weber, M. (1978) *Economy and society*. Berkeley, CA: University of California Press.

Weck, R.L., Paulose, T., and Flaws, J.A. (2008) 'Impact of environmental factors and poverty on pregnancy outcomes'. *Clinical Obstetrics and Gynecology* 51: 349–59.

Weiner, H. (1992) *Perturbing the organism: The biology of stressful experience*. Chicago, IL: Chicago University Press.

Wilkinson, R., and Pickett, K. (2009) *The spirit level: Why more equal societies almost always do better*. London: Penguin.

World Health Organization (2008) Closing the gap in a generation: Health equity through action on the social determinants of health. *Final report of the Commission on Social Determinants of Health*. Geneva: WHO.

World Health Organization (2014) *Review of social determinants and the health divide in the WHO European region: Final report* (2nd edition). Copenhagen: WHO, Regional Office for Europe.

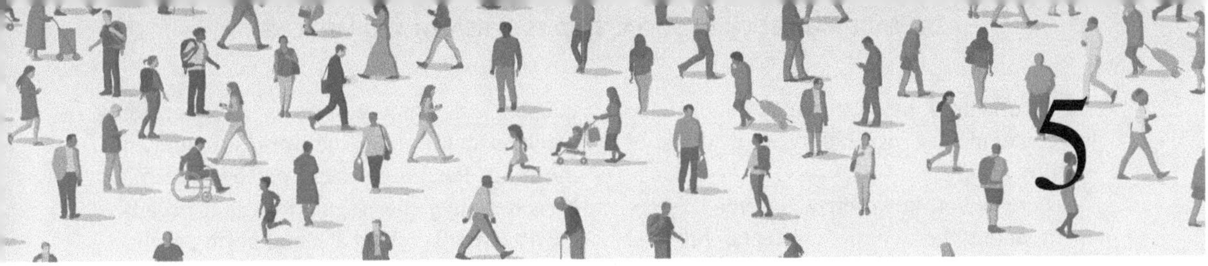

5

The History of the Changing Concepts of Health and Illness: Outline of a General Model of Illness Categories

Bryan S. Turner

INTRODUCTION: A TYPOLOGY OF HEALTH CONCEPTS

Concepts of health and illness stand at the core of the social values of human society because they express many of our fundamental assumptions about the meaning of life and death, and address the basic vulnerability of all human existence. A description of health, therefore, tends necessarily to offer a description of 'the good life' as a moral state of affairs. Although we attempt in the social sciences to avoid the confusion between description and evaluation, in ordinary usage these separate notions tend to merge because the description of an average state of affairs provides a convenient, if limited, measure of conventional morality. Additionally, the conception of illness as disease is derived from the old French word *aise* meaning 'comfort' (to strengthen or fortify), and disease indicates that an illness involves discomfort or lack of ease. The discomfort of disease is the loss of power we experience in otherwise comfortable or homely situations. Discomfort and disease both express our subjective sense of alienation, which follows the disempowerment of illness, while 'normal' provides a lay benchmark for things that are both healthy and moral (King 1982: 119).

In this chapter, I pay attention to the connections between health, well-being and human flourishing, and refer to the legacy of the Greek idea of *Eudaimonia* that played a major role in Western thought from Aristotle to modern times. For Aristotle (2011), *Eudaimonia* is the ultimate goal of all human activity and is achieved within a flourishing *polis*, and hence Aristotle uses *Eudaimonia* to describe individual and collective existence. *Eudaimonia*, somewhat misleadingly translated as 'happiness,' has remained at the core of much contemporary discussion of health, happiness and well-being. For example, Steven Pinker (2018: 264) in *Enlightenment Now* briefly acknowledges the legacy of Aristotle and comments 'happiness has become a major topic in the social sciences.' As I shall observe, happiness (or flourishing) has become a major issue in contemporary psychological theories of healthy ageing.

There is not, however, widespread agreement about these basic concepts. Medical terms are frequently used as metaphors to describe society, as in a 'sick society,' or to categorize deviancy in individuals, as in a 'sick mind.' Corporations or national economies that are financially sound are often referred to as being 'healthy.' Because they involve struggles over the moral significance of life, concepts of health tend to be highly contested. Conceptions of health tend to merge into or be based on fundamental religious and moral views about existence. Differences in orientations towards health reflect or express basic structural and cultural differences in power relations in society. Thus there is little consensus about what constitutes 'health' and 'illness,' or about 'happiness' and 'well-being' which are 'essentially contested concepts,' because their employment 'inevitably involves endless disputes about their proper uses' (Gallie 1956: 169).

Thus, it is not possible to give an authoritative account of the history of these concepts. It is more appropriate to talk in the plural about the histories of the many conceptualizations of human well-being and suffering. For simplicity's sake, I start with a general model of the historical development of concepts of health and illness. I argue that beliefs about health and illness in traditional or pre-modern societies were inextricably caught up with notions of purity and danger. As Mary Douglas (1966) has demonstrated, early notions of pollution and taboo were not about hygiene because there was simply no knowledge about such principles; concepts about scientific hygiene simply did not exist. The dietary prescriptions of the Old Testament are recommendations about religious not hygienic behavior. In other words, medical concepts were directed at the health of the soul rather than the body.

A taboo, which divides the world into acceptable/not acceptable in terms of the couplet edible/not edible, is a conceptual mechanism for giving the world structure and meaning. People got sick, not because of a breach of hygienic regulations, but because they had transgressed a social norm or taboo that separated the sacred from the profane. Sickness and health were often associated with taboos about bodily fluids where contact, for example with menstrual blood, could cause illness in an individual or disaster for a tribe. For instance, Polar Inuit explained personal misfortune, illness, and failure to catch food in terms of transgressions of taboos (typically surrounding the ritualistic organization of menstruation). These misfortunes and sicknesses were treated through shamanistic practices, where a 'confession' took place to purify the individual and the group (Hepworth and Turner 1982: 71).

In such a system of meaning, sickness was associated with evil forces that attacked human beings through, for instance, witchcraft and demonic possession. Concepts of illness functioned within a cosmology of good and evil forces, and were explanatory devices that described, and possibly justified, evil and misery. Notions of illness have typically been set within a system of beliefs that attempts to explain and justify the presence of human disease and suffering (as a theodicy). When people fall victim to disease and sickness, there is almost inevitably the question: Why me? Concepts of health and disease have typically provided an answer to that type of question. The dominant assumptions of disease, misfortune and suffering in traditional societies were located within a discourse of a sacred world. One possible conclusion is that with the process of modernization health and illness were transferred to more secular paradigms and eventually became embraced by various scientific discourses. However, there are many problems with any simple notion of a uniform modernization process. There is ample evidence that exorcism and so-called rites of deliverance are widely used in response to mental suffering and belief in the devil and possession have increased in recent years (Giordan and Possamai 2018). Religious values and institutions also play a significant role in mainstream health care. For example, Padre Pio (Saint Pio of Pietrelcina), who was famous in his life time for the stigmata on his body, has become the driving force behind a successful private hospital and research center (The Casa Sollievo della Sofferenza) at San Giovanni Rotondo in southern Italy (Luzzatto 2010).

Yet, even traditional medical systems have considerable complexity and ambiguity. For example, Andrew Cunningham (1997) notes that there were radical differences among Plato, Aristotle, Erasistratus, and Galen as to the nature of the human body, its functions and structure, and the purpose of medicine. There is also no neat point in history where secular views came to dominate. While the anatomical works of Versalius were assumed to have paved the way towards scientific medicine, Versalius retained a religious view that the ultimate role of medicine was to reveal the hand of God in Nature.

The history of medical concepts is inevitably tied to changing notions of the human body. In Western medicine, disease entities became increasingly differentiated and disease states more specified as the human body was itself differentiated into its component parts. Microbiology offered an account of viruses invading the body without overt connection to the moral or religious status of the individual. As scientific concepts of disease replaced traditional notions of the quasi-religious state of illness, the status of the medical professional increased, and the status and role of traditional healers (medicine men, wise women, and midwives) decreased (Flint 1989). There was, in addition, a differentiation between physical and mental health, relying on a basic division between mind and body. This mind/body dualism was associated with the empiricist revolution in philosophy, Cartesian rationalism. The notion of 'mental illness' was subsequently elaborated by separate developments in clinical psychology, psychiatry, and psychoanalysis (Foucault 1971). These developments had major consequences for the training of doctors and the curricula of medical faculties, and medical faculties were increasingly separated physically and culturally from the main body of the university (Brosnan and Turner 2009). Finally, the social sciences of health and illness were themselves part of the growing complexity of the contemporary model of sickness, where medical sociology, for instance, distinguishes among various levels, like the illness experience in the individual, cultural categories of sickness at the social level, and health-care systems at the societal level (Turner 1995: 5).

Increasing secularization characterized the development of health and illness concepts, the rise of scientific theories of health, the separation of mental and physical illness, the erosion of traditional therapies by scientific practices (a process that also involved the colonization of indigenous belief systems), and the differentiation of categories into specific micro-notions. The domain assumptions of health and illness phenomena became predominantly secular, but medical notions continued to evoke and be connected with paradigms of both religious and moral behavior. For example, there is still a professional and lay tendency to blame people for their illness, and thus attribute moral responsibility for health status. Western societies often 'psychologized' cancer by believing that at least some specific cancers result from the fact that people cannot or will not express themselves emotionally; blaming them for their cancer because they do not manage their emotions effectively (Sontag 1978). The idea that the feckless individual is the cause of his or her own misfortune and poor health rather than the structure of society became more dominant as government health policies since the 1970s were increasingly based on neo-liberal economic models. Neo-liberal economics support: deregulating markets; reducing the role of the state; cutting taxes; and promoting privatization to stimulate economic growth. Critics argue that these changes produced growing income inequality, low wages, unaffordable housing, and health inequalities (Harvey 2007).

The authority of doctors trained in secular and scientific medicine was not passively accepted by the lay public; alternative medical systems have always thrived alongside Western allopathic medicine. In the twentieth century, there was a revival of alternative systems of medicine and widespread criticism of the claims of allopathic medicine. The growth of alternative and complimentary medicine is in part a consumer response to the cost of health care in a deregulated market environment, and in part a response to the fact that, while modern medicine has been very successful in the treatment of acute illness, it has been less successful in response to chronic conditions like diabetes and ailments that accompany ageing. There are considerable philosophical and ethical problems with the notion of 'scientific medicine,' which cannot be regarded as a single, unified, and complete account of disease. In short, we cannot accept a theory of medicine as the inevitable march of reason resulting in the final triumph of enlightenment in the form of rational science over traditional notions of well-being.

A TYPOLOGY OF MEDICAL SYSTEMS

With these caveats in mind, this chapter is organized as a simple conceptual structure. I argue (see Figure 5.1) that health concepts can be analyzed along two dimensions: the sacred/profane domain and the collective/individual orientation to health and illness. First, the causes and treatment of disease can be set within a religious framework in which the ultimate explanations of illness are sought in non-natural causes (like divine punishment), and being sick is seen in moral terms, where human beings are held to be responsible for their illness. Alternatively, human illness is explained in natural terms by reference to causal agents such as germs or viruses, and individual humans are not held morally responsible for viral infections. Second, disease can be seen in individual terms like one's genetic legacy and where one is born, or the causes of human suffering and disease are explained in collective terms by reference to poor environmental conditions, low educational provision, poverty, and so forth. Combining these two dimensions produces a four-cell property-space to illustrate this approach. I stress that this framework is heuristic and I recognize that theories of health and illness may well combine various dimensions from my four-cell model. For example, healthy lifestyle theory combines structural variables (such as living conditions, class and age), socialization and experience, and life choices (or agency) (Cockerham 2005).

The growth of collectivist and secular assumptions about health and illness was characteristic of the public health movements of the nineteenth century, when radicals like Friedrich Engels, Edwin Chadwick, and Rudolf Virchow identified the causes of human disease in the deprivations and alienation of the working class in squalid slums within a rapidly expanding urban environment. Disease was a collective and secular condition of social existence in emergent capitalism, where morbidity and mortality rates were directly related to the quality of the food supply and income per capita. In the twentieth century, similar concepts of health and illness were embraced by Marxist medical sociologists like Howard Waitzkin (1983) and Vincente Navarro (1976), and by radical historians of medicine such as Henry E. Sigerist and his students (Fee and Brown 1997). While social reformers have treated disease as an effect of social deprivation, eugenics policies under national socialism in Germany and similar medical strategies in Stalinist Russia attempted to control the health of society by collective, secular approaches to reproduction to remove biological 'defects' from society (Weindling 1989). In addition, there was the eugenics movement in Britain in the early decades of the twentieth century

Sacred	Profane	
Saintly Sickness	Allopathic Medicine	Individual
Sickness Taboos	Social Medicine	Collective

Figure 5.1 Typology of domain assumptions

and the Swedish Society for Racial Hygiene was formed in 1909. These approaches to disease are very different from the individualist/secular concepts that form the basis of allopathic medical approaches, described above. Illness and disease in this paradigm are seen as consequences of malfunctions in the human organism that are produced by infections. Treatment is based on allopathic strategies that attempt to control these infections through medical interventions (for example, drugs, rest cure, or surgery). Health is improved by personal hygiene, isolation from germs and viruses, and the presence of a highly trained cohort of professional doctors with the support system of universities, medical faculties, and general hospitals. Within this individualistic and specialized context, private health insurance is a crucial responsibility of patients if they want effective responses to their acute conditions. By contrast, some argue socialized medical health encourages a lack of responsibility on the part of the individual and increases the burden of the 'undeserving poor' on the taxpayer and the state. Socialized medicine in the American context was regarded as a political threat to the fundamental values of individualism (Porter 1997). In terms of social Darwinism, the survival of the fittest was the only safe guide to public policy.

Medical paradigms, which operate on the basis of a religious belief system and from an individualistic perspective, include the ascetic practices of monastic religious orders, where diet and abstinence were thought to be simultaneously beneficial to soul and body. Illness was linked to the fundamentally evil nature of fallen man in creation, but human beings were exhorted to strive against evil through a 'government of the body' (Turner 1992). Such medico-religious paradigms can also assume more collectivist forms. Taboos attempt to regulate human behavior in the interests of society as a whole, because individuals who disregard ritualistic prohibitions bring misfortune and disease upon the whole community. Shamanistic medical rituals are illustrations of this sacred and collectivist orientation.

I propose that in Western societies there has been a historical trend, starting with the scientific revolution in the late sixteenth and early seventeenth centuries, away from collectivist/sacred conceptions towards individualistic/profane perspectives, which parallels the rise of scientific professional medicine. However, this dominant paradigm is constantly challenged by both collectivist/secular social medicine and by alternative medical paradigms that draw upon various religious legacies. For both the individual and society, various paradigms can exist simultaneously. For example, it is not uncommon to find that a person with cancer may seek out both chemotherapy and homeopathy in a desperate attempt to find a cure.

'Traditional' Medical Systems

In traditional, non-literate, and small-scale societies, disease is symbolic of the relationships between the sacred and the profane world.

Diagnosis and healing are both undertaken within a sacred context. According to Émile Durkheim in *The Elementary Forms of Religious Life* (2001), the belief systems of so-called 'primitive' society were based on a profound dichotomy between the everyday world of practical utilitarian activities and the sacred world, which is organized around religious phenomena that are set apart and forbidden. Human illness and disease provide a bridge between these two worlds because sacred values are revealed to humans via the extraordinary states of consciousness, which are associated with disease. Hence, according to Henry E. Sigerist (1951: 127):

> the primitive does not distinguish between medicine, magic and religion. To him they are one, a set of practices intended to protect him against evil forces. Spirits inhabit the objects of his environment. The ghosts of the dead are hovering over the village. The transcendental world is real to him, and he partakes in it when he dreams and his soul leaves the body temporarily and has intercourse with the spirits.

While Sigerist's summary is still valuable, there are real limitations to this account. First, as Sigerist acknowledged, even in pre-modern society there was, alongside the religious belief system, a realm of practical medical interventions based on experience and experiment. For example, in ancient Egypt, which was already a complex society with a literate culture, Egyptian medicine combined a religious cosmology with an 'empirical-rational medicine.' This understanding of Egyptian medicine was revealed by research in 1922 by James H. Breasted of the so-called 'Papyrus Edwin Smith.' These documents show, among other things, that Egyptian court physicians relied on elementary diagnostic and prescriptive practices that were grounded in observations, case studies, and pragmatic responses to illness through the use of herbs, diets, bed rest, and other mundane approaches. It suggests that, while religious belief systems were important, physicians did not confuse religious meaning with mundane medical interventions (Zucconi 2006).

Similar conclusions can be drawn from the extensive anthropological debate about magic, religion, and science. For example, Bronislaw Malinowski (1948) argued, based on his fieldwork, that Trobriand Islanders systematically distinguish between magic, which attempts to regulate the environment through ritual, and religion, which is an expression of belief. When Trobriand fishermen were involved in outer lagoon fishing – which was considered dangerous – they regularly resorted to magic. In these societies, magic functions to give some structure and predictability to uncertain and dangerous contexts. Religion, by contrast, is the cultural vehicle for general social values. Similar conclusions follow from the work of E. Evans-Pritchard (1937), whose fieldwork showed how human beings believe they are surrounded by risk and uncertainty threats that become the basis for witchcraft beliefs. These dangers are often the products of social conflicts and tensions, wherein accusations of witchcraft, for example, indicate interpersonal conflicts. Divination, which is important in explaining illness, has the important social function of allocating blame and responsibility. Thus, 'disease categories' function in a context of social uncertainty as explanations of misfortunate.

Greek Medicine

In Western philosophy, Greek civilization is often taken as the cradle, not only of democratic institutions, but also of natural science and rational inquiry. Certainly, Greek traditions played a major role in shaping medical ethics and practice. The notion of the Hippocratic Oath itself was fundamental to the evolution of professionalism in medical etiquette and practice. While the Greek tradition contained a mixture of rational scientific and religious perspectives and practices, generally speaking, Greek medicine represents a secular orientation to health and illness because health was seen as a consequence of natural causes. The humoral theory of disease, which survived into the modern period, was derived from the secular tradition of Empedocles, to whom the humoral theory is credited. The world was conceived in terms of four basic elements (fire, water, air, and earth), four qualities (hot, cold, dry, and damp), four humors (blood, phlegm, yellow bile, and black bile), and four personality types (sanguine, phlegmatic, choleric, and melancholic). In this humoral theory, the body was imagined as a hydraulic system in which illness represented a lack of balance (Turner 1996). For instance, melancholia was a consequence of an excess of black bile. Greek therapeutics consisted of bloodletting, diet, exercise, and bed rest, which were designed to restore the equilibrium of the system. In the Greek system, the reproductive processes that involved a sexual act were compared to a convulsion or fermentation; sex involved heating up the organism (Foucault 1986).

Aristotle (384–322 BCE) played a major role in the history of Western medicine in which he is often credited with the basic ideas of evidence-based medicine. For Aristotle, the humoral theory had to conform to both theory and observation. Aristotle sought to explain how the basic elements that constitute matter undergo change and to understand the body Aristotle performed animal dissections. Disequilibrium in the balance between the basic elements was the cause of disease. Aristotle's world view was secular and his influence was found throughout much of the history of scientific medicine in the West in the work of William Harvey (1578–1657).

When medical historians examine Aristotle's contributions to the rise of scientific medicine, they typically focus on Aristotle's contributions to biology especially the three volumes that were composed on the island of Lesbos: *History of Animals*, *Generations of Animals* and *Parts of Animals* (Modell 2010). A better understanding of Aristotle's views on medicine, politics and ethics comes via his discussion of *Eudaimonia* as an answer to questions about the purpose of human life. To grasp his argument, we need to uncover his basic question, namely, what is the measure of human excellence that defines humans as humans rather than as something else – the *ergon* of human beings? What separates us from animals? For Aristotle, in terms of sleep, nutrition and sexual intercourse, nothing separates us from animals. It is rather how we use or misuse our bodies that occasions moral praise or condemnation. As a result of this approach, happiness – the ultimate aim of all human life – is connected to purposeful activity directed at well-being. Virtuous activity in humans leading to happiness revolves around three criteria: being complete or final, self-sufficient, and choice-worthy. By considering the peculiar 'function' or *ergon* of the human being, he arrives at the preliminary definition of *Eudaimonia* as 'a certain activity of the soul in accord with complete virtue' (Aristotle 2011: 1102a5). He then further analyses the issue by taking up the question of how *Eudaimonia* is related to 'external goods' and chance. He concludes the first book, before moving on to a thorough analysis of various individual virtues, with the notion that, while the virtuous person is not beholden to chance, his happiness is. Keeping in mind that 'virtue' is connected to 'virility', human life is subject to chance events over which we have little or no control, but the virtuous citizen faces adversity with fortitude. Only at the end of life can we say that a citizen had enjoyed *Eudaimonia*.

These notions of balance also reflected the basic premise of Aristotle's ethics in which 'the good life' was one that avoided the excesses of both hedonism and asceticism. In these medical regimes, diet played an especially important role. The word *diaita* indicated a way of life, a regimentation or regime, or a government. Medical prescriptions for good living covered a variety of activities, including leisure, nutrition, lifestyle, and sexuality. These regimes were based on secular assumptions about medicine and the role of the physicians, who attempted to distinguish themselves from popular medicine, which included leech craft and magic. For example, the Hippocratic treatise on *The Sacred Disease* argued that epilepsy was not brought about by sacred causes, but could be understood within the naturalistic framework of the four humors.

Greek medical tradition also revealed the tension between an individualistic and a collectivist approach. René Dubos (1959) recalls the struggle between Hygeia and Asclepius. The former was associated with the virtues of a rational life in a pleasant and healthy environment. In Rome she was known as *Salus*, or general well-being, from which we derive notions like 'salubrious' and 'salutary.' Asclepius, the first physician, by contrast, did not teach wisdom as a response to illness, but found therapies in the study of plants and herbs. As the mythology of these figures evolved, Asclepius eventually appears as a self-confident young god in the company of two maidens – Hygeia from whom we derive the notion of hygiene, and Panakeia from whom we derive the concept of panacea. From these gods, a division in medicine developed that I define in terms of a collectivist (hygienic) approach and an individualistic (Asclepian) perspective. Hygeia points towards a communal and preventive approach that recommends a rational lifestyle in a salubrious environment, whereas Asclepius promotes an interventionist medicine that restores health by directly treating the ailments of an individual.

MEDICINE AND THE WORLD RELIGIONS

The Greek legacy of Galen (129–99 AD), Hippocrates (born 460 BCE), and Aristotle shaped medieval practice and laid the foundations for the emergence of secular medicine. Hippocrates, whose theory of medicine described the idea of crisis as the turning point in the process of an illness, held to a secular view of medicine. This Greek legacy often came to the West via the medium of the Abrahamic religions (Judaism, Christianity, and Islam). In the Abrahamic faiths, there was often a tension between the Greek legacy and prophetic monotheism grounded in revelation. Thus, early Christianity was a Hellenizing force whose language was Greek, but whose basic notions of man and God were Hebraic (O'Leary 1949). These tensions were also present in Christian responses to health and illness.

This Judeo-Christian legacy was deeply ambiguous with respect to the importance and role of secular ideas about health and illness. New Testament theology, especially St Paul's interpretation of that tradition, was based on assumptions about the punishment of the flesh. These attitudes were particularly prominent in the early Church's attitudes towards women and sexuality, where marriage was at best regarded as a necessary evil against the corrupting presence of sexual desire. We must also keep in mind that the early Church expected and hoped for the end of the world in a messianic system that predicted the Second Coming of Christ as an end to human suffering and sinfulness. Given the anticipation of the end of human history, there was no strong motivation to invest in either human society or individual happiness.

As the anticipation of the Second Coming largely disappeared in the official position of the Roman Church, there emerged a clear division between lay people who lived in the world (and experienced its sinfulness) and those (monks, nuns, and priests) who devoted their lives to God and His works. Hence, lay people married to reproduce, while religious people 'married' Jesus in order to obtain grace. This division of labor created a system of exchange whereby the charisma of grace, which was stored up in the Church and handed on to the religious, was transferred to the (sinful) laity through such means as baptism, communion, and confession. A metaphorical parallel developed between health and grace, in which the healing grace of the body of Christ, for example, was transferred to the people through the Eucharistic feast. This metaphorical exchange of gifts 'traded' on an etymological similarity between salvation and *salus* (salutation and health). Christianity came to adopt a model in which the religious were responsible for both the health of the body and the salvation of the soul.

The ascetic doctrines of Christianity treated the body as a means of human education through suffering. Disease and discomfort are inevitable in this world because the body, as the vessel of the soul, is corrupted by the Fall from Grace in the narrative of Adam's disobedience. However, through this suffering human beings can come, through humility and pain, to a better understanding of God and themselves. The lives of the saints revealed this ambiguity towards the sinfulness of human embodiment (Turner 1997a). Disease is a corruption that indicates the sinfulness of human kind, but also creates the occasions of insight and knowledge, with a characteristically ambiguous status. It could simultaneously indicate a charismatic status through divine election and indicate the sinfulness of the victim. These contradictions are summarized in Christian theology under the notion of theodicy, which is any attempt to explain and justify God as a merciful and all-powerful being, who loves and occasionally punishes human beings.

This ambiguity was characteristic of the Church's response to plagues and the control of epidemics. While the spread of plague was a sign of human sinfulness, religious institutions had an obligation to care for the sick and the poor. Christian houses for plague victims and leprosaria expressed this religious obligation through acts of charity. Medieval religious houses provided an institutional model of care from which evolved a secular means of poor relief and medical support. The word 'hospital' derives from the Latin adjective *hospitalis*, relating to *hospites* (guests). Early religious houses were 'hospices' (spitals) for pilgrims, and eventually evolved into hospitals in the modern sense. Between 1066 and 1550, 700 spitals were created in the British Isles, and spitals for leprosy emerged around 1078 as so-called 'lazar houses.' Leprosy declined after 1315 partly because of the Black Death (1346–50), which produced a profound crisis of theodicy in the West. Similar developments had taken place in the thirteenth century in the Islamic world, for example in the Divrigi Hospital in Baghdad.

Christian asceticism and the institutions of charity were both responses to this profound theological condemnation of the human body as flesh and as the conduit of evil into the soul (Turner 1991). Because the Fall of Man was blamed on the weakness of Eve, Christian theology was basically patriarchal, and its negative view of women was reinforced by the legacy of Greek philosophy and medicine. For example, Aristotle had noted that women may occasionally achieve orgasm, but their fluids were not seminal. The womb was simply a vehicle within which male sperm produced another human being. Greek medical manuals, which the Fathers of the Church inherited, were written to assist male fertilization and, by implication, control women's bodies. Christian patriarchy can be regarded as a continuation of the attitude of classical authors to women and reproduction in which Christianity contributed a more potent and far-reaching doctrine of sinfulness (Rousselle 1988). The mortification of the flesh by the female religious became a form of 'holy anorexia' by which the saints could paradoxically accept the patriarchal authority of the Church and at the same time assert their own spirituality (Bell 1985).

As the Roman Church became established as part of the dominant political institutions of the medieval period, sin became both regulated and commercialized by the practice of confession and indulgences. Both sinfulness and illness were treated within this network of monetary exchanges, whereby sinful lay people secured their salvation in the next world and health in this world.

This commercialization of the sacred was challenged by Luther and Calvin. The Reformation retained a conception of the total depravity of man and took away the conventional means of grace (baptism, eucharist, and confession) by which that sinfulness had been managed. The consequences of this emphasis on the individual, the authority of the written word, and the criticism of conventional religion produced both uncertainty and individualism, which contributed eventually to the rise of the seventeenth-century scientific revolution and the erosion of medieval notions of disease and depravity.

EMPIRICAL RATIONALISM AND THE GROWTH OF EXPERIMENTAL MEDICINE

In sociology, we are familiar with the argument that the ascetic and individualistic ethic of the Calvinistic sects had an 'elective affinity' with the emergent culture of competitive capitalism (Weber 2002). Alongside the growth of capitalism in the seventeenth century, the development of experimental medicine was founded on the rationalism of Descartes (1596–1650), and Newton (1643–1727) through the work of the physician Herman Boerhaave (1668–1738). Just as early capitalism assumed an individualistic and ascetic orientation, so the medical revolution of the seventeenth century assumed an individualistic, rational, and experimental ethos. There was an important convergence in values and practice between the religious Reformation and the scientific Renaissance, keeping in mind that contemporary historical analysis of the rise of science tends to dispute the notion of any simple 'disenchantment' of the world (Josephson-Storm 2017).

With regard to Newton's alleged 'scientific atheism,' modern research has shown how Newton was involved in alchemy and various esoteric societies (like the Rosicrucians) and held to metaphysical assumptions and presuppositions about the natural world (Figala 2004). More confidence can be placed in interpretations of Descartes and the foundations of modern experimental rationalism by attempting, through a thought experiment, to exclude religious and irrational dimensions from philosophy. His rationalism attempted to find a point of certainty that was beyond further doubt. His solution was the famous individualist slogan, 'I think, therefore I am.' The force of this claim is to give a primacy to cognitive rationalism over emotions and feelings, but it also gives a focus on individual truths. Furthermore, it establishes a foundation for the separation of mind and body, which characterized Western thought from the seventeenth century. Descartes was not entirely successful in establishing his own brand of rationalist philosophy in the universities, being replaced by an empirical philosophy that was probabilistic, mechanical, and Newtonian. Hence, by the end of the seventeenth century, rationalist medicine was neo-Newtonian. However, Cartesian rationalism as a system remained a profoundly influential doctrine whereby Cartesian secularism became a potent aspect of medical belief. It required a simple and complete separation between mind and body. Thus, Cartesian materialism was highly compatible with a mechanistic and materialist vision of reality.

Cartesian rationalism was combined with Newtonian physics in the quest for a mathematical system to express the laws that governed the processes of the human body. Physicians sought to create a medical system that would have the same elegance and simplicity as the Newtonian laws of gravity. In the seventeenth century, physicians such as Archibald Pitcairne (1652–1713) were part of a scientific network stretching from Edinburgh through Oxford to Leiden. This scientific network wanted to give medical theory mathematical precision (Guerrini 1989). The theory was referred to as 'principiia medicinae theoreticae mathematicae'; its influence was considerable. Newtonian mathematics became influential in the work of George Cheyne (1671–1743), whose publications on diet greatly influenced the eighteenth-century London elite (Turner 1992). Cheyne offered medical advice to the London coffeehouse elite who, like Cheyne, were often victims of obesity. For Cheyne, the principal causes of melancholy were connected with the excessive consumption of food, drink, and tobacco.

The iatromathematicians of the period interpreted God to a clock maker who was in a general way responsible for the functioning of the Newtonian universe, but who did not intervene through revelation into the lives of human beings. There was little space here for a compassionate Saviour on the cross. William Harvey (1578–1657) had discovered the principles of the circulation of the blood, validating the doctrine of circulation on Aristotelian and teleological grounds. His *De Circulatione* of 1649 gave further authority to this view of the human body as a mechanical pump whose flows and tides could be measured mathematically by exact calculation. The machine might need a soul to start the motor, but there was little room for a reflexive mind in this mechanical universe. We should not exaggerate the secular dimension of medical practice in the seventeenth century. Medical interventions were still typically set within a broader moral and religious framework. In prescribing a dietary regime to control the machine, Cheyne was following a long line of Christian physicians who sought to regulate the soul through a diet of the body. His views on a disciplined life to control the nerves appealed to John Wesley, the founder of Methodism, who, in his *Primitive Physick* of 1752, provided a methodical version of the medical regime. Also, the moral significance of the seventeenth-century anatomy lesson should not be underestimated. Comparative anatomy had always raised questions of conscience, because it was either thought to spy on God's secret principles of the universe, or it was thought to be a vain and pointless quest for ultimate causes. From a Christian point of view, if the body is merely flesh, can the anatomical inquiry reveal anything of God's purpose? Anatomy had, as a result, remained a conservative area of medical science, where it continued to be dominated by, for example, Galen's text *On the Conduct of Anatomy*. Anatomy began to change eventually with the work of Andreas Vesalius (1514–64) who, through experimentation on human beings, broke away from the scholastic conformity to the Galenic tradition.

In the seventeenth century, the anatomy lesson continued to function as a moral lesson. In the work of anatomists like Andreas Laurentius (1558–1609), the anatomy section encouraged the observer to 'know thyself' and to embrace the feeling that 'there, but for the grace of God, go I.' These sentiments are well illustrated in the famous 1632 painting by Rembrandt, 'The Anatomy Lesson of Dr Tulp,' which shows Dr Nicolaas Tulp in the Waaggebouw standing over the sectioned body of the criminal Aris Kint. The light and shadow employ the realism of Caravaggio, but the picture has many iconic features pointing to Christian truths about the frailty and finitude of humans. For example, behind the figure of Tulp there is on the wall behind the anatomy lesson a Christian symbol of the shell. Hence, the anatomy lesson continued to be part of a moral discourse about sinfulness and judgement within the new framework of scientific experiment, which stood at the core of the seventeenth-century scientific revolution.

MENTAL HEALTH AND THE PANOPTIC GAZE

In this chapter I am primarily concerned with concepts of physical health, but it is important to touch briefly on the issue of mental health. Contemporary sociological analysis of medical systems has been profoundly influenced by the work of Michel Foucault (1926–84), who contributed to the study of madness, French post-revolutionary medicine, the medical responses to sexual deviance, and the history of Christian attitudes to health and illness.

Foucault (1971) identified a break in the middle of the seventeenth century when large numbers of people were confined to detention in such places as the General Hospital in Paris. Because the definition of madness was broad and vague, detention functioned as a way of imposing government or regulations on the poor, needy, and incompetent. 'Madness' is seen by Foucault as a regulatory discourse for the management of large populations. A second break occurred in the eighteenth century when 'madness,' as an indefinite concept, began to give way to modern notions of 'mental illness.' Whereas madness, as in the notion of *folie* or foolishness in Shakespeare's King Lear, was historically associated with divine insight and creativity, mental illness became a technical discourse that overtly attempts to distance itself from more traditional notions of possession, violence, and creativity. In *folie*, reason and madness could communicate, but the modern notion of insanity has domesticated and neutralized the old forces of jest and foolishness. This new conception of mental illness required a new setting, and Foucault traced the evolution of psychiatry alongside the institutional growth of the modern asylum, which applied the principles of panoptic surveillance from Benthamite utilitarianism to the management of the mentally ill (Foucault 1977).

The point of Foucault's history of the categories of mental health was to criticize the dominant discourse of psychiatry, which analyzed the history of its own profession as the triumph of reason over witchcraft. Foucault noted that, as with medieval responses to witchcraft, psychiatry involved various forms of 'governmentality' to regulate individuals whose behavior was in various ways 'deviant.' Foucault's approach directed attention to the function of concepts of disease and illness as components of a larger system of social regulation. Although they used different assumptions and methods, there is some similarity between Foucault and Thomas Szasz (1961, 1970), who questioned the role of psychiatry in eroding individual and human rights. For Szasz, the differences between the liberal West and the communist East had been exaggerated because in both social systems medical practices, such as electroconvulsive therapy, could be used to control political dissidents. Foucault and Szasz and others in the social sciences of medicine raised fundamental questions about the alleged neutrality and reliability of scientific methods and concepts in the management of human affairs insofar as the medicalization of deviance removed the right of an individual to rational debate. The attempt to treat homosexuality as a mental disease is another illustration.

THE NINETEENTH CENTURY: THE STRUGGLE WITH INFECTION

Although the nineteenth century is seen in official histories of medicine as the great triumph of the scientific revolution, it also disguised a profound struggle between individualistic allopathic medicine and social medicine. At the core of this debate was, on the one hand, the great success in scientific responses to infection through such techniques as vaccination, and, on the other, the great social needs of the urban population and the growth in social science responses through, for example, the development of town planning. The classic illustration of these differing approaches is the historical conflict between human suffering and illness as the effects of environmental pollution and social degradation versus a medical response to the isolated individual via a theory of disease entities. These differences are particularly important in the historical analysis of such epidemics as tuberculosis (Szreter 1988). Were the major improvements in health a consequence of medical intervention to control disease through vaccination, or were the improvements in health a function of rising standards of living? The nineteenth century produced monumental social investigations into the conditions of the poor, which continue to influence contemporary social responses to health and illness.

Throughout Europe, there were major social attempts to control infections through the political manipulation of urban conditions to improve hygiene. For example, in the Netherlands from 1840 to 1890, the Hygienists were a group of medical practitioners who embraced the view that the health of the nation was determined by public health (Houwaart 1991). The Hygienists rejected attempts to centralize public health at the level of the state and supported some devolution of health care. The movement illustrates the fact that medical and political reform tend to go together, because the Hygienists were very much a product of the 1848 liberal revolutions, which were characteristic of Germany and France. In their medical views, they rejected assumptions about contagion and traditional methods of describing diseases by their external aspects, which characterized early nineteenth-century epidemiology. These concepts were focused on ontology. For the Hygienists, diseases were not entities that flourish and die following environmental changes, but rather were caused by anatomical and physiological relations in the body. Through their standardization of disease classification, they were able to collect more effective statistical evidence on morbidity and mortality. After 1850, they came to accept the *Bodentheorie* (ground or soil theory) of Max von Pettenkofer (1818–1901), the professor of hygiene, who claimed that epidemics were caused by soil pollution. His reputation was based on his analysis of the south German cholera epidemic of 1854. The cholera germ was a product of the soil, not the human intestine, and von Pettenkofer offered a technical solution, namely a reconstruction of urban water systems in order to regulate water levels. The *Bodentheorie* was well suited to the political culture of post-revolutionary Europe, because it implied a technical, rather than a political response to epidemics.

This illustration of public health in nineteenth-century Netherlands took place within the broader context of the debate about contagion. The notion that disease was passed from one person to another by infective organisms through contagion can be traced back to responses to pestilence in previous centuries. The author of Leviticus recognized that leprosy and gonorrhea were transmitted by contagion and had therefore to be quarantined – a name derived from *quarantina* or the 40-day period of isolation required of people entering Italian ports, who were thought to be infected by disease. The alternative view of epidemics was that they are caused by atmospheric influence or 'epidemic miasma.' Epidemics were thought to be caused by bad air – *mal aria*. Although the notion of miasma has long been discredited, it pointed to the role of poor living conditions and lack of hygiene as causes of illness. However, miasma as a theory was undermined in the nineteenth century by the discovery of the living organisms that produced many diseases. The theory of contagion by infective organisms also led, after much professional resistance, to the conclusion that disease was also spread by doctors from one patient to another. The work of Ignaz Semmelweis (1818–65), from the General Hospital in Vienna, in the 1860s was significant in the development of hygienic practices in the treatment of women during labor and delivery. Through observation, Simmelweis concluded that puerperal fever infection was spread by his own students from dead infective material. Cleanliness and hand washing in a solution of chloride of lime reduced mortality rates by more than 6 per cent. The scientific principles behind these practical procedures were eventually supplied by Joseph Lister, building on the tradition of Louis Pasteur and Robert Koch. These advances made possible a much safer environment for the practice of surgery and contributed to the containment of infections following hospitalization (Youngson 1979).

Despite the resistance of the medical profession to the scientific discoveries of Semmelweis and Lister, the advances in medical science made possible the growth of the medical profession as a 'learned profession' driven by the cutting-edge of scientific advance. It also contributed to the 'mirage of health' as a Utopia of modern consciousness.

THE TWENTIETH CENTURY: THE RISE OF THE MEDICAL FACULTY

The twentieth century was the context for radical changes in medicine. In these changes, one cannot separate transformations of the concepts of health and illness from the development of the role of professional medicine. Medical power and social knowledge are necessarily combined, and the transformation of the university curriculum indicates shifting balances in authority between different professional groups and institutions. The reform of the medical curriculum is an important guide to such changes. The triumph of allopathic, individualist, and secular medicine over social or environmental, and homeopathic medicine is symbolized by the publication of the Flexner Report on *Medical Education in the United States and Canada* in 1910. Abraham Flexner argued that scientific medicine required an intensive and protracted university-based training in the fundamental natural science curriculum. The immediate implication was that only wealthy students from the upper classes could engage in the lengthy university training necessary for professional entry into medical roles (Berliner 1984). This development had the effect of limiting the flow of Black students, women, and the working class into the medical faculty, and the recruitment of these groups into the profession showed no sign of improvement in North America until after 1970 (Mumford 1983).

The Flexner Report recognized and authorized the social dominance of a research-oriented scientific medicine in which the biological sciences, along with laboratory training, provide the foundation of medical understanding. Medicine was increasingly specialized in terms of its knowledge base, and there was a division of labor around the separate organs or functions of the body. The new breed of scientific doctors were specialists in the biological functioning of the human body.

This scientific corpus of medical knowledge was also associated with the evolution of the medical faculty within the university system as a separate, high-cost, research faculty with its own unique authority and eventual dominance over the academic board. Medical faculties were increasingly separate spatially and academically from the rest of the university. This physical separation reinforced the social solidarity of the medical faculty and effectively isolated the medical curriculum from other parts of the university. Specialization and sub-specialization intensified the technical aspects of the scientific discourse of medicine, which was later associated with the rapid growth of physiology and pharmacology (Perrin and Perrin 1984). These curriculum changes laid the foundation of the golden age of twentieth-century scientific medicine from 1910 to 1950, in which Flexnerian reforms were dominant in North America and Europe. The growing importance of the general hospital was also associated with the rising social status of medicine. Improvements in hygiene, sanitation, and nursing resulted in declining morbidity and mortality rates, thereby making hospitals safe for their middle-class clients. The growth of scientific medicine, the research medical faculty, and the evolution of the hospital were the principal factors in a distinctive period of medical professionalism, where the medical associations controlled entry into the medical occupational cluster (Larson 1977). There were eventually complementary processes of professionalism in dentistry, pharmacy, nursing, and many other para-professional groupings. These social changes ushered in the era of the medical-industrial complex

(Ehrenreich and Ehrenreich 1970) and fostered a new wave of social criticism directed at the negative consequences of the 'medicalization' of society and the growth of iatrogenic illness (Illich 2001).

Some analysts have argued that since the 1970s there has been a profound transformation of health-care systems associated with a decline in the centrality of professional medicine and its professional autonomy (Starr 1982). The decline of medical dominance has also been associated with the erosion of social security schemes and centralized welfare states, along with the commercialization of medical provision. As the insurance companies began to influence debates and policies about health funding, the professional autonomy of the medical profession became constrained. Governments have also turned to a mixture of preventive medicine, third-sector finance, and public health policies to support self-regulation. These economic and political crises in health care are closely related to the greying of the population and the spiraling cost of health care. These political and economic changes have focused the attention of medical sociologists on what Foucault called 'governmentality' (Turner 1997b).

THE GREYING OF THE WEST

By the second half of the twentieth century, there was a general agreement that the great epoch of infectious disease had come to an end. Medical historians and epidemiologists like McKeown (1979) could argue that the infectious scourges of the previous century (tuberculosis, measles, whooping cough, and venereal disease) had virtually disappeared with improvements in housing, water supply, food, and education. McKeown's thesis demonstrated the importance of environmental and social causes in the decline of mortality rates, especially among children. Tuberculosis was declining steadily from the 1830s before the use of bacillus Calmette-Guerin vaccination and the introduction of drug treatment like streptomycin in 1944, paraminosalicylic acid in 1946, and isoniazid in 1952. The drug treatment of TB had a profound effect on mortality rates. Whereas 900 girls died from TB in England and Wales in 1946, only nine died in 1961. These improvements, according to McKeown, were the consequences of socio-economic improvements that enhanced the general health status of the population.

Social inequality and poverty are now regarded as major determinants of individual health, with marked differences in morbidity and mortality among social classes, as demonstrated in Great Britain by the publication of the Black Report (Townsend and Davidson 1982). Social medicine, as a result, has often been closely connected with political radicalism, because it has concluded that poverty causes illness, and therefore the remedy has to be sought in social change, if necessary, of a revolutionary character. In Great Britain, the new discipline of social medicine was advanced by radicals like John Ryle, who in 1942 became the first professor of social medicine (Porter 1997). In North America, the debate about the social causes of illness and disease was promoted by medical sociologists like Howard Waitzkin, who explored the notion of 'the second sickness' – a disease of the body produced by social injustice (Waitzkin 1983; Waitzkin and Waterman 1974)

Demographic change has been among the most important forms of social change in the twentieth century. In response to public anxiety about over population, the modern theory of population was originally developed by Warren Thompson (1929) and Kingsley Davis (1945), who described the process as a 'demographic transition.' The lag between declining death rates and birth rates explained population growth. This simple model of one demographic transition was later abandoned as demographers came to realize that the so-called demographic transition set in motion a series of transformations of family life, household composition, age structure, and the urban environment. It is now possible to consider a second demographic transition when population does not achieve an equilibrium. Instead, fertility rates are now critically low and many governments are confronted by declining and ageing populations that are resistant to policy interventions. Many societies in Europe and Asia are now faced by a demographic crisis as they fall well below the Total Fertility Rate of 2.2 live births. Low fertility presents many advanced societies with specific economic and political problems that are now compounded by ageing in which a life expectancy in the high 70s is not unusual.

As Western societies became more affluent, geriatric illnesses like diabetes came to dominate the demography of advanced societies. In terms of social knowledge, these changes were accompanied by the rise of social gerontology, which remains an incoherent domain of theory relating to both individual and cohort ageing (Green 1993). The greying of the population has also given rise to a general debate about the effects of age dependency on the capacity of societies to provide care for the elderly. The new social gerontology has begun to chronicle a wide range of new infirmities and misfortunes waiting for human beings who have successfully survived into later life, in particular Alzheimer's disease, which is present in 20 per cent of the population over age 85.

Although geriatric illness has not enjoyed the same status as heroic medical intervention in acute diseases, there has been considerable interest in a range of degenerative conditions. For example, there has been a medicalization of 'women's complaints,' especially menopause. The existence and consequences of premenstrual tension, the universality of menopause, and the existence of the sexual drive in old age are extensively debated. Some anthropologists have denied that menopause is universal, claiming that maturation for women in many societies, including Japan, is not accompanied by hot flushes, tension, and irritability (Lock 1993). Medical responses to the menopause, like estrogen replacement therapy, have been equally controversial, with accusations that similar ageing processes in men have been ignored or neglected. Indeed, many men's activist groups argue that, given the political importance of feminism, men's diseases like prostate cancer have been neglected. Prostate cancer is the second leading cause of death from cancer for older men in the United States.

The greying of the population in the United States, where in 2010 more than 16 per cent were over age 62 (United States Census Bureau 2011), has resulted in important political conflicts over illness categories. With medicalization, there is a tendency to treat ageing as a disease which, with profound medical interventions (cosmetic surgery, hormone replacement therapy, organ transplants, and coronary bypass surgery), can be partially arrested. While the rich and famous have attempted to deny ageing and death, mainstream grey politics have challenged the assumption that immobility, memory loss, and an erosion of libidinal interest are inevitable consequences of ageing (Friedan 1993).

By the 1970s it was assumed that the conquest of disease in Western societies would require the development of drugs that would delay or manage old age. As medical attention moved from acute to chronic diseases, preventive medicine and health education would contribute to the containment of diabetes and heart disease. This complacency was shattered in the 1980s by the emergence of the HIV/AIDS epidemic, which was first reported in 1979–80 and which spread rapidly among the homosexual communities of North America, Europe, and Australia. The epidemic has, and will have, a major economic impact on Third World societies and in those communities (like societies with a significant element of Islamic fundamentalism) that refuse to recognize the presence of HIV-positive communities in their midst.

The virus was eventually reported in 130 countries and carried by millions. In North

America, it was originally confined to the homosexual communities of the West Coast and New York. In Australia, approximately 80 per cent of new cases were reported in Sydney, the gay capital of the continent. However, the virus spread to heterosexual couples and to hypodermic drug users who failed to observe the necessary etiquette of not sharing needles. The epidemic often gave rise to hostile moral condemnation of gay men, demonstrating once more the intimate connection between medical and moral discourses.

I refer to the HIV/AIDS phenomenon as an 'epidemic' partly to indicate its complexity. One does not die of AIDS but from the cluster of conditions (like pneumonia) to which it gives occasion. AIDS is a medical condition that promotes a spectrum of illnesses and discomforts, so the categorization of AIDS requires other opportunistic infections. The constellation of signs and symptoms in the context of HIV infection is termed the AIDS-related complex or ARC. In short, AIDS is socially constructed of the multiplicity of illnesses and malignancies that opportunistically flourish within a depleted immune system. Given the complexity of the condition, it is not surprising that a wealth of social metaphors also opportunistically multiplied. Susan Sontag (1989) suggests that AIDS shares with medieval plagues the notion of an invasion, but it is also organized around notions of pollution resulting from personal perversity.

Sexually transmitted diseases have forced society to rethink policies towards infectious disease, but they also demonstrated once more that medical understanding can never be easily separated from moral assumptions about normal behavior. AIDS has also indicated that the future development of human health will inevitably and inextricably be part of a more general process of cultural globalization. In previous centuries, while plagues and epidemics were spread by migration and trade in the world, diseases were somewhat specific to geographical niches. With the growth of world tourism and trade, the global risk of infectious disease has spread rapidly. Influenza epidemics now spread almost instantaneously. There is widespread anxiety about the development of a variety of new conditions that are difficult to diagnose and to classify, complex in their functions and diffusion, and resistant to rapid or conventional treatments. The list of such conditions includes the eruption of newly discovered diseases like hantavirus, the migration of diseases to new areas (like cholera in Latin America), diseases produced by new technologies (like toxic shock syndrome and Legionnaires' Disease), and diseases transmitted from animals to humans. These problems have, along with ebola, Marburg virus, Lassa fever, and swine flu, generated a concern for 'the coming plague' (Garrett 1995). This concern was borne out in early 2020 by the arrival of the COVID-19 pandemic.

These fears have been associated with the perception that we now face a new generation of hazards and risks that arise from the global pollution of the atmosphere and the environment. These global hazards gave rise to a new theory of society in the work of Ulrich Beck (1992), who argued that with modernization we have moved into an uncertain and precarious social condition called the 'risk society.' As society becomes more sophisticated, the potential risks from scientific experiments increase, especially where medical innovations are inadequately regulated. Indeed, as societies become more deregulated and subject to market discipline, the scale of risks and hazards increases. Many critical commentators claim that the damage from the thalidomide drug, the spread of 'mad cow disease,' and the speculation surrounding the causes of Creutzfeldt Jacob's Disease (CJD) are evidence of the arrival of a risk society where medical interventions and experimentations are increasingly out of control.

The contemporary opioid epidemic in the United States and beyond represents an even greater crisis in terms of addiction, treatment and mortality (Alexander, Frattarolis, and

Gielen, 2017). In the 1990s the pharmaceutical companies argued that patients would not become addicted to opioid painkillers and, as a result, health-care workers prescribed them at a higher rate. By 2017 opioid addiction was identified by HHS (Health and Human Services) as a public health emergency with 130 people dying per day as a consequence of opioid addiction. Misuse and overdosing are common problems as 2.1 million people now have an opioid use disorder. The social groups who are affected by opioid abuse are diverse: people living in rural communities, Native Americans, the working class and teenagers. Whereas heroin users are typically stigmatized, opioid addiction is less subject to moral criticism. Opioids have had an impact on sporting communities, where sports injuries were regularly treated with such painkillers, which unwittingly resulted in addiction. Education, treatment, and control of such a diverse community of victims are difficult and expensive.

CONCLUSION: THE PHILOSOPHY OF MEDICAL SCIENCE

Providing a history of medical concepts automatically raises questions about the ontological character of disease states; to indicate that any phenomenon has a history is to imply a relativistic view of reality. In this chapter, I traced, through a heuristic typology of disease concepts, the broad parameters of medical change in Western societies. In so doing, I have taken for granted a range of analytical issues concerning disease. It would be important in a more detailed approach to distinguish carefully among the experiences of sickness, the social behavior patterns associated with disease, the social roles that people are expected to perform in such circumstances, and the disease categories by which medical science describes a range of physical and mental malfunctions. In this history of concepts of health and illness, I have been primarily concerned with expert systems of knowledge and belief.

Medical sociology has often embraced 'social constructionism' as a platform for its research. This perspective is said to entail three dimensions. First, the meanings of social reality are neither fixed nor intrinsic, but rather they are the product of human interaction. The meanings of social reality emerge out of the constant flux of social exchange. Second, these meanings can never be taken for granted because they are constantly contested in everyday interactions. Third, human beings are self-reflexive about these meanings and constantly intervene to discuss and to change them (Levine 1992: 186). Such a perspective has been useful in studying the processes by and through which patients and doctors negotiate the meaning or significance of illness. This perspective also goes on to argue that the meanings of illness at the microsocial level are also conditioned by, and impact upon, the more general systems that surround health and illness concepts. At this general level, concepts of health and wellbeing become inextricably connected to fundamental notions of self-identity (Herzlich and Pierret 1987).

Although from a sociological point of view this constructionist argument is persuasive, it is in many respects a limited view of scientific beliefs. A critic of this orientation might argue that, while lay beliefs and everyday assumptions about health and illness are indeed the products of everyday experiences of being sick, the clinical categories of disease that arise from close scientific inspection and doctors' observations of symptoms are not socially constructed and do not change significantly over time. One version of this argument would be to claim that some concepts of disease are more socially constructed than others (Turner 1992: 106). What people say or believe about a disease changes over time, but the clinical condition itself is relatively timeless. Thus, Ilza Veith (1981: 222) claims that Hippocrates' clinical description of mumps could easily be identified and confirmed by a contemporary general practitioner; she argues that 'what is unchanged is disease. What did change, however, is the way in which disease was looked upon.' Our understanding of this contrast can be facilitated by Lester King (1982: 149), who suggests a useful distinction between a clinical entity and a disease entity. A clinical entity (from *kline* or bed) is a configuration or pattern that is observed by a doctor in (a bedside) interaction with a patient. The concept is thus linked to the practice of medicine. A disease entity is 'knowledge about' a condition that is produced by doctors' observations, statistical information, and laboratory tests. As a disease entity becomes scientifically established, it may well radically alter a clinical identity. Any textbook of medicine is, in essence, a collection of theories of disease entities. Thus, if we compare Thomas Sydenham's seventeenth-century description of puerperal fever with Hippocrates' description, we find a remarkable convergence. What is being described (the clinical condition of the fever) is relatively constant, but the theory behind the description has changed considerably. Theories change over time, because they are produced by changes in domain assumptions, the reorganization of university curricula, professional competition between scientists, new discoveries from laboratory trials, and so forth.

It is not contradictory, therefore, to hold both that there is a clinical reality (fever or mumps) which is captured in the 'classic descriptions of disease' that doctors handed down over the centuries (King 1982: 152), and that theories and concepts of health and illness vary considerably over time, being influenced by general social values, fashion, and changing social circumstances. It is in the strong program of the sociology of knowledge and in the social studies of science tradition that one finds research that attempts to demonstrate that these fundamental concepts of science are socially produced. However, clinical entities are also socially produced by the fact that, for example, doctors are trained to recognize the signs and symptoms that announce the presence of fever or mumps. To say that fever is socially produced is not to say that it is a 'fiction,' or that it does not exist, or that it could be conjured up by the doctor as a magician pulls a rabbit from a hat. However, the signs and symptoms of fever in a clinical setting are mediated through and by the experiences and training of physicians, and these physicians are the products of specific and local medical cultures.

From a social science perspective, we can summarize the principal issues in contemporary understandings of the concepts of health and illness in the following manner. Regardless of the epistemological difficulties surrounding the notion of disease entities, there is widespread agreement that conceptions of disease have changed radically. It is no longer accepted that there is a universal taxonomy of disease or that medical categories are neutral. The general theories of health and illness that explain the medical condition of humanity are shaped and organized around the dominant ideologies and beliefs of a culture (its domain assumptions). Medical categories are not neutral, because they typically carry and house the metaphors of a society by which praise and blame are allocated. In addition, the nineteenth-century search for the specific etiologies of every disease, in which each disease has its own cause, has been abandoned. Disease is now seen to have multiple, interactive causes and therefore no simple single cure is possible or desirable. As we have seen, the AIDS epidemic is a good illustration of this complexity. In this respect, Bachelard, Canguilhem, and Foucault have influenced social science approaches that generally accept some version of the argument that sciences develop through revolutionary paradigm shifts, and that scientific theories are socially constructed.

At the everyday level, social experiences of illness are equally shaped and constructed by cultural assumptions and social relationships. At this level of lay beliefs, there is a continuing tendency to see illness experiences within a moral framework of blame and responsibility, a framework that attempts to help individuals, in a predominantly secular environment, to answer questions about life and death. The growing literature, both lay and professional, on death and dying is one indication of the fact that despite, or because of, the erosion of the authority of traditional religious institutions, rituals, and beliefs, ordinary individuals need to find some meaning for the seemingly trivial nature of the passage from birth to the grave (Nuland 1994).

Finally, I have also claimed that medical understanding of disease and illness needs to be considered within the broader parameters of well-being and happiness or *Eudaimonia*. Empirical science might well argue that happiness is too vague and subjective to be a valuable concept. However, happiness studies have flourished in psychology and many governments now have gross domestic happiness as a criterion of social and political success. Happiness was a basic idea of utilitarianism in the assumption that the aim of any liberal government would be to secure the greatest happiness of the greatest number. While nineteenth-century utilitarianism may have gone out of favor, consequentialism remains a potent measure of successful or unsuccessful societies. Consequentialism is normally applied to the behavior of individuals, but it is a highly relevant measure of government success or failure. Unlike deaths from sexually transmitted disease, the opioid epidemic is a serious indictment of pharmaceutical industry and the unintended effects of its use. *Eudaimonia* or human well-being offers us a valuable measure of the success or otherwise of medical science and its implementation.

REFERENCES

Alexander, G.C., Frattaroli, S, and Gielen, A.C. (2015) *The prescription opioid epidemic; an evidence-based approach*. Baltimore: Johns Hopkins Bloomberg School of Public Health.

Aristotle (2011) *Nicomachian Ethics*. A new translation by Robert C. Bartlett and Susan D. Collins. Chicago, IL and London: University of Chicago Press.

Beck, U. (1992) *Risk Society: Towards a New Modernity*. London: Sage.

Bell, R.M. (1985) *Holy Anorexia*. Chicago, IL and London: University of Chicago Press.

Berliner, H.S. (1984) 'Scientific medicine since Flexner', in J.W. Salmon (ed.), *Alternative Medicine, Popular and Policy Perspectives*. London: Tavistock, pp. 30–56.

Brosnan, C., and Turner, B.S. (eds.) (2009) *Handbook of the Sociology of Medical Education*. London: Routledge.

Cockerham, W.C. (2005) 'Health lifestyle theory and the convergence of agency and structure'. *Journal of Health and Social Behavior* 46(1): 51–67.

Cunningham, A. (1997) *The Anatomical Renaissance: The Resurrection of the Anatomical Projects of the Ancients*. Aldershot: Scolar Press.

Davis, K. (1945) 'The world demographic transition'. *Annals of the American Academy Political and Social Science* 237(January): 1–11.

Douglas, M. (1966) *Purity and Danger: An Analysis of Concepts of Pollution and Taboo*. London: Routledge & Kegan Paul. http://dx.doi.org/10.4324/9780203361832

Dubos, R. (1959) *Mirage of Health: Utopias, Progress and Biological Change*. London: George Allen & Unwin.

Durkheim, E. (2001) *The Elementary Forms of Religious Life*. A new translation by Carol Cosman. New York: Oxford University Press.

Ehrenreich, B., and Ehrenreich, J. (1970) *The American Health Empire: Power, Profits and Policies*. New York: Random House.

Evans-Pritchard, E.E. (1937) *Witchcraft Oracles and Magic among the Azande*. Oxford: Oxford University Press.

Fee, E., and Brown, T.M. (eds) (1997) *Making Medical History: The Life and Times of Henry E. Sigerist*. Baltimore, MD and London: The Johns Hopkins University Press.

Figala, K. (2004) 'Newton's Alchemy', in I.B. Cohen and G.E. Smith (eds), *The Cambridge Companion to Newton*. Cambridge: Cambridge University Press, pp. 370–386.

Flexner, A. (1910) *Medical Education in the United States and Canada,* New York: Carnegie Foundation, Bulletin No.4.

Flint, V.J. (1989) 'The early medieval "Medicus," the saint – and the enchanter'. *Social History of Medicine* 2(2): 127–46. http://dx.doi.org/10.1093/shm/2.2.127

Foucault, M. (1971) *Madness and Civilization*. London: Tavistock.

Foucault, M. (1977) *Discipline and Punish: The Birth of the Prison*. London: Tavistock.

Foucault, M. (1986) *The Care of the Self*. New York: Random House.

Friedan, B. (1993) *The Fountain of Age*. New York: Simon & Schuster.

Gallie, W.B. (1956) 'Essentially contested concepts'. *Proceedings of the Aristotelian Society* 56: 167–98.

Garrett, I. (1995) *The Coming Plague: Newly Emerging Diseases in a World Out of Balance*. London: Virago.

Giordan, Giuseppe, and Possamai, Adam (2018) *Sociology of Exorcism in Late Modernity*. Basingstoke, UK: Palgrave Macmillan.

Green, B.S. (1993) *Gerontology and the Construction of Old Age: A Study in Discourse Analysis*. New York: Aldine de Gruyter.

Guerrini, A. (1989) 'Isaac Newton, George Cheyne and the "Principia Medicinae"', in R. French and A. Weir (eds), *The Medical Revolution of the Seventeenth Century*. Cambridge: Cambridge University Press, pp. 222–45. http://dx.doi.org/10.1017/CBO9780511897078.009

Harvey, D. (2007) *A Brief History of Neoliberalism*. New York: Oxford University Press.

Hepworth, M., and Turner, B.S. (1982) *Confession: Studies in Deviance and Religion*. London: Routledge & Kegan Paul.

Herzlich, C., and Pierret, J. (1987) *Illness and Self in Society*. Baltimore, MD and London: The Johns Hopkins University Press.

Houwaart, E.S. (1991) *De hygienisten: Arisen, staaat and volksgezondheid in Nederland 1840–1890*. Groningen: Historische Uitgeverij.

Illich, I. (1976) *Medical Nemesis: The Expropriation of Health*. New York: Random House.

Illich (2001) *London Marion Boyars*.

Josephson-Storm, J.A. (2017) *The Myth of Disenchantment: Magic, Modernity and the Birth of the Human Sciences*. Chicago, IL: University of Chicago Press.

King, L.S. (1982) *Medical Thinking: A Historical Preface*. Princeton, NJ: Princeton University Press.

Larson, M.S. (1977) *The Rise of Professionalism: A Sociological Analysis*. Berkeley, CA: University of California Press.

Levine, M.P. (1992) 'The implications of the constructionist theory for social research on the AIDS epidemic among gay men', in G. Herdt, and S. Lindenbaum (eds), *The Time of AIDS: Social Analysis, Theory and Methods*. Newbury Park, CA: Sage, pp. 185–98.

Lock, M. (1993) *Encounters with Aging: Mythologies of Menopause in Japan and North America*. Berkeley, CA: University of California Press.

Luzzatto, Sergio (2010) *Padre Pio: Miracles and Politics in a Secular Age*. New York: Metropolitan Books.

Malinowski, B. (1948) *Magic, Science and Religion and Other Essays*. Glencoe, IL: Free Press.

McKeown, T. (1979) *The Role of Medicine: Dream, Mirage or Nemesis?* Oxford: Basil Blackwell.

Modell, S.M. (2010) 'Aristotelian influence in the formation of medical theory'. *The European Legacy* 15(4): 409–24.

Mumford, E. (1983) *Medical Sociology: Patients, Providers and Policies*. New York: Random House.

Navarro, V. (1976) *Medicine under Capitalism*. New York: Prodist.

Nuland, S.B. (1994) *How We Die*. London: Random House.

O'Leary, D.L. (1949) *How Greek Science Passed to the Arabs*. London: Routledge & Kegan Paul.

Perrin, E.C., and Perrin, J.M. (1984) 'Anti-intellectual trends and traditions in academic medicine', in W.A. Powell and R. Robbins (eds), *Conflict and Consensus: A Festschrift in Honor of Lewis A. Coser*. London: Collier-Macmillan, pp. 313–26.

Pinker, Steven (2018) *Enlightenment Now: The Case for Reason, Science, Humanism and Progress*. London: Allen Lane.

Porter, D. (ed.) (1997) *Social Medicine and Medical Sociology in the Twentieth Century*. Amsterdam: Rodopi.

Rousselle, A. (1988) *Porneia: On Desire and the Body in Antiquity*. Oxford: Basil Blackwell.

Sigerist, H.E. (1951) *A History of Medicine* (Vol. 1). Oxford: Oxford University Press.

Sontag, S. (1978) *Illness as Metaphor*. New York: Vintage.

Sontag, S. (1989) *AIDS and its Metaphors*. London: Allen Lane.

Starr, P. (1982) *The Social Transformation of American Medicine*. New York: Basic Books.

Szasz, T. (1961) *The Myth of Mental Illness*. London: Paladin.

Szasz, T. (1970) *The Manufacture of Madness*. New York: Harper & Row.

Szreter, S. (1988) 'The importance of social intervention in Britain's mortality decline c. 1850–1914: a reinterpretation of the role of public health'. *Social History of Medicine* 1(1): 1–37. http://dx.doi.org/10.1093/shm/1.1.1

Thompson, W. (1929) 'Population'. *American Journal of Sociology* 34(6): 959–75.

Townsend, P., and Davidson, N. (1982) *Inequalities in Health*. Harmondsworth: Pelican Books.

Turner, B.S. (1991) *Religion and Social Theory* (2nd edition). London: Sage.

Turner, B.S. (1992) *Regulating Bodies: Essays in Medical Sociology*. London: Routledge. http://dx.doi.org/10.4324/9780203214183

Turner, B.S. (1995) *Medical Power and Social Knowledge* (2nd edition). London: Sage. http://dx.doi.org/10.4135/9781446250426

Turner, B.S. (1996) *The Body and Society* (2nd edition). London: Sage. http://dx.doi.org/10.4135/9781446214329

Turner, B.S. (1997a) 'The body in Western society: social theory and its perspectives', in S. Coakley (ed.), *Religion and the Body*. Cambridge: Cambridge University Press, pp. 15–41.

Turner, B.S. (1997b) 'From governmentality to risk: some reflections on Foucault's contribution to medical sociology', in A. Petersen and Robin Bunton (eds), *Foucault, Health and Medicine*. London: Routledge, pp. ix–xxi.

United States Census Bureau (2011) *Age and Sex Composition: 2010*. Washington, DC: US Department of Commerce.

Veith, I. (1981) 'Historical reflections on the changing concepts of disease', in A.L. Caplan, H.T. Engelhardt, and J.J. McCartney (eds), *Concepts of Health and Disease: Interdisciplinary Perspectives*. London: Addison-Wesley, pp. 221–30.

Waitzkin, H. (1983) *The Second Sickness: Contradictions of Capitalist Health Care*. New York: Free Press.

Waitzkin, H., and Waterman, B. (1974) *The Exploitation of Illness in Capitalist Society*. Indianapolis, IN: Bobbs-Merrill.

Weber, M. (2002) *The Protestant Ethic and the Spirit of Capitalism*. A new translation by Stephen Kalberg. Los Angeles, CA: Roxbury Publishing.

Weindling, P. (1989) *Health Race and German Politics between National Unification and Nazism, 1870–1945*. Cambridge: Cambridge University Press.

Youngson, A.J. (1979) *The Scientific Revolution in Victorian Medicine*. Canberra: Australian National University Press.

Zucconi, Laura M. (2006) 'Medicine and religion in Ancient Egypt'. *Religion Compass* 1(1): 26–37.

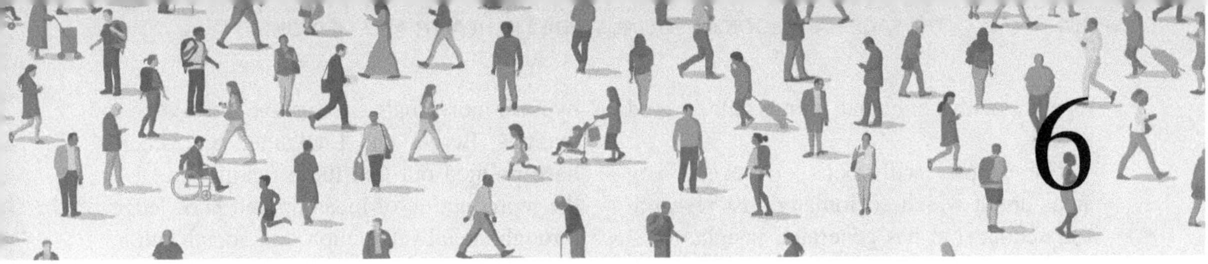

6

The Sociomaterial Nature of the Body and Medicine

Deborah Lupton

INTRODUCTION

This chapter examines the sociomaterial nature of ideas, knowledge, practices and experiences of health and medicine in Western societies, using an interdisciplinary approach. The central argument of the chapter is that health, illness and disease, and health care may all be viewed as more-than-human phenomena that bring together human bodies with nonhuman actors and objects in assemblages that are constantly changing. It is therefore important not only to analyze the nature of their social and cultural representation and the symbolic meanings that surround them, but also the practices, other living things, items and places/spaces in and with which health- and medical-related experiences are generated. Such an approach is important because it can elucidate the lived experience of health, illness and healthcare, highlighting the material and embodied dimensions of what it is like to engage in practices to protect or improve health and experience illness or medical treatment from the layperson's standpoint.

In addressing these issues, the perspectives of sociomaterialist theory and research are employed. Sociomaterialism is a term used to describe a range of theoretical perspectives developed over the past few decades in social and cultural theory. The term encompasses work undertaken in such theoretical approaches as new materialisms, affect theory, actor-network theory, assemblage theory, science and technology studies, environmental humanities, and critical posthumanities. These perspectives draw on and develop the work of a range of theorists, including Spinoza, Foucault, Deleuze and Guattari, Latour, Haraway, and Barad. Sociomaterialism builds on social constructionist approaches to health and medicine, but with greater emphasis on people's embodied practices and engagements with things. The concept of assemblage is often employed in sociomaterialism theory to denote the gatherings that eventuate when humans come together with nonhuman things, places and spaces.

The chapter will focus on several key areas about which sociomaterialist research and scholarship has generated insights concerning the nature of human embodiment in relation to health and medicine, thus serving to illustrate the epistemological and methodological tenets of this approach. The term embodiment is used here to describe the daily lived experience for humans of both having a body and being a body. Humans perceive the world as embodied subjects with particular arrangements of limbs, sensory organs, capacity for memory, vulnerability to disease, and so on. All knowledge is therefore developed through the body as it relates to other human bodies, other living creatures and with non-living things, including medical and digital technologies (Csordas 1990; Leder 1992; Merleau-Ponty 1962). From a sociomaterialist perspective, our identities are interbound with the dynamic processes of embodiment in the context of more-than-human worlds, including incidents of pain, illness, disease and medical care.

FOUNDATIONS OF SOCIOMATERIALISM

The social constructionist perspective as applied to analyzing health, illness, and medicine was initially strongly influenced by writers on phenomenology, cultural anthropology, and the sociology of knowledge who addressed the questions of how shared notions of reality are created through acculturation and social relationships. The work of Berger and Luckmann (1967) on the social nature of knowledge and its role in constituting reality and social life has been particularly influential for social constructionism in sociology. They argued that humans and their social world exist in a dialectical relationship in which each creates the other. Although the material and social worlds are experienced by most individuals as objective, pre-existing realities, Berger and Luckmann and others have pointed out that these realities involve the reproduction of meaning and knowledge through social interaction and socialization, and rely upon shared definitions. They emphasize that because of the continually constructed nature of reality, its meanings are precarious and subject to change.

Many of the more recent scholars taking a social constructionist approach have drawn upon the work of poststructuralist theorists, particularly the writings of Foucault on power, knowledge, practice and discourse. Poststructuralism builds upon the earlier work of writers like Berger and Luckmann. Poststructuralism sees the social world, knowledge, meanings, practices and notions of reality as contingent and dynamic rather than fixed. It draws particular attention to the role played by language and action in constituting notions of reality, including our understanding and experience of embodiment. The concept of discourse brings together language, visual representation, practice, knowledge, and power relations, incorporating the understanding that language and visual imagery are implicated with power relations and the construction of knowledge and practices about phenomena. The concept is commonly used in poststructuralist writings to denote the patterns of ways of thinking, making sense of, talking or writing about, and visually portraying phenomena such as the human body, medical and nursing practices, sexuality and reproduction, illness, disease, and death.

From the poststructuralist perspective, discourse is viewed as a form of social practice; a mode of action as well as a mode of representation (Fairclough 1992: 63). Cultural analysts adopting a poststructuralist perspective argue that there is an inescapable relationship between power, knowledge, discourse, and what counts as 'truth.' Discourses are both delimiting, structuring what it is possible to say, do or even think, and productive, generating new ways of thinking and acting. Discourses bring into being, make visible, render malleable, useful, functional, or dysfunctional, and differentiate between various types of bodies. For some theorists, the human body itself is seen as a text that is 'written' upon by discourses and practices. This is a dynamic and synergistic process, by which culture is made and remade by people's embodied actions and language at the same time as cultural practices and language are inscribed on the body (Csordas 1990). Grosz, for example, refers to the body as an 'inscriptive surface', which various adornments, practices, and actions mark more or less permanently (Grosz 1994: 138).

Binary oppositions based on cultural norms and assumptions are frequently adopted in discourse on embodiment in the attempt to make distinctions between bodies: for example, the female and the male body, the young and the old body, the normal and the deviant body, the homosexual and the heterosexual body, the thin and the fat body, the healthy and the ill or diseased body, the sane and the mad body – to name a few. Specific discourses relating to phenomena may be identified, such as a discourse of hope in relation to cancer, a discourse of nature in relation to alternative therapies or a discourse of science in relation to Western medicine. Some discourses seek to challenge binary oppositions: for example, the discourses of non-binary, gender-queer or fluid genders that overturn and complicate gendered binaries.

These discourses may be articulated and acted upon in a range of contexts, from patients' lay explanations and beliefs about their illness, to news reports of an illness or disease, medical textbooks and curricula – and in more recent times, blogs, smartphone applications ('apps'), YouTube and TikTok videos, or social media discussions about experiences of health and illness. A discourse, however, is sited within a broader matrix of sociocultural and historical meaning and thus extends beyond its context. For example, the discourse of science, as it is expressed in relation to medicine in contemporary Western societies, has a long history, developing over the last few centuries as science and medicine has – as systems of knowledge emerged and developed. A number of underlying assumptions derived from a broader Western tradition of thought contribute to the discourse of science in medicine. These include the assumptions that the mind is separate from the body, nature is separate from society and culture, nature/truth is universal, individuals are distinct from society and culture, and illness is a threat to rationality (Gordon 1988; Kirmayer 1988; Stein 1990).

In the twenty-first century, in which notions of fate have largely been replaced by modernist ideals of order and certainty over the chaos of illness and disease, the discourse of science in medicine has a particular resonance, as it appeals to contemporary beliefs in the efficacy of the rationalist approach to containing disorder (Lupton 2012). For example, this discourse has been evident in responses to the COVID-19 pandemic in Western countries. The pandemic has created high levels of disruption to everyday life and social relationships as well as health and medical challenges across the world. In public discourses (such as news media coverage and public health campaigns) on how best to control the spread of the novel coronavirus, the reliance on scientific medicine and individual responsibility in measures for pandemic management (the importance of practicing hygiene and quarantine measures, the quest for an effective vaccine) is evident. There has been less attention paid to the socioeconomic dimensions of the COVID-19 crisis and the sociocultural determinants of health: for example, the greater risk of serious illness posed to people of color who contract COVID-19, and to those who must leave their homes to continue to work or who otherwise have no source of income (Bhatia 2020; Rambaree and Nässén 2020). In other words, COVID-19 is just as much a social, cultural and economic crisis as it is a health crisis, requiring cultural understanding and social policy knowledge and interventions (Lupton 2020; Lupton and Willis 2021).

The discourses that tend to dominate over others are those emerging from powerful individuals or social groups, helping to further their interests in shaping the ways in which phenomena are represented. The discourse of science in medicine relies, in part, on the assumption that it is politically and culturally neutral, unlike some other knowledge, such as that articulated in lay or alternative therapy discourses (Rapp 1990). The discourse of science serves to underpin the powerful and high-status role of orthodox medical practitioners, who claim that their system of knowledge is superior to that of other health-care providers. Dominant discourses, however, are constantly subject to challenge. While, for example, the discourse of science may currently dominate understanding of the body and health states in Western societies, it may be challenged by the counter discourses expressed by proponents of alternative therapies, who use the discourse of beneficent nature to oppose what they see as being the objectifying nature of scientific approaches in medicine (Lupton 2012).

The emphasis on language and discourse that dominated sociological theory in the late twentieth century has been supplemented since the turn of this century by a greater emphasis placed on the role and agency of affective forces and material objects in human experience. This sociomaterialist perspective still acknowledges the importance of language, discourse and other forms of representation (such as images or sound), but it devotes more attention to the distribution of agencies between humans and nonhumans when they come together in assemblages.

One important source of inspiration for sociomaterialism is the early philosophy of Baruch Spinoza, who wrote about human embodiment and selfhood in the mid-seventeenth century. Scholars have returned to Spinoza's insights, which opposed Descartes' binary between mind and body. Spinoza's conceptualization of affect has been particularly influential in contemporary affective theory and new materialisms scholarship. For Spinoza, affect was considered a dynamic, distributed force that is shared across human bodies, and is therefore transpersonal (Slaby et al. 2019). The philosophy of Deleuze and Guattari takes up this approach to affect, positioning it as a force that could impel or constrain action and movement. Affect from this perspective moves between human bodies. It includes, but is not limited to, emotion and embodied feelings and sensations. Deleuze and Guattari (1987) characterize affective forces as both affecting others and having the capacity to be affected. For Deleuze and Guattari, it is important to understand not what the human body is, but what it can do. An integral element of this understanding is identifying the affects that are generated in and through bodies: 'either to destroy that body or be destroyed by it, either to exchange actions and passions with it or to join with it in composing a more powerful body' (Deleuze and Guattari 1987: 257). As this quotation implies, affects can be productive and destructive, composed with other affects and other bodies and always shared and distributed forces. Affective forces are also generated with nonhuman creatures and things. In their power and vibrancies, affective forces are integral to agencies, including more-than-human agencies.

Indigenous and First Nations peoples' cosmologies reach much further back than the European philosophy of Spinoza. Their philosophies of human embodiment and selfhood are traditionally more-than-human, contrasting with contemporary Western beliefs that tend to make a strong division between nature and culture, humans and nonhumans, and living and non-living things. Indigenous and First Nations peoples' cosmologies place great emphasis on the interembodiment of humans with other living creatures and the natural physical world in understanding the nature of human existence. This understanding goes well beyond recognition of the social determinants of health. It sees specific geographical attributes of place and space, including soil, rocks, bodies of water, terrain, flora and flora as coming together with humans to generate states of health and well-being. These cosmologies view the nonhuman attributes of place and space as generating and distributing agencies with the people who inhabit and move through them. When relational connections between people and nonhumans are disrupted or broken, illness and feelings of unease result that have negative impacts for humans and nonhumans (Bawaka Country et al. 2015; Ravenscroft 2018; Todd 2016).

Actor-network theory, led by the scholarship of Bruno Latour (2005), has played an influential role in identifying how nonhuman things work with humans to generate agency as part of networks. Rather than focus entirely on the meanings and actions of humans, actor-network theory directs greater attention to nonhuman actors (Michael 2016). As the term suggests, actor-network theory builds on poststructuralist theory to examine the ways in which all actors (often described as 'actants') in relational networks engage with each other. These networks are considered to be both material and conceptual. Actants include nonhuman things such as ideas and language as well as material objects. For this reason, actor-network theory is often described as a 'material-semiotic' approach (Michael 2016). It is argued that nonhuman actants do not generate agencies by themselves, but rather through relational actor-networks involving humans. It is through these networks and relationships of actants that scientific (including medical) knowledges and practices are constituted. In the case of medical knowledge and practices, these actants can include medical and laboratory technologies, pharmaceuticals, medical journals and textbooks, conferences, mechanical aids, therapies and the ideas and practices associated with these things (Bearman and Ajjawi 2018).

Feminist materialism theorists have also made a major contribution to understanding the entanglements of humans and nonhumans. For scholars such as Donna Haraway (2016), Karen Barad (2007), Jane Bennett (2009) and Rosi Braidotti (2019), humans are always more-than-human as they move through their lives. Here again, from this theoretical position, agencies are viewed as generated with and through human and nonhuman assemblages. In taking a feminist perspective, these scholars are more interested in the political dimensions of more-than-human worlds than are many actor-network theorists: not only with regard to gender, but also other disadvantaged and marginalized social groups. Feminist materialism scholars are interested in the micropolitical dimensions of more-than-human encounters and identifying in whose interests they serve. These scholars have focused in particular on humans' relationships with things in the natural environment. Adopting a very similar stance to that put forward by Indigenous and First Nations peoples, feminist materialism thought emphasizes the relational connections between people and the natural physical world. Haraway (2003) uses the term 'nature-cultures' to encapsulate these entanglements.

These sociomaterial perspectives build on previous work on the sociology and anthropology of the body that developed in the late twentieth century. Not only do they devote greater attention to the role of affective forces, relational connections and physical things, they also highlight the intersections between biology and culture. The notion that researchers should focus on 'how matter is made to matter', as Barad (2003) puts it, underpins much of this scholarship. Another important emphasis offered in this scholarship is that health and illness states are always dynamic and emergent rather than stable, depending on the human and nonhuman elements that come together at any given moment and in specific temporal and spatial contexts (Andrews 2019).

THE BODY AND NOTIONS OF HEALTH AND ILLNESS

Writings in the sociology, anthropology, philosophy, geography, and history of the human body have made important contributions to understanding the ways in which embodied experience changes across historical periods and social and cultural contexts. People's own experiences of the body – the sensations they feel, the perceptions they make through their bodies – are also important, however. The body is not simply passively inscribed by discourses. Rather, bodily experience and perception themselves contribute to the production and reproduction of discourses, just as discourses and practices shape the ways in which bodies are thought about and experienced. People learn about and know the world through and with their bodies. Social studies of health meanings and experiences, therefore, have increasingly incorporated a focus on their sensory dimensions (Andrews 2019; Lupton and Maslen 2018).

Distinct changes, as well as congruities, in ways of thinking about and representing the body, health, and illness have been identified by cultural analysts. In medieval and Renaissance Europe, for example, very little was known about the internal constituents and workings of the body, for dissections were banned as blasphemous (Muchembled 1985: 26). It was thought that illness and disease entered the body through the skin and bodily orifices. Pre-modern Europeans took care not to allow water – especially hot water – to touch the body, for this was thought to open the skin to unhealthy miasmas, or vapours, bearing disease. They believed that the body could best be protected against such vapours by wrapping oneself in tightly woven clothing, reinforcing the 'closed' nature of the body (Thomas 1997; Vigarello 1988).

Concepts of body image as they relate to health have shifted significantly even within the past century, incorporating centuries-old ideas as well as bringing in new ideas from other cultures, or introduced by scientific or medical discoveries about the body. According to Martin (1994), in the 1940s and 1950s concepts of health in American society tended to represent the body as a castle or fortress, with distinct openings that required protection from external invaders. She notes that following the mid-nineteenth century sanitary reform movement in England and the United States, hygiene became a dominant strategy for defending the body from the 'germs' that sought to enter through its orifices and subsequently cause disease. During the 1960s and 1970s, however, the notion of the body as harboring an interconnected immune system developed, drawing on changing scientific medical knowledge about immune response.

Contemporary notions of the body and health states, as Martin's work demonstrates, combine centuries-old ideas relating to body openings and hygiene with newer ideas concerning the microlevel of bodily function. The body image, therefore, may be understood as a complex intertwining of traditional and novel understandings of the ways in which the body functions and relates to other bodies, objects, and spaces that produces possible ways of thinking about and living in the body. As noted earlier in the chapter, the discourses of scientific medicine are very dominant in contemporary understanding of, and practices related to, the body, health, illness, and disease. The result of this dominance is that the ways in which individuals in Western societies tend to think about health, illness, health care, and their own bodies is very much influenced by the discourses and practices of scientific medicine.

Medical knowledge, however, is just as subject to change and variation as are other systems of knowledge, including lay knowledge. Comparative analyses of medical discourses and practices in different cultural settings often reveal the ways in which the same knowledge system (in this case, scientific medicine) is understood and practiced in strikingly different ways. Rather than see scientific medicine as a singular entity, therefore, it has been argued that it should be viewed as 'a plurality of biomedicines that are socially and culturally situated' (Good 1995: 462). While a series of overarching paradigms that serve to unite biomedicine may be identified, it is taken up in a variety of different cultural contexts, in which such factors as the economic system, assumptions about the doctor–patient relationship, new technologies, and ideas about health and illness, among other elements, shape its manifestations.

A major intervention into the creation and distribution of medical knowledge has been instigated by the emergence of a plethora of digital technologies that assist people to find and share health and medical information (Lupton 2017a). While many popular websites still rely on and present the views of medical science, such as WebMD and government health department sites, new digital media have made a major contribution to the development and distribution of peer-to-peer medical knowledge. Mobile media and ubiquitous Wi Fi services emerging since the early years of the twenty-first century have led to a massive expansion of user-led content creation and sharing (John 2017). Where once lay people had recourse mostly to sources of health and medical information published in self-help books, newsletters or email distribution groups, the emergence of patient support websites, blogs, online discussion forums and social media communities since the early days of the internet has created many more opportunities for lay people to both create and share information about health and medicine. Digital platforms such as Facebook and Twitter allow people to communicate with others and develop condition-specific communities. Content curation-sharing platforms like YouTube and TikTok generate huge quantities of visual materials that present both medical experts and lay people discussing and demonstrating medical care and therapies (Lupton 2017a).

Hundreds of thousands of health and medical apps are available for health consumer use on the two major app stores, Apple App Store and Google Play (Lupton 2014, 2017a). As critical analyses of these apps have shown, they tend to take an individualist approach to preventive health, suggesting that people should take responsibility for managing their health. App developers often seek to promote techno-utopian imaginaries about the potential of these technologies to improve health and well-being (Lupton 2014; Lupton and Jutel 2015). Other studies have highlighted the increasingly important role played by visual digital media in communicating health-related experiences. Popular social media and content-sharing platforms like Facebook, Instagram, Tumblr, Reddit, TikTok, and YouTube, rely on the power of images to generate interest, attention and sharing as part of the 'like economy' (Gerlitz and Helmond 2013) and 'sharing economy' (John 2017) of digital media.

Lay people are now able to readily use their smartphones to take images of themselves and others and share these to almost limitless audiences online. New digital media and devices have led to a greater visibility of non-normative bodies and practices that in previous eras received little public exposure. Images of fat bodies, people living with disabilities or amputated limbs, queer and transgendered bodies, women with mastectomies, people receiving chemotherapy, those engaging in restricted eating or excessive eating, and many other non-normative bodies can now be readily uploaded to blogs, websites or social media platforms. YouTube even provides a forum for videos showing women giving birth and people engaging in do-it-yourself surgical procedures (Lupton 2017a). TikTok, a platform used mostly by young people, has a huge array of short videos made by users about health issues: including self-diagnosis of conditions such as ADHD, autism and mental health disorders.

While the affordances of digital media and devices offer many opportunities for publics to find, share and create medical information as well as provide important peer support, the widespread use of the internet as a health resource has caused disquiet on the part of the medical profession and some health consumer groups. Actively searching online and generating and sharing personal health data can also cause difficulties and tensions in the doctor–patient relationship. The medical profession often supports the ideal of the digitally engaged patient, but can demonstrate considerable ambivalence about the threat to medical authority that online information (often characterized as 'Dr Google') or self-generated biometrics can present (Lupton 2013a). The notion of 'cyberchondria' has been used in the medical literature to suggest that health and medical advice on the internet can create unfounded anxiety. The sheer plethora of information available online can be confusing and difficult to navigate. Patients are therefore often called on to engage in acts of negotiation of information when they visit their doctors, assessing to what extent their doctor wants or expect them to seek out, act on and share their health-related information (Maslen and Lupton 2019).

Of greater concern, lay people offering tutorials on 'do it yourself' surgery or creating or sharing bogus, inaccurate or misleading health advice can exacerbate rather than improve ill-health (Lupton 2017a). There have been a number of highly publicized cases where health or lifestyle 'influencers' with a large following of sometimes desperate people looking for a solution for their health problem, have been proven to be frauds (Baker and Rojek 2020). During the emergence of the COVID-19 pandemic, there was a plethora of misinformation (sometimes described as an 'infodemic') circulating on the internet: particularly in social media sites such as Facebook, Instagram, YouTube, Twitter and Reddit (Baker et al. 2020).

THE MEDICAL GAZE AND THE ROLE OF TECHNOLOGY

The discourses and practices of medical knowledge produce and work on specific kinds of bodies. One way in which they do so is through the use of spatial and temporal dimensions. Many of Foucault's writings devote attention to the material as well as discursive dimensions of human existence. His well-known concept of the Panopticon, the building designed to ensure that prisoners could easily be viewed from all sides by guards who were able to remain hidden from view, underpins his insights into how people learn to conduct self-discipline as an ethical practice of selfhood if they feel that they could potentially always be under surveillance. Foucault's *Birth of the Clinic* (1975) outlines the ways in which the architecture of the medical clinic and certain practices of physicians led to a change in the way human bodies were understood and treated. In the context of the clinic or hospital, the body of the patient becomes subject to the medical gaze. For Foucault (1975), it is through the medical gaze that the patient's body is constructed as a particular archetype of illness. The medical gaze is a product of a dominant discourse in scientific medicine that champions the importance of expert medical practitioners using visual cues to assess and monitor patients' bodies.

This approach to diagnosing and treating the ill body is a result of changes that took place in the late eighteenth and early nineteenth centuries, in which scientific medicine emerged, reliant on systematic measurement and identification of visible signs of disease and comparison. The fields of pathology and anatomy, employing the hitherto taboo practice of dissection of human bodies, began to underpin medical knowledge, opening to the medical gaze what was previously hidden (Armstrong 1983; Foucault 1975). Where once physicians relied on a patient's account of their symptoms to diagnose illness, they now add technologies such as stethoscopes and X-rays to construct their knowledge of the body by seeing or listening to what is going on inside it (Armstrong 1984). As part of the processes of medical examination, diagnosis and treatment, patients are brought into a visibility that differentiates and judges them, comparing them to a norm and attempting to restore them to that norm.

Medical surveillance and treatment practices, therefore, perform a disciplinary function upon the body of the patient, reading the body as docile and productive, the product of medical discourse and power. The use of the term 'disciplinary' in this context does not necessarily imply an interaction that involves punishment or coercion, but rather conveys the sense that patients' bodies, usually voluntarily, conform to and are shaped by medical practices and knowledge. So, too, are patients incited by medical practitioners and other health-care workers to reveal their experiences and feelings as part of diagnostic and treatment routines. This is a dominant aspect of the discourse of 'patient-centred medicine', which has become viewed as the most appropriate approach for health-care workers to interact with their patients (Osborne 1994). This transfer of knowledge about the body and the self, however, is very much one-way: doctors and other health-care workers do not reveal their bodies to patients, and rarely do they reveal their private feelings and thoughts. The medical gaze, therefore, is not reciprocated.

In the clinic, a range of medical technologies is brought to bear to monitor and measure bodily signs, to diagnose and 'bring into visibility' the body of the patient. This is the apotheosis of the extension of the medical gaze into the interior of the body. The various technologies available to survey and visually document aspects of the human body – such as magnetic resonance imaging, X-rays, ultrasounds, CT scanners, nuclear tracing, and electrocardiograms – present different nuances and representations of the body. These accounts are subject to expert interpretation, as are diagnostic tests of sample tissue (Atkinson 1995). The medical gaze may itself be internalized by patients in some cases, changing their perceptions of their bodies. Lay people may come to see themselves differently via their interaction with medical technologies. The experience of interacting with medical technologies may lead to a sense of disruption of body image that is distressing. For example, those who undergo a diagnostic screening test, such as for HIV, or prostate, cervical, or breast cancer, often find themselves entering a liminal state when waiting for the result. When previously they may have had no signs or symptoms of disease, once having undertaken the diagnostic test they are forced to reconsider the notion of themselves as 'healthy' (Lupton 2012).

A significant collection of research drawing on actor-network theory has developed to investigate the ways in which medical care and human embodiment are understood with the interventions of technologies. Annemarie Mol is one such scholar. Her book *The Body Multiple* (Mol 2002) presents an ethnographic analysis of how the diagnosis and treatment of atherosclerosis is carried out in a Dutch hospital. She shows that bodies are multiple in these contexts because of the different practices and knowledges that come to bear on this disease. An anatomical dissection of a human body with atherosclerosis sees the disease as a different phenomenon, and treats it accordingly, compared with a physician conducting a medical examination of a living patient with the disease. A patient's lived experience of the condition is different again – and this may change over time. The ontologies of atherosclerosis, Mol argues, depends on these networks of practices, knowledges and technologies. No body, no object and no disease, therefore, is singular – they are always multiple. In the language of actor-network theory, these phenomena are enacted: brought into existence and field of visibility via these networks.

With the expansion of digital health technologies designed for self-monitoring bodily functions and activities, the affordances of visibility offered by medical technologies are now available to some extent as part of everyday life. The figure of the 'digitally engaged patient' has emerged, involving an emphasis on lay people actively seeking health and medical information using online searches or apps and acting on it to engage in self-care and promote their health. Patients with chronic health conditions are often expected to use home monitoring devices to track bodily functions such as heart rate or blood glucose (Lupton 2017a). Elderly people wanting to age-in-place are encouraged to use 'smart' technologies such as movement-sensing devices, cognitive fitness games and step-tracking apps to ensure their safety and wellbeing (Katz and Marshall 2018). Apps are available to help people engage in self-diagnosis and thereby potentially avoid a visit to a medical professional (Lupton and Jutel 2015).

Beyond these therapeutic uses of digital technologies, the developers of health and medical apps and wearable devices such as fitness bands and smartwatches promote their use for self-tracking biometrics such as body temperature, pulse, steps taken, calories burned, food intake and sleep patterns (Lupton 2016). The Apple Watch is marketed as both a fitness tracker and a medical device: 'part guardian, part guru', as the Apple website puts it. Not only does the Watch have sensors that monitor wearers' movement patterns to track their exercise levels, it sends notifications to remind people to stand and move around if they are recorded as sitting for too long. It can detect heart rates that are deemed too low, too high, or too irregular and send wearers a warning notification. It can even detect falls and send carers messages to notify them.

Such everyday (albeit expensive) technologies perform many of the functions that were once relegated to clinical technologies that were interpreted by trained medical professionals. They bring human bodies into new fields of visibility to lay users, who are charged with making sense of the data that are generated and calculating how to best respond to this detailed information about themselves. These engagements can often be redolent with affective forces that can open up or close down agencies. While 'good' metrics can be encouraging and inspire feelings of confidence and being in control, when the numbers are not 'good', people can respond with disappointment, frustration or annoyance and feel less motivated to continue self-monitoring (Lupton 2016, 2017a; Maslen and Lupton 2019). There are also significant personal data privacy issues raised by the use of apps and wearable devices to monitor users' bodies, activities and health states. Many apps have been generated to manage COVID-19 across a range of countries, including those designed to provide information about how to limit the spread of the coronavirus, to help people self-diagnose, to assist in contact tracing and in some countries (for example, China), to prevent people from entering public spaces if they are designated as contagious or a close contact of someone who is infected with the virus. Questions have been raised about the infringement of privacy or restrictions on freedom of movement some of these apps facilitate: particularly when citizens cannot challenge the automated decisions made by the software (Kitchin 2020; Yu 2020).

ASSEMBLAGES OF HEALTH

In recent social and cultural theory, an interest in the ways in which place and space operate to shape practices and notions of selfhood and embodiment has developed. These writings go beyond a focus on language in acknowledging the importance of physicality, motion, and the material world. Space and place are understood as constructed through sociocultural processes rather than as objective and given. Kearns and Joseph (1993: 712) refer to this approach as a sociospatial rather than a geometric view of space. Previous writings, particularly in cultural geography, referred to 'therapeutic landscapes' (Bell et al. 2017), but current scholarship drawing on new materialism theories now often refers to 'assemblages of health' (Andrews 2019). These perspectives have been adopted in medical geography and the sociology and anthropology of health and illness to explore how spatial and temporal dimensions interact in producing and reproducing the discourses and practices and, thus, the meanings and experiences of health, illness, and medical care. Again, the writings of Foucault have been influential here, particularly in relation to his writings on the role played by the Panopticon in monitoring the inmates of public buildings such as prisons, schools, and hospitals, thus bringing them into a specific field of visibility. Such features of medical care as the architecture of the clinic or hospital, the physical layout of operating theatres, and the bodily movements and interactions of medical staff and patients within the bounded spaces of the clinic/hospital have been studied (see, for example, Armstrong 1988; Fox 1997; Hirschauer 1991).

As noted earlier, Indigenous and First Nations philosophies of embodiment and health acknowledge the importance of the ecological context in which humans move and live. In this mode of thinking, human life, states of health and illness are constituted by more-than-human assemblages. Relational connections with other people, other living things and with non-living things are central to the affective forces that contribute to health and well-being. Feelings of comfort, confidence, well-being and good health emerge from humans' engagements with the nonhuman, as do those of distress, injury and illness. Indigenous and First Nations peoples often refer to a disconnection with the land of their relatives and ancestors caused by colonization as a primary source of ill-health and loss of well-being (De Leeuw 2015; Lines and Jardine 2019). When they feel part of their land (being 'on Country' as many Aboriginal Australians term it) and strongly connected with their traditions of engaging with the nonhuman elements of their land, Indigenous and First Nations peoples feel stronger, more resilient and in better health (Kingsley et al. 2018). For First Nations peoples in the Yukon area of Canada, for example, water is respected as a more-than-human person: a living entity or relative, and they have a sacred responsibility to care for it. In return for caring for waterways and bodies of water, humans are bestowed with the health- and life-giving properties of clean water. This ontological perspective contrasts with the settler view of water as a resource for human use. It emphasizes the reciprocal and shared nature of human–nonhuman health and well-being (Wilson and Inkster 2018).

A greater emphasis on the ways in which features of landscapes contribute to health and well-being is evident in some literatures focusing on Western societies. Cultural geographers have called attention to the powerful therapeutic properties of green or blue (involving bodies of water such as lakes, rivers and seas) landscapes (Bell et al. 2017). Feminist materialism scholars also seek to highlight these dimensions of health and illness. In a discussion on soil–human entanglements, for example, Puig de la Bellacasa (2019) draws attention to the vital forces of these enactments, seeking to recuperate their animated nature as part of strengthening humans' relations of care with and through the soil. As she argues, such re-enlivening of soil–human relations benefits humans as much as it does the earth.

A subfield of the sociology of health and illness, entitled 'materialities of care', takes a sociomaterialist perspective that often draws on actor-network theory. These researchers employ an ethnographic approach to understanding the ways in which people engage with objects as part of caring for their own bodies or those of other people, and how medical knowledges are put into action (Buse et al. 2018a). In one such study, researchers accompanied nurses visiting the homes of elderly Dutch people requiring care. The researchers observed the ways these nurses carefully observed the elderly people's movements around their homes, the state of cleanliness and order in the home, whether people's gardens had been attended to, and other aspects to assess the health and well-being of their patients (van Hout et al. 2015). Other research has investigated laundry practices in British care home settings and the role of clothing in dementia care (Buse et al. 2018b). Such studies make visible the mundane and often unnoticed material cultures of health care, and the ways in which health and medical care is distributed across a range of domains beyond the clinic (Buse et al. 2018a).

Some researchers have taken up insights from feminist materialism and applied them to health and medical care. For example, Fullagar (2020) examines the ways in which recovery from significant mental distress (such as depression or anxiety) involving an assemblage of things and practices: including human care, pharmaceuticals, biochemicals, engagements with other animals and living things, spatial geographies, and practices such as exercise and meditation. Fullagar argues that recovery is constituted through the relations made between these more-than-human assemblages. It is a performative and dynamic process rather than complete event, a gathering of forces and agencies rather than a cognitive process located within the individual. From this perspective, recovery is a continuing enactment of bodyminds rather than a fixed state of being.

Sociomaterial analyses have also highlighted the important role of digital media as spaces for generating affective forces and agencies. They have shown that the opportunity to make relational connections with other people is an integral affordance of social media, helping people feel less alone and to share insights from their experiences with others. These practices can be particularly important for people who are living with marginalized or stigmatized conditions such as mental illness, restricted eating or chronic health conditions (Maslen and Lupton 2019; McCosker and Hartup 2018). The physical isolation forced on people in many countries due to COVID-19 lockdown restrictions highlighted the importance of using technologies such as messaging and video calling apps on their phones, as well as social media interactions, to alleviate loneliness and emotional distress (Watson et al. 2021).

THE CIVILIZED BODY AND THE LOGIC OF CONTROL

One of the most dominant logics organizing ways of thinking and acting in Western societies at the end of the twentieth century is that of control. Individuals constantly engage in activities in the quest for control over their lives. It is believed that most aspects of life are malleable and amenable to the exertion of will. We see ourselves as a continuing unfinished project, requiring work and effort to shape and improve, seeking to impose order and certainty upon what is perceived to be a chaotic, uncertain, disorderly world. Foucault (1988) referred to such practices as the 'technologies of the self'. The technologies of the self involve the voluntary internalization of norms governing appropriate behaviour in the interests of achieving the best possible self, including the quest for self-knowledge, self-mastery, and self-care (Lupton 1995; Rose 1996). Engaging in the technologies of the self involves seeking out and employing knowledge and the constant making of choices.

Nowhere is this desire for control more evident than in the ways in which people conceptualize embodiment, health, and illness. For the late-modern individual, the body is viewed as signifying the self and demonstrating one's capacity for self-knowledge, self-mastery, and self-care. The ideal body is that which is tightly contained, its boundaries stringently policed, its orifices shut, kept autonomous, private, and separate from other things and other bodies (Bordo 1993; Shilling 1993). Good health and 'normal functioning' of the body is commonly viewed in contemporary Western societies as the product of careful self-regulation and self-discipline. Behaviours that are seen to be linked to 'lifestyle' choices and therefore under the control of individuals, such as alcohol consumption, cigarette smoking, diet, physical exercise, and sexual activity, have been singled out in public health campaigns. Such campaigns exhort members of the 'target' audience to engage in 'body maintenance' activities (Featherstone 1991). Under the discourse of self-control, citizens are urged to turn the medical gaze upon themselves, and engage in such technologies of the self as monitoring their own bodies and health states and taking preventive action in accordance with medical and public health directives (Herzlich and Pierret 1987; Lupton 1995; Petersen and Lupton 1996).

The notion of the 'civilized' body, emerging in early modern Europe, is particularly important to contemporary understandings about the ideal body (Elias 1978; Shilling 1993). The 'civilized' body is understood to be that which is self-controlled, which is autonomous and self-regulated. Its boundaries are kept contained from the outside world and from others. In contrast to this ideal notion is the 'grotesque' or 'uncivilized' body, the body that lacks self-control and self-discipline and is constantly breaching its boundaries. The body that is suffering pain or illness, that is deformed or disabled, that is dying, tends to conform far more closely to the 'grotesque' body than the 'civilized' body.

A further perspective drawn from anthropological and psychoanalytic theory is that which acknowledges the ways in which individuals construct a sense of body boundaries and define themselves as self in opposition to 'other'. This perspective has provided insights for those scholars who are interested in how such notions as 'health', 'illness', and 'risk' are used to deal with central anxieties and fears about contamination, the blurring of bodily boundaries and death. The work of anthropologist Mary Douglas has been highly influential in our understanding of the symbolic role played by body image and notions of the body boundaries. In her book *Purity and Danger* (1966), Douglas argued that the human body serves a conceptual means of distinguishing between self and 'other'. Just as the body is seen to have defined boundaries between 'inside' and 'outside', with rules regulating what matter comes in, what comes out, and in which ways, all human societies construct understandings of which people and things belong 'inside' and which should be maintained 'outside'. All humans, as they are socialized into their cultures, learn the appropriate cultural norms about how to police and control their bodily boundaries.

The orifices of the body constantly present a challenge to individuals to exert control over the movement of bodily fluids from 'inside' to 'outside'. In Western societies, we are particularly disgusted by notions of the inside of the body and the slimy viscera, organs, and fluids it contains. Actions or accidents that expose this inside matter break down the boundaries between 'inside' and 'outside' that we are exhorted since early childhood to preserve as part of our accomplishment and maintenance of the 'civilized' body. Hence, 'The disgust that arises when the body is sliced open with a knife or pierced with a bullet is more than just a function of the muck that pours out, it is a function primarily of the inappropriateness of destroying the integrity of the body's seal' (Miller 1997: 58).

In infancy and extreme old age and in illness or some forms of disablement, these bodily boundaries are constantly breached. Other bodily changes, such as pregnancy and menopause, may also involve loss of control over the body. The appearance of reviled body fluids at socially 'incorrect' times or places demonstrates a frightening and disturbing loss of such rational control, signalling a return to a state of bodily chaos of infancy. The dribbling, incontinent elderly or disabled body is a nightmarish vision for its childishness and its supposed loss of humanity. Unlike the ideal of the 'civilized' body, the ill or dying body, the body in pain, the deformed or disabled body is that which lacks control. It is also that which lacks autonomy because it is dependent on others, and that which constantly threatens to breach its boundaries through pain, spasms, or the expulsion of bodily fluids at 'inappropriate' times. Such bodies arouse disgust because they bring the 'inside' of the body 'outside'. Ill, disabled, or dying people are the 'other', those from whom the healthy, young, and able-bodied seek, often unconsciously, to differentiate themselves because of the fears, anxieties, revulsion, and dread they harbour of the incipient chaos and dissolution of their own bodies.

Grosz (1994) has taken up Douglas's writings to analyze the symbolic nature of bodily fluids, with a particular focus on gender implications. She claims that because the female body is conceptualized as more marginal, indeterminate, fluid, borderline, and liminal, as seeping fluids that are considered to be 'dirty' and therefore as less controlled, it is viewed as more dangerous, defiling, and diseased than the male body (Grosz 1994; see also Heywood 1996). Indeed, femininity has been strongly associated with both embodiment and disease. Women's bodies have been traditionally portrayed in medical and other discourses as inferior to men's bodies: as smaller, frailer, weaker, and more disorderly, and as more defective and more prone to illness (Bordo 1993; Ehrenreich and English 1974).

So, too, other types of bodies have been typically represented, both in medical and more popular discourses, as 'inferior' because they are regarded as being unable to properly regulate their body boundaries. These include black or brown bodies, homosexual bodies, ageing bodies, gender-diverse and working-class bodies. Comaroff (1993) has shown, for example, how nineteenth-century British colonialist and medical discourses in South Africa portrayed black Africans as inherently dirty and diseased, as 'savage' rather than 'civilized', and as both morally and physically degenerate. Standing for normality and self-discipline is the white, heterosexual, youthful, middle-class, masculine body. The male body is culturally represented as ideally invulnerable, disciplined, strong, contained, healthy, and physically able, and therefore as more 'civilized' than other bodies (Petersen and Lupton 1996).

The emphasis that is currently placed in Western societies on the importance of the regulation and disciplining of the self and the body has implications for how ill people are conceptualized in moral terms. In the 'new morality' of preventive health, falling ill has become viewed as a sign of moral failure, a source of blame. States of health, therefore, are inherently associated with moral meanings and judgements (Crawford 1994; Greco 1993; Herzlich and Pierret 1987; Lupton 1995; Stein 1990). Not to engage in risk-avoiding behaviour is considered 'a failure of the self to take care of itself – a form of irrationality, or simply a lack of skilfulness' (Greco 1993: 361). In contemporary Western societies, notions of the ideal body conflate health, beauty, youth, and normality. Health tends to be culturally linked to beauty, erotic attraction, and truth as well as morality, and illness and death to ugliness, grotesquerie, falsity, repulsion, and immorality (Lupton 2012, 2013b). Very old bodies, ill bodies, disabled bodies, and fat bodies are either stigmatized in mass media representations, or else are simply absent, treated as unworthy of portrayal because they are deemed to be deviant, unsightly, or dependent (Featherstone and Wernick 1995). In contrast, bodies that are tightly-contained, sparse of flesh, youthful, and toned are considered to represent the moral worth of self-discipline and attractiveness (Lupton 2018; Walseth and Tidslevold 2020).

Susan Sontag wrote about the contemporary moral meanings of illness in her important essay *Illness as Metaphor*, first published in 1978. She points out that 'Nothing is more punitive than to give a disease a meaning – that meaning being invariably a moralistic one' (Sontag 1989: 58). As she observes, cancer is commonly viewed as being caused by the repression of emotion, afflicting those who are sexually repressed, inhibited, unspontaneous, incapable of expressing anger (1989: 21). Like leprosy in medieval times, cancer evokes the meanings of horror, contamination, corruption, and blame. Sontag argues that these meanings also influence the type of treatment given to cancer patients and the words used to describe both the disease and its treatment. Cancer treatment is 'aggressive', used to 'attack' the cancer that has 'invaded' the body, 'bombarding' the body with radiation. With the use of these military metaphors, the patient's body becomes thought of, and treated, as a battleground (1989: 64–65).

In the decades since Sontag's essay was first published, cancer has also become strongly linked to such activities as cigarette smoking, a diet high in animal fat, sun exposure, and in the case of breast cancer, bearing children late in life or not at all (Kerr et al. 2018). People with cancer (and other illnesses) are also expected to be 'heroes' and to 'battle' with their illness and exert will-power to overcome it. Not to do so is considered to 'give in' to the 'enemy', relinquishing the attempt to regain the 'civilized' body from the chaotic ill body (Kerr et al. 2018). Here again, the COVID-19 crisis is an exemplar of how rules and norms about bodily deportment is conducted in response to a major infectious disease outbreak, and the stigmatization that can result when people are deemed to have 'broken' the rules of hygiene, quarantine or physical distancing (Atlani-Duault et al. 2020).

People with significant, disabling and life-threatening conditions often seek to regain control of the uncertainties associated with their conditions by seeking out information voraciously. Online discussion forums and social media are frequently used by people with cancer, chronic health conditions, disabilities, and other serious diseases as a way of seeking to take back control of their bodies and lives by sharing information as well as providing and receiving emotional support (Maslen and Lupton 2019; McCosker and Darcy 2013). Sometimes members of these online networks and communities seek to challenge the moralistic meanings that are associated with 'losing the battle' with cancer. People living with metastatic breast cancer have written accounts of their experiences on blogs, published YouTube videos and shared treatment experiences and advice on Facebook groups and with their Instagram followers. In so doing, they have sought to engage in activism to help others with their condition advocate on their own behalf and to draw public attention to the experiences of people who are dying from cancer as an alternative to the 'heroic survivor' discourse (Jacobson 2018).

Digital media can also provide opportunities for people with non-normative bodies to confront negative portrayals of their bodies in the popular media. Fat- and body-positive activists, for example, have used platforms such as blogs and websites to present images of fat bodies in empowering ways (Lupton 2018). People with disabilities or eating disorders similarly use social media sites to connect with each other and challenge stigmatizing discourses and imagery (Lupton 2017a). However, social media and other digital media can also be sites for the vilification of people who have non-normative bodies. Fat people, for example, are continually held up to ridicule and fat-shaming in YouTube videos, online forums and memes (Lupton 2017b).

CONCLUDING COMMENTS

As this chapter has demonstrated, much research and scholarship relating to the sociocultural representations and meanings of health, medicine, and the body has been published in recent decades. It has been particularly invigorated by the incorporation of poststructuralist and sociomaterialist perspectives and a growing interest in the sociology and history of the human body. One of the most important insights of sociocultural analyses is the identification of the link between knowledge, discourse, practices, power, and notions of reality in the context of more-than-human relationships. Their value lies in challenging the status quo by deconstructing taken-for-granted perspectives and representations, and in the process producing new ways of seeing, thinking, and acting.

Social constructionist and sociomaterialist analyses conducted thus far have provided a richness of material that challenges the objectivist perspective on medicine and the body that reigns in medicine. Much scope remains for further inquiries into how lay people understand their bodies in relation to the dominant discourses and practices emerging from such influential institutions as medicine and public health, and how digital health technologies are contributing to the capacities of lay people to monitor and learn about their bodies, communicate their experiences with each other and challenge medical authority. Continuing investigations into people's engagements with digital technologies and their role in creating and sharing health and medical knowledges among peer-to-peer networks, particularly as new digital media and devices are constantly developed and marketed to publics. It is important to continue to recognize the role played by different social groups and spatial locations in people's engagements with these technologies, and to identify the specific more-than-human contexts in which these relationships and connections take place.

REFERENCES

Andrews, G.J. (2019) Health geographies II: The posthuman turn. *Progress in Human Geography* 43: 1109–1119.

Armstrong, D. (1983) *Political Anatomy of the Body: Medical Knowledge in Britain in the Twentieth Century*. Cambridge: Cambridge University Press.

Armstrong, D. (1984) The patient's view. *Social Science and Medicine* 18: 737–744.

Armstrong, D. (1988) Space and time in British general practice. In M. Lock and D. Gordon (eds), *Biomedicine Examined*. Dordrecht: Kluwer, pp. 207–225.

Atkinson, P. (1995) *Medical Talk and Medical Work: The Liturgy of the Clinic*. London: Sage.

Atlani-Duault, L., Ward, J.K., Roy, M., Morin, C., and Wilson, A. (2020) Tracking online heroisation and blame in epidemics. *The Lancet Public Health* 5: e137–e138. https://doi.org/10.1016/S2468-2667(20)30033-5

Baker, S., and Rojek, C. (2020) *Lifestyle Gurus: Constructing Authority and Influence Online*. Cambridge: Polity Press.

Baker, S., Wade, M., and Walsh, M. (2020) The challenges of responding to misinformation during a pandemic: content moderation and the limitations of the concept of harm. *Media International Australia* 177: 103–107.

Barad, K. (2003) Posthumanist performativity: Toward an understanding of how matter comes to matter. *Signs* 28: 801–831.

Barad, K. (2007) *Meeting the Universe Halfway: Quantum Physics and the Entanglement of Matter and Meaning*. Durham, NC: Duke University Press.

Bawaka Country, Wright, S., Suchet-Pearson, S., et al. (2015) Working with and learning from Country: Decentring human author-ity. *Cultural Geographies* 22: 269–283.

Bearman, M., and Ajjawi, R. (2018) Actor-network theory and the OSCE: Formulating a new research agenda for a post-psychometric era. *Advances in Health Sciences Education* 23: 1037–1049.

Bell, S.L., Wheeler, B.W., and Phoenix, C. (2017) Using geonarratives to explore the diverse temporalities of therapeutic landscapes: Perspectives from 'green' and 'blue' settings. *Annals of the American Association of Geographers* 107: 93–108.

Bennett, J. (2009) *Vibrant Matter: A Political Ecology of Things*. Durham, NC: Duke University Press.

Berger, P., and Luckmann, T. (1967) *The Social Construction of Reality: A Treatise in the Sociology of Knowledge*. London: Allen Lane.

Bhatia, M. (2020) COVID-19 and BAME Group in the United Kingdom. *The International Journal of Community and Social Development* 2: 269–272.

Bordo, S. (1993) *Unbearable Weight: Feminism, Western Culture, and the Body*. Berkeley, CA: University of California Press.

Braidotti, R. (2019) A theoretical framework for the critical posthumanities. *Theory, Culture & Society* 36: 31–61.

Buse, C., Martin, D., and Nettleton, S. (2018a) Conceptualising 'materialities of care': making visible mundane material culture in health and social care contexts. *Sociology of Health & Illness* 40: 243–255.

Buse, C., Twigg, J., Nettleton, S., et al. (2018b) Dirty linen, liminal spaces, and later life: Meanings of laundry in care home design and practice. *Sociological Research Online* 23: 711–727.

Comaroff, J. (1993) The diseased heart of Africa: Medicine, colonialism, and the black body. In S. Lindenbaum and M. Lock (eds), *Knowledge, Power and Practice: The Anthropology of Medicine and Everyday Life*. Berkeley, CA: University of California Press, pp. 305–329.

Crawford, R. (1994) The boundaries of the self and the unhealthy other: reflections on health, culture and AIDS. *Social Science & Medicine* 38: 1347—1365.

Csordas, T.J. (1990) Embodiment as a paradigm for anthropology. *Ethos* 18: 5–47.

De Leeuw, S. (2015) Activating place: Geography as a determinant of Indigenous peoples' health and well-being. In M. Greenwood, S. De Leeuw and N.M. Lindsay (eds), *Determinants of Indigenous Peoples' Health: Beyond the Social*. Toronto: Canadian Scholars, pp. 90–103.

Deleuze, G., and Guattari, F. (1987) *A Thousand Plateaus. Schizophrenia and Capitalism*. Minneapolis, MN: University of Minnesota Press.

Douglas, M. (1966) *Purity and Danger: An Analysis of Concepts of Pollution and Taboo*. London: Routledge & Kegan Paul.

Ehrenreich, B., and English, D. (1974) *Complaints and Disorders: The Sexual Politics of Sickness*. London: Compendium.

Elias, N. (1978) *The Civilizing Process*. New York: Urizen.

Fairclough, N. (1992) *Discourse and Social Change*. Cambridge: Polity Press.

Featherstone, M. (1991) The body in consumer culture. In M. Featherstone, M. Hepworth and B. Turner (eds), *The Body: Social Process and Cultural Theory*. London: Sage, pp. 170–196.

Featherstone, M., and Wernick, A. (1995) Introduction. In M. Featherstone and A. Wernick (eds), *Images of Aging: Cultural Representations of Later Life*. London: Routledge, pp. 1–15.

Foucault, M. (1975) *The Birth of the Clinic: An Archaeology of Medical Perception*. New York: Vintage Books.

Foucault, M. (1988) Technologies of the self. In L. Martin, H. Gutman, and P. Hutton (eds), *Technologies of the Self*. London: Tavistock, pp. 16–49.

Fox, N. (1997) Space, sterility and surgery: Circuits of hygiene in the operating theatre. *Social Science and Medicine* 45: 649–657.

Fullagar, S. (2020) Diffracting mind–body relations: Feminist materialism and the entanglement of physical culture in women's recovery from depression. In J. Newman, H. Thorpe and D. Andrews (eds), *Sport, Physical Culture, and the Moving Body: Materialisms, Technologies, Ecologies*. New Brunswick, NJ: Rutgers University Press.

Gerlitz, C., and Helmond, A. (2013) The like economy: Social buttons and the data-intensive web. *New Media & Society* 15: 1348–1365.

Good, M.-J.D. (1995) Cultural studies of biomedicine: An agenda for research. *Social Science and Medicine* 41: 461–473.

Gordon, D. (1988) Tenacious assumptions in Western medicine. In M. Lock and D. Gordon (eds), *Biomedicine Examined*. Dordrecht: Kluwer, pp. 19–56.

Greco, M. (1993) Psychosomatic subjects and the 'duty to be well': Personal agency within medical rationality. *Economy and Society* 22: 357–372.

Grosz, E. (1994) *Volatile Bodies: Toward a Corporeal Feminism*. Sydney: Allen and Unwin.

Haraway, D. (2003) *The Companion Species Manifesto: Dogs, People, and Significant Otherness*. Chicago, IL: Prickly Paradigm.

Haraway, D. (2016) *Staying with the Trouble: Making Kin in the Chthulucene*. Durham, NC: Duke University Press.

Herzlich, C., and Pierret, J. (1987) *Illness and Self in Society*. Baltimore, MD: Johns Hopkins University Press.

Heywood, L. (1996) *Dedication to Hunger: The Anorexic Aesthetic in Modern Cultures*. Berkeley, CA: University of California Press.

Hirschauer, S. (1991) The manufacture of bodies in surgery. *Social Studies of Science* 21: 279–319.

Jacobson, S. (2018) Among the metavivors: Social media and illness narratives of Stage IV breast cancer patients. *Catalyst: Feminism, Theory, Technoscience*, 4. Available at: https://catalystjournal.org/index.php/catalyst/article/view/29631.

John, N. (2017) *The Age of Sharing*. Cambridge: Polity Press.

Katz, S., and Marshall, B.L. (2018) Tracked and fit: FitBits, brain games, and the quantified aging body. *Journal of Aging Studies* 45: 63–68.

Kearns, R., and Joseph, A. (1993) Space in its place: Developing the link in medical geography. *Social Science and Medicine* 37: 711–717.

Kerr, A., Ross, E., Jacques, G., et al. (2018) The sociology of cancer: A decade of research. *Sociology of Health & Illness* 40: 552–576.

Kingsley, J., Munro-Harrison, E., Jenkins, A., et al. (2018) 'Here we are part of a living culture': Understanding the cultural determinants of health in Aboriginal gathering places in Victoria, Australia. *Health & Place* 54: 210–220.

Kirmayer, L. (1988) Mind and body as metaphors: Hidden values in biomedicine. In M. Lock and D. Gordon (eds), *Biomedicine Examined*. Dordrecht: Kluwer, pp. 57–94.

Kitchin, R. (2020) Civil liberties or public health, or civil liberties and public health? Using surveillance technologies to tackle the spread of COVID-19. *Space and Polity* 24: 362–381.

Latour, B. (2005) *Reassembling the Social: An Introduction to Actor-Network-Theory*. Oxford: Clarendon Press.

Leder, D. (1992) A tale of two bodies: The Cartesian corpse and the lived body. In D. Leder (ed.), *The Body in Medical Thought and Practice*. Dordrecht: Kluwer, pp. 17–35.

Lines, L.-A., and Jardine, C.G. (2019) Connection to the land as a youth-identified social determinant of Indigenous Peoples' health. *BMC Public Health*, 19. Available at: https://bmcpublichealth.biomedcentral.com/articles/10.1186/s12889-018-6383-8.

Lupton, D. (1995) *The Imperative of Health: Public Health and the Body*. London: Sage.

Lupton, D. (2012) *Medicine as Culture: Illness, Disease and the Body*. London: Sage.

Lupton, D. (2013a) The digitally engaged patient: Self-monitoring and self-care in the digital health era. *Social Theory & Health* 11: 256–270.

Lupton, D. (2013b) *Fat*. London: Routledge.

Lupton, D. (2014) Apps as artefacts: Towards a critical perspective on mobile health and medical apps. *Societies* 4: 606–622.

Lupton, D. (2016) *The Quantified Self: A Sociology of Self-Tracking*. Cambridge: Polity Press.

Lupton, D. (2017a) *Digital Health: Critical and Crossdisciplinary Perspectives*. London: Routledge.

Lupton, D. (2017b) Digital media and body weight, shape, and size: an introduction and review. *Fat Studies* 6: 119–134.

Lupton, D. (2018) *Fat* (2nd edition). London: Routledge.

Lupton, D. (2020) Special section on 'Sociology and the Coronavirus (COVID-19) Pandemic'. *Health Sociology Review* 29: 111–112.

Lupton, D., and Jutel, A. (2015) 'It's like having a physician in your pocket!' A critical analysis of self-diagnosis smartphone apps. *Social Science & Medicine* 133: 128–135.

Lupton, D., and Maslen, S. (2018) The more-than-human sensorium: Sensory engagements with digital self-tracking technologies. *The Senses and Society* 13: 190–202.

Lupton, D., and Willis, K. (2021) (editors) *The COVID-19 Crisis: Social Perspectives*. Abingdon: Routledge.

Martin, E. (1994) *Flexible Bodies: Tracking Immunity in American Culture from the Days of Polio to the Age of AIDS*. Boston, MA: Beacon Press.

Maslen, S., and Lupton, D. (2020) Enacting chronic illness with and through digital media: A feminist new materialist approach. *Information, Communication & Society* 23: 1640–1652.

McCosker, A., and Darcy, R. (2013) Living with cancer: Affective labour, self-expression and the utility of blogs. *Information, Communication & Society* 16: 1266–1285.

McCosker, A., and Hartup, M. (2018) *Turning to online peer forums for suicide and self-harm support: 'It does help having you guys'*. Melbourne: Swinburne Social Innovation Research Institute.

Merleau-Ponty, M. (1962) *Phenomenology of Perception*. London: Routledge and Kegan Paul.

Michael, M. (2016) *Actor-network Theory: Trials, Trails and Translations*. London: Sage.

Miller, W. (1997) *The Anatomy of Disgust*. Cambridge, MA: Harvard University Press.

Mol, A. (2002) *The Body Multiple: Ontology in Medical Practice*. Durham, NC: Duke University Press.

Muchembled, R. (1985) *Popular Culture and Elite Culture in France, 1400–1750*. Baton Rouge, LA: Louisiana State University Press.

Osborne, T. (1994) Power and persons: On ethical stylisation and person-centred medicine. *Sociology of Health and Illness* 16: 515–535.

Petersen, A., and Lupton, D. (1996) *The New Public Health: Health and Self in the Age of Risk*. Sydney and London: Allen and Unwin/Sage.

Rambaree, K., and Nässén, N. (2020) 'The Swedish Strategy' to COVID-19 pandemic: Impact on vulnerable and marginalised communities. *The International Journal of Community and Social Development* 2: 234–250.

Rapp, R. (1990) Constructing amniocentesis: Maternal and medical discourses. In F. Ginsburg and A. Tsing (eds), *Uncertain Terms: Negotiating Gender in American Culture*. Boston, MA: Beacon Press, pp. 28–42.

Puig de la Bellacasa, M. (2019) Re-animating soils: Transforming human–soil affections through science, culture and community. *The Sociological Review* 67: 391–407.

Ravenscroft, A. (2018) Strange weather: Indigenous materialisms, new materialism, and colonialism. *The Cambridge Journal of Postcolonial Literary Inquiry* 5: 353–370.

Rose, N. (1996) *Inventing Our Selves: Psychology, Power, and Personhood*. Cambridge: Cambridge University Press.

Shilling, C. (1993) *The Body and Social Theory*. London: Sage.

Slaby, J., Mühlhoff, R., and Wüschner, P. (2019) Affective arrangements. *Emotion Review* 11: 3–12.

Sontag, S. (1989) *Illness as Metaphor! AIDS and its Metaphors*. New York: Anchor.

Stein, H. (1990) *American Medicine and Culture*. New York: Routledge.

Thomas, K. (1997) Health and morality in early modern England. In A. Brandt and P. Rozin (eds) *Morality and Health*. London: Routledge, pp. 15–34.

Todd, Z. (2016) An Indigenous feminist's take on the ontological turn: 'Ontology' is just another word for colonialism. *Journal of Historical Sociology* 29: 4–22.

Vigarello, G. (1988) *Concepts of Cleanliness: Changing Attitudes in France since the Middle Ages*. Cambridge: Cambridge University Press.

van Hout, A., Pols, J., and Willems, D. (2015) Shining trinkets and unkempt gardens: On the materiality of care. *Sociology of Health & Illness* 37: 1206–1217.

Walseth, K., and Tidslevold, T. (2020) Young women's constructions of valued bodies: Healthy, athletic, beautiful and dieting bodies. *The International Review for the Sociology of Sport* 55: 703–725.

Watson, A., Lupton, D., and Michael, M. (2021) Enacting intimacy and sociality at a distance in the COVID-19 crisis: The sociomaterialities of home-based communication technologies. *Media International Australia* 178: 136–150.

Wilson, N.J., and Inkster, J. (2018) Respecting water: Indigenous water governance, ontologies, and the politics of kinship on the ground. *Environment and Planning E* 1: 516–538.

Yu, A. (2020) Digital surveillance in post-coronavirus China: A feminist view on the price we pay. *Gender, Work & Organization* 27: 774–777.

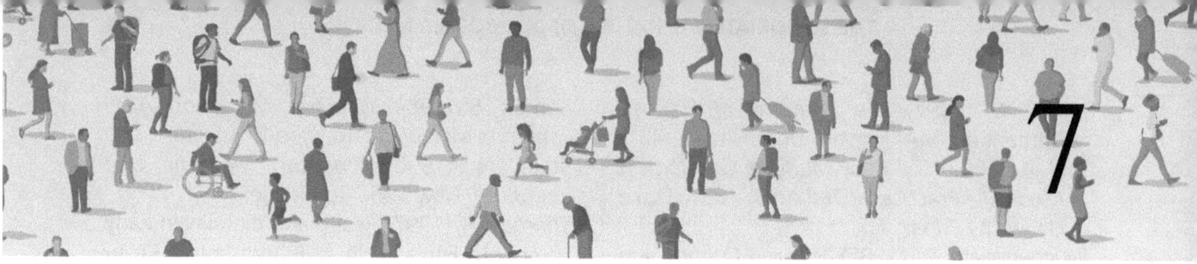

7

Network Analysis: The Social Bridge to Health

Douglas A. Luke and Beth Prusaczyk

INTRODUCTION

Despite the dominance of the medical model of health in the 20th and 21st centuries (Engel 1977), we have always understood that health is very much socially determined. Family and peer influences on smoking and diet; the role of social support on longevity and quality of life; social class and income inequality influencing access to health care; social isolation as a risk factor for depression and suicide; neighborhood influences on the risk of experiencing violence – these are just some of the examples of how social factors are involved with individual, community, and population health. Just as the medical model presupposes certain theories and methods for studying health, we must use other theories and methods if we want to incorporate the social into our understanding of health (Frank & Mustard 1994). The purpose of this chapter is to introduce an important and useful scientific paradigm for studying health, *network science*, and the concomitant set of research methods, *social network analysis*. The chapter starts with an explanation of what network science is, and how it is connected to health. The middle section explores how networks are implicated in infectious disease transmission and prevention, chronic disease, health care delivery, and public health organization. Finally, network analytic methods are briefly discussed.

What are Network Science and Social Network Analysis?

Two definitions are particularly useful for this chapter. First, network science is the use of relational and structural theories to study network representations of complex physical, biological, and social systems. Network science is inherently multidisciplinary, spread across many fields, including genetics, biology, psychology, sociology, political science, public health, engineering, and computer science. Second, *social network analysis* is the set of analytic tools used to explore and model network data, made up of network members (nodes) related to one another via some type of social relationship (ties).

Networks are all around us. Networked systems can be found at every level of organization, from genes, proteins, and cells at the lower end, to networks of organizations, nations, and cultures at the higher end. Biological networks of genes, protein interactions, and inter-cellular communication account for much of human development, physiology, and human disease. The human brain is now viewed as a complex network, or *connectome* (Sporns 2012). Similarly, human diseases and their underlying genetic roots are connected as a *diseasome* (Barabási 2007). Humans naturally organize themselves in socially networked systems. Families, broader kinship ties, neighborhoods, and communities organize themselves in networked systems of relationships. Businesses and other social institutions operate via complex inter-organizational systems of trade, influence, and partnerships (Luke & Harris 2007). Networks are a fundamental way by which the universe is organized and how humans function and thrive.

Exploring and influencing human networks requires alternative scientific theories, methods, and data. Network science is a multidisciplinary set of biological, social, and health theories that view human behavior, health, and disease through relational and structural lenses. Moreover, traditional data collection and analytic approaches are inadequate for studying networked systems. Network data are comprised of information about the relationships (ties) that connect the members (e.g., people, organizations, proteins, etc.) of the network. This implies that networked data are inherently non-independent. Customary statistical assumptions of independence of observations mean that traditional statistical modeling (e.g., general and generalized linear models) cannot be used to analyze network data. Instead, analytic approaches that are appropriate to study dyads, local network structures, network subgroups, and entire networks must be developed and used.

What is the Connection between Networks and Health?

Our experience and a long history of empirical research suggest that physical health, mental health, and societal health are strongly associated with social systems and social connections. How, specifically, might this work? That is, what are the underlying causal mechanisms that create the 'bridge' from the social to health?

Lisa Berkman has presented the most detailed conceptual model for network drivers of health (Berkman et al. 2000). Social networks mediate and moderate the influence of broader cultural, socioeconomic, and physical contexts – and in turn shape a wide variety of psychosocial mechanisms and psychophysical pathways leading to health conditions and outcomes. This can be seen in Figure 7.1, which has been adapted from Berkman's original model (Luke et al. 2017). More specifically, social networks influence their members in two broad ways (Borgatti & Halgin, 2011). First, the networks serve to shape the flow of some resources to the individual members. The resource could be money, health information, social support, etc. Second, the structural position of a person within a social network is important. For example, persons who are in more isolated positions in a network are at greater risk for certain types of health outcomes (e.g., earlier death after a cancer diagnosis).

Berkman's socio-ecological model is being confirmed in a number of ways. One recent and exciting example comes from Schmälzle and colleagues (2017). They conducted experiments where participants were either excluded or included in a 'ball-tossing' social game. They then conducted fMRI (brain) scans and looked for distinctive neuronal network patterns. They were able

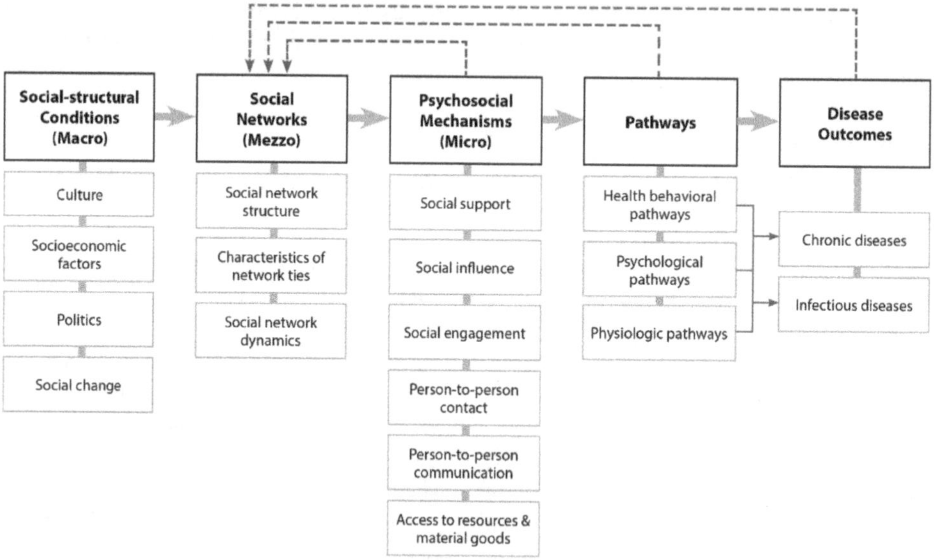

Figure 7.1 An ecological model of social networks and health (adapted from Berkman et al. 2000)

to identify relationships between the participants' friendship networks, their level of exclusion in the experiments, and connectivity patterns in their brains. That is, they demonstrated a pathway between social structure and brain connectivity (Figure 7.2).

NETWORKS IN INFECTIOUS DISEASE

The success of both an infectious disease's spread and its control relies on social networks. This includes not only an individual's immediate social network – their friends, family, colleagues, acquaintances, and other individuals they know and routinely interact with – but also the network of the places they visit and the activities they do where they interact with unknown individuals. An infectious disease thrives on these interactions and its spread can often be traced with great detail through these networks. Because of this, social networks are also critical to the infection control practices employed by public health professionals. An early example of this was during a cholera outbreak in London in 1853 when physician John Snow suspected that contaminated water consumption was the source of transmission and began tracing infected individuals' social and geographic relational structures, specifically their use of various water pumps located in neighborhoods with high rates of cholera. He identified a single pump where a majority of the individuals who became infected early in the outbreak got their water. He hypothesized that this pump was a network hub in the infection outbreak, with many infected individuals connected to it. To test his hypothesis, he convinced officials to disable the pump and upon doing so the outbreak quickly ended. Since 1853, many have built upon Snow's pioneering work to improve and expand the use of network analysis for infectious disease control.

The Impact of Networks on Disease Spread

Due to the ease in which they are transmitted, infectious diseases have plagued cities,

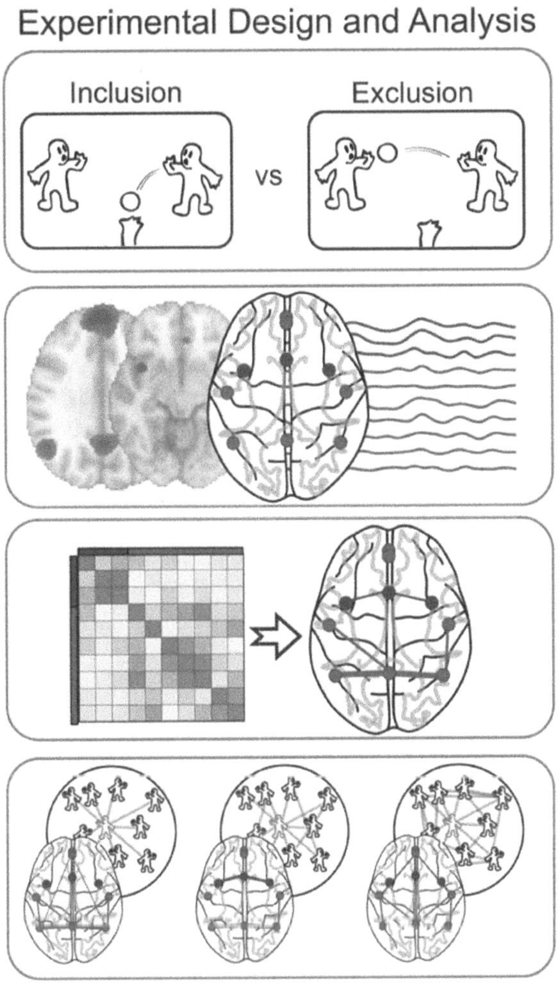

Figure 7.2 Schematic showing how social network factors affect brain network patterns (Schmälzle et al. 2017; Copyright 2017 National Academy of Sciences)

countries, and the world for hundreds of years. Like in the case of cholera and Snow, network analysis has been used to varying degrees in many of these outbreaks. In the early 20th century, when there was still relatively little known about the pathogenesis or transmission of tuberculosis, doctors and public health professionals understood the importance of social networks both in terms of its spread and its treatment. As an airborne disease, cholera spreads more easily in densely populated areas compared to more sparsely populated areas. Neighborhoods with high population density which had many people living in extremely close quarters, such as tenements, saw more transmission than neighborhoods with more single-family residences. The former were primarily neighborhoods for the low-income, low-skilled, or immigrant communities, while the latter were for more wealthy, middle-to-upper-class residents. When physicians realized that the social networks of low-income, low-skilled, and immigrant communities were connected through employment as servants or other service workers to those of the middle and upper classes, a greater emphasis was placed on identifying, counting, and tracing cases (Davis 2000).

This early and crude use of contact tracing has since become more refined (Herrera 2016) and equitable, and is now one of the most critical tools in the armamentarium of infectious disease prevention. Contact tracing, also known as a contact investigation, is the systematic process of identifying individuals (the contacts) exposed to an infectious disease through contact with an infected individual. This analysis of an infected individual's social network includes multiple factors, such as the extent of the disease in the infected index patient, the intensity of an exposure (based on duration, proximity, setting, etc.), the underlying health and immune competence of the contact, and more (CDC report, Taylor 2005). Across the world, contact tracing has increased tuberculosis detection rates, decreased the time to treatment, and helped in the early detection of multidrug-resistant tuberculosis cases (Tian et al. 2013; Kasaie et al. 2014).

While tuberculosis has been around for thousands of years, more novel infectious diseases can also be combatted using network analysis. Those studying the more recent epidemics of Severe Acute Respiratory Syndrome (SARS), Influenza A (H1N1), and the Ebola virus have utilized network analysis during the epidemic to both mitigate the spread, and retrospectively to better understand how the disease was transmitted and what lessons can be learned to apply to future outbreaks (Meyers et al. 2005; Cauchemez et al. 2011; Saurabh & Prateek 2017). Those studying the global COVID-19 pandemic have also utilized network analysis in various ways to understand and mitigate the virus's spread. One emerging application of network analysis with these more recent outbreaks, that has grown exponentially with the COVID-19 pandemic, is the use of social media data for network analyses. The use of social network data collected from Facebook was shown to correlate with the spread of SARS-CoV-2 in early hotspots (Kuchler et al. 2020). In the Wuhan province of China, researchers used the location data of Twitter users to correlate and predict the spatiotemporal spread of COVID-19 globally (Bisanzio et al. 2020).

This novel use of social media data in network analysis has also been applied to more chronic infectious diseases such as human immunodeficiency virus (HIV). In one study of men who have sex with men, those whose closest social network members included an individual met through social media were significantly more likely to have engaged in HIV risk behaviors in the past and more likely to engage in them in the future, compared to individuals who did not have close network members from social media (Holloway et al. 2015).

The Impact of Networks in the Era of COVID-19: Attitudes, Knowledge, and Interventions

The network analyses for infectious diseases described above primarily focus on how the networks facilitate person-to-person transmission of the disease. There is another body of network analysis and infectious disease research that examines the role of an individual's social network on their knowledge, beliefs, attitudes, and opinions on infectious diseases, current outbreaks, real or potential vaccines, and more. Much of this work has been done on the role of social networks during the COVID-19 pandemic. Researchers found that social media users' social networks contributed to the spread of misinformation (Ahmed et al. 2020; Depoux et al. 2020), and that this misinformation hampered the public health response. Others found that the number of Facebook friendships between two locations was associated with how those areas responded to mobility restrictions. The stronger the connection between the two areas based on the number

Box 7.1 Social networks and COVID-19 contact tracing

Contact tracing, an important tool in the infectious disease control armamentarium, is, at its core, a form of network analysis. It has been used around the world to mitigate the spread of COVID-19 and continues to be a critical practice even as vaccines are distributed.

Nagarajan and colleagues (2020) used network analysis methods to analyze the contact tracing data of 1,959 patients diagnosed with COVID-19 in India. Using measures of degree and betweenness centrality as well as sub-group analyses, the authors were able to identify "influential" patients and 19 sub-groups that contributed to almost two-thirds of all transmissions in the network.

While Nagarajan and colleagues analyzed contract tracing data using network analysis methods, Firth and colleagues (2020; see also Figure 7.6) used a publicly available network dataset to simulate, or model, contact tracing. The network dataset, which was created prior to the COVID-19 pandemic, was specifically for modeling infectious disease dynamics. The authors used this network dataset to simulate various mitigation strategies, such as contact tracing, and found that tracing the contacts of contacts, as opposed to tracing only the contacts themselves, led to a reduction in the size of outbreaks. However, this also led to nearly half of the population being quarantined at a single point in time, which would not be a feasible strategy in practice. By using existing network data to simulate infectious disease control practices, the most promising mitigation practices are able to be implemented first with less risk, thus, ideally, improving overall pandemic control.

of Facebook friendships, the more likely the two areas were to have similar compliance responses, even when those areas were geographically distant and had different restriction policies. This suggests that the opinions and attitudes towards the mobility restrictions of those in an individual's social network influenced that individual's behavior (Charoenwong et al. 2020). In the case of HIV and other sexually-transmitted diseases, the influence of an individual's social network on their attitudes and behavior has been well documented, including towards both risk and treatment (Latkin et al. 2003; Kohler et al. 2007; Pilowsky et al. 2007; Bogart et al. 2016).

Because of this documented influence of social networks on infectious diseases, numerous network interventions have been designed and tested. In the case of COVID-19, researchers suggest using the Popular Opinion Leader intervention, which has been shown to be effective in the context of HIV, to train an identified social network opinion leader to disseminate risk reduction strategies (Quinn 2020). Others have used modeling techniques to simulate the effect of network approaches at "flattening the curve" of the COVID-19 pandemic (Block et al. 2020). Block and colleagues' work demonstrated that even in networks with the same size and number of ties, overall network structure can strongly affect the time-course of a disease outbreak like COVID. In addition, they showed how social distancing can break-up social networks, resulting in greater protection from infection risk (Figure 7.3). In an attempt to prevent COVID-19 transmission in the workplace, researchers tested a social network-based intervention that identifies employees who are likely to trigger an outbreak based on characteristics such as sharing offices or participating on the same boards as core nodes. Then, researchers design prevention interventions that address these core nodes (Gallardo et al. 2020).

NETWORKS IN CHRONIC DISEASE

Cancer and Heart Disease

Historically, one of the most consistent network findings in chronic disease has been the association of social isolation and integration with mortality. Starting with the Alameda County study (Berkman & Syme 1979), a

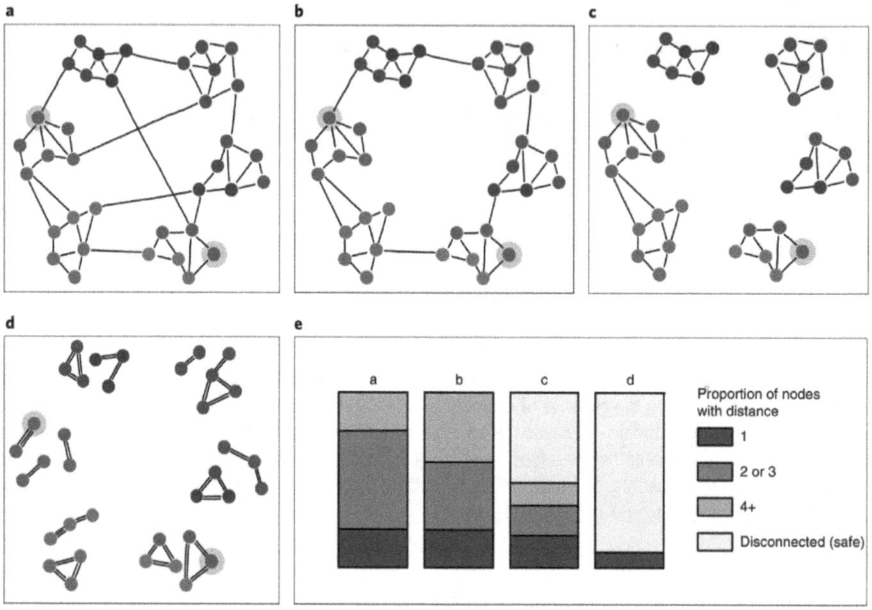

Figure 7.3 Potential infectious protective effects of successive tie-reduction strategies (Block et al. 2020; reprinted with permission)

Distances calculated from a specific node to the nearest "infected" node (denoted by a shaded circle).

long series of large-scale population studies have identified social isolation as a significant general predictor of higher morbidity and mortality from ischemic heart disease, cancer, as well as other chronic conditions such as respiratory diseases (Berkman 1995). Most of these studies relied on simple self-reported measures of personal social network size and degree of social support received; thus, they have little to say about specific causal mechanisms linking social network structures to disease outcomes. In addition to general social support, larger social network size (as well as being married) has been shown to be associated with greater cancer survival rates (Pinquart & Duberstein 2010).

Although we still do not know much about the precise mechanisms that link social network characteristics to the risks for developing cancer and heart disease, research over the past 20 years has started to shed light on two particular pathways: the link between social isolation and chronic disease survival, and the relationship between network characteristics and risk reduction strategies such as cancer screening. Reynolds and Kaplan, with their analyses of the Alameda County study data, were among the first to show that social isolation affects cancer survival rates, but not cancer incidence rates (Reynolds & Kaplan 1990). Since then, a number of studies have confirmed the positive benefits on survival of chronic diseases of social integration (Berkman et al. 2000; Pinquart & Duberstein 2010). These effects are often quite large. Kroenke and colleagues, in their analyses of the Nurses' Health Study (NHS) data, found that women who were socially isolated were more than two times as likely to die from breast cancer than socially integrated women (Kroenke et al. 2006). Another study from the NHS looked more broadly at health-related quality of life; they found that socially isolated women had significantly lower quality of life measures after a breast cancer diagnosis and reported that these effects were larger than tumor size or treatment characteristics (Michael et al. 2002). Most of these studies used quite general measures of network characteristics, often not more than the size of a person's social network. One exception is a study by Villingshøj and colleagues that included measures of social network contact frequency (Villingshøj et al. 2006). Clearly more studies are needed that move beyond simple network size counts as predictors of chronic disease survival.

The second prominent line of research has focused on the role of social networks in chronic disease risk reduction strategies such as cancer screening, genetic testing, and health communications. Over 20 years ago, Allen and colleagues showed that social norms (perceptions that screening was normative among one's peers) were predictive of breast cancer screening among women, but not simple measures of network size (Allen et al. 1999). Using more varied network measures that included both network size and contact frequency, Suarez and colleagues showed that older Mexican-American women with stronger social networks were more likely to get Pap smears and mammograms (Suarez et al. 1994). More recently, Koehly and colleagues showed that family social network characteristics are predictive of the likelihood that two family members will talk to one another about genetic testing for hereditary colorectal cancer (Koehly et al. 2003).

Smoking

In terms of chronic disease risk factors, social network analysis has been used most frequently to study smoking, tobacco use, and tobacco control. Network analysis has been used primarily to address two broad sets of tobacco control questions: how social networks influence individual tobacco use; and how community, state, national, and international tobacco-control systems are structured. Although it has long been known that there are strong peer and family influences on smoking behavior, much of the early empirical work on the social influences on smoking ignored the relational aspect, focusing instead on general social support, familial characteristics, or psychological processes (Biglan et al. 1995). Smoking behavior, especially smoking initiation, is, however, inherently relational and has a network aspect. Almost all people who start smoking do so before they are 18 years old, and when they start, they typically get their first cigarettes from another person, usually a friend or family member (Flay et al. 1994).

Network analysis has been a very powerful approach to studying social and relational influences on smoking behavior. Ennett and Bauman (1993) were among the first to apply this strategy, showing that adolescents who were most isolated from their peers were more likely to smoke. Isolates were identified as having little or no interaction with peers and higher odds of being a current smoker. Clique members, or groups of adolescents who spend more time with each other than with others, and liaisons, who interact with others but not a specific group, both had lower smoking rates.

Other network studies have shown that having a best friend who smoked positively influenced outsiders to smoke but did not show the same influence with those who were part of a friendship group (Aloise-Young et al. 1994). Another study confirmed that there is an accumulation of risk-takers in isolated positions and that individuals in isolated positions drifted towards risk-taking groups, while clique members shifted from non-risk-taking behaviors to risk-taking behaviors over time (Pearson & West 2003).

Gradually, network studies of tobacco use have started to use more sophisticated methods that allow testing of richer structural and causal hypotheses. For example, Alexander and colleagues (2001) conducted an important study that demonstrated an interaction between social network characteristics and school context on the likelihood of smoking. Specifically, they found that popular students (defined in network terms) were more likely to smoke in schools with high smoking prevalence and less likely to smoke in schools with low smoking prevalence (Alexander et al. 2001). Another complex interaction of social environment and network position was recently found by Ennett and colleagues (2008). In their study, they identified an interaction between the number of friends who smoked and the betweenness centrality of the adolescent on the smoking involvement of that adolescent. Essentially, teens who were more centrally positioned in their friendship networks were less likely to be involved in smoking even when they had more friends who smoked. They proposed the interpretation that teens with higher social status (i.e., greater centrality) may have more resources to withstand the influence of friends who smoke. Scientists are also starting to identify potential specific network causal mechanisms for smoking behavior. For example, Lakon and colleagues (2010) suggest that networks influence smoking by structuring flows of emotional support.

Obesity and Physical Activity

Social networks are also implicated in other chronic diseases, including obesity. In an influential network study using data from the Framingham study, Christakis and Fowler (2007) suggested that obesity is "contagious" – participants in the Framingham study were shown to be 57% more likely to become obese if they also had a friend who became obese within a certain time period. Although there have been some methodological critiques of this work (Cohen-Cole & Fletcher 2008; Lyons 2011), its visibility has helped propel further work elucidating the social network mechanisms that may influence obesity (and other chronic disease risk factors).

For example, we know that physical activity behavior is often socially shared (e.g., sports in high school) and that this behavior can directly or indirectly affect weight status. Valente and colleagues (2009) pursue this line in their study of friendship network influence on obesity of adolescents. They found that friendship ties were significantly more likely to occur between teenagers who were of the same weight, compared to those with different weights (Valente et al. 2009). Using more sophisticated exponential random graph model (ERGM) analysis of the much larger National Longitudinal Study of Adolescent Health, Schaefer and colleagues found that non-overweight adolescents (as measured by BMI) tended to avoid forming friendship ties with overweight peers (Schaefer & Simpkins 2014). Although it is challenging to study network effects *on* obesity, it is somewhat easier to assess how networks influence the behavioral risk factors *for* obesity, such as physical activity and diet. For example, adolescents who report spending more time with friends in physical activity are more likely themselves to be physically active (Voorhees et al. 2005). In general, physical activity and exercise to reduce obesity can be enhanced via social networks – for example, participating in a car-pool social network has been shown to predict exercise adherence (Gillett 1988).

NETWORKS IN PUBLIC HEALTH AND HEALTH CARE DELIVERY

The process of delivering health care at the most basic level involves the dyad of the patient and the provider. However, the patient and the provider are part of their own personal networks, the patient and the provider may be part of insurance networks, the provider is part of a network with other providers, and the hospital or clinic is often part of a network with other hospitals or clinics. The interconnectedness of health care delivery makes network analysis a valuable methodology for understanding and improving the delivery process.

Patient Networks

Network analysis has been used to study the impact of patients' networks on their access to care, treatment behaviors, clinical outcomes, and more. Often these studies use ego-centric network analysis. Figure 7.4 represents the ego networks of stroke patients, with the top network (a) representing a smaller network with only strong ties and the bottom network (b) representing a larger network with more weak ties. The researchers found that patients with smaller networks (a in Figure 7.4) were paradoxically more often delayed in arriving at the hospital (Dhand et al. 2019). Similar findings have been shown in cardiac arrest patients (Alonzo 1986).

The networks of patients have also been associated with their attitudes, beliefs, and behaviors towards treatment. One study

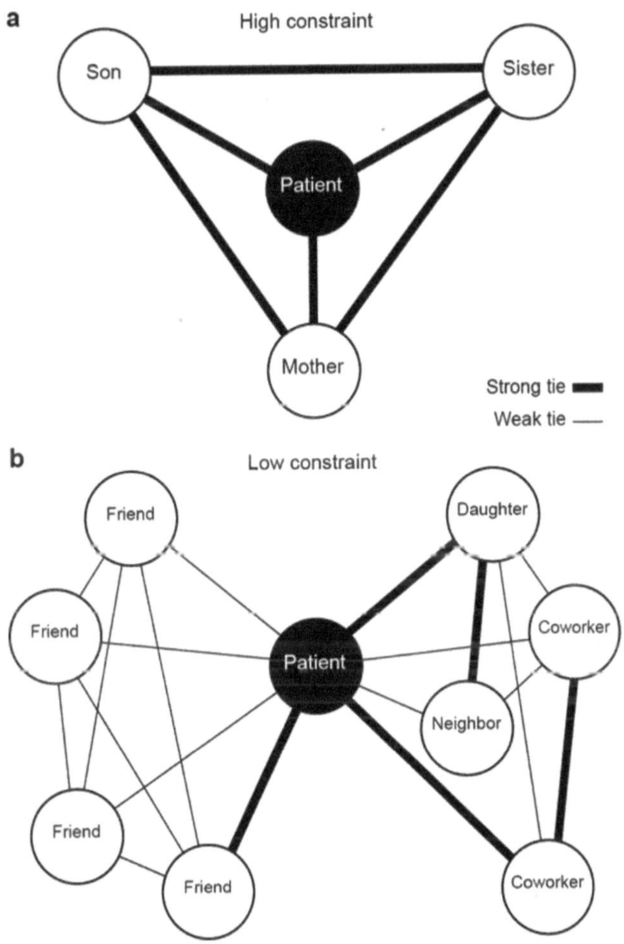

Figure 7.4 Ego-centric networks of stroke patients (monochrome version adapted from Dhand et al. 2019; licensed under the Creative Commons Attribution 4.0 International License, http://creativecommons.org/licenses/by/4.0/)

a. A high constraint, smaller ego patient network with only strong ties. b. A low constraint, larger ego patient network with majority weak ties. The ego is represented by the node in the middle marked "Patient" and the thick lines indicate strong ties and the thin lines indicate weak ties.

of patients with asthma and allergic rhinitis investigated who in their networks was influential in their asthma management decisions. They found that while physicians and other providers were the most commonly reported network members to influence patients' asthma management decisions, non-health care network members also influenced patients' decisions (Cvetkovski et al. 2019). In another study, researchers used the metrics of patients' networks (e.g., betweenness, in-strength, etc.) to predict whether a patient completes or drops out of treatment for depression or anxiety. By using network metrics as predictors in regression models, they found four network characteristics that improved the predictive model, suggesting that collecting information on patients' social networks could be useful in identifying those at risk for attrition (Lutz et al. 2018).

Patients' networks have also been used to understand patients' clinical outcomes. Among patients with serious mental illness, networks that were large, centralized, and homophilous were associated with greater continuity of care, while smaller, centralized, and heterophilous networks were associated with greater social integration (e.g., employment, family relationships, friendships, etc.) (Lorant et al. 2017). In a study of patients with multiple sclerosis, a patient's physical function was found to be associated with their social network structure among patients with multiple sclerosis. Similar to the study predicting treatment attrition for depression or anxiety, in this study, network metrics were entered into multivariable models predicting patients' functional outcomes and the results found that larger network effective size was associated with better physical function and higher network constraint was associated with worse physical function (Levin et al. 2020).

Networks of Providers

Perhaps the most common use of network analysis for health care delivery is among providers. Studies include those on providers' information and decision-making networks (where they seek out and receive information, advice, and support) and of provider teams (both formal and informal, large and small, intra-disciplinary and cross-disciplinary) (Chambers et al. 2012; Bae et al. 2015; Benton et al. 2015; Sabot et al. 2017). One study found that the communication network patterns for nursing units were associated with patient safety and quality outcomes, specifically that more communication was not always associated with better outcomes (Effken et al. 2011). This finding is similar to another network study of hospital discharge teams which found that networks with fewer bidirectional ties were associated with fewer readmissions (Prusaczyk, Kripalani & Dhand 2019).

Networks of Health Organizations and Public Health Systems

A third way in which network analysis can be used to study health care delivery is among inter-organizational health care networks, such as hospital-to-hospital patient transfers or health care systems that own multiple hospitals, clinic practices, home health agencies, and long-term care facilities, or public health networks. The role of geographic location or proximity in health care organization networks has been studied both among hospitals and community clinics. A study of 32 hospitals in Orange County, California, found that geographic proximity was not the primary factor associated with patient-sharing (Lee et al. 2011) while a different study of rural breast cancer care providers found that geographic proximity was the strongest factor associated with patient-sharing (Prusaczyk et al. 2019). In yet another study, geographic proximity was found to be significantly associated with hospital competition and/or cooperation, controlling for organizational characteristics such as size, the volume of activity, perceived quality advantage, and perceived productivity (Mascia & Di Vincenzo 2013).

Public health organizations and systems have also been studied using network analysis. This analysis often studies how different levels (e.g., the organizations, the network/system, and the community) interact or how different types of interaction (e.g., sharing information and resources, collaborating on projects or initiatives, sharing funding, etc.) operate (Provan & Milward 2001; Provan et al. 2005; Valente et al. 2008). For example, in an analysis of five state tobacco control programs, the networks of contact, productivity, money flow, and more were studied (Mueller et al. 2004). The results showed that all states had hierarchical networks where lead agencies served as the hubs of money flow, contact, and more, but that statewide coalitions brought financial stability to the network that allowed for many highly productive relationships. The importance of position in a public health network was also found in a study of organizations involved in a children's health initiative. While a hierarchical pattern was again found, Valente and colleagues (2008) also revealed that an organization's perception of how well the coalition functioned was associated with where an organization fell within that hierarchy. Central organizations that had many opportunities to collaborate across the coalition were more likely to perceive the coalition as well-functioning compared to organizations on the periphery with little opportunity to collaborate. While this hierarchical structure may seem to have a negative effect here, a recent study of community organizations involved in a cardiovascular disease prevention campaign found that a hierarchical structure and high network-level betweenness centrality were associated with achieving program goals (Garney et al. 2020).

NETWORK METHODS FOR THE HEALTH AND SOCIAL SCIENCES

Network analysis comprises a wide variety of analytic techniques. Like any other rich analytic tradition, these network analytic tools can be used for exploratory data analysis, hypothesis building and testing, and more formal model development. Most network analysis techniques fall into one of three broad categories: visualization, network description, and network modeling.

Visualization

A primary product of network analysis, and often the first step of network exploration, is the network diagram. Network diagrams are information graphics that depict the network members (often called nodes) and the relationships that connect them to one another (called ties). Network diagrams are not just pretty pictures; they are analytic tools that can convey important structural properties of a system. For example, consider Figure 7.5, which depicts the sexual transmission network of 'Patient Zero' in the early days of the HIV/AIDS epidemic (Luke & Stamatakis 2012; adapted from Auerbach et al. 1984)[1]. The pattern of ties displays the transmission route of the outbreak, and the judicious use of node labeling and coloring tells a rich story of biology, sexuality, disease, and transportation. These types of disease transmission network visualizations revolutionized how epidemiologists both modeled and observed disease outbreaks, starting in the mid-1980s.

Network Description

Network scientists have developed a multitude of network descriptive statistics that are used to summarize important characteristics and aspects of social networks. These characteristics fall into a few broad categories, including network position (e.g., centrality), local network structure (e.g., transitivity), network sub-groups and communities (e.g., modularity), and overall network structure (e.g., density) (Newman 2010). This only hints at the diversity of descriptive methods that can be used by network scientists. In

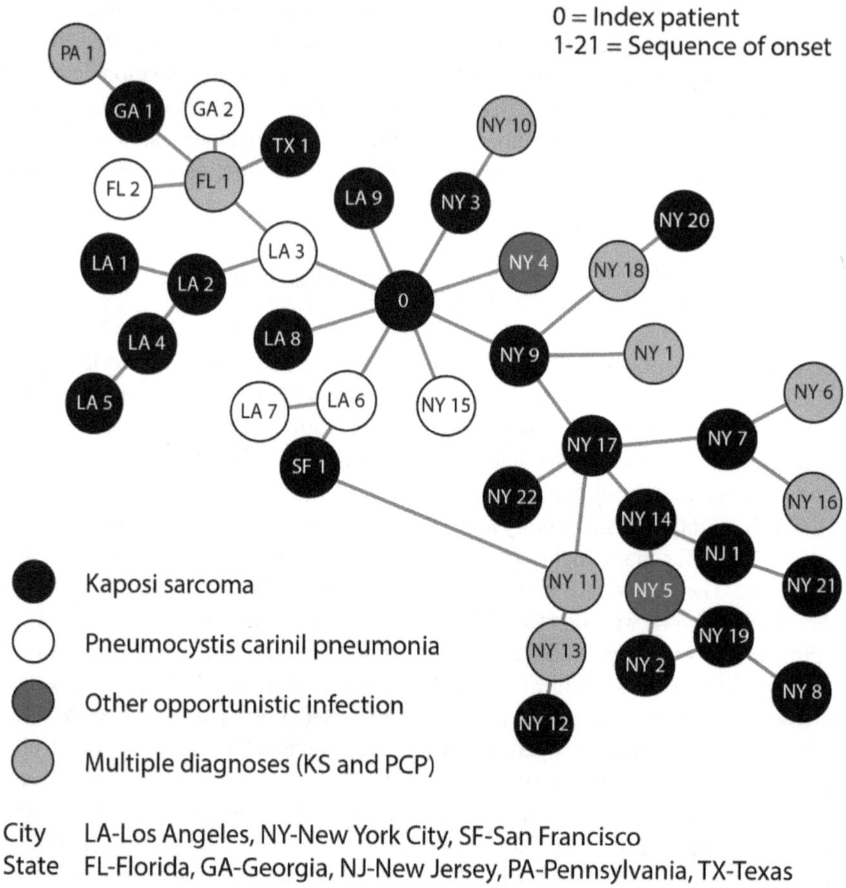

Figure 7.5 Early HIV/AIDS disease transmission network (Luke & Stamatakis 2012; reprinted with permission)

addition to the more basic network descriptions of node location, local structure, subgroups, and overall network characteristics, network analysts can use more advanced techniques to study multiple networks, multiple types of network ties within the same network (e.g., examining trust, friendship, and sexual contact ties within a school), multilevel networks, and how networks change over time (Luke 2015).

Network Modeling

Until recently, network analysis was restricted to visualization and simple description, due to limitation in statistical network theory and computational power. However, in the past few decades there has been rapid development and application of mathematical, statistical, and dynamic network modeling techniques. Theoretical and mathematical models have been developed that help explain fundamental structural properties of real-world social networks, as well as how those networks form. A particularly important theoretical development is the discovery that many real-world networks have heavy-tailed degree distributions that approximately follow a power law. These are typically called *scale-free* networks. Scale-free networks have a distinctive

Table 7.1 Characteristics of social network data

Data Type	*Description*	*Required?*
Nodes	List of nodes in the network	Required
Ties	List of ties connecting the nodes	Required
Node attributes	Characteristics of the nodes	Optional
Tie attributes	Characteristics of the ties	Optional
Metadata	Other information about the entire network	Optional

pattern where most nodes have a small degree (number of connections), while a few nodes have much larger degrees. For example, sexual contacts in human social networks are scale-free (Liljeros et al. 2001).

New advances in statistical modeling of social networks have been one of the most important aids to empirical network research. Exponential random graph models (ERGMs) can be used to develop and test hypotheses about the likelihood of tie formation in cross-sectional social networks (Goodreau 2007; Harris 2013). This means that we can build predictive models that allow us to examine how characteristics of network members, characteristics pairs of members (dyads), and local structural properties (such as transitivity) affect characteristics of the overall social network. These modeling approaches have started to be used more widely in the social sciences and public health, such as in examining the predictors of collaboration among tobacco control networks (Luke et al. 2010).

Valid techniques for modeling network dynamics have also been developed that allow for predictive models of network changes over time (Snijders et al. 2010). These models have important implications for studying social processes, social networks, and health. For example, these types of models have been used to disentangle for the first time the effects of social selection from social influence on how friendship networks and health behavior co-evolve (Mercken et al. 2010).

Social Network Data

Social networks are made up of social objects (e.g., people, hospitals) that are interconnected in some way (e.g., friendship, patient transfers). Therefore, network data must minimally contain information on the network members (i.e., nodes) and their relationships (i.e., ties) (see Table 7.1). In addition to these basic requirements, social network data analyzed using specialized network software will often contain other descriptive information about the nodes and the ties, called attributes. For example, network datasets may contain information on network members such as age or gender. Network ties also can have attributes, so in addition to a network tie indicating whether patients are transferred between two hospitals, the network data may also contain the number of those patients. This is a type of tie strength.

Social network data can be obtained from a myriad of sources. In the health sciences, network data collected through surveys or in-person interviews are probably most common (e.g., Dhand et al. 2019). Disease transmission networks, such as those constructed during the recent COVID-19 pandemic, are based on contact tracing activities that typically included individual interviews. Recent work by Firth and colleagues (2020) simulated control strategies such as contact tracing and quarantine in individuals' social networks (Figure 7.6).

Network data can also be obtained through direct observation, for example in the study of classroom social interactions (Martinez et al. 2003). However, network data can also

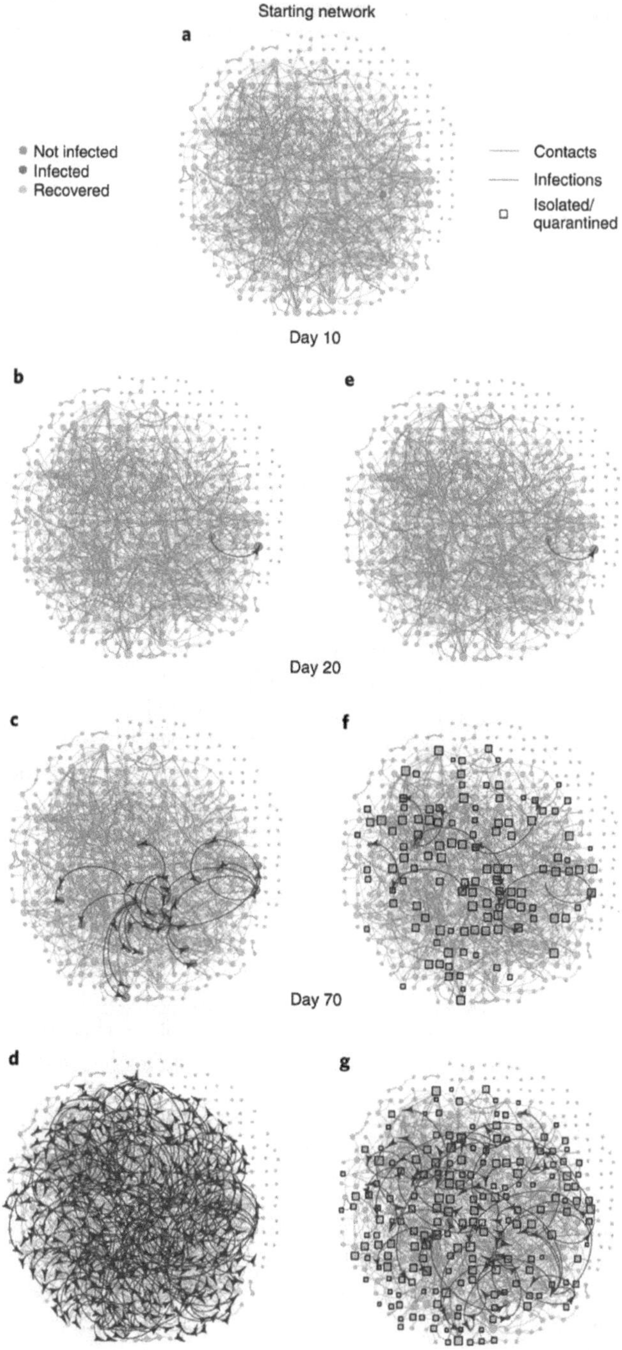

Figure 7.6 Simulating strategies to mitigate the spread of SARS-CoV-2 in social networks (Firth et al. 2020; reprinted with permission)

be created and obtained by using a wide variety of administrative, electronic, data mining, and textual sources. For example, email records are really a type of social network where one person is connected to another through their emails (McCallum et al. 2007). Administrative records of group membership or meeting attendance can be used to produce affiliation data, from which network ties can be inferred and analyzed (Borgatti & Halgin 2011). More details on the collection and management of network data are provided by Adams (2019).

SUMMARY

The world is organized in networks, from our brains to our interconnected webs of animals and organisms, to our information systems. Our social world is similarly interconnected; in fact, it is those connections between people, organizations, communities, and nations that define the concept of 'social.' It is no surprise, then, that much of health is socially driven. It is still surprising to many people to hear that social connections and relationships are the most important predictors of happiness, well-being, and quality of life (Vaillant 2008; Headey et al. 2013).

Berkman and others have articulated how social networks are implicated in maintaining health, structuring disease transmission, and shaping how health care and public health systems support individual and public health. COVID-19 has provided a comprehensive (and devasting) example of how social networks act as 'health conduits.' First, interpersonal networks are the primary avenue for disease transmission. Information networks (both formal and informal) shape individual decision-making around health behavior and risk mitigation. Organizational networks support or hinder everything from national and community pandemic preparedness, distribution of health resources (e.g., vaccines), emergency health care access, and dissemination and implementation of evidence-based protection policies (e.g., social distancing, use of personal protective equipment).

Network science has emerged as the primary paradigm, disciplinary field, and analytic approach for studying connections in complex social systems. As such, it is also an important tool for both studying social drivers of health, and using social information to intervene and hopefully improve individual and population health. Or, as John Donne much more powerfully pointed out more than 400 years ago, "No man [sic.] is an island entire of itself; every man is a piece of the continent, a part of the main."

Note

1 (It is important to note that recent investigations have revealed that the use of the term 'patient zero' is actually a misnomer, and this mis-labeling is based on a typo where a capital 'O', was replaced with a numeric 0. The capital 'O' was meant to refer to the source of the local HIV infection from 'outside' of California (Worobey, et al. 2016).)

REFERENCES

Adams, J. (2019). *Gathering social network data*. London: Sage.

Ahmed, W., Vidal-Alaball, J., Downing, J., & Seguí, F. L. (2020). COVID-19 and the 5G conspiracy theory: social network analysis of Twitter data. *Journal of Medical Internet Research*, *22*(5), e19458.

Alexander, C., Piazza, M., Mekos, D., & Valente, T. (2001). Peers, schools, and adolescent cigarette smoking. *Journal of Adolescent Health*, *29*(1), 22–30.

Allen, J. D., Sorensen, G., Stoddard, A. M., Peterson, K. E., & Colditz, G. (1999). The relationship between social network characteristics and breast cancer screening practices among employed women. *Annals of Behavioral Medicine*, *21*(3), 193–200.

Aloise-Young, P. A., Graham, J. W., & Hansen, W. B. (1994). Peer influence on smoking initiation during early adolescence: a comparison of group members and group outsiders. *Journal of Applied Psychology*, *79*(2), 281.

Alonzo, A. A. (1986). The impact of the family and lay others on care-seeking during life-threatening episodes of suspected coronary artery disease. *Social Science & Medicine*, *22*(12), 1297–1311.

Auerbach, D. M., Darrow, W. W., Jaffe, H. W., & Curran, J. W. (1984). Cluster of cases of the acquired immune deficiency syndrome: patients linked by sexual contact. *The American Journal of Medicine*, *76*(3), 487–492.

Bae, S. H., Nikolaev, A., Seo, J. Y., & Castner, J. (2015). Health care provider social network analysis: a systematic review. *Nursing Outlook*, *63*(5), 566–584.

Barabási, A. L. (2007). Network medicine – from obesity to the "diseasome". *The New England Journal of Medicine*, *357*(4), 404–407.

Benton, D. C., Pérez-Raya, F., Fernández-Fernández, M. P., & González-Jurado, M. A. (2015). A systematic review of nurse-related social network analysis studies. *International Nursing Review*, *62*(3), 321–339.

Berkman, L. F. (1995). The role of social relations in health promotion. *Psychosomatic Medicine*, *57*(3), 245–254.

Berkman, L. F., Glass, T., Brissette, I., & Seeman, T. E. (2000). From social integration to health: Durkheim in the new millennium. *Social Science & Medicine*, *51*(6), 843–857.

Berkman, L. F., & Syme, S. L. (1979). Social networks, host resistance, and mortality: a nine-year follow-up study of Alameda County residents. *American Journal of Epidemiology*, *109*(2), 186–204.

Biglan, A., Duncan, T. E., Ary, D. V., & Smolkowski, K. (1995). Peer and parental influences on adolescent tobacco use. *Journal of Behavioral Medicine*, *18*(4), 315–330.

Bisanzio, D., Kraemer, M. U., Bogoch, I. I., Brewer, T., Brownstein, J. S., & Reithinger, R. (2020). Use of Twitter social media activity as a proxy for human mobility to predict the spatiotemporal spread of COVID-19 at global scale. *Geospatial Health*, *15*(1).

Block, P., Hoffman, M., Raabe, I. J., Dowd, J. B., Rahal, C., Kashyap, R., & Mills, M. C. (2020). Social network-based distancing strategies to flatten the COVID-19 curve in a post-lockdown world. *Nature Human Behaviour*, *4*(6), 588–596.

Bogart, L. M., Wagner, G. J., Green Jr, H. D., Mutchler, M. G., Klein, D. J., McDavitt, B., ... & Hilliard, C. L. (2016). Medical mistrust among social network members may contribute to antiretroviral treatment nonadherence in African Americans living with HIV. *Social Science & Medicine*, *164*, 133–140.

Borgatti, S. P., & Halgin, D. S. (2011). On network theory. *Organization science*, *22*(5), 1168–1181.

Borgatti, S. P., & Halgin, D. S. (2011). Analyzing affiliation networks. *The Sage handbook of social network analysis*, *1*, 417–433.

Cauchemez, S., Bhattarai, A., Marchbanks, T. L., Fagan, R. P., Ostroff, S., Ferguson, N. M., ... & Pennsylvania H1N1 Working Group. (2011). Role of social networks in shaping disease transmission during a community outbreak of 2009 H1N1 pandemic influenza. *Proceedings of the National Academy of Sciences*, *108*(7), 2825–2830.

Chambers, D., Wilson, P., Thompson, C., & Harden, M. (2012). Social network analysis in healthcare settings: a systematic scoping review. *PloS One*, *7*(8), e41911.

Charoenwong, B., Kwan, A., & Pursiainen, V. (2020, April 13). *Social connections with COVID-19-affected areas increase compliance with mobility restrictions.* Available at SSRN: https://ssrn.com/abstract=3574560

Christakis, N. A., & Fowler, J. H. (2007). The spread of obesity in a large social network over 32 years. *New England Journal of Medicine*, *357*(4), 370–379.

Cohen-Cole, E., & Fletcher, J. M. (2008). Is obesity contagious? Social networks vs. environmental factors in the obesity epidemic. *Journal of Health Economics*, *27*(5), 1382–1387.

Cvetkovski, B., Tan, R., Kritikos, V., Yan, K., Azzi, E., Srour, P., & Bosnic-Anticevich, S. (2019). Exploring the Asthma Network in people with allergic rhinitis utilizing an egocentric social network analysis. *Pulmonary Therapy*, *5*(2), 235–245.

Davis, A. L. (2000). A historical perspective on tuberculosis and its control. *Lung Biology in Health and Disease*, *144*, 3–54.

Depoux, A., Martin, S., Karafillakis, E., Preet, R., Wilder-Smith, A., & Larson, H. (2020). The pandemic of social media panic travels faster than the COVID-19 outbreak. *Journal of Travel Medicine*, *27*(3). Epub ahead of print 2020. doi: 10.1093/jtm/taaa031.

Dhand, A., Luke, D., Lang, C., Tsiaklides, M., Feske, S., & Lee, J. M. (2019). Social networks and risk of delayed hospital arrival after acute stroke. *Nature Communications*, *10*(1), 1–8.

Effken, J. A., Carley, K. M., Gephart, S., Verran, J. A., Bianchi, D., Reminga, J., & Brewer, B. B. (2011). Using ORA to explore the relationship of nursing unit communication to patient safety and quality outcomes. *International Journal of Medical Informatics*, *80*(7), 507–517.

Effken, J. A., Gephart, S. M., Brewer, B. B., & Carley, K. M. (2013). Using* ORA, a network analysis tool, to assess the relationship of handoffs to quality and safety outcomes. *Computers, Informatics, Nursing: CIN*, *31*(1), 36.

Engel, G. L. (1977). The need for a new medical model: a challenge for biomedicine. *Science*, *196*(4286), 129–136.

Ennett, S. T., & Bauman, K. E. (1993). Peer group structure and adolescent cigarette smoking: a social network analysis. *Journal of Health and Social Behavior*, 226–236.

Ennett, S. T., Faris, R., Hipp, J., Foshee, V. A., Bauman, K. E., Hussong, A., & Cai, L. (2008). Peer smoking, other peer attributes, and adolescent cigarette smoking: a social network analysis. *Prevention Science*, *9*(2), 88–98.

Frank, J., & Mustard, J. (1994). The Determinants of Health from a Historical Perspective. *Daedalus*, *123*(4), 1–19. Retrieved July 6, 2021, from http://www.jstor.org/stable/20027264

Firth, J. A., Hellewell, J., Klepac, P., Kissler, S., Kucharski, A. J., & Spurgin, L. G. (2020). Using a real-world network to model localized COVID-19 control strategies. *Nature Medicine*, *26*(10), 1616–1622.

Flay, B. R., Hu, F. B., Siddiqui, O., Day, L. E., Hedeker, D., Petraitis, J., ... & Sussman, S. (1994). Differential influence of parental smoking and friends' smoking on adolescent initiation and escalation and smoking. *Journal of Health and Social Behavior*, *35*(3), 248–265.

Gallardo, E. C., de Arroyabe, J. C. F., & Arranz, N. (2020). Preventing internal COVID-19 outbreaks within businesses and institutions: a methodology based on social networks analysis for supporting occupational health and safety services decision making. *Sustainability*, *12*(11), 1–16.

Garney, W. R., Patterson, M. S., Garcia, K., Muraleetharan, D., & McLeroy, K. (2020). Interorganizational network findings from a nationwide cardiovascular disease prevention initiative. *Evaluation and Program Planning*, *79*, 101771.

Gillett, P. A. (1988). Self-reported factors influencing exercise adherence in overweight women. *Nursing Research*, *37*(1), 25–29.

Goodreau, S. M. (2007). Advances in exponential random graph (p*) models applied to a large social network. *Social Networks*, *29*(2), 231–248.

Harris, J. K. (2013). *An introduction to exponential random graph modeling* (Vol. 173). London: Sage.

Headey, B., Muffels, R., & Wagner, G. G. (2013). Choices which change life satisfaction: similar results for Australia, Britain and Germany. *Social Indicators Research*, *112*(3), 725–748.

Herrera, J. L., Srinivasan, R., Brownstein, J. S., Galvani, A. P., & Meyers, L. A. (2016). Disease surveillance on complex social networks. *PLoS Computational Biology*, *12*(7), e1004928.

Holloway, I. W., Pulsipher, C. A., Gibbs, J., Barman-Adhikari, A., & Rice, E. (2015). Network influences on the sexual risk behaviors of gay, bisexual and other men who have sex with men using geosocial networking applications. *AIDS and Behavior*, *19*(2), 112–122.

Kasaie, P., Andrews, J. R., Kelton, W. D., & Dowdy, D. W. (2014). Timing of tuberculosis transmission and the impact of household contact tracing: an agent-based simulation model. *American Journal of Respiratory and Critical Care Medicine*, *189*(7), 845–852.

Koehly, L. M., Peterson, S. K., Watts, B. G., Kempf, K. K., Vernon, S. W., & Gritz, E. R. (2003). A social network analysis of communication about hereditary nonpolyposis colorectal cancer genetic testing and family functioning. *Cancer Epidemiology and Prevention Biomarkers*, *12*(4), 304–313.

Kohler, H. P., Behrman, J. R., & Watkins, S. C. (2007). Social networks and HIV/AIDS risk perceptions. *Demography*, *44*(1), 1–33.

Krauss, M., Mueller, N., & Luke, D. (2004). Interorganizational relationships within state tobacco control networks: a social network analysis. *Preventing Chronic Disease*, *1*(4), A08–A08.

Kroenke, C. H., Kubzansky, L. D., Schernhammer, E. S., Holmes, M. D., & Kawachi, I. (2006). Social networks, social support, and survival after breast cancer diagnosis. *Journal of Clinical Oncology*, *24*(7), 1105–1111.

Kuchler, T., Russel, D., & Stroebel, J. (2020). *The geographic spread of COVID-19 correlates with structure of social networks as measured by Facebook (No. w26990)*. Cambridge, MA: National Bureau of Economic Research.

Lakon, C. M., Hipp, J. R., & Timberlake, D. S. (2010). The social context of adolescent smoking: a systems perspective. *American Journal of Public Health*, *100*(7), 1218–1228.

Latkin, C. A., Forman, V., Knowlton, A., & Sherman, S. (2003). Norms, social networks, and HIV-related risk behaviors among urban disadvantaged drug users. *Social Science & Medicine*, *56*(3), 465–476.

Lee, B. Y., McGlone, S. M., Song, Y., Avery, T. R., Eubank, S., Chang, C. C., … & Huang, S. S. (2011). Social network analysis of patient sharing among hospitals in Orange County, California. *American Journal of Public Health*, *101*(4), 707–713.

Levin, S. N., Riley, C. S., Dhand, A., White, C. C., Venkatesh, S., Boehm, B., … & Levine-Bc, L. (2020). Association of social network structure and physical function in patients with multiple sclerosis. *Neurology*, *95*(11), e1565–e1574; doi: 10.1212/WNL.0000000000010460

Liljeros, F., Edling, C. R., Amaral, L. A. N., Stanley, H. E., & Åberg, Y. (2001). The web of human sexual contacts. *Nature*, *411*(6840), 907–908.

Lorant, V., Nazroo, J., Nicaise, P., & Title107 Study Group. (2017). Optimal network for patients with severe mental illness: a social network analysis. *Administration and Policy in Mental Health and Mental Health Services Research*, *44*(6), 877–887.

Luke, D. A. (2015). *A user's guide to network analysis in R*. Cham, Switzerland: Springer.

Luke, D. A., Dhand, A., & Carothers, B. J. (2017). Social network analysis. In A. M. El-Sayed & S. Galea (Eds.), *Systems science and population health*, pp. 113–126. Oxford: Oxford University Press.

Luke, D. A., & Harris, J. K. (2007). Network analysis in public health: history, methods, and applications. *Annual Review of Public Health*, *28*, 69–93.

Luke, D. A., Harris, J. K., Shelton, S., Allen, P., Carothers, B. J., & Mueller, N. B. (2010). Systems analysis of collaboration in 5 national tobacco control networks. *American Journal of Public Health*, *100*(7), 1290–1297.

Luke, D. A., & Stamatakis, K. A. (2012). Systems science methods in public health: dynamics, networks, and agents. *Annual Review of Public Health*, *33*, 357–376.

Lutz, W., Schwartz, B., Hofmann, S. G., Fisher, A. J., Husen, K., & Rubel, J. A. (2018). Using network analysis for the prediction of treatment dropout in patients with mood and anxiety disorders: a methodological proof-of-concept study. *Scientific Reports*, *8*(1), 1–9.

Lyons, R. (2011). The spread of evidence-poor medicine via flawed social-network analysis. *Statistics, Politics and Policy*, *2*(1).

Martınez, A., Dimitriadis, Y., Rubia, B., Gómez, E., & De La Fuente, P. (2003). Combining qualitative evaluation and social network analysis for the study of classroom social interactions. *Computers & Education*, *41*(4), 353–368.

Mascia, D., & Di Vincenzo, F. (2013). Dynamics of hospital competition: social network analysis in the Italian National Health Service. *Health Care Management Review*, *38*(3), 234–247.

McCallum, A., Wang, X., & Corrada-Emmanuel, A. (2007). Topic and role discovery in social networks with experiments on enron and academic email. *Journal of Artificial Intelligence Research*, *30*, 249–272.

Mercken, L., Snijders, T. A., Steglich, C., Vartiainen, E., & De Vries, H. (2010).

Dynamics of adolescent friendship networks and smoking behavior. *Social Networks*, *32*(1), 72–81.

Meyers, L. A., Pourbohloul, B., Newman, M. E., Skowronski, D. M., & Brunham, R. C. (2005). Network theory and SARS: predicting outbreak diversity. *Journal of Theoretical Biology*, *232*(1), 71–81.

Michael, Y. L., Berkman, L. F., Colditz, G. A., Holmes, M. D., & Kawachi, I. (2002). Social networks and health-related quality of life in breast cancer survivors: a prospective study. *Journal of Psychosomatic Research*, *52*(5), 285–293.

Mueller, N., Krauss, M., & Luke, D. (2004). PEER REVIEWED: Interorganizational relationships within state tobacco control networks: a social network analysis. *Preventing Chronic Disease*, *1*(4).

Nagarajan, K., Muniyandi, M., Palani, B., & Sellappan, S. (2020). Social network analysis methods for exploring SARS-CoV-2 contact tracing data. *BMC Medical Research Methodology*, *20*(1), 1–10.

National Tuberculosis Controllers Association. (2005). Guidelines for the investigation of contacts of persons with infectious tuberculosis. Recommendations from the National Tuberculosis Controllers Association and CDC. *Morbidity and Mortality Weekly Report. Recommendations and Reports*, *54*(RR–15), 1–47.

Newman, M. (2010). *Networks: an introduction*. Oxford: Oxford University Press.

Pearson, M., & West, P. (2003). Drifting smoke rings. *Connections*, *25*(2), 59–76.

Pilowsky, D. J., Hoover, D., Hadden, B., Fuller, C., Ompad, D. C., Andrews, H. F., ... & Latkin, C. (2007). Impact of social network characteristics on high-risk sexual behaviors among non-injection drug users. *Substance Use & Misuse*, *42*(11), 1629–1649.

Pinquart, M., & Duberstein, P. R. (2010). Associations of social networks with cancer mortality: a meta-analysis. *Critical Reviews in Oncology/Hematology*, *75*(2), 122–137.

Provan, K. G., & Milward, H. B. (2001). Do networks really work? A framework for evaluating public-sector organizational networks. *Public Administration Review*, *61*(4), 414–423.

Provan, K. G., Veazie, M. A., Staten, L. K., & Teufel-Shone, N. I. (2005). The use of network analysis to strengthen community partnerships. *Public Administration Review*, *65*(5), 603–613.

Prusaczyk, B., Kripalani, S., & Dhand, A. (2019). Networks of hospital discharge planning teams and readmissions. *Journal of Interprofessional Care*, *33*(1), 85–92.

Prusaczyk, B., Maki, J., Luke, D. A., & Lobb, R. (2019). Rural health networks: how network analysis can inform patient care and organizational collaboration in a rural breast cancer screening network. *The Journal of Rural Health*, *35*(2), 222–228.

Quinn, K. G. (2020). Applying the popular opinion leader intervention for HIV to COVID-19. *AIDS and Behavior*, *24*(12), 3291–3294.

Reynolds, P., & Kaplan, G. A. (1990). Social connections and risk for cancer: prospective evidence from the Alameda County Study. *Behavioral Medicine*, *16*(3), 101–110.

Sabot, K., Wickremasinghe, D., Blanchet, K., Avan, B., & Schellenberg, J. (2017). Use of social network analysis methods to study professional advice and performance among healthcare providers: a systematic review. *Systematic Reviews*, *6*(1), 208.

Saurabh, S., & Prateek, S. (2017). Role of contact tracing in containing the 2014 Ebola outbreak: a review. *African Health Sciences*, *17*(1), 225–236.

Schaefer, D. R., & Simpkins, S. D. (2014). Using social network analysis to clarify the role of obesity in selection of adolescent friends. *American Journal of Public Health*, *104*(7), 1223–1229.

Schmälzle, R., O'Donnell, M. B., Garcia, J. O., Cascio, C. N., Bayer, J., Bassett, D. S., ... & Falk, E. B. (2017). Brain connectivity dynamics during social interaction reflect social network structure. *Proceedings of the National Academy of Sciences*, *114*(20), 5153–5158.

Snijders, T. A., Van de Bunt, G. G., & Steglich, C. E. (2010). Introduction to stochastic actor-based models for network dynamics. *Social Networks*, *32*(1), 44–60.

Sporns, O. (2012). *Discovering the human connectome*. Cambridge, MA: MIT Press.

Suarez, L., Lloyd, L., Weiss, N., Rainbolt, T., & Pulley, L. (1994). Effect of social networks on cancer-screening behavior of older Mexican-American women. *JNCI: Journal of the National Cancer Institute*, *86*(10), 775–779.

Tian, Y., Osgood, N. D., Al-Azem, A., & Hoeppner, V. H. (2013). Evaluating the effectiveness of contact tracing on tuberculosis outcomes in Saskatchewan using individual-based modeling. *Health Education & Behavior*, *40*(1 suppl), 98S–110S.

Vaillant, G. E. (2008). *Aging well: Surprising guideposts to a happier life from the landmark study of adult development*. London: Hachette UK.

Valente, T. W., Coronges, K. A., Stevens, G. D., & Cousineau, M. R. (2008). Collaboration and competition in a children's health initiative coalition: a network analysis. *Evaluation and Program Planning*, *31*(4), 392–402.

Valente, T. W., Fujimoto, K., Chou, C. P., & Spruijt-Metz, D. (2009). Adolescent affiliations and adiposity: a social network analysis of friendships and obesity. *Journal of Adolescent Health*, *45*(2), 202–204.

Villingshøj, M., Ross, L., Thomsen, B. L., & Johansen, C. (2006). Does marital status and altered contact with the social network predict colorectal cancer survival? *European Journal of Cancer*, *42*(17), 3022–3027.

Voorhees, C. C., Murray, D., Welk, G., Birnbaum, A., Ribisl, K. M., Johnson, C. C., … & Jobe, J. B. (2005). The role of peer social network factors and physical activity in adolescent girls. *American Journal of Health Behavior*, *29*(2), 183–190.

Worobey, M., Watts, T. D., McKay, R. A., Suchard, M. A., Granade, T., Teuwen, D. E., … & Jaffe, H. W. (2016). 1970s and 'Patient 0'HIV-1 genomes illuminate early HIV/AIDS history in North America. *Nature*, *539*(7627), 98–101.

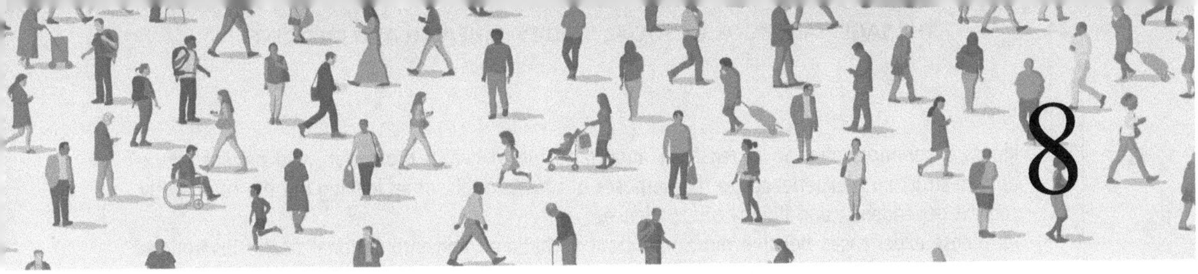

8 Personal Experience of Illness

Christine Holmberg and Martina Breuning

INTRODUCTION

Box 8.1 What you learn from this chapter

- Personal experiences of illness are expressions of social experiences that develop at the nexus of collective experiences, cultural representations, and embodied subjectivities. They are shaped by political, social, and economic frameworks and are represented through language and objects.
- Direct access to 'pure' experience is not possible. We need a description of an individual's inner processes, which can represent the subjective inner experience to the outer world. These verbal or non-verbal representations of experience can be observed and studied.
- Such representations consist of personal or public stories (narratives), pictures, tales, and the arts. They provide unique insights into the cultural and social shaping of lives, as they are themselves formed by cultural and social templates and normative standards.
- Personal illness experiences are an important part of "everyday life" and are presented in different contexts (private and public), with different aims and effects.
- Illness experiences shape and are shaped by other people's experiences, both proximal and distant.
- Understanding personal experiences of illness sheds light on how vulnerability is culturally and socially shaped, and how individuals and society cope with uncertainty, including healthcare seeking.
- Increasingly, both verbal and non-verbal expressions of personal illness experiences are present in the public realm. Such sharing of one's experiences can empower people to manage their illness in a self-assured way and to make their own decisions along their navigations through the medical field.
- The social sciences know many different methods of collecting illness experiences, most importantly narrative interviews and ethnographies.

(Continued)

(Continued)

- Illness experiences play an increasingly important role in health promotion, and patient education, re-structuring experiences to the purposes of professionals, often leaving out the complexitiy, context-dependency, and fluidity of experience.
- As illness experiences become more important to national and international health institutions, standardized measures such as patient-reported outcomes and patient-reported experiences have been developed. While they are useful, their limitations need to be carefully considered. Reducing experience to a number necessarily leaves out the context which is so crucial in making experience. Thus, such measures should always be complemented with open methods that allow us to explore the context and social world of experiences.

> It was a hot summer's day. I was going along a road and it was dry and hot. I was walking in the shade, slowly, plodding home after school. And suddenly I noticed a strange burning feeling of tension that took over. It was as if some force was pulling me this way and another force was pulling me the other way. Forces pulled in all directions. It made me totally immobile. Very strong forces. And then I had a picture – when you close your eyes in sunlight it becomes red with sparkles, just like a sparkler. It seemed like in physics, with a plus and minus pole between which the iron shavings align. And then there was a sound, the bang of a bell and the sound of waves moving outwards. Finally, I heard someone say my name. Then I fell and everything vanished. Obviously someone found me and then I found myself on the couch in the living room of our family home. Everyone was scared and I was exhausted. It is a very private experience. You don't know where the voice is coming from. Sometimes I read of others' experiences of near death. Perhaps this is similar. You have no choice.

This is how Barbara, a 54-year-old woman living in southern Germany, who has had epilepsy since her youth, describes the experience of her first seizure at the age of 15. She had to cope with tonic-clonic convulsive seizures until she was in her mid-twenties; since that time, she has been seizure-free. Why the seizures stopped we do not know. Barbara has two possible explanations: she has trained a lot in meditation practice, which may have had an effect; or she believes that she might have suffered from a type of epilepsy that stops after puberty. After completing school, she started to work as an actress. Today she is working in the medical-therapeutic field. Barbara has an unusual eloquence when describing her seizures. Her story is a mighty one in which forces and powers play a key role. She describes a seizure as a process from which there is no escape, and she uses metaphors from physics to describe her feelings during a seizure. To put her experiences into words, she refers to things she already knew; her background as a German schoolgirl, for instance, is revealed through her choice of metaphors and references.

Another key feature of personal experiences of illness – as opposed to medical or biological descriptions, or epidemiological or statistical representations – is revealed in Barbara's account. Barbara's experience is not a pathological one, nor is it a discourse of normality or present-day norms. It is rather a powerful description of bodily sensations. There is not yet a medical label on the experience, and thus the social consequences of the diagnosis are not (yet) present. The account deals solely with the bodily experience that Barbara encountered as a teenager. This is why this, and other personal accounts of illness experience, help us to understand illness beyond the master narratives of medicine and medical definitions. This in turn enables us to learn about what illness may consist of, and how illness, society, and culture interact with each other to make up an illness experience.

WHAT IS AN ILLNESS EXPERIENCE?

Personal experiences of illness develop out of complex processes of becoming, from what the phenomenologist James calls "pure experience." Such pure experience begins prior to its organization into distinctive contents, forms, and structures (James 1996; Throop 2003). It consists of a sensory immediacy, which is radically subjective and hidden from an empirical gaze. If we follow phenomenological philosophers such as Dilthey, Merleau-Ponty, and others (Dilthey & Rickmann 1976; Merleau-Ponty 2012 [1945]; Desjarlais & Throop 2011) experience is understood as a constant process of becoming in which modes of perception, social relations, things, and events form lived experiences, which through the interpretation of such stimuli, become palpable in conceptualizations, verbalizations, and narrations. Embodied sensations are the base of experiencing.

Personal experiences of illness – as a phenomenon to be studied by social scientists – evolve from a radically subjective mode into an interpretation and ordering of the encountered stimuli within the lived body. Such interpretations are embedded in the values, assumptions, ideals, and norms of the lived-in lifeworld, which is made up of experiences as much as it informs them. The structure of experiencing is both the immediacy of temporal flux and its reflective assessment embedded in the pre theoretical and familiar world we live in, which consists of culturally elaborated systems of significant symbols, "webs of significance" (Geertz 1973; Throop 2003, see also Holmberg 2018, for a summary). Social ordering and cultural assumptions structure our innermost experiences and intertwine with what is considered personal. This involves processes of differentiation, such as between the inner and outer worlds, self and other, the perception and understanding of things (Merleau-Ponty 2012 [1945]). Understanding such sensations as illness, which eventually leads to an illness experience, is not fixed but is a becoming, a becoming that is shaped by time, events, and place. The interpretive frame of experiencing is an ever-changing one.

Scholars of medical anthropology introduced the analytical distinction between disease and illness. This distinction aims to highlight the social and personal embedding of illness and its particularities in contrast to biomedical knowledge and understandings of health and disease. As Seeman and Kleinman (2000: 231) put it, disease in the early phase of medical anthropology was considered "the practitioner's construction of patient complaints in the technical terminology of a particular healing system." It was located in the body, in its cellular and molecular processes that can be investigated in the laboratory. In contrast, illness is understood as what is felt by the afflicted person. As anthropology turned its gaze also on the study of biomedicine as a cultural system (Del Vecchio 1995; Frankenberg 1980; Lock & Gordon 1988; Young 1982), the concepts of illness and disease became more fluid. Disease as a discrete entity to be studied in isolation is one of the "tenacious assumptions of biomedicine" explored by Gordon (1988) and elaborated further by others (e.g. DelVecchio, Good 1994; Singer 2004).

Thus, from a social science perspective, neither illness nor disease are given; they are interconnected and are made by the medical, social, and cultural frameworks in which the normal and the abnormal are shaped. To understand illness experiences in their cultural and social complexity, one needs to dig beyond given cultural differentiation strategies in order to investigate how vulnerabilities are fluid as well as culturally fixed in discourses of the normal. More recently, an analytical differentiation of sensations from symptoms has been suggested to guide an understanding of how symptoms, understood as the signs that guide an individual to seek help in a medical system, come into being. Such processes have been called "symptomatization" (Risør 2011: 22).

The process of symptomatization is what interconnects illness and disease and makes it a lived experience embedded in the social world (see Andersen et al. 2010; Brandner et al. 2014, Gijsbers van Wijk & Kolk 1997; Hay 2008). Scholars have distinguished between sensations and senses on the one hand, and symptoms on the other, to understand the making of illness experiences. Sensations consist of changes in sensual experiences in particular socio-cultural contexts. Sensations signify the initial phase when a person becomes aware of her or his embodied being in the world, which in our everyday lives and interactions tends to remain hidden. Hay (2008) considers this process to be relational and tentative, in which different socio-cultural frameworks are drawn upon in the consideration of what may become a symptom. In an analysis of the illness experiences of women diagnosed with ovarian cancer in Germany, Brandner et al. (2014) describe what they call a "triggering process" of healthcare seeking. Bodily sensations sometimes come to the fore of experience which is then normalized and returned to the subconscious. However, when they come to the fore more often, the normalizing processes needs reassuring social information from others. Particularly when everyday activities become increasingly difficult, the normalizing procedures are transformed into an understanding of the sensations as signs of pathology. Often there was a triggering event that led the women in this study to seek out healthcare services, in order to further explore the sensations as symptoms. Such triggering events could be peers who urge healthcare seeking, a change in one's social responsibilities, e.g., the death of the person one cares for or retirement, or the inability to do everyday tasks, e.g., getting dressed, putting on shoes, or household chores.

It was the anthropologists Andersen and Risør (2014) who investigated how sensations and the experiencing of disease through symptoms are interconnected. Societal power relations and systems of knowledge condition symptomatization (Risør 2011; see also Martinez-Hernandez 2000). In the above-mentioned study of women with a diagnosis of ovarian cancer in Germany, for example, Brandner et al. (2014) show that how and when healthcare was sought out to initiate a diagnosing process was a gendered experience. The researchers demonstrate how the consideration of a bodily sensation as abnormal was in itself insufficient to seek healthcare; rather, additional pathways had to open up for the women to act on their bodily sensations; these are to be found in some change in their everyday lives. In particular, the women's experiences were full of competing social responsibilities, such as balancing work and caring for families, which influenced their healthcare seeking behavior. These are examples of experiences from the initial phase of what then becomes a personal illness experience: bodily sensations that come to the fore, that turn into something out of the ordinary and pathological, that needs an expert system to deal with further, which leads into a diagnostic process and a naming of the sensation as some disease. There are many other processes following in the course of illness, for example, decisions about and experiences with different treatments, termination of treatment, seeking out different medical systems for care, and social adaptions with the illness.

Such illness trajectories are mediated by social and cultural norms and responsibilities, as well as by tacit knowledge. Furthermore, they are embedded in former biographical experiences and will undergo a change in reaction to alterations of the subjects' biography. Such experiences are always embodied, as Barbara's description above of her first seizure so pointedly describes. Finally, experiencing – as a constant process of becoming – is always primordial and in constant flux in terms of sensory immediacy (see Desjarlais & Throop 2011; Holmberg 2018).

The close study of these processes and this understanding of the personal experience of illness offers us a window into "subjunctivizing reality" (Bruner 1986: 26), which refers to the ways in which the indeterminacy of reality, and the uncertain and frightening aspects of illness, are shaped and kept at bay. The analysis of illness experiences provides a rich and varied window into cultural perceptions and understandings of disease and illness, as much as into how societal mechanisms work to support, value, or exclude individual experiences. Personal experiences of illness are an important source for social science scholars to understand how social order and cultural assumptions structure our innermost experiences and intertwine with what is considered personal. They thereby reveal the power relations that make illness experiences as much as the political, economic, and social frameworks.

ILLNESS EXPERIENCES AND THEIR REPRESENTATION

The personal illness experience as an inner subjective process is shaped by the cultural and social context in which it occurs. Studying illness experiences faces a general problem, however: direct access to the inner world of individuals, to "pure experience," is not possible. We need a vehicle to study individual experiences; we need a description of the inner processes that can represent the subjective inner experience to the outer world. In the example below, Katharina, a woman in her late twenties, describes her experience of having generalized seizures in her childhood and youth. Today the seizures have stopped and she works as a teacher.

> Then I would fall down and so on. But I don't know about that anymore, I was never conscious then. And I had this jerking and stiffening. And I only remember that I would then always wake up somewhere where there were people sitting around me, my parents or strangers or sometimes the doctor. And that I couldn't speak, but I was there, and everyone was asking me for my name. And I always knew my name, but I couldn't say it, and that always bothered me (laughing). Because I knew exactly what my name is. It took a while then until I could speak again. And then I often had a really strong headache, but not always, I then slept very long. So then I was out of it. Then I would sleep for surely five hours, so really long. And I thought – so, what I really did not like about the seizures (laughing) was really always this stage of awakening. When all the people were standing around and were watching: is she here now, is she not here yet? Also sometimes even when I could speak again. One is simply so tired and – yes, but nevertheless I am not stupid (laughing).

In this young woman's description of her seizures, the characteristics of, and the differences between, a possibly "pure" experience and a representation of an experience can be seen. Katharina describes losing consciousness during a seizure. She then explains what happened during the seizure itself as "jerking and stiffening." This latter explanation cannot be her own subjective description, since during seizures she was unconscious and could not see or describe what was happening. She could not use her own senses, which would normally help her to grasp what she was experiencing. But of course, others had told her about it, so she could fill in the gaps in her own description of the event. She then goes on to talk again from her own perspective, describing the awakening, being unable to speak, the headache. When she describes her need to sleep following a seizure, there seems to be a mixture between her own subjective perspective and information from others; for instance, when she says "So then I was out of it," she positions herself in a passive role, and it is not clear what she feels in this situation. The next sentence, "Then I would sleep for surely five hours, so really long," reveals a kind of uncertainty about how long she would actually sleep for; the wording "surely" illustrates this. Katharina's multifaceted description shows that we do not form the representations of our experiences alone from pure experience; rather, they are – sometimes more, sometimes less – representations in which observations from others are integrated. We can see clearly how such representations are formed by social and cultural frameworks.

As we have shown above, there is a gradient between pure experience, as understood by James (1996), and its objectification into personal experiences of illness and health.

Katharina's story is a clear example of why and how pure experience cannot be the research object of social studies of experience; the objects of our research are therefore representations of experience. These representations can be encountered through personal or public stories (narratives), pictures, tales, and the arts. They provide unique insights into the cultural and social shaping of lives, as they are themselves formed by cultural and social templates and normative standards. Barbara's representation above, for example, was formed from knowledge she had acquired from studying physics at school. Reflective forms of experiencing develop in interaction with the material, cultural, and social environment. The specific characteristics of the environment can influence the representations.

People with illness experiences often have to encounter a specific environment, the medical field, in which people have specific roles, such as patients and doctors, as we have described above. In their role as patients, people listen to the doctors' knowledge and learn about their disease. In patients' stories, we can observe the influence of interactions with medical professionals on the representation of illness experiences. Often in their choice of wording – "the side effects are worse," "the pain was an 8 on a scale of 1 to 10," "my blood pressure was high" – we can see how patients' words stem from the medical context, indicating that they have learned certain expressions and interpretations through their interactions with doctors. For many possible reasons, patients include medical terms in their representations of their illness. These medical terms are dependent on the cultural and social frame they live in. In an early study on epilepsy in Turkey, Good and DelVeccio Good (1994) show how different interpretive frames are used simultaneously. These different frames do not present a conflict but are rather closely tied to the uncertain nature of experiencing seizures. Thus, one of the authors' interviewees went both to a physician and a *hoca*, a Muslim cleric and healer; in this patient's representations, both scientific and religious interpretive frames were at work at different times, which allowed for the two frames to co-exist.

In addition to the influence of the medical explanatory system, there are many more cultural and social norms which influence the representations of our illness experiences. In the next example, David describes his problems with gender-related expectations and illness. He is 26 years old and works as a nurse. His first seizure happened when he was 17. When he takes his medication, he is seizure-free. In the interview extract below, he recounts his difficulty in imagining a partner to be his "guardian" in the event that he would have a seizure.

> It's just difficult for me to talk about this. Because, I don't know – one feels then just so – yes, degraded, somehow just degraded. So, then I don't feel one hundred percent like a man. It is a limitation. So, as I have said, if I would find a woman someday, that she would then not think of me as a man. That she – somehow attacks me in my maleness (laughs) and says: "Be careful, you can't do this, you are not allowed to do that." There I am attacked in my maleness somehow. These are things that I think about sometimes. I am then really scared to tell my [future] wife about this [having epilepsy]. How will she handle this? Then she will have to protect me somehow (laughs). Do you know what I mean? That doesn't work. That's the way I normally think, but there's nothing to be done about it. That's just the way it is.

In David's case, the social norms of gender roles in the particular society he lives in influence his attitude towards partnership and epilepsy.: He is born and lives in Germany, but his family stems from the Middle East. He thus has a diverse cultural background that influences his attitude towards partnership and epilepsy. He imagines his future wife having to take care of him and protect him against harm from a seizure, but this protective behavior is incompatible with – indeed it "attacks" – his own sense of what it means to be a man.

Cultural frameworks inform illness representations. Such frameworks underlie historical and social changes. For a long time, epilepsy was connected in (Western) scientific discourse with "insanity" (Schneble 1987). Representations of illness experiences in a German context therefore often include a reference to the speaker's mental sanity – see Katharina's text, where she stresses that she is "not stupid" – in order to counter this negative association. Experiencing disease is highly circumstantial and historically embedded. Stigma, for example, was historically an important aspect of understanding the experience of epilepsy (see Goffman 1963; Scambler & Hopkins 1986; Schneider & Conrad 1980). The emphasis has since shifted, however, so that in 2012, the experience of epilepsy in a British cohort of young people saw fear as the most dominant emotion: fear of harm through a seizure and fear in the anticipation of a seizure (Ryan & Raisanen 2012).

Illness experiences are influenced by and change across time and place. However, they are also highly contextualized through the particular context in which the representation takes place. The narrators that share illness experiences are driven by their own motivations and intentions, which depend on the occasion of the representation. In the examples of people with epilepsy given above, the narrators are telling their stories for a German website on illness experiences (*krankheitserfahrungen*) called krankheitserfahrungen.de (DIPEx Germany). The website offers emotional and practical support for patients with a variety of conditions. In an evaluation study, we asked participants of the website project why they had participated, in particular what had motivated them to do so (Lucius-Hoene et al. 2013). The main stated motivation was the desire to help others cope with their illness; other motivations were to give something back to society, to be able to be part of a bigger idea, to make patients' voices heard, and to tell doctors how it feels to be ill. This motivation possibly led to the selection of motivating and helpful experiences. Although the narrators did not conceal difficult topics, they did try to end their stories with a hopeful message or to put them into perspective.

Cultural and social frameworks not only form representations of experiences, they also influence experiences in a more fundamental way. If we know that a specific social norm defines the experience as "not normal," then we cannot position ourselves neutrally in the representation or meaning-making of our experience. So, the social norms surrounding, and the medical knowledge about, epileptic seizures influence the ways in which a person experiences his or her own seizures; for example, when awakening from unconsciousness with the feeling of being embarrassed, as described by Katharina above. Katharina's own feelings are influenced by the social reactions of others, who are perhaps caring for her but are also standing over her and making her an object of their care. She describes this situation as awkward, and to explicate this she does not say much about the consequences of the seizure, such as headache, dizziness, or pain, but rather emphasizes that she is not "stupid," as if the others staring at her are thinking that she could be. Her experiential knowledge of the social reactions and judgements of others seems to influence her own feelings in this experience and she feels awkward.

Both experience and its representations are intertwined and embedded in the social and cultural context. Kleinman et al. (1995) conducted a study about experiences of epilepsy in rural and urban regions in China. The study aimed to gather the collective experiences of people with epilepsy. The author nevertheless found that people with epilepsy in China live in many different "local worlds" and that these different social worlds influence the ways in which they experience their illness. The numbers from epidemiological studies counting cases of remission and compliance with treatment refer to another social reality than the experiences of patients themselves; epidemiology takes into account probabilities, whereas patients refer to an individual, socially-embedded presentation of reality. Patients and their families are connected in their experiences of financial consequences, the impact on social and moral status, and their perspectives regarding the future. Indeed, studying personal experiences of illness enables a particular window into the presence of suffering in people's lives and worlds. A detailed analysis of illness experiences can bring to the fore the institutional formations and structural conditions that "either increase or diminish the negative force of suffering" (Wilkinson & Kleinman 2016: 17). War, famine, and political conditions all shape illness experiences and shed light on the social suffering that is introduced through power relations and political conditions (Biehl & Petryna 2013; Das et al. 2001).

FORMS OF ILLNESS REPRESENTATIONS

The representations of experiences that we construct can exist in different formats. One main form of representations are narratives or stories, which we use to structure and form our representations. They allow us to add meanings and evaluations to the description of experiences, and are easy to share with others. There is an increasing number of both verbal and non-verbal expressions of personal illness experiences present in the public realm. Besides narratives, these mostly consist of visual representations such as paintings or photographs. In presenting our experiences, we are not completely free to decide on which format we choose: there are experiences or occasions that do not "fit" into a narrative or we cannot put them into words. Some emotional and sensual experiences are, for example, better presented in an embodied format, such as dance or acting. In everyday life, we transfer our experiences, not just verbally but also through our facial and body expressions, and our voices. As Toombs (1992: 64) has shown, illness expresses itself in a "change in the body's gestural display." When we are in pain, for example, we may not be able to stand upright, we may move slower than usual, and others will notice a change in our "body style," the usual way we move and present ourselves (ibid.). This too can reveal elements and characteristics of the illness experience. Narratives or stories are the most common form of representing experience.

We organize much of our mental representations of experiences in narrative form when we exchange with others orally and through writing. Sarbin, one of the founders of narrative psychology, describes the omnipresence of narratives in human life: "Human beings think, perceive, imagine and make moral choices according to narrative structures … the narrative allows for the inclusion of actors' reasons for their act, as well as the causes of happening" (Sarbin 1986: 8). When the social sciences took a "narrative turn" in the late 1980s, narratives became the subject of a new theory of knowledge, a new epistemology (Murray 2003). What had previously been dismissed as supposedly unscientific subjectivity that cannot offer access to knowledge was recognized for its potential to offer access to another dimension of reality, namely individual and collective lifeworlds. This change was prompted by the rise of constructivism, the idea that reality is constructed by the observer from his or her perspective, limited and influenced by presumptions, expectations and values (Camic et al. 2003). Following these constructivist theories, it was recognized that narratives do not represent an accurate image, copy, or reproduction of events, but can rather be seen as a reconstruction of events from a subjective point of view, including personal explanations, evaluations, and contextual information (Bruner 1990). Narratives provide insight into the ability of human beings to combine events and meaning. Next to the cognitive paradigm of human behavior, Bruner added a narrative paradigm that understood the self as a narrative and meaning-forming being.

Illness narratives are subject to the same characteristics as all narratives, but they also have special challenges: in the case of chronic illness, for instance, the situation is ongoing, and therefore the narrators face the difficulty of bringing the narrative to an end without knowing the outcome of the story themselves (Hydén 1997). Through the loss of physical integrity, narrators of illness experiences also have to accomplish the task of integrating ongoing changes in their self-image. Particularly in the case of sudden illnesses, the feeling of a biographical disruption is often described, dividing life into a before and after the onset of illness (Bury 1982).

The reconstruction of the illness chronology and the narrative arrangement of events into a logical timeline can help people to overcome the biographical break caused by disease (Hydén 1997; Lucius-Hoene 2002). Arthur Frank (1997), a medical sociologist, describes the occurrence of disease as a shipwreck that interrupts one's relationship to one's own body, to oneself, and to others. By talking about their experiences with a disease, people integrate these experiences into their lives and restore coherence. There is "the need of ill people to tell their stories, in order to construct new maps and new perceptions of their relationships to the world" (Frank 1997: 3). Accordingly, these narratives deal with personal themes concerning questions of guilt and shame, the mourning of loss and autonomy, and responsibility in disease situations. The stories that emerge from experiences of illness are thus often designed in such a way that makes it possible to consider open questions about meaning, future perspectives, and reorientation (Frank 1997: 3; Kleinman 1988). Illness narratives offer a different perspective on ways of experiencing illness and of connecting the experiences to one's own life stories and values. In their moral positioning and negotiations, these narratives provide information about subjective needs, resources, hardships, attempts at coping, and constructions of meaning (Lucius-Hoene & Deppermann 2004; Lucius-Hoene 2013).

Experiences of health and illness are always in flux. Representing experiences through narratives allows for a flexibility in engaging with one's experiences through "reading" what happens and imagining a range of possibilities and points of view, which all equally present a mosaic of an illness experience at one point or another. Illness narratives, Good and DelVeccio Good (1994) argue, are told in a subjunctive mode because they remain in becoming. Different endings, causalities, and trajectories may be interrogated through narrative snippets that allow for the continued change and uncertainty of illness to be interrogated by those affected by it.

REPRESENTATIONS OF ILLNESS EXPERIENCES IN PRIVATE AND PUBLIC CONTEXTS

After the narrative turn in the late 1980s, illness experiences became the subject of many research disciplines (see Murray 2003). In recent years, there have been new developments in studies of personal illness experiences, since such narratives are now almost omnipresent in social media, media coverage, and health policy. There seems to be a second narrative turn of a pragmatic origin, which focuses not on the epistemological aspects but on the fact that narratives are very convincing and suitable for conveying messages (Lucius-Hoene, Holmberg, & Meyer 2018). The vast number of public illness experiences available today opens up a new field for social studies of illness experiences, but also makes it difficult to consider the social and cultural context of these representations. In the following, we try to draw a map of locations and types of context where illness experiences occur today in private and public life.

Private Context and Everyday Life

In our private everyday lives, we are used to sharing our illness experiences with significant others. We use narratives in everyday life to explain our experiences to others and ourselves. Self-narrating serves to establish coherence and a timeline in our own inner organization of everyday life. Narrating to others serves to enable social support and understanding. We are also confronted with the illness experiences of others who tell us their stories. In these encounters, the context depends on the social and cultural background of the persons involved and the private occasion of the representation of the illness experience.

The exchange of illness experiences between peers is a specific occasion of sharing one's own illness experience. The two or more participants share a space of understanding in which the commonalities (and differences) of the experiences and common understandings become important. This has long been acknowledged as helpful, as exemplified by the proliferation of self-help groups since the 1960s. The Internet offers new opportunities for people to exchange information via blogs, forums, and social media (Sillence et al. 2014). New platforms for patient narratives have been created, each of which is specified through its specific design and target audience (see e.g. Yu, Taverner, & Madden 2011, for social media use by young patients; Mazanderani, O'Neill, & Powell 2013, for YouTube as a presentation platform for patients; Sillence & Bussey 2017, for online self-help groups). These platforms also enable new cultural forms, such as those offered by online and virtual communication media, in which the presentation of illness experiences presents an important venue for acknowledging and transforming suffering.

Aside from the communal sharing and transforming of one's own experiences through social media and internet resources, these venues also (re-)shape others' experiences. Experiences of others appear to be relevant in the areas of support, relationships, personal health management, the communication of one's own illness, and visualization of the illness and its consequences, as Ziebland and Wyke (2012) suggest. With regard to the information needs of patients, some studies have shown that patients seek both medical facts and "experiential knowledge" (Blödt et al. 2018; Haase et al. 2018; Lamprell & Braithwaite 2018) to cope with disease in everyday life (Engler et al. 2016).

Medical Professional Context

Conveying one's experiences is also an important part in healthcare seeking. There it plays a role for the medical systems to categorize the experiences into palpable and treatable entities. In a traditional doctor–patient interaction, typically the patient tells his or her story to give the doctor important information about symptoms and the course of the illness, but also about his or her personal life situation. The illness story then may be formed by the specific patient–doctor relationship, where the doctor is the expert and the patient is seeking advice. Difficulties sometimes arise because doctors and patients have different reference systems: the doctor observes the illness as a discrete "disease," a biomedically constructed problem that has to be treated correctly in order to achieve (in the best case) healing; the patient, on the other hand, generally refers to his or her "illness" as a lived experience that is formed by many influences in his or her social and cultural background. Generally speaking, medical systems are embedded in cultural worlds. Healing relationships need a common understanding of what the problem and its solution may be. In biomedical encounters, this means that physicians need a common ground with their patients for their diagnosis to be accepted (Holmberg 2005, 2010).

As Toombs (1992: 11) describes in her phenomenological analysis of the patient–doctor interaction, the physician sees the illness as a "collection of physical signs and symptoms which define a particular disease state. He or she thematizes the illness as being a *particular* case of multiple sclerosis...." The doctor's illness story is not about his or her own illness experience, but rather represents his or her learned knowledge, as well as experiences with the application of this knowledge, mainly gathered through interactions with patients. The patient, on the other hand, is more concerned about the illness's consequences in everyday life and, as we have seen, tries to grasp his or her sensual and bodily experiences and represent them in the illness story. Both doctor and patient relate to different kinds of mindsets that are connected to the representation of illness experience; as the doctor connects to his or her scientific knowledge about the disease in general, the patient connects to his or her own lived experiences, bodily experiences, and autobiographical background or story.

The occasions and situations for presenting illness experiences depend on the cultural and social environment and background. Spaces for the representation of illness experiences depend on the cultural frame and technical-cultural possibilities, depending on the social and political practices of sharing experiences. In some cases, these spaces are reduced to almost nothing due to social practices of coping with an illness or the stigma related to an illness. In a study in Cameroon with people with epilepsy, for instance, the participants told Allotey and Reidpath (2007) that they were advised not to engage in too many activities: they had to stay at home, and should not work or have sexual intercourse. The experience of the illness thus excluded them from work, social activities, and partnership. In this case, there seemed to be almost nowhere for them to share their experiences because of the social practices.

TELLING ONE'S STORY: VULNERABILITY AND EMPOWERMENT

The uncertainty of illnesses – especially chronic illnesses – leads to the use of a subjunctive mode (Good 1994; Good & DelVecchio Good 1994) in the stories people tell; at other times, the narratives are stories of chaos (Frank 1997). People seem to feel the need to tell their stories, to construct coherence, or to explain their world of experiences to others. In this way, illness narratives can have a healing effect (Bury 1982; Frank 1997; Lucius-Hoene 2002); they can help us to cope with the changes and consequences of illness. But narratives can also fail: sometimes it is not possible to tell the whole story, to convey the experience in a coherent form. These "broken narratives" can result from linguistic difficulties due to injury, illness, or psychological factors, as for example trauma experiences. The non-coherent parts of illness experiences can be shown in non-verbal forms of expression, such as silences and breaks (Kokanovich & Stone, 2018). But as we have shown above, the representations of our experiences are formed by social and cultural influences. In this way, the narratives of illness are influenced by culturally-formed meta-narratives. In the case of fragmented experiences, these meta-narratives can make it difficult to tell stories; the narratives thus become "silenced" (Kokanovich & Stone 2018).

On the other hand, stories also offer a chance to connect one's own experiences to collective experiences. In telling his or her own story, a narrator often uses plots and metaphors from other stories, either classical or collective. These "companionship stories" (Frank 2016) can help us through times when it is not possible to tell our own story in a coherent way. They also allow us to feel connected and not alone.

Stories in this sense can empower people to manage their illness in a self-assured way and to make their own decisions along their navigations through the medical field. Telling one's story and understanding one's illness experience, in a public way, has led to what Rabinow

(1996) has coined "biosocial communities." Making experiences public has become a dominant cultural form in which self-help groups, grassroots movements, and pharmaceutical companies all shape the terrain of illness experiences (e.g. Klawiter 2008). These public narratives change the political landscape in which illness experiences take place and re-order who should take responsibility for disease and for cure. For example, the militaristic language used in cancer research has spilled over into the public sphere and in-patient organization movements such as the "pink ribbon" movement and the notion of the "breast cancer survivor" celebrating women with breast cancer publicly as "heroes" (King 2006; Sulik 2010). The suffering underlying these public stories, however, remains silent. Such master narratives structure others' experiences and shape societal fears and vulnerabilities (Press et al. 2000).

Art and photography have become an increasingly common medium for expressing illness experiences publicly. In the second half of the twentieth century, for instance, a number of people engaged in such forms of communication as: creating images to express their experiences of epilepsy (https://ahrc.ukri.org/research/readwatchlisten/imagegallery/visualising-the-conditions-and-experiences-of-seizures/, accessed 11.08.2019); using body painting to express women's experiences of breast cancer (e.g. www.ifitshipitshere.com/the-breast-cancer-awareness-body-paint-project/, accessed 11.08.2019), while the HIV/AIDS pandemic in sub-Saharan Africa has led to an outpouring of theater and arts projects aimed at representing the experiences of society and the devastation that the epidemic has caused. Such venues for expressing experiences are powerful means not only to convey suffering, but more importantly to transform suffering.

USING STORIES: PROFESSIONAL APPLICATIONS

Next to the social movements of patients, there has been a recent development in the professional medical field: today, representations of illness experiences play a role not only in the dyad of patient–doctor interactions but in many areas of healthcare and prevention (Lucius-Hoene, Holmberg, & Meyer 2018). Illness experiences are increasingly being used in illness prevention, health promotion, and patient education (Graaf, Sanders, & Hoeken, 2016), with the high persuasiveness of such narratives being used to initiate behavior change. Decision aids for patients in certain medical situations is another area where illness experiences are being used (Bekker et al. 2013; Entwistle et al. 2011; Shaffer & Zikmund-Fisher 2013). In health policy, representations of illness experiences are used as arguments for certain preventive measures or to generate concern and sympathy for particular patient groups (Grob & Schlesinger 2018; Meisel & Karlawish 2011). In the training and further education of health professionals, illness experiences are used to increase empathy and to improve patient orientation and illness knowledge (Gidman 2013; Haigh & Hardy 2011; Snelgrove, Tait & Tait 2016). Finally, illness experiences are in some instances used for quality assurance and the development of healthcare services using experience-based co-designs (Robert et al. 2015). In this approach, patient narratives are collected, evaluated, and, for example, passed on to the teams of institutions as part of the development or evaluation of care services, in order to initiate a discourse on patient issues and to promote patient orientation (Locock et al. 2014).

In these new applications of illness experiences, the professionals take possession of – one could even say they usurp – patient experiences for their own purposes, using their potential to convince and convey messages to patients. To construct these types of applications, professionals usually have to select parts of the original representations, because it is not possible to use or publish an entire illness experience. The ambiguity of patient narratives makes it possible to exert enormous influence here; in the selection of experiences for a preventive measure aimed at changing health behavior, for example, experiences of frustration or the failure of patients may be disposed of. In these new representations, the context of the illness experience is therefore left out.

These new applications build their own context, where the particular representation of the illness experience is motivated by the purpose of its application. Part of the background of the original experience is sometimes presented as a possibility for users to identify with the presented experiences; for example, if patient users of a decision aid seek experiences of people with their own cultural background, age, gender, etc. In this case, the cultural or ethnic background of the patient in a video offering a representation of his or her illness experience can be chosen by the app designer in order to offer the users many options to identify with and thus to better convey the message. In most of these applications, however, it is not possible to know the whole context of the experience, because we only get to see snippets of the original representation.

Illness experiences are used here without their original context, to support the new context of their application in the medical field. The motivations and interests of the professionals influence the representations through the selection of specific parts and the context in which they are shown. They may also influence the representation in its formation; in the pursuit of certain goals – e.g. the promotion of health behavior – professionals may design a survey situation in order to obtain data that are as goal-compliant as possible. These processes determine the ways in which the narrators of illness experiences assume their roles and thus also the content of the representations of illness experiences. Thus, the representations of illness experiences that are enclosed in professional applications are different from other representations of a person's experiences that he or she may present in a private context or in social movements; they are framed in a new context and the motivations of both narrator and professionals have influenced the formation.

APPROACHES TO STUDYING ILLNESS EXPERIENCES

There are many methods in the social sciences that are used to collect illness experiences, from interviews, ethnographies, collections of speech, pictures, geography, and dates, to standardized surveys. We highlight some of the main fields of collection methods, knowing that there are many more and that the methodological discussion about the possibility (and impossibility) of grasping experience is a much broader and more complex one.

Currently, illness experiences in the social sciences are mostly collected through narrative interviews. There are different forms of interviews with varying degrees of openness, from open interviews that start with an open-ended initiating question to semi-structured interviews that are guided by prepared questions covering fields of interest for the research topic. The interviews conducted with people with epilepsy, which provided the accounts above, for instance, were semi-structured and started with the open question: "Could you tell me when you suspected for the first time that something was different, that you might have epilepsy?"

In many studies, semi-structured interviews are applied, as these allow the narrator to tell his or her own story. Afterwards, the interviewer can ask more open-ended questions that have been prepared in an interview guideline covering fields of interest specific to the research topic. To elicit narratives, the interview situation typically provides specific features: the questions are open-ended to allow the narrator to decide upon his or her own preferences regarding which experiences he or she would like to share, while the interviewer demonstrates his or her understanding – without interfering in the narrative – and creates a space to allow the narrator to develop his or her story (see Lucius-Hoene, Adami, & Koschack 2015; Ziebland 2013). Narratives can also be collected from written presentations, such as blogs or social media contributions. Finally, in some research fields, it is more helpful to collect narratives in focus groups, which allow for the involvement of more people who would possibly not participate if they had to do so alone (Kitzinger 2013).

Ethnography is the most comprehensive approach to understanding illness experiences, as it particularly investigates how differentiation of normality and abnormality are constructed in local and trans-local practices. Rather than a method, it represents an entire research strategy and epistemology that used the idea of the making things unfamiliar to understand their embeddedness in particular cosmologies and everyday practices (e.g. Stroeken 2012). Thus, through ethnographic approaches one learns how illness experiences are embedded in structural power relations (Biehl & Petryna 2013). As a research strategy, it uses all available forms of data to understand and re-construct a phenomenon in ethnography.

As patients' experiences are becoming increasingly important for governing institutions, a range of standardized forms of capturing experiences have been developed. One such possibility for collecting standardized patient experiences are patient-reported outcome measures (PROMs) and patient-reported experience measures (PREMs). PROMs aim to collect subjective measures of treatment outcomes, such as symptom improvement. They are based on statistical methods to ensure comparability within a population, and thus no open questions or information on individual experiences are included (Jenkinson & Fitzpatrick 2013). A PREMs survey, on the other hand, aims to record patients' experiences with regard to variables of healthcare, such as waiting times and experienced quality of communication, in a standardized and quantifiable way (Beattie et al. 2015; Graham & Woods 2013). Data like this is collected through large national surveys. Some of these survey instruments also describe patients' views of healthcare actors: how do they (doctors, therapists, nursing staff) behave and what characteristics do they have? Despite their usefulness, however, other aspects that are relevant for successful treatment are disregarded in these surveys: PREMs, for instance, do not capture what the actions of healthcare providers provoke in patients and how patients process their experiences.

Another dimension that we miss if we reduce experience to a number is the context. As we have shown above, representations of experiences are always influenced by the social context. In Kleinman's study in rural and urban China (Kleinman et al. 1995), we can see the interconnections between family life, individual experiences, and collective social suffering. These would not be represented in standardized collection methods. Such methods take out the context that makes experience. Thus, if such quantitative methods are to be used, they at least should be complemented with open methods that allow us to explore the context and social world of experiences.

CONCLUSION: THE COMPLEXITIES OF EXPERIENCE AND THEIR FLUIDITY

The complexity of experiences cannot be easily anticipated and change with the interpretive frame both in time and place. Personal experiences of illness are an important window into the manifold power structures that make up individual lives and societies. Different layers of fear around bodily, psychological, and social experiences characterize the experience of illness. Fear and worry are the emotional signals of feeling vulnerable in a particular context. These are formed and influenced by social and cultural frameworks, as well as by particular power structures. At the same time, experiences can only be captured through their representations, which are context-bound and can be told in many different ways in time and place.

In the extended application of illness experiences nowadays, the aim is to use illness experiences to convey messages (such as behavior change in public health campaigns), to investigate healthcare in order to identify barriers from the patients' perspective, or to study the effects of medical action on the empowerment of patients (Entwistle et al. 2012; Ryan et al. 2014). This pragmatic approach to using illness experiences has led to a partial neglect of the epistemological background, and the overlooking of the importance of understanding illness experiences as embedded in a particular time and place, which allows for an understanding of power relations and structures as much as of cultural and social frameworks. Illness experiences represent subjective realities, and as Biehl and Petryna (2013) have lamented, ethnographies and subjective realities regularly "die" as evidence in evidence-based policy making in global health. This makes it even more important to work through the epistemological grounding of experience and the power relations involved in shaping them.

Representations of illness experiences express the vulnerability *and* empowerment of individuals at the same time. Making illness experiences public can lead to the empowerment of individuals and the shaping of new social groups. But it can also lead to the creation of powerful master narratives to which individuals' experiences have to align. This can become a threat if a person cannot tell his or her story in a socially and culturally anticipated way, which can in turn lead to "broken stories" (Kokanović & Stone 2018) and psychological stress for the narrator.

REFERENCES

Allotey, P. and Reidpath, D. (2007) Epilepsy, culture, identity and well-being: A study of the social, cultural and environmental context of epilepsy in Cameroon. *Journal of Health Psychology* 12(3): 431–443.

Andersen, R.S., Paarun, B., Vedstedt, P., Bro, F. and Söendergaard, J. (2010) "Containment" as an analytical framework for understanding patient delay: A qualitative study of cancer patients' symptom interpretation processes. *Social Sciences & Medicine* 71: 378–385.

Andersen, R.S. and Risør, M.B. (2014) The importance of contextualization: Anthropological reflections on descriptive analysis, its limitations and implications. *Anthropology & Medicine* 21(3): 345–356.

Bekker, H.L., Winterbottom, A.E., Butow, P., Dillard, A.J., Feldman-Stewart, D. and Fowler, F.J. (2013) Do personal stories make patient decision aids more effective? A critical review of theory and evidence. *BMC Medical Informatics and Decision Making* 13(Suppl 2). Online first, 29 November 2013. DOI: https://doi.org/10.1186/1472-6947-13-S2-S9.

Beattie, M., Murphy, D.J., Atherton, I. and Lauder, W. (2015) Instruments to measure patient experience of healthcare quality in hospitals: A systematic review. *Systematic Reviews* 4: 97.

Biehl, J. and Petryna, A. (eds) (2013) *When People Come First: Critical Studies in Global Health*. Princeton, NJ: Princeton University Press.

Blödt, S., Kaiser, M., Adam, Y., Adami, S., Schultze, M., Müller-Nordhorn, J. and Holmberg, C. (2018) Understanding the role of health information in patients' experiences: Secondary analysis of qualitative narrative interviews with people diagnosed with cancer in Germany. *BMJ Open*. Epub ahead of print 12 March 2018. DOI: https://doi.org/10.1136/bmjopen-2017-019576.

Brandner, S., Müller-Nordhorn, J., Stritter, W., Fotopoulou, C., Sehouli, J. and Holmberg, C. (2014) Symptomization and triggering processes: Ovarian cancer patients' narratives on pre diagnostic sensation experiences and the initiation of healthcare seeking. *Social Sciences & Medicine* 119: 123–130.

Bruner, J.S. (1986) *Actual Minds, Possible Worlds*. Cambridge, MA: Harvard University Press.

Bruner, J.S. (1990) *Acts of Meaning*. Cambridge, MA: Harvard University Press.

Bury, M. (1982) Chronic illness as biographical disruption. *Sociology of Health and Illness* 4(2): 167–182.

Camic, P.M., Rhodes, J.E., and Yardley, L. (2003) Naming the stars: integrating qualitative methods into psychological research. In P.M. Camic, J.E. Rhodes and L. Yardley (eds), *Qualitative Research in Psychology: Expanding Perspectives in*

Methodology and Design. Washington, DC: American Psychological Association, pp. 3–15.

Das, V., Kleinman, A., Lock, M.M., Ramphele, M. and Reynolds, P. (eds) (2001) *Remaking a World: Violence, Social Suffering and Recovery*. Berkeley, CA: University of California Press.

Del Vecchio Good, M. (1995) *American Medicine: The Quest for Competence*. Berkeley, CA: University of California Press.

Desjarlais, R. and Throop, C. (2011) Phenemenological approaches in anthropology. *Annual Review of Anthropology* 40: 87–102.

Dilthey, W. and Rickmann, H.P. (1976) *W. Dilthey: Selected Writings*. Cambridge: Cambridge University Press.

Engler, J., Adami, S., Adam, Y., Keller, B., Repke, T., Fügemann, H., Lucius-Hoene, G., Müller-Nordhorn, J. and Holmberg, C. (2016) Using others' experiences: Cancer patients' expectations and navigation of a website providing narratives on prostate, breast and colorectal cancer. *Patient Education and Counseling* 99(8): 1325–1332.

Entwistle, V.A., Firnigl, D., Ryan, M., Francis, J. and Kinghorn, P. (2012) Which experiences of health care delivery matter to service users and why? A critical interpretive synthesis and conceptual map. *Journal of Health Services Research & Policy* 17(2): 70–78.

Entwistle, V.A., France, E.F., Wyke, S., Jepson, R., Hunt, K., Ziebland, S. and Thompson, A. (2011) How information about other people's personal experiences can help with healthcare decision-making: A qualitative study. *Patient Education and Counseling* 85(3): 291–298.

Frank, A.W. (1997) *The Wounded Storyteller: Body, Illness, and Ethics*. Chicago, IL: University of Chicago Press.

Arthur W. Frank (2016) *"Truth Telling, Companionship, and Witness: An Agenda for Narrative Bioethics,"* Hastings Center Report 46, 3: 17–21. DOI: 10.1002/hast.591

Frankenberg, R. (1980) Medical anthropology and development: A theoretical perspective. *Social Science and Medicine* 14(4): 197–207.

Geertz, C. (1973) *The Interpretation of Cultures: Selected Essays*. New York: Basic Books.

Gidman, J. (2013) Listening to stories: Valuing knowledge from patient experience. *Nurse Education in Practice* 13(3): 192–196.

Gijsbers van Wijk, C.M.T. and Kolk, A.M. (1997) Sex differences in physical symptoms: The contribution of symptom perception theory. *Social Science & Medicine* 45: 231–246.

Goffman, E. (1963) *Stigma: Notes on the Management of Spoiled Identity*. Englewood Cliffs, NJ: Prentice-Hall.

Good, B.J. (1994) *Medicine, Rationality and Experience: An Anthropological Perspective*. Cambridge: Cambridge University Press.

Good, B.J., and Del Vecchio Good, M.J. (1994) In the subjunctive mode: Epilepsy narratives in Turkey. *Social Science & Medicine* 38(6): 835–842.

Gordon, D.R. (1988) Tenacious assumptions of biomedicine. In M. Lock and D.R. Gordan (eds), *Biomedicine Examined*. Dordrecht: Springer, pp. 19–56.

Graaf, A., Sanders, J. and Hoeken, H. (2016) Characteristics of narrative interventions and health effects: A review of the content, form, and context of narratives in health-related narrative persuasion research. *Review of Communication Research* 4: 88–131.

Graham, C. and Woods, P. (2013) Patient experience surveys. In S. Ziebland, A. Coulter, J.D. Calabrese and L. Locock (eds), *Understanding and Using Health Experiences. Improving Patient Care*. Oxford: Oxford University Press, pp. 81–93.

Grob, R. and Schlesinger, M. (2018) When public and private narratives diverge: Media, policy advocacy, and the paradoxes of newborn screening policy. In G. Lucius-Hoene, C. Holmberg and T. Meyer (eds), *Illness Narratives in Practice: Potentials and Challenges of Using Narratives in Health-related Contexts*. Oxford: Oxford University Press.

Haase, K.R., Gifford, W., Holtslander, L. and Thomas, R. (2018) Managing cancer experiences: An interpretive description study of internet information use. *Cancer Nursing* 42(5): 53–63.

Haigh, C. and Hardy, P. (2011) Tell me a story: A conceptual exploration of storytelling in healthcare education. *Nurse Education Today* 31(4): 408–411.

Hay, M.C. (2008) Reading sensations: Understanding the process of distinguishing "fine" from "sick". *Transcultural Psychiatry* 45: 198–229.

Holmberg, C. (2005) *Diagnose Brustkrebs: Eine Ethnografische Studie über Krankheit Und Krankheitserleben*. Frankfurt: Campus Verlag.

Holmberg, C. (2010) Klinisches Emplotment – Erfolgreiche Arzt-Patienten-Beziehungen?! In C. Witt (ed.), *Der gute Arzt aus interdisziplinärer Sicht: Ergebnisse eines Expertentreffens*. Essen: Natur und Medizin KVC Verlag, pp. 141–156.

Holmberg, C. (2018) What's in a name. In G. Lucius-Hoene, C. Holmberg and T. Meyer (eds), *Illness Narratives in Practice: Potentials and Challenges of Using Narratives in Health-related Contexts*. Oxford: Oxford University Press.

Hydén, L.C. (1997) Illness and narrative. *Sociology of Health & Illness* 19(1): 48–69.

James, W. (1996) *Essays in Radical Empiricism*. New York & Lincoln, NB: University of Nebraska Press.

Jenkinson, C. and Fitzpatrick, R. (2013) Patient reported outcomes. In S. Ziebland, A. Coulter, J.D. Calabrese and L. Locock (eds), *Understanding and Using Health Experiences: Improving Patient Care*. Oxford: Oxford University Press, pp. 72–80.

King, S. (2006) *Pink Ribbons, Inc.: Breast Cancer and the Politics of Philanthropy*. Minneapolis, MN: University of Minnesota Press.

Kitzinger, J. (2013) Using focus groups to understand experiences of health and illness. In S. Ziebland, A. Coulter, J.D. Calabrese and L. Locock (eds), *Understanding and Using Health Experiences: Improving Patient Care*. Oxford: Oxford University Press, pp. 49–59.

Klawiter, M. (2008) *The Biopolitics of Breast Cancer: Changing Cultures of Disease and Activism*. Minnesota, MN: University of Minnesota Press.

Kleinman, A. (1988) *The Illness Narratives: Suffering, Healing, and the Human Condition*. New York: Basic Books.

Kleinman, A., Wang, W.Z., Li, S.C., Cheng, X.M., Dai, X.Y., Li, K.T. and Kleinmann, J. (1995) The social course of epilepsy: Chronic illness as social experience in interior China. *Social Science & Medicine* 40(10): 1319–1330.

Kokanović, R. and Stone, M. (2018) Listening to what cannot be said: Broken narratives and the lived body. *Arts and Humanities in Higher Education* 17(1): 20–31.

Lamprell, K. and Braithwaite, J. (2018) When patients tell their own stories: A meta-narrative study of web-based personalized texts of 214 melanoma patients' journeys in four countries. *Qualitative Health Research* 28(10): 1564–1583.

Lock, M. and Gordan, D.R. (eds) (1988) *Biomedicine Examined*. Dordrecht, The Netherlands: Springer.

Locock, L., Robert, G., Boaz, A., Vougioukalou, S., Shuldham, C. and Fielden, J. (2014) Using a national archive of patient experience narratives to promote local patient-centered quality improvement: An ethnographic process evaluation of "accelerated" experience-based co-design. *Journal of Health Services Research & Policy* 19(4): 200–207.

Lucius-Hoene, G. (2002) Narrative Bewältigung von Krankheit und Coping-Forschung. *Psychotherapie und Sozialwissenschaft* 4(3): 166–203.

Lucius-Hoene, G. (2013) Constructing perspectives as positioning resources in stories of the self. In C. Holler (ed.), *Rethinking Narrative Identity: Persona and Perspective*. Amsterdam: Benjamins, pp. 85–101.

Lucius-Hoene, G., Adami, S. and Koschack, J. (2015) Narratives that matter: Illness stories in the "third space" of qualitative interviewing. In F. Gygax and M.A. Locher (eds), *Narrative Matters in Medical Contexts across Disciplines*. Amsterdam: John Benjamins, pp. 99–116.

Lucius-Hoene, G. and Deppermann, A. (2004) *Rekonstruktion narrativer Identität: Ein Arbeitsbuch zur Analyse narrativer Interviews*. Wiesbaden: VS Verlag für Sozialwissenschaften.

Lucius-Hoene, G., Groth, S., Becker, A.K., Dvorak, F., Breuning, M. and Himmel, W. (2013) Wie erleben Patienten die Veröffentlichung ihrer Krankheitserfahrungen im Internet? *Die Rehabilitation* 52(3): 196–201.

Lucius-Hoene, G., Holmberg, C. and Meyer, T. (eds) (2018) *Illness Narratives in Practice. Potentials and Challenges of Using Narratives in Health-related Contexts*. Oxford: Oxford University Press.

Martinez-Hernandez, A. (2000) *What's behind the Symptom? On Psychiatric Observation and Anthropological Understanding*. Amsterdam: Harwood Academic.

Mazanderani, F., O'Neill, B. and Powell, J. (2013) "People power" or "pester power"? YouTube as a forum for the generation of evidence and patient advocacy. *Patient Education and Counseling* 93(3): 420–425.

Meisel, Z.F. and Karlawish, J. (2011) Narrative vs evidence-based medicine – and, not or. *JAMA* 306(18): 2022–2023.

Merleau-Ponty, M. (2012 [1945]) *Phenomenology of Perception*. Abingdon: Routledge.

Murray, M. (2003) Narrative psychology and narrative analysis. In P.M. Camic, J.E. Rhodes and L. Yardley (eds), *Qualitative Research in Psychology: Expanding Perspectives in Methodology and Design*. Washington, DC: American Psychological Association, pp. 95–112.

Press, N., Fishman, J.R., Koenig, B.A. (2000) Collective fear, individualized risk: The social and cultural context of genetic testing for breast cancer. *Nurse Ethics* 7(3): 237–249.

Rabinow, Paul (1996) *Essays on the Anthropology of Reason*. Princeton, NJ: Princeton University Press.

Risør, M.B. (2011) The Process of Symptomization. Clinical encounters with functional disorders. In S. Fainzang and C. Haxaire (eds), *Of Bodies and Symptoms: Anthropological Perspectives on their Social and Medical Treatment*. Tarragona: Publications URV, pp. 21–37.

Robert, G., Cornwell, J., Locock, L., Purushotham, A., Sturmey, G. and Gager, M. (2015) Patients and staff as codesigners of healthcare services. *BMJ (Clinical Research Ed.)* Epub ahead of print 10 February 2015. DOI: https://doi.org/10.1136/bmj.g7714.

Ryan, M., Kinghorn, P., Entwistle, V.A. and Francis, J.J. (2014) Valuing patients' experiences of healthcare processes: Towards broader applications of existing methods. *Social Science & Medicine* 106: 194–203.

Ryan, S. and Raisanen, U. (2012). The brain is such a delicate thing - an exploration of fear and seizures among young people with epilepsy. *Chronic Illness* 8(3): 214–224.

Sarbin, T.R. (ed.) (1986) *Narrative Psychology: The Storied Nature of Human Conduct (Praeger special studies)*. New York: Praeger.

Scambler, G. and Hopkins, A. (1986) Being epileptic: Coming to terms with stigma. *Sociology of Health and Illness* 8(1): 26–43.

Schneble, H. (1987) *Krankheit der ungezählten Namen: Ein Beitrag zur Sozial-, Kultur- und Medizingeschichte der Epilepsie anhand ihrer Benennungen vom Altertum bis zur Gegenwart*. Bern: Huber.

Schneider, J.W. and Conrad, P. (1980) In the closet with illness: Epilepsy, stigma potential and information control. *Social Problems* 28(1): 32–44.

Seeman, D. and Kleinman, A. (2000) Personal experience of illness. In G. Albrecht, R. Fitzpatrick and S.C. Scrimshaw (eds), *The Handbook of Social Studies in Health and Medicine*. London: Sage.

Shaffer, V.A. and Zikmund-Fisher, B.J. (2013) All stories are not alike: A purpose-, content-, and valence-based taxonomy of patient narratives in decision aids. *Medical Decision Making: An International Journal of the Society for Medical Decision Making* 33(1): 4–13.

Sillence, E. and Bussey, L. (2017) Changing hospitals, choosing chemotherapy and deciding you've made the right choice: Understanding the role of online support groups in different health decision-making activities. *Patient Education and Counseling* 100(5): 994–999.

Sillence, E., Hardy, C., Harris, P.R. and Briggs, P. (2014) Modeling patient engagement in peer-to-peer healthcare. *WWW '14 Companion: Proceedings of the 23rd International Conference on World Wide Web*. Epub ahead of print. DOI: https://doi.org/10.1145/2567948.2576937.

Singer, M. (2004) The social origins and expressions of illness. *British Medical Bulletin* 69(1): 9–16.

Snelgrove, S., Tait, D.J.R. and Tait, M. (2016) Teaching psychology to student nurses: The use of "Talking Head" videos. *Research in Learning Technology* 24(1): 30891.

Stroeken, K. (2012) *Moral Power: The Magic of Witchcraft*. Oxford & New York: Berghahn Books.

Sulik, G. (2010) *Pink Ribbon Blues: How Breast Cancer Culture Undermines Women's Health*. New York: Oxford University Press.

Throop, C. (2003) Minding experience: An exploration of the concept of "experience" in the early French anthropology of Durkheim, Lévy-Bruhl, and Lévi-Strauss. *Journal of the History of the Behavioral Sciences* 39(4): 365–382.

Toombs, S.K. (1992) *The Meaning of Illness: A Phenomenological Account of the Different Perspectives of Physician and Patient*. Dordrecht: Springer Netherlands.

Wilkinson, I. and Kleinman, A. (2016) *A Passion for Society. How We Think about Social Suffering*. Berkeley, CA: University of California Press.

Young, A. (1982) *The Anthropologies of Illness and Sickness*. Palo Alto, CA: Annual Reviews.

Yu, J., Taverner, N. and Madden, K. (2011) Young people's views on sharing health-related stories on the Internet. *Health & Social Care in the Community* 19(3): 326–334.

Ziebland, S. (2013) Narrative interviewing. In S. Ziebland, A. Coulter, J.D. Calabrese and L. Locock (eds), *Understanding and Using Health Experiences: Improving Patient Care*. Oxford: Oxford University Press, pp. 38–48.

Ziebland, S. and Wyke, S. (2012) Health and illness in a connected world: How might sharing experiences on the internet affect people's health? *The Milbank Quarterly* 90(2): 219–249.

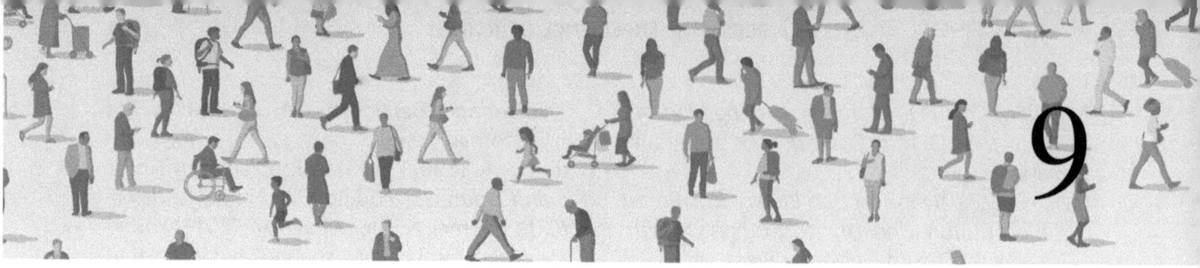

9

Anthropological Approaches to Food and Nutrition

Miguel Cuj and Susan C. Scrimshaw

"People eat food, not nutrients." (King 2003: p. 2116)

INTRODUCTION

This chapter examines the anthropological approaches to food and nutrition. It focuses on people's relationships to food from cultural perspectives and how these perspectives impact individual, familial and community behaviors surrounding food and nutrition, including beliefs and behaviors surrounding food procurement, production, and consumption, which in turn affect nutritional status. It also provides examples of community responses to nutrition programs. The focus of this chapter is more on individual behaviors in low-income communities than on affluent or Middle-class populations. It complements Chapter 29 in this volume, *Connecting Human Health to Nature Health: The Bridging Potential of Sustainable Food Systems*, by Stephan Rist and Theresa Tribaldos, which deals with food at the macro levels of production, access, health equity and environmental sustainability. This chapter also complements Chapter 2 in this volume, *Cultural Variation in the Experience of Health and Illness*, by Pamela Erickson and Cynthia Frank, which includes health belief systems, some of which relate to food. The discussion of social determinants in the Introduction and in Chapter 3 by Zambrana et al., *The Intersectional Impact of Race, Class, Ethnicity, and Place on Social Determinants of Health across the Life Course*, are also fundamental to concepts discussed in this chapter.

Anthropological frameworks and methods provide vital pragmatic instruments to understand food beyond the traditional lens of clinical nutrition science which focuses on nutrients, measurement of their value, and nutrient intake. Anthropological contributions to our understanding of behaviors surrounding food and nutritional status come from the traditional four fields of anthropology – archeology, linguistics, cultural anthropology, and physical anthropology. Archeology studies foods produced or hunted and consumed in the past, including the domestication of plants and animals. Linguistics helps us understand how health, food and nutritional status are described and classified within language, which in turn reveals cultural attitudes and practices. Cultural anthropology describes attitudes, beliefs and practices surrounding food in contemporary cultures, and is at the core of this chapter. Physical anthropology contributes to our understanding of nutritional status through measurement of growth and other metabolic processes.

This chapter highlights the cultural issues of food. Understanding food consumption has global implications for the broader view of nutritional status in relation to individual and population health. While under-nutrition remains a problem in many parts of the world, over-nutrition and poor nutrition has played a role in the epidemiologic transition from morbidity and mortality related primarily to infectious diseases to the impact of chronic and non-communicable diseases (NCDs), a shift that is especially pronounced in low- and middle-income countries. The cultural context of food includes culturally and linguistically shaped attitudes towards food, food preparation and safety, intra-household food allocation, perceptions of the role of food in health and illness and ways of perceiving, describing, and classifying food. Food procurement, or how food is obtained, is also influenced by factors such as economic status, culture, and food availability. Food production at the household and community levels is also culturally influenced.

THE ANTHROPOLOGY OF FOOD AND NUTRITION

Nutritional anthropology is the study of food and nutrition from evolutionary, behavioral, social, and cultural perspectives, and how these interact in the production of nutritional health at the individual, community, and population levels (Johnston 1987). Nutritional anthropology also fuses issues past and present, local, and global, and biological and cultural in order to provide a comprehensive understanding of food and nutrition in cultural context. In this sense, nutritional anthropology is the interplay between human biology, economic systems, cultural perceptions and practices, nutritional status, and food security, and how this complex assemblage affects human populations (Karaman 2008). The anthropological study of food and culture over the past 20 years has evolved to take on broad topics such as food, culture, power, and gender (Chrzan and Brett 2017; Counihan 1999). Anthropologists collect data about how people in diverse cultures live, as often as possible documenting the words of the people, via participant observation, as well as informal and structured interviews, and direct observation (Bernard 2017; Herman and Bentley 1993; Scrimshaw and Hurtado 1987). Anthropologists analyze those data to help us understand human behavior regarding food, accounting for the variety of perspectives expressed by the research participants. These analyses can reveal patterned and structured systems of values based on underlying cultural logic. These value systems are shifting, flexible, and dynamic as cultures are continually changing in response to external and internal forces. Food, as discussed here, goes beyond clinical nutritional definitions of biological and chemical aspects of food, specifically macro- and micro-nutrients. The nutrition sciences also look at areas such as measurements of dietary nutrient intake, nutritional status of individuals and populations, access to food, actual dietary behaviors, and disparities in diet/dietary patterns and health outcomes. Anthropological approaches allow food to be seen as a principal medium for social interaction and reciprocity, with underlying layers of cultural meaning. Food thus becomes part of the construction and creation of group and individual identity through the interaction of native language and cultural practices (Hastorf 2016; Riley and Paugh 2018). Anthropological methods and theoretical understandings can not only improve the accuracy in measurement of dietary behaviors through direct and participant observation, but also allow for understanding of the meanings that underlie these behaviors.

A fundamental concern in the study of culture in food and nutrition is that people eat food, not nutrients, as noted by several scholars that focus on food (Food and Agriculture Organization 1992; Hastorf 2016; Hawkins 2007; Neuenswander and Arnold 1977; Staller and Carrasco 2009; Staller, Tykot, and Benz 2016). Western biomedicine's essentialism defines food as a set of macronutrients (protein, carbohydrates, and fat) and micronutrients (vitamins and minerals), that cause disease when elements of the diet are inadequate or over-abundant (Nestle 2007; Yates-Doerr 2010, 2012, 2015b). Much of nutritional science addresses the biochemical processes of nutrients in the human body (Scrinis 2013), particularly their impact on human development, growth of children, and health. The contemporary bio-language of food describes, for example, how proteins are constituted for amino acids, the fats are constituted for essential and non-essential fatty acids, carbohydrates are constituted for carbons and oxygens atoms, and vitamins and minerals are constituted for chemical elements. Bio-language is a coded system where food is defined as three groupings – nutri-metrics (metrics of nutrients), statistics (population metrics of food issues), and biological and chemical language (biomarkers). This kind of bio-language allows the medicalization of food through the ability to understand and use numbers – quantitative methodologies – to study food and its interaction with health. Due to the classic approach of laboratory nutrition science which focuses on metrics to understand food, these bio-western elements can only be measured and understood by metrics (calories, grams, milligrams).

Nutrimetrics methods are the different forms of measuring food, in numerical units, for example by the number of calories. Nutrimetrics is another form of bio-language where numbers become the main way to describe food. This notion promotes the idea that people eat numbers and quantities rather than food. The numerical language with regards to food creates an environment where numbers shape the identification of food. This quantification provides a mental image which promotes a dominant paradigm of abstract characteristics as a way to approach food. It is a widespread view by some nutritionists that food can only be interpreted in calories and grams because these elements can be measured as impacting biological and metric dimensions in the body of a human being. These concepts overlook the value of socio-cultural relations of food where food becomes meaningful through cultural perceptions and language, for example, the cultural and linguistic value of maize to Guatemalan Maya people.

A focus on cultural elements is only one way to approach the topic of food. Nutritional deficiency has been recognized as being associated with specific foods that have high cultural importance. For example, both cultural significance and a nutritional deficiency could be attributed to maize in Mesoamerican population. Maize has lysine and tryptophan deficiency; both are essential amino acids to human nutrition. But cultural practices in food preparation have solved this problem with the addition of lime to corn in the preparation of ground corn for tortillas, a daily Maya food, and tamales, *atole* (a corn-based beverage) and other preparations based on maize (Parker et al. 1998; N.S. Scrimshaw et al. 1957; N.S. Scrimshaw et al. 1960). Understanding these practices has led to international applications of the principle of combining foods to create complete proteins in culturally acceptable ways (Caballero 1988; Tartenac 2000).

FOODWAYS

Foodways has emerged as an umbrella term for the understanding of cultural attitudes, beliefs and behaviors related to food and nutrition. The journal *Food and Foodways* is devoted to this area of scholarship. Foodways is one of the main topics in contemporary medical and food/nutritional anthropology theory because it has global implications for transitions around human food access in the current era of climate change. Foodways refers to an integrated system of practices, attitudes, and beliefs that surround the consumption and production of food. The anthropology of food has expanded to include the social and cultural conditions of foodways, including sociolinguistics, gender, and food behaviors. This concept also embraces how people use their language and culture in relating to food to conceptualize and to interact with social, cultural, and economic factors to express food identity, gender, and agency through their sustenance (Bennett, Smith, and Passin 1942; Camp 1982; Cuj, Sattler, and de Beausset 2020; Kittler and Sucher 2012; Mintz and Du Bois 2002; Riley and Paugh 2018; Staller and Carrasco 2009; Staller et al. 2016). As discussed earlier, while a large portion of food studies focuses on the production and industry of food, another aspect of the scientific community focuses on the biological and consumption mechanisms of food such as nutritional science, metrics of nutrients, and dietetical knowledge (Kittler and Sucher 2012; McGarvey 2009; Nestle 2007; Scrinis 2013; Yates-Doerr 2010, 2012, 2015a, 2015b).

Foodways also have global implications for the contemporary epidemiologic transition from infectious diseases such as smallpox and tuberculosis to chronic non-communicable diseases (NCDs) like diabetes, a shift that is especially pronounced in low- and middle-income countries (Black et al. 2013; Di Cesare et al. 2013; Ramirez-Zea et al. 2014; Tapela et al. 2019). As a consequence, poor nutrition leads to poor health outcomes that contribute to the prevalence of NCDs, including malnutrition, cancer, diabetes, obesity, metabolic syndrome, and hypertension. NCDs cause 41 million deaths each year and account for an estimated 71% of all deaths globally (Nestle 2007; Patel 2012; Patel and Moore 2017; World Health Organization 2021; Yates-Doerr 2010, 2012, 2015a, 2015b).

LANGUAGE AND FOOD

The meaning and symbolism of food emerge from the intersection of a particular structure of language, cultural identities, and the material realities of food. The way that we speak and conceptualize the discourse of food comes from the structure of specific language and cultural behaviors. Language, which is itself a product of culture, embodies the spiritual, symbolic, seasonal, and agricultural meanings of food in each culture. From this perspective, looking separately at food, culture, and language alone is insufficient. Food and language complement each other to generate foodways in indigenous communities (Riley and Paugh 2018). Foodways are a critical part of the anthropology of food and nutrition because they incorporate how people use language to conceptualize and interact with social, cultural, and economic factors to express their sustenance and nourishment (Boerboom 2015; Hosking 2010; Karrebæk, Riley, and Cavanaugh 2018; Kittler and Sucher 2012; Mintz and Du Bois 2002; Staller and Carrasco 2009).

First, language through food encompasses the way in which people express personal and socio-cultural meanings through their food habits. Second, language about food allows us to focus our attention on how food becomes a topic of both everyday discourse and ideological discourse. Third, language around food demonstrates that language is used in specific ways around food involving its production, marketing, preparation, and its consumption. This shows how communication is interwoven with food in various settings. Finally, language as food demonstrates how discourse is often viewed and consumed like a substance (Boerboom 2015; Hastorf 2016; Karrebæk et al. 2018; Riley and Cavanaugh 2017; Riley and Paugh 2018; Staller and Carrasco 2009).

Anthropological frameworks about food focus on categorizing, organizing, and labeling, for example, food as a process of culture that follows cultural models through linguistic classifications. It establishes that there is a certain relationship between the grammatical categories of language that a person speaks and the way in which the person acts regarding food. These approaches emphasize the importance of language and culture as a whole (Binder and Smith 2013; Chatterjee 1969; Chrzan and Brett 2017; Duranti 1997; Riley and Cavanaugh 2017). Extant frameworks based on food studies can inform the operationalization between foodways, how humans produce, exchange, consume, and think about food, and discourse, how humans use language for everyday speech as well as its ideological, meaning, symbolism, and shaping of identity.

CULTURAL CONCEPTS OF FOOD

While contemporary clinical nutritional scholarship defines food through the lens of western biomedicine, as discussed above, indigenous peoples' conception of food diverges from conventional western food biological logic (Harvey 2008, 2013; Huber and Sandstrom 2001; Saravia 2006). Western biomedical food logic has been mobilized by scientific, rational norms. Conversely, indigenous peoples' understandings of food are often delegitimized as mere customs, myths, beliefs, and stories (Good and McDowell 2015; Goodman 2001). Food concepts reflect cultural diversity since food-related beliefs and behaviors are based on cultural thoughts about the food landscape that may differ from western logic (Chen 2008; Solomon 2015, 2016). This means that food beliefs and behaviors can support multi-ethnic and multilingual rationality about food diversity through understanding local language, indigenous knowledge, and social settings surrounding food. For most cultures, producing and consuming food is not only a means of funneling nutrients into the body. Instead, food operates as a meaningful set of symbols, practices, and beliefs through which we express who we are, how we relate to one another, and how we feel about the world in which we live. The semiotic and semantic values are constructed partly through discourse about food. These features differ from the bio-language model.

Culturally derived food beliefs and practices have functional implications beyond mere nourishment. Acceptable foods vary widely from culture to culture. Plants and animals (including avians, insects, fish, shellfish, etc.) that are considered food in one culture are considered unacceptable to eat in others. Food that is consumed raw, or both raw and cooked in some cultures must be eaten only cooked in others. In some instances, it has been argued belief systems around food are functional in that forbidden foods may carry risks such as infection (e.g. trichinosis or tapeworm in pork) or food poisoning (e.g. raw vs cooked). Recent examples of SARS, Ebola and COVID-19 are indications of the risks of consuming food that may transmit infections. Diseases latent in animal populations such as bats and monkeys can mutate to infect humans when contact with animals increases as wild animals are used for food (Baize et al. 2014; Li et al. 2020). It has also been suggested that following cultural and/or religious norms around food serve to reinforce the culture and keep people together. The importance of keeping Kosher in traditional Judaism, Halal in the Muslim tradition, avoiding eating beef in the Hindu religion, vegetarianism for Buddhists and strict veganism for Jains can serve both protective and cultural reinforcing functions (Douglas and Gross 1981).

In many cultures, food is perceived as being able to cause illness through its role in the hot and cold belief system; through spoiled foods, dirty foods, or raw foods; and by combining the wrong foods (Logan 1977; Manderson 1987; S.C.M. Scrimshaw and Hurtado 1988; S.C.Scrimshaw and Lane 2020). For example, sweets are implicated as a cause of worms in children and children who eat mud or dirt are viewed as risking illness. Foods may also cause problems if eaten at the wrong time of day, such as "heavy" foods at night (Saravia 2006).

The hot and cold belief system, first recorded in the Hippocratic Corpus (circa 40 BCE) was then further developed by Galen in the second century (Millar and Lane, 1988). It was studied and further developed by Islamic scholars, such as Ibn Sina (known as Avicenna, in Latin), and may also have developed independently in India and China, as well as among the indigenous peoples of the Americas (Foster 1953; Manderson 1987). It now permeates cultures around the world and it is usually referred to by social scientists as humoral medicine, because the qualities hot, cold, wet, and dry applied to fluids (or humors in the original Greek and East Indian conceptions) in the body. The hot/cold concept of balance is particularly important in Asian, Latin American, and Mediterranean cultures. In the hot and cold belief system, food is seen as crucial in maintaining a healthy body. It is believed that illness can occur if food upsets the body's humoral balance, such as eating hot or heavy foods at night, or breastfeeding while upset (the milk will be hot from the emotions and make the baby ill) (Scrimshaw and Hurtado 1988). "Hot" does not always refer to temperature; instead, it can describe a symbolic quality, for example when it is attributed to such foods as beef and pork, which in some cultures are regarded as hot regardless of the physical temperature at which they are consumed, whereas fish may be seen as cold even when cooked and served warm. To complicate matters, classification of foods into hot/cold and heavy/light can vary from community to community, even within the same cultural groups. Hot and cold food beliefs are tied to other aspects of the Hippocratic humoral body balances tradition. For example, the concept of "doing the month" after childbirth in Chinese culture involves using foods as well as other practices to prevent cold from harming the body during this vulnerable period (Pillsbury 1978).

Food beliefs affect behaviors designed to prevent illness and are also used in treatment of illness to attempt to restore balance. For example, in Central America, some diarrheas in children are viewed as hot, and protein-rich "hot" foods such as meats are withheld, aggravating the malnutrition that may be present and may be exacerbated by the diarrheal disease (S.C.M. Scrimshaw and Hurtado, 1988). Figure 9.1 shows the classification of perceived causes of diarrheal disease in infants and young children in Central America and includes foods as a cause in a number of instances. Figure 9.2 shows a range of culturally described treatments for diarrheal disease in infants and young children. By far the most frequent treatment was giving the patient some form of fluid. This finding led to the recommendation that a culturally acceptable way to encourage rehydrating infants and young children would be to suggest adding oral rehydration salts (ORS) to fluids already being given to treat diarrhea. (S.C. Scrimshaw and Hurtado 1988).

An extensive literature describes food beliefs and practices worldwide, which have important implications in public health (Chrzan and Brett 2017; Hastorf 2016; Herman and Bentley 1993; Kittler and Sucher 2012; Riley and Paugh 2018; Staller and Carrasco 2009). Foods are described, labeled, evaluated, and acted upon in the context of culture. In this sense, the cultural context of food is complex, and includes knowledge, beliefs, art, morals, laws, customs, and any other capabilities acquired by humans as members of society to make sense of food.

	Mother						Food					Tooth eruption	Fallen fontanel	Fallen stomach	Evil eye	Stomach worms	Cold enters stomach	Disentery
	Hot			Emotional														
CAUSE	Physical activity	Hot foods	Pregnancy	Anger	Sadness	Fright	Bad food	Excess	Does not eat on time	Quality: Hot	Quality: Cold							
SYMPTOMS All types have watery and frequent stools				Very dangerous			Flatulence, feeling of fullness					Tooth eruption	Green with mucus	Sunken fontanel vomiting; green in color	Fever	Worms	White in color	Blood in stools, "urgency": color is red or black
TREATMENT	Not breastfeeding when hot	Mother changes diet	Breastfeeding stops	Home, drugstore, Injectionist, witch, spiritist			Home, fold curer					None	Folk curer		Folk curer	Drugstore, home, folk curer	Folk curer	Home. drugstore, health post

Figure 9.1 Taxonomy of diarrhea

Source: S. C. M. Scrimshaw and E. Hurtado, *Rapid Assessment Procedures for Nutrition and Primary Health Care: Anthropological Approaches to Improving Program Effectiveness (RAP)* (Los Angeles: UCLA Latin America Center, 1987), p. 26. Reprinted with permission of the Regents of the University of California.

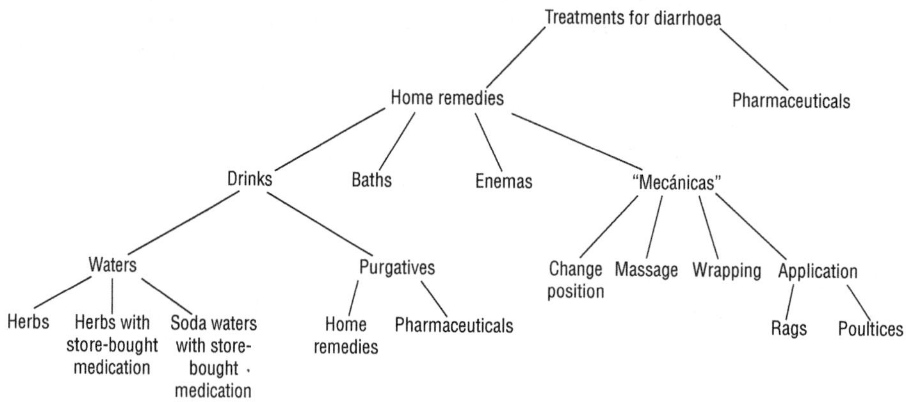

Figure 9.2 Taxonomy of treatments for diarrhea

Source: S. C. M. Scrimshaw and E. Hurtado, *Rapid Assessment Procedures for Nutrition and Primary Health Care: Anthropological Approaches to Improving Program Effectiveness (RAP)* (Los Angeles: UCLA Latin America Center, 1987), p. 26. Reprinted with permission of the Regents of the University of California.

FOOD PRODUCTION

Chapter 29 in this volume, *Connecting Human Health to Nature Health: The Bridging Potential of Sustainable Food Systems*, discusses the shift away from small-scale food production to large-scale agricultural production and food distribution and the need to re-establish the balance between food production, distribution, and environmental sustainability. It provides the framework for noting here that food production exists in many forms and at many levels around the world. The vast majority of the world's farms are small or very small (Meyfroidt 2017; Samberg et al. 2016). Worldwide, farms of less than one hectare account for 72% of all farms but control only 8% of all agricultural land. Farms between one and two hectares account for 12% of all farms and control 4% of the land. In contrast, only 1% of all farms in the world are larger than 50 hectares, but they control 65% of the world's agricultural land (International Labor Organization 2018).

Subsistence farming and small farms remain an important source of food for families around the world, particularly in rural areas. What is grown or raised (in the case of animals) and how it is produced are influenced not only by climate, soil conditions and the availability of water, but also by culturally influenced modes of production and choices around what to produce. People produce what they prefer to eat and what they can sell. As an example of the deep meaning of foods discussed earlier in this chapter, for a Maya in Guatemala who owns even the smallest amount of land, it is considered essential to grow some *milpa*, which is maize (corn). In addition to subsistence farming, families, often the women in the family, maintain small plots in rural or suburban areas, sometimes even in urban areas. There, they can grow a few vegetables and herbs to supplement the family diet, and sometimes raise a few chickens or ducks and even other animals like rabbits, pigs and goats. In the Andean highlands, guinea pigs are also raised. These animals not only serve as a source of income and protein, they consume garbage, thus reducing the environmental impact of food waste.

In looking at food production, gender differences in roles should be noted. These range from the roles of women in maintaining small garden plots and raising a few animals, to gender roles in bartering and selling food which is produced. In many instances, women prepare food for sale and sell it on the streets or in small markets. In describing research on a Guatemalan coffee plantation, Mary Scrimshaw noted that women made food such as tamales to sell at local soccer games and to people waiting in line on payday (Cosminsky and M.W. Scrimshaw 1980). During a 2000 concert tour on the part of a Chicago chorus to rural Costa Rica, one of us (Scrimshaw) noted that food sellers, most of them women, would gather outside the concert venues to sell their wares. The market women of Africa are famous, and similar entrepreneurs are seen around the world (Kawarazuka, Béné and Prain 2017; Levin et al. 1999; Otoo et al. 2012).

Thus, examining the relationships between culture, food and nutrition needs to include food production at both macro- and micro-levels. It also needs to include the roles of many of the social determinants of health discussed in the Introduction to this volume and in several other chapters, including Chapter 29 on *Connecting Human Health to Nature Health: The Bridging Potential of Sustainable Food Systems*. In particular, environmental, educational and economic issues impact heavily on food production.

FOOD PROCUREMENT

The concept of food procurement refers to understanding who gathers/grows/buys food for the family and how culture shapes this. It should also be noted that there are differences in access to food between and within large urban areas, small towns and rural areas. Social determinants again come into play here, through factors such as transportation, economic resources, an understanding of food and nutrition, and food distribution systems. Even in high-resource countries such as the USA, there has been much discussion around "food deserts," areas in large urban areas where foods are expensive, and fresh, good quality food is virtually unobtainable (Walker, Keane, and Burke 2010). Food insecurity (Barett 2010) around the world has been exacerbated by the economic impact of COVID-19, which has resulted in large increases in unemployment and under-employment (Pereira and Oliveira 2020; Wolfson and Leung 2020).

There are gender differences in roles and strategies (Levin et al. 1999; S.C. Scrimshaw and Lane 2020). Often, those who do the food preparation, usually women, select and purchase or barter for food. In some instances, men share this role; in other instances, men make larger purchases while women make smaller ones (Cosminsky and M.W. Scrimshaw 1980). Sometimes people purchase in larger quantities and then re-sell to friends and neighbors, particularly in remote areas where access and transportation are issues. In many low-income communities, only a few households may have items such as refrigerators. These families often purchase perishable food such as butter and milk in quantities, and then re-sell to neighbors in smaller amounts. Small purchases are not just influenced by factors like refrigeration, but also economic constraints. Anthropologist Sol Tax was the first to describe what he called "the penny economy," where people purchase items in very small quantities because that is what they can afford at the time (Tax 1963).

While food procurement is dependent on economic resources and access, it is also influenced by cultural attitudes, as discussed earlier. Food quality, food types, and convenience are all important. For example, a case study based on a rapid (focused) ethnographic study in Africa that was conducted before introducing a new infant cereal provided essential information for the program to introduce the cereal, avoiding spending time and money on a fortified food product that would not be accepted. The study showed that the problem in acceptance would not be around the fact that the infant feeding product was fortified, but instead, the study revealed the reality

> that a food that must be cooked, however briefly, is *unlikely* to be chosen over instant foods that do not require cooking. Busy mothers will spend more money to purchase prepared cooked cereals from a street vendor or buy small packets of instant cereal that can be mixed with water rather than cooking a cereal themselves. This was extremely important guidance, as it showed that the cereal planned for introduction would need to be modified so that it would not require cooking if it was to be a success. (S.C. Scrimshaw and Lane, 2020: 65)

FOOD PREPARATION

Food preparation is also influenced by culture. In most cultures, women are the most involved in food preparation, although this is increasingly shared by men in some countries. Ironically, while food preparation at home has traditionally been considered women's work, for decades high-level professional cooking was considered a male domain, particularly in the western world. This is now changing, with the emergence of many successful woman chefs.

It is beyond the scope of this chapter to go into the details of how food preparation affects the nutritional values of foods, but this has been well documented and is a source of continuing research. Not only do hot and cold temperatures affect the quality of food, so do combinations of food. Additions of salt, sugar, and fats alter the nutritional value of foods. Combinations of foods are also important, as in the previous example of the nutritional quality of maize being improved by the addition of lime. Around the world, combinations of plant-based foods can create meals complete with needed proteins (Caballero 1988; Parker et al. 1998; N.S. Scrimshaw et al. 1957; N.S. Scrimshaw et al. 1960). These combinations traditionally are culturally influenced, but are becoming more intentional as understanding of their value increases.

Culture also influences safe food handling and storage, which, along with food preparation, are learned by each generation. Food safety involves the temperatures at which food is prepared and stored, cleanliness of preparation surfaces and implements, how long food is left at warm temperatures before storage after preparation or serving, how long food is kept after it has been procured or prepared, and many similar variables. These depend on knowledge and practices, but also on economic factors and living conditions. Economic factors and living conditions impact the availability and quality of refrigerators, stoves and other cooking devices and food preparation surfaces and implements, as well as water and cleaning supplies.

INTRA-HOUSEHOLD FOOD DISTRIBUTION

Food is not allocated equally within households (Engle and Nieves 1993; S.C.M. Scrimshaw 1990). Portion size and quality and the order in which people eat are influenced by age, gender and other cultural designations of status. In many societies, adult males, particularly the male head of household, eat first and are allocated the most and best food. After them, the elders and children are served, while women often are served or eat last. Male children may be served before female children in some cultures. Some foods may be reserved only for some family members. Some family members can take food whenever they want, others have to wait for it to be given to them.

Box 9.1 K'iche' Maya culture, language and food

MIGUEL CUJ

While the splendor of Mayan heritage is celebrated in Guatemala, the history of the rural Maya population is still largely unwritten. According to the Guatemalan Instituto Nacional de Estadistica (National Institute of Statistics of Guatemala), 40% of the total population is indigenous Mayan, representing 23 linguistic groups, with different languages and cultures. K'iche' Mayan is the largest group in terms of number of speakers, with about a million in total. Most of the K'iche' Mayan ethnic group lives in the Western Highlands of Guatemala in the departments of Quiche, Totonicapán, Quetzaltenango, Sololá, and other regions. Most K'iche' speak their native language and a variable amount of Spanish, but some isolated rural communities speak only K'iche' Maya.

The social, cultural, military, and political conditions of Guatemala are the result of a complex history of colonialism, armed conflict, and various natural disasters as well as the current public health crisis. These elements provide a framework for a broad understanding of the context in which the rural Maya population lives at a heightened risk for food insecurity, health disparities, and lack of economic and educational opportunities. For many indigenous Maya, access to electricity, food, and potable water is limited. In fact, 51% of the population has no access to sanitation. In the dry season, water arrives by truck once or twice per week, which makes regular washing difficult (ICEFI 2015). With public transportation restricted, communities struggle to access the most basic goods, such as soap or food, from local markets. Given the reality in Guatemala that 20% of households with children suffer from diarrheal disease, 33% of households with children have respiratory infections, and nearly 50% of all children are chronically malnourished, many individuals are living with already compromised immune systems which leaves them especially susceptible to infections (CENSO 2018; ENSMI 2015; ICEFI 2015).

In Maya culture, food serves as more than a nutritional substance. Food is the cornerstone of religious, cultural, linguistic, agricultural, and social life. Maya people have classified food into three major categories: food for people, food for otherworld inhabitants, and food for the soul. These categories include topics such as feasting, fasting, healing, corn-based food, non-corn-based food, and forbidden foods. In the same way, the Maya designate plants into four categories delimiting cultural significance: cultivated plants, protected plants, wild-based useful plants, wild-based insignificant plants. Also, the Maya population operates within an intricate system to categorize the food based on the experience and sense of hot or cold and wet or dry, as described earlier in this chapter. Additionally, the Maya population has language structure categories about food groups with regards to feeding and eating: solid corn food base, solid non-corn food base, spicy food, liquid food including drinks and hot beverages, break or mealtimes food, and side meal food (Cuj, Grabinsky, and Yates-Doerr 2020; Food Agriculture Organization 1992, 2011; Harvey 2013; Hawkins 2007; Hull 2010; Neuenswander and Arnold 1977; Searcy 2011; Staller and Carrasco 2009; Staller et al. 2016; Taube 1989; Yates-Doerr 2015b). These categorizations demonstrate the complex roles of foodways within many spheres of cultural and language ideation.

In Mayan culture, maize is not just a staple food providing nutritional substance, it is also the mainstay for sustaining religious, linguistic, and agriculture life (Food Agriculture Organization 1992; Staller et al. 2016). Maize is sustenance and forms the basis for the cultural, agronomic, and ecological organization of Maya communities (Staller and Carrasco 2009; Staller et al. 2016). The distinctive cultural elements around maize production, transformation, and consumption are revealed by examining the uses of maize as food, especially food and beverages that have symbolic meaning. The categorization of maize (*ixim*) in the Maya language has specific meanings, for example, *saq ixim* (white maize), *q'an ixim* (yellow maize), *q'eq ixim/me'ix ixim* (black maize), *mari'y ixim/raxwa'ch ixim* (blue maize). The semantics and logic of maize can shed light on fundamental elements that support communal connections in Maya area. The language of maize influences the logistics of the Maya people: the root word *ixim* is combined with other Maya words as a lexical couplet, for example, *iximulew* (*ixim*: maize, *ulew*: land = land of the maize) and *Iximche' (ixim*: maize, *Che'*: tree = maize tree). Even the Popol Wuj, a written account of the origins of K'iche' Mayan people transmitted orally for generations, describes the great importance of maize in the identity of the Maya population. Maize is not a crop but a deep cultural symbol intrinsic to daily life. Maize is inextricably tied to the quotidian lives of the Maya people. As the basic grain, it shapes daily meals and its growing cycle influences the timing of festivals. The image and shape of maize is a ubiquitous component of the material expression of food in a Maya lexical.

The language of food embraces the Maya civilization from ancient times to the current Maya population in Mesoamerica. In this regard, language revitalization in the Maya population through the language of food is an opportunity to understand the cultural context of food dynamics over time and how these impact food production and consumption. Food and language contribute to the foundation of the identity of the Maya population in Mesoamerica. Since ancient times, the Maya population has used language to describe and classify food. Both written and spoken traditions around food have endured, maintaining the legacy of this civilization from early ancient to current times. Maya civilization developed a communication system that became one of the early writing systems in the world (Demarest and Demarest 2004; Scarre and Fagan 2016). These linguistic roots are thought to have originated from a common ancestral language called Proto-Mayan, which was spoken since ancient times by inhabitants of Mesoamerica. Mayan languages spread through one-third of the territory of Mesoamerica. Linguistic documentation points out that the Proto-Mayan language emerged around 2000 BCE (Early Pre-classic 2000 BCC to 1000 BCE). The Proto-Mayan words that refer to maize – "ixim" and "wa" – have been registered over time from the classic period of the Maya civilization to current modern Maya people (Staller and Carrasco 2009; Staller et al. 2016; Taube 1989). This means that both foodways and language have a deep cultural heritage in the Maya population.

A clear example of how language becomes a health issue is seen in the dissemination of health policies and guidelines. For example, governmental institutions, such as the Guatemalan Ministry of Health, have made efforts to implement national food guidelines for Guatemala (Pan American Health Organization/Ministerio de Salud Publica de Guatemala 2014). One of the objectives of these guidelines is to improve the nutritional status of people at the rural community level. Although designed for a multicultural Guatemalan population (Maya and non-Maya people), these guidelines are developed purely from a western nutrition science paradigm and only published in Spanish rather than in indigenous languages. The cultural aspects of Mayan models regarding experiences of health are rarely, if at all, considered. As a result, these cultural barriers have negative implications for preventing and treating nutritional problems. Not only are the Guatemalan Food Guidelines only written in Spanish while the Mayan communities speak local Mayan languages, these languages are generally not written. Additionally, as a result of poor access to education, a significant proportion of the adult population does not know how to read and write in Spanish. Indigenous women, who are traditionally in charge of preparing meals, are the most vulnerable to educational exclusion. This reality represents a significant language, social, and gender barrier to communicating the information contained in the guidelines. In short, the nationally approved health and nutrition guidelines are based on a western policy structure and world view that may lead to an increase in inequalities in health status among the Mayan population. In this way, language can serve as a significant barrier to accurate dissemination of information related to food and nutrition in the K'iche' population.

Recent research (Cuj, Sattler, and de Beausset. 2020) has found that K'iche' women often describe K'iche' food categories in ways that are framed by the K'iche' Mayan language and influence food consumption. Maya languages have food logics that categorize food based on *wa* (food corn-based), *riki'l* (food non-corn-based), *kunel* (seasoning) *xaq* munil (snacks) *xaq kaqatijo* (refreshment food), and *meq'in* (hot beverage). These features explain food behavior that are different from concepts of food from western nutrition science as biological concepts that focus on macronutrients (protein, carbohydrates, and fat) and micronutrients (vitamins and minerals). Those concepts do not have translation or meaning in the K'iche' language. These findings indicate that nutrition guidelines should attend not only to other people's cultures, but to what might be called "cultures of nutrition." Understanding cultures of nutrition can lead to strategies for how culture, language, and logic of food of K'iche' people could operate within the field of nutrition science based on an adaptive approach to developing guidelines. Such culturally based approaches should be especially useful for handling the diversity within nutrition science and for engaging situations where many different cultures of nutrition collide, as is the case of the Maya population.

CONCLUSIONS

It is important to bridge the gap between the cultural and sociolinguistic aspects of indigenous foodways, and biomedical, nutritional, and related scientific studies in order to encourage a more in-depth understanding of how food is actually produced, obtained, prepared, distributed in households and communities, and consumed. The social determinants of health, discussed in chapters throughout this volume, also strongly impact food production, access, preparation and consumption. Nutritional science can tell us about the composition of food and the biological impacts of dietary practices at both the individual and population levels. In order to fully measure actual practices, it is essential to include a deep cultural understanding of foodways along with anthropological methodologies that facilitate more accurate measures of what people actually do, and what motivates them. These understandings can then lead to more effective ways to implement the findings from both the nutritional and the behavioral sciences to improve people's access to food, along with improved production and improved diets.

REFERENCES

Baize, S., Pannetier, D., Oestereich, L.,... Günther, S. (2014). Emergence of Zaire Ebola Virus Disease in Guinea. *New England Journal of Medicine* 371, 1418–1425. DOI: 10.1056/NEJMoa1404505.

Barrett, C.B. (2010). Measuring Food Insecurity. *Science* 327(5967), 825–828.

Bennett, J.W., Smith, H.L., and Passin, H. (1942). Food and Culture in Southern Illinois: A Preliminary Report. *American Sociological Review* 7(5), 645–660. https://doi.org/10.2307/2085690.

Bernard, H.R. (2017). *Research Methods in Anthropology: Qualitative and Quantitative Approaches* (6th edition). Lanham, MD: Rowman and Littlefield.

Binder, P.-M., and Smith, K.. (2013). *The Language Phenomenon: Human Communication from Milliseconds to Millennia*. Springer Science & Business Media.

Black, Robert E. et al. (2013). Maternal and Child Undernutrition and Overweight in Low-Income and Middle-Income Countries. *Lancet* 382(9890), 427–451. https://doi.org/10.1016/S0140-6736(13)60937-X.

Boerboom, S. (2015). *The Political Language of Food*. Lanham, MD: Lexington Books.

Caballero, B. (1988) Nutritional Implications of Dietary Interactions: A Review. *Food and Nutrition Bulletin* 10(2), 9–20.

Camp, C. (1982). Foodways in Everyday Life. *American Quarterly* 34(3), 278–289. https://doi.org/10.2307/2712779.

CENSO de Guatemala. (2018). *Portal de Resultados Del Censo 2018*. Instituto Nacional de Estadistica de Guatemala. Available at: www.censopoblacion.gt/. Accessed October 10, 2019.

Chatterjee, Margaret. (1969). "Language as Phenomenon." *Philosophy and Phenomenological Research* 30(1), 116–121. https://doi.org/10.2307/2105926.

Chen, Nancy N. 2008. *Food, Medicine, and the Quest for Good Health: Nutrition, Medicine, and Culture*. Columbia University Press.

Chrzan, J., and Brett, J. (2017). *Food Culture: Anthropology, Linguistics and Food Studies*. Oxford: Berghahn Books.

Cosminsky, S., and Scrimshaw, M.W. (1980). Medical Pluralism on a Guatemalan Plantation. *Social Science and Medicine, Part B: Medical Anthropology* 13(4), 267–278.

Couninhan, C. (1999). *The Anthropology of Food and Body: Gender, Meaning and Power*. London: Routledge.

Cuj, M., Grabinsky, L., and Yates-Doerr, E. (2020). Cultures of Nutrition: Classification, Food Policy, and Health. *Medical Anthropology*. Online first, December 4. DOI: 10.1080/01459740.2020.1826475.

Cuj, M., Sattler, M., and de Beausset, S. (2020). Maya K'iche' Food Groups and Implications for Guatemalan Food Guidelines. *Food and Nutrition Bulletin* 41(2), 261–274. https://doi.org/10.1177/0379572120912161.

Demarest, Arthur, and Demarest Demarest Arthur Andrew. 2004. *Ancient Maya: The Rise and Fall of a Rainforest Civilization*. Cambridge University Press.

Douglas, M., and Gross, J. (1981). Food and Culture: Measuring the Intricacy of Rule Systems. *Social Science Information* 20(1), 1–35.

Di Cesare, Mariachiara, et al. (2013). Inequalities in Non-communicable Diseases and Effective Responses. *The Lancet* 381(9866), 585–597.

Duranti, Alessandro. (1997). *Linguistic Anthropology*. Cambridge University Press.

Encuesta nacional de salud materno infantil de Guatemala (ENSMI). (2015). *Instituto Nacional de Estadística (Guatemala), Macro International, and Demographic and Health Surveys*.

Food Agriculture Organization of the United Nations (FAO). (1992). *Maize in Human Nutrition*. Rome: FAO.

Food Agriculture Organization of the United Nations (FAO). (2011). *Cultura y Prácticas Alimentarias en Totonicapán*. Fondo para el Logro de los Objetivos de Desarrollo del Milenio. Guatemala: FAO.

Foster, G.M. (1953). Relationships between Spanish and Spanish-American Folk Medicine. *Journal of American Folklore* 66, 201–217.

Good, Byron, and Andrew McDowell. (2015). "Belief, Anthropology Of." In *International Encyclopedia of the Social & Behavioral Sciences (Second Edition)*, edited by James D. Wright, 493–497. Oxford: Elsevier. https://doi.org/10.1016/B978-0-08-097086-8.12024-0

Goodman, David. (2001). "Ontology Matters: The Relational Materiality of Nature and Agro-Food Studies." *Sociologia Ruralis* 41(2): 182–200. https://doi.org/10.1111/1467-9523.00177.

Harvey, T.S. (2008). "Where There Is No Patient: An Anthropological Treatment of a Biomedical Category." *Culture, Medicine and Psychiatry* 32(4): 577–606. https://doi.org/10.1007/s11013-008-9107-1.

Harvey, T.S. (2013). *Wellness beyond Words: Maya Compositions of Speech and Silence in Medical Care*. USA. Albuquerque, NM, University of New Mexico Press.

Hastorf, Christine A. (2016). *The Social Archaeology of Food: Thinking about Eating from Prehistory to the Present*. Cambridge: Cambridge University Press. https://doi.org/10.1017/9781316597590.

Hawkins, John Palmer. (2007). *Health Care in Maya Guatemala: Confronting Medical Pluralism in a Developing Country*. Norman, OK: University of Oklahoma Press.

Herman, E., and Bentley, M. (1993). *Rapid Assessment Procedures to Improve the Household Management of Diarrhea*. Boston, MA: International Nutrition Foundation for Developing Countries.

Hosking, Richard. (2010). *Food and Language: Proceedings of the Oxford Symposium on Food and Cooking*. Oxford: Oxford Symposium.

Huber, Brad Richard, and Alan R. Sandstrom. 2001. *Mesoamerican Healers*. University of Texas Press.

Hull, Kerry. (2010). An Epigraphic Analysis of Classic-Period Maya Foodstuffs. In John Staller and Michael Carrasco (eds.), *Pre-Columbian Foodways: Interdisciplinary Approaches to Food, Culture, and Markets in Ancient Mesoamerica* (pp. 235–256). New York: Springer. https://doi.org/10.1007/978-1-4419-0471-3_9.

International Labor Organization. (2018). www.globalagriculture.org. Accessed February 13, 2021.

Instituto Centro Americano de Estudios Fiscales (ICEFI). (2003). *Cuanto Invierte el Estado en los Pueblos Indigenas*. ICEFI press.

Instituto Centro Americano de Estudios Fiscales (ICEFI). (2003). *Cuanto Invierte el Estado en los Pueblos Indigenas*. ICEFI press.

Johnston, Francis E. (1987). *Nutritional Anthropology*. New York: A.R. Liss.

Karaman, O. (2008). A New Philosophy of Society: Assemblage Theory and Social Complexity by Manuel DeLanda. *Antipode* 40(5), 935–937.

Karrebæk, Martha Sif, Riley, Kathleen C., and Cavanaugh, Jillian R. (2018). Food and Language: Production, Consumption, and Circulation of Meaning and Value. *Annual Review of Anthropology* 47(1), 17–32. https://doi.org/10.1146/annurev-anthro-102317-050109.

Kawarazuka, N., Béné, C., and Prain, G. (2017). Adapting to a New Urbanizing Environment: Gendered Strategies of Hanoi's Street Food Vendors. *Environment & Urbanization (IIED)* 30(1), 233–248.

King, C. K. 2003 *Doris Howes Calloway* (1923–2001). *The Journal of Nutrition* 133(7):2113–2116. doi:10.1093/jn/133.7.2113.

Kittler, Pamela Goyan, and Sucher, Kathryn. (2012). *Food and Culture* (6th edition). Belmont, CA: Wadsworth/Cengage Learning.

Levin, C.E., Ruel, M.T., Morris, S.S., Maxwell, D.G., Armar-Klemesu, M., and Ahiadeke, C. (1999). Working Women in an Urban Setting: Traders, Vendors and Food Security in Accra. *World Development* 27(11), 1977–1991.

Li, X., Song, Y., Wong, G., and Cui, J. (2020). Bat Origin of a New Human Coronavirus: There and Back Again. *Sci China Life Sci* 63(3), 461–462.

Logan, M. H. (1977). Anthropological Research on the Hot-Cold Theory of Disease: Some Methodological Suggestions. *Medical Anthropology* 1(4), 87–112.

Manderson, L. (1987). Hot-Cold Food and Medical Theories: Overview and Introduction. *Social Science and Medicine* 25(4), 329–330.

Meyfroidt, P. (2017). Mapping Farm Size Globally: Benchmarking the Smallholders debate. *Environmental Research Letters* 12(3), 1002.

Millar, M.I., and Lane, S.D. (1988). Ethno Ophthalmology in the Egyptian Delta: An Historical Systems Approach to Ethnomedicine in the Middle East. *Social Science and Medicine* 26(6), 651–657.

Mintz, Sidney W., and Du Bois, Christine M. (2002). The Anthropology of Food and Eating. *Annual Review of Anthropology* 31(1), 99–119. https://doi.org/10.1146/annurev.anthro.32.032702.131011.

Nestle, Marion. (2007). *Food Politics: How the Food Industry Influences Nutrition and Health*. Berkeley, CA: University of California Press.

Neuenswander, Helen L., and Arnold, Dean E. (1977). *Cognitive Studies of Southern Mesoamerica*. USA: Duncanville, TX, SIL Museum of Anthropology.

Otoo, M., Ibro, G., Fulton, J., and Lowenberg-Deboer, J. (2012). Micro-Entrepreneurship in Niger: Factors Affecting the Success of Women Street Food Vendors. *Journal of African Business* 13(1), 16–28.

Pan American Health Organization/Ministerio de Salud Publica de Guatemala (2014). *Guias Alimentarias para Guatemala Recomendaciones para una Alimentacion Saludable*. Guatamala City: Ministerio de Salud Publica de Guatemala.

Parker, M.E., Schroeder, D.G., Begin, F., and Hurtado, E. (1998). Maternal Preferences for Consistency of Complementary Foods. *Food and Nutrition Bulletin*, 19(1), 6–12.

Patel, Raj. (2012). *Stuffed and Starved: The Hidden Battle for the World Food System*. New York: Melville House.

Patel, Raj, and Moore, Jason W. (2017). *A History of the World in Seven Cheap Things: A Guide to Capitalism, Nature, and the Future of the Planet*. Los Angeles, CA: University of California Press.

Pereira, M., and Oliveira, A.M. (2020). Poverty and Food Insecurity may Increase as the Threat of COVID-19 Spreads. *Public Health Nutrition* 23(17), 3236–3240.

Pillsbury, B.K. (1978). "Doing the Month": Confinement and Convalescence of Chinese Women after Childbirth. *Social Science and Medicine, Part B: Medical Anthropology* 12, 11–22.

Ramirez-Zea, Manuel, Kroker-Lobos, Maria F., Close-Fernandez, Regina, and Kanter, Rebecca. (2014). The Double Burden of Malnutrition in Indigenous and Nonindigenous Guatemalan Populations. *The American Journal of Clinical Nutrition* 100(6), 1644S–1651S. https://doi.org/10.3945/ajcn.114.083857.

Riley, Kathleen C., and Cavanaugh, Jillian R. (2017). Tasty Talk, Expressive Food. *Semiotic Review*. https://semioticreview.com/ojs/index.php/sr/article/view/1.

Riley, Kathleen C., and Paugh, Amy L. (2018). *Food and Language: Discourses and Foodways across Cultures*. Abingdon, UK: Routledge.

Scarre, Chris, and Brian M. Fagan. 2016. *Ancient Civilizations*. Routledge

Samberg, L.H., Gerber, J.S., Ramakutty, N., Herrero, M., and West, P. (2016). Subnational Distribution of Average Farm Size and Smallholder Contributions to Global Food Production. *Environmental Research Letters* 11(12), 4010.

Saravia, María Teresa Mosquera. (2006). *Lógicas y racionalidades: entre comadronas y terapeutas tradicionales*. Instituto de Estudios Interétnicos, Universidad de San Carlos de Guatemala.

Scrimshaw, N.S., Bressani, R., Behar, M., Wilson, D., and Arroyave, G. (1960). A Low-cost Protein Rich Vegetable Mixture for Human Consumption. *Proceedings of the Federation of the American Society of Experimental Biology* 19, 320.

Scrinis, Gyorgy. (2013). *Nutritionism: The Science and Politics of Dietary Advice*. New York, Columbia University Press.

Scrimshaw, N.S., Squibb, R.L., Bressani, R., Behar, M., Viteri, F.E., and Arroyave, G. (1957). Vegetable Protein Mixtures for the Feeding of Infants and Young Children. In W.H. Cole (ed.), *Amino Acid Malnutrition, XIII Annual Protein Conference* (pp. 28–46). New Brunswick, NJ: Rutgers University Press.

Scrimshaw, S.C.M. (1990). Combining Quantitative and Qualitative Methods in the Study of Intra-household Resource Allocation. In B.L. Rogers and N.P. Schlossman (eds.), *Intra-household Resource Allocation: Issues and Methods for Development and Policy Planning. Food and Nutrition Bulletin Supplement* 15. Tokyo, Japan: United Nations University Press.

Scrimshaw, S.C.M., and Hurtado, E. (1987). *Rapid Assessment Procedures for Nutrition and Primary Health: Anthropological Approaches to Programme Improvement*. Los Angeles, CA: UCLA Latin American Center/Tokyo: United Nations University/New York: UNICEF.

Scrimshaw, S.C.M., and Hurtado, E. (1988). Anthropological Involvement in the Central American Diarrheal Disease Control Project. *Social Science and Medicine* 27(1), 97–105.

Scrimshaw, S.C., and Lane, S.D. (2020). Culture, Behavior, and Health. In M.H. Merson, R.E. Black, and A.J. Mills (eds.), *Global Health: Diseases, Programs, Systems, and Policies* (4th edition, pp. 43–74). Burlington, MA: Jones and Bartlett Learning.

Solomon, Harris. 2015. "Unreliable Eating: Patterns of Food Adulteration in Urban India." *BioSocieties* 10(2): 177–193. https://doi.org/10.1057/biosoc.2015.10.

Solomon, Harris. (2016). *Metabolic Living: Food, Fat, and the Absorption of Illness in India*. Duke University Press.

Searcy, M. (2011). *The Life-Giving Stone: Ethnoarchaeology of Maya Metates*. Tucson, AZ: University of Arizona Press.

Staller, John, and Carrasco, Michael. (2009). *Pre-Columbian Foodways: Interdisciplinary Approaches to Food, Culture, and Markets in Ancient Mesoamerica*. New York: Springer Science & Business Media.

Staller, John, Tykot, Robert, and Benz, Bruce. (2016). *Histories of Maize in Mesoamerica: Multidisciplinary Approaches*. Abingdon, UK: Routledge.

Tapela, Neo M., et al. (2019). Integrating Noncommunicable Disease Services into Primary Health Care, Botswana. *Bulletin of the World Health Organization* 97(2), 142–153. https://doi.org/10.2471/BLT.18.221424.

Tartanac, F. (2000). Incaparina and Other Incaparina-based Foods: Experience of INCAP in Central America. *Food and Nutrition Bulletin*, 21(1), 49–54.

Taube, K.A. (1989). The Maize Tamale in Classic Maya Diet, Epigraphy, and Art. *American Antiquity* 54(1), 31–51.

Tax, Sol, (1963). *Penny Capitalism: A Guatemalan Indian Economy*. Chicago, IL: University of Chicago Press.

Walker, R.E., Keane, C.R., and Burke, J.G. (2010). Disparities and Access to Healthy Food in the United States: A Review of Food Deserts Literature. *Health & Place* 16(5), 876–884.

Wolfson, J.A., and Leung, C.W. (2020). Food Insecurity During COVID-19: An Acute Crisis with Long-term Health Implications. *American Journal of Public Health* 110(12), 1763–1765.

World Health Organization (WHO). (2021). *Non-Communicable Diseases Report*. Geneva: WHO. Available at: www.who.int/news-room/fact-sheets/detail/noncommunicable-diseases.

Yates-Doerr, Emily. (2010). Measured Meals: Nutrition in America. *Gastronomica: The Journal of Food and Culture* 10(4), 98–99.

Yates-Doerr, Emily. (2012). The Weight of the Self: Care and Compassion in Guatemalan Dietary Choices. *Medical Anthropology Quarterly* 26(1), 136–158. https://doi.org/10.1111/j.1548-1387.2011.01169.x.

Yates-Doerr, Emily. (2015a). The World in a Box? Food Security, Edible Insects, and "One World, One Health" Collaboration. *SSM Social Science & Medicine* 129, 106–112.

Yates-Doerr, Emily. (2015b). *The Weight of Obesity: Hunger and Global Health in Postwar Guatemala*. Los Angeles, CA: University of California Press.

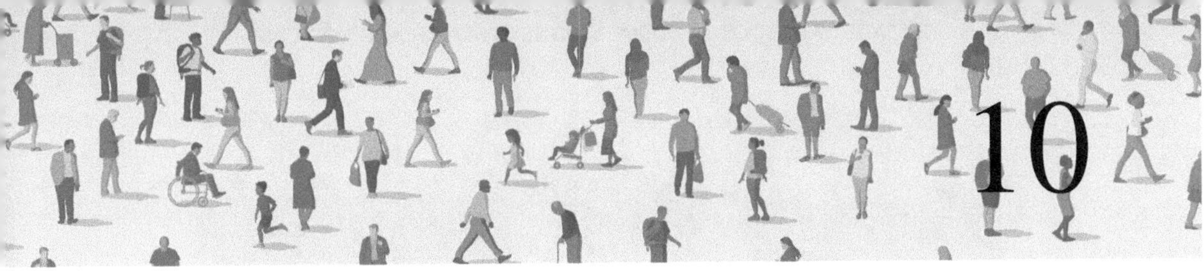

10

Community Engaged Learning: Community Health and Learning through Service in Sri Lanka

Suzanne M. Gaulocher, Tumisang Ramarea, Vinya Ariyaratne, and N. Ewen Wang

INTRODUCTION

Community Engaged Learning (CEL) is a pedagogical practice that integrates community organizations and undergraduate students in a course with common goals and activities (Annette 2002; Bandy 2016; Campus Compact 2020; Preskill & Brookfield 2009; Trickett et al. 2011). Community Engagement in a course involves preparation, critical reflection, high impact practice, academic rigor, reciprocal partnerships, shared goals, and actions that create change and promote equity (Chávez et al. 2008; Trickett et al. 2011). Community Engaged Learning helps to educate future professionals who will understand, respect and work with communities. It can also serve to improve relationships between academic institutions and communities if done correctly.

This chapter uses a case study to provide a tool for people thinking about integrating a Community Engaged Learning portion into an existing course, creating a new course or working with students in Community Engaged Scholarship. The process the case study course followed, though time-consuming, integrated ethical and effective practices working with students and community partners. It is the hope of the authors that this chapter provides a framework, resources, tips and lessons learned that may benefit the creation or evolution of Community Engaged Learning courses.

For this course, a Community Engaged Learning pedagogical practice was used intentionally to allow students to work together in a structured way to address social issues, learn skills, improve gaps in knowledge around social determinants of health, apply theoretical content and engage in community development work with a community partner (Rooks & Rael 2013; Tinto 2020). Alongside the community-based work, students were engaging in critical reflection and examining complex issues and social determinants of health. Community engagement in a course is meant to create collaborative and reciprocal relationships between universities and communities while "...instilling in

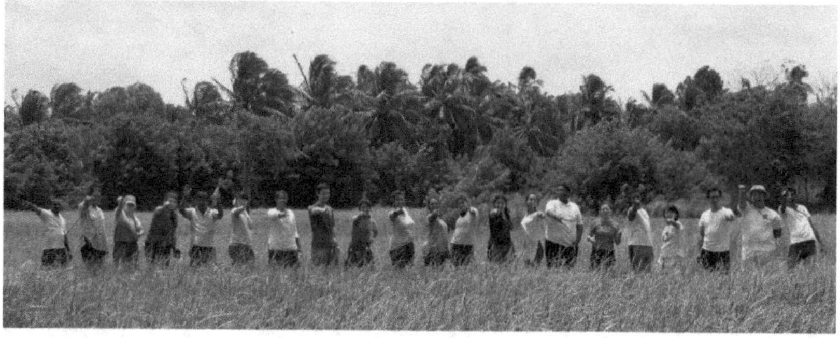

Figure 10.1 Participants in Community Engaged Scholarship Course

students the values of community and social responsibility" (Neururer & Rhoads 1998: p.321.

Community Engaged Learning (hereafter CEL) continues to grow as a pedagogical practice at the college level, with increased focus on how to improve this practice, and for good reason (Ash & Clayton 2009; Eby 1998; Saltmarsh 2005; Scott 2015; Trudeau & Kruse 2014). If not done well, this practice has the potential to reinforce stereotypes, power relationships and exploitation (Hartman et al. 2014). As such, this community engaged global health course was taught intentionally to allow time for preparation, in-country learning and critical reflection. It spanned nine months, over a three-quarter sequence, taught at a private university in California in the spring, summer and fall of 2016. *Community Health and Learning Through Service in Sri Lanka* is a course that integrated four distinct approaches: (1) CEL pedagogy, (2) Participatory Photo Mapping, (3) sustainable development through the lens of Social Determinants of Health (SDH) and social justice, and (4) positive community impact, specifically highlighting community–campus partnerships from a cross-cultural perspective.

Through the CEL pedagogy, intentional integration of SDH and social justice oriented this class towards a focus on social and environmental causes of health inequities (Lane et al. 2019; National Academies of Sciences, 2016). The World Health Organization defines Social Determinants of Health as:

> "the conditions in which people are born, grow, work, live, and age, and the wider set of forces and systems shaping the conditions of daily life. These forces and systems include economic policies and systems, development agendas, social norms, social policies and political systems. The social determinants of health are mostly responsible for health inequities. (World Health Organization 2019)

Framing this course within context through academic learning, reflection and collaboration with a community partner allowed for a deeper understanding of the issues that academic learning alone could not achieve. As future professionals, it was important that the students not only be exposed to SDH, but apply their learning in context. People who are going to work on anything that has to do with health in any way need to be health citizens. WHO's Health in All Policies affirms that in order to effectively address SDH, "the health sector needs to understand the imperatives of other sectors and form common understanding of health, its determinants and broader societal well-being or quality of life" (WHO 2019). The experience with our community partner created deep learning opportunities for students, faculty and partners (Brandy 2016). CEL integrated with health sciences is especially useful in addressing and eliminating health disparities and building health equity (Sabo et al. 2015). Students who work to solve social issues collaboratively with communities and reflect upon those processes adapt skills, knowledge and attitudes that may influence increased civic engagement when they start their careers (Rooks & Rael 2013). In order to effectively implement the solutions developed by population health science in every area of interest noted, it is important to educate a workforce that can effectively collaborate with vulnerable communities (Hartman et al. 2018).

Community Partner

Our course partnered with a non-governmental organization called Sarvodaya in the country of Sri Lanka. Sri Lanka was chosen as the site for this course due to previous collaboration and partnerships. Sarvodaya is a Sri Lankan organization that draws from Buddhist and Gandhian philosophies to mobilize communities towards improved development. Through this partnership, students and partners co-created a short community-based participatory research project using Participatory Photo Mapping (hereafter PPM), an ethnographic, collaborative method that is based on mutual trust between community and campus partners to identify community strengths and barriers to health, broadly defined (Dennis et al. 2009; Lane et al. 2011).

Significance of the Chosen Location and Relevance to the Course Content

This class was taught in the United States and in Sri Lanka as a collaborative community–university partnership. Sri Lanka (formerly Ceylon) is an island country in Southeast Asia, home to many ethnicities and languages. It is rich in tropical rain forests, with 25 hotspots of biodiversity. In terms of religion, Sri Lanka is 70% Buddhist, yet is home to many Hindus,

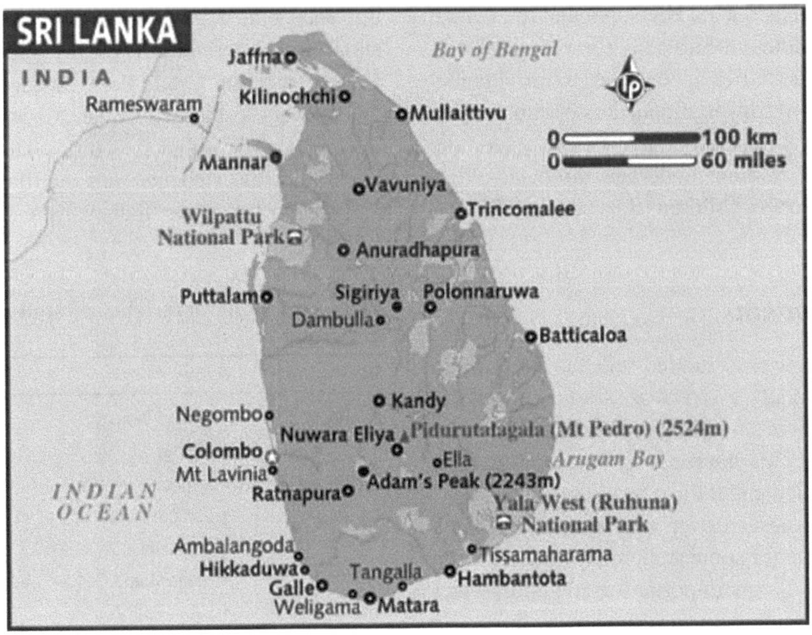

Figure 10.2 Map of Sri Lanka*

*Source: www.mapsopensource.com/sri-lanka-map.html
www.mapsopensource.com is licensed under a Creative Commons

Muslims and Christians. Sri Lanka has the oldest democracy in South East Asia.

Although it is considered a developing country, Sri Lanka is second only to the Maldives in South Asia in terms of per capita income and GDP growth, sustaining a successful plantation economy, including cinnamon, rubber and Ceylon tea. However, economic, educational and health disparities continue to exist across the country. Government and grassroots-level health care providers provide a substantial amount of health prevention and treatment, creating a population-level impact on positive health outcomes.

Our community-based partner, Sarvodaya's (meaning literally "progress of all") philosophy draws from Buddhism and Gandhian thought. Sarvodaya is Sri Lanka's largest people's organization, with 60 years of experience. It is comprised of 25 district offices, 10 specialist Development Education Institutes and over 100,000 youth mobilizing for peace (Sarvodaya 2020). It serves as an international role model and has a presence not only in Sri Lanka, but also in Nepal and the United States. Although Sarvodaya is recognized in multiple countries, it continues to provide ideological and inspirational leadership locally. Sarvodaya Suwasetha serves orphaned and destitute children, underage mothers, elders and pre-school children (Sarvodaya 2020).

The Students

This course was funded and taught through the university's overseas studies program, which offers several overseas experiences for students. This course was awarded funding that supplemented the cost to students, eliminating a cost barrier that may have been prohibitive for some students to participate in the class. It was important to the course faculty that no student be turned away due to an inability to pay for the course. The course was founded within a framework of social justice, and decisions were made through that lens from the beginning of the class to the end. Because of this overarching focus on addressing injustice, it made sense to approach the student selection as such.

In order to take an overseas course, students submit a lengthy application, including essays describing why they want to participate in the program, how the program will build on their education, how they plan to prepare for the in-country experience, and what challenges they expect may arise. For this course in particular, and because it was the only CEL class offered through the program, students had to answer additional questions about their personal interest in community and global health and provide three examples of how international CEL is reciprocal to the communities we came into contact with on our trip. Sixty-nine students applied to take this class with space for only 15 students (due to the hardship of selecting students, we asked for and were granted an additional slot). The selection process included both faculty members. Both faculty members read each and every application and selected our top students and then compared our lists. Next, faculty met with the 30 top-ranking students for small group interviews. These top students were ranked based on Grade Point Average (GPA), the answers to their essay questions, personal interest, and fit within the cohort. Through the interviews, the students were narrowed down and 16 undergraduate students were selected.

Table 10.1 Characteristics of student participants

Students: 16	*Majors: 11*
• 5 Frosh	• Human Biology
• 6 Sophomores	• Biology
• 4 Juniors	• Symbolic Systems
• 1 Senior	• Computer Science
	• Environmental Systems
	• Feminist and Gender Studies
	• Public Policy
	• Music
	• Science, Technology and Society
	• Management Science & Engineering
	• Product Design

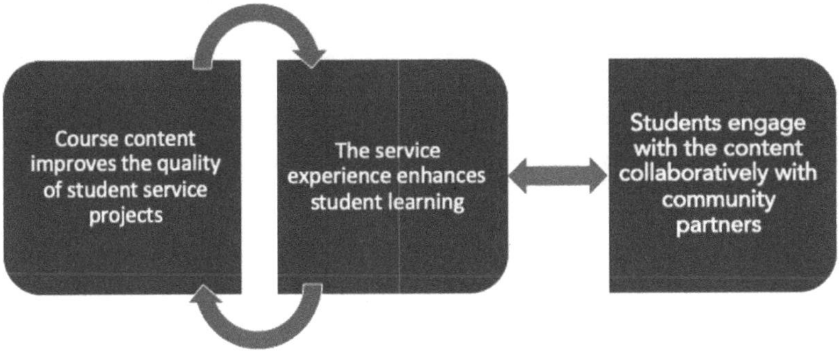

Figure 10.3 Course design

It was the intention of both faculty members not only to create a cohort with a range of student interests, but to include students from a variety of majors and to pull people outside of the health disciplines (WHO 2019). Teaching SDH to students exclusively in the health sciences was not our goal. We wanted students from different disciplines to take what they had learned into their own disciplines and future careers as a way to systematically address health inequity from a transdisciplinary perspective.

In addition, because the partnership with humanitarian organizations, such as Sarvodaya, is based on a collaborative relationship, it was our aim that our partners engage as co-educators in the learning experience with our students (see Figure 10.3). This course encouraged students to identify themselves as agents of social change, and to use the experience of community engagement to address injustice in communities and to explore solutions to complex humanitarian issues both locally and internationally.

This class emphasized the intersection between human and environmental systems with a focus on approaches that integrate these systems as a way of protecting biodiversity and promoting human health. Our students had an opportunity to meet high-level health officers and public health providers, such as doctors, along with grassroots providers, like midwives, village-level providers, water specialists, etc. depending on their own academic focus.

OUR MODEL – FOCUS ON EQUITY AND SOCIAL JUSTICE

We used the United Nations Sustainable Development Goals (see Figure 10.4) in addition to SDH as a way to teach students about the importance of equity in community development. The World Health Organization states that "the SDGs provide a comprehensive blueprint for human development and for systematically addressing the social determinants of health" (WHO 2019). The SDGs are multidimensional and multi-sectoral policy interventions that disrupt the status quo and build up or on policies that positively impact health. This powerful tool allows students to view overlapping and complex health issues within the context of other development goals, and the international community. The SDGs have targets and indicators that are evidence-based, community-driven and range from short- and long-term goals. Each student selected a health topic and one SDG and completed a robust literature review, key informant interviews and observation, and completed a research paper.

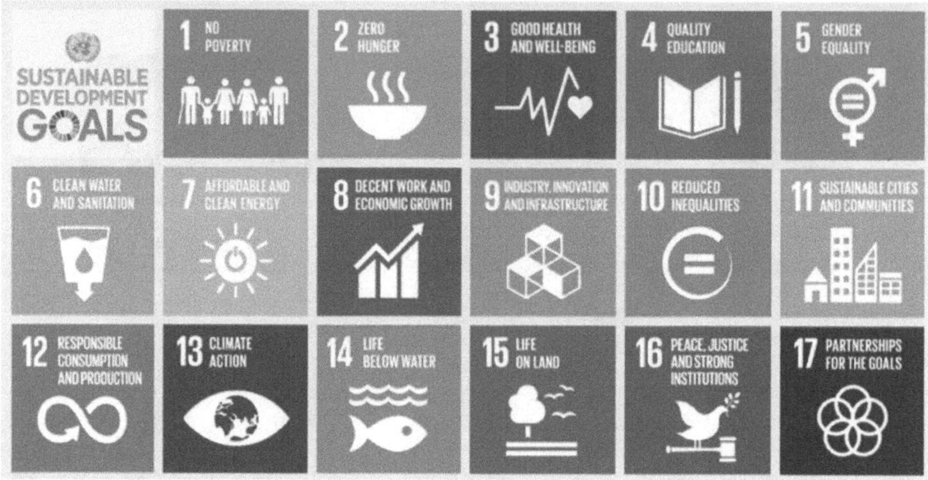

Figure 10.4 Sustainable Development Goals*

**Source*: United Nations Sustainable Development (2020)

Through planning and preparation, the faculty designed the class to teach students about the interaction between health and culture, environment and community in the historical, diverse and seemingly contradictory setting of rural Sri Lanka. In order to do this correctly, the faculty felt it was important to properly prepare students prior to the in-country class, as well as work with students as they re-entered the United States after the in-country class (see Figure 10.5). Through shared learning and open exploration of opinions and ideas, learning was participatory and transgressive for all involved. This chapter will cover each of the three main components of this model: Preparation, Application and Critical Reflection.

Preparation

The first phase was to prepare the faculty by identifying ethical frameworks, engaging a social justice mindset and identifying goals that met the need of our community partner, students and faculty together. As noted

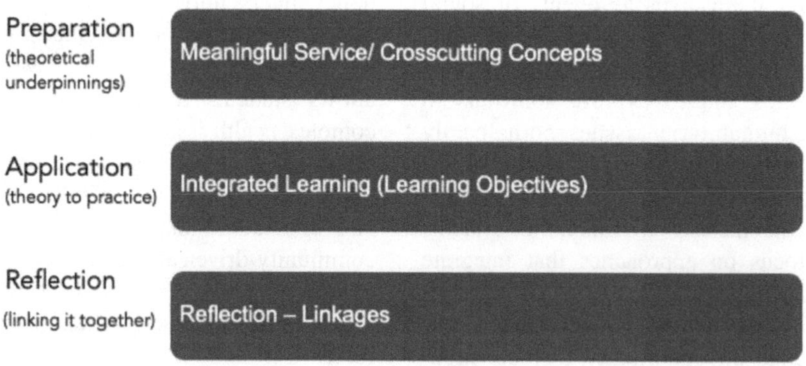

Figure 10.5 Main course components: preparation, application and critical reflection

earlier, Community Engaged Learning, done poorly, can reinforce prejudices and stereotypes (Hartman et al. 2014) and it was the intention of the faculty to teach a class that encourages didactic learning and constructivist pedagogical practice (Chávez et al. 2008; Hartman 2018; Hung & Khine 2006). In order to inspire socially minded students, faculty recognized the need to frame the entire class through didactic processes and experiences.

The student preparation phase was taught the spring before the in-country experience. Students and faculty met once a week and course topics ranged from etiquette, culture, expectations, reflection. The executive director of our partner organization travelled to meet with the students as part of a larger trip to the US. This course was the first opportunity for students to meet each other, our community partner and the faculty and teaching assistant.

With CEL courses, it is important to lay an ethical foundation early on. Ethics is not static, it's through exposure to differences and other ways of being and doing that we form our values and beliefs. Cultural competency isn't enough, as it implies that once you achieve competence, there is no need for further growth. A big part of the reflective component of this course was to reflect on experiences and practice cultural humility, understanding and competence (Allwright et al. 2019; Lane et al. 2019; Yeager & Bauer-Wu 2013). Cultural humility is the practice of self-reflection and mindfulness in interactions in order to implement "meaningful and ethical projects to better address health disparities" (Yeager & Bauer-Wu 2013: p.8). To begin, this class was introduced to the Principles of Ethical and Effective Service to get students thinking about areas of ethical considerations and to reflect on how public service can have a positive impact through collaboration between community partners and the campus community (see Figure 10.6) (Principles of Ethical and Effective Service 2020). In addition to integrating the Principles of Ethical and Effective Service, students began to explore topic ideas within the United Nation's Sustainable Development Goals and do research on those topics.

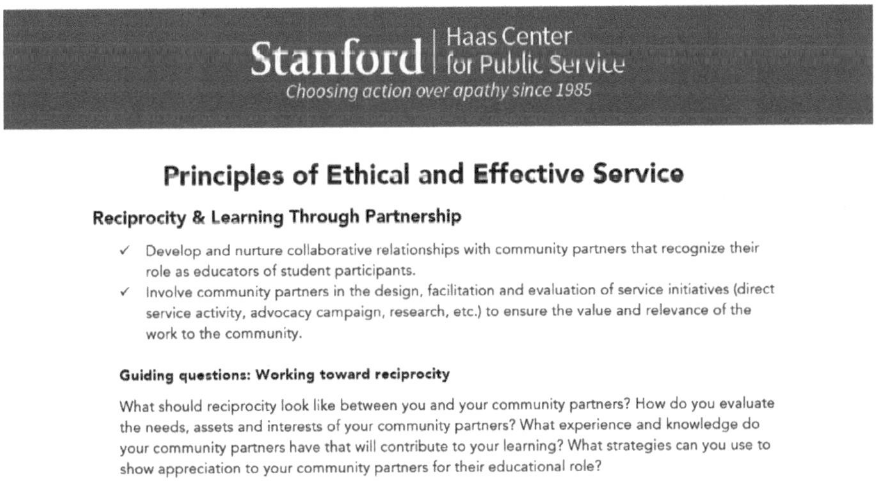
Stanford | Haas Center for Public Service

Choosing action over apathy since 1985

Principles of Ethical and Effective Service

Reciprocity & Learning Through Partnership

- ✓ Develop and nurture collaborative relationships with community partners that recognize their role as educators of student participants.
- ✓ Involve community partners in the design, facilitation and evaluation of service initiatives (direct service activity, advocacy campaign, research, etc.) to ensure the value and relevance of the work to the community.

Guiding questions: Working toward reciprocity

What should reciprocity look like between you and your community partners? How do you evaluate the needs, assets and interests of your community partners? What experience and knowledge do your community partners have that will contribute to your learning? What strategies can you use to show appreciation to your community partners for their educational role?

Figure 10.6 Stanford Principles of Ethical and Effective Service

Excerpted from Stanford University's *Principles of Ethical and Effective Service*, which include Reciprocity & Learning Through Partnerships, Clarity Expectations & Commitment, Respect Diversity, Preparation, Safety & Wellbeing, Reflection & Evaluation and Humility, and are used as a way to frame engagement and alignment with scholarship and community work (Principles and Ethical and Effective Service 2020).

For example, if a student wanted to research clean water and sanitation, they would begin in the spring semester preparation course and would be knowledgeable on the topic prior to landing in Colombo.

Application

Our course began and ended in Moratuwa, a suburb of Sri Lanka's capital, Colombo. The group made a loop through the central part of the country, staying in three of the five cities that make up Sri Lanka's 'Cultural Triangle'. A list of all the sites visited is listed in the Appendix at the end of this chapter. This three-week long course allowed students to engage with international partner organizations in a unique culture outside of the traditional classroom setting. Course objectives included: (1) engaging in a respectful, collaborative relationship with a community partner, (2) placing the service-learning experience within a broader context of humanitarian issues relevant to the community, (3) acknowledging the differences in backgrounds, worldviews and social contexts within the community, and (4) producing a final deliverable to the community partner that was context-specific and meets the needs of the community, while demonstrating accumulated knowledge from both the classroom and the community.

This experiential learning course immersed students in rural Sri Lankan life and engaged students in the basic elements of the holistic grassroots development strategy of the village-based Sarvodaya Movement, with a special focus on implications for individual, family and village health. The course curriculum aimed to teach students how to articulate and evaluate how Sarvodaya creates a comprehensive and integrative approach to global and community development and health. In order to do this, students were expected to identify indicators of a healthy community by visiting program sites, including preschools, organic farms, refugee settlements, Shanti Sena (youth peace brigades) and Eco Villages (sustainable rural development). It was important that students be able to articulate multiple approaches towards development and health through first-hand observation of different levels of health initiatives in Sri Lanka.

Student assessment of micro and macro health programs (grassroots to grass tops) across the country began with readings and interviews with the leaders within Sarvodaya. Using the framework of asset-based community development, students explored topics such as: nutrition, maternal and child health, water, prevention and treatment of violence, traditional healing and meditation in the context of ethnic and religious diversity, poverty, recovery from natural disaster and civil war. Students then prepared a presentation and presented their topic to the seminar participants prior to the onset of the in-country experience.

SHRAMADANA

A key strategy used by Sarvodaya for community development is Shramadana, which translate as "the gift of labor". The Sarvodaya Shramadana movement is a participatory development strategy and focuses on sustainable development or working with communities that have experienced a disaster. Throughout the three weeks, students, faculty and community members engaged in work that helped out a community, such as planting coconut trees or repairing the local Buddhist Temple. The role of Shramadana and its adoption into economic and community development is intentionally meant to remove social and economic injustice and free people from exploitation. It is deliberate community action meant to transform communities and build equity among community members (Sarvodaya 2020). Participating in the Shramadana allowed students to integrate their academic component through learning about health, culture, environmental sustainability, the importance of historical contexts and community development.

Participatory Photo Mapping

Participatory Photo Mapping is a tool that blends community participation, narratives and photographs with a focus on place. It combines photographs, maps and narratives in order to explore people's experience of place and to communicate this experience to community stakeholders and decision-makers. This proven methodology strengthens local voice and a sense of community (Dennis et al. 2009). Exploring issues of health within the context of place has the potential to create a more comprehensive snapshot of community health (Dennis et al. 2009). There is increasing attention on the relationship between place and health, particularly in disadvantaged communities (i.e. geographies), and that participation and collaboration with community members, public health professionals, urban planners and researchers all work together, and health outcomes improve (O'Brien et al. 2011). Working across sectors helps identify and address the multiple factors that affect health in places (Stokols et al. 2003). The PPM approach is meant to specifically address health in the context of place, emphasizing where people live, work and play as an important context within which individuals, families and groups experience aspects of life that affect health. In PPM, participants are given cameras and asked to take pictures of the places in their community that stand out in terms of a specific issue. Researchers and practitioners walk along with the participants, allowing for observation and relationship building (Carpiano 2009). After the picture-taking session, participants view the photos on the wall or on a computer and talk about each image. The maps and photographs document a direct observation to places in the community (John et al. 2012). Recommendations are compiled, vetted and delivered to the community, and an action plan is put in place.

Box 10.1 Participatory Photo Mapping (PPM)

PPM's aims to contribute to community–university participatory action research in four major ways:

1. Contribute a tool that captures attitudes and perceptions of people as they navigate an environment.
2. Develop products used to communicate with policy and decision-makers.
3. Communicate findings to a broad audience.
4. Create actionable processes in which community members take a part in mobilizing and engaging calls to action. (Dennis et al. 2009)

Our community partner asked our group to facilitate PPM with community members in the village of Pahalagama, the location of our village stay. Students and faculty spent part of this trip in home stays with families. Students were paired up and lived with one family for five days. Not only is this a proven technique to help outsiders understand a community, the families were compensated for home stays, so it is a source of income for community members (Schroeder et al. 2009; Shiri 2015). This allowed us to easily come together each day to work together on the Shramadana as well as the Participatory Photo Mapping project. The entire group participated in a photo mapping project with village residents. We worked with the leaders of the village. They asked the people of the village to gather and take pictures of what they found healthy about living in their village and what they'd like to see improve. Three different groups went out on foot (see Figure 10.1) and took pictures. After the pictures were deposited into a computer, students in the class were taught qualitative research analysis, including coding and assessing the photos according to place. Their lesson included addressing bias in the analysis process by coding the data with multiple people and using a comparative analysis method and vetting with community members (Glaser 1965; Hewitt-Taylor 2001). Using electronic documents with both the photographs and matched narratives generated by community members, the students coded by highlighting both key phrases and images. They noted in the margins where they made interpretations about the data. The photos were shared back with the people of the village and narratives were captured through a translator and vetted with Sarvodaya leadership. The main finding from this PPM project was unhappiness with litter around a beloved tank (reservoir) that provided beauty, bathing and water to this village. The results of the PPM project were to share findings with Sarvodaya Leadership, strategize with them on solutions, and raise money for signage for the village in order to reduce litter and appropriately dispose of trash.

Picture	Narrative	Narrative Code	Parent Code
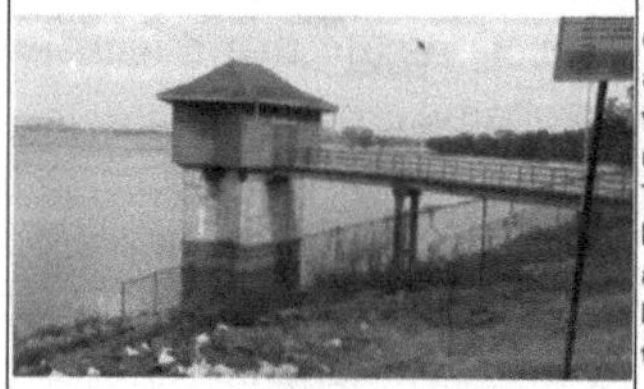	There are two rivers that meet. This is an example of environmental pollution - it's known as south bank. This rubbish is not put here by the villagers but by tourist that come to see the reservoir. This is something very precious to us and it is being destroyed is a pity and we feel very sad about it. Below that is the place were a lot of farmers get the water to water their crops = irrigation system.	Two rivers Meet South bank Rubbish Tourists "This is something very precious to us and it's being destroyed." Feel sad Farmers Water crops Irrigation system	Litter Tourism Environmental pollution Livelihood

This is an example of how students coded data and identified themes from the study. The photo is coded and the narrative is attached to that exact image using constant comparative method (Olson et al. 2016). Through this iterative process, themes are identified, shared back with community partners, and the themes are modified based on suggestions. The themes are then presented as recommendations to our community partner.

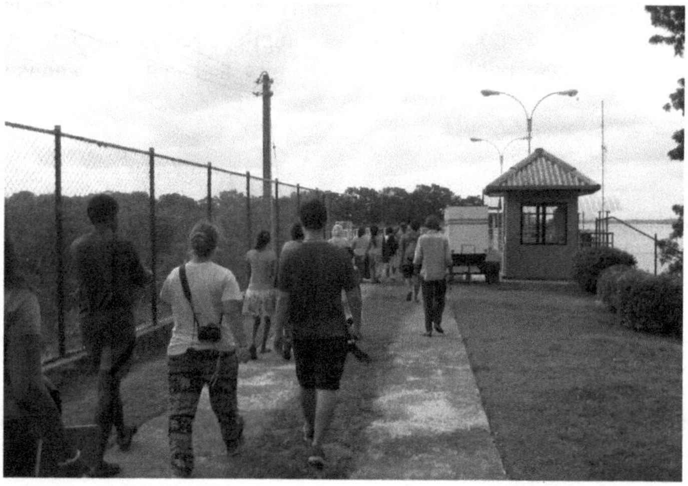

Students and partners walking around the village to identify supports and barriers to healthy living. Our partners really wanted to focus on the local tank (water reservoir), and issues surrounding that included: safety, bathing, environmental pollution, tourism, and livelihood.

Figure 10.7 Data collection and coding

Critical Reflection

Critical reflection within the group as well as on their own was also a major component of the course experience. Critical reflection happened in two parts: (1) daily reflection while in Sri Lanka (both individual writing time and group reflection), and (2) the fall term re-entry reflection course. While in country, reflection sessions were integrated into the daily routine, which allowed students to process their experiences as they related to their own interests and the greater understanding of the health practices of the Sri Lankan people. Reflection is the "intentional consideration of an experience in light of particular learning objectives" (Hatcher & Bringle 1997: p.153). The goal of reflection for this class was to provide ongoing opportunities for students to critically examine their experiences and make connections to course content. It also helped faculty gain insight into student projects and learning. This practice became so important that, even after long days in Shramadana or in the classroom, students and faculty would gather to reflect. The faculty introduced the reflection at the beginning of the course and the students took it over after the first few sessions. Student-led reflection allowed students to take a leadership role in the process. Opportunities to critically reflect on the CEL experiences is essential in helping students recognize how to break down systems of power and privilege, oppression and exploitation, and how not to reinforce it (Asghar & Rowe 2017). Reflection offered up rich discussions of power, privilege, the civil war in Sri Lanka, exploitation, inequity, LGBTQ+ issues across cultures, sustainable development, poverty, collectivism vs. individualism, gender and sexism, just to scratch the surface. It was through reflection that students and faculty had the chance to talk about the hard parts of the course, address misconceptions that often come up in CEL classes regarding helping people perceived to be less privileged, and the importance of reciprocity.

CASE STUDY: ONE STUDENT'S EXPERIENCE

I spent the two years prior to Stanford away from my native Botswana, far from my family and everything I was familiar with. I was fortunate enough to attend the United World College of Costa Rica, one of a group

Box 10.2 Reflection

We integrated opportunities to reflect throughout all phases of this experience. In addition, after modeling how in-person group reflections work, each student had an opportunity to lead a group reflection. Reflection prompts ranged from writing poetry, sharing an item that represented one's identity, art, writing a gratitude letter, co-creating a rap song, and identifying aspects of the trip that were difficult or challenging or a surprise or delight. Each student was given a journal and in addition to daily reflection, students were given time to write in their journal throughout the trip. The teaching team took part in both activities.

The re-entry reflection course was identified as a necessary component of overseas service as a way of deepening academic linkages (Pagano & Roselle 2009). This class was unique in this requirement. Upon return to the USA, students and faculty met once per week for eight weeks to process the trip. The faculty recognize that CEL experiences are meant to expose students to unique opportunities to better understand the world around them (Mitchell et al. 2015; Pagano & Roselle 2009). This is where the linkages solidify. For eight weeks students and faculty met and began each session with meditation at the student's request. Sessions were framed around the Sustainable Development Goals, exploring bias and stigma, identity and how the experience impacted future goals. Many of the students in the course were pre-medical and described the experience as shifting attitudes about health, wellness, disparity and equity. The experience was transformative in that it allowed students to engage in a critical examination of their own beliefs and values and how that shifted throughout the nine-month experience. The purposeful inclusion of this third component cannot be emphasized enough.

of schools that hope to use education as a tool to unite the world. In those two years I was inspired that I could be an agent of change in the world. As such, when I came into Stanford, I had an eye out for service opportunities. There is no scarcity of service opportunities at Stanford, with the Haas Center for Public Service dedicated to connecting students with Service-Learning opportunities. The Community, Health and Learning through Service in Sri Lanka class stood out to me for a few reasons. First, the country of Sri Lanka was faced with a kidney disease crisis and having lost my childhood best friend to kidney disease in 2014, I was curious to learn how accessible was care and treatment options for those affected. Second, I saw this as an opportunity to explore possible answers to economic poverty, inequality, and access to basic health care. At the time I was convinced I was going to be the President of Botswana in the future, and since these were also problems that existed there, I hoped the experience would give me insights on how to approach health provision in a similar country.

After submitting the application and completing a group interview, I found myself sitting in the preparatory class at the Stanford Medical School campus. It was a different world for me. Not only because the Medical School campus is located far from the rest of the campus, but also because as a Mathematical and Computational Science major, the small size of the class and the format was very different from the large lecture halls I was used to. The class equipped us with some knowledge to better prepare for the experience. We were introduced to the Stanford University's Principles of Ethical and Effective Service (see Figure 10.6). While my service experiences from the United World College of Costa Rica had elements of these principles, being introduced to them more formally like this framed the experience in a new way for me. It enabled me to see service as a means of learning. We also got to hear from Dr Vinya Ariyaratne, who introduced us to our community partner: Sarvodaya. After his presentation, I could not wait for the summer so we could travel to Sri Lanka. He had spoken of their Shramadana model of community development and I was anxious to witness this in action during our in-country experience.

I landed in Colombo one morning. Although the airline had mistakenly left my bags in Dubai, I did not care much because I was excited about being in Sri Lanka at last. As we drove to our arrival location, I realized I was also nervous. I was not friends with any one of the other students coming on the trip. I worried about fitting in. Our preparatory class in the spring had met only once a week and that was not enough time for me to build strong friendships with my classmates. But within hours of my arrival, we were all joking together over an afternoon cup of tea. I was pleasantly surprised at how well the group came together so seamlessly. The teaching team had done a great job of selecting our cohort. Each person, although different, was unified by a spirit of generosity. As we rotated the leadership of our daily reflection activities, we supported each other and shared our creativity, as we processed the experience. It was an enriching experience.

With all the preparation we had done, I could not imagine how the experience would unfold. I do not remember what my expectations were going into the experience, but I can confidently say they were exceeded. Every community we interacted with on our three-week excursion around the country was generous to us: they shared their food, their space, and their knowledge. Not even the language barrier could stop the bidirectional flow of experiences. The highlight for me was the village-stay and being welcomed into the Shramadana. Loading sand onto the tractor-drawn trailer from the river was fulfilling in ways I cannot imagine. Of all the things I could offer, in that moment the community of Pahalagama needed my muscle power. Working alongside them and seeing their determination to solve their development needs themselves, I was inspired. In my village in Botswana, we have an expectation that development issues are for the government to solve. This is in spite of having a history of the collective solution of community problems. I was witnessing something magical. I could not help but wonder how they were able to do it? For everyone to come together, give what they could, and build their communities one brick at a time. That is magical!

Three weeks is too short, and it is too long. It was short as we could not spend an extended period of time with the very communities that opened their homes to us. But it was long because service learning is not for the faint at heart. Even with all the preparation we had, learning about community and health can be a lot to handle. For this very reason, I am grateful for the reflections we shared as a group. Upon our return back to the United States, we met once a week for a quarter to process the insights from our time in Sri Lanka. We also worked on a fundraising campaign and sent the money back to the community in Pahalagama to use in resolving the issue of littering around their sacred water tank. That issue had been identified during our collaboration with the community on a Participatory Photo Mapping project. It was gratifying to know that the work we did with the community was continuing even long after we had left. It felt like a satisfying close to the experience.

Our service-learning trip had been a success, but as we continued on with our lives back at Stanford, my heart and mind were back in Sri Lanka. I wanted to go back. I had to find out what made community-driven development work with Sarvodaya. I applied for and was awarded a Cardinal Quarter Fellowship from Stanford to return to Sri Lanka to work with Sarvodaya. It was also an opportunity to apply the service-learning lessons from the previous visit. Based on my skillset and their need, I worked on a database system project for Sarvodaya. The database was to store details of the over 3,000 community-based organizations they work with, making it easy to get in contact with any one of them. I also worked with the Executive Director of Sarvodaya reviewing and testing their online systems. Working with the Executive Director was my favorite part of the ten-week fellowship. We went on field trips to interact with Sarvodaya Community Organizations. I learned a lot. For example, the experiences I got on the role of Sarvodaya Development Financing and community-based microfinance schemes inspired me to change my major to Management Science and Engineering, focusing on Finance and Decision Analysis. To this day, this experience is one of the most defining of my academic career.

LESSONS LEARNED

Because this course spanned nine months, it gave students, faculty and partners a lot of time to interact and learn from each other. In addition, due to the reflective nature of this course, faculty were able to collect information through observation and written experiences that could be used to better inform future courses. The students felt the prep course could have provided more information on the Sri Lankan culture, people, customs, etc. They also felt that the number of units (credits towards their graduation) were too few given the amount of work that was expected of them. Even so, they felt the three-week time period in the country was too short and would have liked more time in Sri Lanka. They also informed their faculty that they would have liked a larger group project and less focus on their individual research papers.

The case study illustrates the impact that CEL can have both on individuals and on the community. The student in our case study applied for and received funding to return to the community and developed a database for the community in concert with community members. The student also changed their major as a result of the experience.

The harder lessons involved the relationship between the faculty and the community partner. Sarvodaya as an organization emphasizes the tourism component as a way of creating revenue. This created a disconnect between the faculty's goal that the course be academically rigorous and the partner's interest in showing students and faculty places they loved about their country. As a result, there was a lot of sight-seeing and a dialectic between partners wanting to show students (and students wanting to see) unique parts of Sri Lanka. The difficulty being the cost (many Sri Lankans don't visit some of the sites we visited due to transportation barriers and entry fees).

Sarvodaya is very active in a large number of both Buddhist and non-Buddhist communities. The village where we stayed happens to be a Buddhist Sinhala village. If the option/time was there in the program to experience a non-Buddhist community, that could have been easily arranged. For other University groups we have done this as a routine. In the future, faculty will arrange to engage with both Buddhist and non-Buddhist communities.

CONCLUSIONS

Students in college are increasingly interested in international experiences that are aligned with their academic studies (Pagano & Roselle, 2009). This course was far from perfect and stimulated dialogue about the actual process of Community Engaged Learning in the college setting. The faculty struggled with some components, such as the possibility of reinforcing privilege, perpetuating stereotypes or even dealing with corruption within a different cultural context. The students and faculty together were central in processing these difficult concepts and due to the careful consideration and the daily reflection, students and faculty were equipped with tools and skills to grapple with their own biases and to work through tough concepts.

The three-phased curriculum was essential to its success. Building solid and ongoing partnerships with Sarvodaya also proved to be central to the success of the program. The specific project of photo-mapping provided a way to help the community identify a problem and institute solutions. It is important for both student learning and community-engaged projects that relationships and trust be built over time. Since the culmination of this class, students and faculty have remained connected with community partners, raised funds for the community, and collaboratively presented process and outcomes at three conferences internationally and in the USA.

APPENDIX: ALL SITES VISITED IN THE THREE-WEEK COURSE

1 Moratuwa – Moratuwa sits on the western coast of the island and is a short bus ride (1 hour) to Sri Lanka's capital of Colombo (to the north). It is home to Sarvodaya headquarters.
2 Anuradhapura – Faculty and students visited the dry-zone of Anuradhapura and learned about agricultural practices and volunteered on an organic farm. This ancient capital has public health care and education systems, extensive irrigation systems, and advanced agriculture and health practices.
3 Home stay and Shramadana was held in Pahalagama in Anuradhapura District.
4 Kandy – The scenic city of Kandy's temperate climate offers a respite from the extreme temperatures that dominate the island. It is home to the most sacred Buddhist temple.
5 Bandaragama – Faculty and students spent two days at this learning center to engage in reflection and participate in a final seminar to present their project. Bandaragama is in the small, secluded town in the south east of the island in a Sarvodaya learning center.
6 Unawatuna – To celebrate the end of the course and to relax after an intense trip, students and faculty spend a few days in the well-known tourist attraction of South Beach at the most southern region of Sri Lanka.

ACKNOWLEDGEMENTS

The authors would like to thank Sarvodaya for their guidance, commitment, and support of students throughout the years and during the writing of this manuscript. We are also thankful for our host families of Pahalagama for our continued connections and friendships. Finally, the authors would like to express gratitude for the editors, especially Susan Scrimshaw and Sandra Lane, for the gentle guidance, support and mentorship as this chapter was being developed.

REFERENCES

Allwright, K., Goldie, C., Almost, J., & Wilson, R. (2019). Fostering positive spaces in public health using a cultural humility approach. *Public Health Nursing*, *36*(4), 551–556.

Annette, J. (2002). Service learning in an international context. *Frontiers: The Interdisciplinary Journal of Study Abroad*, *8*(1), 83–93.

Asghar, M., & Rowe, N. (2017). Reciprocity and critical reflection as the key to social justice in service learning: A case study. *Innovations in Education and Teaching International*, *54*(2), 117–125.

Ash, S. L., & Clayton, P. H. (2009). Generating, deepening, and documenting learning: The power of critical reflection in applied learning. *Journal of Applied Learning in Higher Education*, *1*(1), 25–48.

Bandy, J. (2016). *What is service learning or community engagement*. Center for Teaching, Vanderbilt University. Available at: https://cft.vanderbilt.edu/guides-subpages/teaching-through-community-engagement.

Campus Compact, 2020. (2020). https://compact.org/who-we-are/.

Carpiano, Richard M. (2009). Come take a walk with me: The "Go-Along" interview as a novel method for studying the implications of place for health and well-being. *Health & Place*, *15*(1), 263–272.

Chávez, V., Duran, B., Baker, Q. E., Avila, M. M., & Wallerstein, N. (2008). The dance of race and privilege in CBPR. *Community-based participatory research for health: From process to outcomes*, 91–105.

Dennis Jr, S. F., Gaulocher, S., Carpiano, R. M., & Brown, D. (2009). Participatory photo mapping (PPM): Exploring an integrated method for health and place research with young people. *Health & Place*, *15*(2), 466–473.

Eby, J. (1998). *Why service-learning is bad*. Available at: www1.villanova.edu/content/dam/villanova/artsci/servicelearning/WhyServiceLearningIsBad.pdf, accessed on January 10, 2021.

Glaser, B. G. (1965). The constant comparative method of qualitative analysis. *Social Problems*, *12*(4), 436–445.

Hartman, E., Kiely, R. C., Friedrichs, J., & Boettcher, C. (2018). *Community-based global learning: The theory and practice of ethical engagement at home and abroad*. Sterling, VA: Stylus Publishing, LLC.

Hartman, E., Paris, C. M., & Blache-Cohen, B. (2014). Fair trade learning: Ethical standards for community-engaged international volunteer tourism. *Tourism and Hospitality Research*, *14*(1–2), 108–116.

Hatcher, J. A., & Bringle, R. G. (1997). Reflection: Bridging the gap between service and learning. *College Teaching*, *45*(4), 153–158.

Hewitt-Taylor, J. (2001). Use of constant comparative analysis in qualitative research. *Nursing Standard*, *15*(42), 39.

Hung, D., & Khine, M. S. (Eds.). (2006). *Engaged learning with emerging technologies*. Dordrecht, The Netherlands: Springer.

John, D. H., McCahan, B., & Gaulocher, S. (2012). Partnering to enable active rural living: Pearl project. *Journal of Rural Social Sciences*, *27*(3), 4.

Lane, S., Rubinstein, R., Narine, L., Back, I., Cornell, C., Hodgens, A., ... & Suk, W. (2011). Action anthropology and pedagogy: University–community collaborations in setting policy. *Human Organization*, *70*(3), 289–299.

Lane, S. D., Rubinstein, R. A., Schimpff, T. R., Keefe, R. H., Jennings-Bey, T., Leed, S. R., ... & Satterly, L. B. (2019). Bringing in the community: A university–community endeavor to teach marital and family therapy students about community-based violence and trauma. *Contemporary Family Therapy, 41*(2), 147–156.

LCME Accreditation Standards. (n.d.). Available at: www.iaomc.org/lcme.htm, accessed on July 6, 2016.

Mitchell, T. D., Richard, F. D., Battistoni, R. M., Rost-Banik, C., Netz, R., & Zakoske, C. (2015). Reflective practice that persists: Connections between reflection in service-learning programs and in current life. *Michigan Journal of Community Service Learning, 21*(2), 49–63.

National Academies of Sciences, Engineering, and Medicine (NASEM). (2016). *A framework for educating health professionals to address the social determinants of health*. Washington, DC: National Academies Press.

Neururer, Julie, & Rhoads, R. A. (1998). Community service: Panacea, paradox, or potentiation. *Journal of College Student Development, 39*(4), 321–330. https://files.eric.ed.gov/fulltext/EJ831374.pdf.

O'Brien, Matthew J., & Whitaker, Robert C. (2011). The role of community-based participatory research to inform local health policy: A case study. *Journal of General Internal Medicine, 26*(12), 1498–1501.

Olson, J. D., McAllister, C., Grinnell, L. D., Gehrke Walters, K., & Appunn, F. (2016). Applying constant comparative method with multiple investigators and inter-coder reliability. *Qualitative Report, 21*(1).

Pagano, M., & Roselle, L. (2009). Beyond reflection through an academic lens: Refraction and international experiential education. *Frontiers: The Interdisciplinary Journal of Study Abroad, 18*, 217–229.

Petkar, P. M., Kumar, N. V., & Fattepur, G. (2016). Augmentation of learning through the use of simulation tools and techniques in under-graduate metal forming course. *Journal of Engineering Education Transformations [S.l.]*, January. doi:10.16920/jeet/2016/v0i0/85692. Available at: www.journaleet.org/index.php/jeet/article/view/85692, accessed on January 10, 2021.

Preskill, S., & Brookfield, S. D. (2009). *Learning as a way of leading: Lessons from the struggle for social justice*. San Francisco, CA: Jossey-Bass.

Principles of Ethical and Effective Service. (2020). https://haas.stanford.edu/about/about-haas-center/principles-ethical-and-effective-service, accessed on January 18, 2020.

Rooks, R. N., & Rael, C. T. (2013). Enhancing curriculum through service learning in the social determinants of health course. *Journal of the Scholarship of Teaching and Learning, 13*(2), 84–100.

Sabo, Samantha, et al. (2015). Service learning: A vehicle for building health equity and eliminating health disparities. *American Journal of Public Health, 105*(S1), S38–S43.

Saltmarsh, J. (2005). The civic promise of service learning. *Liberal Education, 91*(2), 50–55.

Sarvodaya. (2020). *Sarvodaya Collected Works: Introduction*, www.sarvodaya.org/collected-works-vol-1, accessed January 31, 2020.

Schroeder, K., Wood, C., Galiardi, S., & Koehn, J. (2009). First, do no harm: Ideas for mitigating negative community impacts of short-term study abroad. *Journal of Geography, 108*(3), 141–147.

Scott, C. (2015). *The Futures of Learning 3: What kind of pedagogies for the 21st century?* Education Research and Foresight Working Papers. UNESCODOC Digital Library, https://unesdoc.unesco.org/ark:/48223/pf0000243126, accessed January 10, 2021.

Shiri, S. (2015). The homestay in intensive language study abroad: Social networks, language socialization, and developing intercultural competence. *Foreign Language Annals, 48*(1), 5–25.

Stokols, D., Grzywacz, J. G., McMahan, S., & Phillips, K. (2003). Increasing the health promotive capacity of human environments. *American Journal of Health Promotion, 18*(1), 4–13.

Stokols, Daniel. (2006). Toward a science of transdisciplinary action research. *American Journal of Community Psychology, 38*, 63–77.

Tinto, V. (2020). Learning better together. In Jones, A., Olds, A., & Lisciandro J. G. (Eds.), *Transitioning students in higher education: Philosophy, pedagogy and practice* (pp. 13–24). New York: Routledge.

Trickett, E. J., Beehler, S., Deutsch, C., Green, L. W., Hawe, P., McLeroy, K., … & Trimble, J. E. (2011). Advancing the science of community-level interventions. *American Journal of Public Health*, *101*(8), 1410–1419.

Trudeau, D., & Kruse, T. P. (2014). Creating significant learning experiences through civic engagement: Practical strategies for community-engaged pedagogy. *Journal of Public Scholarship in Higher Education*, *4*, 12–30.

United Nations Sustainable Development. (2020). *About the Sustainable Development Goals – United Nations Sustainable Development*. New York: United Nations. Available at: www.un.org/sustainabledevelopment/sustainable-development-goals/, accessed on July 27, 2020.

World Health Organization. (2019). *Social determinates of health*. Geneva: WHO. Available at: www.who.int/health-topics/social-determinants-of-health#tab=tab_1, accessed on August 20, 2020.

Yeager, K. A., & Bauer-Wu, S. (2013). Cultural humility: Essential foundation for clinical researchers. *Applied Nursing Research*, *26*(4), 251–256.

PART 2

Lived Experiences

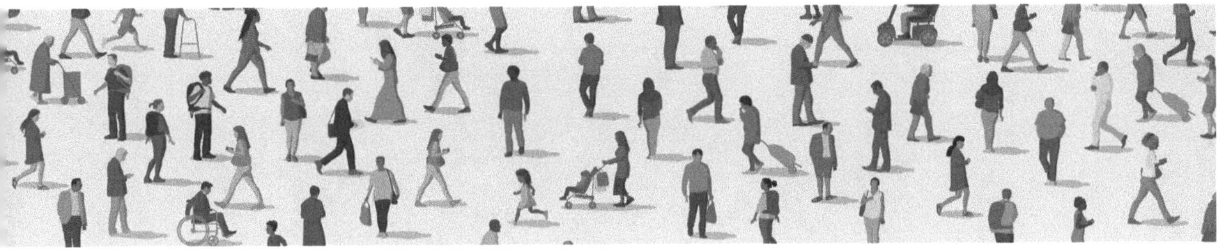

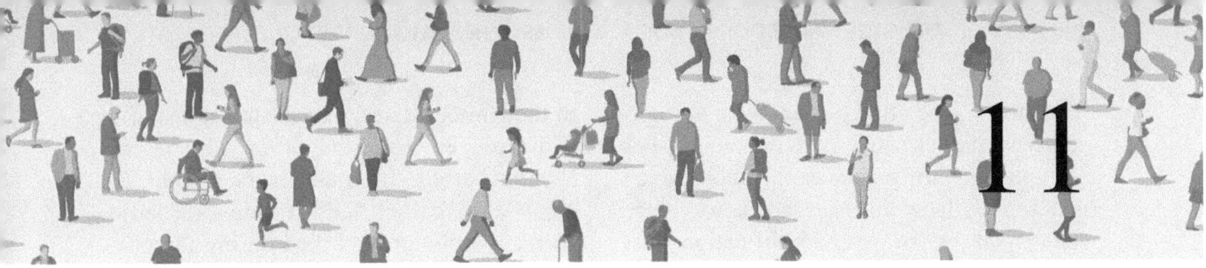

11

Historical Trauma and Epigenetics

Wencheng Zhang, Gary Rodziewicz, Margaret Voss, and Sandra D. Lane

INTRODUCTION

In this chapter, we address three well-known famines: the Irish potato famine (1846–47), the Dutch 'hunger winter' at the end of World War II (1944–45), and the China famine (1959–62). Each of those tragedies caused significant population loss and many of the survivors experienced ongoing adverse health conditions, with premature death. In the sections below, we first review the causes and consequences of the three famines. Next, we examine what is known about the population-level changes in the three famines with regard to:

1. Whether vulnerable members of the population are more likely to die. The famine in this regard could be considered an evolutionary "selective pressure" that influences the survival of those who are genetically predisposed to the efficient use and conservation of food energy, and thus better able to cope with severe malnutrition (the "thrifty-gene" and "thrifty phenotype" hypotheses (Neel, 1999; Stipp, 2011).
2. How survivors may accrue molecular modifications to their existing genetic code from prevailing environmental and dietary conditions. These changes occur above the level of the gene (are epigenetic), are heritable, and may alter the expression of individual genes in response to stressors such as diet, illness, or starvation. Epigenetic modifications can turn genes on, off, or act as molecular dimmer switches, making the affected individual more reactive to stress or altering their metabolic response to specific nutrients. Epigenetic molecular modifications may be inherited for generations (Pembrey et al., 2014).
3. How cultural changes after a famine may affect food-related and other behaviors.

There are limitations in our analyses: Less is known about the Irish famine since the survivors themselves were impoverished and often lacked literacy. The two 20th-century famines (the Dutch hunger winter and the China famine) have the most documentation and scientific evidence and are discussed in greater depth. Furthermore, with regard to the potential genetic differences in post-famine populations (i.e., thrifty-gene, thrifty-phenotype, and epigenetics), the science is evolving rapidly. For example, the thrifty-gene explanation, which is described later in this chapter, was once abandoned as an oversimplification that lacked sufficient evidence to support it, but elements of it have been recently reconsidered (Prentice et al., 2008; Reddon, 2018; Hollstein et al., 2019). Epigenetics, a rapidly growing area of science, makes reevaluation of this hypothesis a timely topic. Epigenetics is the study of changes in gene expression patterns that arise from molecular modifications to the genome. Although these modifications do not alter the underlying DNA sequence, they can influence the amount of protein made from a particular gene sequence. A large body of work now supports the supposition that early-life exposure to dietary factors and maternal stress can increase the likelihood of developing disease and poor health outcomes later in life. What we discuss in this chapter outlines these findings regarding the three famines, but our chapter does not entirely cover all recent developments in epigenetics.

THE IRISH FAMINE (1846–47)

In 1846 the potato crop in Ireland became infected with a fungus that turned the potatoes black and inedible. A second crop failure in 1847, caused as the first by a fungal blight, hit the already malnourished population hard (Shaw-Taylor, 2020). Many of the vulnerable, impoverished Irish residents succumbed from malnutrition in the first year, but in the famine's second year outbreaks of typhus and cholera proved especially fatal to those whose immune systems were compromised by protein malnutrition.

The double-whammy of starvation, followed by infection, was further worsened by English governmental policies that failed to halt the carnage. An estimated one million died, and another million emigrated to the United States, Canada, and Australia (Edwards & Williams [1956] 1997). In Boston harbor, Irish survivors arrived on what were called "coffin ships" because so many onboard had died during the passage and the surviving passengers looked like corpses walking off the ships (Puleo, 2020).

Bantry, a rural village in County Cork, was among the worst affected areas; over 60% of the residents lined up to receive food rations provided by welfare organizations (Geary, 2018). In one Cork workhouse in 1847, overflowing with impoverished starving people, there was one death per hour, to the extent that normal burial customs broke down, and the dead were put into the ground with slabs of rough wood at night when others could not see (Mulraney, 2018). An American ship captain, who arrived in Cork with food aid, gave a first-hand account of the suffering:

> Hovels crowded with the sick and dying, without floors, without furniture, and with patches of dirty straw covered with still dirtier patches and shreds of humanity… (Mulraney, 2018, p. 1)

In addition to the American government food aid, the Native American Choctaw Nation shipped food to Ireland. Irish scholars argue that, for the most part, England ignored the starving (Lynch, 2018). Some prominent English policy-makers sought to use the famine to clear the land of poor people (Kelly, 2012). For example, Sir Charles Edward Trevelyan, who led the governmental response to the famine, blamed the starving people for their suffering: "The real evil with which we have to contend is not the physical evil of the Famine but the moral evil of the selfish, perverse and turbulent character of the people" (Keneally, 2011, p. 65). Even at the height of the famine, income-producing food crops were being exported out of Ireland for profit, leading some scholars to accuse the English government and major landowners of genocide (Kelly, 2012). In 1997, then UK Prime Minister Tony Blair apologized for England's role (Marks, 1997, p. 2):

> The famine was a defining event in the history of Ireland and Britain. It has left deep scars. That one million people should have died in what was then part of the richest and most powerful nation in the world is something that still causes pain as we reflect on it today. Those who governed in London at the time failed their people.

In addition to the one million Irish deaths, historians estimate that an additional one million emigrated to the United States, Canada, and Australia as a result of the famine (called the Gorta Mor, meaning the Great Hunger in Gaelic), of an original Irish population of 6 million (Kelly, 2012).

Irish historian Oonagh Walsh called attention to an increase in schizophrenia among famine survivors, which she argued resulted from epigenetic changes arising from the famine (Walsh, 2016; Smith, 2017). Psychiatric scholars provided support for Walsh's hypothesis by charting the 87% increase of psychiatric patients admitted to facilities in Ireland following the famine as supporting the contention that survivors of the famine experienced higher rates of schizophrenia (Walsh, 2012). Anthropologist Nancy Scheper-Hughes' studies in Ireland (mid-1970s) and among homeless mentally ill Irish Americans in South Boston (circa 1980), trace the cultural patterns of schizophrenia and other severe mental illness among people several generations after the famine (Scheper-Hughes, 1987, 2001). If Oonagh Walsh's contention is correct, Scheper-Hughes' research participants may have had elevated rates of schizophrenia due to the famine.

DUTCH HUNGER WINTER OF 1944–45

In the winter of 1944–45, the Nazi government of Holland cut off food supplies to the entire western half of the country, causing a severe famine called Hongerwinter in Dutch (Heijmans et al., 2008). On average, the Dutch people consumed 667 kilocalories per person per day (range 400–800) (van der Zee, 1998). This famine began in late 1944 and was relieved only in May 1945 with the Allied liberation. During this time, health services were still functioning. For example, pregnant women could visit their doctors for prenatal care, which was documented as usual, a fact that allowed researchers to study this issue in depth. The Dutch Hunger Winter of 1944–45 has probably the best documentation of who was affected, when, and how. Record-keeping was detailed enough to classify individuals into those who were conceived during the famine, and those who had later prenatal life (i.e., were born) during the famine. An estimated 18,000 to 22,000 people died due to the famine, with the highest death rates in cities where people could not grow their own food. The highest death rate was among elderly (van der Zee, 1998).

Prenatal exposure to the Dutch famine is associated with multiple health consequences in later life. Women who were born during the famine, especially those who were exposed during early gestation, have a higher weight, higher BMI, and an elevated risk of obesity (Ravelli et al., 1976; Ravelli et al., 1999; Lumey et al., 2011). Experiencing the Dutch famine in utero is also associated with early onset of coronary artery disease, and a higher risk of type 2 diabetes, impaired glucose tolerance, and schizophrenia (Susser & Lin, 1992; Ravelli et al., 1998; Painter et al., 2006; Lumey et al., 2009; van Abeelen et al., 2012). The prenatal exposure to the Dutch famine might have intergenerational effects. Children of women who were exposed to the Dutch famine in utero tend to have higher neonatal adiposity, and children of men who were exposed to the Dutch famine prenatally are more likely to be obese than the children whose fathers were not exposed to famine prenatally (Painter et al., 2008; Veenendaal et al., 2013).

There are inconsistent findings regarding how prenatal exposure to the Dutch famine relates to fertility among women. Painter et al. (2008) found that women who were prenatally exposed to the Dutch famine have more children and tend to give birth to their first baby at a younger age. However, an earlier study by Lumey and Stein (1997) did not find significant differences in fertility between famine-exposed women and non-exposed women. Given the high prenatal death rate during the famine, women who gave birth during the famine might have had a higher ability to conceive. This trait might be passed down to their daughters who were born during the famine (Lumey et al., 2011).

THE 1959–61 CHINA FAMINE

The 1959–61 China Famine began in the winter of 1959 and affected all regions of China. Research estimates that 16.5 to 30 million people died prematurely, and an additional 30 million lost or postponed births, making the 1959–61 China Famine the worst in human history (Fung, 2009). The national death rates were 14, 25, and 14 per thousand during the years of 1959, 1960, 1961, respectively, compared with 11 per thousand average mortality rate for 1956–58 (Chen & Zhou, 2007). The average birth rate from 1959 to 1961 was 21.22 per thousand, compared with 32.3 per thousand for 1956–58.

The causes of the famine mainly include adverse weather conditions, high government procurement of grain, and the negative effects of the Great Leap Forward. It is important to understand the social, political, and ecological context of China just before the Great Leap Forward (1958–60). China was a new country, having successfully won its independence in 1949. Mao Zedong, the leader, inherited a country that had experienced a brutal Japanese invasion, a civil war, previous famines, and extensive bombing of its major cities and population centers during World War II. The Great Leap Forward movement aimed to substantially increase the productivity of agriculture and massive industrialization within a short range of time (Li & Yang, 2005). During the movement of the Great Leap Forward, the government procured large amounts of grain from peasants, which left the peasants with inadequate seed stocks to sustain their cultivation. To achieve mass industrialization, the government also diverted labor from agriculture to industry, which led to insufficient workers dedicated to agriculture, further decreasing the production of grain. In addition, a drought, a major locust swarm, an urban-biased food distribution system, and continuous exports of grain before the famine contributed to the famine (Li & Yang, 2005; Fung, 2009). The famine affected rural areas and urban areas in China disproportionately due to the urban-biased food distribution systems, leading to rural residents having much poorer food availability during the famine than their urban counterparts (Chen & Zhou, 2007).

Studies have shown that exposure to the China Famine in early life is associated with an increased risk of metabolic syndrome, schizophrenia, hypertension, diabetes, and hyperglycemia (St Clair et al., 2005; Li et al., 2012; Wang et al., 2015). For example, using a nationwide survey in China, Wang et al. (2015) explored the association between prenatal exposure to famine and the risk of having diabetes in adult life. They found that compared with those born after the famine, fetus-exposed individuals and childhood-exposed individuals have 53% and 82% higher odds of developing diabetes than those who were not exposed, respectively (Wang et al., 2015). Another study among 7,801 retirees from Dongfeng Motor Corporation in China showed that women who were exposed to the China Famine during middle childhood and late childhood had a higher risk of developing type 2 diabetes in their later life. However, the association was not statistically significant among men (Wang et al., 2016).

Several studies have shown that the exposure to famine disproportionally affects women survivors (Wang et al., 2010; Wang et al., 2016). Mortality selection and son preference could partly explain the health inequality in women and men (Mu & Zhang, 2011). During the China Famine, the mortality of males was higher than females, and after the famine, sons tended to receive better caregiving than daughters, which increased the inequality in health outcomes among the famine survivors.

THE EXPLANATIONS FOR THE HEALTH CONSEQUENCES OF FAMINE EXPOSURE

The Thrifty-Gene Hypothesis (Death of the Vulnerable, Survival of the Advantaged)

The thrifty-gene hypothesis was first introduced by geneticist James V. Neel in 1962 to explain the epidemic of diabetes mellitus type 2 in modern times and why certain populations were particularly susceptible to diabetes. The hypothesis was initially proposed to explain the disparity in the prevalence of diabetes between populations. Neel later expanded it to explain the prevalence of obesity and other metabolic syndromes (Neel, 1999).

The hypothesis rests on the mechanism of natural selection. It assumes that there were cycles of feasts and famines in human history. Individuals with so-called "thrifty genes" might be able to absorb and process food efficiently to store fat during times of plenty, with the result of increased survival during famines over those lacking thrifty genes (Neel, 1962). However, the trait of metabolic efficiency could be detrimental in modern times with a constant abundance of food. Thrifty genes could become maladaptive in an environment of plenty because they efficiently store energy in fat to prepare for a famine that may not come.

The thrifty-gene hypothesis has been under debate for 50 years (Hay, 2018). One of the challenges to the thrifty-gene hypothesis is: if the famine was such a powerful force throughout human history, all humans should have become obese; this, however, is not the case. It is difficult to explain the heterogeneity of obesity observed in specific populations within the context of the thrifty-gene hypothesis (Genné-Bacon, 2014). Furthermore, there is limited genetic evidence to support the hypothesis at present (Gosling et al., 2015). For example, Koh et al. (2014) explored whether the thrifty-gene hypothesis could explain the higher risk of type 2 diabetes among East Asians. They compared the genes associated with obesity and type 2 diabetes in East Asians and their European counterparts but did not find supportive evidence for the thrifty-gene hypothesis. The thrifty-gene hypothesis has long been an accepted explanation for the high prevalence of diabetes among the Pacific Island populations. However, there is no direct genetic evidence regarding the known genes associated with diabetes and obesity (Gosling et al., 2015). Several genes that are related to obesity have been found, but the effects of those genes are considered too small to support the thrifty-gene hypothesis (Speakman, 2013).

The Thrifty-Phenotype Hypothesis

Hales and Barker (1992) developed the "thrifty-phenotype hypothesis" to explain the association between low birth weight and higher risks of developing metabolic diseases in adulthood. They proposed that undernutrition in utero and during infancy led to permanent changes in insulin secretion and insulin resistance. They also argued that malnutrition during fetal life has the potential to change the function and structure of the body cells permanently. These changes, along with obesity, aging processes, and physical inactivity, were among the most important factors contributing to type 2 diabetes (Hales & Barker, 2001). Hales and Barker (2001) pointed out that there is a clear relationship between malnutrition in early life and insulin resistance in adult life. However, there was limited evidence supporting the association between maternal malnutrition and impaired insulin secretion in later life.

Hales and Barker (1992) proposed that the malnourished fetus tended to allocate more nutrition to tissues such as the brain, rather than the pancreas. The "thrifty-phenotype hypothesis" further suggests that the discrepancy between the environment in utero (e.g., famine) and the environment in later life (e.g., overnutrition) are the primary drivers of the higher risk of type 2 diabetes. Inadequate insulin secretion and insulin resistance would be less detrimental to those who continue to be malnourished in childhood and adult life. However, if malnutrition as a fetus or as an infant is followed by overnutrition in childhood and adult life, the individual has higher risks of developing glucose intolerance and type 2 diabetes (Hales & Barker, 1992).

Many studies supported the prediction of the thrifty-phenotype hypothesis. For example, Law et al. (1992) showed that people who went through malnutrition in fetal life and infancy tended to store fat in their abdomens and develop abdominal obesity, which thus can increase the risk of cardiovascular diseases and diabetes. This finding was supported by results from a comparison of individuals who were exposed or were not exposed to a famine in early life; when both were limited to the same amount of energy intake and energy expenditure, those with early famine exposure were more likely to develop abdominal obesity. Thus, the famine-exposed group would have a higher risk of developing type 2 diabetes later in life than their non-exposed counterparts. Ravelli et al. (1976) found that exposure to famine during the first half of pregnancy leads to significantly higher obesity rates. Their interpretation of those results was that early famine-exposure might disrupt the development of the hypothalamus, a brain region that regulates food intake and growth, which could cause changes in appetites and weight control. A subsequent study by Ravelli et al. (1999) found that early-life exposure to famine appears to influence the development of central endocrine regulatory systems in women, which could lead to higher BMI and waist circumference in later life.

The thrifty-phenotype hypothesis emphasized that prenatal nutrition and nutrition in the early stages of life are more important than interventions in adult life regarding the prevention of metabolic syndrome (Genné-Bacon, 2014). If this hypothesis holds, more resources should be devoted to prenatal nutrition to reduce the risks of adulthood diabetes and promote the health of the next generation. The fetal origins of adult diseases theory, coined by Barker, has been used in obstetrics to explain how severe distress affecting pregnant women may alter the development of the fetal nervous system (Barker, 2004; Kinsella & Monk, 2009). There is a fetal response to maternal stress that includes both increased heart rate and a more reactive response to stress throughout later life. According to this theory, fetal exposure to maternal stress may explain the increased rates of mental illness in survivors of severe famine (Calkins & Devaskar, 2011). The impact of famine in this regard may be two-fold: first, leading to metabolic changes associated with obesity and type 2 diabetes, and second, priming the fetal nervous system to over-respond to stress in ways that increase the likelihood of psychological difficulties.

Epigenetic Changes

Although many factors contribute to the increased prevalence of health problems in prenatally stressed populations, one possible mechanism tying prenatal stress to poor health outcomes later in life is a stress-induced alteration of epigenetic gene expression during prenatal development. The literal translation of the word epigenetic is "above the gene." It refers to control mechanisms beyond the structure of DNA. Epigenetics can be formally defined as "the study of mitotically and/or meiotically heritable changes in gene function that cannot be explained by changes in DNA sequence" (Riggs et al., 1996, p. 1). What this means in practical terms is that the chemical environment of a cell leaves "marks" on the structure of its DNA that change the way a gene sequence codes for its product, a protein. These "marks" are heritable, even though they do not alter the underlying DNA sequence. One of the best-understood examples of this is the addition of small methyl molecules to the backbone of some regions of DNA, a process known as methylation (Bird, 2007). Without changing the individual's inherited DNA sequences, epigenetic mechanisms can turn up or turn down the expression of existing genes. Environmental conditions during certain stages of gestation and the early postnatal period might influence the expression of genes, leading to permanent changes in body cells (Stöger, 2008).

Reinhard Stöger synthesized the "thrifty-epigenome hypothesis" by combining the thrifty-gene hypothesis and the thrifty-phenotype hypothesis (Stöger, 2008). As mentioned above, Stöger proposed that all human beings had thrifty genes due to the force of evolution, but those thrifty genes were insufficient by themselves to cause the development of obesity and type 2 diabetes. Instead, the susceptibility to type 2 diabetes and obesity was likely determined by epigenetic changes, which resulted from biochemical epigenetic programming during early stages of life.

Epigenetic alterations mainly involve three distinct but interrelated processes within the existing cellular nucleus: DNA methylation, histone modifications, and non-coding RNAs (Desai et al., 2015). These alterations may influence gene expression independently or simultaneously. DNA methylation starts after an embryo implants in the mother's uterine lining, during which time it directs the cells to create the organs of what will become a fetus. Exposure to malnutrition during the very beginning of pregnancy may limit or alter the availability of biochemical compounds that have the potential to permanently "mark" regions of DNA and thereby change subsequent gene expression patterns in the fetus. These changes could alter the function and structure of body cells, leading to metabolic abnormalities in later life (Desai et al., 2015). (Box 11.1 outlines how epigenetic changes result from cellular control mechanisms involved in methylation.)

Box 11.1 How Do Epigenetic Changes Work?

All the information needed to develop a human being from a single cell is contained in the DNA of this original cell. How and when this information is retrieved and used to direct the sequence of events that results in an entire organism is called epigenetics. DNA, the famous double helix of our genetic code, is a string of repeating elements called bases. These four bases (A, T, C, G) store information just like the 1s and 0s of binary computers.

In order to read the information stored in any particular sequence of bases (a "gene"), an exact copy of that gene is made into messenger RNA (mRNA) in a process called "transcription." This mRNA information then directs the assembly of amino acids to form a protein in a process called "translation." This is a cellular version of a 3D printer.

Only about 2% of our DNA is actually transcribed to make mRNA; the other 98% of our DNA controls how that 2% of DNA is transcribed. Epigenetic mechanisms affect how the control regions of DNA (the 98%) direct the transcription of the 2% of DNA that is read and expressed.

One important epigenetic control mechanism is DNA methylation. In humans, this primarily takes the form of adding methyl groups to C (cytosine) bases of DNA. A methyl group attached to DNA is an example of an "epigenetic marker." Various events in the mother's life (e.g., starvation) can change the degree of DNA methylation in the developing fetus. Dietary protein, and its constituent amino acids, are a significant source of methyl groups that attach to DNA. A balanced diet also supplies the coenzymes (vitamins) that make methyl attachment possible. Adding a methyl group to a control region of DNA can slow transcription of the subsequent gene region into mRNA, resulting in fewer copies of that gene. In contrast, adding a methyl group to the DNA in the gene itself can actually increase the transcription of a particular gene. Thus, epigenetic mechanisms can fine-tune exactly how many copies of a gene get made.

Many such epigenetic control systems interact with each other to tune both transcription and translation of any one gene. Now consider how many genes are being controlled like this, and how one gene's proteins can affect the control of any or many other genes. This is the dynamic complexity of epigenetic control in the developing organism.

Heijmans et al. (2008) studied epigenetic DNA methylation patterns in individuals who were prenatally exposed to famine during the Dutch Hunger Winter compared to their unexposed, same-sex siblings. Once they had identified a population of individuals appropriate for a longitudinal study, these researchers sought a reliable gene and epigenetic marker combination that would reflect the stress of maternal starvation.

One of the best-understood epigenetically regulated genes is insulin-like growth factor II (IGF2) (Heijmans et al., 2008). The IGF2 gene produces proteins that are critical for gestation and is sensitive to prenatal stress. In addition to promoting prenatal growth, IGF2 also regulates the formation of pancreatic islet cells, the cells which later in life produce insulin needed for blood sugar control. Heijmans et al. (2008) compared 60 individuals subjected to maternal starvation around the time of conception, 62 individuals subjected to maternal starvation around the time of birth, and a matched set of siblings who were not subject to the same undernutrition. In the individuals whose mothers were starved around the time of conception, IGF2 promoter DNA was methylated around 5% less than in either controls or individuals whose mothers were starved later in pregnancy. This difference was statistically significant. Tobi et al. (2009) provided further evidence for the association between prenatal famine exposure in the Dutch famine and subsequent epigenetic changes, with the strength of the association dependent on the timing of the exposure and the sex of the exposed individuals. They concluded that diet controlled epigenetic regulation of this gene could be a common process among those who were exposed to the famine prenatally.

Studies on animals have found that some epigenetic changes due to malnutrition during pregnancy could be inherited in subsequent generations, a process known as "epigenetic inheritance" (Radford et al., 2014). In Radford et al.'s (2014) study, mice that were subjected to severe undernutrition during the prenatal period had low birth weight and multiple metabolic defects. Those phenotypes were then passed on to the next generation to the offspring of male mice but not female mice.

There is some evidence for the transgenerational influence of prenatal exposure to famine in humans as well. Veenendaal et al. (2013) found that the individuals whose fathers were exposed to the Dutch famine prenatally have higher weight (4.9kg) and higher BMI than the individuals with non-exposed fathers, but mothers who were prenatally malnourished did not seem to affect their children's BMI or body weight differently (Veenendaal et al., 2013). In this study, the average age of the offspring of the famine survivor cohort was 37 years old, so some adverse health outcomes may not yet have appeared. A study in China showed the transgenerational impact of prenatal exposure to famine from the maternal side. Women living in rural areas who were exposed to the China Famine as a fetus give birth to bigger babies – babies with higher weight, length, and birth body mass index (Huang et al., 2010). These associations, however, were not found for women in urban areas who were exposed to the famine as a fetus; this might be because the famine disproportionately affected the rural areas.

One of the implications of epigenetics is that thrifty genes could be "turned off" among subsequent generations if they have sufficient nutrition in utero (Genné-Bacon, 2014). Dolinoy et al. (2007) showed that exposure to the plastic borne chemical bisphenol A (BPA) was associated with the risk of metabolic diseases in mice. However, an enhanced maternal diet during the prenatal period could counteract the DNA methylation caused by exposure to BPA. This suggests that populations that have previously experienced the harmful effects of malnutrition in early life may particularly benefit from nutritional supplementation during pregnancy to offset the current epidemic of metabolic disease.

STRESS, EPIGENETICS, AND TELOMERE LENGTH

The concept of stress was first introduced by Hans Selye (1907–82), who defined it as "the nonspecific response of the body to any demand." (Selye, 1976, p. 15). Some scholars define stress as "conditions where an environmental demand exceeds the regulatory and adaptive capacity of an organism, in particular in the case of unpredictability and uncontrollability" (Koolhaas et al., 2011, p. 1291). Stress is evoked by a stressor, which is "a stimulus that threatens homeostasis" (Koolhaas et al., 2011, p. 1292). We all experience a wide range of stressors every day, such as financial strain, relationship issues, work pressure, and health anxieties; thus, stress is almost ubiquitous in modern life. The deleterious effects of stress are well established and documented by many disciplines. Recent developments in epigenetics further elucidate the influence of stress at the genetic level and the role that stress-induced changes in the epigenome play in health outcomes.

A cornerstone of stress studies is the concept of "homeostasis," which originated from the work of Claude Bernard (1813–78) (Robinson, 2018). Bernard came up with the idea of "milieu interieur," which means that organisms keep their interior environment stable to adapt to the external environment. Bernard had the important insight that all vital systems and organs work together to maintain internal stability (Bernard [1878] 1974; Robinson, 2018). Walter B. Cannon (1871–1945) expanded the work of Claude Bernard and coined the concepts of "Fight or Flight Response" and homeostasis (Cannon, 1932). Cannon's research focused on the transient response of the body to stress, especially the function of adrenaline in regulating the adaptive responses in an emergency (Robinson, 2018). While Cannon mainly examined the transient response to stressors, Hans Selye focused on the impact of chronic stress (Robinson, 2018). Selye's experiments on mice showed that deleterious insults such as exposure to extreme cold, injury, and surgery lead to conditions such as stomach ulcers, enlarged adrenal glands, and damage to the lymphatic system (Selye, 1936). He named this pattern of pathological response to stress "the general adaptation syndrome", which he later renamed as "stress response." Selye was the first to show the involvement of the hypothalamic-pituitary-adrenal axis (HPA) in the stress response. He was also the first to isolate glucocorticoids and identify their role as stress hormones (Szabo et al., 2012).

The works of Bernard, Cannon, and Selye and other early researchers laid the foundation for the study of stress (Robinson, 2018; Tan & Yip, 2018). Building on the pioneering work of these early researchers, contemporary scientists have found that chronic stress is associated with multiple negative physiological responses, including hypertension (Spruill et al., 2018; Caplan et al., 2020), hyperglycemia (van der Kooij et al., 2018; van der Kooij, 2020), stomach cancer (Ulanova et al., 2016; Zhang et al., 2019), metabolic syndrome (Pervanidou & Chrousos, 2012; Bergmann et al., 2017; Branyan et al., 2018), stroke (Ulanova et al., 2016), and other diseases risks. More recently, exposures to prenatal, perinatal and early life stress have all been linked to a broad range of adverse health outcomes, such as low birth weight, neuroendocrine dysfunction, and increased risk of infectious, cardio-metabolic, and psychiatric diseases in later life (Lobel et al., 1992; Kajantie, 2006; Beydoun & Saftlas, 2008; Cottrell & Seckl, 2009; Mastorci et al., 2009; Harris & Seckl, 2011; Nielsen et al., 2011; Vaiserman, 2015).

Prenatal maternal stress (PNMS), in particular, has been linked to increased obesity and metabolic dysfunction in children (Pervanidou & Chrousos, 2012; Cao-Lei et al., 2015). Exposure to high levels of PNMS stimulates the HPA axis. The HPA regulates many physiological systems, including stress responses, energy metabolism, and the immune system. Chronic stress induces the HPA to produce small peptide molecules (adrenocorticotropic hormone and β-endorphin) that stimulate cortisol levels, which in turn influence fetal behavior and subsequent birth outcomes (Sandman et al., 1994; Cao-Lei et al., 2015). The molecular mechanism that links PNMS to postnatal metabolic dysfunction, including increased BMI, central adiposity, and diabetes, is the epigenetic methylation of genes involved in HPA regulated metabolic pathways. PNMS alters DNA methylation patterns for at least 31 genes that influence BMI and regulate the type 1 and type 2 diabetes mellitus pathways (Cao-Lei et al., 2015). Additional genes modified by prenatal stress include several that code for insulin-like growth factor 2 (IGF2), a major fetal growth hormone (Liu et al., 2012); H19, a non-coding RNA molecule involved in the regulation of body weight (Chen et al., 2014); the glucocorticoid receptor NR3C1 involved in the regulation of the HPA (Radtke, 2011; Conradt et al., 2013); and the 11 β -HSD2 gene that produces the stress hormone cortisol (Conradt et al., 2013). In animal models, Park et al. (2008) found that fetal growth restriction is associated with the progressive silencing of Pdx1 gene in rats, elevating the risk of diabetes in adulthood.

Psychosocial stress, by way of increased HPA activity and cortisol secretion, is also known to induce telomere shortening (Epel et al., 2004), a cellular marker of aging (Jiang et al., 2019). Telomeres are repetitive nucleotide sequences found at the ends of all chromosomes. They function as end caps that protect the protein-coding gene sequences of the chromosome from degrading (Blackburn, 2000, 2001), much as the plastic ends of a shoelace protect its structure and function. As a cell divides, its telomeres shorten. Eventually, telomere length will reach a critical point, and the cell will stop dividing or die (Harley et al., 1990).

Shortened telomere length has been reliably linked to many health risks and diseases (Zhao et al., 2013; Haycock et al., 2014; Ridout et al., 2016), including type 2 diabetes, hypertension, and early mortality (Liu et al., 2017). Telomere length can therefore be an indicator of an individual's age and general health. High levels of PNMS have been linked to shortened telomeres in newborns (Entringer et al., 2013; Marchetto et al., 2016). Maternal social adversity and PNMS are both associated with behavioral disorders later in life (Szyf, 2019), and one proposed mechanism is telomere shortening (Simon et al., 2006; Shalev et al., 2013). For example, shortened telomere length has been associated with childhood autism (Li et al., 2014) and depression (Shalev et al., 2013). Racial discrimination can be a major source of PNMS, and within race patterns of discrimination, including low socioeconomic status, gender (female), and race (Black), are all associated with shorter telomere length (Pantesco et al., 2018). Mendez et al. (2014) found that pregnant women that experienced high levels of daily discrimination were more likely to experience preterm birth, while Jones et al. (2017) found in a comparative study that infants born to Black women had earlier gestational age and significantly shorter telomere length in placental tissues. Thus, factors that induce high levels of perinatal stress, including racial discrimination and socioeconomic status, can result in adverse physical and mental health outcomes through epigenetic mechanisms such as telomere shortening.

CULTURAL FOOD-RELATED CHANGES

The experience of starvation or famine has behavioral and psychological consequences for both human and animal subjects. The Minnesota Starvation Experiment (also known as Minnesota Semi-Starvation Experiment) showed that people who experienced starvation had subsequent binge eating, depression, less concentration, and lowered sex drive (Baker & Keramidas, 2003). A study of former prisoners of war (POWs) showed that POWs were more likely to have binge eating disorders compared with combat veterans (Polivy et al., 1994). Those studies suggest that the fear or anxiety of starvation could motivate people to eat more than required to meet their daily energy expenditure. Within a family, the eating disorders of subjects who went through food restriction, starvation, or famine likely influence their family members, especially their children.

The Minnesota Starvation Experiment examined the physiological and psychological consequences of severe and prolonged food restriction and the effects of different rehabilitation diets. The experiment was designed to provide information to help people in Europe and Asia rehabilitate and recover from the starvation experienced during World War II (Brožek, 1995). The experiment was led by Ancel Keys at the University of Minnesota. It began on November 19, 1944 and ended on December 20, 1945. During that time, 36 men aged 22 to 33 years were recruited from the Civilian Public Service to volunteer in the experiment as an alternative to serving in the military.

The experiment had four stages. The first stage was a control phase to establish a baseline for each subject; this lasted 12 weeks. During this time, the subjects consumed approximately 3,200 kilocalories of food per day. Adjustments were made for overweight and underweight subjects to ensure that they all achieved their ideal weight by the end of the first stage. The following 24 weeks comprised the semi-starvation phrase; each subject received a diet of approximately 1,560 kilocalories per day. During this phase of the study, subjects averaged a 25% loss of body mass. The third stage estimated the effects of rehabilitation diets with different combinations of macronutrients (i.e., protein, carbohydrates, and fats) and micronutrients (vitamins and minerals). During the final stage, food consumption was not restricted, but participant behaviors were carefully recorded.

The results of the experiment showed that: (1) severe and prolonged food restriction caused depression and hysteria; (2) subjects who experienced severe starvation were obsessed with food, and they tended to overeat when food intake was not restricted; and (3) the participants reported reduced ability of concentration, comprehension, and judgment, although those effects were not supported by the formal test in the experiment (Baker & Keramidas, 2003). This experiment is a valuable source for understanding the consequences of starvation, and the diet of rehabilitation from starvation or famine. There are behavioral consequences of food restriction – the participants tended to eat more than required to compensate for their daily activities when unlimited food was provided.

Another study on human beings reported on binge eating disorders among former prisoners of war. Polivy et al. (1994) compared binge eating habits in the postwar era between former prisoners of war and combat veterans who were not captured in the war. On average, the combat veterans gained 8.18 lb. during training and the war, while the POWs lost 22.83 lb. due to food restriction in prison. There was no significant difference between the weight of former prisoners and the weight of combat veterans at the time of the postwar study. The results, however, showed that former prisoners were more likely to report more postwar binge eating than combat veterans. Despite the limitations of the dataset, the study showed that food restriction and weight loss could affect binge eating habits in humans.

Based on the results of biocultural studies, it appears that famine survivors are more likely to develop binge eating habits, and these eating behaviors are very likely to influence the eating habits of their offspring. Thus, cultural food-related changes could be a possible explanation of the health consequences of famine exposure. Few studies have examined the diet and eating habits of famine survivors and their families, and the potential intergenerational transmission of eating habits awaits further exploration (Lussana et al., 2008).

There are fewer social science studies of populations undergoing or having experienced famine; many of those studies focus more on the causes than the cultural patterns following famine. Colin Turnbull's (1972) book on the Ik, an ethnic group in Uganda undergoing severe resource deprivation, shocked anthropologists when it was published. Turnbull described how young children formed age cohort groups that banded together to fight off older individuals who would try to steal food from the younger children. Shipton's (1990) review of African famines addresses cultural "coping strategies" that help families to survive food shortages, including women's jewelry as a mobile type of savings, "storing up debts" as an expectation of future reciprocity, and, in severe cases, selling children or infanticide.

CONCLUSION

In this chapter, we reviewed disparate bodies of literature on historical famines and the scientific understanding of the genetic and behavioral changes that result. As we have presented, populations that experience severe famines subsequently have higher rates of chronic diseases and mental illnesses. Those changes involve the death of the vulnerable, making famine a potential form of evolutionary selective pressure. This selection pressure acts on both physical and behavioral traits, resulting in phenotypic changes in subsequent generations.

In the late 20th century, the notion that survivors might deposit more fat on their bodies, compared with those who did not experience famine, was called the "thrifty-gene" hypothesis. While the thrifty-gene explanation has been found to be inadequate, without sufficient evidence of actual genetic changes to support the hypothesis, it led to the search for other explanations, such as the thrifty-phenotype and epigenetic regulation. A key issue that clinicians and nutritionists may find useful is that the prevention of type 2 diabetes in populations that have histories of severe famine, may need to start with maternal nutrition in the first weeks of pregnancy. A second point in our analysis is that such famines do not affect all residents equally. Even in the worst affected areas, some individuals have greater protection. Such privilege can be due to social advantages, such as slightly higher economic resources or family connections.

The evidence for epigenetic changes leading to abdominal obesity, metabolic changes, insulin resistance, and type 2 diabetes is fairly well documented in the literature. Nevertheless, epigenetics is an area of science that is quickly expanding and will likely become more refined in the near future. The evidence of the stress of famine leading to epigenetic changes that make individuals more reactive to trauma and increased risk of schizophrenia or other mental illnesses is similarly developing.

In our review of the social science literature on cultural changes surrounding food in post-famine populations, we have found fewer studies. However, this is an important area. The post-famine food environment in the two 20th-century famines differed significantly from that prior to the famine. The increased availability of food appears to have greatly influenced contemporary overnutrition. How much overnutrition may be due to cultural changes, food hoarding, food anxiety, and child feeding is difficult to pinpoint precisely, but the starvation studies that we reviewed earlier suggest that it could be significant.

REFERENCES

Baker, D., & Keramidas, N. (2003). *The psychology of hunger*. https://www.apa.org/monitor/2013/10/hunger

Barker, D. J. P. (2004). The Developmental Origins of Adult Disease. *Journal of the American College of Nutrition*, 23(sup6), 588S–595S. https://doi.org/10.1080/07315724.2004.10719428

Bergmann, N., Ballegaard, S., Krogh, J., Bech, P., Hjalmarson, Å., Gyntelberg, F., & Faber, J. (2017). Chronic psychological stress seems associated with elements of the metabolic syndrome in patients with ischaemic heart disease. *Scandinavian Journal of Clinical and Laboratory Investigation* 77(7): 513–519.

Bernard, C. ([1878] 1974). *Lectures on the phenomena common to all animals and plants*. Trans. H.E. Hoff, R. Guillemin, & L. Guillemin. Springfield, IL: Thomas.

Beydoun, H., & Saftlas, A.F. (2008). Physical and mental health outcomes of prenatal maternal stress in human and animal studies: a review of recent evidence. *Paediatric Perinatal Epidemiology* 22: 438–466.

Bird, A. (2007). Perceptions of epigenetics. *Nature* 447(7143): 396–398. https://doi.org/10.1038/nature05913

Blackburn, E.H. (2000). Telomere states and cell fates. *Nature* 408: 53–56.

Blackburn, E.H. (2001). Switching and signaling at the telomere. *Cell* 106: 661–673.

Maternal prenatal cortisol predicts infant negative emotionality in a sex-dependent manner. *Physiology & Behavior*, 175: 31–36. https://doi.org/10.1016/j.physbeh.2017.03.017

Branyan, K.W., DeVallance, E.R., Lemaster, K.A., Skinner, R.C., Bryner, R., Olfert, I.M., Kelley, E.E., Frisbee, J.C., & Chantler, P.D. (2018). Role of chronic stress and exercise on microvascular function in metabolic syndrome. *Medicine and Science in Sports and Exercise* 50(5): 957.

Brožek, J. (1995). Bibliographical note on behavioral aspects: on the margin of the 50th anniversary of the Minnesota Starvation-Nutritional Rehabilitation Experiment. *Perceptual and Motor Skills* 81(2): 395–400. https://doi.org/10.1177/003151259508100207

Calkins, K., & Devaskar, S. U. (2011). Fetal origins of adult disease. *Current Problems in Pediatric and Adolescent Health Care*, 41(6), 158–176. PubMed. https://doi.org/10.1016/j.cppeds.2011.01.001

Cannon, W.B. (1932). *The wisdom of the body*. W. W. Norton & Company.

Cao-Lei, L., Dancause, K.N., Elgbeili, G., Massart, R., Szyf, M., Liu, A., Laplante, D.P., & King, S. (2015). DNA methylation mediates the impact of exposure to prenatal maternal stress on BMI and central adiposity in children at age 13½ years: Project Ice Storm. *Epigenetics* 10(8): 749–761. https://doi.org/10.1080/15592294.2015.1063771

Caplan, M., Keenan-Devlin, L.S., Freedman, A., Grobman, W., Wadhwa, P.D., Buss, C., Miller, G.E., & Borders, A.E. (2020). Lifetime psychosocial stress exposure associated with hypertensive disorders of pregnancy. *American Journal of Perinatology* 7(2).

Chen, J., Li, Q., Rialdi, A., Mystal, E., Ly, J., Finik, J., Davey, T., Lambertini, L., & Nomura, Y. (2014). Influences of maternal stress during pregnancy on the epi/genome: comparison of placenta and umbilical cord blood. *Journal of Depression & Anxiety* 3(2).

Chen, Y., & Zhou, L.-A. (2007). The long-term health and economic consequences of the 1959–1961 famine in China. *Journal of Health Economics* 26(4): 659–681. https://doi.org/10.1016/j.jhealeco.2006.12.006

Cottrell, E.C., & Seckl, J. (2009). Prenatal stress, glucocorticoids and the programming of adult disease. *Frontiers in Behavioral Neuroscience* 3: 19.

Conradt, E., Lester, B.M., Appleton, A.A., Armstrong, D.A., & Marsit, C.J. (2013). The roles of DNA methylation of NR3C1 and 11β-HSD2 and exposure to maternal mood disorder in utero on newborn neurobehavior. *Epigenetics* 8(12): 1321–1329.

Desai, M., Jellyman, J.K., & Ross, M.G. (2015). Epigenomics, gestational programming and risk of metabolic syndrome. *International Journal of Obesity* 39(4): 633–641. https://doi.org/10.1038/ijo.2015.13

Dolinoy, D.C., Huang, D., & Jirtle, R.L. (2007). Maternal nutrient supplementation counteracts bisphenol A-induced DNA hypomethylation in early development. *Proceedings of the National Academy of Sciences of the United States of America* 104(32): 13056–13061. https://doi.org/10.1073/pnas.0703739104

Edwards, R. D., & Williams, T. D. (1997). *The Great Famine: Studies in Irish History, 1845–52*. Lilliput Press. (Original work published 1956).

Entringer, S., Epel, E.S., Lin, J., Buss, C., Shahbaba, B., Blackburn, E.H., Simhan, H.N., & Wadhwa, P.D. (2013). Maternal psychosocial stress during pregnancy is associated with newborn leukocyte telomere length. *American Journal of Obstetrics and Gynecology* 208(2): 134.e1–134.e7. https://doi.org/10.1016/j.ajog.2012.11.033

Epel, E.S., Blackburn, E.H., Lin, J., Dhabhar, E.S., Adler, N.E., Morrow, J.D., & Cawthon, R.M. (2004). Accelerated telomere shortening in response to life stress. *Proceedings of the National Academy of Sciences of the USA* 101(49): 17312–17315. doi: 10.1073/pnas.0407162101

Fung, W.W.-Y. (2009). *Early childhood malnutrition and adult obesity: Evidence from the 1959–61 China famine*. Harvard University, Mimeograph. http://cahnrs-cms.wsu.edu/ses/seminars/Documents/PastSeminarsPapers/Obesity_WinnieFung.pdf

Geary, L. (2018). Brutality of Cork's Famine years: 'I saw hovels crowded with the sick and the dying in every doorway.' *Irish Examiner*. https://www.irishexaminer.com/news/arid-20470367.html

Genné-Bacon, E.A. (2014). Thinking evolutionarily about obesity. *The Yale Journal of Biology and Medicine* 87(2): 99–112.

Gosling, A.L., Buckley, H.R., Matisoo-Smith, E., & Merriman, T.R. (2015). Pacific populations, metabolic disease and 'Just-So Stories': a critique of the 'thrifty genotype' hypothesis in Oceania. *Annals of Human Genetics* 79(6): 470–480. https://doi.org/10.1111/ahg.12132

Hales, C.N., & Barker, D.J.P. (1992). Type 2 (non-insulin-dependent) diabetes mellitus: the thrifty phenotype hypothesis. *Diabetologia* 35(7): 595–601. https://doi.org/10.1007/bf00400248

Hales, C.N., & Barker, D.J.P. (2001). The thrifty phenotype hypothesis: type 2 diabetes. *British Medical Bulletin* 60(1): 5–20. https://doi.org/10.1093/bmb/60.1.5

Harley, C.B., Futcher, A.B., & Greider, C.W. (1990). Telomeres shorten during ageing of human fibroblasts. *Nature* 345(6274): 458–460. https://doi.org/10.1038/345458a0

Harris, A., & Seckl, J. (2011). Glucocorticoids, prenatal stress and the programming of disease. *Hormones and Behavior* 59(3): 279–289.

Hay, T. (2018). Commentary: The Invention of Aboriginal Diabetes: The Role of the Thrifty Gene Hypothesis in Canadian Health Care Provision. *Ethnicity & Disease* 28(Suppl 1), 247–252. PubMed. https://doi.org/10.18865/ed.28.S1.247

Haycock, P.C., Heydon, E.E., Kaptoge, S., Butterworth, A.S., Thompson, A., & Willeit, P. (2014). Leucocyte telomere length and risk of cardiovascular disease: systematic review and meta-analysis. *British Medical Journal* 349: g4227. https://doi.org/10.1136/bmj.g4227

Heijmans, B.T., Tobi, E.W., Stein, A.D., Putter, H., Blauw, G.J., Susser, E.S., Slagboom, P.E., & Lumey, L.H. (2008). Persistent epigenetic differences associated with prenatal exposure to famine in humans. *Proceedings of the National Academy of Sciences* 105(44): 17046. https://doi.org/10.1073/pnas.0806560105

Hollstein, T., Ando, T., Basolo, A., Krakoff, J., Votruba, S. B., & Piaggi, P. (2019). Metabolic response to fasting predicts weight gain during low-protein overfeeding in lean men: Further evidence for spendthrift and thrifty metabolic phenotypes. *The American Journal of Clinical Nutrition* 110(3): 593–604. PubMed. https://doi.org/10.1093/ajcn/nqz062

Huang, C., Li, Z., Venkat Narayan, K.M., Williamson, D.F., & Martorell, R. (2010). Bigger babies born to women survivors of the 1959–1961 Chinese famine: a puzzle due to survival selection? *Journal of Developmental Origins of Health and Disease* 1(6): 412–418. https://doi.org/10.1017/S2040174410000504

Jiang, Y., Da, W., Qiao, S., Zhang, Q., Li, X., Ivey, G., & Zilioli, S. (2019). Basal cortisol, cortisol reactivity, and telomere length: a systematic review and meta-analysis. *Psychoneuroendocrinology* 103: 163–172. https://doi.org/10.1016/j.psyneuen.2019.01.022

Jones, C.W., Gambala, C., Esteves, K.C., Wallace, M., Schlesinger, R., O'Quinn, M., Kidd, L., Theall, K.P., & Drury, S.S. (2017). Differences in placental telomere length suggest a link between racial disparities in birth outcomes and cellular aging. *American Journal of Obstetrics and Gynecology* 216(3): 294.e1–294.e8. https://doi.org/10.1016/j.ajog.2016.11.1027

Kajantie, E. (2006). Fetal origins of stress: related adult disease. *Annals of the New York Academy of Sciences* 1083(1): 11–27.

Kelly, J. (2012). *The Graves Are Walking: The Great Famine and the Saga of the Irish People*. Henry Holt and Company.

Keneally, T. (2011). *Three Famines: Starvation and Politics*. Public Affairs.

Kinsella, M.T., & Monk, C. (2009). Impact of maternal stress, depression and anxiety on fetal neurobehavioral development. *Clinical Obstetrics and Gynecology*, 52(3):

425–440. PubMed. https://doi.org/10.1097/GRF.0b013e3181b52df1

Koh, X.-H., Liu, X., & Teo, Y.-Y. (2014). Can evidence from genome-wide association studies and positive natural selection surveys be used to evaluate the thrifty gene hypothesis in East Asians? *PloS One* 9(10): e110974–e110974. https://doi.org/10.1371/journal.pone.0110974

Koolhaas, J.M., Bartolomucci, A., Buwalda, B., de Boer, S.F., Flügge, G., Korte, S.M., Meerlo, P., Murison, R., Olivier, B., Palanza, P., Richter-Levin, G., Sgoifo, A., Steimer, T., Stiedl, O., van Dijk, G., Wöhr, M., & Fuchs, E. (2011). Stress revisited: a critical evaluation of the stress concept. *Neuroscience & Biobehavioral Reviews* 35(5): 1291–1301. https://doi.org/10.1016/j.neubiorev.2011.02.003

Law, C.M., Barker, D.J., Osmond, C., Fall, C.H., & Simmonds, S.J. (1992). Early growth and abdominal fatness in adult life. *Journal of Epidemiology and Community Health* 46(3): 184–186. https://doi.org/10.1136/jech.46.3.184

Li, H., Oldenburg, B., Chamberlain, C., O'Neil, A., Xue, B., Jolley, D., Hall, R., Dong, Z., & Guo, Y. (2012). Diabetes prevalence and determinants in adults in China mainland from 2000 to 2010: a systematic review. *Diabetes Research and Clinical Practice* 98(2): 226–235. https://doi.org/10.1016/j.diabres.2012.05.010

Li, W., & Yang, D.T. (2005). The Great Leap Forward: anatomy of a central planning disaster. *Journal of Political Economy* 113(4): 840–877. https://doi.org/10.1086/430804

Li, Z., Tang, J., Li, H., Chen, S., He, Y., Liao, Y., Wei, Z., Wan, G., Xiang, X., Xia, K., & Chen, X. (2014). Shorter telomere length in peripheral blood leukocytes is associated with childhood autism. *Scientific Reports* 4: 7073. https://doi.org/10.1038/srep07073

Liu, H., Zhou, G., Chen, Q., Ouyang, F., Little, J., Zhang, J., & Chen, D. (2017). Impact of dehydroepiandrosterone sulfate on newborn leukocyte telomere length. *Scientific Reports* 7: 42160. https://doi.org/10.1038/srep42160

Liu, Y., Murphy, S.K., Murtha, A.P., Fuemmeler, B.F., Schildkraut, J., Huang, Z., Overcash, F., Kurtzberg, J., Jirtle, R., Iversen, E.S., Forman, M.R., & Hoyo, C. (2012). Depression in pregnancy, infant birth weight and DNA methylation of imprint regulatory elements. *Epigenetics* 7(7): 735–746. https://doi.org/10.4161/epi.20734

Lobel, M., Dunkel-Schetter, C., & Scrimshaw, S.C. (1992). Prenatal maternal stress and prematurity: a prospective study of socioeconomically disadvantaged women. Health psychology: official journal of the Division of Health Psychology, *American Psychological Association* 11(1): 32–40. https://doi.org/10.1037//0278-6133.11.1.32

Lumey, L.H., & Stein, A.D. (1997). In utero exposure to famine and subsequent fertility: The Dutch Famine Birth Cohort Study. *American Journal of Public Health* 87(12): 1962–1966. https://doi.org/10.2105/ajph.87.12.1962

Lumey, L.H., Stein, A.D., & Kahn, H.S. (2009). Food restriction during gestation and impaired fasting glucose or glucose tolerance and type 2 diabetes mellitus in adulthood: evidence from the Dutch Hunger Winter Families Study. *Journal of Developmental Origins of Health and Disease* 1–S164.

Lumey, L.H., Stein, A.D., & Susser, E. (2011). Prenatal famine and adult health. *Annual Review of Public Health* 32: 237–262. PubMed. https://doi.org/10.1146/annurev-publhealth-031210-101230

Lussana, F., Painter, R.C., Ocke, M.C., Buller, H.R., Bossuyt, P.M., & Roseboom, T.J. (2008). Prenatal exposure to the Dutch famine is associated with a preference for fatty foods and a more atherogenic lipid profile. *The American Journal of Clinical Nutrition* 88(6): 1648–1652. https://doi.org/10.3945/ajcn.2008.26140

Lynch, S. (2018). *Choctaw generosity to Famine Ireland saluted by Varadkar*. https://www.irishtimes.com/news/ireland/irish-news/choctaw-generosity-to-famine-ireland-saluted-by-varadkar-1.3424542

Marchetto, N.M., Glynn, R.A., Ferry, M.L., Ostojic, M., Wolff, S.M., Yao, R., & Haussmann, M.F. (2016). Prenatal stress and newborn telomere length. *American Journal of Obstetrics and Gynecology* 215(1): 94.e1–94.e8. https://doi.org/10.1016/j.ajog.2016.01.177

Marks, K. (1997, June 2). Blair issues apology for Irish Potato Famine. *Independent*. https://www.independent.co.uk/news/blair-issues-apology-for-irish-potato-famine-1253790.html

Mastorci, F., Vicentini, M., Viltart, O., Manghi, M., Graiani, G., Quaini, F., Meerlo, P.,

Nalivaiko, E., Maccari, S., & Sgoifo, A. (2009). Long-term effects of prenatal stress: changes in adult cardiovascular regulation and sensitivity to stress. *Neuroscience & Biobehavioral Reviews* 33(2): 191–203.

Mendez, D.D., Hogan, V.K., & Culhane, J.F. (2014). Institutional racism, neighborhood factors, stress, and preterm birth. *Ethnicity & Health* 19(5): 479–499. https://doi.org/10.1080/13557858.2013.846300

Mu, R., & Zhang, X. (2011). Why does the Great Chinese Famine affect the male and female survivors differently? Mortality selection versus son preference. *Economics & Human Biology* 9(1): 92–105. https://doi.org/10.1016/j.ehb.2010.07.003

Mulraney, F. (2018, May 11). Cork witness recorded shock at poverty and death during the Great Hunger. *Irish Central*. https://www.irishcentral.com/roots/history/cork-city-irish-famine-deaths

Nielsen, N.M., Hansen, A.V., Simonsen, J., & Hviid, A. (2011). Prenatal stress and risk of infectious diseases in offspring. *American Journal of Epidemiology* 173(9): 990–997.

Neel, J.V. (1962). Diabetes mellitus: a 'thrifty' genotype rendered detrimental by 'progress'? *American Journal of Human Genetics* 14(4): 353–362.

Neel, J.V. (1999). The 'Thrifty Genotype' in 1998. *Nutrition Reviews* 57(5): 2–9. https://doi.org/10.1111/j.1753-4887.1999.tb01782.x

Painter, R.C., de Rooij, S.R., Bossuyt, P.M., Simmers, T.A., Osmond, C., Barker, D.J., Bleker, O.P., & Roseboom, T.J. (2006). Early onset of coronary artery disease after prenatal exposure to the Dutch famine. *The American Journal of Clinical Nutrition* 84(2): 322–327. https://doi.org/10.1093/ajcn/84.2.322

Painter, R., Osmond, C., Gluckman, P., Hanson, M., Phillips, D., & Roseboom, T. (2008). Transgenerational effects of prenatal exposure to the Dutch famine on neonatal adiposity and health in later life. *BJOG: An International Journal of Obstetrics & Gynaecology* 115(10): 1243–1249. https://doi.org/10.1111/j.1471-0528.2008.01822.x

Pantesco, E.J., Leibel, D.K., Ashe, J.J., Waldstein, S.R., Katzel, L.I., Liu, H.B., Weng, N., Evans, M.K., Zonderman, A.B., & Beatty Moody, D.L. (2018). Multiple forms of discrimination, social status, and telomere length: Interactions within race. *Psychoneuroendocrinology* 98: 119–126. https://doi.org/10.1016/j.psyneuen.2018.08.012

Park, J.H., Stoffers, D.A., Nicholls, R.D., & Simmons, R.A. (2008). Development of type 2 diabetes following intrauterine growth retardation in rats is associated with progressive epigenetic silencing of Pdx1. *The Journal of Clinical Investigation* 118(6): 2316–2324. https://doi.org/10.1172/JCI33655

Pembrey, M., Saffery, R., Bygren, L.O., Network in Epigenetic Epidemiology, & Network in Epigenetic Epidemiology. (2014). Human transgenerational responses to early-life experience: Potential impact on development, health and biomedical research. *Journal of Medical Genetics* 51(9): 563–572. PubMed. https://doi.org/10.1136/jmedgenet-2014-102577

Pervanidou, P., & Chrousos, G.P. (2012). Metabolic consequences of stress during childhood and adolescence. *Metabolism* 61(5): 611–619.

Polivy, J., Zeitlin, S.B., Herman, C.P., & Beal, A.L. (1994). Food restriction and binge eating: a study of former prisoners of war. *Journal of Abnormal Psychology* 103(2): 409–411. https://doi.org/10.1037/0021-843X.103.2.409

Prentice, A.M., Hennig, B.J., & Fulford, A.J. (2008). Evolutionary origins of the obesity epidemic: Natural selection of thrifty genes or genetic drift following predation release? *International Journal of Obesity* 32(11): 1607–1610. https://doi.org/10.1038/ijo.2008.147

Puleo, S. (2020). Amid Irish potato famine, a ship from Boston embarked on history's first humanitarian mission. *Globe Magazine*. https://www.bostonglobe.com/2020/02/05/magazine/it-is-not-an-everyday-matter-see-nation-starving/

Radford, E.J., Ito, M., Shi, H., Corish, J.A., Yamazawa, K., Isganaitis, E., Seisenberger, S., Hore, T.A., Reik, W., Erkek, S., Peters, A.H.F.M., Patti, M.-E., & Ferguson-Smith, A.C. (2014). In utero effects: in utero undernourishment perturbs the adult sperm methylome and intergenerational metabolism. *Science* (New York), 345(6198): 1255903–1255903. https://doi.org/10.1126/science.1255903

Radtke, K.M., Ruf, M., Gunter, H.M., Dohrmann, K., Schauer, M., Meyer, A., & Elbert, T. (2011). Transgenerational impact of intimate partner violence on methylation in the

promoter of the glucocorticoid receptor. *Translational Psychiatry* 1(7): 1–6.
Ravelli, A.C., van der Meulen, J.H., Michels, R., Osmond, C., Barker, D., Hales, C., & Bleker, O. (1998). Glucose tolerance in adults after prenatal exposure to famine. *The Lancet* 351(9097): 173–177. https://doi.org/10.1016/S0140-6736(97)07244-9
Ravelli, A.C., van der Meulen, J.H., Osmond, C., Barker, D.J., & Bleker, O.P. (1999). Obesity at the age of 50 in men and women exposed to famine prenatally. *The American Journal of Clinical Nutrition* 70(5): 811–816. https://doi.org/10.1093/ajcn/70.5.811
Ravelli, G.-P., Stein, Z.A., & Susser, M.W. (1976). Obesity in young men after famine exposure in utero and early infancy. *New England Journal of Medicine* 295(7): 349–353. https://doi.org/10.1056/NEJM197608122950701
Reddon, H., Patel, Y., Turcotte, M., Pigeyre, M., & Meyre, D. (2018). Revisiting the evolutionary origins of obesity: Lazy versus peppy-thrifty genotype hypothesis. *Obesity Reviews*, 19(11), 1525–1543. https://doi.org/10.1111/obr.12742
Ridout, K.K., Ridout, S.J., Price, L.H., Sen, S., & Tyrka, A.R. (2016). Depression and telomere length: a meta-analysis. *Journal of Affective Disorders* 191: 237–247. https://doi.org/10.1016/j.jad.2015.11.052
Riggs, A.D., Martienssen, R.A., & Russo, V.E.A. (1996). Introduction. In R.A. Martienssen, A.D. Riggs, & V.E.A. Russo, *Epigenetic mechanisms of gene regulation* (pp. 1–4). New York: Cold Spring Harbor.
Robinson, A.M. (2018). Let's talk about stress: history of stress research. *Review of General Psychology* 22(3): 334–342. https://doi.org/10.1037/gpr0000137
Sandman, C.A., Wadhwa, P.D., Dunkel-Schetter, C., Chicz-DeMET, A., Belman, J., Porto, M., Murata, Y., Garite, T.J., & Crinella, F.M. (1994). Psychobiological influences of stress and HPA regulation on the human fetus and infant birth outcomes. *Annals of the New York Academy of Sciences* 739(1): 198–210. https://doi.org/10.1111/j.1749-6632.1994.tb19822.x
Scheper-Hughes, N. (1987). Mental in Southie: individual, family, and community responses to psychosis in South Boston. *Culture, Medicine and Psychiatry* 11(1): 1–25. https://doi.org/10.1007/bf00055009
Scheper-Hughes, N. (2001) *Saints, scholars and schizophrenics*. Berkeley, CA: University of California Press.
Selye, H. (1976). *Stress in health and disease*. Boston, Massachusetts: Butterworth Inc.
Shalev, I., Entringer, S., Wadhwa, P.D., Wolkowitz, O.M., Puterman, E., Lin, J., & Epel, E.S. (2013). Stress and telomere biology: a lifespan perspective. *Psychoneuroendocrinology* 38(9): 1835–1842.
Shaw-Taylor, L. (2020). An introduction to the history of infectious diseases, epidemics and the early phases of the long-run decline in mortality. *The Economic History Review* 73(3): E1–E19. https://doi.org/10.1111/ehr.1301942.
Shipton, P. (1990). African Famines and Food Security: Anthropological Perspectives. *Annual Review of Anthropology* 19(1): 353–394. https://doi.org/10.1146/annurev.an.19.100190.002033
Simon, N.M., Smoller, J.W., McNamara, K.L., Maser, R.S., Zalta, A.K., Pollack, M.H., Nierenberg, A.A., Fava, M., & Wong, K.K. (2006). Telomere shortening and mood disorders: preliminary support for a chronic stress model of accelerated aging. *Biological Psychiatry* 60(5). 432–435.
Smith, M.K. (2017). Did the Irish Famine trigger mental illness in the Irish? *Irish Central*. www.irishcentral.com/news/irish-famine-mental-illness-connection
Speakman, J.R. (2013). Evolutionary perspectives on the obesity epidemic: adaptive, maladaptive, and neutral viewpoints. *Annual Review of Nutrition* 33(1): 289–317. https://doi.org/10.1146/annurev-nutr-071811-150711
Spruill, T.M., Butler, M.J., Thomas, S.J., Tajeu, G.S., Castaneda, S.F., Langford, A.T., Abdalla, M., Blackshear, C., Ogedegbe, G., Sims, M., & Shimbo, D. (2018). Cumulative stress exposure is associated with incident hypertension in African Americans: findings from the Jackson Heart Study. *Circulation* 137(suppl_1): A005–A005.
St Clair, D., Xu, M., Wang, P., Yu, Y., Fang, Y., Zhang, F., Zheng, X., Gu, N., Feng, G., Sham, P., & He, L. (2005). Rates of adult schizophrenia following prenatal exposure to the Chinese Famine of 1959–1961. *JAMA* 294(5): 557–562. https://doi.org/10.1001/jama.294.5.557
Stipp, D. (2011). Linking nutrition, maturation and aging: From thrifty genes to the

spendthrift phenotype. *Aging* 3(2): 85–93. PubMed. https://doi.org/10.18632/aging.100286

Stöger, R. (2008). The thrifty epigenotype: an acquired and heritable predisposition for obesity and diabetes? *BioEssays* 30(2): 156–166. https://doi.org/10.1002/bies.20700

Susser, E.S., & Lin, S.P. (1992). Schizophrenia after prenatal exposure to the Dutch Hunger winter of 1944–1945. *Archives of General Psychiatry* 49(12): 983–988. https://doi.org/10.1001/archpsyc.1992.01820120071010

Szabo, S., Tache, Y., & Somogyi, A. (2012). The legacy of Hans Selye and the origins of stress research: a retrospective 75 years after his landmark brief 'Letter' to the Editor# of Nature. *Stress* 15(5): 472–478. https://doi.org/10.3109/10253890.2012.710919

Szyf, M. (2019). The epigenetics of perinatal stress. *Dialogues in Clinical Neuroscience* 21(4): 369–378. https://doi.org/10.31887/DCNS.2019.21.4/mszyf

Tan, S.Y., & Yip, A. (2018). Hans Selye (1907–1982): founder of the stress theory. *Singapore Medical Journal* 59(4): 170–171. https://doi.org/10.11622/smedj.2018043

Tobi, E.W., Lumey, L.H., Talens, R.P., Kremer, D., Putter, H., Stein, A.D., Slagboom, P.E., & Heijmans, B.T. (2009). DNA methylation differences after exposure to prenatal famine are common and timing- and sex-specific. *Human Molecular Genetics* 18(21): 4046–4053. PubMed. https://doi.org/10.1093/hmg/ddp353

Turnbull, C. (1972). *Mountain People* (1st ed.). Simon and Schuster.

Ulanova, M., Gekalyuk, A., Agranovich, I., Khorovodov, A., Rezunbaeva, V., Borisova, E., Sharif, A.E., Navolokin, N., Shuvalova, E., & Semyachkina-Glushkovskaya, O. (2016). Stress-induced stroke and stomach cancer: sex differences in oxygen saturation. In *Oxygen Transport to Tissue XXXVIII* (pp. 135–140). Cham, Switzerland: Springer.

Vaiserman, A.M. (2015). Epigenetic programming by early – life stress: evidence from human populations. *Developmental Dynamics* 244: 254–265. doi:10.1002/dvdy.24211

van Abeelen, A.F.M., Elias, S.G., Bossuyt, P.M.M., Grobbee, D.E., van der Schouw, Y.T., Roseboom, T.J., & Uiterwaal, C.S.P.M. (2012). Famine exposure in the young and the risk of type 2 diabetes in adulthood. *Diabetes* 61(9): 2255. https://doi.org/10.2337/db11-1559

van der Kooij, M.A. (2020). The impact of chronic stress on energy metabolism. *Molecular and Cellular Neuroscience* p.103525.

van der Kooij, M.A., Jene, T., Treccani, G., Miederer, I., Hasch, A., Voelxen, N., Walenta, S., & Müller, M.B. (2018). Chronic social stress-induced hyperglycemia in mice couples individual stress susceptibility to impaired spatial memory. *Proceedings of the National Academy of Sciences* 115(43): E10187–E10196.

van der Zee, H.A. (1998). *The hunger winter: Occupied Holland 1944–1945*. Lincoln, NB: University of Nebraska Press.

Veenendaal, M., Painter, R., de Rooij, S., Bossuyt, P., van der Post, J., Gluckman, P., Hanson, M., & Roseboom, T. (2013). Transgenerational effects of prenatal exposure to the 1944–45 Dutch famine. *BJOG: An International Journal of Obstetrics & Gynaecology* 120(5): 548–554. https://doi.org/10.1111/1471-0528.12136

Walsh, D. (2012). Did the Great Irish Famine increase schizophrenia? *Irish Journal of Psychological Medicine* 29(1): 7–15 https://doi.org/10.1017/S0790966700017547

Walsh, O. (2016). 'An invisible but inescapable trauma': epigenetics and the Great Famine. In C. Kinealy & J. King (Eds.), *Women and the great hunger* (pp. 173–183). Cork: Cork University Press.

Wang, J., Li, Y., Han, X., Liu, B., Hu, H., Wang, F., Li, X., Yang, K., Yuan, J., Yao, P., Miao, X., Wei, S., Wang, Y., Liang, Y., Zhang, X., Guo, H., Yang, H., Hu, F.B., Wu, T., & He, M. (2016). Exposure to the Chinese famine in childhood increases type 2 diabetes risk in adults. *The Journal of Nutrition* 146(11): 2289–2295. https://doi.org/10.3945/jn.116.234575

Wang, N., Wang, X., Han, B., Li, Q., Chen, Y., Zhu, C., Chen, Y., Xia, F., Cang, Z., Zhu, C., Lu, M., Meng, Y., Chen, C., Lin, D., Wang, B., Jensen, M. D., & Lu, Y. (2015). Is exposure to famine in childhood and economic development in adulthood associated with diabetes? *The Journal of Clinical Endocrinology & Metabolism* 100(12): 4514–4523. https://doi.org/10.1210/jc.2015-2750

Wang, Y., Wang, X., Kong, Y., Zhang, J.H., & Zeng, Q. (2010). The Great Chinese Famine leads to shorter and overweight females in Chongqing Chinese population after 50 years. *Obesity* 18(3): 588–592. https://doi.org/10.1038/oby.2009.296

Zhang, X., Zhang, Y., He, Z., Yin, K., Li, B., Zhang, L., & Xu, Z. (2019). Chronic stress promotes gastric cancer progression and metastasis: an essential role for ADRB2. *Cell Death & Disease* 10(11): 1–15.

Zhao, J., Miao, K., Wang, H., Ding, H., & Wang, D.W. (2013). Association between telomere length and type 2 diabetes mellitus: a meta-analysis. *PLoS One* 8(11): e79993. https://doi.org/10.1371/journal.pone.0079993

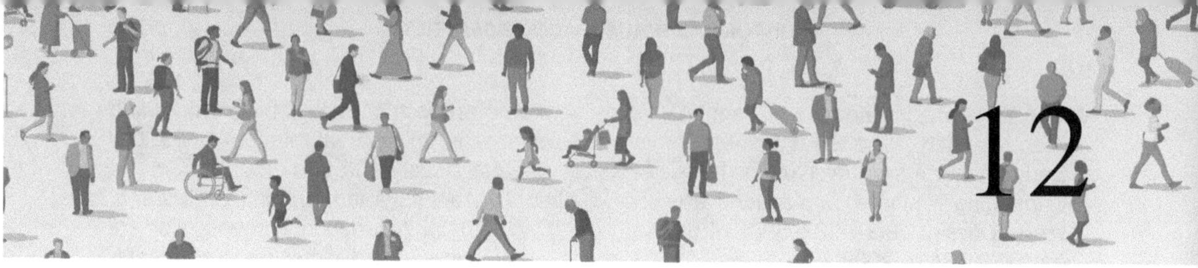

12

Historical Trauma and Health Injustice in Indigenous Communities

Corinne Yawę'nęhà·wi' Abrams and Lois M. Jircitano

INTRODUCTION

Indigenous peoples in North and South America, as well as other colonial settler countries, including in Africa, Asia, Australia, New Zealand, and Greenland, share traumatic historical experiences. Native Peoples have experienced the loss of ancestral lands, language, tradition, and culture, meaning that those who remain today are survivors of attempts at genocide and other atrocities inflicted upon them over centuries. In addition to attempted genocide, this trauma includes murder, exposure to new diseases, robbing of indigenous territory, abrogation of treaties, and attempts destroy their cultures, committed by European migrants. These historical antecedents form the context and social determinants of continuing health injustices in the present day.

This chapter addresses contemporary public health issues faced by Native and aboriginal communities in North America from a social science perspective that emphasizes the role of historical trauma and structural violence among Native and aboriginal groups. In discussing the health disparities among Indigenous Peoples, we focus particularly on obesity and chronic diseases, addictions, and interpersonal violence, all of which have their roots in this tragic trajectory. Because Native Peoples are diverse, the chapter cannot do justice to the health challenges of each group. The chapter therefore focuses predominantly on the **Haudenosaunee Six Nations Confederacy** in New York State and Canada, whose experiences illustrate many of the issues of structural violence that we argue have led to the present situation of poorer health and survival. The Haudenosaunee, called the Iroquois Confederacy among English, Dutch, and French settlers in their territory, means "People of the Longhouse," and comprises the Seneca, Oneida, Onondaga, Cayuga, Mohawk, and Tuscarora, each of which is an individual Nation with its own language and culture, but share many similarities in traditions and religious ceremonies. The chapter also includes case studies of a Haudenosaunee family and of the K'iche' Maya in Guatemala.

HISTORICAL TRAUMA

We begin by exploring the forces of change and social determinants that oppressed and adulterated the unique culture of Indigenous people to undermine the political, social and spiritual lives of American Indians over the centuries (Colden 1958; Twaithes 1899). The resulting negative health influences are the context leading to contemporary health disparities. It is important in the study of chronic illness to understand the relationship linking historical trauma and other traumatic events to the subsequent development of chronic diseases that inordinately affect aboriginal populations. As documented in the sections below, Indigenous Peoples exhibit high rates of diabetes, hypertension, heart disease and kidney failure (Centers for Disease Control and Prevention 2018). Their communities are also compromised by mental health problems, alcohol, and substance abuse, with serious consequences, including early death. A growing body of evidence documents that historical trauma suffered by Native Americans to be a major determinant of health injustice, chronic disease, premature mortality, and mental health problems (Joe and Gauchupin 2012).

This analysis is challenged by the diversity of Native communities and the difficulty of compiling accurate statistical assessments of their populations and health issues. Since the beginning of European contact in the hemisphere that they termed the "new world," dating from 1492, an estimated 56 million Native people have been murdered or indirectly killed by European diseases and continued oppression (Koch et al. 2019). The relatively small population of Native Americans reported in the United States (US) official statistics results in part from mistrust among some Indigenous Nations and Tribes to be counted by the federal government and the fact that Native Peoples are often misclassified as other races, with the result that they are frequently undercounted in census tallies or are misclassified with other races. In addition, Indigenous Tribes are diverse and multicultural, with unique languages, customs, and forms of self-government, making statistical tracking of public health data a challenge. The US Bureau of Indian Affairs acknowledges 578 federally recognized tribes, and there are many more which have lost federal recognition and their ancestral homelands. All have been systemically discriminated against by the federal government through policies of forced assimilation, which attempted to strip Indigenous people of their language and customs (Maresca 2012).

While Native American health statistics today document grave disparities, pre-contact descriptions of Native American people tell a very different story. Accounts by English and Dutch colonial settlers of Native Americans in North America describe tall, robust people. Mid-nineteenth century painter George Caitlin, who created detailed portraits of the Osage Tribe in what is present-day Missouri, described them, in language reflecting the contemporary racism of his time as, "the tallest race of men in North America, either of red or white skins." William Penn (1683) described the Lenni-Lenape, whose land was located in present-day Pennsylvania, as "they are generally tall, streight [sic], well-built, and of singular Proportion; they tread strong and clever." In contrast, the European settlers often had dental caries, loss of teeth, and chronic infections with tuberculosis, shortening their lives and causing significant disability, as well as frequent waves of communicable diseases such as smallpox. Their history of repeated infections rendered the European survivors more resistant to death from such contagions, but also led to stunting in their height for many, as well as skin sores and limping gaits for some. At first contact, the Native Peoples would have appeared much healthier and more robust than the colonial interlopers. However, the many contagious diseases they brought with their ships from Europe devastated the Native people they met.

To understand the historical trauma of present-day Native Peoples, it is necessary to examine the life circumstances of early Indigenous populations in America to learn what hereditary or environmental conditions presented challenges to survival, among which recurrent trauma exposure were prominent. Their histories demonstrate the negative outcomes from persistent intertribal conflict. In addition, some of the widespread social conditions Indigenous people lived through include ongoing exposure to the provision and use of alcoholic substances in the trade economy, exploitation, and manipulation of Indigenous governments to create relinquishment of territories for colonial settler migration, food deprivation and recurrent waves of epidemics among Aboriginal people who were without physical immunity to European diseases.

Foremost, Indigenous culture traditionally featured socio-political interconnectedness, relationship structures organized by family relationships, and clan kinship group recognition. Indigenous people suffered grave traumatization from the high death rates accompanying constant wars, which affected their entire village communities (Richter 1992). After European intrusion, they lived through long periods of food and housing insecurity, theoretically causing sustained internal system damage from exposure to the endocrinology attendant to hyper-alert social conditions. The mental and emotional health of Indigenous societies was imperiled by the exponential increase in alcohol consumption, which instigated individual and familial violence unknown in aboriginal societies, the hallmarks of which exhibited cohesion and ethical behavior (Parker 1968; Pflug 1998). As described in the Haudenosaunee family case history in Box 12.1, the implementation of the boarding school system was a major social determinant of poorer mental health and a huge blow to the psyche of Native children who were removed and institutionalized by federal and state governments working in tandem to begin a forced re-education process designed to rob them of their culture (Brave Heart and Debruyan 1998; Child 1995). Aboriginal children would thus be separated from parents and families during a critical period of child development, and exposed to severe physical punishment, emotional deprivation and sexual violence. Many would die from communicable diseases, in part because they were not given appropriate medical care. Native child burials in school graveyards, miles from family communities, disrupted Traditional Haudenosaunee family observances of caring for the deceased, another experience which would traumatize family relatives seeking to properly care for their child's spirit (Child 1995).

The individual and collective trauma of Indigenous people would last for more than 200 years from early contact in the fur trade economy to the last treaty that established and placed Indigenous Nations and Tribes on small reservation territories, generally located near US Military posts for the security of white settlers (Schoolcraft 1992). The sequestration of the Indigenous people in geographically isolated areas allowed the United States government to ignore the plight of aboriginal people for another 100 years (Lyons, Grinde, and Berkey 1992; Maresca 2012; Richter 1992). Most aboriginals continued to live in primitive conditions, bereft of sufficient housing, limited by a lack of employment and educational opportunities needed to participate in the American labor market. Despite all these constraints, they managed to transfer traditional knowledge across generations, conveying oral histories and teaching essential skills for maintaining a healthy life.

Once the boarding school system emerged with the stated goal as re-educating Indigenous children to indoctrinate American values and beliefs, reservation life changed. Parents and children felt estranged from those students who had adopted philosophies consistent with the White institution. Reservations, subsequently, were often split between the older generation's desire to maintain traditional ways and returning youths seeking to institute cultural disruption that served to rupture the cultural cohesion that was a traditional characteristic of Indigenous people, thus affecting generations of families (Adams 2020). The boarding school experience at its best provided labor market training in agriculture and domestic service. The long-term trauma of those Indigenous children exposed to systemic institutional violence and sexual exploitation was much more damaging to aboriginal societies (Lechner, Cavanaugh, and Bryler n.d.). The sustained personal trauma experienced by Native American children would affect the mental and physical health of aboriginal people for generations to come as returning youths, stripped of their cultural identity and inalterably changed by physical, spiritual and sexual violence, brought their trauma histories back to their home communities. Thereafter, self-medicating behaviors, ingrained alcohol, and later substance abuse, would enter and remain the aboriginal culture to continue the trauma for generations to come.

THE HAUDENOSAUNEE

The Iroquois Confederacy or Haudenosaunee people are a league of Six Nations made up of the Mohawk, Cayuga, Onondaga, Oneida, Seneca, and Tuscarora. In the present day, the League of the Iroquois exists in the northeastern region of the United States within New York State and Southern Ontario, being comprised of a series of reservations (Haudenosaunee Confederacy n.d.). The estimated Native American population of New York State totals approximately 82,000, comprising Six Nations Haudenosaunee members and Natives from other US Tribes, according to the US Census, 2010.

The Haudenosaunee-rich history in this region dates back thousands of years (Haudenosaunee Confederacy n.d.). The Six Haudenosaunee Nations traditionally followed the same political organization and matrilineal line of succession. This system has provided longevity for the organization and cohesion among the Six Nations. Currently, some of the Nations have continued to follow the traditional form of government, including chiefs and clan mothers, and others have chosen to reorganize their political systems into modified ones.

Understanding Indigenous health requires an appreciation of the natural world embodied in Native American epistemology and culture. The connection to Mother Earth and all creation is the fundamental to Native American cultures. The manner in which Native Peoples see and view the world is the element which connects Indigenous Peoples across the globe. Native epistemology, or our knowledge of the world, is heavily based on the linguistic lens through which we traditionally viewed the world. For example, religious ceremonies and tradition evolved around gratitude for the Natural World. Deeply important and central to cultural knowledge are these ceremonies that give thanks to all living things in our world and appreciation of nature enshrined in ceremonies that reverence the four directions, the four beings, changing of the seasons, harvest, birth, and death

The Haudenosaunee traditionally used an oral history; they recorded treaties and other important events by creating Wampum Belts to express the agreements in treaties and as a reminder for future generations of our history. Figure 12.1 is a photograph of the "Two-Row Wampum" that represents a treaty made in 1613 between the Haudenosaunee and the Dutch settlers in what is present-day Northern New York. Native American historian Ray Fadden described how the Dutch originally proposed a kind of parent–child relationship, with the Dutch as the parents (Keefer 2014). The Haudenosaunee's response was:

> We will not be like Father and Son, but like Brothers. [Our treaties] symbolize two paths or two vessels, travelling down the same river together.

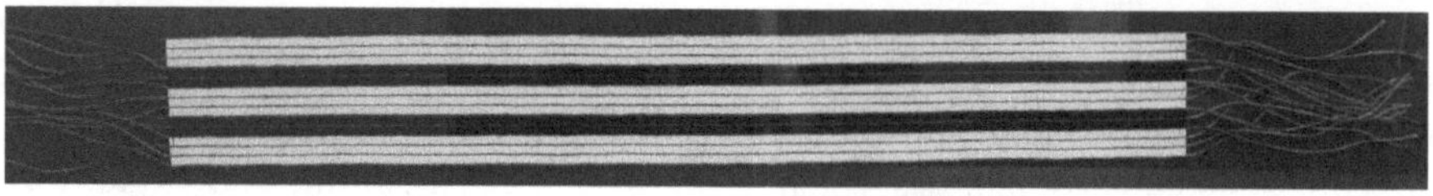

Figure 12.1 The Two-Row Wampum

> One, a birchbark canoe, will be for the Indian People, their laws, their customs, and their ways. The other, a ship, will be for the white people and their laws, their customs, and their ways. We shall each travel the river together, side by side, but in our own boat. Neither of us will make compulsory laws nor interfere in the internal affairs of the other. Neither of us will try to steer the other's vessel. (Keefer 2014)

The Two-Row Wampum, pictured in Figure 12.1, illustrates this side-by-side trajectory of White and Native boats that can be understood without requiring language fluency or literacy. Unfortunately, this treaty, like many others, was abrogated by the European colonial settlers.

The organization of the Iroquois Confederacy was an inspiration for the writing of the US Constitution. Prior to the Constitutional Convention in 1787, John Adams wrote a three-volume report about various forms of governments to provide background to the Convention delegates regarding the potential options for them to consider. This work reviewed the Iroquois Confederacy Longhouse model of consensus building and provided description of other Indigenous governmental approaches (Kickingbird 1987).

Biomedical research refers to this population as American Indian/Alaskan Native (AI/AN). In fact, Native Americans can have strong preferences on what they wish to be called. Tribal titles often have historically been anglicized, and therefore Nation Members may self-identify in their own language. For example, The Navajo Nation formally changed its name to Diné in 1993. Members of this Nation found the word "Navaho" to be inaccurate and rejected the name (Tribal College 1997).

SOCIAL DETERMINANTS OF HEALTH

US Federal Government's approach to Indian Health Care

Indian Health Services (IHS) was established in 1955 by the department of Health and Human Services, previously called the Department of Interior. Throughout the history of the United States, Native American Indians and Alaskan Natives (AIAN) have had a complex history that gave rise to the formation of a health care system for the betterment of AIAN peoples (Maresca 2012). Lack of resources allotted to medical provisions and access to physicians has been an issue since the last treaties were signed with the Indians in 1871. In 1890 the Annual Report for Indian Affairs showed that doctors who worked on reservations were paid $1,028 per year, compared to $2,823 for Army physicians and $2,622 for Navy physicians (Warne and Frizzell 2014).

The health care system's main obstacle in delivering health services is low accessibility for many of the rural and isolated tribal entities, which results in poorer health outcomes for Native Americans living on reservations. Yet, Native Americans who have relocated from their Indigenous territories to live in cities also experience disproportionately high rates of poverty and corresponding morbidities that are well known in public health research to be associated with socioeconomic disadvantage (Ablon 1964; Burhansstipanov 2012).

Politically, there is a complex and lengthy history between the US Federal Government and Tribal Nations dating back to before the ratification of the Constitution. The Nations' distrust of the federal government is substantiated by many occasions of broken treaties and

Box 12.1 A Haudenosaunee family history

CORINNE YAWĘʾNĘHÀ·WIʾ ABRAMS

I am from an Indian reservation within the United States and as a child we did not have running water in our home. My parents had to go to the well and fill up buckets and haul in the water every day. This was not uncommon – my best friend and close neighbor a few houses away did not have water at her home either. We were exceptionally poor. It's an experience that I don't share often because I associate it with the shame that sometimes comes from being a "poor Indian." When I read the article "Historical trauma as public narrative: a conceptual review of how history impacts present-day health" in graduate school I realized that my family and Native Americans suffered from historical trauma (Mohatt et al. 2014). I realized that my shame and suffering with poor living conditions as a child was an outcome of traumatic experiences that affected my parents and grandparents. According to Yoshikawa, Aber and Beardslee (2012), living in poverty can have a negative impact on the health of an individual. Indigenous people worldwide face such difficulties, for example, the average income of Aboriginal Australians only compares to two-thirds of the income of predominantly White general population, according to the Australian Museum (The Australian Museum 2019).

My maternal Great-Great Grandmother was named Florence Lilia Jones, was born and raised on the Cattaraugus Reservation; her father was Horacio Jones, from the Seneca Nation. She and her brother and sister were taken to an Indian Residential School (a boarding school) in Hampton, Virginia. The Indian boarding schools were a European American governmental attempt to change the culture of Native students, to "civilize" and "Christianize" them (Adams 2020; Magagnini 2005). The students' hair was cut, they were given English names, they were not allowed to speak their Indigenous languages. They were subject to harsh corporal punishment for infractions. The motto for one of the boarding schools was, "Kill the Indian, Save the man" (Bear 2008). This horrific experience harmed many of the children, in a way that we now realize can cause life-long trauma and health problems, which we now call ACEs, Adverse Childhood Experiences. A major study from Kaiser Permanente in California found that neglect, abuse, and major losses in childhood increased the likelihood of chronic disease, addiction, and premature death (Felitti et al. 1998). Growing evidence suggests that such ACEs affect the functioning of genes, in a pattern called epigenetics, making the affected children more reactive to stress and potentially leading to increased rates of type 2 diabetes, heart disease, and mental illness (Brockie, Heinzelmann, and Gill 2013).

My paternal Great-Grandmother, Phoebe Rosetta Shenandoah (Hill) Dyaoñnihses, meaning "slow rising moon," was sent to a Friends Quaker Indian boarding school, where they taught things like cooking and cleaning to the girls and all were forbidden from using their Native language. As an adult, she became an Eel Clan Clanmother of the Onondaga Nation and Onondaga Language teacher. She told me that many of the Native American boarding school attendees stopped speaking their language completely and some left their communities, sadly never to return. The loss of the ability to speak their languages is particularly harmful to Native children because those languages are the medium in which Native ceremonies are conducted. Those who are robbed of their languages, and unable to fully participate in the ceremonies, are thus robbed of the psychological comfort of their identities and the grounding of their place in Native American history, cosmology, and world view.

In late 2020, my Grandfather died of COVID-19 at age 80. As described earlier, the coronavirus pandemic has devastated Native communities. My Grandfather Morley A. "Jay" Gaʔohn·taʔ Clause, Jr. had run the local 7clan AA group for over 40 years and helped countless people deal with alcoholism. Many Indigenous Elders like him found social distancing and quarantine difficult because of the interdependent nature of our family, being close to loved ones was valued more than the potential risks from COVID-19 infection. Other Elders live in multigenerational households and also cannot avoid being in close contact with extended family members.

the substandard treatment of AIAN people as Nations. Today, the new problem is the concept of discretionary and mandatory spending as appointed by Congress. Much of spending for AIAN is treated as discretionary, leaving them chronically underfunded and leaving thousands of Native Americans without access to adequate health care. The IHS estimated in 2005 that 25% of spending on AIAN health care comes from other third party sources (Cullen et al. 2019).

IHS Policy to AIAN Health

Socioeconomically, Indigenous populations fare the worst on many different indicators.

Health outcomes are very poor in comparison to the rest of the United States. Unemployment rates are higher on reservations across the United States, including Alaska. Mortality rates due to alcohol-related illness and accidental death is especially alarming. Diabetes mellitus is 300% higher among Indigenous populations compared to the overall population (Burhansstipanov 2012; Joe and Gauchupin 2012).

Historically, treaties were made with Indian Nations who relinquished their land with the promise of health care by the federal government. At the time, this consisted of smallpox vaccination, physicians being made available to Native American Nations and in other ways that helped with public health of Indigenous Peoples. The federal government gave supplies to the Indians to pacify them and fulfill the stipulations of the treaties made with the Indian Nations. These obligations were made in perpetuity and to date many Nations still receive annuities such as cloth, provisions, and medical care, fulfilled today in part by Indian Health Service.

Eligibility and Accessibility of IHS

Access to care is one of the major indicators of quality health care and one of the initiatives taken by the federal government to insure better health outcomes for its people. To be eligible for services, the IHS has strict requirements that patients must meet to acquire coverage. There are two types of IHS facilities: (1) federal facilities that operate outside of the jurisdiction of any Nation, and (2) health facilities that are operated by a Tribe/Nation under a Title IV, Indian Self-Determination Education Assistance Act (ISDEAA) PL-638 (Federal Register 1996). The first requirement is that a person be an enrolled member of a federally recognized tribe (or a descendant in the first or second degree). For health care facilities run by a tribal government, each is then given sole responsibility for establishing the criteria for its members to become enrolled by their tribal entity, which may include blood quantum, and any other conditions established by their tribe.

Tribal governments are also eligible to apply for grant funding for health care, which is often given by organizations like Substance Abuse and Mental Health Services Administration (SAMHSA) or Housing and Urban Development (HUD). However, many of these grants are established in the form of block grants. Consequently, the Indian reservations with the greatest need are not always the recipients of available funds, because they are competitive. It is also important to note that although technically eligible from the perspective of government agreements, Tribal 638 programs are eligible for many grants funded by federal monies, because the IHS is a federal agency it is not elibigible for grants made by federal sources (Warne and Frizzell 2014). The Indian Health Service has significant issues because it is based on a model of discretionary spending by Congress, making the IHS budget one of the first to be cut. As a result, programs that fall under IHS are often drastically underfunded (Maresca 2012).

In a system that is habitually underfunded, it is almost impossible to maintain a high standard of patient care and satisfactory outcomes. Consumer preferences are limited for health care options and the overall structure of the Indian Health Service health care system. In 1976, The Indian Health Care Improvement Act (IHCIA) gave legal authority for the provision of health care to Native Americans in the US. In the Affordable Care Act, the IHCIA was made permanent by President Obama. The Snyder Act, which gave citizenship to Native Americans in 1924, together with IHCIA are the two cornerstone Acts that gave Congress appropriations authority for the Indian Health Service.

Reimbursement for services is given at the Medicaid rate of pay. One common problem is that it is difficult to find specific services, such as mental health services, or specialists who will accept this method of payment. The IHS works in collaboration with State-level Health Systems. For example, in New York State, eligibility levels for the American

Indian Health Program are established through the New York State Department of Health (New York State 2018).

When taking into consideration the funding process of the federal government, it is necessary to have a fundamental understanding of Tribal/Nation governance. As established by numerous treaties throughout the country, Native Americans are considered sovereign Nations when they have a land base. Being cognizant of Tribal protocol and governance issues when creating policy would be effective in creating policy that has relevance to the people being served. As a result of the Tribes/Nations being sovereign, they should not be expected to vote or participate in a "foreign" government's election process. Taking cultural consideration into the needs and wants of Nations is equally important to adequately funding health programs for Native Americans.

MAJOR PUBLIC HEALTH DISPARITIES OF NATIVE AMERICANS

COVID-19 Epidemic

During the SARS-CoV-2 pandemic, Native American communities were disproportionately affected by the virus. According to the Centers for Disease Control and Prevention (CDC), Native Americans have a four-fold increase in relative risk of hospitalization and a 2.6-fold increase in relative risk of death from COVID-19 compared to white people. Nationwide, one in every 475 Native Americans has died from COVID-19 (Tapia 2021). The impact upon Indigenous communities is tremendous, with each passing generation we lose a little bit of the wisdom from our ancestors. For all Indigenous people, elders in our communities are revered for their knowledge and wisdom. Healy and Blue (2021) describe in tragic and vivid detail the impact on Indigenous communities of the loss of healers, religious leaders, those with agricultural knowledge of the ancient ways, and keepers of songs and stories, memories and languages: "It's like we're having a cultural book-burning," said Jason Salsman, a spokesman for the Muscogee (Creek) Nation in eastern Oklahoma (Healy and Blue 2021, A6). During the pandemic access to medical supplies was a burden to Indigenous Nations, when the Seattle Indian Health Board requested medical supplies and personal protective equipment (PPE), they were instead sent body bags for the deceased (Ortiz 2020).

Obesity and Chronic Diseases

Native Americans' health disparities include both type 1 and type 2 diabetes, obesity, hypertension, cardiovascular disease, hyperlipidemia, and some types of cancer (Adamsen et al. 2018; Burhansstipanov 2012; Joe and Gauchupin 2012). Native American Indians are at higher risk of many health disparities resulting from obesity. "National estimates indicate that American Indian (AI) children have higher rates of overweight and obesity than children of other races/ethnicities" (Karanja et al. 2012, 161). Breastfeeding has been shown to reduce childhood obesity as well as reducing the mother's weight after childbirth. Breastfeeding is one simple way that the rates can be reduced in both mother and child and the cost is low. The community health worker program at the Tuscarora Nation strives to have healthy outcomes for mothers and babies: "77% of American Indians initiated breastfeeding but only 42% breastfed at 6-months postpartum" (Rhodes et al. 2008, S46). The goal is to increase the number of mothers who breastfeed their babies at birth and in general to increase the overall health and wellness of mother and child. A substantial amount of research indicates that infancy is a crucial period for the development of obesity (Stettlar 2007). Research has also documented that the benefits for the infant is increased cognitive function and mothers have lower rates of obesity. The World Health Organization (WHO) Collaborative Group found an increase in infant mortality in the first few years of life in infants who were not breastfed. Today, it is recommended to exclusively breastfeed for the first six months of life (Victora and Barros 2000).

The Opioid Epidemic among Native Americans

The prevalence of alcohol and substance abuse in Native communities has resulted in multi-generational social problems and related comorbidities (Hatala, Desjardins, and Bombay 2016). Opioid abuse is a major issue in the United States as a whole, and is a rising public health issue as an increasing number of people become addicted to opiates. Opiates range from endorphins created by the body in response to stress, to prescription pain pills, heroin, and newly derived synthetic opioids such as fentanyl. These molecules act on the central nervous system and opioid receptors throughout the body to relieve pain; they bind to one or more of the three opioid receptors in the body (Lord et al. 1977). Opioid pain relievers are generally safe when taken for a short duration and as prescribed by a doctor, but in addition to relieving pain they may produce euphoria, which makes them a target for misuse. Demographic information available on Native Americans indicates higher drug use as compared to the standard population in the United States, due to a history of discrimination and various social problems. Tribal groups also suffer with opiate addictions at a higher rate than other populations, leading to elevated overdose rates. Nearly 20% of Native Americans currently misuse drugs, including 6% who use prescription drugs non-medically (Office of National Drug Control Policy 2011).

In 2014, The National Survey on Drug Use and Health indicated that the rate of non-medical use of prescription painkillers was slightly decreasing, but consequently the rate of heroin abuse was increasing. This has been attributed to the high cost of prescription opiates and so people are more inclined to abuse the cheaper street drugs (Center for Behavioral Health Statistics and Quality 2015). Though this trend is not specific to the Native American population, it has been shown to be especially dangerous on reservations, as there is limited availability of funds as well as a lack of law enforcement resource (Morales 2015). Another factor that has been shown to contribute is the low employment rates on reservations, which makes them a target for drug cartels to recruit people for drug trafficking and also leads to less money availability. Native Americans also experience high rates of suicide due to their isolation and mistreatment as well as emotional pain from social challenges and unemployment, in addition to the lack of resources to cope with the psychological problems. This can cause Native Americans to resort to opioids (Burhansstipanov 2012; Ernst 2008).

Interpersonal Violence

American Indian women are about four times more likely than non-Native women to experience violent victimization (Evans-Campbell 2008; Rogers and Giroux 2012). This is a serious public health problem due to the short- and long-term negative health outcomes. The prevalence of alcohol and substance abuse (ASA) in Native communities has resulted in multi-generational social problems and trauma-related illness (Burhansstipanov 2012). The origin of Native childhood trauma, which persisted among second- and third-generation survivors of the boarding school experience, has been recognized to continue affecting families due to the parent/child separation, loss of their language and cultural heritage, and eventual reunion with a society from which they had become estranged. The Tuscarora Indian Nation population aligns with this description in that there is significant multi-generational involvement in alcohol and substance abuse, which has caused domestic violence, sexual assault, and child abuse across generations (Rogers and Giroux 2012).

Box 12.2 K'iche' Maya in Guatemala

MIGUEL CUJ

Guatemala, a Central American country, presents a paradox: the same lands that are the mecca of one of the greatest ancient civilizations – the Maya – also are the same lands where the Maya population has suffered repression since the conquest period to current times, thus surviving almost five centuries of conquest. Currently, Guatemala has 22 distinct linguistic Maya groups making up 51% of the population of nearly 18 million in 2020. The Maya of Guatemala have suffered constant attacks, massacres, mass exploitation and discrimination at all levels in the last two centuries.

From 1524 to 1821 conquest and colonial rule created the destruction of a thriving Maya population and culture. The conquest of Guatemala was brutal, prolonged and complex, fraught with intrigue and deception, and not at all clear-cut (Lovell, Lutz, and Kramer 2020). The conquest of Guatemala was made an arduous, protracted affair because of intense political fragmentation that, prior to the conquerors' arrival, had resulted in open hostilities between competing Maya groups. Spanish hegemony put Maya communities under immediate pressure to conform to imperial designs. A fundamental element of the Spaniard conquest was to organize space and to control population movement by founding towns and villages as a colonial model and restricting residents to their communities (Lovell 1988). Thus, the first step for the repression was the colonial model. The largest single element in the colonial population consisted of native Mayas, but transatlantic contact added other important groups to the mix, among them Spaniards, who intermarried to create *ladinos* (as *mestizos* are called in Guatemala). At the center of the colonial economy was the system of *encomienda* and *repartimiento*. The *encomienda* granted Indian labor and tribute in a certain geographical area. The people who held one of these grants could tax Indigenous people and conscript them for labor – in exchange, the holder agreed to maintain order and educate the Indigenous people in Catholicism and the Spanish language. The *encomenderos* exploited the Indigenous people by seizing land, increasing taxes, and forcing the natives into debt bondage. The *repartimiento* was a system that wasn't all together much different. Local magistrates now controlled the distribution of workers and called for a donation of between 2% and 4% of the Indigenous populations that were close to Spanish settlements, who would work as laborers. This institutional style of labor would continue on in different forms for many years (Martinez 1994). In 1821 Guatemala's independence was the result of influences of power which included creoles (people who were born in the New World but were of Spanish descent). Creoles took the local control of the colonial system and repressed the Maya populations under policies that clearly benefited the creole people.

More recently, the Maya people of Guatemala have suffered more than 36 years of severe internal conflict, beginning in 1960 and formally concluding with the signing of the Peace Accords at the end of 1996 (Grandin 2011). The Guatemalan armed conflict hindered development and resulted in multiple human rights violations with approximately 200,000 victims, the majority of which were Maya people (Pion-Berlin 2003; Skaar and Malca 2014). Violations were committed against ethnic Maya Indigenous people and Ladino peasants, who together make up the rural poor. Today's sociopolitical conditions are the result of a complex history of Spanish colonialism, 36 years (1960–1996) of genocidal civil war, and ongoing structural violence. Currently, 2020, Guatemala celebrates the splendor and vibrancy of the Maya to tourists, it harbors ongoing "racial ambivalence" (at best) and more often overt racism towards its Indigenous citizens (Hale 2006). This racial ambience materializes in reduced educational and economic opportunities and increased health disparities for Maya when compared to their Ladino (persons of mixed-ancestry; non-Indigenous) counterparts. Indigenous communities live in a permanent state of precarity. For example, Maya communities may experience stunting rates, due to malnutrition and infection, as high as 75% for children under five (compared to a sorry national stunting rate of 49%) (Black et al. 2013). All these features detailed above describe a long history of repression that is still an everyday experience for the Maya population.

CONCLUSION

Indigenous Peoples work to actively let go of these traumas that have impacted so many aspects of our community and family life. Our ancestors fought for our values, cosmology, truth, and way of life. For all people, resilience and trauma go hand in hand. Our lives are impacted by the generational pain that our ancestors endured as we experience new patterns of trauma as a direct result of the historical traumas. As noted above, the trauma resulting from the boarding school experience continunes to affect families among second- and third-generations. Many Haudenosaunee families reflect this traumatic history with multi-generational involvement in alcohol and substance abuse, contributing to domestic violence, sexual assault, and child abuse across generations.

As the world changes, Haudenosaunee and other Indigenous Peoples live in modern societies with many conveniences and advances in technology and modern medicine; yet they still remember the sacredness of all living things, and the importance of natural cycles and rhythm of the earth. In this regard, we aim to live for peace, righteousness, and the power of the good mind. At present, our people constantly look for ways to preserve our culture, our way of life, and our way of being. It is this aspect of Native American society that is imbued with intelligence, harmony with nature, and sustainability for all living things inhabiting Mother Earth. Our path toward healing and moving beyond hundreds of years of colonization, pain, and loss, includes learning about all of these aspects of creation, of ourselves as spiritual beings. Every Indigenous person was put on the earth to continue to carry on our traditions, languages, and culture so they will be there for the next seven generations that have not yet been born.

REFERENCES

Ablon, Joan. 1964. "Relocated American Indians in the San Francisco Bay area: Social interaction and Indian identity." *Human Organization* 23 (4): 296–304.

Adams, David Wallace. 2020. *Education for Extinction: American Indians and the Boarding School Experience, 1875–1928* (3rd Printing). Kansas City: University of Kansas Press.

Adamsen, C., S. Schroeder, S. LeMire, and P. Carter. 2018. "Education, income, and employment and prevalence of chronic disease among American Indian/Alaska Native Elders." *Preventing Chronic Disease* 15 (170387): e37.

Bear, Charla. 2008. "American Indian boarding schools haunt many." *NPR*. Available at: www.npr.org/templates/story/story.php?storyId=16516865, accessed 1/22/2021.

Black, R.E., C.G. Victora, S.P. Walker, Z.A. Bhutta, P. Christian, M. Onis, M. de Ezzati, S. Grantham-McGregor, J. Katz, R. Martorell, and R. Uauy. 2013. "Maternal and child undernutrition and overweight in low-income and middle-income countries." *The Lancet* 382 (9890): 427–451.

Brave Heart, M.Y., and L.M. Debruyan. 1998. "American Indian Holocaust – healing historical unresolved grief." *American Indian Alaska Native Mental Health Research* 8 (2): 56–78.

Brockie, T.N., M. Heinzelmann, and J.A. Gill. 2013. "A framework to examine the role of epigenetics in health disparities among Native Americans." *Nursing Research and Practice* 23 (Article ID 410395): 1–9.

Burhansstipanov, L. 2012. "Health disparity: the morbidity and mortality picture." In *Health and Social Issues of Native American Women*, edited by J. Joe and F.C. Gauchupin, pp. 79–100. Santa Barbara, CA: Praeger.

Center for Behavioral Health Statistics and Quality. 2015. *Behavioral Health Trends in the United States: Results from the 2014 National Survey on Drug Use and Health*. Washington, DC: Sustance Abuse and Mental Health Services Administration/Department of Health and Human Services.

Centers for Disease Control and Prevention. 2018. *CDC and Indian Country Working Together*. Atlanta, GA: Centers for Disease Control and Prevention.

Child, Brenda. 1995. *Boarding School Seasons, American Indian Families 1900–1940*. Lincoln, NB: University of Nebraska Press.

Colden, Cadwallder. 1958. *The History of the Five Nations Depending on the Province of New York in America (1727)*. Ithaca, NY: Cornell University Press.

Cullen, T., J. Flowers, T. Sequist, H. Hays, P. Biondich, and M. Laing. 2019. "Envisioning health equity for American Indian/Alaska Natives: a unique HIT opportunity." *Journal of the American Medical Informatics Association* 26 (8–9): 891–894.

Ernst, Anthony. 2008. *Environmental Scan, Summary Report*. Washington, DC: Native

American Center for Excellence, Substance Abuse and Mental Health Services, Department of Health and Human Services.

Evans-Campbell, T. 2008. "Historical trauma in American Indian/Native Alaska communities: a multilevel framework for exploring impacts on individuals, families, and communities." *Journal of Interpersonal Violence* 23 (3): 316–338.

Federal Register. 1996. "Indian Self-Determination and Education Assistance Act amendments – BIA, IHS. Notice of proposed rulemaking." *Federal Register* 61 (16): 2038–2077.

Felitti, V.J., R.F. Anda, D. Nordenberg, D.F. Williamson, A.M. Spitz, V. Edwards, M.P. Koss, and J.S. Marks. 1998. "Relationship of childhood abuse and household dysfunction to many of the leading causes of death in adults: The Adverse Childhood Experiences (ACE) Study." *American Journal of Preventive Medicine* 14 (4): 245–258.

Grandin, G. 2011. *The Last Colonial Massacre: Latin America in the Cold War* (Updated Edition). Chicago, IL: University of Chicago Press.

Hale, C.R. 2006. *Más Que Un Indio (More than an Indian): Racial Ambivalence and the Paradox of Neoliberal Multiculturalism in Guatemala*. Santa Fe, NM: School of American Research Press.

Hatala, A., M. Desjardins, and A. Bombay. 2016. "Reframing narratives of aboriginal health inequity: Exploring Cree Elder resilience and well-being in contexts of historical trauma." *Qualitative Health Research* 26 (14): 1911–1927.

Haudenosaunee Confederacy. n.d. *"Who we are: About the Haudenosaunee Confederacy."* Available at: www.haudenosauneeconfederacy.com/who-we-are/, accessed 1/24/2021.

Healy, Jack, and Victor J. Blue. 2021. "Cultural crisis for American Indians as Elders die." *The New York Times*, January 13: A6(L). Available at: https://link.gale.com/apps/doc/A648166411/SPN.SP01?u=nysl_ce_syr&sid=SPN.SP01&xid=9c80a2a3.

Joe, J., and F.C. Gauchupin, eds. 2012. *Health and Social Issues of Native American Women*. Santa Barbara, CA: Praeger.

Karanja, N., M. Aickin, T. Lutz, J.B. Jobe, G. Maupome, and C. Ritenbaugh. 2012. "A community-based intervention to prevent obesity beginning at birth among American Indian children: Study design and rationale for the PTOTS study." *Journal of Primary Prevention* 33 (4): 161–174.

Keefer, Tom. 2014. "A short introduction to the Two Row Wampum." *Briar Patch Magazine*, https://briarpatchmagazine.com/articles/view/a-short-introduction-to-the-two-row-wampum#:~:text=The%20Two%20Row%20Wampum%20is%20one%20of%20the,up%20the%20Hudson%20River%20into%20Kanien%E2%80%99keh%C3%A1:ka%20(Mo), accessed 1/22/2021.

Kickingbird, Kirke. 1987. *Indians and the United States Constitution: A Forgotten Legacy*. Washington, DC: Institute for the Development of Indian Law.

Koch, Alexander, Chris Brierley, Mark M. Maslin, and Simon L. Lewis. 2019. "Earth system impacts of the European arrival and Great Dying in the Americas after 1492." *Quaternary Science Reviews* 207: 13–36.

Lechner, Amanda, Michael Cavanaugh, and Crystal Bryler. 2016. *Addressing Trauma in American Indian and Alaska Native Youth*. Vol. https://aspe.hhs.gov/system/files/pdf/207941/AIANYOUTHTIC.PDF, accessed 1/23/2021, *Mathematica Policy Research Final Report*. Washington, DC: US Department of Health and Human Services.

Lord, J., A. Waterfield, J. Hughes, and H. Kosterlitz. 1977. "Endogenous opioid peptides: Multiple agonists and receptors." *Nature* 267 (5611): 495–499.

Lovell, W. George. 1988. *Surviving Conquest: The Maya of Guatemala in Historical Perspective*. Austin, TX: Latin American Research Review.

Lovell, W. George, Christopher Lutz, and Wendy Kramer. 2020. *Strike Fear in the Land: Pedro de Alvarado and the Conquest of Guatemala, 1520–1541*. Norman, OK: University of Oklahoma Press.

Lyons, Oren, Donald Grinde, Jr, and Curtis Berkey. 1992. *Exiled in the Land of the Free, Democracy, Indian Nations and the U.S. Constitution*. Sante Fe, NM: Clear Light Publishers.

Magagnini, Stephen. 1997. "Long-suffering urban Indians find roots in ancient rituals." *Sacramento Bee*, https://infoweb-newsbankcom.

libezproxy2.syr.edu/apps/news/openurl?ctx_ver=z39.88-2004&rft_id=info%3Asid/infoweb.newsbank.com&svc_dat=AWNB&req_dat=0D0CB6142C34B04A&rft_val_format=info%3Aofi/fmt%3Akev%3Amtx%3Actx&rft_dat=document_id%3Anews%252F0EB0466D1F6E3F5C, accessed 9/7/2021.

Maresca, T.M. 2012. "The impact of Federal Government policies on American Indian and Alaska Native health care." In *Health and Social Issues of Native American Women*, edited by J. Joe and F.C. Gauchupin. Santa Barbara, CA: Praeger, pp. 55–78.

Martinez, Pelaez Severo. 1994. *La Patria Del Criollo: Ensayo De Interpretación De La Realidad Colonial Guatemalteca*. Mexico, MX: Ed. en Marcha.

Mohatt, N.V., A.B. Thompson, N.D. Thai, and J.K. Tebes. 2014. "Historical trauma as public narrative: A conceptual review of how history impacts present-day health." *Social Science and Medicine* 106: 128–136.

Morales, Laurel. 2015. "Many Native American communities struggle with effects of heroin use." *National Public Radio*, Morning Edition. Available at: www.npr.org/2015/05/20/405936140/many-native-american-communities-struggle-with-effects-of-heroin-use, accessed 1/24/2021.

New York State, Department of Health. 2018. *American Indian Health Program in New York State*. New York: New York State Department of Health. Available at: www.health.ny.gov/community/american_indian_nation/, accessed 1/24/2021.

Office of National Drug Control Policy. 2011. *"Collaborating with Native Americans and Alaskan Natives."* Available at: www.whitehouse.gov/ondcp/native-americans-and-alaskan-indians, accessed 10/9/2017.

Ortiz, E. 2020. "Native American health center asked for COVID-19 supplies: It got body bags instead." *NBC News*, www.nbcnews.com/news/us-news/native-american-health-center-asked-covid-19-supplies-they-got-n1200246, accessed 1/24/2021.

Parker, Arthur C. 1968. *Parker on the Iroquois*. Edited by William N. Fenton. Syracuse, NY: Syracuse University Press.

Penn, William. 1683. "The Diversity of Native America: The Middle Colonies." *Digital History*. Available at: www.digitalhistory.uh.edu/disp_textbook.cfm?smtid=3&psid=641, accessed 1/22/21.

Pflug, Melissa A. 1998. *Ritual and Myth in Odawa Revitalization: Reclaiming a Sovereign Place*. Norman, OK: University of Oklahoma Press.

Pion-Berlin, D. 2003. *Civil-Military Relations in Latin America: New Analytical Perspectives*. Chapel Hill, NC: University of North Carolina Press.

Rhodes, K.L., W.L. Hellerstedt, C.S. Davey, P.L. Pirie, and K.A. Daly. 2008. "American Indian breastfeeding attitudes and practices in Minnesota." *Maternal and Child Health Journal* 12: 46–54.

Richter, Daniel K., ed. 1992. *The Ordeal of the Longhouse: The Peoples of the Iroquois League in the Era of European Colonialization*. Chapel Hill, NC, and London: The University of North Carolina Press.

Rogers, Mary, and Jennifer Giroux. 2012. "Domestic violence in American Indian communities: Background, culture, and legal issues." In *Health and Social Issues of Native American Women*, edited by J. Joe and F.C. Gauchupin. Santa Barbara, CA: Praeger, pp. 153–168.

Schoolcraft, Henry. 1992. *Schoolcraft's Narrative Journal of Travels Through the Northwestern Regions of the United States extending from Detroit through the Great Chain of American Lakes to the Sources of the Mississippi River in the Year 1820*. Edited by Mentor L. Williams. Lansing, MI: Michigan State University Press.

Skaar, E., and C.G. Malca. 2014. *Latin American Civil–Military Relations in a Historical Perspective: A Literature Review*. Bergen, NO: CMI (Chr. Michelsen Institute).

Stettlar, N. 2007. "Obesity risk factors and prevention in early life: Pre-pregnancy through infancy." In *Handbook of Obesity Prevention*, edited by S.K. Kumanyika and R.C. Brownson. New York: Springer, pp. 403–428.

Tapia, Rafael. 2021. "Native news picks of the month: COVID-19's toll on Elders and the perspective of one indigenous man." *Partnership with Native Americans*. Available at: http://blog.nativepartnership.org/, accessed 2/23/2021.

The Australian Museum. 2019. *"Indigenous Australia's First People's exhibition*

1996–2015." The Australian Museum, Canberra. Available at: https://australian.museum/about/history/exhibitions/indigenous-australians/?gclid=EAIaIQobChMI2Zyh5I2w7gIVEcDICh35-QhEEAAYASAAEgLi_vD_BwE, accessed 1/19/2021.

Tribal College. 1997. "Navajos change name to Diné College." *Tribal College: Journal of American Indian Higher Education* 9 (1): 30.

Twaithes, Reuban Gold. 1899. *Jesuit Relations – Allied Documents, Travels and Explorations of Jesuit Missionaries in New France.* Cleveland, OH: Burrows Co, Imperial Press.

Victora, C.G., and A.J. Barros. 2000. "Effect of breastfeeding on infant and child mortality due to infectious diseases in less developed countries: A pooled analysis." *The Lancet* 355 (9202): 451–455.

Warne, D., and L. Frizzell. 2014. "American Indian health policy: Historical trends and contemporary issues." *American Journal of Public Health* 104 (Supplement 3): S262–S267.

Yoshikawa, H., J. Aber, and W. Beardslee. 2012. "The effects of poverty on the mental, emotional, and behavioral health of children and youth: Implications for prevention." *American Psychologist* 67 (3): 316–338.

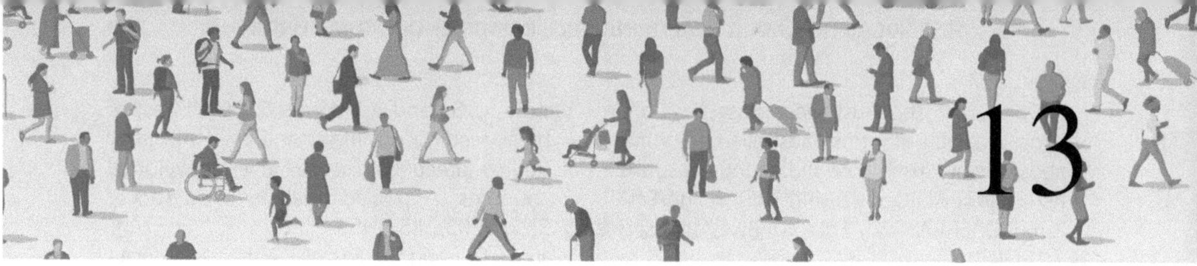

Refugees, Life in Host Communities, and the Health Challenges

Julia McDaniel, Andrea V. Shaw and Jok Madut Jok

INTRODUCTION

This chapter focuses on the health needs of refugees, mainly African refugees who have been resettled into new countries. In helping the refugees settle into a third country, after their perilous journeys of flight, many of the health professionals working with them lack information about these journeys and their impact on the refugees. Therefore, an understanding of these unique challenges that refugees face could improve the quality of care being provided to them. The chapter uses the experiences of African refugees resettled in Syracuse, New York, as a case study to illustrate many of these challenges. (For more information on the circumstances that caused Africans to seek refuge in the global north, see news reports on South Sudan, Democratic Republic of the Congo, and Somalia, as these are the countries most represented in the African refugee populations in Syracuse.) We focus predominantly on health and health care, concerns that the United Nations High Commission for Refugees (UNHCR), the World Health Organization (WHO) and refugee resettlement agencies in the recipient countries have identified as the most daunting area of refugee care, both for the refugees themselves and the providers who struggle with issues of culture, mental health and trauma that influence health-seeking behavior. Additionally, refugees face the social determinants of health risks, such as poor and unsafe housing and lack of transportation, as well as education, and socio-economic inequities (Kang et al., 2019; Love, 2020).

Each of this chapter's three co-authors has encountered these challenges in their work. The first author is a graduate student whose doctoral dissertation deals with refugee women's sexual and reproductive health. The second is a primary care physician who focuses on refugee family care. The third is a refugee who has lived and has navigated the minefields of the complex United States health care system and can attest to the challenges refugees confront every day in search for health.

The chapter reviews the literature on refugee health and the challenges therein, combined with the stories of how refugee families cope and come to terms with their new home in Syracuse, taken from our work. We chronicle the efforts of our physician colleague to care for these families and the personal reflections of the refugees who have managed to adjust to and even thrive in their new setting. We start with a general description of the health challenges that uniquely face refugees, with a view to understanding the circumstances of flight, and a description of the common types of health problems faced on arrival. Then we provide a historical context to the crisis of instability in parts of Africa that gives rise to refugee crises. Lastly, the chapter includes an account of the traumatic history of civil conflict in the new country of South Sudan as a refugee-sending country.

The UNHCR, a multinational agency mandated to aid and protect refugees, reports that more people than ever before have fled their homes in fear for their lives, becoming displaced either within their home countries or across national borders. Global agencies estimate that close to 79.5 million people worldwide have been forcibly displaced. Only 26 million fall in the category of "refugees," i.e., those who have crossed international boundaries seeking safety and registered with the United Nations (UN). The figure of 79.5 million includes registered refugees, registered asylum seekers, and internally displaced people, but fails to account for all migrants who are fleeing persecution or political/economic oppression, which suggests that these numbers underestimate the true global burden (UNHCR, 2020).

Four categories of people leave their traditional territories to seek protection: (1) refugees, (2) internally displaced persons (IDPs), (3) asylum-seekers, and (4) migrants. Their flight from their own regions or countries becomes necessary because their lives or livelihoods are threatened either by the governments or by other powerful groups attacking them or competing for control of resources in a given region.

The stories of each of these groups, however, are often horrific, extending over generations of abuse, racial, religious, or ethnic targeting. The factors forcing people to flee their homelands are many and varied. Many people often flee at a sharp and pointed moment following a long history of oppression. Others are compelled to flee under unspeakable duress, only choosing to leave after they have exhausted every effort to stay in their homes. An Iranian refugee, Dina Nayeri, fled Iran with her family but was forced to leave her father behind. She spent time as a refugee in the United Arab Emirates before being resettled in the United States. Her book chronicling her experiences relates that "…we were so unmoored it was hard to fathom a next step. Maybe that's why every move had been last minute, someone's kindness or a stroke of luck" (Nayeri, 2019: 3).

The stories of those who leave their home countries and enter a refugee camp in a second country are often two-fold. The first is their flight itself, what they saw and what prompted them to flee at that very moment and what they have had to endure along the way. Once they have reached safety, it is often this story of survival that many policy makers in the host country seem to sympathize with, often masking other stories that may be even more daunting to the refugee. The second is about their relatives, perhaps spouses or children, they have left behind in that moment of distress, possibly in an IDP camp. The stories of those left behind can easily become a serious mental and logistical burden on those who have made it across the border. Upon resettlement in a second or third country, the latter story may not be at the surface of the efforts to survive in the new home of refuge, but can be a source of emotional trauma for some refugees, who never stop thinking about those they have left behind. Care agencies are often incapable of resolving that grief, which such refugees may not even share with them, but may greatly affect the ability of the refugee to cope in the new homeland (Miller, 2017).

Table 13.1 Categories of individuals seeking refuge

Term	*Definition*
Refugees	In the 1951 Refugee Convention, a refugee is anyone with "a well-founded fear of being persecuted for reasons of race, religion, nationality, membership of a particular social group, or political opinion, and is thus unable or unwilling to return to their country of origin" (UNHCR, 1951). Those who hold this status of fear and seek protection from the UNHCR or equivalent organizations will be counted as refugees (UNHCR, 2020). Those who flee persecution and live or work in a setting that does not recognize their citizenship (i.e., "undocumented immigrant" in a bordering country) are socially equivalent, but are not counted or protected in the same manner. A refugee registered and counted by UNHCR is placed on a pathway to resettlement, a process that is not influenced or under the control of the individual. For refugees coming to the United States, this timeline is a minimum of two years, an average of a decade, and many times it is 10–20 years before a family is resettled. UNHCR will provide safety and meet basic needs, but the ultimate destination to be resettled in one of 25–35 countries accepting refugees on a given year is a decision made by the host country. In 2019, for every one refugee that was resettled to a third country, three refugees were repatriated to their home country (UNHCR, 2020). Ultimately, the desire to return home and take control of one's life and future outweighs the risk of often returning to face the persecution that one fled. The uncertainty of life in a refugee camp provides little ability to thrive or plan for a future; it is simply a place to survive. Once a country accepts a refugee for resettlement, they are guaranteed a legal path to citizenship (although requirements and supports are country-dependent).
Internally Displaced Persons (IDPs)	Internally Displaced Persons (IDPs) flee the same persecution, economic desperation due to destruction of their property, evisceration of their livelihoods, and dismantling of their social safety nets, but they remain within the borders of their home countries. IDPs have sought protection either with the United Nations or with non-governmental organizations (NGOs), are much more numerous than refugees, and often suffer just as much if not more. It is not always their choice to remain within their country, as their existence can be just as painfully hard as the one experienced by those who leave. Instead, they may be stuck in IDP camps because the choice of leaving is unattainable or obstructed by the circumstances that led to their displacement in the first place. Otherwise, their conditions are nearly identical to those of refugees. The word "refugee," despite its popular use, has a more practical, historically, and spatially contingent meaning, which is that it refers to people who have crossed an international border. And although we are using it in this chapter to refer to the more generic meaning of people who have sought refuge in another country, we would like the reader to keep in mind that refugees are just human beings who flee from terror. The difference between "refugees" and "IDPs" does not reflect the direness of the situations they find themselves in or the extent of their suffering, but rather occurs due to the circumstance of crossing or not crossing a national border. A few minutes of making it across the border in a moment of violent distress or being caught within the country is all it takes to create either refugees or IDPs. How the world's governments treat the refugees versus how they respond to IDPs is also a matter of international conventions and not a measure of the gravity of their circumstances. We mention this here to remind the reader that as we focus on refugees who have made it across a border, refugees may have family members who are IDPs who failed to escape their home country. Leaving loved ones behind may haunt the refugees throughout their journeys.
Asylum seekers	Asylum seekers are individuals who have crossed a border and are requesting legal status and sanctuary in the country in which they are claiming asylum (UNHCR, 2020). Asylum seekers have fled exactly the same circumstances as the refugee and IDP mentioned above, but have landed on the soil of the country they are requesting asylum from. In order to get to this country, by definition the asylum seekers have had sufficient means to travel to that location and need a way to support themselves until their case is reviewed. Without legal status, they are not eligible for most federal benefits in the United States. There are more than 40 countries who accept asylum cases, but not all countries do. Once an asylum case is processed, if this results in a denial, the individual does not have a legal pathway to exist in this country. The timeline for arrival in an accepting host country, filing an asylum case and hearing a decision on that case is often a faster process than the uncertain and prolonged period of time that an individual may remain in a refugee camp, but a final denial will not provide for a legal path forward. This is a risk any asylum seeker takes.
Migrants	Migrants are individuals who have migrated from their home country, often in pursuit of economic opportunity, but also frequently for reasons of persecution, as mentioned for the three parties above. Migrants are forced to provide for themselves as they live outside of a registered and documented system. They may be traveling through one country with a different destination in mind, or they may pursue an asylum case or request citizenship depending on the country they are in. Most are often opportunistically looking for employment to support themselves, their families, or relatives back home who are facing more dire circumstances. Their unofficial status may put them at risk for legal, health, and social concerns as they are not afforded the same rights as are other documented people.

The circumstances that cause a refugee to leave home, the experiences along the way, and the cultural beliefs and attitudes they have carried from their cumulative life experience all contribute to their health needs. Many have fled poorly developed health systems amid conflict and experienced minimal basic supports in a refugee camp, resulting in undiagnosed chronic conditions that cause more morbidity. A lot of education is needed to understand and manage such conditions in a western medicine model that is challenging to navigate for American-born individuals. Low rates of literacy and limited opportunity for education along these uncertain paths compounds low health literacy. Preventative health care is something very few refugees have been exposed to in the systems they come from. Years of experiencing trauma contribute to impaired mental and physical health. Others, once resettled in a third country but still with social and cultural disconnection, may also find themselves in ill health, especially because of the inability to rely on any familiar relations to address such health requirements (Cronkright & Lupone, 2018).

Despite the highest number of forcibly displaced people worldwide, more than 25 million are registered as refugees and awaiting resettlement. In 2019, less than 0.5% of those requesting resettlement were resettled (UNHCR, 2020), leaving millions of people to "survive" in a refugee camp for an uncertain future with little contribution to the local economy or society. In 2019, the Trump administration announced the lowest ceiling on refugee admissions of 18,000 in the financial year 2020, the lowest since the Refugee Act of 1980 (Fabi, 2020). In political debates over public funding used for refugee resettlement, xenophobia and racism have overshadowed the humanitarian call to support vulnerable persecuted populations. "The threat from radical Islamic terrorism is very real, just look at what is happening in Europe and the Middle-East. Courts must act fast!" (Phillips, 2017). Such statements have been used to support the executive orders that President Trump issued, which suspended the refugee program, indefinitely banning refugees from Iran, Iraq, Somalia, Sudan, Syria and Yemen, all of them citizens from majority-Muslim countries, from entering the US in 2017. These political displays stigmatize refugees who arrive with little more than what they can carry, have limited transferable skills after living a decade or more in a camp, and many families that do arrive rely on public assistance in the early years of assimilation. But there is plenty of data nationally (Bahar, 2018) and internationally (Maxmen, 2018) to show that host economies improve and unemployment rates drop where refugees are provided safe havens.

THE CHALLENGE OF CARING FOR REFUGEES

It is important to explain at the outset the nature of health and health care issues that face refugees and communities, agencies and persons who care for them. By reflecting on some of these factors in detail, as demonstrated in medical, public health literature and refugee studies journals, one can paint a clear picture about health as a challenge for refugees. Refugees are known to face the risks of falling sick in transition or while staying in new countries along the way to safety, due to poor living conditions with poor shelter and sanitation or changes in their lifestyle, such as inadequate nutrition and increased stress. Unaccompanied minors and women are at high risk of abuse as they are in vulnerable situations with limited protection during their flight. Apart from the traumatic events that lead to their departure from their homelands, often involving witnessing the death of loved ones and frequent experiences of torture, life in refugee camps in a second country before resettlement adds an uncertain period of time with limited access to health care for refugees in their flight (Gibson-Helm, 2014).

One of these health risks is sexual violence, especially intimate partner violence (IPV), which is a common form of sexual violence experienced by refugee girls and women. More broadly, the term "defines the abuse that occurs between two people in a relationship and includes acts of physical, sexual, and psychological violence committed by a current or former partner" (Wako et al., 2015, p. 1087). Recent standardized, multinational studies have looked at the "emotional, social, and physiological" effects of IPV. The studies revealed that IPV is linked to "a myriad of negative outcomes, including chronic pain, substance abuse, suicidal ideation, reduced sexual autonomy, sexual risk-taking, gynecological disorders, and sexually transmitted infections" (Wako et al., 2015, p. 1088). A 2008 population-based study of Congolese female refugees in two Rwandan refugee camps looked at IPV prevalence among conflict-affected communities. The study was conducted by the American Refugee Committee (ARC) at Gihembe and Nyabiheke refugee camps, where the ARC runs gender-based violence (GBV) prevention programs, mostly serving Congolese refugees. The results showed that "approximately one fifth of the women interviewed (20.1%) reported past year IPV, more than half (52.7%) reported experiencing outsider violence, and 6.4% reported having experienced family violence during the past year" (Wako et al., 2015, p. 1091).

One form of gender-based violence that displaced females may experience is engaging in sex acts in "exchange" for desperately needed food and supplies for their families. This exchange is referred to by researchers as "transactional sex." It is important to note that while many refugee women are forced, whether by family members, circumstances, and/or by patrons, into such sexual acts, other women actively choose to exercise their personal agency to engage in said sex acts. This can be considered an empowering activity where women are able to, for example, contribute to a joint family income and, for that, experience a good deal of pride. However, whether the sex acts are willingly or unwillingly preformed, the practice can result in the spread of sexually transmitted diseases, unintended pregnancy, physical and/or psychological harm, trauma, and other unintended outcomes (Mengesha et al., 2017). (Major news outlets around the world, from BBC, CNN, *The Guardian*, Al-Jazeera, Reuters and Associated Press, have reported extensively on refugees who become so desperate for a variety of needs that they resort to the sale of sex as a way to survive.)

During displacement, there is a strong correlation between transactional sex and the spread of sexually transmitted diseases. Displaced women in some African countries already face an increased risk of HIV contraction since 60% of people living with HIV live in sub-Saharan Africa. Tanaka et al. (2008) researched HIV prevention and HIV infection risk among Congolese refugees in the Nyarugusu refugee camp in Tanzania. The study found that the risk of contracting HIV increased after displacement since the number of refugees engaging in transactional sex increased. The transactional sex was mainly for money or gifts. The focus group discussions (FGD) revealed that transactional sex was common for women between the ages of 30 and 49. The main reason for engaging in such activity was to obtain food for one's family when food rations ran low. As one woman recounted:

> People don't eat well and don't dress properly. Some of us women in this camp, particularly during the period of Ndenga (when food rations from aid agencies run out and before the next distribution arrives), cannot help but leave our husbands inside the house and go out to perform sex in order to obtain food. These women don't know whether their casual partners are HIV infected or not, and when they come home could be directly contaminating their husbands. (Tanaka et al., 2008, p. 438)

While the cultural norms of various African refugee communities are for women to have many children, family planning is often encouraged in humanitarian settings and during resettlement. Still, cultural patterns prevail in these contexts and women continue to have children. Culturally-linked reasons as to why refugee women continue to have children include a need to create more sources of labor, replace lost children from former contexts of war and violence, and/or a desire to have a child born in the West during resettlement. Another instance for having more children is for food security. Since food security in refugee camps is a common concern, women are said to try to have as many children as possible since families are given a food ration card for each member of their family, whether the family member is a baby or an adult. Further, having more children is seen as a source of power among refugee families since that means more labor. As one refugee remarked, "Making many children, in our culture, creates power. For us, children are considered a source of labor. Most refugees arrived here after cruel displacement processes during which many children died" (Tanaka et al., 2008, pp. 441–442).

At the moment of flight, regardless of wherever they end up, as IDPs or in a refugee camp, all the displaced confront serious, often unspeakable distresses, especially with regards to maintaining their health, as their social and cultural networks, which would otherwise undergird the well-being of people, are also dislocated, along with the forced physical displacement. The very fact of their registration as a refugee has often demonstrated their exhaustion of social networks. For example, if they could flee to a neighboring country, stay with a relative and find a safe/legal future path, there would be no reason to face the limited security and unclear future of life in a refugee camp. Studies show that as refugees resettle in their countries of refuge, it is often the re-creation or rebuilding of a semblance of these networks that most preoccupy their minds – how to navigate and utilize the support networks that are offered by the host communities and how to connect with other refugees from the same countries of origin. Sometimes networks are formed because of a shared language and at other times because of the simple comfort of knowing people with a similar physical appearance, similar stories of flight and similar social roles that they once utilized but which they are now unable to use in the new environment (Chagos Refugee Group, 2018). Sometimes the highly traumatic social and political circumstances of flight leave newly resettled refugees seeking entirely different groups with which to recreate social networks, in order to avoid the constant reminders of the past that can re-trigger the traumatic stress from which they fled. Every individual processes traumatic experiences differently and has a unique path to healing, given their own socio-cultural circumstances.

After resettlement, refugees often seek to replicate socio-cultural roles in the new setting. Traditional roles of women transform in the context of forced migration. For instance, global Gender and Development (GAD) assistance programs and policies focus on women's empowerment by providing women access to personal funds, public services, and formal educational opportunities. However, this access to resources, in turn, "erod[es] men's role (as protectors, providers and decision makers, for example) and hence their social position and self-esteem..." (El-Bushra, 2000, p. 4). Moreover, during displacement in Western-run refugee camps and in resettlement, gender roles favoring equity are often encouraged or even forced on women, who sometimes prefer to maintain the traditional roles that they held prior to displacement. People often seek comfort by being connected to a history, a shared experience and intergenerational foundation. Being disconnected from family and from the familiar can be a major risk for depression and other mental health issues. Lastly, within the early years of resettlement, it is not uncommon for young children to overcome language barriers before their parents have the opportunity to do so, and this alters power dynamics in families and contributes to stress on parents and added responsibilities for children.

Once resettled after arriving in an unfamiliar country, refugees often have to spend a good amount of time dealing with issues of their legal status, navigating federal programs to support life at the poverty level, facing discriminatory policies and behaviors, all amid language barriers that make it more challenging to lead a productive healthy life. The US Government requires a Refugee Health Assessment (RHA) upon arrival into the country, which is focused on communicable disease (e.g., tuberculosis (TB), venereal disease), and is not unlike the Public Health Service screening at Ellis Island at the turn of the 20th century (Bateman-House & Fairchild, 2008). Although refugees arrive from many tropical climates with endemic infectious disease risks and, by definition, have a history of trauma, they are more likely to be diagnosed with a previously unrecognized chronic illness than either an infectious disease or mental illness upon arrival. These initial RHAs are set up to connect refugees to a primary care home which accepts their government-issued Medicaid insurance. When the initial months of survival are focused on accessing safe housing, food and social services enrollment, it is often a lower priority for refugees to learn a new model and system of health care unless they are feeling unwell (Berkowitz, 2016).

Refugees are more likely to be diagnosed with a chronic disease than any other infectious or mental health condition (Brown et al., 2020). It is felt that a life of cumulative stressors, poor living environments and subsequent adaptation to more sedentary lifestyles and new foods in the host country contributes to this situation. The complexity of the situation and the limited time refugee patients have to fully adapt to their new environment contributes to less understanding and knowledge of chronic disease and preventative health. This gap in understanding the complexity of the US health care system and possibly having different beliefs often means refugees fail to present for help until their illnesses have become chronic and they have suffered a great deal. Thus, refugee advocates emphasize the importance of making caregivers aware of this particular risk factor. Cancer is reportedly low among refugees, although it has been slowly increasing over the past decade. But when it occurs, it is more likely to be diagnosed at an advanced stage, which can lead to considerably worse health outcomes compared with the host population (Muecke, 1983). The delay in diagnosis is partly due to refugees' lack of familiarity with the formal health care system in the United States and the conflict between the expectations that refugees hold about the health system and beliefs and practices which refugee cultures present.

One reality about refugees is that they often come from countries where the health system is obliterated by war or inherently weak due to a lack of investment by the national government, including the training of personnel, poor facilities, and basic medication, or because corruption has diverted resources that were originally earmarked to improve national health systems. An extended transitional period in a refugee camp may have left refugees with access to a system designed to handle minor acute problems, but with little infrastructure for extensive health evaluation or chronic disease management. This means that by the time the refugees reach safety, they would have had to endure poor sanitation, contaminated water, poor feeding, and limited access to medication or medical care during the journey of refuge. Available health services are limited to public health services offered by the host country. Frontline health care workers may not be aware of the whole health experience during the dangerous migratory journey, so it is important for them to probe the risks for this population (Byrskog et al., 2014).

In 2019, the United Nations High Commissioner for Refugees (UNHCR) reported that there were an estimated 79.5 million individuals globally who were forcibly displaced from their homes (UNHCR, 2020). According to the data available, "51 per cent of the stateless population were women, and 48 per cent were children" (UNHCR, 2020, p. 60). "Data availability for stateless populations is scarce in most countries when it comes to disaggregation by demographic characteristics. In 2019, sex-disaggregated data was available for 28 of the 76 countries reporting on stateless populations, covering 73 per cent of the reported stateless population" (UNHCR, 2020, p. 60). Displaced populations as a whole are more susceptible to a range of illnesses and disease. Health complications include "malnutrition, anaemia, and infectious and parasitic diseases" (Correa-Velez & Ryan, 2012, p. 13). Furthermore, refugees and asylum seekers who are pregnant experience various complications in accessing maternity care during and after displacement. Pregnant refugee women are also susceptible to even more complications, such as "high parity, existing untreated complications related to pregnancy and childbirth, physical and emotional issues related to sexual violence" (Correa-Velez & Ryan, 2012, p. 13).

The trauma of refugee flight and its aftermath after resettling in a new country, has been documented widely (Sigvardsdotter et al., 2016). As described earlier, a particularly difficult issue in terms of the mental health of refugees is grief over loved ones who were unable or unwilling to leave, family members and friends who have "disappeared" or been killed by armed groups, or lost to starvation and disease during flight or in refugee camps prior to resettlement (Jenkins et al., 2002). Psychologist Kenneth Miller suggests that "threats to refugees' mental health extend well beyond exposure to potentially traumatic experiences of war-related violence," including, for example, "post-migration stresses present in the host setting, such as social isolation, poverty, unemployment, overcrowded and unsafe housing, and heightened family violence" (Miller, 2017). A history of an accumulation of traumatic experiences has been found to increase the risk for chronic medical conditions (Sledjeski, 2008). This does not mean that all survivors of traumatic events, such as war, are broken. At times, the focus on war-related Post Traumatic Stress Disorder overshadows the psychological power of resilience and positive experiences to smooth out the traumatic events.

For anyone providing holistic care to refugee patients, it is essential for them to take the time to understand where a refugee is from and where they have been, in addition to the social context in which they have been resettled, in order to support their health.

REFUGEES AND THE HISTORIES BEHIND THEIR FLIGHT

Regardless of their origin, refugees face similar threats that are now widely familiar to anyone who follows global political dynamics, the single most important of which is insecurity. While a significant number of refugees flee due to environmental and climate factors, or because of economic hardships, the vast majority of people who flee across the borders are forced out by socio-political factors such as war, human rights violations, war crimes, genocide and persecution. These include civil wars, violent crime, ethnic or individual targeting such as in cases of human trafficking, and of smuggling of illicit substances that turn violent when transactions go wrong. A brief historical context to the refugee "crisis" in Africa is important here, just to sift through and separate the popular generic descriptions of the reasons why sub-Saharan Africa is said to produce and send massive numbers of refugees to the global north. For example, it is true that countries like South Sudan, Somalia, and Congo are a source of refugees because of contemporary governance failures or ongoing rebellions. But a more rounded view is to look further back in history to the post-colonial states of some 60 years ago. The roots of the refugee problem may be found in the slave trade, colonial occupation and in the legacy of colonialism, long before the emergence of the post-colonial state. Historically, at least dating back 400 years to the slave trade, the trend is that movement was mostly in the direction of global south as European empire were, sending invasion armies, colonists, fortune seekers, missionaries and colonial administrators to Africa, most of it to the detriment of the welfare of the colonized people. The movement of refugees from the global south to the north is one of the few exceptions to this direction of flow.

Whereas the movement of Europeans to Africa was voluntary and invasive, the movement of Africans was forced, whether that was through the slave trade or wars or economic circumstances triggered by the long history of slavery, and imperial invasion or colonialization. However, the indigenous people in the global south were pushed out of their territories, pacified, and ruled, the actions of the colonizers, invaders and slave traders have always created terror, causing the affected people to leave their homes in order to escape violence, political persecution, criminal targeting or genocide (Pries, 2018). To become independent, many African countries had to fight long wars of liberation, provoking vicious colonial counter-insurgency tactics that were saturated with racism, leaving behind a legacy that continues to influence the post-colonial relationships. Racism and violent hegemonic power that were inherently built into colonialism were particularly venomous in creating the colonial state. Racist violence was extreme at the time of conquest, during enforcement of colonial rule and in response to decolonization efforts. The legacy of that history is political instability of the post-colonial state because it was structured in the image of the colonizer. It then proved extremely hard to sustain that structure without using the tools of coercion and violence that the colonizer had used to create the state by forcing ethnic nationalities that had been independent entities into polities that proved unworkable once the empire retreated. Civil wars ensued in many countries soon after decolonization and with them came the flight of Africans into refugee camps. The wars in Sudan, Somalia and Congo became the most spectacular in their destruction of human lives. African intra-state wars fanned by the Cold War geopolitics in Ethiopia and Angola in the 1970s and 1980s also were sources of massive numbers of refugees (Sommers, 2001).

In contemporary times, the plight of refugees is often depicted in the stories we watch on primetime news channels or read in the newspapers in the developed world. These sometimes arouse the pity and sympathy of people living in the global north, but only provoke questions in the minds of very few about the long history that created lopsided relations, where people from the developing world are seen as mere victims of their own local circumstances and the people in the developed world see themselves as saviors, unaware or unwilling to engage with the history of how the world, its people, its resources and its power hierarchies were ordered to the advantage of the global north so long ago. This is a story which is at least partly at the root of why so many Africans desire to migrate or seek refuge in Europe or North America (Davies, 2019).

Today, for example, the Democratic Republic of Congo, which, due to complex causes rooted in the history of the Belgian colonial system, sends out hundreds of thousands of refugees and has been doing so for over 30 years. Most of these fleeing Congolese end up in countries within Central and Eastern Africa, but many make it further, crossing oceans to settle as refugees in Europe and North America. Much of the story being told about their plight and flight focuses more on the political rivalries within the Congo, on the competing militias jockeying for both political power and control of Congo's immense mineral wealth (Human

Rights Watch, 2019). Focusing on these local dynamics, the global media and activist groups paint a simplistic picture of a country whose people have supposedly turned on each other and whose leaders are heartless thieves who are killing their own people over power and money, raping them and forcing them to flee their homeland (Global Conflict Tracker, 2020).

If this image may have a kernel of truth in it, told this way, the story has long ignored the roots of this misery, which are in the times of King Leopold II of Belgium, whose reign wreaked havoc in Congo between 1885 and 1908. The legacy of those times has continued to haunt this country, including the disastrous role of Mobutu Sese Seko's dictatorial reign (1965–97) in further dividing the country and looting its resources, making Congo, a resource rich country, become one of the poorest on the African continent (Hochschild, 1999). Mobutu was imposed on the people of Congo by Western countries, particularly the United States, which saw Congo as a battleground for their "war" with the Soviet Union. In that war, Mobutu became the man for the US, supported with weapons and intelligence, all to the detriment of the Congolese people. This invited foreign corporations to loot Congo's mineral resources in exchange for providing military support to Mobutu so he could continue to bully his people into supporting his government and providing access to foreign mining companies (Stearns, 2011). In other words, stories of African refugees that do not link this experience to the politics of a modern scramble for African minerals by Western corporations are only telling a fraction of a much bigger story. Even though these stories have roots in global politics, the global capitalist system, in racism, exploitation and abuse by colonizers, they are often told in ways that prejudice and cloud the image of Africans in the eyes of Europeans and Americans, such that even the few who make it through the refugee resettlement programs, essentially arrive in Europe or North America with negative stories about the supposed inhumanity of Africa hanging over them.

One might argue that the 107,800 refugees resettled among 26 countries in the global north in 2019 is a mere fraction of what might be owed to those countries, where historical instability involves previous relationships with these same countries.

SOUTH SUDAN AND THE REFUGEE CRISIS: A CASE STUDY

South Sudan's journey to independent statehood presents an illuminating case in terms of the complex web of events and experiences in that drive for freedom which produces refugees and how they cope. It exposes the role of certain global political events that may favor or disadvantage a particular group in terms of resettlement outside Africa. To demonstrate some of the main reasons why people flee their countries and risk the treacherous refugee path to safety, including the resettlement in the global north, it is important to explore the anatomy of the failure of the post-colonial state to reckon with fundamental racial, tribal and religious schisms that the colonial enterprise had sowed and nursed in Africa.

South Sudan is now the world's newest country, attaining its independence in 2011, after close to 192 years of struggle against various colonial hegemonies, from Ottoman Egypt's aspiration to control a large swathe of territory on the Upper Nile as fields from which to harvest slaves, to British Colonial rule, and to post-colonial Arab rule following the end of European empires. It was a long journey indeed, to becoming a sovereign and independent country. Its people fought many wars of resistance to hegemony. However, it was the last four decades of civil war, 1983–2011 and 2013–2020, that we are focusing on, as the main period in that long history which produced many people who became "refugees," so many of them young children, women and people who were rendered disabled by the brutalities of the civil war between Sudan and the people of South Sudan.

Let's start at the time of Sudan's independence from British rule in 1956. British rule had created Sudan out of an amalgam of ethnic nationalities but imposed different policies for the Arab and Muslim north and for the black African south, including concentrating development projects, education, and skills training in the north. But in the dismantling of the British Empire following World War II, the South Sudanese people did not want to remain in this artificial union called Sudan. (The word Sudan, the name of the country, is derived from Arabic Bilad A-Sudan, which means "land of the blacks." In the medieval times, when the word was first use, it is impossible to say whether it had the racial connotations. When the "Arabized Sudanese" began to apply the term, it had a double meaning, namely "the Sudan," the country, and "Aswad," black. In using the term, they synonymized it with the word "Abid," slave.) They saw independence as an end to British colonialism and a potential beginning of an Arab and Islamic colonialism over the south. They proposed various options that could solve the north–south divide, including asking the British to give independence to two countries, one northern and the other southern, instead of leaving behind a polity that was most definitely unviable, given the racism and Islamic bigotry with which the north had treated the south. When Britain left, Sudan plunged into a civil war that would last 17 years, kill half a million South Sudanese and send millions more as refugees to Ethiopia, Uganda, Congo, Central African Republic and other countries across Africa.

Race, specifically racism, had combined with Islam to justify the abduction and enslavement of South Sudanese people as far back as 1821, and it continued well into the British rule. It had played a role in why the British had favored the north during their rule. It should be noted that while the North Sudanese and South Sudanese would all be considered Black in the global north's colonial designation of "races," there is a long history of colorism, where Northerners with somewhat lighter skin tone see themselves as Arabs or Arabized and, based on their assumed superiority, they see Southerners as Black and inferior beings, fit for enslavement, in part justified by their darker coloring. On this basis, the British promoted what was a pre-colonial Arab prejudice in their communications with colonial administrators and in their correspondence with the Colonial Office in London. It manifested itself in how the colonial administrators addressed the "natives," as they called sub-Saharan Africans. Because of this history, there was ground for fear among South Sudanese people that the race and racism that had permeated the various periods of foreign rule were bound to become major factors in the way the more colonially developed north was going to relate to the south once the north took power from the British.

This structural racism was part of the basis for the south demanding a separate country. But the British, having come under pressure to turn to other geostrategic concerns, including the fate of the Suez Canal, hastily handed power over to the north without sorting out the mess they had created in structuring what was essentially two countries into one. The south revolted and the war lasted 17 years, during which time the Sudan Armed Forces (northern army) engaged in unspeakable atrocities in the south. The armies in garrison towns throughout the south applied race and religion as the lens to use in executing the counter-insurgency, just as much as the general northern public had been focused on racism against the south since 1821 when Sudan became a territory of Ottoman Egypt.

Throughout the first civil war 1955–72, the north imposed a near total media blackout and accurate war reportage was a challenge – almost as hard and dangerous as the war itself. For all practical purposes, South Sudan was persecuted in darkness, where no reports or images of atrocities were reaching the rest of the world. Hardly anyone bore witness to the tragedy, except for the dedication of a small number of southern print journalists who committed themselves in the 1960s to bringing the news of the suffering in the region to the attention of the rest of the world. These included reporters for *The Vigilant* and *The Grass Curtain*. Both publications had dedicated themselves to documenting the atrocities taking place at the hands of Sudan Armed Forces stationed in southern garrison towns of Juba, Bor, Malakal, Wau, Aweil, among other areas. Stories of chiefs massacred in Bor, families attacked at a wedding in Wau, attempts to exterminate all the educated South Sudanese in Juba, and mass burials of victims in wells or drowning in rivers all across South Sudan, were just but a few examples of what these publications documented.

There was one very rare film recording made in Equatoria and Bahr el Ghazal by Allan Reed, an American working for the United States Agency for International Development (USAID), in 1971. This makes clear the brutality with which Khartoum had conducted its counter-insurgency, the level of suffering inflicted on the civilians, and the resourcefulness of the southern separatist fighters of that time. The latter's ability to use their meager and rudimentary military supplies to score victories against the well-equipped armed Sudan government forces stood as testament to the level of objective determination to achieve set political goals. This was done without any form of mass media, but through village-to-village mobilization for the war, for the civilians to commit to shouldering the cost of the war and for the political objectives to remain clear. Much less violence was meted out against the civilians in support of war than the Southern Peoples' Liberation Army (SPLA) would do many decades later. The lesson in this history is that documentation of war crimes is a very difficult endeavor, but one that needs to be included in the story of refugees. Then the care agencies in refugee-receiving countries can use these stories to nuance images of refugees as people who come from established lives of their own, which they would not have abandoned had they not been in danger, instead of the prejudiced view that some political leaders propagate for short-term political gains.

During the second civil war in Sudan (1983–2005), two and half million South Sudanese perished through a combination of starvation, due to food blockades, disease, due to the destruction of health facilities, direct combat and a system designed to deny the southern fighters any support base within the south but attacking, killing, displacing and abducting women, young adult males and children for sale into slavery in the north (Jok, 2001).

The Sudan army's war strategy against southern freedom fighters was a mix of the old tactics of hitting at the civilian population – as the fighters came from these communities that were being targeted – to wiping them out, as the more people they could displace the less viable was the opposition's army. But the result was the destruction of property, the maiming of people, the raping of women, and other atrocities. In particular, the approach seemed to operationalize a cultural ethos that sees women as the moral guardians of the society's customs and beliefs and the honor of the community. It appeared that the northern army's leaders believed that the quickest way to humiliate the southern fighters and potentially dislodge them from the south or force them to surrender was to go after "their women." According to this belief and practice, part of the way to defeat an enemy is to attempt to emasculate them, and what better way to do so than to attack, rape and abduct their women?

Another war tactic employed by Sudan's army was the use of the racial and religious identity of the soldier to imbue them with a sense of superiority in terms of intelligence, physical strength and Islamic fervor in defense of Umma, the Islamic state. Various televised or radio-broadcasted army programs, such *Saha al-Fida*, fields of martyrdom, showed Sudan's soldiers in the battlefields of South Sudan, appearing victorious over *Abid* (Arabic for slaves), and this excited many young people to join *Jesh al-Umma*, the nation's defense force, for the killing of *kufar* (Arabic for infidels), during *jihad* (Arabic for holy war) earns the fighter a place in heaven.

This war, fought with such disregard for the Geneva Code of the international laws of war, sent nearly 4 million people into refugee and IDP camps, especially in Uganda, Kenya, and Ethiopia, and even further afield, in Egypt, where some of them sought resettlement in the US, Canada, Australia, New Zealand and in some European countries. There are now about 20,000 South Sudanese in the US, including 4,000 young men and women who were brought there around 1999 from Kakuma refugee camp in northern Kenya. These people had traversed East Africa as part of a group of 100,000 children who had traveled to Ethiopia in late 1980s fleeing war and searching for education. They were recruited and trained by southern liberation fighters but were not deployed for combat. When the dictatorial government of Ethiopia, known as the *derg*, which had hosted and supported South Sudan's liberation fighters, was toppled in 1991, many fled Ethiopia, back into Sudan and were met with Sudan's air force attacking them from the sky. They dispersed in different directions, some dying along the way from hunger, or drowning while trying to cross rivers, or eaten by wild animals. The survivors in this group made it to Kakuma, becoming known as "Lost Boys of Sudan," many of whom were eventually resettled in Syracuse, NY.

Once in the US, the South Sudanese refugees were finally physically safe from the state violence that Sudan's government had exercised, but found themselves battling with similar issues they had experienced in Sudan. African refugees in America, because of the limited resources available to them in their new country, end up in low-income neighborhoods, often predominantly inhabited by people of color who are also marginalized within their own country, or by other refugees from Asia, Eastern Europe or the Middle East. These neighborhoods that take refugees tend to have a relatively higher crime rate than White areas, a greater police presence, rundown housing, and poor business climates, where supermarkets are few and far in-between and employment opportunities are very rare. This means refugees also step into a space that is already racially, socially and economically segregated, often trapping these would-be new Americans into an already volatile situation, sometimes triggering the trauma of war and the poverty of the refugee camps from which they came. The discrepancy between their expectations of life in the US and the realities they find only combines with social isolation, cultural dislocation, the trauma of war and refuge, and separation from family and community to create a burden that affects their health, physical and mental.

Perhaps the exception to this sense of disappointment that so many South Sudanese felt was the lost boys, for these young men were placed with host families who took them in as their adopted children and they almost all excelled in education, getting graduate degrees and finding well-paid jobs. They were then able to transfer money to the families they left behind in Kakuma or back home once the war of liberation ended and South Sudan became an independent state. Others, once resettled in a third country but still with social and cultural disconnection, may find themselves in ill health, especially because of their inability to rely on any familiar relations to address such health requirements (Cronkright & Lupone, 2018).

On the whole, most South Sudanese refugees in America have struggled in terms of finding a solid footing as first-generation immigrants. They are scattered across the US, although there are large communities in US cities like Chicago, Syracuse, San Diego, Sioux Falls, Rochester in Minnesota, Omaha and Lincoln in Nebraska, and Greensborough in North Carolina. The communities face challenges accessing quality health care, including mental health services, and cope with alcohol addiction, teenage delinquency, violence and school drop-out. Why are these things happening? It is easy to see structural racism that affects people of color at play in the case of refugees as well. But Africans don't seem to talk much about race in America because the concept, while prevalent in colonial times, was not part of their contemporary experience before arriving in America. Instead, they tend to see the racial issues that structurally undergird access to health care, education, employment and the justice system as consequences of being new Americans, who are not sufficiently prepared to succeed in this environment. Their history needs to be understood properly by care agencies so these health issues, violence and addiction can be explored from the perspective of the influence of their journeys in their ability to cope with the new setting.

REFUGEES IN SYRACUSE, NEW YORK

The city of Syracuse in Onondaga County, New York State, is a designated "refugee-friendly" city. Syracuse is the fifth largest city in New York State, with a 2018 population of 142,749. The 2018 medium household income is $36,308 compared to the national household income of $63,179, and 31.8% of the residents live at or below the federal poverty level compared to the national average of 11.8%. The city is comprised of 55% European Americans, 29.7% African Americans, 9.3% Hispanic or Latino, 6.8% Asian Americans, 8% Native Americans, and 5.4% who have two or more racial ancestries (US Census Bureau, 2020). Syracuse is classified by the Office of Refugee Resettlement as a "preferred community for refugee resettlement" for the "availability of jobs, affordable housing, receptivity of the local community, specialized services, and the strength of the local agencies including Catholic Charities of Onondaga County and Interfaith Works" (Miller et al., 2016, p. 485). In 2018, of the 1,139 refugees who were resettled in upstate New York, 223 resettled in Onondaga County (Bureau of Refugee Services, 2018). In the past 10 years, Syracuse has welcomed over 7,000 refugees from over 25 countries (New American Economy, 2017). Currently 13.3% of the city's residents are foreign born. They come from such disparate origins as Syria and Iraq, Afghanistan, Nepal, Burma, Somalia, Sudan, South Sudan and Congo. They arrive with a mix of experiences that range from the brokenness of their social relations to language barriers to the unimaginably complex health problems resulting from both the trauma that expelled them from their countries and prolonged illnesses that were not attended to in refugee camps.

The social influences on health are reflective of the population of origin. Additional social influences pile on from the circumstances of their flight and life in a refugee camp. The average refugee family spent a decade in a refugee camp prior to resettlement. While refugee camps are designed to provide safety, there is little room to support growth, development, health, education, and careers. For a young teenager fleeing war, a refugee camp is not a place where educational opportunities abound. For the business owner whose livelihood and savings were destroyed back home, a refugee camp hardly provides an opportunity to restart. For the fractured families who have exhausted linkages to familial supports and find themselves stateless, a refugee camp offers survival supports. Refugee families flee persecution. When they have exhausted a safe means of survival, they turn to a life of being counted, being granted "temporary structures" that may become home for years, of monthly food rations, and limited opportunity for education and health services, all underwritten by an uncertain time when they may be granted a safe future in one of a list of countries whose political leaders will determine their opportunities. Lack of influence over their future and lack of control over their destiny leaves many refugee families with years of uncertainty, layering stress onto family heads who cannot help but feel responsible. The accumulation of stress, with inadequate social or health supports, leads to higher risk for chronic non-communicable diseases (e.g., cardiovascular disease and diabetes) and mental illness in the future. Forty percent of our adult refugee patients settled into Syracuse have not had enough formal education to be literate in their native tongue. Despite these odds that set them up for challenges, these families are resilient. Many come with an attitude that despite the hell they have survived, they are here for the next generation. Their children are repeatedly top performers in city schools and their parents are often more entrepreneurial than the average American family.

While the challenges that face refugees, their host communities and the people who struggle to look after them are immense, they are not unsurmountable. The refugees have proven industrious and are able to transform communities where they settle, making both the moral and the legal case for the appeal of refugee resettlement. The 2030 UN Sustainable Development Goal Agenda recognizes the positive contributions of refugees and migrants for inclusive growth and sustainable development. In Syracuse, resettled refugees boost the local economy by taking jobs in industries like manufacturing and wholesale trade, and by starting their own businesses. In 2014, 1,681 individuals from the refugee and immigrant communities in Syracuse owned their own businesses, collectively earning over $22 million in income. In the years since then, more refugee-owned businesses have opened, most of which were restaurants and convenience stores. Furthermore, in 2014, foreign-born Syracuse residents contributed $1.7 billion to Syracuse's GDP, $89.2 million to Social Security, and $22.4 million to Medicare (New American Economy, 2017).

As the fields of resettled refugee health and health care expand in the West, refugee health trends and statistics are examined to better understand and improve health care for this growing and unique demographic. In Syracuse, two groups have studied the "healthy immigrant effect" on low birth weight and preterm births among immigrants and refugees (Krishnakumar et al., 2011; Miller et al., 2016). The healthy immigrant effect or paradox is defined as a "phenomenon by which immigrants experience more positive health outcomes than the native-born population in developed countries. The strength of this effect appears to be related to country of origin, health outcome, health-care and integration policies of receiving countries, as well as immigration class" (Miller et al., 2016, p. 484). Therefore, the effect looks not only at the health of the refugees before or after resettlement but at a wide amalgamation of various health and social factors from both pre- and post-resettlement periods. The study notes that the healthy immigrant effect has been shown to apply to "a variety of health domains: overall mortality rate, mental health, obesity, and perinatal outcomes such as infant mortality and the incidence of low birth weight and preterm infants" (Miller et al., 2016, p. 484). Further, the effect is "paradoxical" because most immigrants and refugees in the US have lower socio-economic status and thus would presumably have the same health issues associated with other individuals of lower socio-economic status, including fewer "health-promoting behaviors" such as poor diet and exercise. However, the studies ultimately found that infants born to foreign-born parents had less low birth weight than their native-born counterparts (Krishnakumar et al., 2011) and those "born to both foreign-born women and to women from refugee countries had decreased risks of being born preterm compared to infants born to US mothers, controlling for race, late/no prenatal care, maternal age less than 18 years and smoking" (Miller et al., 2016, p. 487).

Potential explanations for these positive birth outcomes include the fact that most refugees who are able to be resettled are usually the younger and healthier members of refugee communities. Additionally, more foreign-born women than US-born women would receive prenatal care, which could be due to the fact that Syracuse, a designated refugee-friendly city, offers a good deal of gratuitous public health care resources for refugees. For instance, refugees have a preliminary health assessment within their first 30 days in Syracuse. Pregnant refugees "are scheduled for prenatal care and typically have their initial visit within 2 weeks, and their appointments are usually scheduled at health centers where interpretive services are available" (Miller et al., 2016, p. 490). Pregnant women also have access to the Syracuse Healthy Start (SHS) program for a variety of pregnancy resources.

The researchers reported that the reasons some foreign-born women did not seek prenatal care were because of preferences for "alternative medicine includ[ing] unfamiliarity with a new healthcare system, general illness, desire to continue traditional practices, and cultural bereavement (i.e., the experience of the uprooted person and loss of old sense of self, social structures, cultural values and meaning)" (Miller et al., 2016, p. 490). Furthermore, general reported health and health care difficulties in refugee pregnancy and childbirth in Syracuse appear to result from complications in patient–provider communication, emotional challenges associated with their previous experiences of refugee flight, injury, and loss of family members.

Sandra Lane discusses how she launched Syracuse Healthy Start (SHS), a branch of the federal Healthy Start program, in 1997, when she worked for the Onondaga County Health Department. To do this, she leveraged anthropological fieldwork to understand community views on maternal and infant mortality in Syracuse. One of the core issues from Lane's findings was that health for women of color in Syracuse is a bigger issue than health care access, since health care does not fix the various other "disease-inducing environments" that are created from systemic racism and the larger structural violence. She adds that:

> Syracuse, a city of fewer than 150,000 residents, has five hospitals providing world-class medical care. Three of these hospitals have labor and delivery services and two feature neonatal intensive care units. Yet, within 2 miles of these sophisticated medical facilities are neighborhoods that have some of the highest rates of infant death in the United States. Clearly, we need to look beyond the clinic and hospital to the neighborhoods, schools, correctional facilities, and policies that create the context in which actual lives are lived. (Lane, 2009, pp. 2–3)

Another key issue that she discovered is that discrimination has many intersecting layers: "discrimination based on poverty and on gender, race, and ethnicity overlaps but it is not the same. Women and people of color with financial resources can afford better health care, food, and homes, but their resources cannot entirely protect them" (Lane, 2009, p. 10).

Another recurring finding from her fieldwork is that responsibility for health and disease should not solely be attributed to individual-level behavior as social determinants and traumatic histories greatly increase poor health and survival even among those with positive health habits. As Lane found, "unsafe, sickness-inducing environments are hard to overcome. History matters and place matters; the context in which people live – their neighborhoods as well as their culture and social institutions – shapes their health behavior" (Lane, 2009, p. 10). Refugees and immigrants settled into this concentrated poverty in Syracuse and with adverse health consequences for these minority communities that are well documented (Central New York Community Foundation, 2018).

CONCLUSION

This chapter has attempted to highlight the health challenges that face refugees once they are resettled in the United States. We have tried to relate these health crises to the violence, the trauma and their memories of flight from countries suffering from war. We have discussed the cultural and social dislocation that accompanies physical displacement from home and how this dislocation causes a constant search for opportunities to recreate the order that used to give meaning to life back in their home countries. Using a social science perspective to tell this story, we aim to arm health providers with an insight into the lives of refugees so that their efforts to assist them do not run into conflict with the perceptions held by the host communities. There is a lot of basic support provided by host communities and public resources, from health insurance through Medicaid to basic food and housing for refugees upon resettlement. The challenge is often one of limited capacity to communicate across cultural barriers between refugees and providers within a system that is very foreign.

In sum, the psychological burden the refugees carry with them due to the perilous circumstances they flee from, low health literacy from prior experiences, lack of exposure to a western medicine model in their previous communities, and a biocultural view of medicine held by many refugee families may raise challenges for providing care to meet the health needs of refugee populations. If health professionals are to be of maximum help to their refugee patients, it is vital that they acquaint themselves as much as possible with their patients' background and circumstances. We recommend that they take on board the history of refugee flight, their views of what they have lost during their movement, and the social and cultural perspective on the host community and vice versa. Schools of health education in the US should continue to incorporate programs that train providers on social medicine and trauma-informed care, to better understand how the social and historical fabric of their patients impacts the health of globally-diverse resettled refugees assimilating into this country.

REFERENCES

Bahar, D. (2018). Why accepting refugees is a win-win-win formula. *Brookings*, June 19. www.brookings.edu/blog/up-front/2018/06/19/refugees-are-a-win-win-win-formula-for-economic-development/ (accessed January 21, 2021).

Bateman-House, A., and Fairchild, A. (2018). Medical examination of immigrants at Ellis Island. *Virtual Mentor* 10(4), 235–241.

Berkowitz, S.A., Fabreau, G.E., Raghavan, S., Kentoffio, K., Chang, Y., He, W., Atlas, S.J., and Percac-Lima, S. (2016). Risk of developing diabetes among refugees and immigrants: a longitudinal analysis. *Journal of Community Health* 41(6), 1274–1281.

Brinlee, M. (2017). "27 outrageous things President Trump actually said." *Bustle*, www.bustle.com/p/27-real-things-trump-has-actually-said-since-becoming-president-37189 (accessed January 21, 2021).

Brown, B., Ramaiya, A., and Cronkright, P. (2020). Chronic disease management. In A. Anamalai (Ed.), *Refugee Health Care* (2nd edition, pp. 143–168). Cham, Switzerland: Springer.

Bureau of Refugee Services. (2018). *Population Data for FFY 2018*. https://otda.ny.gov/programs/bria/documents/population-report.pdf.

Byrskog, U., Olsson, P., Essén, B., and Allvin, M.K. (2014) Violence and reproductive health preceding flight from war: accounts from Somali born women in Sweden. *BMC Public Health* 14, 892. https://doi.org/10.1186/1471-2458-14-892.

Central New York Community Foundation. (2018). How the history of Redlining and I-81 contributed to Syracuse poverty. *CNY Vitals*, https://cnyvitals.org/how-the-history-of-redlining-and-i-81-contributed-to-syracuse-poverty/ (accessed, January 21, 2021).

Chagos Refugee Group. (2018, August 5). *How to Help Refugees Cope with the New Environment*. https://chagosrefugeesgroup.org/2018/08/05/how-to-help-refugees-cope-with-the-new-environment.

Correa-Velez, Ignacio, and Ryan, Jennifer. (2012). Developing a best practice model of refugee maternity care. *Women and Birth* 25(1), 13–22.

Cronkright, P., and Lupone, C.D. (2018). Emotional distress, medical utilization, and disability claims in adult refugees. *Journal of Immigrant and Minority Health* 20(2), 339–344.

Davies, T. (2019). Ruins of empire: refugees, race and the postcolonial geographies of European migrant camps. *Geoforum* 102, 214–217.

El-Bushra, J. (2000). Gender and forced migration. *Forced Migration Review* 9, 4–7.

Fabi, R., Serwer, D., Singh, N.S., Persad, G., Spiegel, P., and Rubenstein, L. (2020). Determining the number of refugees to be resettled in the United States: an ethical and policy analysis of policy-level stakeholder views. *Journal of Immigrant and Refugee Studies*. Published online: https://doi.org/10.1080/15562948.15562020.11747670.

Gibson-Helm, Melanie et al. (2014). Maternal health and pregnancy outcomes among women of refugee background from African countries: a retrospective, observational study in Australia. *BMC Pregnancy and Childbirth* 14(1), 392.

Global Conflict Tracker. (2020). *Violence in the Democratic Republic of Congo*. Council on Foreign Relations. https://www.cfr.org/global-conflict-tracker/conflict/violence-democratic-republic-congo (accessed August 20, 2020).

Hochschild, A. (1999). *King Leopold's Ghost: A Story of Greed, Terror, and Heroism in Colonial Africa*. New York: Houghton Mifflin.

Human Rights Watch. (2019). *Democratic Republic of Congo: Events of 2018*. New York: HRW World Report.

Jenkins, J.H., Kesler, J., Stevenson, J., and Westermeyer, J. (2002). Measuring trauma and health status in refugees: a critical review. *JAMA* 288, 611–621.

Jok, J.M. (2001). *War and Slavery in Sudan*. Philadelphia, PA: University of Pennsylvania Press.

Kang, C., Tomkow, L., and Farrington, R. (2019). Access to primary health care for asylum seekers and refugees: a qualitative study of service user experiences in the UK. *British Journal of General Practice* 69(685), e537–e545. https://doi.org/10.3399/bjgp19X701309.

Krishnakumar, A., Lane, S., Hall, M., Tso, E., Pinto, N., Suk, W., Oberoi, N., Selabi O., and Badawy, Z. (2011). The paternal component of the "healthy migrant" effect: fathers' natality and their infants' low birth weight. *Maternal and Child Health Journal* 15(8), 1350–1355.

Lane, S. (2009). Applying global health lessons to Syracuse, New York. In D. Perlman and A. Roy (Eds.), *The Practice of International Health* (pp. 148–175). Oxford: Oxford University Press.

Love, C. (2020). Welcoming the stranger: refugees in America. *MEDILL Reports Chicago*, https://news.medill.northwestern.edu/chicago/welcoming-the-stranger-refugees-in-america/.

Maxmen, A. (2018). Migrants and refugees are good for economies. *Nature News*, www.nature.com/articles/d41586-018-05507-0 (accessed January 21, 2021).

Mengesha, Z.B., Perz, J., Tinashe, D., and Ussher, J. (2017). Refugee and migrant women's engagement with sexual and reproductive health care in Australia: a socio-ecological analysis of health care professional perspectives. *PLoS One* 12(7). https://doi.org/10.1371/journal.pone.0181421.

Miller, K. (2017). What do refugees leave behind? Loss, grief, and healing among people displaced by war. *Psychology Today*, May 1. https://www.psychologytoday.com/us/blog/the-refugee-experience/201705/what-do-refugees-leave-behind (accessed May 18, 2021).

Miller, L.S., Robinson, J.A., and Cibula, D.A. (2016). Healthy Immigrant Effect: preterm births among immigrants and refugees in Syracuse, NY. *Maternal and Child Health Journal* 20(2), 484–493.

Muecke, M.A. (1983). Caring for Southeast Asian refugee patients in the USA. *American Journal of Public Health* 73(4), 431–438.

Nayeri, D. (2019). *The Ungrateful Refugee: What Immigrants Never Tell You*. New York: Catapult.

New American Economy. (2017). *New Americans in Buffalo and Syracuse*. New York: Partnership for a New American Economy Action Fund.

Phillips, K. (2017). "Radical Islamic terrorism," Trump said over and over. But not in Saudi Arabia. *The Washington Post*, May 22. www.washingtonpost.com/news/the-fix/wp/2017/

05/22/radical-islamic-terrorism-trump-said-over-and-over-but-not-in-saudi-arabia/ (accessed January 21, 2021).

Pries, L. (2018). *Refugees, Civil Society and the State: European Experiences and Global Challenges*. Cheltenham, UK: Edward Elgar.

Sigvardsdotter, E., Malm, A., Tinghög, P., Vaez, M., and Saboonchi, F. (2016). Refugee trauma measurement: a review of existing checklists. *Public Health Reviews* 37(1), doi:10.1186/s40985-016-0024-5.

Sledjeski, E.M., Speisman, B., and Dierker, L.C. (2008). Does number of lifetime traumas explain the relationship between PTSD and chronic medical conditions? Answers from the National Comorbidity Survey-Replication (NCS-R). *Journal of Behavioral Medicine* 31(4), 341–349.

Sommers, M. (2001). *Fear in Bongoland: Burundi Refugees in Urban Tanzania*. Oxford, UK: Berghahn Books.

Stearns, J. (2011). *Dancing in the Glory of Monsters: The Collapse of The Congo and the Great War of Africa*. Philadelphia, PA: Public Affairs.

Tanaka, Y., Kunii, O., Hatano, T., and Wakai, S. (2008). Knowledge, Attitude, and Practice (KAP) of HIV prevention and HIV infection risks among Congolese refugees in Tanzania. *Health & Place* 14(3), 434–452.

UNHCR. (1951). *The 1951 Refugee Convention*. Available at: www.unhcr.org/1951-refugee-convention.html (accessed October 26, 2020).

UNHCR. (2020). *UNHCR – Global Trends 2019: Forced Displacement in 2019*. New York: UNHCR Global Trends 2019. www.unhcr.org/globaltrends2019/ (accessed October 26, 2020).

US Census Bureau. *Syracuse, New York [Internet]*. (2018). [cited February 21, 2020]. Available at: www.census.gov/quickfacts/fact/table/syracusecitynewyork/RHI125218#RHI125218

US Census Bureau. (2020). *Syracuse City, New York. The United States Census Bureau*. www.census.gov/quickfacts/syracusecitynewyork (accessed April 24, 2020).

Wako, E., Elliott, L., De Jesus, S., Zotti, M., Swahn, M., and Beltrami, J. (2015). Conflict, displacement, and IPV: findings from two Congolese refugee camps in Rwanda. *Violence Against Women* 21(9), 1087–1101.

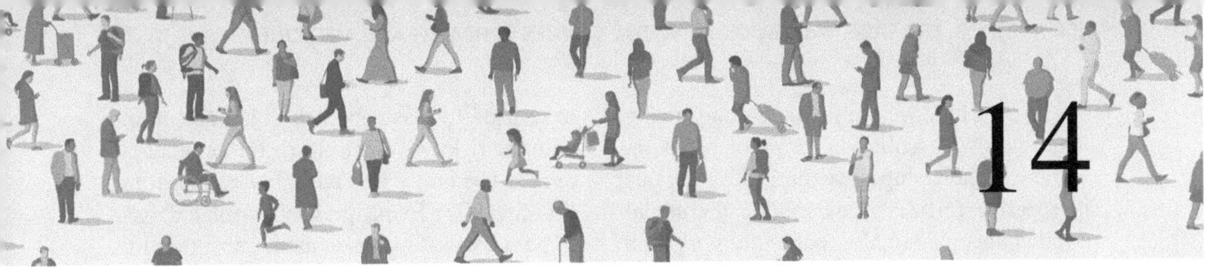

14

Gender and Health

Humayra Mayat, Mariel Rivera, and Sandra D. Lane

INTRODUCTION

This chapter addresses the influence of gender on health from both social science and public health perspectives. The major organizing theme is the interplay of the cultural patterning of gender and the biomedical outcomes that can result. Gender influences life-cycle roles and choices, notably those surrounding reproduction, but it also influences less obvious phenomena such as aging and survival. Gender minorities, including transgender people, also face significant barriers to health care that result in major health disparities within their populations. Rather than an exhaustive listing of the available data, this chapter utilizes case studies, both international and domestic, to illustrate many of the ways that gender influences health. An important caveat is that cross-culturally and within individual cultures, tremendous variation is the norm.

APPROACHES TO THE STUDY OF GENDER, SEX, AND HEALTH

Gender studies have proliferated enormously, but this wealth of published literature has produced more questions than definitive answers. In part, this confusion results from the different premises that scholars bring to the subject. Two main approaches characterize the study of gender and health. The first seeks to understand how culture shapes gender roles, and therefore health perceptions, policy, and research questions; the second relies on epidemiological or clinical measurements of health status, morbidity, and mortality.

Beginning with Mead's landmark studies, *Sex and Temperament in Three Primitive Societies* (1935) and *Male and Female: A study of sexes in a changing world* (1949), anthropological studies have demonstrated how gender roles vary greatly in human societies, and that there is little we can say that is universally feminine or masculine in terms of behavior. Feminist scholarship since the 1970s took this perspective further by examining the social disadvantage of females, particularly women and girls, in the West (di Leonardo 1991).

In much of the social science literature, current understandings distinguish between sex and gender, with sex referring to the biological categories of male and female and gender to the roles into which societies socialize men and women (Los Rios and Gomez 1991; Whitehead and Conaway 1986). This distinction has heuristic value in feminist scholarship, particularly in the many studies of women's social roles that have proliferated (see, for example, Bonvillain 1998; Morgen 1989). The distinctions between sex and gender are also essential in our later discussion on health concerns facing the transgender population. In terms of health, however, it is difficult to separate those aspects governed by social roles from those intricately tied to biomedical health risks. Culturally-patterned gender expectations – such as the drive to be thin – do influence health behavior and health status; for example, some 90% of anorexia nervosa sufferers are female (Leutwyler 1998). Thus, there is utility in understanding gender-influenced illness within a cultural context. However, this can also be harmful to those outside the commonly represented demographic. For example, understanding eating disorders as "female problems" can thus serve as a barrier for correctly diagnosing and treating males in a timely manner. A study from the United Kingdom found that the framing of eating disorders initially led to a failure for many of the men in the study to recognize their behaviors as an illness (Räisänen and Hunt 2014). As a result, many of their habits were already firmly entrenched before they finally sought treatment and this made the habits more difficult to reform.

Social gender norms also shape the context in which individual health behaviors are enacted and the range of choices available (Lane and Millar 1987). Some authors have tried to tease apart the biomedical and cultural risks by controlling for pregnancy-related morbidity and mortality. Fortney and Smith (1997) found pregnancy-related risks to be increased by inadequate transportation, which is a social determinant. It seems at least possible that if men could die of pregnancy risks, emergency transportation might be more available to prevent such tragedies.

Clearly, both culturally-patterned gender behavior and biologically-based risks interact to produce health or illness. Few studies, however, link the examination of the cultural and political construction of gender with rates of actual morbidity and mortality. Some landmark studies that do link the sociocultural, political, epidemiological, and clinical aspects of gender and health are Lock's work on menopause in Japan and in the United States (Lock 1986, 1993) and Inhorn's analysis of infertility in Egypt (Inhorn 1993, 1996). Lock shows that many of the salient features of menopause in the United States, notably hot flashes, do not even have linguistic correlates in Japanese. Inhorn demonstrates that the cultural imperative to have children becomes a quest for infertile women, who undergo expensive and risky treatments in their hope of conceiving.

Within the analysis of how culture shapes gendered health experiences are several overlapping areas of concern. A number of authors address the influence of culturally-defined gender roles on health-promoting behaviors and seeking health-related information. Women's responsibility, in most societies, for the nutrition, health promotion, and hygiene of their families may influence them to take better care of their own health. One study from Canada found that women were more likely to seek information about chronic health diseases like diabetes, obesity and mood disorders than their male counterparts. The study also found that women were more likely to engage in wellness screenings like annual blood pressure checks than their male counterparts (Deeks et al. 2009). Furthermore, a cross-sectional study from

Patrão and colleagues (2017) from Brazil found that women were also more likely than men to pursue healthier lifestyles. Lifestyle in the study was measured as a summation of four variables: tobacco use, alcohol consumption, physical exercise, and nutrition. The influence of social support on both overall health and the pursuit of health-promoting behavior is also a potential factor as women tend to have stronger social supports than men (Denton et al. 2004). In rural Egypt, gender and age were found to influence women's sick-role behavior and access to costly biomedical care (Lane and Meléis 1991; Morsey 1978). Egyptian *baladi*, women's illness stories, as recounted by Early (1993), bring to life the women's struggles to obtain health care for themselves and for their children.

Critical medical anthropology assesses biomedicine as a cultural system, dissecting biomedical discourse and questioning both the categories into which biomedical knowledge is sorted and the increasing use of technology to control women's bodies. Martin (1987) analyzes the language in medical textbooks, in which the female reproductive cycle is described in terms of failure, waste, and loss, whereas male reproductive function is depicted in robustly positive terms. An edited volume on *Gender and Health: An International Perspective* (Sargent and Brettell 1996) presents articles on the cultural construction of premenstrual and menopausal syndromes (Davis 1996) and the hegemony of technology in women's birth choices (Davis-Floyd 1996), which are covered in greater depth in Chapter 24 of this volume by Davis-Floyd and Lim. As the editors describe in their Introduction, much of the reproductive processes in the female life-cycle – especially menstruation, childbirth, and menopause – have been medicalized (Sargent and Brettell 1996). Once transformed into pathologies, their treatment becomes an economic boon to drug companies and physicians.

Another critical perspective, political economy, weighs the impact of gender on health in the context of local, national, or international resource struggles (Singer and Gerdes 1988; Whiteford 1996). Important differences exist between women in industrialized countries and those in less developed areas with regard to morbidity and mortality (Lane and Meléis 1991; Okojie 1994). Morsy (1993) shows how the female research subjects in the internationally-funded Egyptian Norplant trials were denied removal of the implanted contraception devices, which caused them considerable discomfort, despite their frequent requests. The study by Lane et al. (1998) of Egyptian women's access to induced abortion demonstrated how, even where abortion is severely restricted, safety can be purchased. Moreover, the assumption that household resources are evenly allocated by gender has been shown not to be the case by studies that detail the allocation of resources to males and females within families (Bruce 1989; Scrimshaw 1990). Poor women, who cannot afford safety, risk injury and death in ending their unwanted pregnancies.

The second main approach to the study of gender and health attempts to quantify the magnitude of morbidity and mortality afflicting males and females. Since the 1990s, a wealth of information has been compiled to describe women's health status worldwide (United Nations 1991, 1995a, 1995b). With this quantitative data comes the ability to make comparisons between males and females, or between females of different geographical areas. The public recognition of these statistical findings of higher than expected morbidity and mortality for females as compared to males in some countries has pushed policy makers to consider more seriously the welfare of women and girls. *The Programme of Action*, for example, adopted at the 1994 International Conference of Population and Development in Cairo, addressed the higher rates of preventable mortality among young girls and maternal mortality, two issues that became officially "visible" only after the publication of the tragically high rates of their occurrence (United Nations 1995a: 19, 42).

Yet, aggregate statistics often do not provide the kinds of information with which to fashion effective interventions, and even the categories in which the data are collected can be misleading. For example, when the Safe Motherhood initiative began in 1987, the World Health Organization (WHO) and the United Nations Population Fund (UNFPA) alerted the international community to the tragedy of 500,000 women dying each year of pregnancy-related causes. Since then, the global maternal mortality ratio has decreased by 44%, with the worldwide maternal death being closer to 303,000 women as of 2015 (UNICEF 2017). However alarming, this information insufficiently outlines the steps to be taken to remedy the situation. A four-country study (Egypt, Bangladesh, Indonesia, and India) on the severe and life-threatening morbidities that women suffer during pregnancy did point to possible remedies because it combined epidemiological measurements with in-depth analyses of how and why these morbidities occurred (Fortney and Smith 1997). The study found that inadequate transportation and other impediments to access to emergency services were more salient causes of maternal morbidity (and a predictor of mortality) than the oft-cited clinical diagnoses.

MORBIDITY AND SURVIVAL

In most areas around the world, and in most subgroups that have been studied, females report greater morbidity than males, yet they have lower rates of mortality and live longer lives. As discussed in the next section, males in most societies die about seven years before their female counterparts.

In the United States, women more often restrict their activities and stay in bed for illness than men (Verbrugge 1985). Studies on US middle-class adolescents (Goodman and Kagan 1997), the homeless (Ritchey and Mullis 1991), and the elderly in the United States, Jamaica, Malaysia, Bangladesh, and the United Kingdom (Arber and Ginn 1993; Rahman and Fox 1994) all found that women more frequently report illness symptoms. A United States national survey demonstrated that between the ages of 17 and 44 years, and excluding reproductive conditions, women utilize 30% more health care than men (Verbrugge 1985). A Canadian survey, however, found that controlling for pregnancy and other reproductive-based services resulted in nearly equal levels of health care expenditure for males and females (Mustard et al. 1998). However, an accompanying editorial in the *New England Journal of Medicine* argued that because Canadian women outlive men by on average 6.4 years, equal levels of care may not be equitable (J. Haas 1989).

A major portion of the nonreproductive causes of women's excess morbidity is emotional distress and depression. The World Health Organization (2017) found depression to be the "disease burden" in the world, leading to an estimated 50 million years lived with disability (YLD) globally. Depression is also currently the leading cause of global disease burden in women between the ages of 15 and 44 (World Health Organization 2017). These findings have been relatively consistent over the last few decades and thus have inspired numerous studies that attempt to provide explanations for these differences. Gove's (1984) finding that married women have poorer mental health than married men led him to speculate that women's many-role stresses affect them negatively. Verbrugge (1989) subsequently demonstrated that employed women have much less risk of affective and psychological disorder. Support for Verbrugge's findings were provided by a four-country study (Denmark, Finland, Norway, and Sweden), indicating that in families where women are full-time housewives, their morbidity was about 150% that of men; in families where women worked for pay, their morbidity rates were more nearly equal (Haavio-Mannila 1986).

The continued role females hold as caregivers in many societies may also be a contributing factor to their worsened mental health. According to a 2015 report by the National Alliance for Caregiving, 60% of caregivers in the United States are female (National Alliance for Caregiving 2015). Adding to the gender difference, a 2006 meta-analysis further found that when females were caregivers, they provided more hours of care and were more likely to help with caregiving tasks than their male counterparts (Pinquart and Sorensen 2006). This caregiving gap is a significant variable as multiple studies have linked caregiving to worse physical and mental health (Schulz and Beach 1999). Risks for depression, anxiety, and insomnia were particularly high for caregivers of dementia patients as well (Liu et al. 2016). Research conducted in Scotland, England, and the Czech Republic claim that male/female differences in reported malaise and psychological and physical symptoms are much less prevalent than earlier reported, particularly when demographic variables are well controlled (Arber and Ginn 1991; Hraba et al. 1996; MacIntyre and Sweeting 1996).

WHY THE MALE DISADVANTAGE IN SURVIVAL?

At every age, in most regions, males have consistently higher mortality than females (Verbrugge 1985). The female advantage in survival is being somewhat eroded, however, as more women smoke cigarettes. The World Health Organization examined the years of life lost by premature death, combined with the loss of healthy life from disability, in a disability-adjusted life years analysis (DALYs) (World Health Organization 2020) (Table 14.1). Across the board, both globally and among sub-regions, male death and disability is higher than female. India and China are notably among the countries with more comparable ratios due to reasons that will be discussed later in this chapter.

Unresolved is the extent to which males' poorer survival is a biological vulnerability, a product of male socialization, or, perhaps most likely, some combination of both factors. Some of the causes of female protection and male excess mortality are biologically based. Genetic diseases carried on the X-chromosome (such as hemophilia) and the protective effect of female sex hormones for heart disease are clear examples (Global Burden of Disease 2016). Other causes of male excess death – accidents, suicides, homicides, lung cancer, chronic obstructive pulmonary disease, liver cirrhosis, and some heart disease – are associated with health-risk behaviors that are at least in part culturally mediated. Although there is considerable cross-cultural and inter-cultural variation, several generalizations hold for male/female differences in risk-taking in Western countries, and possibly in other countries as well (Verbrugge 1985; Waldron 1994). Males tend to work at occupations and

Table 14.1 DALYs lost per 1,000 population

Region	*Male*	*Female*	*Male/female ratio*
Africa	641	542	1.18
India	401	379	1.06
China	275	257	1.07
Americas	319	258	1.24
Eastern Mediterranean	395	360	1.10
South East Asia	387	354	1.09
European Region	368	297	1.24
World	380	335	1.13

Source: *World Population Prospects 2015* (United Nations 2016).

to pursue leisure activities that also involve risk. Worldwide, males have higher rates of cigarette smoking than females, although this difference is narrowing. Males drive cars more often than females and have higher rates of accidents than females for comparable hours of driving. Males drink alcohol more frequently, and more males use illicit drugs than do females. These risky behaviors are intrinsic to the masculine role in many societies, where less adventuresome males may be stigmatized as weak, or even effeminate. Indeed, it has been suggested that learning to adopt the masculine gender role is in itself a source of psychosocial stress (Eisler and Ward 1988).

The degree to which these behaviors are the product of culturally-shaped male gender roles or are genetically hard-wired is the source of extensive debate. The cross-cultural evidence for male physical risk-taking and violence provides substantial support for a male genetic vulnerability to risky behavior (Blum 1997). What is not at all clear, however, is how much of this propensity is reinforced by culture, or how it might be reined in by deliberate attempts to minimize its harm. One of the authors of this chapter (SDL) served on the Onondaga County (NY) Child Death Review Committee for seven years. This committee reviewed the case reports of many males between the ages of 12 and 17 years whose deaths resulted from risky behavior in bicycle and automobile accidents. Because part of the committee's mandate is to suggest educational or policy interventions to prevent such occurrences in the future, the question of how to protect adolescent males from their own reckless behavior was a key part of the committee's discussions.

Along with a male disadvantage in survival, males are increasingly lagging behind in education. Beginning about 1975 in the United States, the female high school graduation rate outpaced male graduation rates (Murnane and Hoffman 2013). In the first half of the 1970s both 80% of males and females attained high school diplomas. By 2010 the female rate reached 87% while the male rate, which dipped down to 74% in 2000, crept back up to 80% (Murnane and Hoffman 2013). In 2018 in New York State, 87% of females graduated high school, compared with 80% of males (New York State School District Report Card 2018). Females in the United States are attending and graduating from college at numbers that exceed their male peers (Perkins et al. 2004). In 2015, 72.5% of females in the United States were enrolled in a two- or four-year college courses as opposed to 65.8% of men (Kena et al. 2015). This disparity is found in other countries. Between 2015 and 2017, in Canada female high school graduates outpaced their male counterparts by 5.5%, in the Netherlands by 5.2%, and in Israel by 6.8% (OECD 2019). This disparity may be resulting in affirmative action for males. In 2018, Tokyo Medical University in Japan was found to have intentionally lowered the entrance exam scores of female applicants by subtracting 20 points from the score of all female applicants, in order to keep their overall numbers below 30% (Harding 2018). In other science subjects, such as physics and engineering, women outscored men on the college entrance exams, but by falsely lowering the female scores for medical school applicants their scores were lower than their male counterparts.

Recent scholars have attributed this achievement gap to an academic culture that at times frames academic achievement as oppositional to masculinity (Legewie and DiPrete 2014). Other scholars have laid the origins of this gender gap to a hegemonic masculine culture that favors dominance and athleticism over conscientiousness and diligence among males (Hsin 2018). Looking at the data over time shows that male achievement has mostly remained flat at least for high school completion, whereas around the mid-1970s female achievement began to rise. It seems likely that women responded to the increasing opportunities in education and the professions at that time, combined with the availability of effective birth control. Prior to the mid-1970s in the United States many women worked to support husbands to complete their education, while also caring for the house and children (Goldin et al. 2006). However, since education promotes health and survival, the gender educational gap may worsen the existing premature male mortality.

DIFFERENTIAL MORTALITY BY GENDER: CASE STUDIES

The health risks, or health benefits, associated with gender are part of a complex picture in which poverty and ethnic or racial discrimination also interact to influence health status. As will be described, in certain developing societies females have greater rates of malnutrition and less access to health care, resulting in excess female death (McGee 1984). The interaction of male gender, social class, and racial discrimination may also negatively influence health status. In the United States, for example, the interaction of gender and the pervasive social disadvantage facing Black people results in measurable mortality disparities among Black men.

Egypt: Female Gender and Poverty as Synergistic Risks

Amartya Sen, in looking at the disparity in female mortality in Asia and North Africa, claims that, "failure to give women medical care similar to what men get and to provide them with comparable food and social services results in fewer women surviving than would be the case if they had equal care" (Sen 1990: 61). Based on an analysis of aggregate national sex ratios, Sen claims that 100 million women and girls are "missing" worldwide. This section uses Sen's approach with demographic data from Egypt to illustrate the potential mortality effects of gender stratification that favors the survival of males.

As mentioned earlier, more boys than girls are conceived and born, but after that at every age from birth to old age, given equal care, females have better survival rates than males (Sen 1990; United Nations 1989: 19, 1991: 11). In countries where male and female infants receive apparently equal care, for example in Eastern Europe and in Japan, Sweden, and The Netherlands, male infants have between 10% and 30% higher mortality than female infants (Turner 1991). Where females receive fairly equal food and medical care to males, researchers generally expect them to outnumber males in population census counts as well. A recently published study that looked at male:female survival ratios in seven populations under extreme conditions of famine, slavery, and epidemics consistently found higher survival rates among females. This gender gap seems to hinge on early infant mortality – with newborn females better able to handle these conditions than their male counterparts (Zarulli et al. 2018).

In areas where it appears that females receive less food and health care than males, the expected gender ratio is reversed, as shown in Table 14.2. The conditions influencing the premature mortality of females is not simply a result of general poverty. On the contrary, sub-Saharan Africa, cited above, is one of the world's poorest geographical areas. Although poverty plays a role, in cultures where male children and adult males are favored in terms of food, education, health care, and social support, girls and women have higher death rates during childhood and during the childbearing years (Bekele 1980; Chen and D'Souza 1981). In contrast, where women have higher education status and greater economic and

Table 14.2 Gender ratios in areas where males receive greater care

Country	*Females per 100 males*
Afghanistan	93
India	94
Bhutan	89
Pakistan	97
Nigeria	97
China	93

Source: Compiled from *World Population Prospects 2010* (United Nations 2011).

reproductive autonomy, they and their children have greater survival rates (MacCormack 1988; Williamson and Boehmer 1997).

When we examine the population in Egypt by gender, there is a preponderance of males. The 2017, Egyptian census enumerated 93.9 females for every 100 males, or 45,907,309 women out of a total population of 94,798,827 (CAPMAS 2017). If Egyptian gender ratios were similar to those of sub-Saharan Africa, where 50.1% of the population is female, then we would expect there to be 47,494,212 women in Egypt. Subtracting the actual number of women in the Egyptian census from the expected number yields a total of 1,586,903 "missing" women. Worldwide estimates of missing women paint an even darker picture with recent estimates determining that there were up to 126 million "missing women" between 1970 and 2010 (Bongaarts and Guilmoto, 2015). More research is needed to examine mortality by gender in Egypt and elsewhere, but a likely explanation for this disparity in gender ratios is differential mortality of females.

There are, however, other potential explanations for missing females in census data that must be considered. It is possible that some women were simply not counted. In the rural Egyptian hamlet where one of the authors (SL) conducted fieldwork, if one asked a father how many children he had, he would often respond by enumerating only his sons. It was necessary to phrase the question to include daughters as well. Similarly, when interviewing one of the two co-wives of a polygamous man, she would not usually include the other wife or her co-wife's children in her responses. While this may account for some inaccuracies in reporting, it seems unlikely that it would result in large differences. Another possible explanation is selective migration of women. In rural Ireland or in the Philippines, two countries where women leave in search of work abroad, this explanation might make sense. In Egypt, however, women represent a very small percentage of labor migrants. More often it is the women who stay home and the men who leave in search of work.

While a proportion of the overall difference between the numbers of males and females in Egypt might therefore be due to inaccuracies in enumeration, the most likely explanation for the preponderance of men is preventable mortality of girls and women. Figure 14.1 presents a population census, compiled by Rubinstein (Rubinstein 1992),

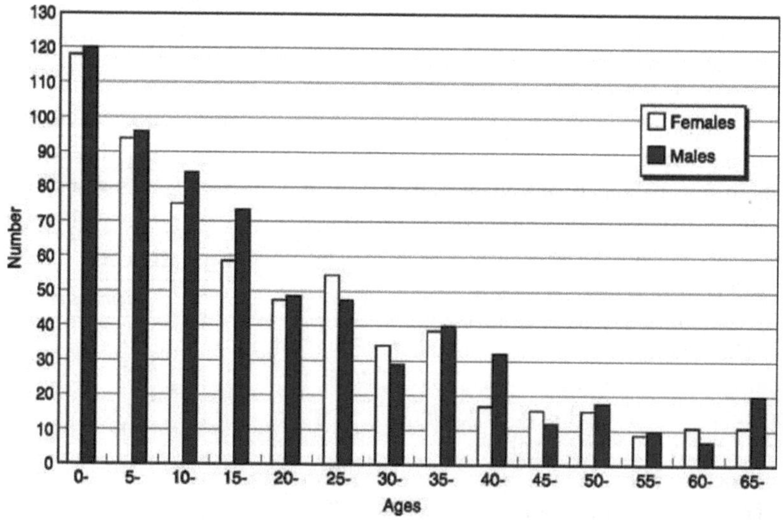

Figure 14.1 Population distribution spring 1991, Ei Youni, Beheira, Egypt

for a rural Egyptian hamlet. In the breakdown of age and gender it is clear that in every age except 20–30 years old (when males are in the military or working abroad as migrant laborers), males outnumber females.

Studies have found that among poor rural and urban Egyptian families, males have greater access to care than females. In a random sample of 25 rural Egyptian households, women were interviewed to determine sources of therapy for eye disease and reasons for the choice of therapy (Lane and Millar 1987). A number of variables (education, innovation, socioeconomic status, belief in microbes as a source of disease, gender, and age) were cross-tabulated with sources of therapy for eye disease. Only two variables, gender and age, were associated with type of therapy. Females were more likely to receive treatment with home remedies only; males were more likely to progress to second-step therapy (treatment by either a traditional or biomedical practitioner). Adults were more likely to receive therapy from a private physician than were children, and adult women who received such therapy were most often mothers of sons. Logistic regression indicated that both gender and age were independently predictive of access to therapy. Thus, the status associated with male gender and advanced age seems to have influenced access to therapy for eye disease. Despite the fact that the most common eye disease in the area, trachoma, is highest among children, and its long-term sequelae overwhelmingly affect women, these groups received the least biomedical therapy.

In poorer Egyptian families, limited food supplies are often directed preferentially toward the boys and men in the family. A study of child health in a squatter settlement outside Cairo found significantly more malnutrition among girls as compared with boys aged two and three (Tekce 1990). Research conducted in villages in the Qalyubeya governorate among children from birth to age six found that one of the risk factors for protein-energy malnutrition was being female (Hemid and El-Mosallami 1978). A number of leading Egyptian experts in nutrition summed up the data on food distribution within rural and poor Egyptian households as: male wage earners receive the largest share, women and children receive a smaller share, and young girls are given the least of all (Galal and Shaheen 1984). Adequate nutrition is the cornerstone of good health and, as these studies make clear, many Egyptian females of all ages suffer from gender-linked undernutrition.

In Egypt, data on the number of deaths are relatively accurate, but population-based data on the causes of death are less reliable because so many people die at home, and family members report the causes of death to the authorities. Therefore, there are insufficient data on the causes of excess female mortality, with the exception of certain conditions such as those affecting child survival and pregnancy-related mortality. The data that are available illustrate that access to care, and probably predisposing malnutrition, play a role in female deaths.

Syracuse, New York: Male Gender and Black Race as Synergistic Risks

In most of the published literature, "gender" means female. Male gender is either assumed to be the norm from which all differences are derived, or ignored altogether. This framing of the male gender as the default is problematic because of the dangerous picture it paints of superior male health. This is concerning since, as mentioned earlier, where gender and social disadvantage intersect, minority males have disproportionate mortality over non-minority males. This paradigm ultimately leaves a critical demographic vulnerable (Heckler 1985). In Syracuse, New York, a demographic analysis – based on vital records data from the 2010 census – of the white and Black populations illustrates what appears to be a considerable disparity in survival between the two groups, particularly among males. Syracuse has a

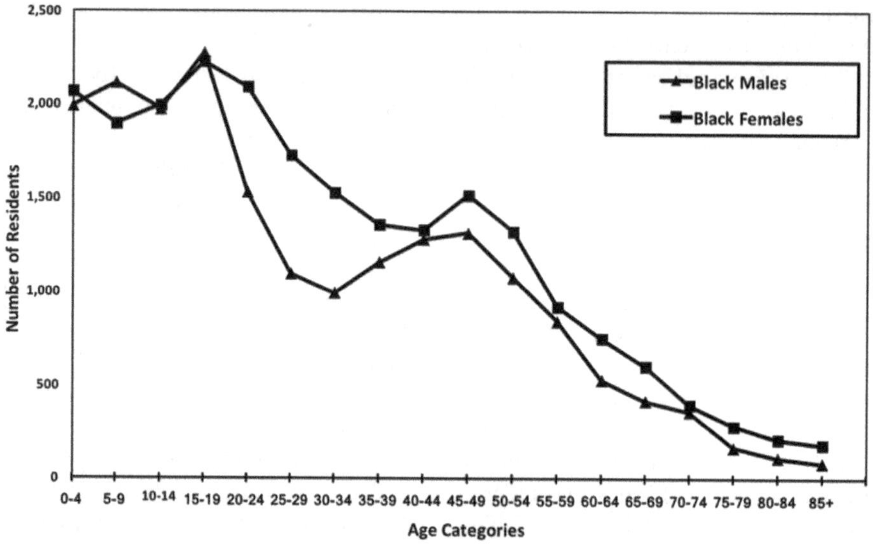

Figure 14.2 Syracuse Black population by age and gender (2010)

population of just over 145,000 with 29% being Black and less than 16% other minority groups. Coale (1991) has said that in all populations, given the larger number of males born and their poorer survival, there is a point of "cross-over" at which time females outnumber males. As illustrated by Figure 14.2, the Syracuse Black population cross-over to fewer males than females begins at age 15. This cross-over age of 15 has not changed since the first edition of this chapter was published with data from the 1990 census. In addition, it seems the Black male age curve has actually become steeper between the ages of 20 and 29 than what was seen in the 1990 census. In the Syracuse white population, the cross-over occurs at age 39. Figure 14.3 presents a comparison of Syracuse Black and white populations. In populations with a younger age structure (higher fertility, lower survival in the older ages), such as that of Syracuse Black population, the cross-over would be expected to occur later. Therefore, the Syracuse Black population exhibits the opposite of what would be expected.

Because the white population has much greater survival past age 65 and the Black population has higher fertility, it would be inaccurate to compare their total populations of males and females. A comparison of the two groups between the ages of 20 and 59 controls somewhat for this bias. Moreover, this age category has social meaning, in that those between these ages are the primary productive and caretaking members of society. In the 2010 census in Syracuse, for every 100 white males there are 100 females; for every 100 Black males there are 127 females. This analysis shows that there is a 21% difference in the proportion of males among the Black and white populations in Syracuse. If we calculate the "expected" number of males, based on the proportion of white males (50%), then there are 2,507 "missing" Black men in Syracuse.

As with the missing Egyptian females, the Black males in the Syracuse study may have been under-counted by census takers, they may have migrated, they may be incarcerated, or they may have died. Recent concerns have been raised about the under-enumeration of minorities in census counts, so this may account for a portion of the missing males. While differential migration of males away from Syracuse does not seem likely,

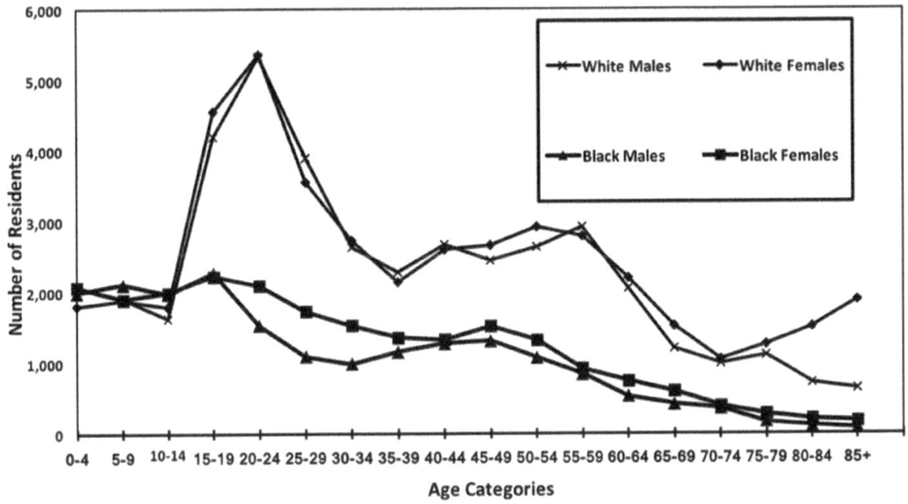

Figure 14.3 Syracuse population by age and gender: Black and white populations (2010)

incarceration is a possible reason for a portion of the missing males. The US Bureau of Justice estimates that 32.2% of Black males born in 2001 will enter state or federal prisons in their lifetimes versus 5.9% of white males (Bonczar 2003). However, an examination of the vital records data on 2010 deaths in Onondaga County (the county in which Syracuse is located) indicates that not only do Black people as a group have much earlier rates of death than the white population, but also Black males have a much steeper rate of death, beginning at about age 20, than either white males or females of either race. From these data it seems evident that a portion of the "missing" Black males have died.

Infant mortality is also a significant cause for excess Black male and female death in this country. An article in the *American Journal of Public Health* estimated that 64,876 babies could have been saved between 1999 and 2013 if the Black–white infant mortality rate had been eliminated (Speights 2017). Recent research has indicated that part of this disparity is inextricably linked to the lack of racial concordance between physicians and their patient population. A study of 1.8 million births between 1992 and 2015 in Florida found that Black newborns were between 39% and 58% less likely to die when their birth was cared for by a Black attending physician (Greenwood et al. 2020). Thus, it becomes clear how the racial and demographic makeup of our health care providers community play a key role in health outcomes.

The difference in Black male mortality may also be a result of more systemic, structural issues related to health care access and insurance coverage. Black people in the United States have consistent gaps in health care over the course of their lives when compared to the white population. For example, Black children under age six are less likely to have seen a health care provider in the last year and have a lower percentage of receiving a full vaccination series than white children (Centers for Disease Control and Prevention 2013). These disparities beginning at a young age point to concerns with health care access. Another major systemic contributing factor in the increase in male deaths may also be attributed to the difference in health insurance rates between races. Prior to the passage of the Affordable Care Act (ACA), the non-elderly Black population had an uninsured rate of 19% compared with 12% for the white population

(Artiga et al. 2017). Since the passage of the ACA, that number has dropped considerably, but the gap persists, with 11.1% of non-elderly Black people lacking health insurance, compared with 7.3% of whites (Artiga et al. 2017). Moreover, while Medicaid provides coverage to low-income women with children, Black men are likely to have less health insurance coverage than Black women.

GENDER-LINKED HEALTH RISKS

In many societies worldwide, the enactment of gender roles, rites of passage, or gendered behavior causes considerable harm or death. In an earlier era, males disproportionately experienced the gender-linked harm of serving in the military during wars. Two examples of gender-linked health risks that disproportionately affect women are: (1) family and sexual violence, and (2) female genital cutting.

Family and Sexual Violence

Intimate partner violence is a major cause of female disability and death worldwide. While both males and females are victims of domestic violence, females are assaulted by domestic partners twice as often as males and are more frequently injured by such assaults (Mankind Initiative n.d.). In the United States, approximately one in four women have experienced severe physical violence by an intimate partner in their lifetime. One in six women have experienced stalking in which they feared that they or someone close to them would be harmed or killed (Smith et al. 2017). Almost three women are killed every day by a current or former partner (Smith et al. 2017). Fifty-five percent of female homicides in the United States are related to partner violence, with the majority being carried out by a male partner (Petrosky et al. 2017). Transgender people are also disproportionately affected by intimate partner violence, often at rates higher than the female identifying population. Thirty-five percent of transgender people in the 2015 National Transgender survey reported physical violence by a partner and more than 50% reported some type of intimate partner violence (James et al. 2016).

Internationally, intimate partner violence also occurs at alarming rates. In Canada, a nationwide survey indicated that one in three women had faced a form of physical violence by an intimate partner (Black et al. 2011). In Costa Rica, half of the 1,388 women attending a primary care clinic reported being physically abused (Heise 1994). In Bolivia, Demographic and Health Surveys from 2003 found that more than 50% of women report lifetime physical intimate partner violence (PAHO/WHO 2012). The United Nations reports that the African continent has the highest rates of physical violence. More than 40% of women in about half of the countries on the continent report having experienced physical violence from an intimate partner (United Nations 2015).

During the 2020 COVID-19 pandemic and subsequent mass quarantine, rates of intimate partner violence escalated globally as well. This situation highlighted the challenging situations that women are forced to navigate in order to maintain their health. Quarantine, while an effective public health measure to guard the public from a communicable illness, also simultaneously exposed vulnerable women to increased violence. The pandemic, physical isolation, economic and social stressors all created a situation that easily triggered rises in intimate partner violence (Gelder et al. 2020). In addition, the pandemic threatened the work of many essential social service groups involved in prevention and protection efforts (UNFPA 2020).

Intersectional and socioeconomic perspectives are also increasingly important when discussing violence and systemic violence against women. The phenomenon of femicide in Latin America is a prime example of this. "Femicide" describes the intentional killing of females because they are female. The term is broader than intimate partner violence as it can refer to the systemic murder of women outside of an intimate relationship (World Health Organization and Pan American Health Organization 2012). Fifty percent of countries in the top 25 for highest femicide rates are located in Latin America, and thus the term "femicide" has become increasingly popular among activist groups in the region. The largest number of femicides occur in Brazil with people in the Black, indigenous, and LGBTQ communities at the highest risk of femicide (IACHR 2015). In addition, non-intimate femicide is seen in the highest rates among women working in stigmatized professions, such as bars and night clubs. Thus, we see the importance of taking demographic realities into consideration when drafting governmental policy to combat violence against the most vulnerable women.

In certain areas family violence takes culturally patterned forms. In India, for example, "bride burning" or "dowry deaths" are a significant concern (Bumiller 1990). Among many groups in India, a prerequisite for marriage is that the bride's family provide her with furnishings, electronic equipment, jewels, and/or cash. In recent years, this dowry has been affected by inflation and is often quite difficult for families of daughters to afford. In some cases, the husband's family's unhappiness with his bride's dowry is the motive behind their dowsing her with kerosene and setting her ablaze. While the custom is probably not new, it has come to public attention since the 1970s through the social action of Indian feminists. Because kerosene is a ubiquitous cooking fuel and fires are common, these deaths are seriously under reported. Nevertheless, in 1987 the Indian government documented 1,786 dowry deaths, which was higher than the death toll due to terrorism in Punjab that year (Bumiller 1990).

"Honor killing" in the Arab world is another culturally-specific type of family violence. Females whose reputations have been compromised by premarital or extramarital relations, even if these are only rumored to have occurred, or by an illegitimate pregnancy, may be killed by the males of her own family – father, brothers, cousins, or paternal uncles – to restore the family's honor. The Egyptian Ministry of the Interior reported that nationally there were 775 cases of homicide in 1988, 49 of which were to "wipe out shame," a euphemism for honor killing (Asharq al-Awsat 1989).

Sexual coercion and rape are also gender-linked health risks that are predominantly perpetrated on females and transgender people. Males are predominately raped by other males and less often by females (Black et al. 2011). As with intimate partner violence, the reported figures are a serious underestimate because of the stigma still attached to being a victim of sexual assault. The United States National Intimate Partner and Sexual Violence survey found that one in five women reported having been raped in their lifetime by either an intimate partner (51.1%) or an acquaintance (40.8%) (Smith et al. 2017). The US 2015 survey of transgender individuals also found that 47% have been sexually assaulted at some point in their lifetime (James et al. 2016).

Forced and coerced sex are risk factors in sexually transmitted diseases (STDs) (Heise 1994) and adolescent pregnancy (Guttmacher 1994). Scholars at the Alan Guttmacher Institute found that in the United States 74% of girls who began intercourse before age 13 had involuntary sex (Guttmacher 1994: 28). In addition, of the women who reported a completed rape in their lifetime, 41% reported it occurring before the age of 18 (Smith et al. 2017).

Female Genital Cutting

Female genital cutting (FGC), or female circumcision, denotes a set of traditional surgeries, usually performed in childhood, that remove part or all of the external genitalia and are conducted primarily on African and some Middle Eastern and Asian women.

Toubia's (1993) two-part scheme of classification divides the procedures into (1) reduction and (2) covering operations. Reduction operations include partial or total clitoridectomy, in some cases with excision of the labia minora. Covering operations (infibulation and pharonic circumcision) involve clitoridectomy, excision of the labia minora, removal of part of the labia majora, and approximation of the wound edges of the remaining labia majora, which heal to form a sheet of skin and scar tissue. The wound edges are held together while healing by suturing or by binding the girl's legs together for up to 40 days (El Dareer 1982). In some cases, a small object is placed in the wound to maintain a small opening for the flow of urine and menstrual blood (El Dareer 1982). The resulting "hood of skin" covers the urinary meatus and most of the vagina (Toubia 1993: 10). Depending on the resulting size, the vaginal opening may need to be widened after marriage to allow sexual intercourse. Deinfibulation, or anterior episiotomy, to release the scar must be performed for childbirth. Women are then reinfibulated, or resutured, after childbirth.

Traditional female genital cutting has been performed on an estimated 200 million women worldwide – the majority of whom underwent the procedure before the age of 15. The majority of these cases have been documented in 29 Eastern and Western African countries, parts of Yemen, and scattered groups in India and Malaysia (UNICEF 2016). Available data show that 90% of the procedures worldwide involve clitoridectomy, while infibulation accounts for about 10% of all procedures (UNICEF 2016).

Concerns with virginity, marriageability, and the husband's sexual pleasure are also commonly stated reasons for performing female circumcision (El Dareer 1982; SHDS 1991). Infibulation provides physical evidence of virginity, and the diminution of a woman's sexual response, caused by removal of clitoris and labia minora, is valued because it is believed that she will then be much less likely to act in a manner that would compromise her family's honor. Many rural and poor urban Egyptians also believe that if a girl is not circumcised her clitoris will grow long like a penis, and thus removal of this potentially masculine organ makes a girl more completely female (Early 1993; Lane and Rubinstein 1996). In areas where different ethnic groups live in close proximity, the tradition can be an important marker of group identity (Gruenbaum 1991). Also common is the belief that female circumcision is required by religion (El Dareer 1982; SHDS 1991). In Egypt and Sudan, both Christians and Muslims (Assaad 1980; SHDS 1991) and in Ethiopia, the Falashas, a Jewish group, have all circumcised young girls (Toubia 1993). Perhaps the most important rationale is that because it is such an ancient and commonly practiced tradition, reduced or infibulated genitals are simply considered normal. Indeed, when villagers in Sudan, Egypt, or Mali have discussed the custom with female Western researchers, they have been shocked to discover that the female researchers have not themselves been circumcised (Dettwyler 1994; Gruenbaum 1982; Lane and Rubinstein 1996).

In a great number of cases, the genital cutting is performed without anesthesia or sterile instruments. The immediate direct adverse health effects include hemorrhaging, shock, infection, pain, urinary retention, and damage to the urethra or anus (Toubia 1994). Septicemia, tetanus, and urinary infections result, as well as acute urinary retention due to fear of the pain of urinating through the open wound. The range of long-term physical complications and health effects due to the procedures are considerably more severe with covering operations than with reduction operations, and include repeated urinary tract infections, urethral or bladder stones, excessive scar tissue formation, dermoid cysts, and obstructed labor (Toubia 1994). After infibulation, the urinary meatus is covered by the "hood" of skin, making urination occur more slowly, which makes a woman more prone to urinary tract infection and to the formation of stones (El Dareer 1982). Among infibulated women, scarring and the need for an anterior episiotomy for childbirth and frequently resulting tears, fistulae, and chronic pelvic infections, are likely contributors to infertility and the very high rates of maternal mortality in Sudan and Somalia (Toubia 1985). Sexual and psychological problems include dyspareunia or painful intercourse, diminished sexual response, depression, and anxiety.

Pelvic inflammatory disease from chronic infection, and blockage of the fallopian tubes by scar tissue can cause infertility. In a study conducted in Khartoum Hospital, Rushwan (1980) found that infibulation is an important cause of pelvic inflammatory infection in Northern Sudan. As mentioned earlier, vesico-vaginal fistulae and recto-vaginal fistulae are potentially disabling consequences of childbirth (Toubia 1985). The prolonged obstructed labor from which these fistulae result can be due to the extensive scar tissue caused by infibulation.

Gender Minorities

The health disparities that affect gender minorities are a significant area of research that is under-studied. This section will deal in particular with the health concerns present among transgender people because of a number of issues including: structural barriers to health care, discrimination and harassment, STI prevalence, substance abuse and mental health issues.

Transgender refers to people with a gender expression, gender identity, or behavior that differs from the social norm of their biological sex. It is estimated that about 1 million individuals in the United States, or 0.3% of the population, identify as transgender (Flores 2016). Due to their existence outside of what is viewed as sociocultural norms about gender, transgender individuals have a particular set of physical and mental health needs, which are complicated by prejudices against the transgender community (Stroumsa 2014). Thus, health policy and research developed with the transgender community in mind must address concerns that go beyond an illness-focused model that focuses on treating sexually transmitted infections and HIV/AIDs. Rather, the viewpoint must be broader and encompass structural and social issues – that leave transgender people vulnerable – as well as unique health issues that are prevalent within their communities (Mule et al. 2009).

The lack of awareness around transgender health care is linked both to the absence of transgender health issues taught at most medical schools as well as a general discomfort among older physicians in dealing with this population (Obedin-Maliver et al. 2011). Consequently, there is a limited availability of physicians who focus or are comfortable with providing health care for transgender individuals (Stroumsa 2014). This is unfortunate because it reveals gross inadequacies in care received by this population. While the focus of transgender health care should not be limited to HIV and STIs, these parameters offer a good example on how the medical profession has done a disservice to transgender individuals. An estimated 14% of transgender women in the United States are HIV positive; however, nearly two-thirds of transgender individuals that were surveyed in the Behavioral Risk Factor Surveillance System from 2014 to 2015 reported never having had an HIV test (Centers for Disease Control and Prevention 2015).

To compound matters, the language health care professionals use to discuss the stressors faced by transgender youth and adults has only recently evolved in the medical literature. In the United States this evolution is seen clearly in the recent edition of the *Diagnostic and Statistical Manual of Mental Disorders* (DSM). The DSM is an authoritative manual for psychiatric diagnoses in the United States. The manual classifies and describes mental disorders and is relied on heavily by health care professionals, insurance companies, pharmaceutical companies, policy makers and others. However, it was only in the most recent DSM-5 that "gender identity disorder" was removed in favor of "gender dysphoria" (American Psychiatric Association 2013). The terminology signaled a shift in the medical community from framing transgender as a disorder in favor of focusing more on "dysphoria" experienced by the individuals. The new diagnosis was meant to focus on the social anxiety and distress that can occur in some people due to the incongruence between a person's gender identity and biological sex.

Thus, the new diagnosis served two purposes. The replacement of gender-identity-disorder with dysphoria was meant to remove the connotation that identifying as a gender opposite from one's biological sex was a disorder in itself. Thus, focusing on the symptom of dysphoria was hoped to help in reducing the stigma. The American Psychiatric Association (APA) further defended the need for listing gender dysphoria at all by arguing that removing the condition as a potential diagnosis may actually serve as a barrier for care. Treatment options like counseling and hormone replacement therapy often require a diagnosis before they can be covered by insurance. Thus, having a condition listed in the DSM-5 was important to help maintain care for transgender individuals (Zucker et al. 2013).

Due to the barriers that transgender people face with accessing medical care, they are often unable to meet health-related needs in connection to gender affirming surgery or hormone therapy (Stroumsa 2014). The National Center for Transgender Equity and the National Gay and Lesbian Task Force conducted a landmark large-scale national survey of more than 7,500 transgender people in 2008 in the United States to establish the issues faced by transgender people, including within health care. The study found that 28% of respondents reported verbal harassment; 19% reported being denied health care by a provider due to their gender identity; 28% reported postponed care, including preventative care, because of disrespect and discrimination. These structural barriers of care contribute to a situation that makes it difficult for transgender individuals to receive adequate care for their health needs. Insurance policies also complicate matters as they often exclude these procedures and may even deem them medically unnecessary (James et al. 2016). Additionally, insurance coverage frequently denies coverage of sex-specific care that differs from the gender identity on documents (Padula et al. 2016). Transgender individuals, specifically low-income and people of color, also report higher rates of prejudice in accessing care than other gender minorities (James et al. 2016).

Transgender men and women in the United States also have the highest prevalence of lifetime suicide attempts at 41%. This number is in stark contrast to the 4.6% rate in the general population (Haas et al. 2014). Research into the causes of increased suicide attempts and mental health issues among gender minorities has increasingly looked toward the social stress model. The social stress model posits that the increased mental health disorders in minority groups may stem from the added societal stressors that come with being a member of a stigmatized minority group (Reisner et al. 2014).

The high levels of stigma, bias, violence, and harassment experienced by transgender people thus contribute to the increase in mental health disparities in this population. These factors are also highly contributory to increased substance use, unemployment, and homelessness within this population (Valentine and Shipherd 2018). However, recent studies on socially transitioned transgender youth supported in their identities have normal levels of depression for their age groups and only marginal increases in anxiety (Olson et al. 2016). Changes like the use of a transgender person's chosen name that affirm their chosen identity were also correlated with reduced depressive symptoms and suicidal ideation among transgender youth (Russell et al. 2018). There were also lower rates of substance abuse among transgender youth who reported decreased bullying in social settings (Olson et al. 2016). These findings taken together further demonstrate the numerous benefits and importance of social and familial support of transgender people in order to mitigate future adverse health outcomes.

Power and Policy

Discussions of gender's influence build upon critical assumptions about the power imbued in, or available to, a given gender – almost universally male – and the lesser power to which females have access. However, as Inhorn (1996: 10) asserts in her review of the multiple scholarly usages of both power and patriarchy, the terms are variously and often loosely applied (in this discussion of power and gender, we draw on Inhorn's analysis of patriarchy and power). Largely taking an imperialist perspective, Weber views power as involving prestige and the authority to impose one's will (Gerth and Mills 1958: 160). In addition to his claim of the hegemonic power of discourse, Foucault sees power as interwoven in kinship, family, and sexuality relations (Gordon 1980). Handwerker's more materialist argument defines power as access to resources (Handwerker 1990: 1). Nelson (1974) suggests that in the Arab world female deference to male authority is publicly demonstrated, but in the privacy of the family, power is often negotiated.

All of these definitions of power can be found in the examination of gender and health. Idealized visions of women's bodies that proliferate in magazines and on television, combined with advice on how to achieve the look, represent a hegemonic discourse involving the creation of abnormalities that can be corrected through medical intervention – liposuction for cellulite, breast augmentation, or pharmaceutical diet aids. The widespread prohibitions against women and girls consuming protein-rich meat, described by Simoons (1967) in *Eat Not This Flesh*, represent significant barriers of female access to health-promoting resources. The high fertility rate in societies where women's status depends at least in part on the number of children, especially sons, to whom she gives birth, is a bid for power. Among Palestinian women in the West Bank, high fertility contributes toward nationalist aspirations as well (Peteet 1991: 185).

The high value placed on sons over daughters, combined with the technology to detect and abort female fetuses, has resulted in some areas in measurable decreases in the number of girls born. This phenomenon was seen quite starkly in the sex ratios that developed in China during their one-child-policy between 1979 and 2015. According to the United Nations World Population Prospective (United Nations 2011), between 2005 and 2010, China's sex-ratio at birth had been stable at a skewed rate of 120 male births to 100 female births (United Nations 2015). Women in gender-stratified societies often actively seek to enhance their access to power and resources – for themselves, their children, or their families – through reproductive strategies. While the women may not be passively acted upon, nor uniformly compelled into obedience by men, the restrictions on female gender severely constrain their options. The personal health consequences of their strategies, moreover, may be disability or death from pregnancy-related risks. The societal consequences of the skewed sex ratios present in China's population seems to have partly contributed to the increase in crime rates and violence in the country since these excess males have entered adulthood (Hesketh and Xing 2006).

National and international goals in the field of reproductive health have evolved considerably over the last few decades. From the beginning of the public funding of family planning programs in the 1960s, through the 1980s, the dominant metaphor guiding these efforts was population control. The thrust of this development work was aimed at controlling what was perceived to be the unruly fertility behavior of poor women, at home and abroad (Ward 1986). It was not until the late 1980s when a critical mass of women achieved positions of influence as health professionals, researchers, and policy makers that there was a paradigm shift in how to approach reproductive health (Lane 1994).

A major accomplishment of these efforts was the hard-won acceptance of reproductive health, human rights, and women's empowerment as the dominant paradigm at the 1994 International Conference on Population and Development, held in Cairo, Egypt. Reproductive health – a women- and family-centered approach to research, policy, and programs – focuses instead on quality of care, access to services, choice, confidentiality, dignity, and comfort (Germain and Ordway 1989). Accordingly, the Population Council's Middle East Working Group defines reproductive health as, "The ability of women to live through reproductive years and beyond with reproductive choice, dignity, and successful childbearing, and to be free of gynecological disease and risk" (Zurayk 1991).

The 1984 Mexico City policy, instituted by US President Ronald Reagan in 1984 and reinstated by every Republican president following him, including President Trump, demonstrates a clear example of the influence of US internal policy conflicts over the actions and policies of local actors and non-governmental organizations (NGOs). Known as the Gag Rule, the policy mandates that NGOs certify that they do not perform or promote abortion in order to receive global family planning assistance from the United States. Under the Trump administration in 2017, the policy was expanded to include most other global health assistance. These new regulations were a significant blow to many NGOs because while US Family Planning Assistance encompassed about $600 million of foreign US aid, the new regulations now applied to up to $7.4 billion of foreign global health aid (Kaiser Family Foundation 2019). The policy is a prime example of how major powers can dictate global health policies based on their own ideological preferences.

The critical mass of women gaining power has resulted in policy changes. Through the efforts of Representative Patricia Shroeder, National Institutes of Health (NIH) Director Dr Bernadine Healy, and others, the NIH created the Office of Research on Women's Health in 1990. The goal of this new agency was to redress inattention to women's health needs, in part through an initial allocation of $500 million over ten years to the Women's Health Initiative study (Cotton 1992; Pinn 1994). After significant lobbying, in 1993, the NIH also passed the Revitalization Act that legally mandated the inclusion of women and minorities into clinical studies (Mazure and Jones 2015). The significant increase of women going into medical careers as physicians thus may also continue to have a lasting impact on female health.

Policy changes are quite apparent in the United States' approach to the lesbian, gay, bisexual, transgender (LGBT) populations as well. In this case, it seems rapidly evolving public opinion along with lobbying efforts may have ultimately helped influence policy changes. In 2010, the NIH commissioned the Institute of Medicine (IOM) to examine the research gaps present among the LGBT population and set an agenda to advance their health needs (Coulter et al. 2014). In 2013, the Supreme Court went one step further in the landmark case *United States v. Windsor*, which ultimately struck down the Defense of Marriage Act (DOMA) and ruled that bans on same-sex marriages were unconstitutional.

Part of these changes may have been due to evolving public perceptions. A Pew Research Center poll in 2004 demonstrated that 61% of people opposed same-sex unions. However, as of 2019, that number has significantly decreased, down to a minority of 31% (Pew Research Center 2019). This occurrence signaled a massive shift on the policy level of the treatment of the LGBT population in the United States.

CONCLUSION

The data in this chapter make it clear that gender influences health status, social roles, culturally patterned behavior and access to both nutrition and health care. The biological aspects of risk are so intertwined with the social, cultural, political, and economic life experiences that to separate these factors seriously distorts the analysis.

Widespread gender stratification favoring males negatively affects the health of females and gender minorities in many societies, and on many levels in society. On a macro/policy level, allocation of resources for health concerns is influenced not only by cultural assumptions about gender, the number of women in positions of authority, public opinion, and even ideological preferences on the part of the actors providing monetary aid. On the family level in many countries, unequal distribution of food and resources critically affects the health of women and girls.

Yet, despite having less access to power, and despite the disproportionate numbers of women in poverty, women have lower mortality and greater longevity than men do in most countries. A significant cause of the excess male mortality is risk behavior (reckless driving, substance abuse, and intentional injury) that is at least in part a product of male socialization, and a large cause of female death and disability is male violence. Gender minorities also suffer from excess mortality due to widespread structural health disparities in accessing care and the widespread social discrimination faced by the community.

The cultural aspects of gender combine synergistically with economic disadvantage and racism to dramatically increase health risks among some groups. The vast differences in health status between the citizens of developed and developing countries result in large measure from economic disparities. Even in less developed areas such as Egypt, however, where gender stratification favors male survival, girls and women from wealthier families are much less affected. Similarly, among the Black population in Syracuse, poverty exacerbates the social disadvantage in ways that hit hardest on men in their productive years. Gender concerns must therefore be assessed in the context of resource allocation, resource equity, and ethnic and racial discrimination.

REFERENCES

American Psychiatric Association (2013) *Diagnostic and Statistical Manual of Mental Disorders* (5th edition). DSM-5. Washington, DC: APA.

Arber, Sara, & Ginn, J. (1991) The invisibility of age: Gender and class in later life. *The Sociological Review*, 39(2): 260–291.

Arber, Sara, & Ginn, J. (1993) Gender and inequalities in health in later life. *Social Science and Medicine* 36: 33–46.

Artiga, S., Orgera, K., & Damico, A. (2017) *Changes in Health Coverage by Race and Ethnicity since Implementation of the ACA, 2013–2017*. Retrieved from: www.kff.org/disparities-policy/issue-brief/changes-in-health-coverage-by-race-and-ethnicity-since-implementation-of-the-aca-2013-2017/.

Asharq al-Awsat (1989) *Asharq al-Awsat (a London-based weekly Arabic language newspaper)*, 1 March.

Assaad, M.B. (1980) Female circumcision in Egypt: Social implications, current research, and prospects for change. *Family Planning* 11(1): 3–16. doi: 10.2307/1965892.

Bekele, M. (1980) Social and economic factors affecting women's health. *Assignment Children* 49/50: 63–79.

Black, M.C., Basile, K.C., Breiding, M.J., Smith, S.G., Walters, M.L., Merrick, M.T., Chen, J., & Stevens, M.R. (2011) *The National Intimate Partner and Sexual Violence Survey (NISVS): 2010 Summary Report*. Atlanta, GA: National Center for Injury Prevention and Control, Centers for Disease Control and Prevention. Retrieved from: www.cdc.gov/violenceprevention/pdf/nisvs_report2010-a.pdf.

Blum, D. (1997) *Sex on the Brain: The Biological Differences between Men and Women*. New York: Viking.

Bonczar, T.P. (2003) *The Prevalence of Imprisonment in the U.S. Population, 1974–2001*. Washington, DC: US Department of Justice.

Bongaarts, J., & Guilmoto, C.Z. (2015) How many more missing women? Excess female mortality and prenatal sex selection, 1970–2050. *Population and Development Review* 41(2): 241–269.

Bonvillain, N. (1998) *Women and Men: Cultural Constructs of Gender*. Upper Saddle River, NI: Prentice Hall.

Bruce, J. (1989) Homes divided. *World Development* 17(1): 979–991. doi: 10.1016/0305-750X(89)90162-9

Bumiller, E. (1990) *May You be the Mother of a Hundred Sons*. New York: Ballantine.

CAPMAS (Central Agency for Public Mobilization and Statistics) (2017) *Annual Report*. Cairo: CAPMAS.

Centers for Disease Control and Prevention (2013a) *Years of Potential Life Lost before Age 75 for Selected Causes of Death, by Sex, Race, and Hispanic Origin: United States, Selected Years 1980–2011*. Atlanta, GA: Centers for Disease Control and Prevention. Retrieved from: http://cdc.gov/nchs/hus/contents2013.htm.

Centers for Disease Control and Prevention (2015) *Behavioral Risk Factor Surveillance System Survey Questionnaire*. Atlanta, GA: Centers for Disease Control and Prevention. Retrieved from: www.cdc.gov/brfss/annual_data/annual_2015.html.

Chen, L.C., & D'Souza, S. (1981) Sex bias in the family allocation of food and health care in rural Bangladesh. *Population Development Review* 7(1): 55–70. doi: 10.2307/1972764.

Coale, A. (1991) Excess female mortality and the balance of sex in the population: An estimate of the numbers of missing females. *Population and Development Review* 17(3): 517–523.

Cotton, P. (1992) Women's health initiative leads way as research begins to fill gender gaps. *Journal of the American Medical Association* 267: 469–473. doi: 10.1001/jama.1992.03480040013002.

Coulter, R.W., Kenst, K.S., Bowen, D.J., & Scout, D.J. (2014) Research funded by the National Institutes of Health on the health of lesbian, gay, bisexual, and transgender populations. *American Journal of Public Health* 104(2): e105–e112. doi:10.2105/AJPH.2013.301501.

Davis, D. (1996) The cultural constructions of the premenstrual syndromes. In C.F. Sargent & C.B. Brettell (eds), *Gender and Health: An International Perspective*. Upper Saddle River, NJ: Prentice Hall.

Davis-Floyd, R. (1996) The technocratic body and the organic body: Hegemony and heresy in women's birth choices. In C.F. Sargent & C.B. Brettell (eds), *Gender and Health: An International Perspective*. Upper Saddle River, NJ: Prentice Hall.

Deeks, A., Lombard, C., Michelmore, J., & Teede, H. (2009) The effects of gender and age on health related behaviors. *BMC Public Health* 9(1). doi:10.1186/1471-2458-9-213.

Denton, M., Prus, S., & Walters, V. (2004) Gender differences in health: A Canadian study of the psychosocial, structural and behavioural determinants of health. *Social Science & Medicine* 58(12): 2585–2600. doi:10.1016/j.socscimed.2003.09.008.

Dettwyler, K. (1994) *Dancing Skeletons: Life and Death in West Africa*. Prospect Heights, IL: Waveland Press.

di Leonardo, M. (1991) *Gender at the Crossroads of Knowledge: Feminist Anthropology in the Postmodern Era*. Berkeley, CA: University of California Press.

Early, E. (1993) *Baladi Women of Cairo: Playing with an Egg and a Stone*. Boulder, CO: Lynne Rienner.

Eisler, R., & Ward, C. (1988) Masculine gender-role stress: Predictor of anger, anxiety and health-risk behaviors. *Journal of Personality Assessment* 52(1): 133–141. doi: 10.1207/s15327752jpa5201_12.

El Dareer, A. (1982) *Woman, Why do You Weep?* London: Zed Press.

Flores, A.R., Herman, J.L., Gates, G.J., & Brown, T.N.T. (2016) *How Many Adults Identify as Transgender in the United States?* Los Angeles, CA: The Williams Institute.

Fortney, J., & Smith, J. (1997) *The Base of the Iceberg: Prevalence and Perceptions of Maternal Morbidity in Four Developing Countries*. Triangle Park, NC: Family Health International.

Galal, O., & Shaheen, F. (1984) The state of food and nutrition in Egypt. In O. Galal & E.K. Amine (eds) *Nutrition Workshop on Identification and Prioritization of Nutritional Problems in Egypt*. Cairo: UNICEF and Egyptian Ministry of Health.

Gelder, N.V., Peterman, A., Potts, A., Odonnell, M., Thompson, K., Shah, N., & Oertelt-Prigione, S. (2020) COVID-19: Reducing the risk of infection might increase the risk of intimate partner violence. *E Clinical Medicine* 21, 100348. doi:10.1016/j.eclinm.2020.100348

Germain, A., & Ordway, J. (1989) *Population Control and Women's Health: Balancing the scales*. New York: International Women's Health Coalition and the Overseas Development Council.

Gerth, H.H., & Mills, C.W. (1958) *From Max Weber: Essays in Sociology*. New York: Oxford University Press.

Global Burden of Disease (GBD) (2016) 2015 Mortality and Causes of Death Collaborators. Global, regional, and national life expectancy, all-cause mortality, and cause-specific mortality for 249 causes of death, 1980–2015: A systematic analysis for the Global Burden of Disease Study 2015 [published correction appears in *Lancet* 389(10064), 7 January 2017: e1]. *Lancet* 388(10053): 1459–1544. doi:10.1016/S0140-6736(16)31012-1.

Goldin, C., Katz, L.F., & Kuziemko, I. (2006) The homecoming of American college women: The reversal of the college gender gap. *Journal of Economic Perspectives* 20(4): 133–156.

Goodman, E., & Kagan, J. (1997) Influences of gender and social class on adolescents: Perceptions of health. *Archives of Pediatrics and Adolescent Medicine* 151: 99–104.

Gordon, C. (1980) *Power/Knowledge: Selected Interviews and Other Writings 1972–1977: Michel Foucault*. New York: Pantheon.

Gove, W.R. (1984) Gender differences in mental and physical illness: The effects of fixed roles and nurturant roles. *Social Science and Medicine* 19: 77–91.

Greenwood, B.N., Hardeman, R.R., Huang, L., & Sojourner, A. (2020) Physician–patient racial concordance and disparities in birthing mortality for newborns. *Proceedings of the National Academy of Sciences*, 117(35): 21194–21200. doi:10.1073/pnas.1913405117

Gruenbaum, E. (1982) The movement against clitoridectomy and infibulation in the Sudan: Public health and the women's movement. *Medical Anthropology Newsletter* 13(2): 4–12. doi: 10.1525/maq.1982.13.2.02a00020

Gruenbaum, E. (1991) The Islamic movement, development, and health education: Recent changes in the health of rural women in central Sudan. *Social Science and Medicine* 33: 637–645.

Guttmacher, A. (1994) *Sex and Americas Teenagers*. New York and Washington, DC: Alan Guttmacher Institute.

Haas, A.P., Rodgers, P.L., & Herman, L.J. (2014) *Suicide Attempts among Transgender and Gender Non-conforming Adults: Findings of the National Transgender Discrimination Survey*. Los Angeles, CA: American Foundation for Suicide Prevention and the Williams Institute.

Haas, J. (1989) The cost of being a woman. *New England Journal of Medicine* 338(23): 1694–1695. doi: 10.1056/NEJM199806043382312.

Haavio-Mannila, E. (1986) Inequalities in health and gender. *Social Science and Medicine* 22: 141–149.

Handwerker, W.P. (1990) Politics and reproduction: A window on social change. In W. Penn Handwerker (ed.), *Births and Power: Social Change and the Politics of Reproduction* (pp. 1–38). Boulder, CO: Westview Press.

Harding, R. (2018) Japanese medical school admits rigging exams to favor men. *CNBC Financial Times* [online], August 9. www.cnbc.com/2018/08/09/japanese-medical-school-admits-rigging-exams-to-favor-men.html.

Heckler, M.M. (1985) *Black and Minority Health. Report of the Secretary's Task Force*. Bethesda, MD: US Department of Health and Human Services.

Heise, L.L. (1994) Gender-based violence and women's reproductive health. *International Journal of Gynecology and Obstetrics* 46: 221–229. doi: 10.1016/0020-7292%2894%2990239-9.

Hemid, G.A., & El-Mosallami, M.A. (1978) An epidemiological study of energy protein malnutrition in a rural community in Egypt. *Journal of the Egyptian Medical Association* 61: 9–10.

Hesketh, T., & Xing, Z.W. (2006). Abnormal sex ratios in human populations: Causes and consequences. *Proceedings of the National Academy of Sciences* 103(36): 13271–13275. doi:10.1073/pnas.0602203103.

Hraba, L., Lorenz, F., & Pechacova, Z. (1996) Gender differences in health: Evidence from the Czech Republic. *Social Science and Medicine* 43(10): 1443–1451.

Hsin, A. (2018) Hegemonic gender norms and the gender gap in achievement: The case of Asian Americans. *Sociological Science* 5: 752–774. doi:10.15195/v5.a32.

Inhorn, M. (1993) *Quest for Conception*. Philadelphia, PA: University of Pennsylvania Press.

Inhorn, M. (1996) *Infertility and Patriarchy: The Cultural Politics of Gender and Family Life in Egypt*. Philadelphia, PA: University of Pennsylvania Press.

Inter-American Commission on Human Rights Report 2015, *Organization of Inter-American States*. https://www.oas.org/en/iachr/.

James, S.E., Herman, J.L., Rankin, S., Keisling, M., Mottet, L., & Ana, M. (2016) *The Report of the 2015 U.S. Transgender Survey*. Washington, DC: National Center for Transgender Equality.

Kaiser Family Foundation (2019) *The Mexico City Policy: An Explainer*. Retrieved from: www.kff.org/global-health-policy/fact-sheet/mexico-city-policy-explainer/.

Kena, G., Musu-Gillette, L., Robinson, J., Wang, X., Rathbun, A., Zhang, J., Wilkinson-Flicker, S., Barmer, A., & Dunlop Velez, E. (2015) *The Condition of Education 2015 (NCES 2015–144)*. Washington, DC: U.S. Department of Education, National Center for Education Statistics. Retrieved from: http://nces.ed.gov/pubsearch.

Lane, S.D. (1994) From population control to reproductive health: An emerging policy agenda. *Social Science and Medicine* 39: 1303–1314.

Lane, S.D., & El-Mouelhy, M.T. (1998) Buying safety: The economics of reproductive risk and abortion in Egypt. *Social Science and Medicine* 47(8): 1089–1099.

Lane, S.D., & Meléis, A. (1991) Roles, work, health perceptions and health resources of women in rural Egypt. *Social Science and Medicine* 33: 1197–1208.

Lane, S.D., & Millar, M.I. (1987) The hierarchy of resort reexamined: Status and class differentials as determinants of therapy for eye disease in the Egyptian Delta. *Urban Anthropology* 16: 151–182.

Lane, S.D., & Rubinstein, R.A. (1996) Judging the other: Responding to traditional female genital surgeries. *Hastings Center Report* 26(3): 31–40.

Lane, S.D., El-Mouelhy, M.T., & Jok, J.A. (1998) 'Buying safety: The economics of reproductive risk and abortion in Egypt' *Social Science and Medicine* 47(8):1089–1099.

Legewie, J., & DiPrete, T.A. (2014) The high school environment and the gender gap in science and engineering. *Sociology of Education* 87(4): 259–280. https://doi.org/10.1177/0038040714547770.

Leutwyler, K. (1998) *'Dying to be thin'*. *Women's Health* 9(2): 16–19.

Liu, S., Li, C., Shi, Z., Wang, X., Zhou, Y., Liu, S., & Ji, Y. (2016) Caregiver burden and prevalence of depression, anxiety and sleep disturbances in Alzheimer's disease caregivers in China. *Journal of Clinical Nursing* 26(9–10): 1291–1300. doi:10.1111/jocn.13601.

Lock, M. (1986) 'Ambiguities of aging: Japanese experience and perceptions of menopause'. *Culture, Medicine and Psychiatry* 10:23–47. http://dx.doi.org/10.1007/BF00053261.

Lock, M. (1993) *Encounters with Aging: Mythologies of Menopause in Japan and North America*. Berkeley, CA: University of California Press.

Los Rios, R., & Gomez, E.(1991) *'Women in health and development: An alternative approach'*, Paper presented at the University of Rochester, New York Fourth International Women's Conference, 10 April, 1991.

MacCormack, C. (1988) Health and the social power of women. *Social Science and Medicine* 26(7): 677–683.

MacIntyre, S., & Sweeting, H. (1996) Gender differences in health: Are things really as simple as they seem? *Social Science and Medicine* 42(4): 617–624.

Mankind Initiative (n.d.) www.mankind.org.uk/statistics/ (accessed May 28, 2020).

Martin, E. (1987) *The Women in the Body: A Cultural Analysis of Reproduction*. Boston, MA: Beacon Press.

Mazure, C.M., & Jones, D.P. (2015) Twenty years and still counting: Including women as participants and studying sex and gender in biomedical research. *BMC Women's Health* 15(1): 94–110. doi:10.1186/s12905-015-0251-9.

McGee, L. (1984) Introduction: Child survival and sex differentials in the treatment of children. *Medical Anthropology* 8(2): 81–83.

Mead, M. (1935) *Sex and Temperament in Three Primitive Societies*. New York: William and Morrow.

Mead, M. (1949) *Male and Female: A Study of Sexes in a Changing World*. New York: William and Morrow.

Morgen, S. (ed.) (1989) *Gender and Anthropology: Critical Reviews for Research and Teaching*, Washington, DC: American Anthropological Association

Morsy, S. (1978) Sex roles, power, and illness in an Egyptian village. *American Ethnologist* 5: 137–150. doi:10.1525/ae.1978.5.1.02a00100.

Morsy, S. (1993) Bodies of choice: Norplant experimental trials on Egyptian women. In *Norplant: Under Her Skin*. Amsterdam: Women's Health Action Foundation.

Mule, N.J., Ross, L.E., Deeprose, B., Jackson, B.E., Daley, A., Travers, A., & Moore, D. (2009) Promoting LGBT health and wellbeing through inclusive policy development. *International Journal for Equity in Health* 8(18): 1–11. doi:10.1186/1475-9276-8-18.

Murnane, R.J., & Hoffman, S. (2013) Graduations on the rise. *Education Next: The Journal* 13(4). www.educationnext.org/graduations-on-the-rise/.

Mustard, C., Kaufert, P., & Mayer, T. (1998) Sex differences in the use of health care services. *New England Journal of Medicine* 338: 1678–1683. doi: 10.1056/NEJM199806043382307.

National Alliance for Caregiving (2015) *Caregiving in the US*. Washington, DC: The National Alliance for Caregiving (NAC) and the AARP Public Policy Institute.

Nelson, C. (1974) Public and private politics. Women in the Middle-Eastern world. *American Ethnologist* 1(3): 551–563. doi: 10.1525/ae.1974.1.3.02a00100.

Obedin-Maliver, J., Goldsmith, E., Stewart, L., White, W., Tran, E., Brenman, S., Wells, M., Fettrman, D.M., Garcia, G., & Lunn, M. (2011) Lesbian, gay, bisexual, and transgender-related content in undergraduate medical education. *Journal of the American Medical Association* 306(9): 971–977.

OECD (2019) *Education at a Glance 2019: OECD Indicators*. Paris: OECD Publishing.

Okojie, C. (1994) Gender inequalities of health in the Third World. *Social Science and Medicine* 39: 1237–1247.

Olson, K.R., Durwood, L., Demeules, M., & Mclaughlin, K.A. (2016) Mental health of transgender children who are supported in their identities. *Pediatrics* 137(3): e20153223. doi:10.1542/peds.2015-3223.

PAHO/WHO (2012) *Violence against Women in Latin America and the Caribbean: A Comparative Analysis of Population-based Data from 12 Countries*. Retrieved from: www.paho.org/hq/index.php?option=com_content&view=article&id=8175:2013-violence-against-women-latin-america-caribbean-comparative-analysis&Itemid=41342&lang=en

Padula, W.V., Heru, S., & Campbell, J.D. (2016) Societal implications of health insurance coverage for medically necessary services in the U.S. transgender population: A cost-effectiveness analysis. *Journal of General Internal Medicine* 31(4): 394–401. doi:10.1007/s11606-015-3529-6.

Patrão, A.L., Almeida, M.D., Matos, S.M., Chor, D., & Aquino, E.M. (2017) Gender and psychosocial factors associated with healthy lifestyle in the Brazilian Longitudinal Study of Adult Health (ELSA-Brasil) cohort: A cross-sectional study. *BMJ Open* 7(8): e015705. doi:10.1136/bmjopen-2016-015705.

Perkins, R., Kleiner, B., Roey, S., & Brown, J. (2004) Transcript studies: The High School Transcript Study: A decade of change in curricula and achievement, 1990–2000. *PsycEXTRA Dataset*. doi:10.1037/e492142006-002.

Peteet, J.M. (1991) *Gender in Crisis: Women and the Palestinian Resistance Movement*. New York: Columbia University Press.

Petrosky E, Ertl A, Sheats KJ, Wilson R, Betz CJ, Blair JM. Surveillance for Violent Deaths National Violent Death Reporting System, 34 States, Four California Counties, the District of Columbia, and Puerto Rico, 2017. *MMWR Surveill Summ*. 2020 Dec 4;69(8):1–37. doi: 10.15585/mmwr.ss6908a1. PMID: 33270620; PMCID: PMC7713989.

Pew Research Center (2019) *Changing Attitudes on Same-Sex Marriage*. Washington, DC: Pew Research Center. Retrieved from: www.pewforum.org/fact-sheet/changing-attitudes-on-gay-marriage/www.pewforum.org/fact-sheet/changing-attitudes-on-gay-marriage/.

Pinn, V. (1994) The role of the NIHs office of research on women's health. *Academic Medicine* 69: 698–702. doi: 10.1097/00001888-199409000-00003.

Pinquart M., & Sörensen, S. (2006) Gender differences in caregiver stressors, social resources, and health: An updated meta-analysis. *The*

Journals of Gerontology Series B: Psychological Sciences and Social Science, 61: 33–45.

Rahman, O., & Fox, K. (1994) Gender differences in adult health: An international comparison. *Gerontologist* 34: 463–469. doi: 10.1093/geront/34.4.463.

Räisänen, Ulla & Hunt, Kate (2014). The role of gendered constructions of eating disorders in delayed help-seeking in men: A qualitative interview study. *BMJ open*. 4. e004342. 10.1136/bmjopen-2013-004342.

Reisner, S.L., Greytak, E.A., Parsons, J.T., & Ybarra, M.L. (2014) Gender minority social stress in adolescence: Disparities in adolescent bullying and substance use by gender identity. *The Journal of Sex Research* 52(3): 243–256. doi:10.1080/00224499.2014.886321.

Ritchey, F., & Mullís, J. (1991) Gender differences in health risks and physical symptoms among the homeless. *Journal of Health and Social Behavior* 32: 33–48. doi: 10.2307/2136798.

Rubinstein, R. (1992) *Household and behavioral factors affecting the prevalence of blinding trachoma in the Egyptian delta*. A paper presented at the annual American Anthropological Association meeting, San Francisco, CA, 6 December.

Rushwan, H. (1980) Etiological factors in pelvic inflammatory disease in Sudanese women. *American Journal of Obstetrics and Gynecology* 136: 877–879.

Russell, S.T., Pollitt, A.M., Li, G., & Grossman, A.H. (2018). Chosen Name Use Is Linked to Reduced Depressive Symptoms, Suicidal Ideation, and Suicidal Behavior Among Transgender Youth. *The Journal of adolescent health : official publication of the Society for Adolescent Medicine*, *63*(4), 503–505. https://doi.org/10.1016/j.jadohealth.2018.02.003.

Sargent, C.F., & Brettell, C.B. (eds) (1996) *Gender and Health: An International Perspective*. Upper Saddle River, NJ: Prentice Hall.

Schulz, R., & Beach, S.R. (1999) Caregiving as a risk factor for mortality. *Journal of the American Medical Association* 282(23): 2215. doi:10.1001/jama.282.23.2215.

Scrimshaw, S.C.M. (1990) Combining quantitative and qualitative methods in the study of intra-household resource allocation. In B.L. Rogers & N.P. Schlossman (eds), *Intra-household Resource Allocation: Issues and Methods for Development and Policy Planning. Food and Nutrition Bulletin Supplement 15*. Tokyo, Japan: United Nations University Press.

Sen, A. (1990) More than 100 million women are missing. *New York Review of Books*, December 29: 61–66.

SHDS (1991) *Sudan Demographic and Health Survey 1989/1990*. Khartoum, Sudan and Columbia, MD: Department of Statistics, Ministry of Economic and National Planning and Institute for Resource Development.

Simoons, F. (1967) *Eat Not this Flesh: Food Avoidances from Prehistory to the Present*. Madison, WI: University of Wisconsin Press.

Singer, M., & Gerdes, G. (1988) Culture, critical theory, and reproductive illness behavior in Haiti. *Medical Anthropology Quarterly* 2: 370–385. doi: 10.1525/maq.1988.2.4.02a00060.

Smith, S.G., Chen, J., Basile, K.C., Gilbert, L.K., Merrick, M.T., Patel, N., et al. (2017) *The National Intimate Partner and Sexual Violence Survey (NISVS): 2010–2012 State Report*. Atlanta, GA: National Center for Injury Prevention and Control, Centers for Disease Control and Prevention.

Speights, J.S., Goldfarb, S.S., Wells, B.A., Beitsch, L., Levine, R.S., & Rust, G. (2017) State-level progress in reducing the Black–White infant mortality gap, United States, 1999–2013. *American Journal of Public Health* 107(5): 775–782. doi:10.2105/ajph.2017.303689.

Stroumsa, D. (2014) The state of transgender health care: Policy, law, and medical frameworks. *American Journal of Public Health* 104(3): e31–e38. doi:10.2105/ajph.2013.301789.

Tekce, B. (1990) Households, resources, and child health in a self-help settlement in Cairo, Egypt. *Social Science and Medicine* 30: 929–940.

The New York State Education Department (NYSED) (2018). https://data.nysed.gov/, accessed 10/10/20.

Toubia, N. (1985) The social and political implications of female circumcision: The case of Sudan. In E. Fernea (ed.), *Women and the Family in the Middle East* (pp. 148–159). Austin, TX: University of Texas Press.

Toubia, N. (1993) *Female Genital Mutilation: A Call for Global Action*. New York: Women Ink.

Toubia, N. (1994) 'Female circumcision as a public health issue' *New England Journal of Medicine* 33: 712–16 http://dx.doi.org/10.1056/NEJM199409153311106.

Turner, R. 'Over the past 30 years, most developed countries have had substantial declines in infant mortality' *Family Planning Perspectives* 23: 139–40. http://dx.doi.org/10.2307/2135828.

UNFPA (2020) *Impact of the COVID-19 pandemic on family planning and ending gender-based violence, female genital mutilation and child marriage*. UNFPA Interim Technical Note. 27 April. Available at: www.unfpa.org/sites/default/files/resource-pdf/COVID-19_impact_brief_for_UNFPA_24_April_2020_1.pdf.

UNICEF (2016) *Female Genital Mutilation/Cutting: A Global Concern*. New York: UNICEF.

UNICEF (2017) *Maternal Mortality*. New York: UNICEF.

United Nations (1989) *World Population Prospects 1988*. New York: United Nations

United Nations (1991) *The World's Women 1970–1990: Trends and Statistics*. New York: United Nations.

United Nations (1995a) *The World's Women 1995: Trends and Statistics*. New York: United Nations.

United Nations (1995b) Population and Development: Programme of Action adopted at the International Conference on Population and Development, Cairo, 5–13 September 1994. New York: United Nations.

United Nations (2011) *World Population Prospects 2010*. New York: United Nations.

United Nations (2015) *The World's Women 2015: Trends and Statistics*. New York: United Nations.

United Nations (2016) *World Population Prospects 2015*. New York: United Nations.

Valentine, S.E., & Shipherd, J.C. (2018) A systematic review of social stress and mental health among transgender and gender non-conforming people in the United States. *Clinical Psychology Review* 66: 24–38. doi:10.1016/j.cpr.2018.03.003.

Verbrugge, L. (1985) Gender and health: An update on hypotheses and evidence. *Journal of Health and Social Behavior* 26: 156–182. doi: 10.2307/2136750.

Verbrugge, L.M. (1989) The twain meet: Empirical explanations of sex differences in health and mortality. *Journal of Health and Social Behavior* 30: 282–304. doi: 10.2307/2136961.

Waldron, I. (1994) What do we know about causes of sex differences in mortality? A review of the literature. *The Sociology of Health and Illness*. New York: St. Martin's Press.

Ward, M. (1986) *Poor Women, Powerful Men: Americas Great Experiment in Family Planning*. Boulder, CO: Westview Press.

Whiteford, L. (1996) Political economy, gender and the social production of health and illness. In C.F. Sargent & C.B. Brettell (eds), *Gender and Health: An International Perspective*. Upper Saddle River, NJ: Prentice Hall.

Whitehead, T.L., & Conaway, M.E. (1986) *'Introduction'*, in T.L. Whitehead, and M.E. Conaway (eds), Self, Sex, and Gender in Cross-Cultural Fieldwork. Urbana and Chicago: University of Illinois Press, 1–14.

Williamson, J.B., & Boehmer, U. (1997) Female life expectancy, gender stratification, health status, and level of economic development: A cross-national study of less developed countries. *Social Science and Medicine* 45: 305–317.

World Health Organization (WHO) (2017) *Depression and Other Common Mental Disorders, Global Health Estimates*. Geneva: World Health Organization. Available at: http://apps.who.int/iris/bitstream/10665/254610/1/WHO-MSD MER-2017.2-eng.pdf.

World Health Organization (2020) *Disability-Adjusted Life Year (DALY)*. Geneva: World Health Organization. Available at: www.who.int/healthinfo/global_burden_disease/metrics_daly/en/ (accessed on May 27, 2020).

World Health Organization & Pan American Health Organization (2012) *Understanding and Addressing Violence against Women: Femicide*. Geneva: World Health Organization. Available at: https://apps.who.int/iris/handle/10665/77421.

Zarulli, V., Jones, J.A., Oksuzyan, A., Lindahl-Jacobsen, R., Christensen, K., & Vaupel, J.W. (2018) Women live longer than men even during severe famines and epidemics. *Proceedings of the National Academy of Sciences* 115(4): e882–e840. doi:10.1073/pnas.1701535115.

Zucker, K.J., Cohen-Kettenis, P.T., Drescher, J., Meyer-Bahlburg, H.F., Pfafflin, F., & Womack,

W.M. (2013) Memo outlining evidence for change for gender identity disorder in the DSM-5. *Archives of Sexual Behavior* 42(5): 901–914. doi:10.1007/s10508-013-0139-4.

Zurayk, H. (1991) *Reproductive health and reproductive morbidity*. A paper presented at a Seminar on Measurement of Maternal and Child Mortality, Morbidity, and Health Care: Interdisciplinary Approaches. International Union for the Scientific Study of Population, Committee on Population and Health, and the Center for Applied Demography, Institute of Statistical Studies and Research, Cairo University, 4–7 November 1991.

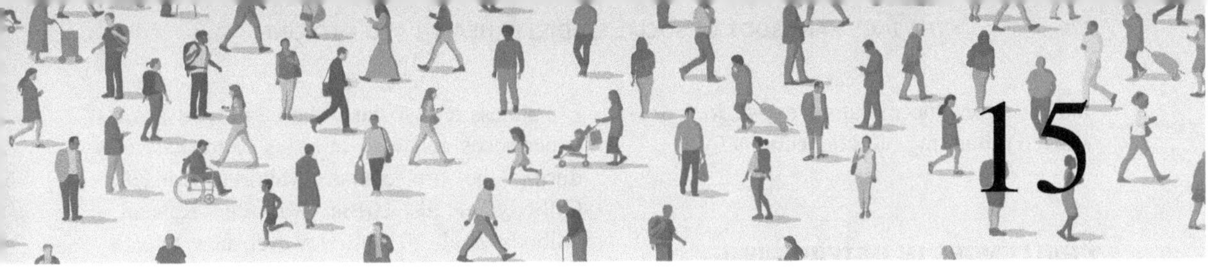

A Public Health Approach to Loneliness and Isolation among Older Adults

Thomas Prohaska, Roger O'Sullivan, Gerard Leavey, and Annette Burns

> A guy needs somebody to be near him. A guy goes nuts if he ain't got nobody. Don't make no difference who the guy is, long's he's with you. I tell ya, a guy gets lonely an' he gets sick. (*Of Mice and Men*, Steinbeck [1937] 1994)

INTRODUCTION

While loneliness and social isolation may be as old as civilization, our understanding of these remains limited. There is widespread concern regarding a perceived increase in social isolation and loneliness and its negative impact on health and well-being in older adults. There has also been an exponential growth in research, interventions, policy and programs designed to alleviate the burden of loneliness and social isolation.

In this chapter, we compare different types of loneliness and social isolation and highlight issues relating to measurement, definitions and types. We explore findings on the risk factors for loneliness and isolation, from potentially causal to basic associations, and the impact on individuals and society. We also examine systematic reviews and meta-analyses of interventions and summarize the state of evidence on interventions focused on loneliness and social isolation. We critique examples of programs addressing loneliness and isolation and conclude with recommendations for research design, policy responses and the role of public health approaches in addressing isolation and loneliness.

In the course of completing this chapter, a new life-threatening pandemic has profoundly affected health and well-being both locally and globally. The full impact of the coronavirus/COVID-19 will not be known for years to come. Directly and indirectly, we have come to realize how fragile life and the social fabric we take for granted are. Widely expressed norms for social engagement have been threatened. We are becoming more aware of the health risk of the virus and increasingly the financial risks, but also how much we depend on each other for survival. Our challenge is to engage in physical distancing without feelings of social isolation and loneliness accelerating as we look forward to rebuilding our connections.

CHALLENGES IN DETERMINING THE EXTENT OF LONELINESS AND ISOLATION

A challenge for researchers, government agencies and policy advocates working in this field is to raise awareness of this important public health issue without reinforcing age-based stereotypes and misperceptions. Prior to the COVID-19 pandemic, we read media reports of an epidemic of loneliness especially among older people.[1] The Health Resources and Services Administration (HRSA) in the USA and the United Kingdom Government, among many others, have also referred to loneliness as an epidemic (Holt-Lunstad et al. 2017). However, given the lack of consensus regarding the definition and measurement of loneliness and the lack of historical surveillance data, it is impossible to conclude that loneliness among older adults is an epidemic (Fried et al. 2020; Hawkley et al. 2019; Victor et al. 2002).[2] While we must take seriously the well-being of those experiencing chronic loneliness, it is also important to note that most older adults will not experience chronic loneliness. A further challenge is the changes which naturally occur over time for humans. Loneliness and social isolation are not static experiences and vary in terms of trajectories during the life course (Valtorta, Kanaan, Gilbody et al. 2016a; Valtorta, Kanaan, Gilbody et al. 2016b). However, new threats and challenges, such as the life-threatening impact of the COVID-19 pandemic on older adults and added restrictions and physical distancing have yet to be fully determined. The new reality suggests that many more people will experience loneliness, social isolation and risk for depression may increase (O'Sullivan, 2021a).[3]

DEFINITIONS OF LONELINESS AND ISOLATION

As stated above, the challenge in determining the prevalence of loneliness and isolation is due in part to how researchers operationally define and measure these phenomena. The terms "social isolation" and "loneliness" are distinct concepts but are often used interchangeably (O'Sullivan 2019a; Valtorta and Hanratty 2012). Evidence suggests that isolation and loneliness are not highly correlated and differ in terms of physical and mental health profiles (Coyle and Dugan 2012; Kotwal et al. 2021; Perissinotto 2018). As demonstrated in Figure 15.1, there is a .20 correlation between loneliness and social isolation.

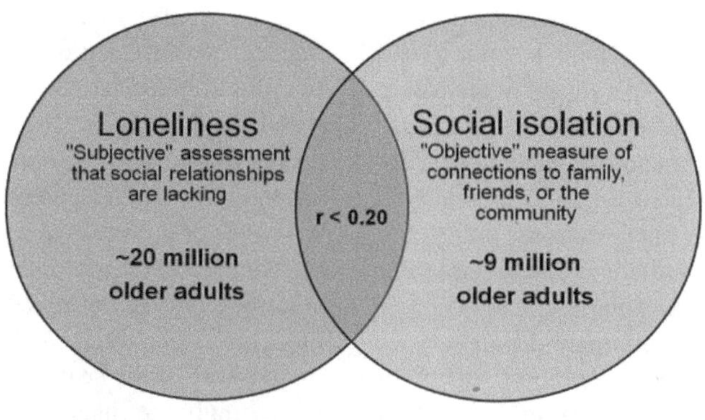

Figure 15.1 Intersection of loneliness and isolation

Loneliness

Loneliness can be defined as a subjective negative experience that results from inadequate meaningful connections (Fried et al. 2020; Prohaska et al. 2020). It is an aversive emotion linked to a lack or loss of meaningful companionship and engagement. Loneliness has also been defined by Peplau and Perlman as "the unpleasant experience that occurs when a person's network of social relationships is deficient in some important way, either quantitatively or qualitatively" (de Jong Gierveld 1998: 73). The experience of loneliness is both personal and subject to interpretation. Cattan et al. (2005: 42) describe loneliness as "the subjective unwelcomed feeling of lack or loss of companionship." What these definitions have in common is an expression of perceived unmet need.

Three main types of loneliness have been identified: social, emotional and existential. Social loneliness is the perceived lack of an acceptable social network, i.e. a wider circle of friends and acquaintances that provide a sense of belonging, companionship and community (Weiss 1973). Emotional loneliness describes the absence of a significant other with whom a close emotional attachment is formed (e.g. a partner or best friend). Existential loneliness describes feeling separate from other people and society – a void within, and being aware of one's own mortality, e.g. a sense of longing that cannot be sated through any type of social interaction; despite solid relationships, the person still feels empty (Fried 2019, personal communication). Existential loneliness also has connotations with alienation, the sense of being disconnected from society, community and culture. The growth of consumerism and secularism in Western societies may play a role in the prevalence of loneliness among older people at an existential level as well as at social network level (see risk factors section).

O'Sullivan (2019a) set out four context-based frequencies of loneliness. *Transient loneliness* can occur at a time of change in one's life, such as bereavement, retirement, moving, becoming a caregiver. *Situational loneliness* is associated, for example, with certain times of the year or instances where loneliness comes to the fore (e.g. an anniversary of losing a spouse or significant other, Christmas or summer holidays). *Occasional loneliness* describes a feeling that comes and goes – one could say this is a natural part of being human. Finally, *chronic/persistent loneliness* is where one feels lonely all or most of the time. Based on an analysis of longitudinal patterns of self-reported feeling "often" lonely, a small percentage of people remain in this category. These frequencies of loneliness reflect duration but not intensity of experience.

Social Isolation

Social isolation is more than just the absences of interaction with others; it is also a lack of *significant others* who provide meaningful social and emotional support and connections (Cacioppo and Patrick 2008). Nicholson (2009: 1346) defined social isolation as "a state in which the individual lacks a sense of belonging socially, lacks engagement with others, has a minimal number of social contacts and they are deficient in fulfilling and quality relationships."

Social isolation relates to the quantity of relations, social interactions, social support structures and engagement with wider communities and activities. It is measured in terms of the size of one's network and frequency of interactions with the same. In understanding social isolation objectively, one examines primary groups (family, friends, and neighbours) and secondary social groups (clubs, churches, work). Emotional isolation, meanwhile, describes a situation in which a person with a large social network may still feel emotionally disconnected. This could be due to a specific issue for which they may need to connect with others who have the same lived experience, e.g. a specific disease or trauma.

Solitude

Sometimes solitude is included in conversations on loneliness and isolation, although it is generally characterized as voluntary. People can seek solitude as a positive and beneficial experience. Benefits which have been attributed to solitude include freedom, creativity, intimacy, and spirituality (e.g. in the case of nuns or monks) (Long and Averill 2003). Even within monastic life, however, the motivations and experiences of solitude are complex and replete with ambiguities as to a personal sense of agency and its benefits (Durà-Vilà and Leavey 2017).

GLOBAL PREVALENCE OF LONELINESS AND SOCIAL ISOLATION

Younger people also experience loneliness. A BBC global online survey, with over 55,000 responses, found that 16–24 year-olds were "often" or "very often" lonely more frequently than any other age group. Overall, 40% of respondents aged 16–24 reported feeling lonely "often" or "very often", while only 29% of people aged 65–74 and 27% of people aged over 75 reported the same (Victor 2018). These statistics are based on a self-selecting internet survey, and therefore do not claim to be representative of population prevalence. However, other surveys report similarly high levels of loneliness among young adults (Luhmann and Hawkley 2016).

Loneliness rates differ globally. Yang and Victor's (2011) study of loneliness was across age groups and across 25 European nations, which were aggregated into three clusters: Northern European, Eastern European and Russia. The study was based on data from the European Social Survey (total sample size 47,099, age range 15–101) and the "self-rating" loneliness scale. They found that, with the exception of Denmark, loneliness levels are higher among older age groups and that the prevalence of loneliness appeared to increase with age. However, Russia and Eastern European nations had the highest proportions of lonely people (about 10–34% for different age groups) and Northern European nations the lowest (mostly below 6%). The findings suggest that loneliness among older adults is lower in social democratic countries and higher in countries with less well-developed social security systems and resources, suggestive of the importance of welfare regimes (including pensions, social security schemes and health care) (Fokkema et al. 2011). Moreover, the former Soviet bloc countries have undergone radical economic and social transformation with high levels of outward youth migration, depleting many rural areas and leaving older residents isolated.

Recent surveys comparing the United States, United Kingdom, and Japan revealed significant differences in the prevalence of loneliness and social isolation (DiJulio et al. 2018). Loneliness among people aged 50+ years in the US (16%) was notably less than that reported in the UK (25%) and Japan (21%). The proportion of those who experienced loneliness for more than ten years was considerably higher in Japan compared to the US and the UK (35%, versus 20% and 22% respectively). It should be noted that Japan has gone through a period of societal change in the last several decades, particularly among older women living alone (Fukukawa 2011; Muramatsu and Akiyama 2011). The Japanese word *kodokushi* refers to the phenomenon of older adults dying alone (solitary death) and remaining undiscovered for a long period of time (Fukukawa 2011). While there was no discussion here as to the reason for the considerably higher prevalence of loneliness among older persons in Japan (Fukukawa 2011), it is noted that people living in single-person households is currently 26.7% for the general population but over 40% among older Japanese citizens. Also, Japanese seniors living alone increased by 600% between 1985 and 2015.[4]

Finally, Table 15.1 provides a summary of levels of loneliness reported in four surveys across Northern Ireland, Ireland, England and the USA. The studies were based on comparable age groups and measures of loneliness. There was considerable consistency in reported levels of loneliness across the four studies. Overall, the prevalence of reporting feeling lonely "often" was low (between 5% and 11%) and the majority of the respondents reported feeling lonely "hardly ever/never". As can be seen in Table 15.1, Northern Ireland, Ireland and England found the lowest proportions of older adults reporting feeling lonely "often" (5% to 8%). Findings from the US Health and Retirement Survey (HRS 2010) meanwhile were somewhat higher for "feeling alone often" at 11%.

While various studies reveal interesting differences in the prevalence of loneliness across developed countries, different scales or single-item measures of loneliness may have been used. Also, some studies have further combined these with socio-demographic aspects, such as living alone and marital status, under the umbrella term of isolation/loneliness. This can make it difficult to corroborate findings across studies from different countries and groups on rates of loneliness. This is also a limitation in the measures of social isolation and the varying indicators of isolation can differ widely both across and within disciplines. The resulting uncertainties highlight the need for standardized measures as well as incorporating broader macro social, economic and environmental influences on loneliness.

THE IMPACT OF LONELINESS AND SOCIAL ISOLATION

Two of the earliest and commonly used measures for social isolation are the Berkman-Syme Social Network Index (Berkman and Syme 1979) and the Lubben Social Network Scale (Lubben 1988). In a seminal article by Berkman and Syme (1979), the association between community ties and all-cause mortality was examined using longitudinal data from the Alameda County 1965 Human Population Laboratory study in the US. It assessed a broad array of socio-demographic measures, including marital status, sociability (number and frequency of contacts with children, close relatives, and friends), church group membership, and membership in other community organizations. This community-based longitudinal study followed a cohort of 6,928 adults over a nine-year period. The authors found that those with fewer social and community ties were at significantly higher risk for all-cause

Table 15.1 Comparison of loneliness across studies of people aged 50+

Location	*Year*	*Study*	*Age group*	*Level of loneliness*
N. Ireland	(W1 collected 2014–16)	NICOLA	50+	5% "often" felt lonely, while 28% felt lonely "some of the time" with the remainder (67%) reporting they "hardly ever or never" feel lonely.
Ireland	(W1 collected 2009–11)	TILDA	50+	6% "often" felt lonely, while 29% felt lonely "some of the time" with the remainder (65%) reporting they "hardly ever or never" feel lonely.
England	Loneliness at W3 (2006)	ELSA	50+	8% "often" felt lonely, while 24% felt lonely "some of the time" with the remainder (68%) reporting they "hardly ever or never" feel lonely. (W3 Aged 50+ [2006])
USA	Loneliness first added 2002	HRS	51+	In 2010, 11% reported feeling "alone" often, 33% reporting feeling alone some of the time with the remainder (56%) reporting feeling alone hardly ever of never.

mortality than persons who had greater engagement with community and social ties. The relative risk ratio for mortality was comparable by gender when controlling for the protective and risk factors noted above. Lubben established a social network scale (Lubben Social Network Scale (LSNS), Lubben 1988) for a state-wide home care program to measure perceived social support from family and friends. The LSNS assesses the size, closeness, and frequency of contacts in a respondent's social network (including both kin/family and non-related individuals). Lubben (2018) has indicated that social researchers commonly examine social networks through a lens measuring participation in social activities, whereas clinical researchers usually focus on primary social groups. It is important to recognize not only the varying indicators of isolation, but also how they can differ widely both across and within disciplines. The distinction between primary (family, friends, neighbours) and secondary social groups (clubs, churches, work) is important in understanding discrepancies in findings across different scales.

The work of Townsend (1957) on the lives of older people in East London remains relevant in understanding loneliness and isolation. He suggested that while desolation and isolation are related, the underlying reason for loneliness in later life was likely desolation (e.g. recently deprived of a meaningful relationship by death, illness or migration) rather than isolation (cut off from family and society). The implications of the above findings on the factors associated with loneliness among older people also suggest that several of the correlates may change (e.g. marital status, gender) and identifying the etiology (root cause) for loneliness in individuals may be challenging for those trying to set in place policy or service solutions. However, distinctions such as desolation versus isolation versus existential loneliness are critical in the development of tailored interventions based on the sources contributing to loneliness.

RISK AND PROTECTIVE FACTORS FOR LONELINESS

Risk factors associated with loneliness among older persons are typically based on cross-sectional data rather than longitudinal studies or randomized control trials. The findings are often conflicting or cannot be replicated across studies. Nevertheless, they can be broadly categorized as follows: socio-demographic characteristics; lifestyle factors, including health practices; and community and environmental factors. There are both individual and wider societal factors that appear to have implications for one's risk of loneliness. Commonly cited individual socio-demographic risk factors include age (older), gender (female), childlessness, poverty, education, income, personality and psychosocial (e.g. trust, anxiety, neuroticism, self-esteem), widowhood, LGBTQ being a caregiver, migration. Lifestyle behavioural risk factors include excessive alcohol/drug misuse, reduced physical activity and smoking. Other risk factors associated with loneliness include chronic health issues such as difficulties in hearing, mobility, vision and cognitive impairment. We note, however, that the variation in measurement, many cross-sectional studies and mixed evidence on risk factors overall make it quite difficult to draw strong conclusions regarding risk factors for loneliness.

Socio-demographic Risk Factors

The American Association of Retired Persons (AARP) conducted a nationwide survey with over 3,000 older persons age 45 and older in 2010 to provide a descriptive profile of risk factors associated with loneliness (Wilson and Mouton 2010).[5] Based on the UCLA 20-item scale, persons who scored 44 or greater (35%) were identified as being lonely (Wilson and Mouton 2010). The survey revealed that loneliness was lower among women (34%) compared to men (37%), while higher income, being retired, and longer time being married were also associated with lower rates of loneliness. Those who reported higher levels of spirituality and engagement in community activities were less likely to report being lonely, while poor health, lower formal education, insufficient sleep and lack of social interactions were all associated with greater loneliness. One unique finding in the AARP study was that almost 70% reported that they could not identify the root cause (Wilson and Mouton 2010). O'Sullivan (2019a) noted a socioeconomic gradient, in population data in Northern Ireland between those who reported being often lonely compared to those who reported never or rarely feeling lonely. This is consistent with the AARP report on loneliness among older adults, in which 45% of adults in the lowest income category (less than $25,000 per annum) were lonely compared to 29% in the highest income category ($75,000 or more per annum) (Wilson and Moulton 2010). This area of socioeconomic inequalities and loneliness requires considerable further examination both nationally and internationally.

Gender Differences

Research on older adults often suggests that women may be more susceptible to loneliness than men (Demakakos et al. 2006; Pinquart and Sörensen 2001). However, the opposite has also been reported (Hawkley, Hughes et al. 2008; Tesch-Romer et al. 2013), as has the need to adjust for potential confounders such as age, marital status and household composition (de Jong Gierveld 1998; Wenger et al. 1996). Further research into gender differences is needed.

Environmental Risk Factors

The relationship between environment and loneliness has received scant attention. Aspects such as low population density in rural locations and/or living in an impoverished neighbourhood, lack of transportation, and perceived crime may deter community engagement (Satariano et al. 2010). Thus, an association between environmental barriers and walking difficulties has been linked to loneliness among older adults (Rantakokko et al. 2014). Rantakokko et al.'s (2014) community survey of 848 older adults in Finland revealed that perceived environmental barriers had both a direct effect on loneliness as well as an indirect effect as a result of perceived loss of autonomy. The Finnish and American studies both conclude that environmental barriers may have similar detrimental influence on loneliness. Although not intervention based, the findings highlight the importance of environmental barriers, and person–environment fit may be useful in addressing loneliness.

The specific type of loneliness experienced is also a consideration. As previously noted, there appears to be a paucity of information as to risk factors associated with existential loneliness, except for death and end-of-life care. However, existential loneliness has also been identified among patients with cancer, women with HIV, and mothers of chronically ill children (Ettema et al. 2010). It is assumed that a life-threatening event is the major risk factor initiating the onset of existential loneliness. However, a qualitative study in Sweden assessed 20 patient/family dyad communications in palliative home care settings to determine triggers of existential loneliness and found that when patients were in need of support but were left alone or when the patients were treated disrespectfully or contact with patients was avoided, existential loneliness was experienced (Sand and Strang 2006).

Data from the English Longitudinal Study on Ageing (Gale et al. 2018) concur with findings of many other relevant studies (Pinquart and Sörensen 2001; Savikko et al. 2005), showing that the risk factors for high rates of loneliness are related to being aged 80 years or more, low levels of wealth, not living with a spouse or partner (and not being married), having no friends and not having a close relationship with any of one's children. They also point out that the association between relationships and loneliness contains a qualitative dimension: those who have a very close relationship with their partners, who feel close to at least one of their children, who have frequent communication with their children, and who have at least two close friends, report the lowest rates of loneliness.

Ethnic Minority and Migrant Status

A discussion of individual risk factors for loneliness, especially when these have been found within cross-sectional studies, detracts from the complex, intersectionality of these factors and the need for more life-course, stratified and narrative studies of how people become lonely, incrementally or circumstantially.

One potential source of illumination in terms of loneliness journeys could be the variation and life experiences involved within migration. In Western settings, poor mental health is commonly reported by people from minority ethnic and migrant communities. However, there are well-documented associated risk factors among these populations that contribute to racial and ethnic difference in the use of mental health services (e.g. poor housing, racism and discrimination, under-employment and economic deprivation) (Bamford et al. 2021; Chun-Chung et al. 2003). Less delineated perhaps are the similar if not identical determinants and pathways of common mental disorders and loneliness and how these may intersect. Based on Berry's work on acculturation strategies (integration, assimilation, separation and marginalization), other evidence reinforces the point that marginalized migrants may be the loneliest (Klok et al. 2017; Leavey et al. 2004). Leavey et al. (2004) note that early life experiences, culture and personality, social and occupational opportunities and problems based on gendered employment sectorization, may have contributed to a greater risk of loneliness among older Irish men than Irish women; pathways to loneliness for other migrant groups and for other Irish cohorts will be different. The risk of loneliness among return migrants is also being increasingly documented (Barrett and Mosca 2013; Curran et al. 2019; Leavey et al. 2007). Research and policy should therefore be mindful of the heterogeneity among ethnic minority and migrant groups and cohorts when considering risk factors and potentially useful interventions.

Consumerism, Secularism, and Religion

The growth of consumerism and secularism in Western societies may also play a role in the prevalence of loneliness among older people at an existential level as well as at a social network level. Religion is argued to have a health buffering effect through communality and may provide the individual with an existential direction and purpose, protective against loneliness. Moreover, religious beliefs can sustain individuals through times of crisis, such as bereavement and trauma (Pargament 1997). However, while religion may provide a degree of social capital, protective against loneliness, religious beliefs and doctrines can also be excluding (e.g. LGBT individuals).

Health Consequences of Loneliness and Social Isolation

There is a considerable body of research documenting the association between the experience of loneliness, poor health, and quality of life. However, in much of the literature it is not clear whether loneliness causes these or whether poor health and a declining quality of life are triggers for loneliness or whether there might be a more complex bidirectional relationship at play. Similar to research on risks, research on the impact of loneliness and social isolation can be organized into three levels of evidence: cross-sectional associations, longitudinal designs, and intervention studies. Loneliness and social relationships have been linked to a wide variety of health-related outcomes, including mortality (Holt-Lunstad et al. 2010; Steptoe et al. 2013), cognitive and mental/emotional health, health behaviours (Coyle and Dougan 2012), and health care utilization (Burns et al. 2020; Gerst-Emerson and Jayawardhanc 2015).

As highlighted in Fried et al. (2020) and Prohaska et al. (2020), evidence suggests associations between loneliness and poor health, including depression and anxiety, non-communicable diseases (e.g. cardiovascular disease), health behaviours (e.g. smoking), stress, sleep, cognition, and premature mortality (with the evidence especially strong for depression). Findings from the 2010 National Survey of Adults 45+ by the American Association of Retired Persons, reported association between levels of loneliness and measures of health and well-being. It revealed that over half of those feeling lonely reported anxiety, depression, and alcohol/drug abuse (Wilson and Moulton 2010).

While loneliness and social isolation share common associations with health and well-being, the methods to address the underlying causes of both may be very different. For example, in cases in which loneliness and depression are experienced, it is not sufficiently clear if one preceded the other or whether there is a synergistic or additive effect of having both. Evidence from studies with longitudinal designs provides greater support of a causal relationship between loneliness and poor health. These longitudinal cohort studies report higher risk for adverse health outcomes compared to those who are not lonely. This includes greater risk for dementia (Wilson et al. 2007). A meta-analysis of 148 studies (N = 308,849) with a mean follow-up period of 7.5 years revealed "individuals with adequate social relationships have a 50% greater likelihood of survival compared to those with poor or insufficient social relationships" (Holt-Lunstad et al. 2010). Data from the English Longitudinal Study of Ageing (ELSA) found loneliness and social isolation are associated with poor health practices, such as diet, smoking, and activity level (Steptoe et al. 2013).

Beyond health, impacts on health care use, while often cited, are not as well established for both loneliness and social isolation. However, Burns et al. found that among older adults in Ireland after adjusting for health and health behaviours, male loneliness did not appear to influence contact with emergency admissions or general practitioner visits, while older women who reported loneliness had slightly elevated rates of General Physician visits, meaning older women experiencing loneliness appear to visit their GP a little more often irrespective of health, health behaviours or social isolation (Burns et al. 2020).

INTERVENTIONS

While there is a growing body of inferential evidence as to the health consequences of loneliness among older adults, there is a paucity of evidence demonstrating cause, efficacy and effectiveness of loneliness interventions, i.e. we must invest in more robust research using standardized validated measures and adjusting for key potential confounders, mediators, and moderators to assess if the currently reported associations are to be evaluated independently. An under standing of the social determinants, causal pathways, and trajectories of loneliness and isolation could help prevention and facilitate early intervention as well as the targeted matching of interventions to individuals currently experiencing loneliness. The global response to the need for services, programs and policy designed to prevent the onset of loneliness and minimize the harmful adverse effects of loneliness are key issues for individuals and government alike.

What we know about loneliness is still developing, but we do know that positive healthy relationships matter, as does building social support, and physical and psychological resources. In terms of preventing loneliness, we know that people who report less loneliness and those who are more socially active and engaged with networks have a more positive outlook on later life (Pikhartova et al. 2016). The challenge in developing loneliness interventions is to identify the most relevant risk factors and to determine the mutability of the risks. In cases such as death of a spouse or being a prisoner, it may be possible to attenuate the isolation or loneliness by addressing the social circumstances and/or the psychological barriers/impacts. This suggests that interventions to address loneliness and social isolation may require a comprehensive assessment of the loneliness and isolation profile.

In the last few years, there has been a growth of policy and programme initiatives to address loneliness and social isolation in communities. In the UK, *A Connected Society: A Strategy for Tackling Loneliness – Laying the Foundations for Change* was published in October 2018 and a Minister for Loneliness was appointed. In the US, the National Academies of Sciences, Engineering, and Medicine has set up a special committee to examine the problem, focusing on how social isolation and loneliness impact health outcomes in adults aged 50 and older, particularly among low-income, underserved, and vulnerable populations.

There is a broad range of interventions (one-to-one or group interventions) that aim to address loneliness, such as befriending schemes or social clubs. The primary objective in response to loneliness and isolation among older adults is to develop programs, services, and interventions that minimize or prevent the experience of loneliness and social/emotional isolation, and are often focused on helping people make social contact. It is assumed that accomplishing this objective would reduce exposure to the harmful health risks and consequences associated with loneliness. While the response has been overwhelmingly well intentioned, there is little, if any, evidence that current interventions are effective in reducing loneliness, and success, where observed, has been modest (Cattan and White 1998; Findlay 2003). Systematic reviews and meta-analyses have examined the effectiveness of interventions on loneliness and social isolation. Findlay (2003) conducted an evaluation of the effectiveness of interventions targeting social isolation over a 20-year period and concluded that there is little evidence that they are successful. He provides recommendations for improvement, including outcome evaluations, pilot studies, and assessment of cost and cost-effectiveness.

More recently, a comprehensive review of interventions that target loneliness and or social isolation was conducted to determine effectiveness (Gardiner et al. 2018). Of the studies published between 2003 and 2016, 38 met the inclusion criteria for review. The authors note that while several of the programs reviewed showed some success, the evidence was weak. An assessment of program intervention content revealed that the most effective strategies were those that used a community developmental approach and productive engagement. To add to the complexity, study design also appears to play a role. A 2011 meta-analysis by Masi et al. examined interventions to reduce loneliness and found that single-group pre-post and non-randomized comparison studies yielded larger mean effect sizes than randomized comparison studies. Within this the most successful interventions were those that addressed maladaptive social cognition (Masi et al. 2011). A review of good practice in relation to tackling loneliness among older people reveals that there is a lack of a strong comparative, analytical evidence base for the approaches currently being used. Listing approaches is much easier than determining their effectiveness (Cattan et al. 2005).

In 2015, the Institute of Public Health in Ireland report noted that most loneliness interventions and programs reviewed lacked an evidence base and required an evaluation culture (Harvey and Walsh 2016). Likewise, Victor et al.'s (2018) review found no evidence that those initiatives reviewed to address loneliness actually work. Often loneliness interventions tend to be weighted towards simply providing opportunities for social contact even though this may not be the answer to the person's loneliness (Victor et al. 2018). In summary, a stronger evidence base is required for loneliness interventions in order to assess effectiveness and to help explore new approaches to tackling the issue. We propose that a community-based public health approach may provide a platform and ingredients for success.

PUBLIC HEALTH APPROACH TO LONELINESS AND ISOLATION

The principles of public health provide a useful framework to understand and investigate the causes and consequences of loneliness and social isolation as well as interventions which may be helpful. Public health is a population-based discipline which strives to promote and protect health and well-being. Unlike other health disciplines, public health's focus is on primary prevention and in identifying and addressing the root causes of health problems. It is designed to identify risk factors to health, including the role of the individual, the environment and the broader social context in which they live. Public health uses a systematic approach to health that includes individuals, communities, and organizations. By definition, public health aims to provide the maximum benefit for the largest number of people and asks questions relevant to the issues of loneliness and isolation (Prohaska et al. 2012). Our understanding of loneliness and social isolation emanate from major sources: research, practice and policy as well as, increasingly, the media. Unfortunately, all three approaches (research, practice and policy) to loneliness have progressed somewhat independently and are often unaware of the findings and progress of each. What is needed is a coordinated and interactive strategy to address loneliness across research, policy and practice. A public health approach to loneliness has considerable potential for advancing our understanding and addressing loneliness and social isolation. Loneliness can be viewed as a form of widespread social health disparity. A public health approach emphasizes primary prevention and population-based strategies to promote health. It is based on the biopsychosocial model and a focus on both upstream and downstream determinants of population health. A public health approach recognizes the role of the individual's life course, living conditions, communities, socioeconomic factors and broader ecological factors affecting health (see Figure 15.2).

Furthermore, community-based public health programs focus on conducting programs that are evidence-based and focus on translating research to practice. Reach, effectiveness, implementation, adoption, and long-term maintenance or sustainability must all be taken into account (Glasgow et al. 1999; Prohaska and Etkin, 2010; Prohaska et al. 2012).

Translation of research into evidence-based community programs is a process in which accumulation of effective research interventions helps shape community interventions. The process also flows from practice to research. This reciprocal process between research and practice has the potential to lead to program improvement. Below is a summary of the research questions which are key to informing the process of research to practice (Prohaska et al. 2000):

- What is the incidence and prevalence of loneliness and social isolation among specific populations of older adults?
- What are the consequences of loneliness on the health and well-being of older adults?
- What are the mechanisms and antecedents (e.g. psychological, environmental, societal systems) contributing to loneliness among older persons?

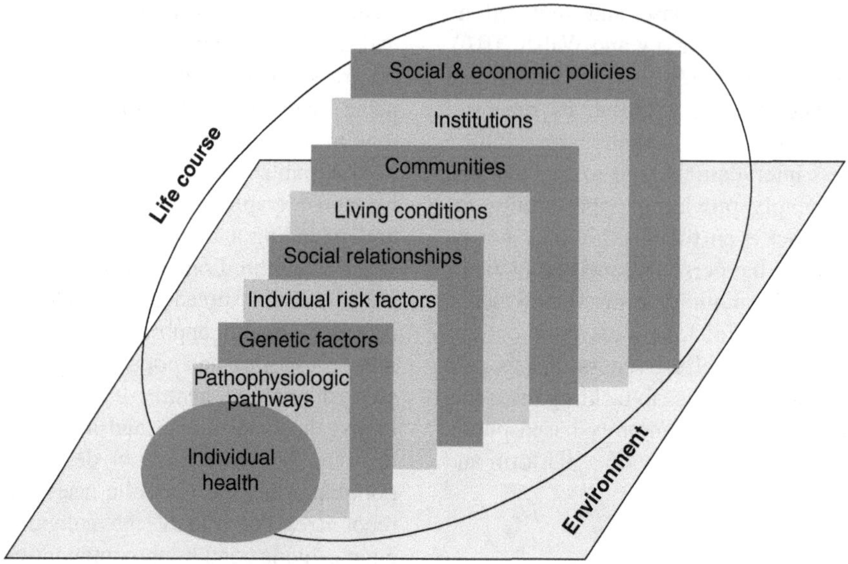

Figure 15.2 Upstream and downstream determinants of population health

- Can we intervene on these risks for loneliness among older persons?
- Can we successfully translate and disseminate these loneliness programs/interventions into the community and do the benefits of these strategies outweigh the costs?

The current state of the field provides sufficient evidence that loneliness is prevalent among specific populations of older adults, although considerably more evidence is needed in terms of identifying specific populations at risk. There is more than sufficient evidence that loneliness is associated with a wide array of adverse health outcomes, including all-cause mortality (Steptoe et al. 2013). However, research demonstrating causal (rather than associated) adverse health effects on health should be emphasized. While there is a considerable number of interventions, meta-reviews of interventions reveal a lack of high-quality evidence to review (lack of large randomized controlled trials in varied populations with long follow-ups and inconsistent measurement of loneliness) resulting in a paucity of documented impact. While there has been considerable progress in the development of community-based programs to address loneliness, relatively few have resulted in an evidence-based review or documented the therapeutic elements and the actual impact of the program on loneliness. Meta-analyses of loneliness interventions conclude that few interventions to address loneliness result in broad dissemination and sustainability. Having a loneliness intervention that is effective across multiple at-risk populations is key, as is the process of identifying critical components to ensure that loneliness interventions are based on relevant theory and a well-defined therapeutic component (Prohaska et al. 2000). The RE-AIM, framework is a useful tool for Public Health Action for researchers, program planners, evaluators and policy development as well as program modification (Glasgow et al. 1999). RE-AIM is an acronym for Reach, Effectiveness, Adoption, Implementation and Maintenance, and has considerable potential relevance to this work on loneliness and social isolation. It provides a method for determining the public health impact of loneliness programs and strategies on how to transition from highly controlled randomized studies to community-based interventions for loneliness and social isolation. The RE-AIM framework provides five aspects to consider in evaluating implementation: determining the *Reach* of the program (often measured in terms of number of participants and continued participation); *Effectiveness* and efficacy are measured in terms of the impact on targeted outcomes. *Adoption* focuses on settings and/or practitioners initiating the program. *Implementation* addresses adherence to the program components, thereby reducing program drift. *Maintenance* of the program refers to continued participation in the program. Thus, the public health impact of programs can be evaluated in terms of success in all five constructs of the RE-AIM model.

As noted throughout, we view loneliness and social isolation as impacting all segments of society and as all-encompassing social and socioeconomic determinants of health. We have also noted specific risk factors and that loneliness and isolation appear to impact some segments of society more so than others, e.g. those of lower socioeconomic status and younger adults. Frieden's Health Impact Pyramid is a well-known model for determining the impact of different types of programs (Frieden 2010; see Figure 15.3). Variations of the Health Impact Pyramid have been applied to public health programs and strategies. At its base, socioeconomic factors are noted and reflect broad social determinants of health. Examples applied to loneliness in older adults may include ageism and a lack of social roles for older adults. Frieden's Health Impact Pyramid also offers guidance in determining what strategies will have the greatest impact. Strategies located towards the bottom of the pyramid are said to have the greatest population impact, while those at the top are the most focused.

At Level 1 it is necessary to address issues of poverty, education, inequalities, ageism, housing and set in place policy to address these structural factors that impact upon loneliness in older adults. Level 2 focuses on healthy choices, making it easier to connect with groups in the community, changing working environments and increasing opportunities for trust building. Level 3 is about protective interventions, such as public awareness campaigns that address stigma and stereotypes around loneliness, valuing volunteering, and community involvement and participation. Level 4 focuses on group and individual interventions, tailored to individual need, e.g. men's sheds, befriending, etc. Finally, Level 5 refers to specialized

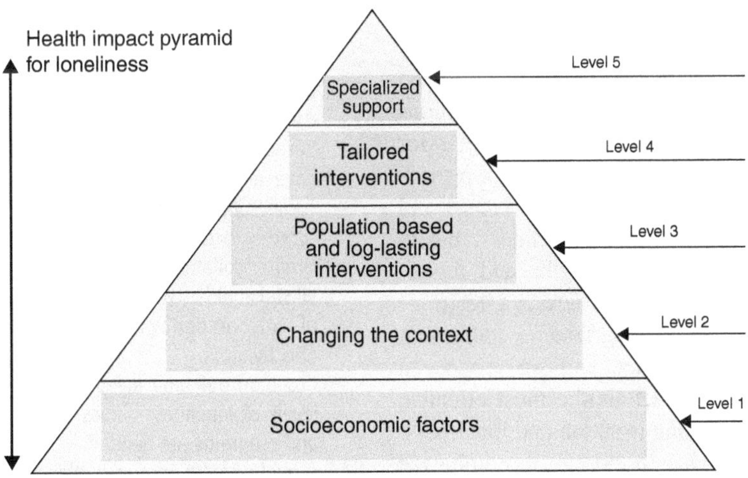

Figure 15.3 A public health approach to loneliness

interventions that require input and support from health professionals.

To be effective (and long term), a public health approach to loneliness must ensure there are appropriate policy frameworks and legislation in place that address the root causes of loneliness and tackle issues around the built and natural environment, workplaces, housing models, transport, as well as funding to support community-based programs. Supporting healthy choices, challenging ageism and the causes of ageism and the stigma around loneliness is fundamental. Foundation services are crucial in helping to identify people who need help who are lonely, as are community navigators who can help direct people towards support or towards exploring opportunities in their local area and how they might become involved with other people, groups and activities. Finally, direct interventions must be tailored to the individual, be these group or individual programs. Tailored in this case means that one must identify the type of loneliness, its duration, and understand and address the root cause(s) of loneliness for this person.

CONCLUSION

This chapter has considered the similarities and differences between different types of loneliness and social isolation and highlighted issues relating to measurement, definitions and types, and the related challenges for researchers, policy makers and service providers. We provided findings on the causal and associated risk factors of loneliness, health consequences and the strengths and limitations of evidence to date. There is a dearth of evidence on effective programs for addressing loneliness and isolation, and we propose a public health approach as the most effective model for addressing isolation and loneliness.

To conclude, it is important to emphasize that feeling lonely or being isolated are not static experiences for most and the vast majority of older people are neither lonely nor isolated. However, for those who are lonely or isolated, we need to provide support and address the root causes of their loneliness or isolation. Research, policy and the practice community will all benefit from a greater pooling of expertise and knowledge exchange in this area. Our societies are changing and we need to more fully understand and address the causes and consequences of loneliness and isolation not just in later life but across the life cycle. New and unique challenges have emerged during the pandemic. This has also been matched by growing levels of interest, compassion and care towards those experiencing loneliness and social isolation. There is now an opportunity to set in place public health policies and programs to address the causes and consequences of loneliness and social isolation (O'Sullivan et al 2021b). Finally, it is important to emphasize and remember that much of what we do to help older people who are lonely or isolated will benefit everyone.

Recommendations

1 Healthy People 2020[6] does not include loneliness and social isolation as a content area for focus. While Social Determinants of Health is noted in Healthy People 2020, loneliness and social isolation cannot be adequately addressed under this category. Loneliness should be included as a content area by 2030.
2 Researchers, practitioners and policy advocates have all contributed to making loneliness and social isolation visible to the community. However, success to date has been largely independent. Greater collaboration and coordination between all stakeholders would facilitate the development of intervention programs with documented effectiveness.
3 Common outcome measures and assessment of levels of loneliness across interventions, studies and programs are needed.
4 A public health approach which sets the research process in line with policy and programs to understand pathways is required.

5 The COVID-19 pandemic has highlighted we need to build the evidence base in the area of loneliness and social isolation e.g., greater attention to environmental risk factors including transportation, housing, access to social environments, and walkability.

Notes

1 For example, www.upi.com/Health_News/2020/09/14/Poll-finds-surge-in-loneliness-among-older-adults-during-pandemic/4751600096309/; www.bbc.co.uk/news/uk-42887932;https://time.com/5833681/loneliness-covid-19/

2 Based on the limited surveillance type data we do have, chronic loneliness (often/always) among adults aged 65 and over in the UK appears to be stable at 8-9% since the 1940s (Victor et al. 2002).

3 This chapter was written prior to the COVID-19 pandemic and although not covered here, we recognize new and unique challenges have subsequently emerged and therefore should be addressed by a public health approach, as set out in this chapter.

4 However, it should also be noted that, as discussed above, differences in measurement are common when it comes to loneliness and isolation (Prohaska et al. 2020).

5 The 2018 report also found 35%; see www.aarp.org/content/dam/aarp/research/surveys_statistics/life-leisure/2018/loneliness-social-connections-2018.doi.10.26419-2Fres.00246.001.pdf

6 In the US, data-driven national objectives are set to improve health and well-being over the next decade. See https://health.gov/healthypeople

REFERENCES

Bamford, J., Klabbers, G., Curran, E., Rosata, M., and Leavey, G. (2021). Social capital and mental health among black and minority ethnic groups in the UK. *Journal of Immigrant Minority Health* 23, 502–510. Online first 4 July 2020. https://doi.org/10.1007/s10903-020-01043-0

Barrett, A., and Mosca, I. (2013). Social isolation, loneliness and return migration: evidence from older Irish adults. *Journal of Ethnic and Migration Studies* 39(10), 1659–1677.

Berkman, L., and Syme, L. (1979). Social networks, host resistance, and mortality: a nine-year follow-up study of Alamedia County Residents. *American Journal of Epidemiology* 109(2), 186–204.

Burns, A., Leavey, G., Ward, M., and O'Sullivan, R. (2020). The impact of loneliness on healthcare use in older people: evidence from a nationally representative cohort. *Journal of Public Health*. Online first 22 June, 1–10.

Burns, A., Leavey, G., and O'Sullivan, R. (2021). Loneliness and Healthcare Use in Older Adults: Evidence From a Nationally Representative Cohort in Northern Ireland—A Cross-Sectional Replication Study. *Frontiers in public health*. 2021 May 5;9:470.

Cacioppo, J. T., and Patrick, W. (2008). *Loneliness Human Nature and the Need for Social Connection*. New York: Norton.

Cattan, M., and White, M. (1998). Developing evidence-based health promotion for older people: a systematic review and survey of health promotion interventions targeting social isolation and loneliness among older people. *Internet Journal of Health Promotion* 13(2), 1–9.

Cattan, M., White, M., Bond, J., and Learmouth, A. (2005). Preventing social isolation and loneliness among older people: a systematic review of health promotion interventions. *Ageing & Society* 25(1), 41–67.

Cornwell, E. Y., and Waite, L. J. (2009). Social disconnectedness, perceived isolation, and health among older adults. *Journal of Health and Social Behavior* 50(1), 31–48.

Coyle, C. E., and Dugan, E. (2012). Social isolation, loneliness and health among older adults. *Journal of Aging and Health* 24(8), 1346–1363.

Curran, E., Rosato, M., Cooper, J., McGarrigle, C. A., and Leavey, G. (2019). Symptom profiles of late-life anxiety and depression: the influence of migration, religion and loneliness. *Depression and Anxiety* 36(9), 824–833.

de Jong Gierveld, J. (1998). A review of loneliness: concept and definitions, determinants and consequences. *Reviews in Clinical Gerontology* 8(1), 73–80.

Demakakos, P., Nunn, S., and Nazroo, J. (2006). Loneliness, relative deprivation and life satisfaction. In Banks, J. and Breeze, E., Lessof, C., and Nazroo, J. (eds.), *Retirement, Health and Relationships of the Older Population in*

England: The 2004 English Longitudinal Study of Ageing (Wave 2). (pp. 297–338). London: The Institute for Fiscal Studies.

DiJulio, B., Hamel, L., Muñana, C., and Brodie, M. (2018). *Loneliness and Social Isolation in the United States, the United Kingdom, and Japan: An International Survey*. San Francisco, CA: Kaiser Family Foundation. http://files.kff.org/attachment/Report-Loneliness-and-Social-Isolation-in-the-United-States-the-United-Kingdom-and-Japan-An-International-Survey

Durà-Vilà, G., and Leavey, G. (2017). Solitude among contemplative cloistered nuns and monks: conceptualisation, coping and benefits of spiritually motivated solitude. *Mental Health, Religion & Culture* 20(1), 45–60.

Ettema, E., Derksen, L., and van Leeuwen (2010). Existential loneliness and end-of-life care: a systematic review. *Theoretical Medicine and Bioethics* 31, 141–169.

Findlay, R. A. (2003). Interventions to reduce social isolation amongst older people: where is the evidence? *Ageing & Society* 23(5), 647–658.

Fokkema, T., de Jong Gierveld, J., and Dystra, P. A. (2011). Cross-national differences in older adult loneliness. *The Journal of Psychology, Interdisciplinary and Applied* 146(1–2), 201–228.

Fried, L. P., Prohaska, T., Burholt, V., Burns, A., Golden, J., Hawkley, L., Lawlor, B., Leavey, G., Lubben, J., O'Sullivan, R., Perissinotto, C., van Tilburg, T., Tully, M., and V. C. (2020). A unified approach to loneliness. *The Lancet* 395(10218), 114.

Frieden, T. (2010). A framework for public health action: The Health Impact Pyramid. *American Journal of Public Health* 100(4).

Fukukawa, Y. (2011) Solitary death: a new problem of an aging society in Japan. *Journal of the American Geriatrics Society* 59(1), 174–175.

Gale, C.R., Westbury, L., and Cooper, C. (2018). Social isolation and loneliness as risk factors for the progression of frailty: the English Longitudinal Study of Ageing. *Age and Ageing*. May 1; 47(3), 392–397.

Gardiner, C., Geldenhuys, G., and Gott, M. (2018). Interventions to reduce social isolation and loneliness among older people: an integrative review. *Health and Social Care in the Community* 26(2), 147–157.

Gerst-Emerson, K., and Jayawardhanc, J. (2015). Loneliness as a public health issue: the impact of loneliness on health care utilization among older adults. *American Journal of Public Health* 105(5), 1013–1019.

Glasgow, R. E., Vogt, T. M., and Boles, S. M. (1999). Evaluating the public health impact of health promotions: the RE-AIM framework. *American Journal of Public Health* 89(9), 1322–1327.

Harvey, B., and Walsh, K. (2016). *Loneliness and Ageing: Ireland, North and South. A Summary*. Dublin: Institute of Public Health in Ireland.

Hawkley, L. C., Masi, C. M., Berry, J. D., and Cacioppo, J. J. (2006). Loneliness is a unique predictor of age-related difference in systolic blood pressure. *Psychology and Aging* 21, 152–164.

Hawkley, L. C., Hughes, M. E., Waite, L. J., Masi, C. M., Thisted R. A., and Cacioppo, J. T. (2008). From social structural factors to perceptions of relationship quality and loneliness: the Chicago Health, Aging, and Social Relations Study. *The Journals of Gerontology: Series B* 63(6), S375–S384.

Hawkley, L. C., Wroblewski, K., Kaiser, T., Luhmann, M., & Schumm, L. P. (2019). Are U.S. older adults getting lonelier? Age, period, and cohort differences. *Psychology and Aging*, *34*(8), 1144–1157. https://doi.org/10.1037/pag0000365

HM Government. *A connected society: A strategy for tackling loneliness–laying the foundations for change*. Department for Digital, Culture, Media and Sport, London. 2018.

Holt-Lunstad, J., Robles, T. F., and Sbarra, D. A. (2017). Advancing social connection as a public health priority in the United States. *American Psychologist* 72(6), 517.

Holt-Lunstad, J., Smith, T. B., and Layton, J. B. (2010). Social relationships and mortality risk: a meta-analytic review. *PLoS Medicine* 7(7), e1000316.

Kaplan, G.A. (2004). What's wrong with social epidemiology, and how can we make it better?. *Epidemiologic Reviews* 26(1), 124–135. Oxford: Oxford University Press.

Klok, J., van Tilburg, T. G., Suanet, B., Fokkema, T., Huisman, M. (2017). National and transnational belonging among Turkish and Moroccan older migrants in the Netherlands:

protective against loneliness? *European Journal of Ageing* 14(4), 341–351.

Kotwal, A. A., Cenzer, I. S., Waite, L. J. et al. (2021). The epidemiology of social isolation and loneliness among older adults during the last years of life. *Journal of the American Geriatrics Society.* 1–11. https://doi.org/10.1111/jgs.17366

Leavey, G., Rozmovits, L., Ryan, L., and King, M. (2007). Explanations of depression among Irish migrants in Britain. *Social Science & Medicine* 65(2), 231–244.

Leavey, G., Sembhi, S., and Livingston, G. (2004). Older Irish migrants living in London: identity, loss and return. *Journal of Ethnic and Migration Studies* 30(4), 763–779, doi: 10.1080/1369183041000169960З

Long, C. R., and Averill, J. R. (2003). Solitude: an exploration of benefits of being alone. *Journal for the Theory of Social Behaviour* 33(1), 21–44.

Lubben, J. E. (1988). Assessing social networks among elderly populations. *Family & Community Health: The Journal of Health Promotion & Maintenance* 11(3), 42–52.

Lubben, J. E. (2018). *Isolation and loneliness – a US perspective*. Presentation at Loneliness in Later Life: Interventions – What Works? 5–7 December. Belfast, Northern Ireland.

Luhman, M., and Hawkley, L. C. (2016). Age differences in loneliness from late adolescence to old age. *Developmental Psychology*. 52(6), 943–959.

Masi, C. M., Chen, H.-Y., Hawkley, L. C., and Cacioppo, J. T. (2011). A meta-analysis of interventions to reduce loneliness. *Personality and Social Psychology Review* 15(3), 219–266.

Marmot, M., Allen, J., Goldblatt, P. et al. (2010). *Fair society, healthy lives: strategic review of health inequalities in England post 2010*.

Muramatsu, N., and Akiyama, H. (2011). Aging society preparing for the future. *The Gerontologist* 51(4), 425–432.

Nicholson Jr, N. R. (2009). Social isolation in older adults: an evolutionary concept analysis. *Journal of Advanced Nursing* 65(6), 1342–1352.

O'Sullivan, R. (2019a). The Age of Loneliness? *Annual Public Health Lecture*. Féile An Phobail, 6 August. Belfast, Northern Ireland.

O'Sullivan, R. (2019b). *Loneliness and Isolation: Policy, Practice and Politics*. Presentation at the Social Isolation and Loneliness: Health Consequences and Policy Implications conference, 25 October. Dublin.

O'Sullivan, R., Burns, A., Leavey, G., Leroi, I., Burholt, V., Lubben, J., Holt-Lunstad, J., Victor, C., Lawlor, B., Vilar-Compte, M., Perissinotto, C.M., Tully, M.A., Sullivan, M.P., Rosato, M., Power, J.M., Tiilikainen, E., Prohaska, T. R. (2021a). Impact of the COVID-19 Pandemic on Loneliness and Social Isolation: A Multi-Country Study. Int. J. Environ. Res. Public Health 2021, 18, 9982. https://doi.org/10.3390/ijerph18199982

O'Sullivan, R., Lawlor, B., Burns, A., Leavey, G. (2021b). Will the pandemic reframe loneliness and social isolation? Lancet Health Longev, 2, e54–e55.

Pargament, K. I. (1997). *The Psychology of Religion and Coping: Theory, Research, Practice*. New York: Guilford Press.

Perissinotto, C. M. (2018). *The role of the health professional in loneliness assessments*. Presentation at Loneliness in Later Life: Interventions – What Works? 5–7 December. Belfast, Northern Ireland.

Pikhartova, J., Bowling, A., and Victor, C. (2016). Is loneliness in later life a self-fulfilling prophecy? *Aging & Mental Health* 20(5), 543–549.

Pinquart, M., and Sörensen, S. (2001). Influences on loneliness in older adults: a meta-analysis. *Basic and Applied Social Psychology* 23(4), 245–266.

Prohaska, T., and Etkin, K. (2010). External validity and translation from research to implementation. *Generations* 34(1), 59–65.

Prohaska, T., Peters, K., and Warren, J. (2000). Health behavior: from research to community practice. In Albrecht, G., Ray Fitzpatrick, R., and Scrimshaw, S. C. (eds.), *The Handbook of Social Studies in Health and Medicine* (pp. 359–373). London: Sage Publications.

Prohaska, T., Smith-Ray, R., and Glasgow, R. E. (2012). Translation and dissemination of evidence-based programs. In Prohaska, T., Anderson, L. A., and Binstock, R. H. (eds.), *Public Health for and Aging Society* (pp. 162–180). Baltimore, MD: The Johns Hopkins University Press.

Prohaska, T., Burholt, V., Burns, A. et al. (2020). Consensus statement: loneliness in older adults, the 21st century social determinant of health? *BMJ Open* 10(8), e034967. doi: 10.1136/bmjopen-2019-034967.

Rantakokko, M., Iwarsson, S., Vahaluoto, S., Portegijs, E., Viljanen, A., and Rantanen, T. (2014). Perceived environmental barriers to outdoor mobility and feelings of loneliness among community-dwelling older people. *Journal of Gerontology* 69(12), 1562–1568.

Sand, L., and Strang, P. (2006). Existential loneliness in a palliative home care setting. *Journal of Palliative Medicine* 9(6), 1376–1387.

Satariano, W. A., Ivey S. L., Kurtovich, E., Kealey, E., Hubbard A. E., Bayles C. M., Bryant, L., Hunter, H. H., and Prohaska, T. R. (2010). Lower-body function, neighbourhoods, and walking in an older population. *American Journal of Preventive Medicine* 38(4), 419–428.

Savikko, N., Routasalo, P., Tilvis, R. S., Strandberg, T. E., and Pitkälä, K. H. (2005). Predictors and subjective causes of loneliness in an aged population. *Archives of Gerontology and Geriatrics* 41(3), 223–233.

Steinbeck, J. (1994). *Of Mice and Men*. New York: Penguin Books.

Steptoe, A., Shankar, A., Demakakos, P., and Wardle, J. (2013). Social isolation, loneliness, and all-cause mortality in older men and women. *Proceedings of the National Academy of Sciences* 110(15), 5797–5801.

Tesch-Romer, C., Wiest, M., Wurm, S., and Huxhold, O. (2013). Loneliness trends in the second half of life: results from the German Ageing Survey (DEAS). *Zeitschrift für Gerontologie and Geriatrie* 46(3), 237–241.

Townsend, P. (1957). *The Family Life of Old People: An Enquiry in East London*. London: Routledge & Kegan Paul.

Valtorta, N., and Hanratty, B. (2012). Loneliness, isolation and the health of older adults: do we need a new research agenda? *Journal of the Royal Society of Medicine* 105(12), 518–522.

Valtorta, N., Kanaan, M., Gilbody, S., et al. (2016a). P39 Changes in loneliness and social isolation over time in adults aged over 50: the English Longitudinal Study of Ageing. *Journal of Epidemiology and Community Health* 70: A70. https://jech.bmj.com/content/70/Suppl_1/A70.2

Valtorta, N. K., Kanaan, M., Gilbody, S., Ronzi, S. and Hanratty (2016b). Loneliness and social isolation as risk factors for coronary heart disease and stroke: systematic review and meta-analysis of longitudinal observational studies. *Heart* 102(13), 1009–1016.

Victor, C. R. (2018). *Loneliness – a UK Perspective: what we know, what we think we know and what we don't know*. Presentation at Loneliness in Later Life: Interventions – What Works? 5–7 December. Belfast, Northern Ireland.

Victor, C. R., Mansfield, L., Kay, T., Daykin, N., Lane, J., Duffy, L. G., Tomlinson, A., and Meads, C. (2018). *An Overview of Reviews: The Effectiveness of Interventions to Address Loneliness at All Stages of the Life-course*. London: What Works Centre for Wellbeing.

Victor, C. R., Scambler, S. J., Shah, S., Cook, D. G., Harris, T., Rink, E., and De Wilde, S. (2002). Has loneliness amongst older people increased? An investigation into variations between cohorts. *Ageing & Society* 22, 585–597.

Weiss, R. S. (1973). *Loneliness: The Experience of Emotional and Social Isolation*. Cambridge, MA: MIT Press.

Wenger, G. C., Scott, A., Davies, R., and Shahtahmasebi, S. (1996). Social isolation and loneliness in old age: review and model refinement. *Ageing & Society* 16(3), 333–358.

Wilkinson, R., & Pickett, K. (2009). *The Spirit Level: Why More Equal Societies Almost Always Do Better*. London: Allen Lane.

Wilson, C., and Moulton, B. (2010). *Loneliness among Older Adults: A National Survey of Adults 45+*. Prepared by Knowledge Networks and Insight Policy Research. Washington, DC: AARP.

Wilson, R., Krueger, K., Arnold, S., Schneider, J., Kelly, J., Barnes, L., Tang, Y., and Bennett, D. (2007). Loneliness and risk of Alzheimer's disease. *Archives of General Psychiatry* 64, 234–240.

Yang, K., and Victor, C. R. (2011). Age and loneliness in 25 European nations. *Ageing & Society* 31(8), 1368–1388.

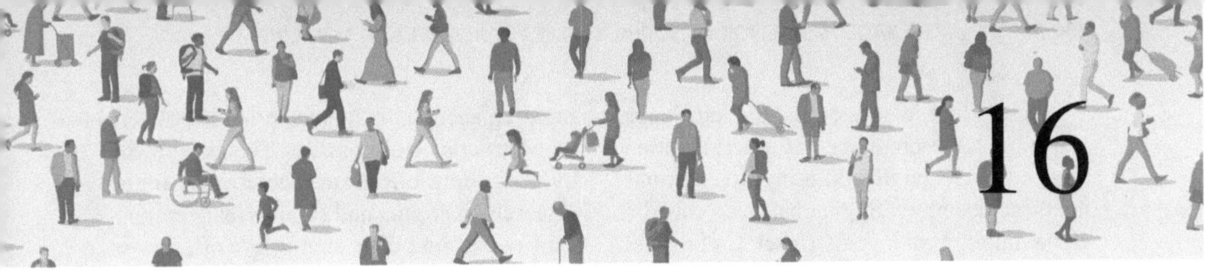

16

Mental Illness, the Global Landscape of Stigma, and the Power of Social Relationships

Bernice A. Pescosolido and Bianca N. Manago

INTRODUCTION

Mental illness stands among the most prevalent and disabling health problems globally. Affecting more than 1 billion people, mental health disorders represent 7% of all disability-adjusted life years (DALYs) worldwide (Rehm and Shield 2019). In fact, rivaling cardiovascular and circulatory diseases, depressive disorders represent the second leading cause of years living with a disability (IHME 2018). No region of the world is spared; but not surprisingly, mental illness takes a greater toll on individuals who live in areas of conflict where anxiety, depression, and post-traumatic stress disorder affect over 20% of the population (Charlson et al. 2019; Sagar et al. 2020; Vos et al. 2012). Overall, though often misquoted or misunderstood, a "one in four" prevalence rate translates into one-quarter of the US, and one quarter of the global, population experiencing a diagnosable, but not necessarily chronic, mental health problem *at some point in their lifetime* (World Health Organization 2001).

While there is some debate about whether mental illnesses are on the rise or just in line with population increases, the relative burden of these disorders has increased in the past decades, and has become even more of a concern as natural disasters and pandemics have become a routine part of the human experience (McGinty et al. 2020; Simon, Saxe and Marmar 2020; Whiteford, Ferrari and Degenhardt 2016). Further, there is general agreement that the global burden is underestimated due to the way that diseases and deaths are classified (e.g., overlap between psychiatric and neurological disorders, the contribution of severe mental illness to associated-cause mortality such as suicide; *The Lancet* 2016). Even with these considerations, the staggering effect of mental illness on global populations can be captured by noting that, in 2017, the number of affected people in India alone stood at 197.3 million across diagnoses, including 45.7 million with depression and 44.9 million with anxiety (GBD 2017 Disease and Injury Incidence and Prevalence Collaborators 2018).

What is not contested is the challenge that stigma, the prejudice and discrimination attached to mental illness, brings to confronting these disorders. Stigma has been called a global public health crisis (Insel, Collins and Hyman 2015). It stands as a primary obstacle to: addressing the mental health treatment gap (Rehm and Shield 2019; Sartorius and Schulze 2005; Wainberg et al. 2017); to providing adequate care to people with mental illness for other, physical, health problems; reducing the staggering, shortened life expectancy reported in many countries; and dismantling a range of barriers to recovery (US Department of HHS 1999). All in all, individuals with mental illness, their families, and even those who provide care not only face the challenges of mental health disorders, but they also confront shame, rejection, and marginalization, which they often experience as more destructive than the illness (The Lancet 2016).

In short, stigma is pervasive and pernicious. It can infiltrate the self, the family, the health care system and the community. While most often thought of in terms of negative and isolating personal interactions, stigma finds its way into institutions, including medicine, where psychiatric resources are not commensurate with its toll; where people with mental health problems are often not welcomed in intensive care units or emergency rooms; where aspiring health care personnel are discouraged from pursuing mental health specialties; and where research resources pale in comparison to similarly prevalent diseases. In turn, the stigmatization of mental illness results in secrecy and shame in families, a staffing crisis in high-income countries, a near absence of help in middle- and low-income ones, and fewer advances in treatment than in others areas with similar or even lower disease burden (Patel et al. 2018).

In this chapter, we attempt to provide a conceptual map to the nature, research, and efforts to address the stigma attached to mental illness. We begin with a brief lexicon reflecting current thinking and research on stigma and an even briefer historical background on this research agenda, though we provide pointers to more detailed discussions. This is followed by describing efforts to theoretically frame research on stigma and summarizing empirical findings on public stigma. We offer novel cross-national findings on what is considered the primary lever to reduce stigma – previous contact with people with mental illness. National trends and efforts to reduce stigma conclude the chapter.

WHAT IS STIGMA?

As a term, stigma is familiar, over-used, and often misused. While few have ever dismissed its relevance as a phenomenon, the term has been discussed, debated, disparaged by a former director of the National Institute of Mental Health and Neurosciences (NIMHANS) as "silly", and seen by a former president of the American Psychiatric Association as "dissipating" (Goin 2004; Insel 2014). We stay with a common usage of stigma as the prejudice and discrimination attached to devalued statuses, in this case mental health status (see reviews of the concept in Grinker 2020; Link and Stuart 2017; Pescosolido 2013; Pescosolido and Martin 2015). As laid out in Table 16.1, stigma begins with a stereotype consisting of characteristics that are applied, in blanket fashion, to all those labelled with the status. As such, it ignores their individuality, their value, and their humanity. Having a stigma trips a set of attitudes (e.g., not like me), beliefs (e.g., neither competent nor intelligent), and opinions (e.g., not suitable for employment, marriage). While these are most often negative, they can sometimes be positive (e.g., people with bipolar disorder are extraordinarily creative). In all cases, however, they are erroneous in their homogeneity and, most often, in fact. Yet, because individual cases that circulate through gossip in communities or through reports in the media fit the stereotype, stigma is reinforced.

Table 16.1 The basics of stigma

Stigma ⟶	*Prejudice* ⟶	*Discrimination*
Stereotype Attribution of a set of characteristics	Negative (often) and positive (sometimes) attitudes	Behaviors
Fixed, apply to all members of the marked group	Knowledge: MI = bad character Beliefs: MI = Dangerousness Attitudes: MI = Unsuitable employees, supervisors, marriage partners	Reject, exclude, isolate... Coerce, restrain, arrest... Not hire, promote, date, rent to...

Stigma can target perceptions of the underlying cause of mental illness (e.g., attributions such as bad or weak character), what "these" people are like (e.g., unpredictable), what they deserve (e.g., care, concern, or shunning), and how society, writ large, should respond to them (e.g., provide or deny government or medical assistance). In turn, prejudice translates into greater likelihood of discrimination, including exclusion (e.g., from employment), removing the rights of citizenship (e.g., voting), taking away individual decision-making (e.g., forced/assisted medication), and denying basic freedom (e.g., involuntary commitment, 72-hour holds) (e.g., see Corrigan, Markowitz and Watson 2004).

Figure 16.1, from the US National Academics of Sciences, Engineering, and Medicine's report on stigma (NASEM 2016), lays out the many layers and types of stigma. *Stigma* was originally conceived of as a "mark" that identifies the marked person as "outside the norm" in a particular time and place. Its origin in Ancient Greece arose from the need to separate the conquered (and subsequently enslaved people) from the conquerors who were phenotypically like the citizens of Greece. To do so, enslaved people were permanently branded by burning their flesh, a mark that was intended to signal these persons' devalued status as property and as less than truly human (Hinshaw 2006). In contemporary society, that mark may be physical (e.g., skin color, visible disabilities) or socio-cultural (e.g., ethnic background, religion), it may be concealable (e.g., mental illness, asthma, HIV-infected) or visible (e.g., person in a wheelchair, cleft palate), and may be conferred by informal (e.g., gossip) or formal (e.g., diagnosis) means.

The *process of* stigmatization reflects the way that a particular status comes to have the mark of stigma. That process is dynamic across historical periods, within and among different societies, and even across a person's life (Goffman 1963). Link and Phelan (2001) lay out a number of steps in that process – noting and marking difference, linking difference to negative stereotypes, defining, supporting and enforcing "us" versus "them", and producing material and nonmaterial consequences. Stigma is not present or absent, it exists on a continuum, and it has multiple dimensions. As such, there is an entire stigma *complex* (Pescosolido and Martin 2015: 101; see Figure 16.1).

Stigma exists at three main levels – the individual with the mark, the population where communities can respond differentially to the person with the mark, and the institutional level where the structures in society harass, deny, and exclude individuals. There are also many types and categorizations of stigma, which sometimes produces confusion. First, individuals can internalize the definition of their status as "less than". That *self-stigma* can have a wide variety of consequences, including self-isolation and self-loathing, but, as Thoits (2011) points out, individuals can also resist, redefine, and refuse to accept discrimination as justifiable. Second, as Goffman (1963) saw the essence of stigma as embedded in and materialized through social interaction, *public stigma* represents the prejudice and discrimination that exists in cultural contexts, large and small, in

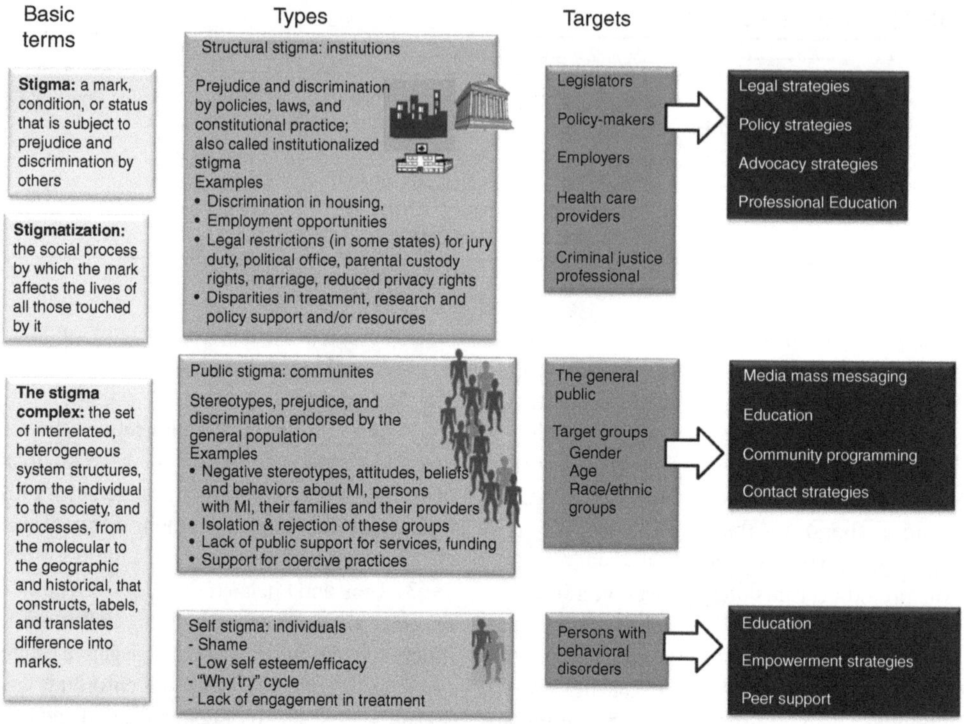

Figure 16.1 The basics of stigma

Source: Adapted from NASEM 2016, used with permission

which individuals live their lives. Third, policies, laws, and even organizational routines can entrench ways of interaction and providing (or denying) access to resources to those labelled as "other" (i.e., *structural stigma*; Hatzenbuehler 2018).

The richness of stigma research, as well as part of its confusion, is that these three general types have spawned many forms, such as perceived, endorsed, and experienced stigma (Pescosolido and Martin 2015; see Table 16.1). For example, providers who care for people with mental illness can experience a lack of respect or fear of contagion from patients and even from colleagues in other areas of medicine (i.e., stigma toward providers, also called associational or courtesy stigma). They can also knowingly or unknowingly avoid certain kinds of patients (e.g., borderline personality disorder) or provide messages in treatment that diminish individuals' efforts at recovery (e.g., provider-based stigma) (Charles 2013).

The general findings and lessons of stigma research are better understood when researchers clarify what kinds of stigmas, individuals, and consequences they are targeting. This is key because the target of anti-stigma programming can be very different depending on the configuration of levels, types and forms, requiring different approaches and messages (NASEM 2016; Stuart, Arboleda-Flores and Sartorious 2012; see final section for more detail).

A BRIEF RESEARCH HISTORY

Erving Goffman's research in the 1960s is heralded as the beginning of research on the stigma of mental illness. Ironically, his observations on mental hospitals barely mentioned stigma; yet his descriptions of the process of stripping identity, the mortification of self, or the irrevocable loss of roles in a federal psychiatric hospital vividly portrayed stigmatization (Goffman 1961: 128, 158, 159). But it was his later general work, *Stigma* (1963), where he provided the now standard definition of stigma, an accounting of basic types, and theoretical fundamentals that are still widely used in research and practice (see Pescosolido 2015 for more detail).

Two efforts preceded and scaffolded research on the stigma of mental illness. The first was the theoretical and empirical work on race, most notably, Allport's (1954) path-breaking work on intergroup relations and Williams' (1947) work on prejudice (see Dovidio, Glick and Rudman 2005; Pettigrew and Tropp 2000). The second set was commissioned by the US federal government, where joint congressional committees asked for data on what Americans knew about mental illness and what they did when they experienced it. The first nationally representative study of Americans' knowledge of and attitudes toward mental illness was conducted by the National Opinion Research Center (now NORC) at the University of Chicago. It documented the inability of Americans to recognize mental illness and to see mental health problems beyond psychosis (Star 1955). At about the same time, the University of Michigan's Institute for Social Research fielded the first wave of the *Americans View Their Mental Health* nationwide survey. It provided critical information on public understandings of and response to mental illness, including if they had "ever anticipated having a nervous breakdown" and what they did in response (Gurin, Veroff, and Field 1960). In 1976, the survey was repeated on a new representative sample, finding positive attitudinal change but little behavioral change regarding the low use of mental health professionals for all groups (Kulka, Veroff, and Douvan 1979; Veroff, Douvan, and Kulka 1981; see Pescosolido and Martin 2007 for more detail).

The social science dialogue on stigma was intimately connected to the advent of labeling theory and the "myth of mental illness" (Scheff 1966; Szaz 1961). Basic arguments centered on ideas that mental illnesses were really "problems of daily living," that diagnoses were really attempts to control deviant behavior, and that the label itself produced internal and external conformity to social scripts, producing chronic mental illness. In the end, path-breaking research on individuals with serious mental illness (e.g., Link et al. 1989's modified labeling theory) concluded that labels did not "produce" chronic mental illness, but did result in stigma and devastating effects on individuals' lives.

While research on stigma continued, the focus waned across disciplines through the 1970s and 1980s. However, and without clear explanation, a resurgence of interest on mental illness began cross-nationally, primarily in high-income countries (e.g., in the US, Phelan et al. 2000; Martin, Pescosolido and Tuch 2000; in the UK, Crisp et al. 2000; in Germany, Angermeyer, Daeumer and Matschinger 1993; in Australia, Jorm et al. 1997; in Canada, Stuart and Arboleda-Florez 2001) and, a bit later, in middle- and low-income countries. Much of the impetus came from the leadership of Norman Sartorius, a Croatian psychiatrist, who in his various positions as director of the World Health Organization's Division of Mental Health and president of important organizations (e.g., World Psychiatric Association, WPA) brought renewed and powerful attention to stigma (e.g., Sartorius and Schulze 2005; see also US Department of Health and Human Services 1999). In the US, for example, from 1996 to 2018, a series of modules on the US General Social Survey, now referred to as the US National Stigma Studies (NSSs), focused on the public stigma of mental illness, measuring perceived attributions, stereotypes, help-seeking, and behavioral predispositions (see Pescosolido 2013). In low-incomes countries, the concern with the stigma attached to HIV/AIDS predominated, producing a large body of research (see the special collection on: Stigma Research and Global Health, *BMC Medicine* 2019, volume 17). In total, by the beginning of the 21st century, there were new theoretical frameworks (e.g., the FINIS model, Pescosolido, Martin et al. 2008; the Attribution Model, Corrigan et al. 2003; the Theory of Fundamental Causes, Hatzebuehler et al. 2013), new methodological approaches and measures (Link at al. 2004; see next section), and reviews of findings (Link and Phelan 2001). This was matched by new programs (e.g., the Rosalynn *Carter Fellowships* for Mental Health Journalism, established in 1995; the WPA's Open the Door Programme, Sartorius 1997) and larger scale efforts to change stigma (e.g., the UK's "Time to Change" program, Henderson and Thornicroft 2009; see NASEM 2016 for a summary).

One Theoretical Approach

The Framework Integrating Normative Influences on Stigma (FINIS, Pescosolido, Martin et al. 2008) brought together ideas and empirical findings from a range of disciplines with relevant theories. As a systems science approach, the underlying assumption (i.e., stigma is embedded in many connected individual and societal systems) emphasizes interdependence and interactions, increasing concerns for unintended consequences. FINIS begins with Goffman's insights that understanding stigma requires a language of social relationships and how those relationships are embedded in structural contexts. As depicted in Figure 16.2, FINIS emphasizes interaction at the interface of individuals and communities. On the model's left-hand side, social characteristics of the individual and of the situation shape both the evaluation of the targeted person's behavior and the probability that others can easily identify a person with mental illness. When the target person holds several devalued statuses, the greater the likelihood that others will see the situation as serious, will label it, and will stigmatize the individual. Greater social distance between the target person and the observer translates into either protection from stigma (if the target person has more social power) or greater stigma (for those with relatively less social power). However, while FINIS acknowledges the importance of structural contexts, including organizations, media, and larger cultures, stigma may be different for individuals of different social classes, race/ethnicities, and genders (see Kim and Sasaki 2014; Krendl et al. 2006). On the model's right-hand side, stigma is seen as embedded in a larger cultural context that shapes the extent to which stereotyping exists, the nature of social cleavages that define "others," and the way that different groups accept, reject, or modify dominant cultural beliefs. Research has shown that these larger cultural context shapes individual experiences. For example, media images, which reify or counter popular stereotypes, also vary cross-nationally (Olafsdottir 2007) and over time (Wahl, Wood and Richards 2002), influencing individuals' attitudes and behaviors (see summary of cross-level research below).

Once the label is affixed, the stigmatizing consequences can be complicated. Being formally labeled may simultaneously initiate greater social support from one's social network while producing greater rejection and discrimination by acquaintances and strangers (Perry 2011). It allows access to services but opens the door to prejudice and discrimination (Rosenfield 1997). And, as has been discussed above, stigma can shape treatment decisions and outcomes, by both patients and providers. Together, these forces have broad effects on life chances. Finally, stigma can permeate and reverberate back on the community, its institutions, and the population. When stigma is a significant source of stress and social disadvantage, it can have substantial effects on population health, similar to other social determinants, such as discrimination based on socioeconomic status (SES) and race/ethnicity (Hatzenbuehler et al. 2013).

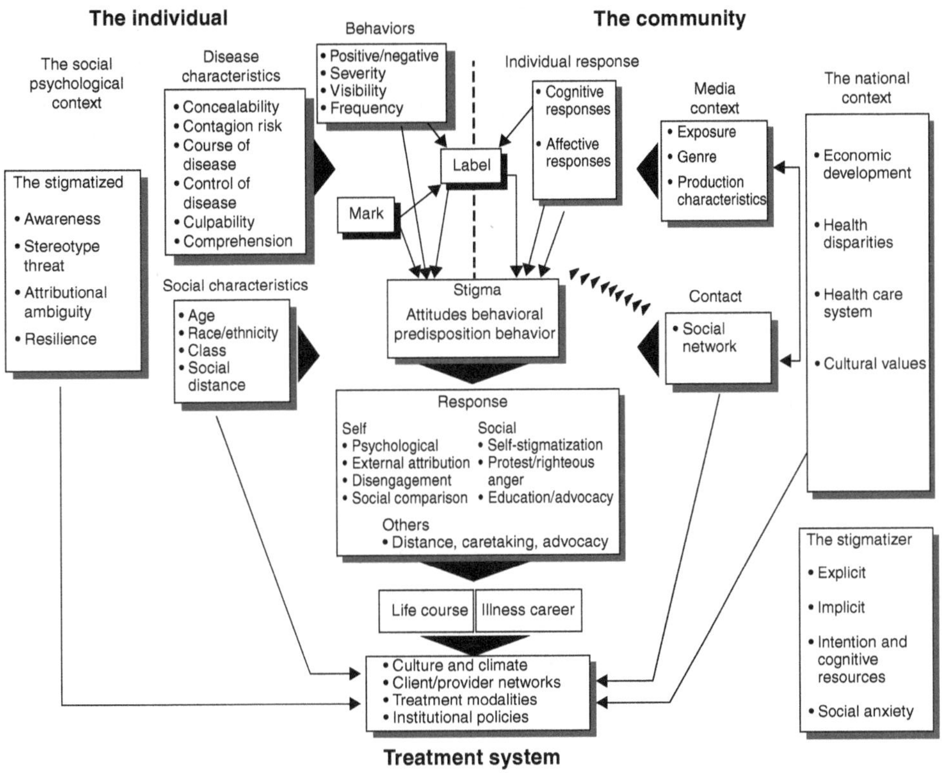

Figure 16.2 The FINIS model of stigma (Pescosolido, Martin et al. 2008)

GLOBAL LEVELS OF STIGMA

Getting a cross-national picture of the stigma of mental illness is difficult. Many small-scale, convenience-sample reports, that use one of three main methodological approaches, provide some global insights, although data that allow rigorous cross-national comparison are relatively rare. The ethnographic approach typically uses observational and deep field methods to understand local meanings, experiences, and effects of stigma. The survey approach uses mail, face-to-face, or web instruments to gather data on the larger cultural profile of groups (e.g., persons "with," the public, or target groups such as providers or employers). The psychological approach employs experimental or "implicit" methods to uncover levels, levers, and unconscious aspects of stigma (see Littlewood, Jadhav and Ryder 2007; Major and O'Brien 2005; Teachman, Wilson and Komarovskaya 2006). Each approach has strengths and limitations, and together they have provided a deep understanding of stigma. However, each approach has provided limited cross-national data. For example, while researching the stigmatization of mental illness among medical students in Croatia or in Portugal (Filipcic et al. 2003; Telles-Correia et al. 2015), dental students in India (Madhan et al. 2012), or nursing students in Singapore (Chang et al. 2017) has a distinct relevance for local training, the reliance on convenient student samples for examining stigma generally has limited utility for understanding population-level stigma profiles. What we do know, no matter which group is studied, which methods are employed, or what country is targeted, is that stigma has not dissipated.

Our focus on public stigma here will rely primarily on nationally representative population studies. Where the sampling frame is virtually unknowable (e.g., stigma experiences of persons with mental illness), we will target studies expressly designed to compare stigma cross-nationally. Not surprisingly, then, much of what we know of public stigma's global profile comes from high-income countries where the resources to do broad-based, representative data collection is greater. In this section, we will review the surprisingly consistent findings from those countries, summarize findings from expressly designed comparative international studies on population or "persons with" data, and discuss those rare studies that link the stigma larger context to personal experiences. Following this, we present novel data to illustrate stigma differences across 17 countries and stigma's association with previous contact, considered a prime lever of stigma change.

Similarities across Independent, High-income Country Studies

Based on a series of studies done in the UK, the US, Germany, and Australia, a set of stigma findings more or less describe public stigma in high-income, primarily Western, countries. Table 16.2 summarizes both "good news" and "bad news" (Pescosolido 2013). On the positive side, most respondents recognize mental illness (e.g., in Australia, over 70% correctly identified a case), but many fewer could identify specific disorders (just under 40% recognize the case as depression; Jorm et al. 1997). Further, most respondents across these studies attributed mental illness to scientific causes (including genetics, chemical imbalance, stress) rather than moral ones (e.g., "bad character," less the case for addictions; Pescosolido et al. 2010). In addition, more respondents reporting a willingness to talk to family and friends about mental health problems (Swindle et al. 2000). Across the board, support for help-seeking appears to be high,

Table 16.2 Summary of findings from population-based studies in high-income countries

"Good News"	• Public has become more knowledgeable about mental illness (familiarity with MI beyond psychosis, greater endorsement of neuro-biological cause, fewer endorsement of moral causes) • More individuals reporting a willingness to talk to family and friends about mental health problems • Increasingly high endorsement of formal sources of care • Research is beginning to show decreases in population levels of stigma, although effects are modest with societies changing slowly
"Bad News"	• Stigma levels are high (~50% of the population) • People respond more negatively to alcohol and drug issues than mental illness, and, this is one area where moral attributions are trending in the direction of more stigmatizing (i.e., "bad character) • Levels of perceiving people with mental illness as "dangerous" remain high and, for schizophrenia, are trend in the wrong direction • While endorsement of neurobiological attributions has increased, there is no connection to lower levels of stigma, and a backlash may be in evidence regarding beliefs about genetic attributions
Major Considerations	• There are clear differences in the response to different mental health problems, with schizophrenia eliciting more stigmatizing responses than depression, with notable East Asian exceptions • There is also a clear gradient of response – the more intimate the venue (e.g., marriage, work closely on the job), the more individuals endorse social distance • Stigma toward child mental health problems elicit much lower levels of stigma than adult problems; however, child/adolescent depression is the exception • Both the label (i.e., respondents agreeing that the situation is a mental illness) and the behaviors (i.e., different types of mental illness described in vignettes) are significantly associated with stigmatizing responses

and in some cases, reaching ceilings and approximating levels reported by mental health professionals, despite continued low actual service use (in the UK, Crisp et al. 2000; in the US, Pescosolido et al. 2010; in Australia, Jorm, Christensen and Griffiths 2006).

Within countries, the response to mental illness appears to vary by the diagnosis/problem and the type of interaction. In nearly all societies, perhaps with the exceptions of China and Japan, the stigma attached to schizophrenia is greater than to depression, and this appears to be a level of difference rather than a qualitatively different phenomenon. Finally, in all high-income countries where asked, perceptions of dangerousness and unpredictability are associated with more stigmatizing responses, while reports of having had previous contact with people with mental illness was associated with lower levels of stigma types (e.g., in Germany, Angermeyer and Matschinger 2003; in Canada, Thompson et al. 2002; in the US, Pescosolido Olafsdottir et al. 2008; and in Japan, Krendl and Pescosolido 2020).

Perhaps the most notable finding is the *lack* of association between holding scientific, medical beliefs about underlying causes of mental illness and the endorsement of stigmatizing attitudes. A major assumption underlying many efforts to reduce stigma relies on the contention that when individuals see mental illness as a "disease," the associated blame, shame, and rejection will dissipate. But a review of 33 studies, primarily in the Global North, concluded that "biogenetic attributions" were not associated with more tolerant attitudes; in fact, there was sometimes a backlash (mostly with schizophrenia) where such attributions were associated with greater stigma endorsements by the general population (Angermeyer et al. 2011; see also Pescosolido et al. 2010; Phelan 2005). This finding has fundamentally changed the way many providers, advocates, and researchers think about stigma change.

Findings from Cross-nationally Coordinated Studies

Comparative stigma studies are rare for obvious reasons, including cost, access, coordination logistics, and methodological limits. However, two kinds have been done: those that focus on the perceptions and experiences of people with mental illness, targeting clinics or advocacy groups for respondents; and those that focus on the reaction of the general population to those individuals, using statistical sampling methods to ensure representativeness.

Research on "Persons With"

A multi-site face-to-face, cross-sectional survey undertaken in 35 countries combined the efforts of the European Union (EU)-funded ASPEN (Anti Stigma Programme European Network) study and the INDIGO-Depression (International Study of Discrimination and Stigma for Depression) research network. Together, data were collected in 19 sites in 18 European countries and 20 sites in 17 countries, which included high-income (e.g., Canada, Australia) and middle-income (e.g., India, Brazil, Egypt, Nigeria) countries. Local research staff identified people attending specialist outpatient or day care (public or private sector) with a diagnosis of major depressive disorder in the last year, with over 1,000 individuals completing a depression screener (DISC-12). Of those, just under 80% reported experiencing discrimination in at least one area of life and reported this as a factor in decisions not to pursue opportunities (e.g., 37% not initiating close personal relationships, 25% not seeking employment, 20% not seeking further education/training). Those who had more severe illnesses or poorer social functioning, had been hospitalized, or kept their diagnosis a secret were more likely to report stigmatizing experiences and restricting their opportunities. Signaling the power of self-stigma to affect lives, fewer than half of the respondents who anticipated discrimination reported actual experiences (Lasalvia et al. 2013).

Another 27-country study also leveraged the INDIGO Research Network, finding that over 90% of 700 individuals with diagnoses of schizophrenia reported discriminatory experiences and most (over 70%) felt a need to conceal their mental health status (Thornicroft et al. 2009). Finally, data on experiences of stigma from over 1,000 individuals diagnosed with bipolar disorder or depression, who were members of a national, mental health, non-governmental advocacy organization, completed a mail survey. Referred to as the GAMIAN-Europe study, over 70% of individuals reported moderate/high perceived discrimination and one-fifth reported moderate/high levels of self-stigma. Yet, a majority (around 60%) also reported moderate/high stigma resistance or moderate/high empowerment (Brohan et al. 2010). In 2019, the UK stigma research group, involved in both the INDIGO and GAMIAN studies, concluded that "stigma and discrimination are universal, that they are reversible, and that there are some variations in their manifestations across cultures" (Thornicroft et al. 2019: 229).

Research on Public Stigma

Two major cross-national efforts used population-based sampling methods to approximate representation of each country as a whole. The first is European-based, fielded in 2006 and again in 2010, funded by the European Union in concert with World Health Organization, as part of the Eurobarometer Studies (see European Commission, TNS Opinion and TNS Social 2006, 2010). Short face-to-face interviews were conducted with nearly 30,000 individuals aged 15+ years old in 27 EU countries at each time point. A basic question, designed to measure stigma by asking respondents if they would find it difficult to talk to someone with mental health problems, revealed an extraordinary range from a low of 6% in Cyprus to a high of 52% in Lithuania. Overall, countries newer to the EU (new member states, or NMS12) reported higher levels of stigma than the original EU countries (EU15). Much of the data are reported overall for all countries, for example, that 45% agree/strongly agree that people with mental health problems are dangerous; even more (over 68%) say that they are unpredictable. Mirroring the findings described above in the Western national studies, the levels of stigmatizing attributions are quite low (between 7% and 16%) compared to measures of acceptance, contact, or exclusion (Evans-Lacko et al. 2012).

The second effort is the Stigma in Global Context–Mental Health Study (SGC–MHS), funded by the US National Institutes of Health's Fogarty International Center and Office for Behavioral and Social Science Research. Drawing on the International Social Survey Program (ISSP) platform, trained interviewers conducted face-to-face interviews in 17 countries (Table 16.3). By leveraging the ISSP infrastructure and using its well-developed set of standardized socio-demographic measures, the SGC–MHS team was able to focus in more detail on developing and including stigma measures (seven types and 27 items) and a novel vignette approach to eliciting stigma responses in the SGC–MHS instrument (overall SGC–MHS response rate = 65%).

Specifically, following the US National Stigma Studies, the SGC–MHS employed vignettes coupled with a unique translation approach. The vignette strategy provided respondents with an unlabeled case description (rather than items about, for example, "people with mental illness"). The case was consistent with symptoms meeting criteria for standard psychiatric diagnoses (see Box 16.1). While sidestepping many controversies over psychiatric diagnoses, vignettes avoid giving labels (i.e., "mental illness") which leave the referent subject to a wide variety of respondent interpretation and provides the possibility of examining the public's recognition of mental illness (Martin, Pescosolido, and Tuch 2000; and see Angermeyer and Dietrich 2006 on vignettes). While the interview schedule was not decentered (Smith 2004), a meeting of representatives from all

Box 16.1 The Stigma in Global Context-Mental Health Study

The SGC–MHS conducted face-to-face interviews with nationally representative samples of adults on every continent. Participants were provided a vignette describing an individual with schizophrenia and asked about their willingness to interact with that person across six social settings, including work, neighborhood, and marriage into the family. Vignettes randomly varied characteristics, including a second stigmatized condition that constituted an "outgroup" (e.g., race/ethnicity/region) in that society (details can be found at: https://icmhsr.sitehost.iu.edu/sgcmhs.html). Participants were asked, among other things, to identify the condition as labeling has been shown to affect stigma. A social distance score was then created, enumerating participants' willingness to interact with the individual described in the vignette and examined based on characteristics presented.

Schizophrenia. John/Mary [White]/Tyrone/Shontell [Black] is a White/Black man/woman. Up until a year ago, life was pretty okay for John/Mary/Tyrone/Shontell. But then things started to change. He/she thought that people around him/her were making disapproving comments and talking behind his/her back. John/Mary/Tyrone/Shontell was convinced that people were spying on him/her and that they could hear what he/she was thinking. John/Mary/Tyrone/Shontell lost his/her drive to participate in his/her usual work and family activities and retreated to his/her home, eventually spending most of his/her time on his/her own. John/Mary/Tyrone/Shontell became so preoccupied with what he/she was thinking that he/she skipped meals and stopped bathing regularly. At night, when everyone else was sleeping, he/she was walking back and forth at home. John/Mary/Tyrone/Shontell was hearing voices even though no one else was around. These voices told him/her what to do and what to think. He/She has been living this way for six months.

Depression. John/Mary [White]/Tyrone/Shontell [Black] is a White/Black man/woman. For the last several weeks, John/Mary/Tyrone/Shontell has been feeling really down. He/she wakes up in the morning with a sad mood and a heavy feeling that sticks with him/her all day long. He/she isn't enjoying things the way he/she normally would. In fact, nothing gives him/her pleasure. Even when good things happen, they don't seem to make John/Mary/Tyrone/Shontell happy. The smallest tasks are difficult to accomplish. He/she finds it hard to concentrate on anything. He/she feels out of energy, out of steam, and cannot do things he/she usually does. And even though John/Mary/Tyrone/Shontell feels tired, when night comes, he/she can't go to sleep. John/Mary/Tyrone/Shontell feels pretty worthless, very discouraged, and guilty. John's/Mary's/Tyrone's/Shontell's family has noticed that he/she has lost appetite and weight. He/she has pulled away from them and just doesn't feel like talking.

countries increased engagement and enhanced the translation process from standard translation–back translation to adding a cultural translation with a native speaker who had no mental health or survey training (Boyer, Pescosolido and Medina 2008). Though with clear limitations, the rigorously monitored, collaboratively constructed, and culturally informed approach allows a reasonable, comparative examination of the cultural landscape of stigma in 17 countries that touched every inhabited continent.

SGC–MHS analyses focused on similarities and differences in levels of stigma between countries. The earliest findings revealed large variations in cross-national stigma but more modest differences in geographic areas such as western Europe. The SGC–MHS supported past findings that stigma levels varied by problem type and was not sufficiently understood by examining the socio-demographic characteristics of respondents (e.g., education predicting lower endorsement of stigma) (Olafsdottir and Pescosolido 2011; Pescosolido, Olafsdottir et al. 2008). However, using a different approach, the SGC–MHS asked two novel questions: (1) Does a lack of knowledge, an unwillingness to include individuals with mental health problems in civil society, or concerns about treatment stand in the way of recovery? (2) Is there a "backbone" of larger cultural beliefs, attitudes, and opinions about mental illness that presents the greatest challenges to individuals, families, and providers? The results suggested that, with some clear

Table 16.3 The countries included in the stigma in global context – Mental Health Study (SGC–MHS)

Abbreviation	*Full Name*	*Flag*	*Continent*	*N*
ARG	Argentina	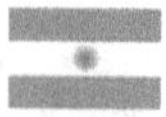	South America	1420
BE	Belgium		Europe	1166
BGD	Bangladesh	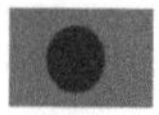	Asia	1501
BRA	Brazil	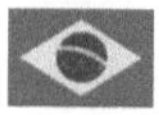	South America	1522
BGR	Bulgaria	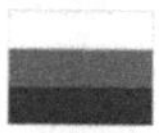	Europe	1121
CH	China		Asia	5620
CYP	Cyprus		Europe	804
DEU	Germany		Europe	1255
ESP	Spain	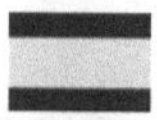	Europe	1206
GBR	Great Britain		Europe	1030
HUN	Hungary		Europe	1252
ISL	Iceland	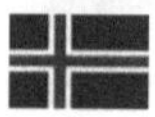	Europe	1033
KOR	South Korea		Asia	1003
NZL	New Zealand		Australia	1020
PHL	Philippines		Asia	1200
USA	United States	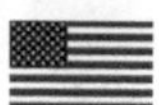	North America	1425
ZAF	South Africa	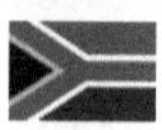	Africa	1550
			Total N:	**18,342**

exceptions the embrace of neurobiological causes, the acceptance of the utility of medical providers, and the evaluation of severity are widespread. Stigma is not as much lodged in mental health literacy as in the potential for discrimination. What stood out even more was that, even in countries with low overall stigma levels, a core of prejudicial beliefs exists among more than half of each country's population for depression and two-thirds of their populations for schizophrenia. These issues targeted aspects of life that were more intimate (reject as an in-law, see potential for violence toward self, unpredictable) or ones that tapped authority-based statuses (not care for children, not teach children). Other forms of prejudice that were high but not reaching these consensus levels included that the vignette persons were not suitable to supervise others in the workplace, are hard to talk to, and are less productive than others.

Linking Stigma and Country Context

What is perhaps most interesting in international stigma research is not only that it provides data on national stigma levels, and correlates, but also that it explores links between country profiles, stigma levels, and outcomes for individuals with mental illness. For example, until recently, a common cultural myth surrounding stigma maintained that traditional, deep, and rich community ties purported to characterize social life in low- and middle-income countries (as opposed to truncated, superficial ones in modern societies), produced lower stigma and greater acceptance of people with mental illness. However, analyses from the SGC–MHS found no support for this "developing" versus "developed" country correlate of the WHO's International Studies of Schizophrenia's provocative finding of better schizophrenia outcomes in Nigeria and India than in the US or Great Britain (Pescosolido et al. 2015; Hopper and Wanderling 2000). Although the WHO researchers' preliminary, limited analyses of the stigma hypothesis did not support the nostalgic myth (i.e., finding the difference to be more likely related to treatment contexts across sites), this does not dismiss the importance of "moral worlds" or everyday cultural practices (Hopper et al. 2007 book). Rather, what may shape stigma and its effects cross-nationally may not be tied to a crude "developed versus developing" distinction. In fact, where there was any relationship between measures of stigma and level of development, the SGC–MHS documented lower stigma in countries where more of the GDP is spent on public health (Pescosolido et al. 2015). Further, within the narrower confines of the European Union, analyses of the Eurobarometer data (described earlier) reveal that those countries with higher levels of income inequality and unemployment are those where the population endorses more stigmatizing attitudes and reports lower use of services from specialty or general providers (Bracke, Delaruelle and Verhaeghe 2019; Verhaeghe, Bracke and Pattyn 2010). These findings align with other research that supports the contention that countries with higher levels of public stigma have greater reported levels of stigmatizing experiences, a reluctance to seek care, and a higher suicide rate (Evans-Lacko et al. 2012; Mojtabi 2010; Schomerus et al. 2015).

A more recent approach offers a curiously different set of findings. A survey of Worldwide Web users (596,712 over 1.7 years) in 229 countries asked individuals whether they had a daily interaction with someone with mental illness, whether they associated mental illness with violence, and whether individuals with mental illness could recover. Stigma levels were lower here than in any of the studies reported above and, also to the contrary, reported significant differences between respondents in "developed" and "developing" countries. However, since the participants were reported to primarily be young, educated, English speaking males, there are questions about the representativeness of these findings for studying global differences (Seeman et al. 2016).

An Illustration: Social Distance and Personal Contact in 17 Countries

The results above provide a research summary but fail to offer a visual, detailed sense of stigma cross-nationally. Most cross-national research examines structural-level factors that contribute to stigma. Here, we examine how the prevalence of individual-level contact with those with mental illness maps onto the amount of stigma in each country.

Using data from the SGC–MHS, Figures 16.3, 16.4, and 16.5 display basic data on the most common operationalization of stigma, social distance (Link et al. 2004), and the individual-level correlate thought to be the most robust, i.e., previous personal contact (Couture and Penn 2003). Specifically, respondents were asked to indicate how willing they would be to move next door, make friends, spend an evening socializing, start working closely on the job, have as in-law, and have a group home with people like the vignette person in the neighborhood. After dichotomizing each response as yes (1) or no (0), the responses were summed, with higher numbers indicating a desire for greater social distance. The scales were averaged by country for the schizophrenia and depression vignettes. "Contact" with mental illness represents the proportion of people in the country (by vignette) who report either having or knowing someone with a mental illness.

Figures 16.3 (depression) and 16.4 (schizophrenia) show that the individual-level relationship, documented in so many research reports, between contact and stigma also exists at the country level. Figure 16.3 summarizes the amount of desired social distance from the vignette character with depression, ranging from the country with the least desired social distance (Brazil) to the country with the most desired social distance (Bangladesh). It also summarizes the amount of contact by country (for those who saw the depression vignette) with the least reported contact (China) to the country with the most reported contact (Iceland). For schizophrenia (Figure 16.4), there is a wide range of rejection across countries with the lowest average level of desired social distance (Brazil) to the country with the most desired social distance (Cyprus) and also a wide range of personal contact with persons with mental illness (lowest in China, highest in Iceland).

For both schizophrenia and depression, there are middle-income countries, such as Bangladesh and Philippines; also high levels in countries in the former Soviet Union (e.g., Bulgaria and Hungary); and the lowest rates in countries as diverse as Germany, Argentina, South Africa, and Brazil. There is no evidence of regional clustering of stigma (e.g., Global North vs. Global South; east vs. west). The broadly similar placement of countries around the spiral suggests that the response to different mental illness is more similar within countries than across different mental health problems. In 15 of the 17 countries, respondents desire significantly more social distance from the character in the schizophrenia vignette than the character in the depression vignette (China and Bangladesh stand as exceptions, details on request).

A comparison of the two figures for depression reveals inverse mirror images with significant correlation between contact and social distance ($r = -0.597$, $p<0.05$), but the alignment is far from perfect with Iceland and the US, in the moderately low levels of stigma endorsement, reporting the highest rates of previous contact. Roughly, the countries with the highest levels of desired social distance also report lower levels of contact (e.g., Cyprus, Philippines , Bangladesh). but China stands out as an exception, with low levels of contact but more middling stigma levels. These patterns are similar for schizophrenia, the inverse relationship between contact and desired social distance, apparent in the depression vignette, is also present here ($r^2 = -0.596$, $p<0.05$).

Figure 16.5 may reveal an important and novel finding in both cases. For both depression and schizophrenia, the relationship at the aggregate level appears to be vaguely non-linear. That is, as the percentage of the population who reports previous contact increases, social distance decreases *to a point*. Somewhere in the 50% range, the stigma reducing effect of contact levels off. So, for the US, Belgium, Iceland, New Zealand, and Great Britain, where between 60% and 80% of the country has had contact with persons with mental illness, the

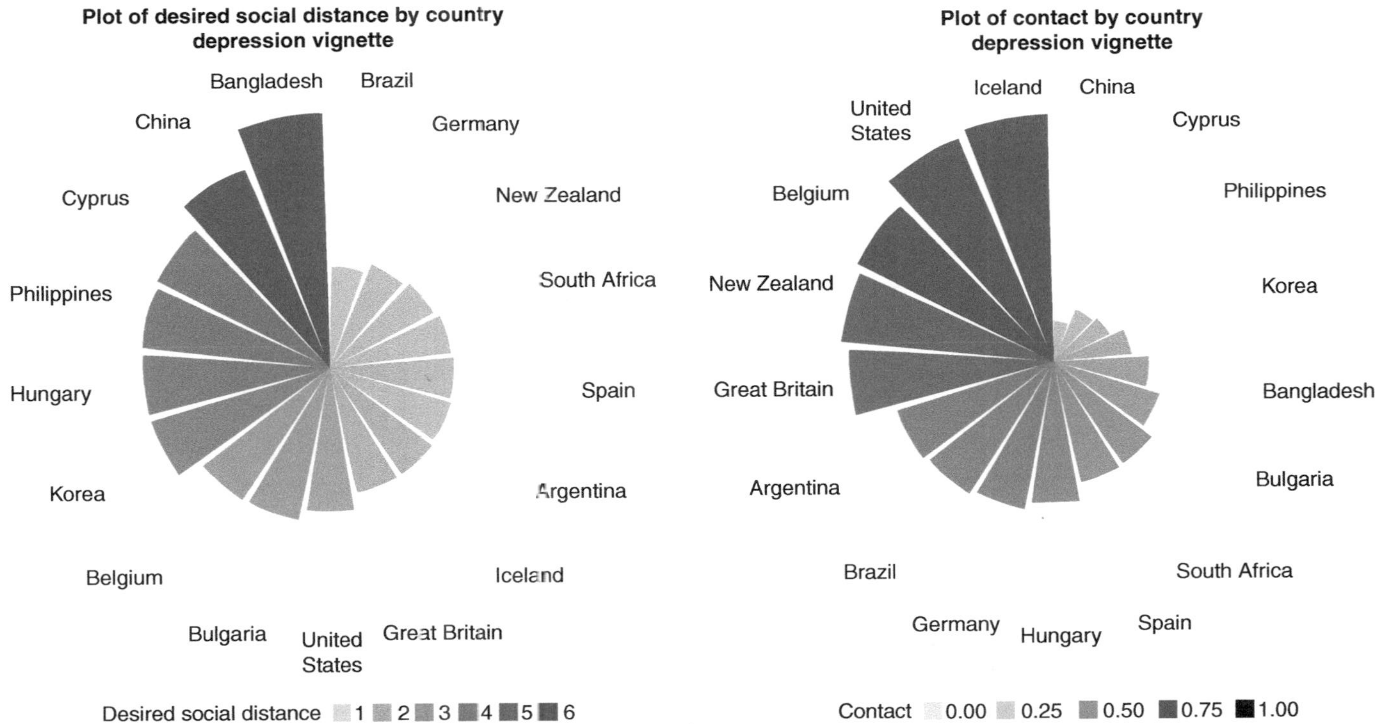

Figure 16.3 Summary of desired social distance and amount of contact by country – depression vignette

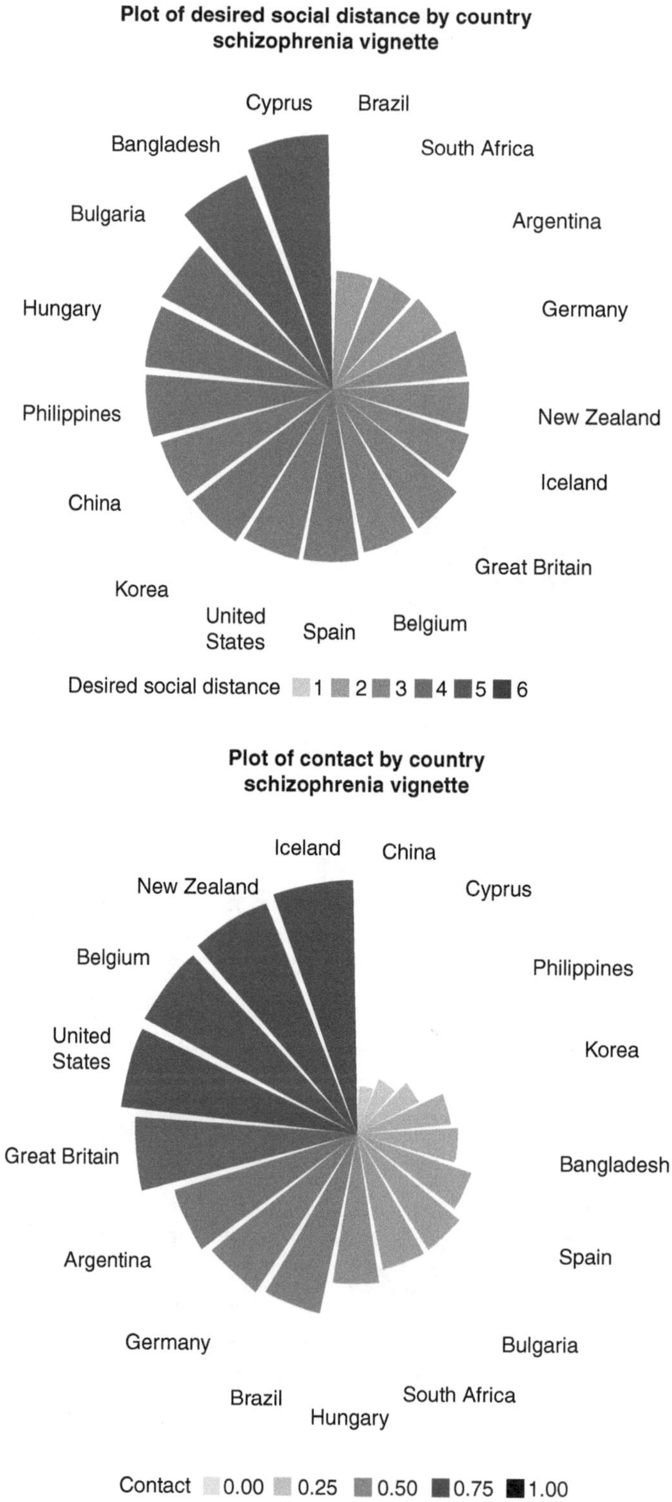

Figure 16.4 Summary of desired social distance and amount of contact by country – schizophrenia vignette

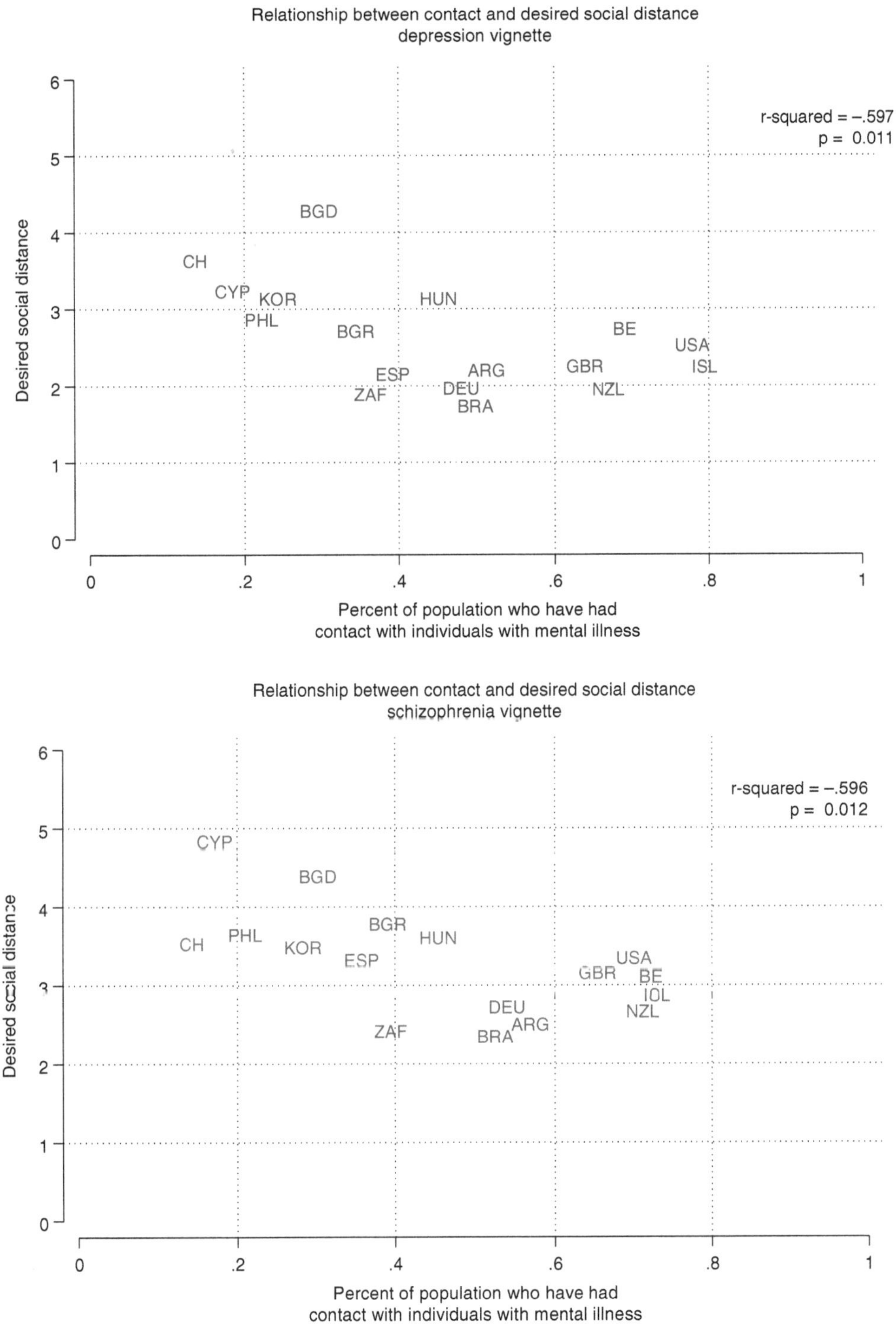

Figure 16.5 Relationship between contact and desired social distance – depression and schizophrenia vignettes

aggregate stigma profile is no better than in countries like Spain or South Africa, where only about 40% of the population reports previous contact. With the few cases in the SCG–MHS, a curvilinear specification did not reach significance. Yet, the suggestion remains that contact, like scientific attributions before it, may have unanticipated limits as a tool of stigma reduction.

HAS PUBLIC STIGMA SHIFTED? NATIONAL TRENDS

There are only a few countries, again most in the Global North, where population trend data on public stigma are available. Some of these are aligned with national anti-stigma efforts; others are not. In one of the earliest studies, Jorm and colleagues (2006) documented an improvement in recognition of depression and schizophrenia and greater endorsement of the use of multiple services (mental health professionals, medications, psychotherapy, mental hospital) admission over an eight-year period (1995–2001). In Germany, where the most consistent monitoring of stigma has been done, Angermeyer and Matschiner (2005) analyzed data across two population surveys (1990 and 2001), reporting that the public believed that stigma towards people with mental illness was decreasing, especially among those with greater knowledge about psychiatric care. However, responses endorsing discrimination by employers or in intimate relationships showed no change. A later survey, updating trends to 2011, documented the same population perception that stigma toward people with mental illness was decreasing. However, at this point, not only were attitudes unchanged, but in some case, has worsened. This was also the case in an analysis of trend data in England and Scotland from 1994 to 2003, where some improvement in attributions were documented alongside increasing stigma around social exclusion (Mehta et al. 2009). In the US, a decade of change (1996–2006) in the NSSs showed an increase in mental health literacy (attributions and care endorsements), but no change in social distance, signaling the "disease like any other" findings described earlier (Pescosolido et al. 2010). The most recent follow-up, in 2018, is showing mixed results, with public stigma toward depression decreasing. Specifically, the desire for social distance decreased across social circumstances including working on the job, having as a friend, and marrying into the family (Pescosolido et al. In Press). However the 2018 NSS reveals a drift toward more public perception of the potential for violence among the vignette characters overall and schizophrenia reaching significance (Pescosolido, Manago and Monahan 2019).

The most detailed trend data come from the UK where two different national campaigns, Changing Minds and Time to Change, collected nationally representative data in 1998, 2003 and each year between 2007 and 2013. The initial study (Crisp et al. 2005) reported a small but significant decrease in stigma that had initial high endorsements, including perceptions that individuals with some mental illnesses are dangerous, "different than us," and "hard to talk to". There was little improvement in areas where stigma was already low (e.g., "not improved if treated," "selves to blame"). As shown in Figure 16.6 below, the Time to Change effort used the data from the 2013 and added the yearly data, documenting significant increases in positive attitudes toward prejudice and exclusion, but not for tolerance or support for community care (Z score 0.01, -0.01 to 0.03, $p = 0.27$). Overall, the authors concluded that change was "significant and moderate" (Evans-Lacko et al. 2014a).

In 2012, a systematic review of all existing, national, population-based, rigorous studies on mental illness-related beliefs and attitudes in the general population analyzed time trends for representative national studies with a follow-up interval of at least two years. Of the six studies that met strict inclusion

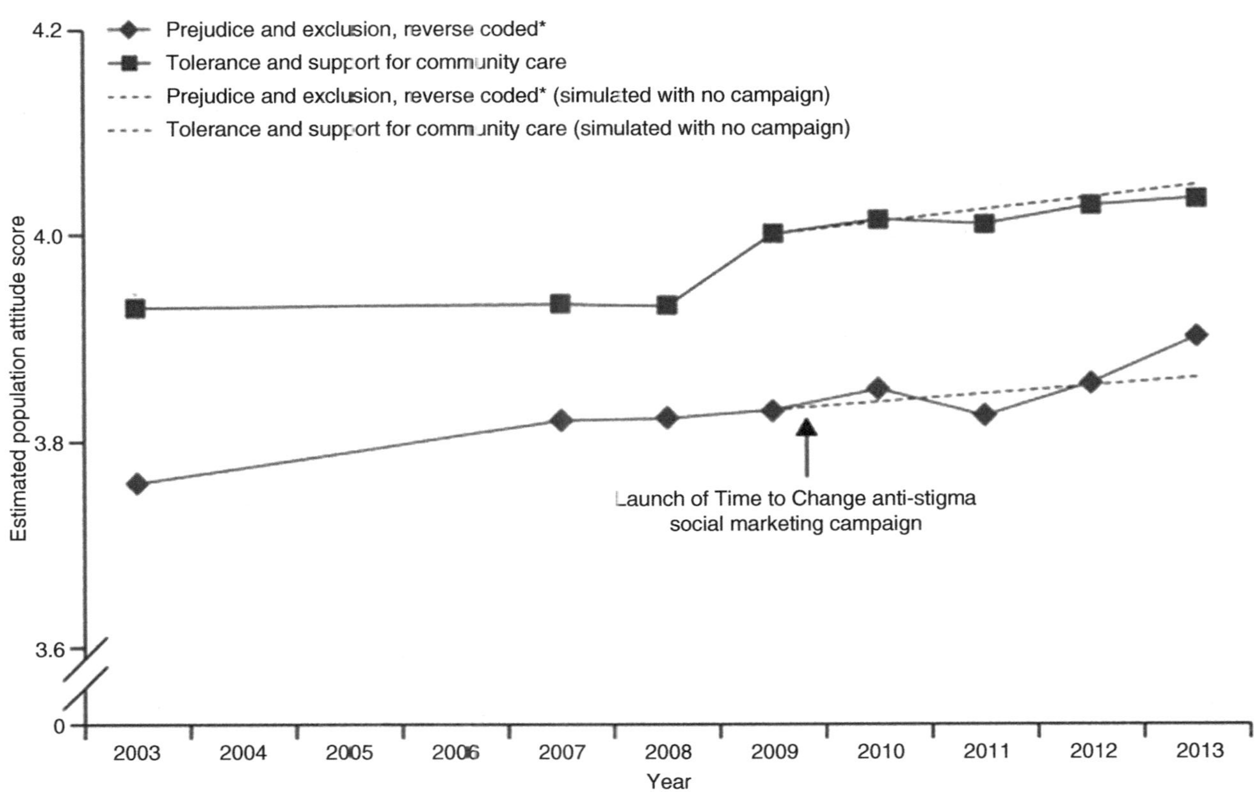

Figure 16.6 Population attitude trends across England 2003–13

Source: Evans-Lacko et al. 2014a (used with permission) – higher numbers indicate more positive attitudes.

criteria, the analyses supported the two major findings hinted at above. First, there is a general cross-national trend to improved mental health literacy, measured by issues such as endorsement of scientific, medical (rather than moral) causes of mental illness. Second, few positive changes in prejudice are in evidence, and in some cases, this has become worse (Schomerus et al. 2012). We would add to this, looking at Figure 16.6 and from our own research, three considerations – societies change slowly in terms of core values and perceptions, are subject to fluctuations in other areas of social life (e.g., economic downturns), and cannot be separated from overall liberalizing or conservatizing trends toward social issues in general.

CONCLUSION: EFFORTS TO CHANGE AND GAPS TO FILL

The number and types of individual-level interventions are too numerous and diverse to review. There are, however, a set of widely shared ideas about change. For example, Thornicroft et al. (2016) contend that some promising, group-level anti-stigma inventions decrease self-stigma and increase empowerment; that for some target groups (e.g., students) interventions show stigma decrease; and that when anti-stigma programming includes personal contact, the results are more likely to be effective. Corrigan, Kuwabara and O'Shaughnessy (2009) adds that educational efforts are most effective for younger age groups; protest often backfires in effect; and contact is the most potent potential lever, whether face-to-face or in some video format. As described earlier, we believe that the "disease like any other" tag line may be useful in improving the public's health knowledge but rarely transfer over to reducing prejudice or discrimination and is unlikely to lower stigma, at least in the Global North.

Such conclusions are not surprising because they correspond to what is known about intervention studies in general. Specifically, one-shot interventions rarely have longer-term effects with initial benefits appearing to extinguish over even short periods of time. According to the 2016 National Academy of Sciences, Engineering and Medicine report, *Ending Discrimination against People with Mental Illness and Substance Use Disorders: The Evidence for Stigma Change*, national programs with sufficient resources and a longer time frame appear to have more lasting, but slow to appear, effects (see the NASEM 2016 summary of *Like Mind, Like Minds* in New Zealand' *See Me*, in Scotland, *Time to Change* and *Opening Minds* in Canada). Yet, researchers involved in some of these programs raise concerns. As noted earlier, the documented effects are not consistently positive. In *Paradigms Lost: Fighting Stigma and the Lessons Learned*, a seasoned team of researchers and providers identified a number of common assumptions that, in the past, were used as foundations to build anti-stigma programs. They lay out "myths", recommending the abandonment of "familiar but ineffective approaches" (Stuart, Arboleda-Florez and Sartorius 2012: 36). In the end, they argue for a focus on local efforts, ones that target issues that consumers raise, and ones that attack the structural stigma they see as perpetuating inequality.

Further, nearly everyone who has been involved in these issues, especially in the US, laments the lost power of a concerted and collaborative effort to share what is known, what is available, and what might be built cumulatively. The NASEM (2016) report calls for national leadership and coordination that could better deploy resources, amplify efforts, and increase effectiveness even as efforts are tailored for sites and specific populations. Some have called into question the scalability of "personal contact" approaches; others have abandoned the idea of changing cultures in favor of improving individual lives (Pescosolido 2020). However, the rare but incredibly important research summarized above that links larger context to individual experiences suggests that empowering individuals and changing culture are not likely to improve stigma unless they are done in tandem (see also Rao et al. 2019).

While several limitations have been described above, some merit repeating while others need to be considered. As Evans-Lacko et al. (2014b), point out, even in Europe, research to date has targeted Northwest Europe. A broad and deep understanding of global stigma remains beyond our reach at this point. Further, we have only a limited understanding of "intersectional stigma", the convergence of multiple stigmatized identities within a person or group; of how and where mental illness figures in; and of how to address their joint effects on health and well-being. While inquiry into the intersections of race, class, and gender serves as the historical and theoretical basis for intersectional stigma, there is little consensus at present on how best to characterize and analyze intersectional stigma, or on how to design interventions to address this complex phenomenon (Turan et al. 2017). Finally, we do not know if the blatant prejudice and discrimination that is attached to mental illness will be replaced by new, and more subtle forms as we have seen with regard to racism (Rabinowitz et al. 2009).

The conclusion of what we know about mental illness stigma is that what most, if not all, research shares is the call for "enlightened opportunism" (Stuart, Arboleda-Florez and Sartorius 2012), that is, taking every opportunity to fight stigma to improve the lives of those affected in any way. Since stigma remains widespread, incredibly resistant to change, and subject to considerable backsliding in the face of other social crises, evidence represents the most solid foundation for interventions with defined goals. These goals target a focus on recovery, leveraging the power of peer-based strategies, and not only changing "hearts and minds" but policies and practices targeting discrimination. Essential ingredients include, but are not limited to, grassroots inclusion from the beginning, diverse levels of effort, and sustained and sustainable endeavors (NASEM 2016).

The bottom line is that no *single* anti-stigma approach is best. Eliminating stigma will require an "all hands on deck" approach, using qualitative and quantitative data to understand stigma and stigma change for different problems in different settings, over time, and in response to interventions and general social change (Weiss and Ramakrishna 2006). Even as The Lancet Commission on Global Mental Health and Sustainable Development (Patel et al. 2018) recognizes that anti-stigma efforts have different starting points, their call for mental health services to be an essential, integrated component of universal health coverage in order to reduce the global burden of disease and disability, requires the elimination of the stigma attached to persons with mental illness, to providers who care for them, and to policies that exclude them (Patel et al. 2018). Nothing has brought forth the need for new research and anti-stigma vigilance more than the intersectional implications from the reemergence of infectious disease, the global pandemic represented by COVID-19, and the vision of a future where borders matter less than ever for health and well-being. Individuals with severe mental illness may be among the most vulnerable populations affected by this changing landscape given their greater comorbidities, lower household resources, residential instability, smaller social networks, and susceptibility to discrimination in the medical sector in the best of times (Kahl and Correll 2020; Thornicroft, Rose and Kassam 2007).

REFERENCES

Allport, G. E. (1954). *The Nature of Prejudice*. Garden City, NY: Doubleday.

Angermeyer, M. C., Daeumer, R., & Matschinger, H. (1993). Benefits and risks of psychotropic medication in the eyes of the general public: Results of a survey in the Federal Republic of Germany. *Pharmacopsychiatry*, *26*(4), 114–120.

Angermeyer, M. C., & Dietrich, S. (2006). Public beliefs about and attitudes towards people with mental illness: A review of population studies. *Acta Psychiatrica Scandinavia*, *113*(3), 163–179.

Angermeyer, M. C., Holzinger, A., Carla, M. G., & Schomerus, G. (2011). Biogenetic explanations and public acceptance of mental illness: Systematic review of population studies. *British Journal of Psychiatry*, *199*, 367–372.

Angermeyer, M. C., & Matschinger, H. (2003). The stigma of mental illness: Effects of labelling on public attitudes towards people with mental disorder. *Acta Psychiatrica Scandinavia*, *108*(4), 304–309. doi:10.1034/j.1600-0447.2003.00150.x

Angermeyer, M. C., & Matschinger, H. (2005). Causal beliefs and attitudes to people with schizophrenia. *British Journal of Psychiatry*, *186*, 331–334.

Boyer, C. A., Pescosolido, B. A., & Medina, T. R. (2008). *Issues in Understanding Mental Illness and Its Measurement: Global Problems, Local Manifestations and the Issue of Labeling*. Paper presented at the International Conference on Survey Methods in Multinational, Multiregional, and Multicultural Contexts, Berlin, Germany.

Bracke, P., Delaruelle, K., & Verhaeghe, M. (2019). Dominant cultural and personal stigma beliefs and the utilization of mental health services: A cross-national comparison. *Frontiers in Sociology*, *4*, 40. Retrieved from www.frontiersin.org/article/10.3389/fsoc.2019.00040

Brohan, E., Elgie, R., Sartorius, N., Thornicroft, G., & GAMION-Europe Study Group. (2010). Self-stigma, empowerment and perceived discrimination among people with schizophrenia in 14 European countries: The GAMIAN-Europe study. *Schizophrenia Research*, *122*(1–3), 232–238.

Chang, S., Ong, H. L., Seow, E., Chua, B. Y., Abdin, E., Samari, E., & Subramaniam, M. (2017). Stigma towards mental illness among medical and nursing students in Singapore: A cross-sectional study. *BMJ Open*, *7*(12), e018099. doi:10.1136/bmjopen-2017-018099

Charles, J. L. K. (2013). Mental health provider-based stigma: Understanding the experience of clients and families. *Social Work in Mental Health*, *11*(4), 360–375. doi:10.1080/15332985.2013.775998

Charlson, F., van Ommeren, M., Flaxman, A., Cornett, J., Whiteford, H., & Saxena, S. (2019). New WHO prevalence estimates of mental disorders in conflict settings: A systematic review and meta-analysis. *The Lancet*, *394*(10194), 240–248. doi: https://doi.org/10.1016/S0140-6736(19)30934-1

Corrigan, P. W., Kuwabara, S. A., & O'Shaughnessy, J. (2009). The public stigma of mental illness and drug addiction: Findings from a stratified random sample. *Journal of Social Work*, *9*(2), 139–147.

Corrigan, P. W., Markowitz, F. E., & Watson, A. C. (2004). Structural levels of mental illness stigma and discrimination. *Schizophrenia Bulletin*, *30*(3), 481–491. doi:10.1093/oxfordjournals.schbul.a007096

Corrigan, P. W., Markowitz, F. E., Watson, A. C., Rowan, D., & Kubiak, M. A. (2003). An attribution model of public discrimination towards persons with mental illness. *Journal of Health & Social Behavior*, *44*(2), 162–179.

Couture, S., & Penn, D. L. (2003). Interpersonal contact and the stigma of mental illness: A review of the literature. *Journal of Mental Health*, *12*, 291–305.

Crisp, A., Gelder, M., Goddard, E., & Meltzer, H. (2005). Stigmatization of people with mental illnesses: A follow-up study within the Changing Minds campaign of the Royal College of Psychiatrists. *World Psychiatry*, *4*(2), 106–113.

Crisp, A. H., Gelder, M. G., Rix, S., Meltzer, H. I., & Rowlands, O. J. (2000). Stigmatization of people with mental illness. *British Journal of Psychiatry*, *177*(1), 4–7.

Dovidio, J. F., Glick, P., & Rudman, L. (2005). *On the Nature of Prejudice: Fifty Years after Allport*. New York: Wiley-Blackwell.

European Commission, TNS Opinion and TNS Social. (2006). *Special Eurobarometer 248: Mental Well-being*. Brussels: European Commission. Retrieved from https://ec.europa.eu/commfrontoffice/publicopinion/archives/ebs/ebs_248_en.pdf

European Commission, TNS Opinion and TNS Social. (2010). *Special Eurobarometer 345: Mental Health. Part 1: Report*. Brussels: European Commission. Retrieved from https://ec.europa.eu/commfrontoffice/publicopinion/archives/ebs/ebs_345_en.pdf

Evans-Lacko, S., Brohan, E., Mojtabai, R., & Thornicroft, G. (2012). Association between public views of mental illness and self-stigma among individuals with mental illness in 14 European countries. *Psychological Medicine*, *42*(8), 1741–1752. doi:10.1017/S0033291711002558

Evans-Lacko, S., Corker, E., Williams, P., Henderson, C., & Thornicroft, G. (2014a). Effect of the Time to Change anti-stigma campaign on trends in mental-illness-related public stigma among the English population in 2003–13: An analysis of survey data. *The Lancet Psychiatry*, *1*(2), 121–128. doi:10.1016/S2215-0366(14)70243-3

Evans-Lacko, S., Courtin, E., Fiorillo, A., Knapp, M., Luciano, M., Park, A. L., & Thornicroft, G. (2014b). The state of the art in European research on reducing social exclusion and stigma related to mental health: A systematic mapping of the literature. *European Psychiatry*, *29*(6), 381–389. doi:10.1016/j.eurpsy.2014.02.007

Filipcic, I., Pavicic, D., Filipcic, A., Hotujac, L., Begic, D., Grubisin, J., & Dordevic, V. (2003). Attitudes of medical staff towards the psychiatric label "schizophrenic patient" tested by an anti-stigma questionnaire. *Collegium Antropologicum*, *27*(1), 301–307.

GBD 2017 Disease and Injury Incidence and Prevalence Collaborators. (2018). Global, regional, and national incidence, prevalence, and years lived with disability for 354 diseases and injuries for 195 countries and territories, 1990–2017: A systematic analysis for the Global Burden of Disease Study 2017. *Lancet*, *392*(10159), 1789–1858. doi:10.1016/s0140-6736(18)32279-7

Goffman, E. (1961). *Asylums: Essays on the Social Situation of Mental Patients and Other Inmates*. Garden City, NY: Anchor.

Goffman, E. (1963). *Stigma: Notes on the Management of Spoiled Identity*. New York: Simon & Schuster.

Goin, M. K. (2004). Presidential Address. *American Journal of Psychiatry*, *161*, 1768–1771.

Grinker, R. R. (2020). Autism, "stigma," disability: A shifting historical terrain. *Current Anthropology*, *61*(S21), S55–S67. doi: 10.1086/705748

Gurin, G., Veroff, J., & Feld, S. (1960). *Americans View Their Mental Health: A Nationwide Survey*. New York: Basic Books.

Hatzenbuehler, M. L. (2018). Structural stigma and health. In B. Major, J. F. Dovidio, & B. G. Link (Eds.), *The Oxford Handbook of Stigma, Discrimination, and Health*. New York: Oxford University Press.

Hatzenbuehler, M. L., Phelan, J. C., & Link, B. G. (2013). Stigma as a fundamental cause of population health inequalities. *American Journal of Public Health*, *103*(5), 813–821.

Henderson, C., & Thornicroft, G. (2009). Stigma and discrimination in mental illness: Time to Change. *The Lancet*, *373*(9679), 1928–1930. doi: https://doi.org/10.1016/S0140-6736(09)61046-1

Hinshaw, S. P. (2006). *The Mark of Shame: Stigma of Mental Illness and an Agenda for Change*. Oxford: Oxford University Press.

Hopper, Kim, Glynn Harrison, Aleksandar Janca, and Norman Sartorius. (2007). *Recovery from Schizophrenia: An International Perspective*. Oxford: Oxford University Press.

Insel, T. R. (2014, March 31). Commentary: Stubbornly high suicide rate. *Christianity Today*. Retrieved from www.ctlibrary.com/ct/2014/march-web-only/rick-warren-saddle-back-mental-health.html

Insel, T. R., Collins, P. Y., & Hyman, S. (2015). Darkness invisible: The hidden global costs of mental illness. *Foreign Affairs*, *94*(1), 127–135.

Institute for Health Metrics and Evaluation (IHME). 2018. *"Findings from the Global Burden of Disease Study 2017."* Seattle, WA: IHME.

Jorm, A. F., Christensen, H., & Griffiths, K. M. (2006). Changes in depression awareness and attitudes in Australia: The impact of beyondblue: The national depression initiative. *Australian and New Zealand Journal of Psychiatry*, *40*(1), 42–46. doi:10.1080/j.1440-1614.2006.01739.x

Jorm, A. F., Korten, A. E., Jacomb, P. A., Christensen, H., Rodgers, B., & Politt, P. (1997). Mental health literacy: A survey of the public's ability to recognize mental disorders and beliefs about treatment. *Medical Journal of Australia*, *166*(4), 182–186.

Kahl, K. G., & Correll, C. U. (2020). Management of patients with severe mental illness during the coronavirus disease 2019 pandemic. *JAMA Psychiatry*, *77*(9), 977–978. doi:10.1001/jamapsychiatry.2020.1701

Kim, H. S., & Sasaki, J. Y. (2014). Cultural neuroscience: Biology of the mind in cultural contexts. *Annual Review of Psychology, 65*, 24.21–24.28.

Krendl, A. C., Macrae, C. N., Kelley, W. M., Fugelsang, J. A., & Heatherton, T. F. (2006). The good, the bad, and the ugly: An fMRI investigation of the functional anatomic correlates of stigma. *Social Neuroscience, 1*(1), 5–15.

Krendl, A. C., & Pescosolido, B. A. (2020). Countries and cultural differences in the stigma of mental illness: The East–West divide. *Journal of Cross-Cultural Psychology, 51*(2), 149–167. doi:10.1177/0022022119901297

Kulka, R. A., Veroff, J., & Douvan, E. (1979). Social class and the use of professional help for personal problems: 1957 and 1976. *Journal of Health and Social Behavior, 20*(1), 2–17.

Lasalvia, A., Zoppei, S., Van Bortel, T., Bonetto, C., Cristofalo, D., Wahlbeck, K., & Thornicroft, G. (2013). Global pattern of experienced and anticipated discrimination reported by people with major depressive disorder: a cross-sectional survey. *Lancet, 381*(9860), 55–62. doi:10.1016/s0140-6736(12)61379-8

Link, B. G., Cullen, F. T., Struening, E. L., Shrout, P. E., & Dohrenwend, B. P. (1989). A modified labeling theory approach to mental disorders: An empirical assessment. *American Sociological Review, 54*, 400–423.

Link, B. G., & Phelan, J. C. (2001). Conceptualizing stigma. *Annual Review of Sociology, 27*, 363–385.

Link, B. G., & Stuart, H. (2017). On revisiting some origins of the stigma concept as it applies to mental illnesses. In W. Gaebel, W. Rössler, & N. Sartorius (Eds.), *The Stigma of Mental Illness: End of the Story?* (pp. 3–28). Cham, Switzerland: Springer International.

Link, B. G., Yang, L. H., Phelan, J. C., & Collins, P. (2004). Measuring mental illness stigma. *Schizophrenia Bulletin, 30*(3), 511–541.

Littlewood, R., Jadhav, S., & Ryder, A. G. (2007). A cross-national study of the stigmatization of severe psychiatric illness: Historical review, methodological considerations and development of the questionnaire. *Transcultural Psychiatry, 44*, 171–202.

Madhan, B., Gayathri, H., Garhnayak, L., & Naik, E. S. (2012). Dental students' regard for patients from often-stigmatized populations: Findings from an Indian dental school. *Journal of Dental Education, 76*(2), 210–217.

Major, B., & O'Brien, L. T. (2005). The social psychology of stigma. *Annual Review of Psychology, 56*, 393–421.

Martin, J. K., Pescosolido, B. A., & Tuch, S. A. (2000). Of fear and loathing: The role of disturbing behavior, labels and causal attributions in shaping public attitudes toward persons with mental illness. *Journal of Health and Social Behavior, 41*(2), 208–233.

Mehta, N., Kassam, A., Leese, M., Butler, G., & Thornicroft, G. (2009). Public attitudes towards people with mental illness in England and Scotland, 1994–2003. *The British Journal of Psychiatry, 194*, 278–284.

McGinty, E. E., Presskreischer, R., Han, H., & Barry, C. L. (2020). Psychological distress and loneliness reported by US adults in 2018 and April 2020. *JAMA, 324*(1), 93–94. doi:10.1001/jama.2020.9740

Mojtabai, R. (2010). Mental illness stigma and willingness to seek mental health care in the European Union. *Social Psychiatry and Psychiatric Epidemiology, 45*, 705–712.

NASEM (National Academies of Sciences, Engineering, and Medicine). (2016). *Ending Discrimination against People with Mental and Substance Use Disorders: The Evidence for Stigma Change*. Washington, DC: The National Academies Press.

Olafsdottir, S. (2007). *Medicalizing Mental Health: A Comparative View of the Public, Private, and Professional Construction of Mental Illness*. (PhD dissertation). Indiana University, Bloomington, IN.

Olafsdottir, S., & Pescosolido, B. A. (2011). Constructing illness: How the public in eight Western nations respond to a clinical description of "schizophrenia". *Social Science & Medicine, 73*, 929–938.

Patel, V., Saxena, S., Lund, C., Thornicroft, G., Baingana, F., Bolton, P., & Unützer, J. (2018). The Lancet Commission on global mental health and sustainable development. *The Lancet, 392*. doi:10.1016/S0140-6736(18)31612-X

Perry, B. L. (2011). The labeling paradox: Stigma, the sick role, and social networks in mental illness. *Journal of Health and Social Behavior, 52*, 460–477.

Pescosolido, B. A. (2013). The public stigma of mental illness: What do we think; what do we know; what can we prove? *Journal of Health and Social Behavior*, *54*(1), 1–21.

Pescosolido, B. A. (2015). Erving Goffman: The moral career of stigma and mental illness. In F. M. Collyer (Ed.), *The Palgrave Handbook of Social Theory for Health and Medicine* (pp. 273–286). London: Palgrave Macmillan.

Pescosolido, B. A. (2020). Stigma as a mental health policy controversy: Positions, options, and strategies for change. In H. Goldman, R. Frank, & J. Morrissey (Eds.), *The Palgrave Handbook of American Mental Health Policy*. Cham, Switzerland: Palgrave Macmillan.

Pescosolido, B.A., Halpern-Manners, A., Luo, L. & Perry, B. (In Press). Shifts in the Public Stigma of Mental Illness in the US, 1996–2018. *JAMA Network Open*.

Pescosolido, Bernice A., Jack K. Martin, Sigrun Olafsdottir, J. Scott Long, Karen Kafadar, and Tait R. Medina. (2015). "The theory of industrial society and cultural schemas: Does the "cultural myth of public stigma" underlie the WHO Schizophrenia Paradox?" *American Journal of Sociology* 121(3), 783–825.

Pescosolido, B. A., Manago, B., & Monahan, J. (2019). Evolving public views on the likelihood of violence from people with mental illness: Stigma and its consequences. *Health Affairs*, *38*(10), 1735–1743. doi:10.1377/hlthaff.2019.00702

Pescosolido, B. A., & Martin, J. K. (2007). Stigma and the sociological enterprise. In W. R. Avison, J. D. McLeod, & B. A. Pescosolido (Eds.), *Mental Health, Social Mirror* (pp. 307–328). New York: Springer.

Pescosolido, B. A., & Martin, J. K. (2015). The stigma complex. *Annual Review of Sociology*, *41*, 87–116.

Pescosolido, B. A., Martin, J. K., Lang, A., & Olafsdottir, S. (2008). Rethinking theoretical approaches to stigma: A framework integrating normative influences on stigma (FINIS). *Social Science & Medicine*, *67*, 431–440.

Pescosolido, B. A., Martin, J. K., Long, J. S., Medina, T. R., Phelan, J. C., & Link, B. G. (2010). "A disease like any other?" A decade of change in public reactions to schizophrenia, depression and alcohol dependence. *American Journal of Psychiatry*, *167*, 1321–1330. doi:10.1176/appi.ajp.2010.09121743

Pescosolido, B. A., Olafsdottir, S., Martin, J. K., & Long, J. S. (2008). Cross-cultural issues on the stigma of mental illness. In J. Arboleda-Florez & N. Sartorius (Eds.), *Understanding the Stigma of Mental Illness: Theory and Interventions* (pp. 19–35). London: John Wiley & Sons.

Pettigrew, T. F., & Tropp, L. R. (2000). Does intergroup contact reduce prejudice? Recent meta-analytic findings. In S. Oskamp (Ed.), *Reducing Prejudice and Discrimination: Social Psychological Perspectives* (pp. 93–114). Mahwah, NJ: Lawrence Erlbaum.

Phelan, J. C. (2005). Geneticization of deviant behavior and consequences for stigma: The case of mental illness. *Journal of Health and Social Behavior*, *46*(4), 307–322.

Phelan, J. C., Link, B. G., Stueve, A., & Pescosolido, B. A. (2000). Public conceptions of mental illness in 1950 and 1996: What is mental illness and is it to be feared? *Journal of Health and Social Behavior*, *41*(2), 188–207.

Rabinowitz, J. L., Sears, D. O., Sidanius, J., & Krosnick, J. A. (2009). Why do white Americans oppose race-targeted policies? Clarifying the impact of symbolic racism. *Political Psychology*, *30*(5), 805–828.

Rao, D., Elshafei, A., Nguyen, M., Hatzenbuehler, M. L., Frey, S., & Go, V. F. (2019). A systematic review of multi-level stigma interventions: State of the science and future directions. *BMC Medicine*, *17*(1), 41. doi:10.1186/s12916-018-1244-y

Rehm, J., & Shield, K. D. (2019). Global Burden of Disease and the impact of mental and addictive disorders. *Current Psychiatry Reports*, *21*(2), 10. doi:10.1007/s11920-019-0997-0

Rosenfield, S. (1997). Labeling mental illness: The effects of received services and perceived stigma on life satisfaction. *American Sociological Review*, *62*(August), 660–672.

Sagar, R., Dandona, R., Gururaj, G., Dhaliwal, R. S., Singh, A., Ferrari, A., & Dandona, L. (2020). The burden of mental disorders across the states of India: The Global Burden of Disease Study 1990–2017. *The Lancet Psychiatry*, *7*(2), 148–161. doi:https://doi.org/10.1016/S2215-0366(19)30475-4

Sartorius, N. (1997). Fighting schizophrenia and its stigma: A New World Psychiatric Association Educational Programme. *British Journal of Psychiatry*, *170*(4), 297.

Sartorius, N., & Schulze, H. (2005). *Reducing the Stigma of Mental Illness: A Report from a Global Programme of the World Psychiatric Association*. Cambridge: Cambridge University Press.

Scheff, T. J. (1966). *Being Mentally Ill: A Sociological Theory*. Chicago, IL: Aldine.

Schomerus, G., Evans-Lacko, S., Rusch, N., Mojtabai, R., Angermeyer, M. C., & Thornicroft, G. (2015). Collective levels of stigma and national suicide rates in 25 European countries *Epidemiology and Psychiatric Sciences, 24*(2), 166–171.

Schomerus, G., Schwahn, C., Holzinger, A., Corrigan, P. W., Grabe, H. J., Carta, M. G., & Angermeyer, M. C. (2012). Evolution of public attitudes about mental illness: A systematic review and meta-analysis. *Acta Psychiatrica Scandinavia, 125*(6), 440–452.

Seeman, N., Tang, S., Brown, A. D., & Ing, A. (2016). World survey of mental illness stigma. *Journal of Affective Disorders, 190*, 115–121. doi: https://doi.org/10.1016/j.jad.2015.10.011

Simon, N. M., Saxe, G. N., & Marmar, C. R. (2020). Mental health disorders related to COVID-19-related deaths. *JAMA, 324*(15), 1493–1494. doi:10.1001/jama.2020.19632

Smith, T. W. (2004). Developing and evaluating cross-national survey instruments. In S. Presser, J. M. Rothgeb, M. P. Couper, J. T. Lessler, E. Martin, & E. Singer (Eds.), *Methods for Testing and Evaluating Survey Questionnaires*. New York: John Wiley & Sons.

Star, S. A. (1955). *The Public's Idea about Mental Illness*. Paper presented at the National Association for Mental Health Conference, Chicago, IL.

Stuart, H., & Arboleda-Florez, J. (2001). Community attitudes toward persons with schizophrenia. *Canadian Journal of Psychiatry, 46*(3), 245–252.

Stuart, H., Arboleda-Florez, J., & Sartorius, N. (2012). *Paradigms Lost: Fighting Stigma and the Lessons Learned*. New York: Oxford University Press.

Swindle, R., Heller, K., Pescosolido, B. A., & Kikuzawa, S. (2000). Responses to "nervous breakdowns" in America over a 40-year period: Mental health policy implications. *American Psychologist, 55*(7), 740–749.

Szasz, T. S. (1961). *The Myth of Mental Illness: Foundations of a Theory of Person Conduct*. New York: Dell Publishing.

Teachman, B. A., Wilson, J. G., & Komarovskaya, I. (2006). Implicit and explicit stigma of mental illness in diagnosed and healthy samples. *Guilford Press Periodicals*. Online March 2006. doi:10.1521/jscp.2006.25.1.75].

Telles-Correia, D., Marques, J. G., Gramaca, J., & Sampaio, D. (2015). Stigma and attitudes towards psychiatric patients in Portuguese medical students. *Acta Médica Portuguesa, 28*(6), 715–719. doi::http://dx.doi.org/10.20344/amp.6231.

The Lancet. (2016). The health crisis of mental health stigma. *The Lancet, 387*(10023), 1027. doi: https://doi.org/10.1016/S0140-6736(16)00687-5

Thoits, P. A. (2011). Resisting the stigma of mental illness. *Social Psychology Quarterly, 74*(1), 6–28.

Thompson, A. H., Stuart, H., Bland, R. C., Arboleda-Florez, J., Warner, R., & Dickson, R. A. (2002). Attitudes about schizophrenia from the pilot site of the WPA worldwide campaign against the stigma of schizophrenia. *Social Psychiatry and Psychiatric Epidemiology, 37*(10), 475–482. doi:10.1007/s00127-002-0583-2

Thornicroft, G., Bakolis, I., Evans-Lacko, S., Gronholm, Petra C., Henderson, C., Kohrt, B. A., & Sartorius, N. (2019). Key lessons learned from the INDIGO global network on mental health related stigma and discrimination. *World Psychiatry, 18*(2), 229–230. doi:10.1002/wps.20628

Thornicroft, G., Brohan, E., Rose, D., Sartorius, N., Leese, M., & INDIGO Study Group. (2009). Global pattern of experienced and anticipated discrimination against people with schizophrenia: A cross-sectional survey. *The Lancet, 373*(9661), 408–415.

Thornicroft, G., Mehta, N., Clement, S., Evans-Lacko, S., Doherty, M., Rose, D., & Henderson, C. (2016). Evidence for effective interventions to reduce mental-health-related stigma and discrimination. *The Lancet, 387*(10023), 1123–1132. doi: https://doi.org/10.1016/S0140-6736(15)00298-6

Thornicroft, G., Rose, D., & Kassam, A. (2007). Discrimination in health care against people with mental illness. *International Review of*

Psychiatry, 19(2), 113–122. doi:10.1080/09540260701278937

Turan, B., Hatcher, A. M., Weiser, S. D., Johnson, M. O., Rice, W. S., & Turan, J. M. J. A. J. P. H. (2017). Framing mechanisms linking HIV-related stigma, adherence to treatment, and health outcomes. *American Journal of Public Health, 107*(6), June 1, 863–869. doi:10.2105/ajph.2017.303744

US Department of Health & Human Services. (1999). *Mental Health: A Report of the Surgeon General*. Rockville, MD: Department of Health & Human Services, U.S. Public Health Service.

Verhaeghe, M., Bracke, P., & Pattyn, E. (2010). *Structural Concomitants of Stigma and Mental Health Service Use: Results from a Cross-national Comparative Multilevel Analysis*. Paper presented at the 15th Symposium EPA, Bergen, Norway. http://hdl.handle.net/1854/LU-1038321

Veroff, J., Kulka, R. A., & Douvan, E. (1981). *Mental Health in America: Patterns of Help-Seeking from 1957 to 1976*. New York: Basic Books.

Vos, T., Flaxman, A. D., Naghavi, M., Lozano, R., Michaud, C., Ezzati, M., & Memish, Z. A. (2012). Years lived with disability (YLDs) for 1160 sequelae of 289 diseases and injuries 1990–2010: A systematic analysis for the Global Burden of Disease Study 2010. *Lancet, 380*(9859), 2163–2196. doi:10.1016/s0140-6736(12)61729-2

Wahl, O. E., Wood, A., & Richards, R. (2002). Newspaper coverage of mental illness: Is it changing? *Psychiatric Rehabilitation Skills, 6*(1), 9–31. doi:10.1080/10973430208408417

Wainberg, M. L., Scorza, P., Shultz, J. M., Helpman, L., Mootz, J. J., Johnson, K. A., & Arbuckle, M. R. (2017). Challenges and opportunities in global mental health: A research-to-practice perspective. *Current Psychiatry Reports, 19*(5), 28. doi:10.1007/s11920-017-0780-z

Weiss, M. G., & Ramakrishna, J. J. L. (2006). Stigma interventions and research for international health. *The Lancet, 367*(9509), 536–538. doi:10.1016/s0140-6736(06)68189-0

Whiteford, H., Ferrari, A., & Degenhardt, L. (2016). Global Burden of Disease studies: Implications for mental and substance use disorders. *Health Affairs, 35*(6), 1114–1120. doi:10.1377/hlthaff.2016.0082

Williams, R. M. (1947). *The Reduction of Intergroup Tensions*. New York: Social Science Research Council.

World Health Organization. (2001). *The World Health Report 2001— Mental Health: New Understanding, New Hope*. Geneva: World Health Organization.

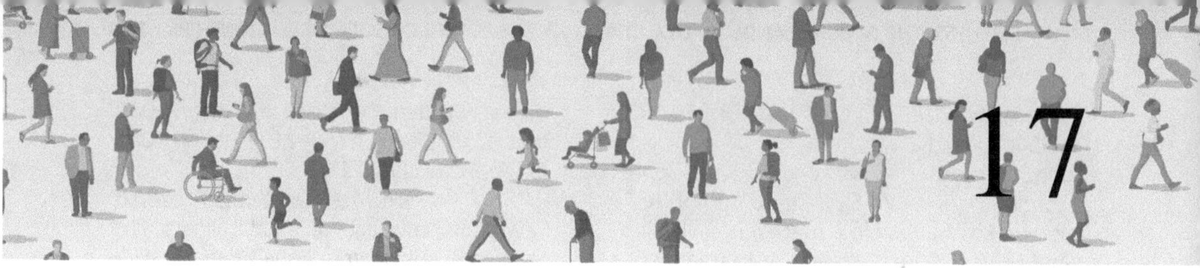

17

From Ableism to *Amplitude*: A Celebration of Dis/ability

Norah A. Schwartz

DISABILITY IN GLOBAL PERSPECTIVE

People with disabilities represent the largest minority group in the world. Today, approximately 1 billion people, or 15% of the world's population, has at least one form of disability (World Health Organization, 2015). Broadly defined, disability includes physical impairments, such as those due to an accident, congenital birth defect, chronic degenerative illness, blindness, deafness, and psychological and developmental learning impairments. Disability transcends age, gender, race, socioeconomic status, nationality and political orientation. According to the World Bank, 80% of people with disabilities live in the "global south", or poorer regions of the world, demonstrating a strong relationship between poverty and disability (World Bank, 2020; World Health Organization, 2018). Approximately 93 million children worldwide under the age of 15 live with a moderate or severe disability. Many more are living with mild disability or degenerative illness (World Health Organization, 2015). People experiencing disability, including children, often remain excluded from fully participating in society due to social and economic barriers, including lack of an accessible physical environment, government services, assistive devices, attendant care and technologies (Fu, Cord & McLain-Nhlapo, 2019).

The vision of the World Health Organization (2015) involves creating a world in which persons with disabilities and their families live in dignity and are able to achieve their full potential. In what Mittler (2015: 86) refers to as a "meta-paradigm shift," the global Convention on the Rights of Persons with Disabilities (hereafter referred to as CRPD) includes persons with disabilities as the primary stakeholders and is monitored by the Committee on the Rights of Persons with Disabilities. Within this shift, persons with disabilities are fully and equally involved as principal stakeholders and change agents in the entirety of the process aimed at improving the quality of life of persons with disabilities (Mittler, 2015: 79). The CRPD profiles the rights allotted to individuals including "the enjoyment of the highest attainable standard of health without discrimination on the basis of disability." Its guiding principles include the right to individual autonomy, freedom to make given choices and independence of persons, as well as the right of children with disabilities to preserve their identities and have access to free and compulsory primary and secondary education. As of July 2021, the text contains 50 Articles and has 163 signatories and 181 parties. The United States is one of the few countries to have signed but not ratified the treaty. Instrumental in its development, Mexico proposed the establishment of an ad hoc committee in 2001 which led to its ratification (United Nations, 2007).

WHODAS: Defining and assessing functionality and disability

The World Health Organization Disability Assessment Schedule (WHODAS) was established for use as a generic instrument to measure disability. Applied worldwide, the WHODAS assesses six physical and psychological domains of disability: one's ability to understand and communicate, get around, take care of one's self, get along with others, participate in life activities (i.e., household, work, and/or school activities), and participate in society (World Health Organization, 2018).

The terms "impairment" and "disability" are often distinguished by disability scholars. Oliver (2013) argues that the issue is not bodily impairment *per se*, but an artifact of the social organization whose aim is to exclude those with non-standard capabilities and those not considered capable of contributing to the capitalist economy. Disability is recognized to be a socially constructed condition (Hahn, 1988). The essence of disability problems lies within the specific environmental systems which do not afford equal rights and opportunities to disabled people; rather than in personal deficiencies of individuals. Ablon (2002:S6) emphasizes that the minority model "highlights the major distinction between the physical or functional impairments people may have and the logistic, social, economic, or political/environmental barriers in their lives that often determine the problems they may experience.

Numerous barriers and disparities contribute to disadvantages experienced by those with disability. Particularly in developing countries, individuals with disabilities experience poorer health status, higher rates of poverty, lower rates of educational achievement and employment, reduced independence and restricted participation within social environments. Stigmatization and bullying are universally significant issues for people with disability around the world (Ablon, 1981, 2008).

FROM ABLEISM TO *AMPLITUDE*: A HISTORY AND CELEBRATION OF DIFFERENCE AND DIS/ABILTY

Ableism: discrimination or prejudice against individuals with disabilities, including stigmatizing and bullying.

Ampletude: a contemporary magazine by and for amputees, placing focus on inclusion through prosthetics and adaptive technology.

As a celebration of dis/ability and difference, this chapter spotlights individuals who display a unique brilliance, talent, penchant for leadership, philosophy of life, or ability to physically take on challenges beyond what might be imagined as humanly possible. It also points up societal barriers that have been either purposefully or inadvertently designed to keep people with disabilities from achieving personal fulfillment and professional success in life, as well as the advocacy and resiliency employed to break down these barriers.

Having worked in the disability field for many years, I have been honored to meet many accomplished and impassioned individuals who live their lives with a sense of dignity, integrity, purpose and resilience – many of whom have become leaders in a field that at some point might be of benefit to each of us, especially as we age. A number of these leaders have risked their lives and taken on government officials at the highest level to advocate for adaptations that are now often taken for granted, such as curb cuts and accessible housing and transportation. On Trevor Noah's popular night-time talk show, Judy Heumann – author, teacher and public speaker – corrected Noah's terminology when he referred to himself as being able-bodied. You are not "able-bodied," she exacted, but "non-disabled", meaning that Trevor Noah, like every other living being, could become disabled at any moment in time and thus qualified to take advantage of the advances that have emerged from the disability rights movement.

The Family Secret

> I visited the State Institution for the mentally retarded and I think that particularly at Willowbrook, we have a situation that borders on a snake pit. (Robert F. Kennedy, 1965)

> We knew nothing about the community and the community knew nothing about us. (Judy Moiseff, ex-resident of Willowbrook, 2013)

I did not meet, nor even know about, my Aunt Mary until I was in college. Now long-buried close to my parents and her mother in a Jewish cemetery in New Jersey, my Aunt Mary spent most of her formative years in a state institution after contracting meningitis as a child. My one surviving aunt, Aunt Sally, still talks about her. Though she does not know the name of the "state institution" in which Aunt Mary was housed, I suspect that Aunt Sally is referring to the Letchworth State School. State "schools" such as Willowbrook, Letchworth and Pennhurst became infamous in the 1970s for the inhumane conditions in which residents were housed and treated.

Sent home to live with my aging grandmother after state institutions became "deinstitutionalized," Aunt Mary's behavior was erratic and marked by temper tantrums. With limited speech and vocabulary, she had difficulty articulating her needs. Many "students" of Willowbrook and other such state run "schools" were non-verbal and thus deemed unintelligent by a society intolerant of and impatient with such differences. Without access to the high-tech communication aids currently available and disability protection laws in place, the voices of those individuals who were institutionalized remained silent and hidden. As a residential supervisor in a group home for adults being deinstitutionalized from Willowbrook, I discovered that temper tantrums are learned, reinforced institutionalized behavior. Given the opportunity and tools to express themselves, at least some of the residents had much to share with a society willing to listen.

When Johnson & Williams (1999), a developmentally disabled man who spent his youth in an institution, met the Executive Director for ARC, USA (formerly the Association for Retarded Citizens) for the first and every time afterwards, he said, "I want to tell you that we have people in institutions who we are worried about. Can you help get them out?" (Johnson & Williams, 1999). An unsung hero of the self-advocacy movement which was started "on behalf of one of the most disenfranchised segments of society," Johnson was recently featured in a *New York Times* obituary section uncovering "remarkable people whose deaths … went unreported in *The Times*" (Rifkin, 2020). As a public speaker, Johnson talked about the physical, psychological and racist abuse that he endured for 13 years while under the care of a Pennsylvania state institution once regarded as "the shame of the nation." Even before a young reporter named Geraldo Rivera used a hidden camera to expose living conditions at the Willowbrook and Letchworth State Schools, a little-known television news reporter named Bill Baldini produced a horrifying five-part portrayal of the Pennhurst State School and Hospital. Johnson was one of the children interviewed in the graphic 1968 documentary, *Suffer the*

Little Children (NBC, 1968). Baldini noted at the time that, "zoos spend more on their wild animals than Pennsylvania spends on its 2,800 patients at Pennhurst." Johnson left Pennhurst in 1971 and later co-authored his autobiography, aptly titled *Lost in a Desert World* (Johnson & Williams, 1999).

As president of the Philadelphia chapter of Speaking for Ourselves and board member of the national Self Advocates Becoming Empowered (SABE), Johnson advocated for the closure of all institutions. SABE's stated mission is: "To ensure that people with disabilities are treated as equals and that they are given the same decisions, choices, rights, responsibilities, and chances to speak up to empower themselves; opportunities to make new friends, and to learn from their mistakes." As part of a delegation that was invited to the White House, Johnson witnessed the landmark signing of the American with Disabilities Act. A strong and articulate public speaker, he would ask his audience, "who's in control?" Urging others to be independent and not to fall victim to dependency, Johnson would state that "the only way to break that barrier is to tell people that you are in control over your own life and in your own ways."

Thanks in part to new technology and self-advocacy groups, we now have access to some of the lived experiences of other ex-"students" of state-run schools. Having experienced first-hand the inhumane conditions and treatment brought to life through Rivera's (cf. Alexandria, 2019) underground reporting, Judy Moiseff (2013), disability advocate and founder of Judy Speaks, was born with cerebral palsy and raised in Willowbrook. Talking through an electronic communication device, she articulates her experience as a young child: "I think that the conditions were so horrible that they crushed our spirits," she said. By openly discussing the living conditions under which she was raised, Moiseff not only validates Rivera's perception of demoralizing surrealism, but she provides us with a rich, though tragic, personal history of the human beings residing there, and who until now had only been seen as two-dimensional waifs.

Generation ADA: "People with disabilities succeed when communities choose to be inclusive"

> People who experience challenges sometimes develop strengths that make them great advocates. (Haben, TEDx Talk, 2014)

Recognized as one of the new faces of disability advocacy, deafblind attorney Haben Girma (2019) introduced President Barack Obama to an audience of disability rights advocates at the White House celebration of the 25th anniversary of the passage of the 1990 Americans with Disability Act (ADA). Among her many achievements, the accessible technology advocate lists the Helen Keller Achievement Award and was included on the Forbes under 30 list. Born in Oakland, California, Girma was guaranteed access to schooling that her older brother, who was born deafblind in Eritrea, had been denied until their family immigrated to the United States.

In her recent memoir, *Haben* (2019: 14), Girma was the first deafblind woman to earn a jurisprudence degree from Harvard Law School. She recalls it as "a sighted, hearing classroom, in a sighted, hearing school, in a sighted, hearing society. They designed this environment for people who can see and hear. In this environment, I'm disabled. They place the burden on me to step out of my world and reach into theirs." Not willing to be bound by the outside world's expectations of a deafblind person, Girma enjoys discovering her own limitations. "Live boldly," she reminds herself. Describing an Alaska adventure in which she climbed an iceberg and slid down the other side, she recalls:

> My arms tremble as I crawl along the ice wall beside Gordon. He guides my hand 4 feet to the left. "This is the edge. It's about a 20 foot drop." He moves my hand to the right. "On this side there is a wall. Stay in the middle and you'll be fine."

> Sam starts shouting.
>
> "He's cheering," Gordon explains.
>
> I smile. So many people would scold me with a persistent chorus of "You can't! You shouldn't! You won't!" But Sam and Gordon are the opposite: not only do they share their Alaskan playground, they cheer me on, too. (Haben, 2019: 193)

Not everybody shares the same sentiment or ability to empathize as Haben's friends. Girma recalls an early act of advocacy when she was confronted with an unsavory situation in college in 2007. Requesting clarification for why cafeteria menus were not being emailed directly to her when she depended on them to make her vegetarian food choices, Haben sent a note to the cafeteria manager. An immediate reply landed in her email box:

> we hope that you understand that this is something that we are trying to help you with, but you also need to understand that this is a service that we are not contracted to provide, and that unlike the college, we do not have people on staff to assist students with special needs. ... It is not reasonable to have an expectation of us that we are not required to do. ... And it is also unreasonable to expect that this assistance will come seamlessly. There will be meals that are missed...

Referring to the Americans with Disabilities Act, a resilient Girma responded as follows with a copy to the school administration: "Bon Appetite has a legal obligation, under the Americans with Disabilities Act, to provide people with disabilities access to its services" (Girma, 2019: 160). Empowered by this minor achievement, Girma then applied and was accepted to Harvard Law School.

With multiple ways for the deafblind community to communicate, including tactile sign language, Girma prefers to work with a translator who types into a wireless keyboard that transfers information directly to her hand-held digital Braille keyboard. Not completely deaf, she hears high-pitch sounds and is able to respond through speech, which allows her more autonomy in her communication. However, Girma has at times found herself being excluded from the credo for which she is an active advocate. Apparently, the editing rooms of *Time Magazine* had not yet been informed that there is "no about us without us":

> TIME Magazine celebrated my disability justice work by including me in TIME 100 Talks, a video series spotlighting influential people. I was surprised and honored. My excitement turned to disappointment when I checked the video – no captions, no audio descriptions, and no transcript. The TIME 100 video featuring me was not accessible to me. (Girma, 2020)

After graduating from Harvard, Girma worked as a public service lawyer in Berkeley. Her salary, she explains,

> is far below what a Harvard Law graduate would typically make, but still exceeds the average income for blind Americans, seventy percent of whom struggle with unemployment. ... In a society that casts people with disabilities as inferior to the non-disabled, having a meaningful job, health insurance, and a law degree feels like a privilege. So I spent hours at my desk working to dismantle our world's barriers. (Girma, 2019: 238)

Representing the National Federation of the Blind, the oldest and largest organization run by the blind, Girma won a lawsuit that ensured that 40 million books and documents would be eligible for viewing and listening for blind and sight-impaired people. Programmed into Scribd's library was a screen read block which prevented sight-impaired people from accessing reading material. Suing Scribd, the self-proclaimed "world's largest collection of e-books and written works," Girma proved that the ADA intended to cover disability access to virtual "places," including the internet. In a stunning victory that opened up a new platform for the ADA, 26-year-old Haben Girma and her colleagues successfully argued to the United States District Court of Vermont that the internet is a "place" and therefore covered under the rules of the ADA.

Currently, Girma travels the world trying to change attitudes toward disability. "Many cultures, including Ethiopian culture, view disability as a curse on the family. Advocates around the world are working to change such attitudes, and I help as best I can" (Shapiro, 2015). Girma's experiences highlight that adults and children are using social media as a tool for self-reflection, communication and a method for explaining their differences and their needs to the outside world.

Disability in the United States

Before the twentieth century, people in the United States with disabilities functioned and contributed as they could within their homes and within the wage labor market. By the late nineteenth and early twentieth century, however, Americans with disabilities began to be viewed as unproductive. Rose writes that:

> Prior to the advent of World War I, individuals in the United States with disabilities lived at home and contributed to the labor market based on their abilities. Due in part to shifting economics, policies and social values, a gradual shift took place in which persons with disabilities became viewed as "unproductive citizens" while essentially being barred from the workplace. With lost access to the workplace, families were relegated to a state of poverty and second-class citizenship, often relying on charity and pity. (Rose, 2017: 111)

By the mid-1960s, it was not unusual for children with physical disabilities to either be showcased on telethons in an effort to demonstrate that they were now able to walk thanks to the generosity of viewers, or institutionalized and kept out of sight. Around this time, Geraldo Rivera exposed living conditions at the Willowbrook and Letchworth State Schools. A poignant and disturbing one-hour documentary produced 25 years later features interviews with family members of those housed in institutions during this time (Fisher, 1997). A new generation of radical and original thinkers, including Ed Roberts and Judy Heumann, demanded transparency and change in the living and working conditions of people with disabilities. This perspective led to the independent living movement and eventually the 1990 passage of the Americans with Disabilities Act (ADA). With simultaneous progress being made in other parts of the world, a global movement toward independent living and disability rights emerged. Judith Heumann, often regarded as the mother of the disability rights movement, later spearheaded the World Institute on Disability.

The Section 504 years: Who is Protected from Discrimination?

The first formal legal protection act was the Rehabilitation Act of 1973. In its entirety, Section 504, Rehabilitation Act of 1973 (29 U.S.C. § 701), is no more than two pages long. Nevertheless, this section of the Rehabilitation Act, or rather the delay in its implementation, was the impetus for the disability rights movement of the 1970s and the precursor to the 1990 passage of the Americans with Disabilities Act. The opening paragraph reads in part: "No otherwise qualified individual with a disability in the United States … shall, solely by reason of his or her disability, be excluded from the participation in, be denied the benefits of, or be subjected to discrimination under any program or activity receiving Federal financial assistance or under any program or activity conducted by any Executive agency or by the United States Postal Service" (US Department of Health and Human Services, 2006).

Persons with disabilities make up the largest minority in the United States. Under Section 504, individuals with disabilities are defined as:

> persons with a physical or mental impairment which substantially limits one or more major life activities. People who have a history of, or who are regarded as having a physical or mental impairment that substantially limits one or more major life activities, are also covered. Major life activities include caring for one's self, walking, seeing, hearing, speaking, breathing, working, performing manual tasks, and learning.

As explained by Kitty Cone, an early and current disability rights advocate, "between 1973 and 1977 no regulations were issued.

… It became clear, through delays and leaks from inside, that the [Section 504] regulations were being seriously weakened in coverage, enforcement, and the whole integration mandate" (Cone, n.d.).

Enter Judy Heumann

> We demonstrated to the entire nation that disabled people could take control over our own lives and take leadership in the struggle for equality. (Judith Heumann, disability rights activist)

Born in the United States to German Jewish immigrants in 1947, Judith Heumann recounts a story about her childhood (Heumann & Joiner, 2020). Upon her recovery from polio at the age of two, the family doctor recommended that her parents "place her in an institution." Not learning about this until she was in her thirties, Heumann claims that this was proposed without malice or foresight. The discrimination by society against her for not being able to walk and the fear that she might spread contagion continued, as did her mother's advocacy to not have her child hidden from society or her rights abnegated (Heumann & Joiner, 2020: xi). Denied access to public school for fear of her being a "fire hazard" and to Hebrew school because "this won't work," Heumann was schooled at home for a few hours each week by a tutor provided by the City of New York. "The idea that I could learn anything meaningful in two and a half hours of instruction a week was, of course, ludicrous" (Heumann & Joiner, 2020: 9). Having a mother who did not understand the meaning of "no," Judy eventually attended public school in New York City, graduated from the Long Island University and attained a master's degree of Public Health from the University of California, Berkeley. In 1970, the proverbial powerhouse of the disability rights movement sued the City of New York for the right to teach – and won her case (Leagle, 2019).

After three years of teaching in the New York City public school system, Judy Heumann became instrumental in the establishment of the Center for Independent Living and the World Institute on Disability in Berkeley. She was appointed the Assistant Secretary of Special Education under President Bill Clinton and worked as a Senior Fellow for the Ford Foundation, among other such notable accomplishments.

The full-length documentary film and winner of the 2020 Sundance Film Festival, *Crip Camp: A Disability Revolution* (Newnham & LeBrecht, 2020) features a young Judy Heumann as a counselor at a specialized camp for youth with a variety of disabilities and disorders around the time of Woodstock. Taking their clues from the civil rights movement of the 1950s and 1960s, this unlikely group of outspoken individuals with disabilities organized and took over the San Francisco federal Health, Education and Welfare Building in 1977. Kitty Cone, one of the major protagonists of the Section 504 sit-in remembers: "At that time, discrimination existed in education, employment, housing, transportation, access to public buildings and other facilities, access to equal medical care and in many other areas."

This San Francisco protest was a major event in the disability rights movement. While not easy to organize a national protest, no less a long-term sit-in, with people with disabilities, the organizers of the San Francisco federal building sit-in determined in advance that "a sit-in meant people would go and stay, until the issue was resolved definitively." Due to lack of transit, support services and so on at the time, limited movement was expected on the part of participants. However,

> the San Francisco federal building sit-in, the only one that endured, lasted 28 days and was critical in forcing the signing of the regulations almost unchanged. It began with a rally outside the federal building, then we marched inside where between 1 and 200 people would remain until the end. The composition of the sit-in represented the spectrum of the disability community with participation from people with a wide variety of disabilities, from different racial, social and economic backgrounds, and ages from adults to kids with disabilities and their parents. We all felt that we

> were acting on behalf of hundreds of thousands of people who were not able to participate, people all over the country who were institutionalized or stuck in other dependency situations. At every moment, we felt ourselves the descendants of the civil rights movement of the '60s. We learned about sit-ins from the civil rights movement, we sang freedom songs to keep up morale, and consciously show the connection between the two movements. We always drew the parallels. About public transportation we said 'we can't even get on the back of the bus'. (Cone, n.d.)

After a long and bitter fight, the essential right to accessible public transportation was won. "We had shown ourselves and the country through network TV that we, the most hidden, impoverished, pitied group of people in the nation were capable of waging a deadly serious struggle that brought about profound social change" (Cone, n.d.).

Amongst the noted actors in the disability rights and independent living movements worldwide is Ed Roberts, founder of the Berkeley Center for Independent Living. Recognized as father of the disability rights movement, Roberts was influenced by the Vietnam War protests and advocated for his right to attend the University of California at Berkeley and live on campus, the same as other students. A placard on the corner of Bancroft and Telegraph Avenues, across the street from the renowned university Sproul Hall, marks the world's first curb cut. A number of years later, Bob Kafka and Stephanie Thomas co-founded the Coalition of Texans with Disabilities and were active participants in American Disabled for Public Transit (ADAPT). In 1987, members of ADAPT formed a human chain link in front of a public bus in Denver, Colorado demanding access to wheelchair lift-equipped buses. It might be difficult to remember that there was a time when public transportation was not accessible to individuals with disabilities. However, it took radical advocacy on the part of people relying on this access to ensure their independence to bring about change. Without their commitment, there would be no accessible public transportation, curb cuts or disabled parking, at the very least.

Judith Heumann concludes her memoir with a quote from Congresswoman Barbara Jordan (Democrat, Texas), who ended her political career early due to multiple sclerosis: "A government is invigorated when each of us is willing to participate in shaping the future of this nation" (Heumann & Joiner, 2020: 211). Black, gay and disabled, the Congressional scholar is remembered for saying that the "the Constitution was written without me in mind." Thanks to advocates like Judy Heumann, the Constitution has become more inclusive. "Challenging the perception of people with disabilities as helpless or objects of pity," Heumann was included in TIME magazine's list of the 100 most influential women of the past century for her activism in the 1997 Section 504 demonstration (TIME, 2020). Heumann is married to Jorge Pineda, a Mexican disability rights activist.

The Capitol Crawl

> The time has come to firmly establish the right of disabled Americans to dignity and self-respect as equal and contributing members of society and to end the virtual isolation of millions of children and adults.
>
> (Senator Hubert Humphrey on the passage of Section 504 of the Rehabilitation Act of 1973)

> Senator, we are not even second-class citizens, we are third class citizens.
>
> (Frank Bowe, deaf, director of American Coalition of Citizens with Disabilities)

Another significant disability rights protest was the Capitol Crawl in March 1990, when disability rights activists left behind their wheelchair and mobility devices to crawl up the 83 steps of the US Capitol in order to demonstrate the need for physical accessibility in public spaces. These demonstrations led to the passage of the Americans with Disabilities Act (ADA), a bipartisan effort crafted by representatives of the Republican and Democratic parties and signed into law by Republican

President George H.W. Bush on July 26, 1990. The umbrella protection of this includes: congenital disabilities, developmental delay, drug addiction, alcoholism, mental illness including depression and anxiety disorders, dyslexia, eating disorders, Alzheimer's disease, autism spectrum, attention deficit disorder, learning disabilities, deafness, blindness, autoimmune disease, cancer, diabetes, heart disease, HIV/AIDS, paraplegia/quadriplegia, degenerative illness, and others.

A Panoply of Conditions, Yet Shared Experiences

Kodi Lee

> We need to stop limiting our children.
>
> (Gabrielle Union, *America's Got Talent* judge)

Savant syndrome expert, Dr Darold Treffert defines savant syndrome as:

> a rare but extraordinary condition in which persons with serious mental disabilities, including autistic disorder, have some "island of genius" that stands in marked, incongruous contrast to overall handicap. As much as 1 in 10 persons with autistic disorder have such remarkable abilities in varying degrees. … Savant skills in autistic persons, rather than being irrelevant and frivolous, can in fact, by "training the talent," serve as a "conduit toward normalization," with an increase in language, social, and daily living skills, providing more independence for the savant overall. (Treffert, 2009: 1351)

When 22-year-old Kodi Lee took to the stage for his live audition on NBC's *America's Got Talent* – the popular globally broadcast amateur talent show – the audience was unsure what to expect. They saw a handsome blind, autistic young man who rocked back and forth, had difficulty pronouncing his name and needed extra time to orient himself to his surroundings and the piano. The minute Kodi started playing the piano, the stunned audience and judges recognized his unique talent. Kodi Lee went on to win the coveted million-dollar prize money and the adulation of audiences around the globe.

Treffert (2009) described Lee as a prodigious musical savant – that is, a person who manifests musical abilities that would be considered extraordinary even in a person who is not autistic. With perfect pitch, timing and audio memory, Kodi Lee is one of only a handful of musical savants known to be alive today. Central to his story is his family's support of his love and passion for music.

Accompanying him everywhere, his mother, Tina Lee, acts as Kodi's guide, surrogate and spokesperson. "When you're autistic," Tina explained to the audience, "it's really hard to do what everybody else does." In a backstage interview, Tina discussed how the non-verbal Kodi would tantrum "like 30 times a day" until he started expressing himself through singing and playing the piano on his own at a very young age. "It actually has saved his life, playing music," she explained.

In 1992, Mary Jeanette Howle wrote that:

> The striking feature of musical savants is the combination of characteristics that are often found in an individual along with musical ability. Blindness (usually retrolental fibroplasia), premature birth, echolalia (a condition in which the individual repeats what is said by other people as if echoing them), and perfect pitch often appear in the same person. Many savants are also autistic (i.e., have poor communication skills) *and seem totally uninterested in anyone but themselves* (emphasis mine). (Howle, 1992: 5)

In a new generation, Tina Lee described Kodi's struggles with self-expression and how advocacy, patience, therapy and musical training helped Kodi express himself and relate to the external world. Rather than being "totally uninterested," Kodi desperately wanted to communicate. In an interview posted on Instagram, Tina Lee recalled that:

> He has all these talents, but he has trouble communicating. … After he started performing, he got it. It really helped us to get his autism under control. He wants to be an entertainer. … He's learned to deal with the emotions, because that's how we taught him…You've got to deal with the people, you've got to socialize with the people. Even though he had this musical talent, he still had all

> of the same behaviors as any autistic child, and every parent asks how do we help them? How do we help them deal with our world? And when I saw that he was an entertainer, that was my cue ...that's what I'm going to use to help him deal. (TalentRecap, 2019)

Kodi Lee's dream of entertaining "thousands of people" was instantly transformed into a global audience of millions through the use of social media. With the help of his family, Lee now reaches audiences through Instagram, TikTok, Facebook and other social media sites for which Haben Girma continues to advocate accessibility. In a heartfelt post, one of Lee's autistic followers wrote: "Thank you for helping humanize autism. I will forever be thankful." Another follower related: "I have autism and people don't realize how powerful our minds and soul can really be." One shared that: "As a person with a disability, it's an ENORMOUS deal that we (neuroatypical people) have representation like this. He's INCREDIBLY TALENTED and is the representation that people like me really need. THIS is how shame is taken away from the concept of having a disability/being neuroatypical."

As Lee continued his journey to become the winner of *America's Got Talent* (2019 season), a beaming judge Gabrielle Union reminded him that just by his presence, he keeps changing the world. Turning to his mother, she emoted, "we need to stop limiting our children!" (TalentRecap, 2019).

In describing her views about how to educate children with autism to an audience at the American Academy of Arts and Sciences (2016), professor, author and public speaker, Temple Grandin, herself autistic, stated that the syndrome "varies from Einstein, who had no language skills at age three to somebody who can't dress themselves. ... I've been out to Silicon Valley. Half the programmers are on the spectrum."

In her YouTube documentary, *Through Our Eyes: Living with Asperger's*, Alyssa Hubber (2015) opens with a clear and concise statement: "I am different from other people." She explains that "I often have a hard time understanding other people, because how I experience the world is different. ... I can't even go out in public sometimes because I am very sensitive to sensory overload."

At the time of writing, Hubber's video has received 3,197 comments, many from people with Asperger's. Street Skater posted that "i cried all through this. 50 and only just realized why i have had trouble fitting in all these years. Sure i have coped through mimicking but i never know or read correctly if others are bored or just wanting to stop talking."

Frank: One Extra Chromosome

Down syndrome is the most common cause of birth defects in humans. Frank Stephens told a captivated audience at the United Nations that, "I am a man with Down syndrome and my life is worth living. ... See me as a human being, not a birth defect ... I need to be valued ... not cured." Children and adults with Down syndrome tend to have weaker immune syndromes and, at the same time, are less prone to certain chronic illnesses, including cancer and heart disease. Actor and self-advocate, Stephens acts as an advocate for scientific research. "When my body was forming, when the first two cells divided, each of them had one extra chromosome. ... Our extra chromosome makes us a blueprint for medical research in areas that include soft tissue cancer, heart disease, immune system disorders and Alzheimer's." Stephens has made a similar declaration to the US Congress, advocating for greater research funding (Fondation Jérôme Lejeune, 2018).

Rachel and Njegoš

"This is my daughter, Rachel Handlin," Jay Handlin (2020) proclaimed in a tweet highlighting a stunning black and white graduation photograph. "Tonight, she earned her full Bachelor of Fine Arts degree in Photography & Media from the prestigious California Institute of the Arts, @CalArts. Rachel has Down syndrome. I am officially the proudest father on the planet."

Rachel Handlin is one of approximately 12 individuals with Down syndrome who is known to have ever earned a bachelor's degree. Down syndrome is characterized by developmental disabilities and other physical issues. Handlin noted that: "out of all the people with Down syndrome in the world, those who've earned a regular college degree are literally about one in a million. That's not because they're the only ones who could do it. They're the ones whose families refused to let their children's futures be denied, who fought unfair odds, social biases, low expectations and systems stacked against them, and somehow managed to win" (Handlin, 2020). Even before receiving her degree in May 2020, Rachel began displaying her photography in museums around the world.

Jay Handlin is not alone in crediting his daughter's success in large part due to family's refusal to let their children's futures be denied. Every one of the individuals portrayed in this chapter was backed by the support of their family and/or community. Interviews conducted by Ablon (2002: S4) revealed that "those who cope successfully with stigmatized health conditions exhibit a commonality of biographical features and ideologies. The most important feature is unconditional family support and clear intrafamily communication.

When asked whether he had any words of encouragement for a daughter entering high school with a system offering only life skills courses, Handlin responded much the same way Judy Heumann and her mother would have responded over 50 years ago:

> Hire a good education rights lawyer if you can; if you can't, find a disability rights org or law school clinical program to help you; fight like hell (w/ or w/o a lawyer); do as much educating as you can outside school. Refuse to take "no" for an answer. And never give up.

Perhaps Haben Girma would be interested in adjudicating such a case.

On the global front, 19-year-old Njegoš Mihajlović, sponsored by Special Olympics (2020b), has become the first person with intellectual disabilities to enrol in a University in Bosnia and Herzegovina. Mihajlović aspires to become a professional trainer in order to transfer his knowledge to people with and without disabilities.

Adaptive Athletes: The 3,000-foot Rock in the Park and Other Stories of Sheer Insanity

> Disability is not simply a physical affair for us; it is our ontology, a condition of our being in the world. (Robert Murphy, *The Body Silent*)

Stephen Wampler, the founder of Camp Wamp for children with disabilities, summited El Capitan, one of the most prestigious and difficult technical rock climbs in the world. In preparation for the climb, Wampler worked out in his local gym six hours a day, six days a week for a year. The climb took a total of five days in the blazing sun. Helped by a team of professional rock climbers, Stephen Wampler, who has severe cerebral palsy, pulled himself up the vertical rock one pull up at a time, for a total of 20,000 pull-ups. Wampler, whose dream is to "inspire kids to achieve what they want out of life," commented after a few days into the climb that he had never been out of his wheelchair for this length of time before (Spitzer, 2020).

Before Wampler, Wellman & Flinn (1992), a Yosemite park ranger who in 1986 was paralyzed from the waist down after a fall in the park, engineered a device that allowed him to summit both Half Dome and El Capitan using only his upper body strength (Wellman & Flinn, 1992). With the assistance of his rock climbing buddies, who have made climbing in Yosemite both their avocation and their vocation, Wellman became the first paraplegic to ascent these routes.

Eric Weihenmayer, who lost his sight as a teenager, not only summited Mount Everest, but the highest mountains on each of the seven continents, known as the Seven Summits, as well. He then kayaked solo down the Colorado River of the Grand Canyon.

Weihenmayer (2001) also founded a mountaineering program for blind youth in the Himalayas. Better known athletes include Michael Phelps, the most decorated Olympian of all time, who was diagnosed with Attention Deficit Hyperactivity Disorder (ADHD). Alex Honnald, the rock-climbing legend who solo-climbed El Capitan in under four hours without the use of a rope and had us sitting on the edge of our chairs, is believed to be on the autistic spectrum. In an article for *outsideonline.com*, Tommy Caldwell, another rock-climbing legend, wrote, "I don't claim to understand the inner workings of Alex's mind, but I know one thing for certain: Alex climbs to live, not to cheat death." A common thread between each of these high achievers is the need to give back to the community. Most, if not all, have founded non-profit organizations serving the disabled population.

Ironmen and the Ironwoman

These stories are emblematic of the many diverse and highly successful individuals with severe disabilities. Among them are athletes, artists, and motivational speakers. Rick Hoyt, together with his father, has traveled around the world participating in racing events and giving motivational speeches. Hoyt was born with spastic paraplegic cerebral palsy, which rendered him non-verbal and unable to implement the use of his muscles. Dick Hoyt, Rick's father and athletic partner described an early trauma: "January 10, 1962, we knew there was something wrong but we didn't know exactly what. The doctor said 'forget Rick, put him away, put him in an institution, he's going to be nothing but a vegetable for the rest of his life'." With the help and support of his family, Hoyt first learned to communicate via a simple manual letter system and later with a communication device similar to the one utilized by physicist, Stephen Hawking. Given the opportunity to express himself, as an adolescent Hoyt stated his desire to do a 5-mile run to raise funds for a recently paralyzed fellow student. After his first race, he discovered his passion for athletics. Like Kodi Lee, Rick Hoyt surpassed everyone's expectations other than his own and his father's. "Dad," he said, "when I'm running it feels like I'm not even handicapped." Despite only being able to raise one arm, Rick Hoyt has completed over 1,000 marathons and multiple triathlons, including the 37 Boston Marathons and two Hawaii Ironman competions. Says Rick Hoyt, "We're Team Hoyt, and we run for the people who think they can't run." Originally with the assistance of his father and later a growing team of athletes who have difficulty keeping up with him, Rick is transferred from his wheelchair to a specially designed bicycle and flotation device for his triathlon races. Rick Hoyt holds a Bachelor's degree in Special Education, lives independently and works as a counselor at Boston University. He is featured in a number of books and co-authored his autobiography. In 1992, the father–son team biked and ran across the United States in 45 days, completing a 3,735 mile trek (Nall, 2002). Rick Hoyt participated in every Boston Marathon between 1981 and 2019. A life-size bronze statue of Dick pushing Rick in his wheelchair, arm raised in victory, graces the starting point of the Boston Marathon. In 2013, Team Hoyt was honored with an ESPY award for athletic endurance and in January 2020 they were inducted into the Triathlon Hall of Fame. After retiring from athletics at the age of 74, Dick Hoyt took on the role of grandmaster of the Boston Marathon. The Hoyts founded the non-profit Hoyt Foundation to help build self-esteem and confidence within the disabled community. Sadly, Rick was hospitalized with pneumonia in 2019 and was unable to participate in the Boston Marathon for the first time in close to 40 years. In 2020, his teammate and close friend, Dr Bryan Lyons, passed away suddenly at the age of 50. At 58 years old, after these tragic events, and in the middle of the protracted COVID-19 pandemic, it is unknown whether Rick Hoyt will continue to pursue his athletic endeavors. Dick Hoyt passed away in 2021 at the age of 80.

Born with proximal femoral focal deficiency – or a shortened leg – Sarah Reinertsen is an icon of adaptive athletes who "live(s) to make a difference." An above-the-knee amputee since the age of seven, Reinertsen (2009) was determined to compete in Ironman after Jim McClaren, fellow amputee and founder of the Challenged Athletes Foundation questioned "whether a girl can do it". Prompted by McClaren's challenge, Reinertsen became the first female and the only above-the-knee amputee to finish the Ironman Triathlon competition in Kona, HI, United States in 2005. In 2018, she completed her second Kona Ironman, taking 24 minutes off her earlier competition time, and while recovering from a broken leg. Reinertsen is one of many spokespeople for the Challenged Athletes Foundation, which sponsors challenged athletes around the world.

Most recently, Chris Nikic, sponsored by Special Olympics (2020a), was inducted into the *Guiness Book of World Records* as the first athlete with Down syndrome to complete an IRONMAN. According to his father, "To Chris, this race was more than just a finish line and celebration of victory. … IRONMAN has served as his platform to become one step closer to his goal of living a life of inclusion and leadership."

Addressing Bullying

Author, and anti-bullying advocate, Lizzie Velasquez@littlelizziev was born with Marfanoid–progeroid–lipodystrophy syndrome, a very rare condition which prevents her from gaining weight. At 68 pounds, she is blind in one eye and has limited vision in the other, which gives her face a distorted appearance. Lizzie has recently become an internet champion to those experiencing bullying and cyberbullying and a role model to those fighting such bullying. Taking to TikTok, Lizzie directly addressed those parents who shared her picture with their children in a "teacher challenge." The parents asked their children if they would like Lizzie to be their teacher. Reacting in horror and dismay to her disfigured appearance, the children are pictured shrieking and the parents laughing, to which Lizzie Velasquez responded by discussing her feelings and educating them about the importance of appropriately respecting physical differences.

Invisible Disabilities/Visible Advocacy

> On a scale of 1 to 10, the pain rates a 15. What makes it even more excruciating is that you can test and look perfectly normal. Viral and bacterial cultures and other indicators can all be negative, making it impossible for you to convince your doctor that you are in agony and in need of help. (Vicki Ratner, MD, Founder and President Emeritus of the Interstitial Cystitis Association)

People with invisible, or so-called "hidden" disabilities often feel that their health issues are dismissed, overlooked, ignored, or misdiagnosed. "But you look good," "you look so healthy," or even "there is nothing wrong with you," are common expressions heard by those who may be suffering from symptoms not evident to the observer. Chronic pain and fatigue can be debilitating, having an effect not only on one's health, but on one's livelihood and sense of self-esteem. Invisible disabilities can include the early stages of degenerative illness, post-traumatic stress disorder (PTSD), deafness, and autoimmune illness such as lupus, fibromyalgia, interstitial cystitis, and vulvodynia. For some, having an invisible disability can leave them feeling as if they are not being truly seen, or at least that their health concerns are not being taken seriously.

The Invisible Disabilities® Association (IDA) states as its mission "to encourage, educate and connect people and organizations touched by illness, pain and disability around the globe." Addressing issues of loneliness and stigmatization, the IDA recognizes that "the frequently invisible nature of illness and pain may lead to disbelief about that illness or pain by those surrounding the person who lives daily with invisible disabilities. This disbelief can lead to misunderstandings, rejection by friends, family and health care providers. It may also lead to accusations of laziness or faking an illness. We are passionate about providing awareness that invisible illness, pain and disabilities are very real!" https://www.businesswire.com/news/home/20210402005238/en/Accelerating-its-Philanthropic-Mission-FashGive-FashWire-Partners-with-Invisible-Disabilities-Association

Non-visible pain can be associated with a physiological genesis, such as a tumor or accident, or psychological one, such as a precipitating traumatic event. The physical pain though real, may lead to a sense of mind–body disintegration and can contribute to fatigue. In the 1980s, fibromyalgia/chronic fatigue syndrome became recognized as a bona fide endemic among strong, driven, middle-class women. Now covered by the ADA, those with invisible disabilities are eligible to receive disability benefits.However, there continues to be a paucity of research or even interest in fibromyalgia/chronic fatigue syndrome. As the long-term effects of COVID-19 among the healthy population become evident, this "invisible" chronic illness is taking on new meaning as scientists search for clues to understand and combat the long-term effects of the virus.

DISABILITY IN THE TIME COVID

We live in trying times. At the time of writing this chapter, the first viral pandemic of the twenty-first century is unfolding around us. COVID-19 received its name because it is a novel corona virus which originated in the year 2019. Its technical name, SARS-CoV-2, makes reference to Severe Acute Respiratory Syndrome because of its severe impact on the lungs. It is becoming evident, however, that COVID-19 not only affects the lungs, but other organs as well. Originating in Wuhan, China, in late 2019 over 1 million cases of COVID-19 were confirmed globally within just a few months. Close to 200 million cases worldwide have been documented so far, as well as over 4 million deaths (https://www.worldometers.info/coronavirus). Because of discrepancies in data collection and analysis, and a current political climate of mistrust of science, the accuracy of these figures is being questioned. With the effects of the pandemic expected to be felt for years to come, the most vulnerable populations are those at highest risk for contracting the illness and suffering severe consequences and death. These populations include the elderly and those with disabilities and co-morbid conditions (Hernandez et al., 2021). Yet, according to the Disability Rights Education & Defense Fund (DREDF), people with disabilities have not been included in the National Academies of Science, Engineering and Medicine's Framework for Equitable Allocation of COVID-19 Vaccine guidance, which is aimed at the equitable allocation of the COVID-19 vaccines (Disability Rights Education & Defense Fund, 2020).

In a recent study involving 5,700 hospitalized patients in New York City (median age, 63 years), the most common comorbidities associated with a COVID-19 diagnosis, were hypertension (56.6%), obesity (41.7%) and diabetes (33.8%) (Richardson, Hirsh, Narasimhan et al., 2020). The Centers for Disease Control and Prevention (CDC) further delineates these risk factors to include chronic lung disease, serious heart conditions, immunocompromised conditions, including cancer treatment, bone marrow or organ transplantation, immune deficiencies, poorly controlled HIV or AIDS, and prolonged use of corticosteroids and other immune weakening medications, obesity, diabetes, liver disease, and those with chronic kidney disease undergoing dialysis. The pandemic seems to be exacerbating economic vulnerability for those already on the lowest vulnerability rungs, including poverty. Tijuana, Mexico, for example, houses the largest border crossing in the world, with cross-border traffic providing a modicum of income for street vendors and beggars with disability lining the lanes between cars. The closing of the border between Mexico and the United States to only "essential travel" is affecting those relying on this traffic for their income, and most have become virtually invisible during this time.

With stay-at-home orders taking place around the world, many more mild cases and at-home deaths are purportedly being undetected and under-reported (Centers for Disease Control and Prevention, 2021a). The global stay-at-home orders can also have the effect of further isolating those who already feel lonely and isolated, especially if they lack access to computers and social networking. Caretakers who cannot follow the physical distancing directives may be at risk of getting sick themselves or of infecting those they attend if either are asymptomatic carriers of the virus. Concomitant to new variants spreading quickly through the world, protests and large public gatherings are taking place, possibly putting those most vulnerable, including those who are not vaccinated due to medical conditions, at even greater risk of exposure. When politics are placed before health, the most vulnerable are often the ones who suffer the most.

The Aftermath of COVID-19 as Invisible Disability

> I used to go to the gym three times a week. [Now,] my physical activity is bed to couch, maybe couch to kitchen. (Athena Akrami, Neuroscientist, University College London)

Older adults and people with underlying and disabling conditions are more likely than others to reside in nursing homes and require hospitalization and are more likely to be subjected to structural inequalities affecting their ability to care for themselves at home should they fall ill. If a triage system is employed, as was discussed at the early stages of the pandemic, those with disabilities could potentially be the least likely to be offered care. Nevertheless, funding to address the needs of people with disabilities is limited. On the 30th anniversary of the passage of the ADA, Fins and Bagenstos (2020) published an op-ed addressing this precarious situation:

> Of the US$3 trillion dollars appropriated in the CARES Act in response to COVID-19 pandemic, less than $1 billion was dispersed to the states to support older people and individuals with disabilities. This neglect of people with disabilities impairs the ADA on its 30th anniversary.

Some individuals with even mild symptoms are becoming 'long-haulers' and are exhibiting long-term symptoms, at times preventing them from returning to a normal life or work. One long-hauler support group member says:

> It has taken control over who Aida used to be pre-COVID ... I have a fog in my brain. I call it 'COVID brain.' That's my term for it ... I forget, sometimes in the middle of my sentence I forget what I'm trying to say. I forget the easiest words. (Gusoff, 2020)

Dr Scott Krakower, a child psychiatrist, has been talking to audiences and describing his own ordeal with COVID-19 as a "COVID long-hauler." Krakower was diagnosed with the virus in April 2020. "Right now I'm okay," he said in one interview, "but I am not going out." Too sick to work after months of fluctuating symptoms, Krakower's lingering symptoms are similar to those of chronic fatigue and fibromyalgia. Due to the novelty of the virus, there is limited information about its long-term effects, and who might be susceptible to them. A cohort study of German patients recently recovered from COVID-19 infection revealed that of 100 patients, 60 (60%) exhibited ongoing myocardial inflammation, independent of pre-existing conditions, severity and overall course of the acute illness, and time from the original diagnosis (Puntmann, Carerj, Wieters et al., 2020).

An informal survey of 1,567 previously healthy long-haulers provides details on the wide-range of long-term and overlapping symptoms, showing that the top ten complaints are similar to those associated with fibromyalgia/chronic fatigue syndrome: 100% fatigue, 66.8% muscle or body aches, 65.1% shortness of breath or difficulty breathing, 59.0%

difficulty concentrating or focusing, 58.5% inability to exercise or be active, 57.6% headache, 49.9% difficulty sleeping, 47.6% anxiety, 45.6% memory problems, and 41.9% dizziness.

As is often the case in fibromyalgia and other non-visible chronic illnesses:

> Their experiences are poorly understood by the medical community and often dismissed by doctors as psychological issues, writes epidemiologist and Covid survivor Margot Gage Witvliet, PhD. … But the aches, pains, and inconveniences are real, according to Witvliet, who had Covid-19 four months ago and is now suffering from tinnitus, chest pain, and heart-racing. (Britt, 2020)

Results from recent studies confirm higher prevalence of specific comorbidities associated with poorer COVID-19 outcomes among people with intellectual disabilities. The authors conclude that people with intellectual disabilities "may be at higher risk of developing more severe outcomes from COVID-19, including death" (Turk et al., 2020: 4). Espinosa (2020: 3) suggests that because of their higher prevalence of autoimmune disorders and increased rates of hospitalization during respiratory viral infections, and higher mortality rates from pneumonia and sepsis, "individuals with Down syndrome are more likely to develop a stronger and more prolonged cytokine storm."

CONCLUSION: "WE ARE NOT YET DONE"

> "I want my civil rights," Paulette Patterson of Chicago stated as she was inching her way to the top. "I want to be treated like a human being."

We are not yet done. At eight years old, Jennifer Keelan left her wheelchair at the bottom of the US Capitol to pull herself up the steps as part of what became known as the Capitol Crawl. At the time, the Capitol was not yet wheelchair accessible and the protesters demonstrated the need for accessible infrastructure. Paulette Patterson just wanted to be treated like a human being. This demonstration led to the passage of the Americans with Disability Act in 1990, the crafting of which Jennifer Keelan and her mother participated (Little, 2020). Keelan is celebrated as one of the faces of the disability rights movement. Nevertheless, 25 years later, she and her mother struggle to find affordable accessible housing and escape bullying.

On the 30th anniversary of the passage of the Americans with Disabilities Act, there is much to celebrate. A blind man summiting Mount Everest is cause for celebration, as is the first female above-the-knee amputee completing the Hawaii Ironman. These accomplishments must be celebrated in light of the long history of disability rights advocacy and in the context of the continuing struggle for the right to live a dignified life. A delightful, accurate and funny YouTube video features actors with disabilities portraying a historic sit-in (Comedy Central, 2020). Yet, these actors still have difficulty finding employment. We have not reached the end of the road in our global fight for rights, equality and inclusion. Judith Heumann visited a boy born with missing arms in India, whose grandmother told his mother not to feed him. That boy, fortunately, was helped by an organization, but many others with disabilities continue to face discrimination and worse. Disparities in access to health care during the COVID-19 pandemic are being acutely experienced among the poorest countries. Nath (2020) suggests that in India, the world's second most populated country:

> People with disabilities who regularly need catheters, caregiver support, cotton wool, urine bags, bandages, medicines, assistive devices, and medical care were badly affected. Lack of funds and the inability to physically travel to get these items due to the lockdown have made life very difficult and even dangerous for disabled Indians.

Adults with disabilities who line up at the Mexico–US border-crossing begging drivers for money are impacted by the restrictions on cross-border travel. People living with chronic pain and fatigue, including those recovering from COVID-19, still do not have their symptoms taken seriously. As Heumann reminds us in her TED Talk, there is still work to be done (Heumann, 2018).

Box 17.1 Me/Cfs: A New Understanding of a Debilitating Mystery

MARY COREY MARCH

Myalgic encephalomyelitis (formerly known as chronic fatigue syndrome) is an extremely misunderstood, underdiagnosed and mistreated condition. People with mild cases can work almost normally and then spend the rest of their time resting. People with the most severe cases can't roll over in bed and need feeding tubes and sensory isolation. Healthy, active people become bedbound overnight (*Unrest* Documentary directed by Jennifer Brea, 2017).

ME/CFS is a debilitating disease syndrome which manifests in multiple pathophysiological changes that affect multiple systems, including immune system abnormalities, cellular metabolism abnormalities, neuroendocrine disturbances and blood pressure or heart rate regulation problems. The causes of ME/CFS are still being investigated, but one of the most common appears to be an autoimmune response to one or more acute viral infections (Centers for Disease Control and Prevention, 2021b).

A deeply flawed and now debunked study (PACE) did an extraordinary amount of damage to people with ME/CFS all over the world (Lubet, 2017; Tuller, 2019). It concluded the condition was psychosomatic and could be treated with cognitive behavioral therapy to convince people they weren't sick and graded exercise to "recondition" their muscles and to break through the "fear" of exercise. New research has revealed that the condition is biological and there are biological treatments (as well as careful pacing), but most doctors are not up on the new research and still follow the PACE protocols. This causes their patients serious damage through exercise that can make them significantly worse. In addition to this, sufferers of ME/CFS are often disbelieved by their doctors, families, friends, insurance companies and cannot get disability allowances. They try to work or contribute to their families and become worse.

I was always hyperactive, literally ADHD. I grew up a competitive gymnast, then a martial artist. Later, I switched to dance and circus. I was generally the strongest, most flexible, most daring person in the room. I was used to pushing through huge amounts of pain and exhaustion on a regular basis my entire life. I had two undergraduate degrees and two master's degrees under my belt, and an active career as an artist. Then came ME/CFS.

I have had CFS/ME for just over four and a half years, but the first year and a half was much milder and I didn't know what was going on. I had a year and a half of lesser symptoms: months in bed feeling sick, randomly not being able to handle sensory or emotional stuff, new bad headaches, sudden weakness, sudden sensitivity to light, noise, even a conversation. I had moments I felt like I needed to sit down or I might fall down. In between I went to my regular workouts and thought maybe I was just getting older. I certainly wasn't at full steam. I collapsed during two of my regular workouts and was fine (if more sore) for others. I pushed through and tried to brush it all off. I thought the hypersensitivity was a new kind of anxiety. Looking back, I don't know how I explained the collapses to myself, but they scared me. I toughed it out.

Then one day, while walking around a fair, I felt strange and terrible. It was an overwhelmed feeling; sensory overload and emotional sensitivity. I also felt physically wrong in an unfamiliar way. I felt like I needed to lay down. By the time I got to the car I was shaking with effort to just walk, and I was crying uncontrollably with the overwhelmed feeling. I felt utterly helpless. An hour later in the car I could barely lift my arms. I had a cold sore. I didn't know it then, but this was probably my "second viral infection" that triggered getting worse.

When I got back home, I was bedbound. Just sitting upright for 15–30 minutes caused sweat to run down my back and made me shake with exertion. I was an artist who couldn't draw a circle. My right hand's handwriting looked worse than my left hand usually did. My hand felt like it was controlled by a broken remote and I was wearing heavy rubber gloves. I had days when I was unable to do more than crawl (with breaks) to the bathroom. I needed breaks brushing my teeth or hair or even chewing food. My brain didn't work – it felt like it was always stuck in neutral. Both my brain and my tongue failed at talking regularly. I took baths instead of showers because I couldn't even sit upright on the floor long enough for a shower. For the first three months, I tried to do things on my best days where I could walk. I would sit on a stool, walk a few feet, sit, walk, etc. Then I would be unable to leave the bed for two weeks. My doctor was testing me for everything, but she initially discarded CFS/ME because she had been taught it was a psychosomatic disease (again, the legacy of the PACE study) and she didn't think that could possibly be the case with me.

During this time, I saw a neurologist at The University of California at San Francisco (UCSF). He gave me the "graded exercise and cognitive behavioral therapy" line (again, the PACE study), but he didn't even *say* CFS. He suggested that my legs were collapsing because "maybe I felt neglected by my husband." I wanted to smack him, but he seemed so sincere and I was too shocked. He implied it would go away if I could get therapy to convince myself I wasn't sick. I was outraged. I saw another neurologist. He was nicer, but also called it a "software problem" (psychological) because he couldn't find a physical problem with existing tests.

(Continued)

(Continued)

In the meantime, I did my own research, self-diagnosed myself with ME/CFS, found out what treatments were being tried and convinced my doctor to try me on Valtrex. She believed me and we tried it. This helped me a HUGE amount and I was suddenly able to walk farther around the house, could brush my hair, etc. After this success, we decided to pursue the CFS/ME line and to get me seen at Stanford (a wait of one and a half years). In the meantime, I made adjustments. I got a wheelchair and wheelchair van. I put chairs in every room in the house. I learned to walk 10 feet and sit, to make one-third of dinner at a time while sitting, and to lie down in between. Pace, pace, pace. I saw another CFS/ME specialist in Los Angeles and he gave me more guidance and supplements. He was able to confirm that it was CFS/ME, and also that I was among the worst cases he had treated. My doctor was able to find drugs to help me sleep and for the horrific headaches. When I was finally seen at Stanford, they also confirmed the CFS/ME diagnosis and went through a variety of drugs until we found three more that helped. At this point I'm taking six prescription drugs related to CFS/ME and about 30–35 supplements. Each one has seemed to raise the floor a little bit along with careful pacing. My trajectory has been gradually up.

These days I can walk freely around the house. I can sit up for two hours on a good day. I can paint again if I'm careful. I can go outside and even travel in the wheelchair. I can usually go into a noisy restaurant without my brain overloading. I can think clearly again. I have to be careful. I pace, I treat my mind just as carefully as my body, but thankfully I have improved. I feel like I owe most of this to my family practice doctor who believed in me and to the Stanford clinic. I hope one day to be able to walk outside freely again. But every day I hear the stories of people made worse by doctors pushing the PACE protocols, or worse, being disbelieved entirely. Every time I leave the house, I confront bias from people who don't understand or are hostile to disability. I get hostile stares from people who think I look too healthy to be in a wheelchair or who resent things like handicapped parking spots. I confront barriers to using the wheelchair, from access to parking to steps and narrow doorways.

Recently, we have learned that many people are suffering with what seems to be ME/CFS post-COVID (Fauci, 2020). This means we have to be even more proactive about treating this serious medical condition with the care and attention it deserves. I continue to work for better understanding and treatment of ME/CFS, and for better understanding and access for those of us with limited mobility.

ACKNOWLEDGEMENTS

The author thanks Drs Joan Ablon and Christine von Glascoe for their thoughtful editing of an earlier version of this manuscript. Thank you, too, to all the amazing, talented and committed individuals and families that I have met over the years who are living and thriving with disabilities. You are my heroes, my role models, my colleagues, my teammates, my friends, and my family. Keep leading the way forward.

REFERENCES

Ablon, J. (1981). Stigmatized health conditions. *Social Science & Medicine. Part B: Medical Anthropology*, 15(1), 5–9.

Ablon, J. (2002). The nature of stigma and medical conditions. *Epilepsy & Behavior*, 3(6), S2–S9.

Ablon, J. (2008). *Brittle Bones, Stout Hearts and Minds: Adults with Osteogenesis Imperfecta*. San Francisco, CA: Jones & Bartlett Learning.

Alexandria, A. (Director). (2019). *Willowbrook: The Last Great Disgrace – Geraldo Rivera 1972 Exposé – Full Short Documentary* [Documentary]. You Tube. (Accessed 5 July 2020).

American Academy of Arts and Sciences (2016, 17 October). *Educating Students Who Have Different Kinds of Minds – Temple Grandin*. [Video file]. YouTube. www.youtube.com/watch?v=8LCrjUL8qU4

Americans with Disabilities Act (1990). *As amended.* Available at: www.ada.gov/pubs/adastatute08.htm. (Accessed 20 July 2020).

Brea, J. (2017) *Unrest Documentary* https://weta.org/watch/shows/independent-lens/unrest

Britt, R.B. (2020, August 14). New survey identifies 98 long-lasting covid symptoms: early research helps quantify coronavirus long-haulers' experiences. *Elemental*. https://elemental.medium.com/new-survey-identifies-98-lo

ng-lasting-covid-symptoms-87935b258a3e. elemental. (Accessed 5 October, 2020).

Centers for Disease Control and Prevention (2021a, April 20). *People at increased risk and other people who need to take extra precautions*. www.cdc.gov/coronavirus/2019-ncov/need-extra-precautions/people-at-higher-risk.html. (Accessed 22 May 2021).

Centers for Disease Control and Prevention (2021b). *Myalgic encephalomyelitis/chronic fatigue syndrome*. www.cdc.gov/me-cfs/healthcare-providers/presentation-clinical-course/etiology-pathophysiology.html. (Accessed 22 May 2021).

Comedy Central (2020, March 25). *Judith Heumann's Fight for Disability Rights (featuring Ali Stroker) – Drunk History*. [Video file]. YouTube. www.youtube.com/watch?v=y505KwHp4O4

Cone, K. (n.d.). Short history of the 504 sit in. *Disability Rights Education & Defense Fund*. (Accessed 4 September 2020).

Couzin-Frankel, J. (2020, July 31). From 'brain fog' to heart damage, COVID-19's lingering problems alarm scientists. *Science*. www.sciencemag.org/news/2020/07/brain-fog-heart-damage-covid-19-s-lingering-problems-alarm-scientists. (Accessed 6 September 2020).

Disability Rights Education & Defense Fund (2020, October 15). *People with disabilities not counted in guidance aimed at equitable allocation of a COVID-19 vaccine*. dredf. https://dredf.org/2020/10/15/people-with-disabilities-not-counted-in-guidance-aimed-at-equitable-allocation-of-a-covid-19-vaccine/. (Accessed 17 November 2020).

Espinosa, J.M. (2020). Down Syndrome and COVID-19: a perfect storm? *Cell Reports Medicine*, 1(2), 100019.

Fauci, A. (2020). Fauci warns about "post-viral" syndrome after COVID-19. *Healthline*. www.healthline.com/health-news/fauci-warns-about-post-viral-syndrome-after-covid-19. (Accessed 22 May 2021).

Fins, J., & Bagenstos, S. (2020, July 26). The Americans with Disabilities Act at 30: a cause for celebration during COVID-19? *The Conversation*. https://theconversation.com/the-americans-with-disabilities-act-at-30-a-cause-for-celebration-during-covid-19-143399. (Accessed 10 September 2020).

Fisher, J. (1997). *Twenty-five Years after Willowbrook*. [Documentary]. City Lights Pictures. www.youtube.com/watch?v=HNLyKW8fCNg. (Accessed 4 September 2020).

Fondation Jérôme Lejeune (2018, March 18). *I Am a Man with Down Syndrome and My Life is Worth. Frank Stephens' speech at the UN Living*. www.youtube.com/watch?v=1d8ocuPrlT8. (Accessed 22 May 2020).

Fu, H., Cord, L., & McLain-Nhlapo, C. (2019, December 3). *A Billion People Experience Disabilities Worldwide – So Where's the Data?* [Blog]. Washington, DC: World Bank. https://blogs.worldbank.org/opendata/billion-people-experience-disabilities-worldwide-so-wheres-data (Accessed 10 September 2020).

Girma, H. (2019). *Haben: The Deafblind Woman Who Conquered Harvard Law*. New York: Twelve. Hachette UK.

Girma, H. (2020). Talking with Time 100 and walking with autonomous robots. *Time 100 Talks*. https://habengirma.com/2020/08/18/talking-with-time-100-and-walking-with-autonomous-robots/. (Accessed 5 September 2020).

Gusoff, C. (2020, July 24). COVID-19 support groups: a life line for survivors suffering panic attacks, memory loss, other lingering symptoms. *CBS New York*. https://newyork.cbslocal.com/2020/07/24/covid-19-support-groups-a-life-line-for-survivors-suffering-panic-attacks-memory-loss-other-lingering-symptoms/. (Accessed 24 July 2020).

Haben (2014). *TEDx Talk: Why I work to remove access barriers for students with disabilities* https://habengirma.com/transcripts/tedx_baltimore_2014.txt

Hahn, H. (1988). The politics of physical differences: Disability and discrimination. *Journal of Social Issues*.

Handlin, J. [@JayHandlin]. (2020, May 15). *This is my daughter, Rachel Handlin. Tonight, she earned her full Bachelor of Fine Arts degree in Photography & Media*. Twitter. https://twitter.com/jayhandlin/status/1261513883413622784. (Accessed 16 May 2020).

Hernandez, S., Manley, B., O'Key, S., & Pettersson, H. (2021, May 22). Tracking COVID-19 Cases in the US. *CNN Health*. www.cnn.com/interactive/2020/health/coronavirus-us-maps-and-cases/. (Accessed 22 May 2021).

Heumann, J. (2018, April 24). Our fight for disability rights – and why we're not done yet. *TED*

Talks. Judith Heumann. [Video file]. YouTube. www.youtube.com/watch?v=uJr4wGcLNsA. (Accessed 22 May 2021).

Heumann, J., & Joiner, K. (2020). *Being Heumann: An Unrepentant Memoir of a Disability Rights Activist*. Boston, MA: Beacon Press.

Howle, M.J. (1992). Musical savants. *Update: Applications of Research in Music Education*, 11(1), 5–7.

Hubber, A. (2015, July 11). *Through Our Eyes: Living with Asperger's*. [Documentary]. [Video file]. YouTube. www.youtube.com/watch?v=2TSlti5bioQ. (Accessed 22 May 2020).

Johnson, R., & Williams, K. (1999). *Lost in a Desert World: An Autobiography*. Philadelphia: Speaking for Ourselves. https://www.leagle.com/decision/1970943320fsupp6231818

Leagle (2019). *Heumann V. Board of Education of the City of New York*. No. 70 Civ. 2166. 320 F.Supp. 623 (1970). www.leagle.com/decision/1970943320fsupp6231818#

Little, B. (2020). https://www.history.com/news/americans-with-disabilities-act-1990-capitol-crawl (Accessed 20 July 2021).

Lubet, S. (2017, March 23). How a study about chronic fatigue syndrome was doctored, adding to pain and stigma. *The Conversation*. https://theconversation.com/how-a-study-about-chronic-fatigue-syndrome-was-doctored-adding-to-pain-and-stigma-74890. (Accessed 22 May 2021).

Mittler, P. (2015). The UN Convention on the Rights of Persons with Disabilities: implementing a paradigm shift. *Journal of Policy and Practice in Intellectual Disabilities*, 12(2), 79–89.

Moiseff, J. (2013, April 1). *My Willowbrook Experience*. [Documentary]. [Video file]. YouTube. www.youtube.com/watch?v=1UCFBjt36rs. (Accessed 22 May 2020).

Murphy, R. *The Body Silent*. 1990 W.W. Norton & Company: New York

Nall, S. (2002). *It's Only a Mountain: Dick and Rick Hoyt, Men of Iron*. St Petersburg, FL: Southern Heritage Press.

Nath, A. (2020, August 18). *COVID Blog: How the COVID-19 Pandemic has Exacerbated Pre-existing Ableism & Difficulties in India*. [Blog]. https://wid.org/2020/08/18/covid-blog-how-the-covid-19-pandemic-has-exacerbated-pre-existing-ableism-difficulties-in-india/

NBC (1968). *Suffer the Little Children*. [Documentary]. [Video file]. NBC 10 Philadelphia. YouTube. www.preservepennhurst.org/default.aspx?pg=26. (Accessed 22 May 2020).

Newnham, N., & LeBrecht, J. (Directors). (2020). *Crip Camp: A Disability Revolution* [Documentary]. Netflix.

Oliver, M. (2013). The social model of disability: thirty years on. *Disability & Society*, 28(7), 1024–1026.

Puntmann, V.M., Ludovica Carerj, Wieters, I., Fahim, M., Arendt, C., Hoffmann, J., Shchendrygina, A., Escher, F., Vasa-Nicotera, M., Zeiher, A.M., Vehreschild, M., & Nagel, E. (2020). Outcomes of cardiovascular magnetic resonance imaging in patients recently recovered from coronavirus disease 2019 (COVID-19). *JAMA Cardiology*, Published online July 27.

Reinertsen, S. (2009). *In a Single Bound: Losing My Leg, Finding Myself, and Training for Life*. Guilford, CT: Globe Pequote Press.

Richardson, S., Hirsch, J.S., Narasimhan, M., et al. (2020). Presenting characteristics, comorbidities, and outcomes among 5,700 patients hospitalized with COVID-19 in the New York City Area. *JAMA*, 323(20), 2052–2059. Online first April 22 2020. doi:10.1001/jama.2020.6775 [Epub ahead of print].

Rifkin, G. (2020, July 21). Overlooked no more: Roland Johnson, who fought to shut down institutions for the disabled. Obituaries. *New York Times*.

Rose, S.F. (2017). *No Right to be Idle: The Invention of Disability, 1840s–1930s*. UNC (University of North Carolina) Press Books.

Shapiro, J. (2015). *She owes her activism to a brave mom, the ADA, and chocolate cake*. www.npr.org/sections/goatsandsoda/2015/07/31/428075935/she-owes-her-activism-to-a-brave-mom-the-ada-and-chocolate-cake. (Accessed 5 October 2020).

Special Olympics (2020a). www.specialolympics.org/stories/news/chris-nikic-shatters-stereotypes-to-become-first-person-with-down-syndrome-to-complete-an-ironman. (Accessed 18 November 2020).

Special Olympics (2020b). www.specialolympics.org/stories/news/special-olympics-athlete-leader-becomes-first-person-with-intellectual-disabilities-to-enroll-in-university-in-bosnia-and-herzegovina. (Accessed 21 November 2020).

Spitzer, Jacques (2020). *Wampler's Ascent* [Documentary].: https://www.imdb.com/title/tt2415838/

TalentRecap (2019). Kodi Lee: Blind autistic singer SHOCKS the world again in the live show! *America's Got Talent 2019*. [Video file]. YouTube. www.youtube.com/watch?v=AlXgLR4wFuU&list=RD7XzfWFWNi1A&index=2

TIME (2020, March 5). 1977: Judith Heumann – 100 women of the year. *TIME Magazine*. https://time.com/5793652/judith-heumann-100-women-of-the-year/ (Accessed 6 September 2020).

Treffert, D.A. (2009). The savant syndrome: an extraordinary condition. A synopsis: past, present, future. *Philosophical Transactions of the Royal Society B: Biological Sciences*, 364(1522), 1351–1357 www.yumpu.com/en/document/view/35875363/savant-syndrome-wisconsin-medical-society

Tuller, D. (2019, February 6). Trial by error: HRA report does not vindicate PACE. *Virology blog*. [Blog]. www.virology.ws/2019/02/06/trial-by-error-hra-report-does-not-vindicate-pace/. (accessed 22 May 2021).

Turk, M.A., Landes, S.D., Formica, M.K., & Goss, K.D. (2020). Intellectual and developmental disability and COVID-19 case-fatality trends: TriNetX analysis. *Disability and Health Journal*, 13(3), 100942.

United Nations. (2007). *General Assembly. Convention on the Rights of Persons with Disabilities: resolution / adopted by the General Assembly* (2007, January 24). www.un.org/development/desa/disabilities/convention-on-the-rights-of-persons-with-disabilities.html. (Accessed 20 July 2020).

US Department of Health and Human Services. *Office for Civil Rights* (2006, June). www.hhs.gov/sites/default/files/ocr/civilrights/resources/factsheets/504.pdf. (Accessed 20 January 2020).

Weihenmayer, Eric (2001). *Touch the Top of the World: A Blind Man's Journey to Climb Farther than the Eye Can See*. New York: Penguin Books.

Wellman, M.R., & Flinn, J.G. (1992). *Climbing Back*. Waco, Texas:WRS Pub.

World Bank (2020, May 15). *Disability Inclusion*. Washington, DC: World Bank. www.worldbank.org/en/topic/disability. (Accessed 20 July 2020).

World Health Organization (2015). *WHO Global Disability Action Plan 2014–2021: Better Health for All People with Disability*. Geneva: World Health Organization.

World Health Organization (2018). *WHO Disability Assessment Schedule 2.0 (WHODAS 2.0)*. Geneva: World Health Organization.

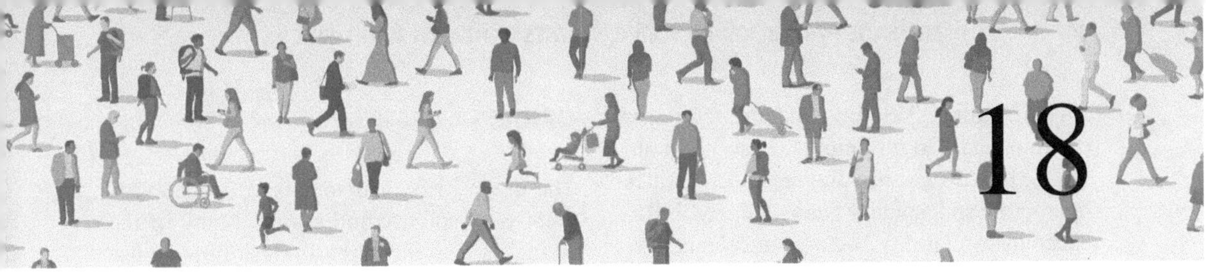

18

Social and Geopolitical Factors Influencing Trends in Substance Use

Dessa Bergen-Cico, David Otiashvili, Irma Kirtadze, and Jay Jeong Hyun Park

Drug use is a complex issue influenced by neurobiological, psychological and sociological factors. This chapter will focus on sociological factors with particular emphasis on socio-political attributes shaping contemporary drug use trends. Whereas alcohol and tobacco are the most commonly used substances on a global scale, they are not the primary focus in this chapter; here we will focus on the broad range of other psychoactive substances. Substance use refers to licit and illicit psychoactive substances including plant-based substances, pharmaceuticals, and the everchanging array of new psychoactive synthetic substances. This chapter highlights the most prominent trends in drug use by category of drugs (amphetamines, cannabis/marijuana, cocaine, opiates/opioids, and new psychoactive substances).

There are three primary policy levels for monitoring and controlling psychoactive drugs: (1) international treaties, (2) federal and state policies, and (3) local or regional policies. We know the most about the prevalence of the drugs used that fall under control of international treaties of the United Nations (UN) Single Convention and those monitored by the World Health Organization (WHO), namely alcohol and tobacco products. The United Nations Office of Drugs and Crime (UNODC) coordinates and monitors drug use trends for amphetamines, cannabis/marijuana, cocaine, and opiates/opioids; however, there are many more psychoactive drugs that are not regulated or monitored by UNODC. There is the broad category of emerging New Psychoactive Substances (NPS) which, if regulated, are generally regulated at the state or federal policy level.

Global estimates for the prevalence of substance use among the adult population are 18% for past 30-day heavy episodic alcohol use; 15% for daily tobacco use; and for past year use 0.8% used amphetamine, 3.8% used cannabis, 0.35% used cocaine and 0.35% used opioids. Age-standardized prevalence rates per 100,000 for dependence are as follows: alcohol dependence 843; 86 for amphetamines; 259 for cannabis; 52.5 for cocaine; and 220 for opioids (Peacock et al., 2018). However, usage and dependence rates by region and country vary and are influenced by availability, socio-political and psychological factors. European regions have the highest prevalence of heavy episodic alcohol and daily tobacco use; and North America has among the highest rates of cannabis, opioid and cocaine dependence. We begin with a broad view of substance use rates by country and region and then we explore the nexus of substance use and conflict analyzing the experiences of the Republic of Georgia and the United States.

CURRENT SUBSTANCE USE TRENDS BY COUNTRY AND REGION

Data on current substance use by country and region for alcohol, amphetamines, cannabis, cocaine, and opioids are presented in Table 18.1. These data indicate past year usage rates standardized by age group 15–64. These data are derived from the best available and most recent, as of 2019, using estimates of use as conferred by the UNODC (2019), which oversees international drug control for amphetamines, cannabis, cocaine, and opiates and some new emerging synthetic psychoactive substances. Note that due to the unavailability of UNODC data for substance use in the Republic of Korea (South Korea), one of our co-authors has translated Korean reports to obtain estimates of information on drug use rates in South Korea where available. In addition to the presentation of usage data for the most common psychoactive substances, we discuss social and geopolitical factors that influence availability, trafficking, and demand for specific drugs by region. These trends are examined in the context of risk factors associated with drug production, routes of administration, and the intersection with drug policy, regional stability, and public health.

OPIOIDS

The usage rates of opioids and opiates vary greatly by country and region. Many of the countries with the highest rates of opiate use are proximate to opium cultivation, and thus the population has greater exposure to raw opium and opiate derivatives (morphine and heroin). Presently, Afghanistan (the Golden Crescent) produces most of the world's opium, followed by Myanmar (and the Golden Triangle), then Mexico and Columbia in descending order (UNODC, 2017). The United Nations recognized illicit drug production as one of the most significant catalysts for conflict in regions of economic instability while political instability is a significant risk factor for drug cultivation, trafficking and use (Bergen-Cico, 2012; UNODC, 2009). Underlying patterns of drug cultivation, production, international trafficking, and domestic consumption have shown dramatic gains following each war opium and heroin are processed in narcotics "labs" throughout Afghanistan and the Northwest Frontier Province (NWFP) of Pakistan where the narco-economy funds families and about 9% of the Afghan population is addicted to opiates. Afghanistan has been mired in conflict for decades, where the trauma and instability have cultivated fertile opium production and addiction. The rate of opiate production in Afghanistan has increased exponentially since 2001 following the start of the United State (US) led Operation Enduring Freedom (OEF). During this same time period opiate use and addiction has increased and reached epidemic rates in the US. The primary sources of opiates (opium and heroin) trafficked and used in the US comes from Mexico and Columbia; heroin use in the US is most likely to be initiated following dependency on prescription opioids (synthetic and prescription and synthetic opiates) (Bergen-Cico, Scholl, Ivanashvili, & Cico, 2016). In the US, the fastest-growing heroin-using demographic groups are women and people with middle to high socioeconomic

Table 18.1 Data on current substance use by region and country

Region and country	*Alcohol liters per capita 15+*	*Amphetamine %*	*Cannabis %*	*Cocaine %*	*Opiates %*	*Opioids %*
		Africa				
Algeria	0.9	0.03	0.53	0.01	0.06	na
Cabo Verde	5.7	na	2.4	0.2	0.18	na
Egypt	0.4	0.48	6.24	0.02	0.44	na
Kenya	3.4	na	1.2	0.1	0.22	na
Morocco	0.6	na	4.22	0.05	0.01	na
Nigeria	13.4	0.24	10.76	0.09	0.7	4.66
Seychelles	12	na	na	na	2.3	na
Sierra Leone	5.7	na	5.42	na	0.17	na
South Africa	9.3	1.02	3.65	1.02	0.41	0.5
Zambia	4.8	0.1	9.5	na	0.37	na
		The Americas				
		Central America				
Belize	6.7	1.35	8.45	0.85	0.3	0.3
Costa Rica	4.8	0	5.18	1.33	0.04	0.79
El Salvador	3.7	0.38	2.03	0.37	0.11	0.14
Guatemala	2.4	0.91	4.8	0.21	0.04	na
Honduras	4	0.84	0.83	0.87	0.15	na
Nicaragua	5.2	0.76	1.07	0.69	0.02	na
Panama	7.9	1.2	0.77	0.1	na	na
		North America & Mexico				
Canada	8.9	0.25	14.73	1.47		0.36
Mexico	6.5	0.2	2.1	0.8	0.18	0.38
United States	9.8	2.95	17	2.4	1.04	5.75
		South America				
Argentina	9.8	na	8.13	1.67	0.07	0.19
Bolivia	4.8	0.5	1.27	0.36	0.07	na
Brazil	7.8	0.3	2.5	1	0.1	0.4
Chile	9.3	0.18	15.1	1.38	0.02	1.22
Colombia	5.8	0.06	3.27	0.7	0.03	na
Ecuador	4.4	0.2	0.67	0.08	0.02	na
Paraguay	7.2	0.51	1.6	0.25	0.03	na
Peru	6.3	0.2	1.03	0.7	0.18	na
Uruguay	10.8	0.04	9.3	1.8	0.06	0.18
Venezuela	5.6	0.47	1.56	0.64	0.03	na
		Asia				
Brunei Darussalam	0.4	0.25	na	na	na	na
Cambodia	6.7	0.6	3.5	na	0.03	na
China	na	na	na	na	0.19	na
Hong Kong SAR	na	0.6	0.4	0.25	0.2	na
India	na	na	na	na	1.42	0.96
Indonesia	0.8	0.56	0.18	0	0.02	0.05
Japan	8	0.3	0.3	na	na	na
Kazakhstan	7.7	na	2.4	na	1.03	1

(Continued)

Table 18.1 (Continued)

Region and country	*Alcohol liters per capita 15+*	*Amphetamine %*	*Cannabis %*	*Cocaine %*	*Opiates %*	*Opioids %*
Laos	10.4	na	0.88	na	0.37	na
Malaysia	0.9	1.39	1.6	na	0.94	na
Myanmar	4.8	0.22	0.94	na	0.8	na
Nepal	2	na	na	na	0.24	na
Philippines	6.6	1.1	1.64	0.07	0.04	0.05
Singapore	2	na	na	na	0.32	0.33
South Korea	10.2	na	0.29	na	na	0.08
Thailand	8.3	1.4	1.2	0.05	0.2	na
Taiwan	7.2	0.6	0.3	na	na	na
Viet Nam	8.3	0.22	na	na	0.53	na
		Europe & Russia				
		Eastern Europe & Russia				
Albania	7.50	0.1	5.6	2.5	0.45	na
Armenia	5.50	0.04	3.5	0.1	0.2	0.16
Azerbaijan	0.8	na	3.5	na	1.5	na
Belarus	11.2	0.35	1.07	0.6	0.76	0.04
Bosnia Herzegovina	6.4	0.5	1.6	0.3	0.3	na
Bulgaria	12.7	0.8	4.2	0.3	0.5	0.3
Croatia	8.9	1	7.9	0.8	0.35	na
Georgia	9.8	0	3.4	na	0.72	1.36
Montenegro	9.80	0.66	1.82	0.62	na	na
Romania	12.60	0.1	3.2	0.2	0.17	0.2
Russian Federation	11.70	0.39	3.49	0.23	1.4	1.03
Serbia	na	0.1	1.6	0.1	0.1	5.15
Ukraine	na	0.3	2.13	na	0.91	na
		Western Europe				
Austria	11.6	0.4	6.4	0.4	0.53	0.53
Belgium	12.1	0.2	4.6	0.63	0.2	0.2
Cyprus	10.8	0.1	2.2	0.2	0.25	na
Czechia	14.4	0.8	9.4	0.1	0.18	2.6
Denmark	10.4	0.6	6.9	0.9	0.52	na
Estonia	11.6	1	6	0.6	1.53	0.7
Finland	10.7	1.1	6.8	0.5	0.41	0.7
France	12.6	0.3	na	1.1	0.52	0.52
Germany	13.4	1.1	6.1	0.6	0.3	0.3
Greece	10.4	na	2.8	0.4	0.23	na
Hungary	11.4	0.45	1.53	0.31	0.13	na
Iceland	9.1	0.78	6.6	1.06	na	na
Ireland	13	0.3	7.7	1.5	0.72	na
Italy	7.5	0.2	9.2	1.1	0.52	0.8
Latvia	12.9	0.3	4.2	0.5	0.49	0.5
Lithuania	15	0.3	2.7	0.1	0.24	na
Luxembourg	13	0.73	5.2	1.04	0.59	na
Netherlands	8.7	1.6	8.7	1.9	0.13	na

Table 18.1 (Continued)

Region and country	*Alcohol liters per capita 15+*	*Amphetamine %*	*Cannabis %*	*Cocaine %*	*Opiates %*	*Opioids %*
Norway	7.5	0.3	3.9	0.6	0.27	na
Poland	11.6	1.7	2.4	1.4	1.7	0.1
Portugal	12.3	0.05	2.7	0.2	0.49	na
Spain	10	0.56	9.5	2	0.21	0.1
Sweden	9.2	0.72	3.4	0.6	1.51	0.53
Switzerland	11.5	0.32	9.09	0.81	0.43	na
United Kingdom	11.40	0.5	6.6	2.3	0.73	na
		Middle East				
Afghanistan	0.20	0	4.28	0	2.65	2.92
Iran	1	0.4	0.58	0.01	3.31	na
Israel	3.8	0.7	2.7	0.6	0.4	0.9
Maldives	2.7	0.1	2.55	0.04	1.34	1.46
Pakistan	0.3	0.08	3.6	0.01	1	2.4
Saudi Arabia	0.2	0.4	0.3	na	0.06	1.5
Turkey	2	0.2	0.3	0.04	na	0.5
		Oceania				
Australia	10.6	1.4	10.4	2.5	0.2	3.3
New Zealand	10.7	1	13.89	0.6	0.1	1.1

status – groups with historically low heroin use (Jones Logan, Gladden, & Bohm, 2015). Concomitant with the increase in Afghan opium cultivation, Europe has also experienced a rise in heroin use. The United Kingdom (Northern Ireland and Great Britain) has the highest opioid overdose death rates in Europe, accounting for 36% of all overdose deaths (EMCDDA, 2016). Behind the US and Afghanistan, Australia has among the highest opioid use rates in the world at 3.3%, which is high not only compared to rates for the Oceanic region, but is high on the global scale.

Much of the heroin in the US and Canada is laced or cross-contaminated with synthetic opioids such as fentanyl, U-47700, AH-792, 1AH-21, and MT-45a, drugs that are 100 to 1,000 times more potent than heroin. Since 2012, overdose death rates in the US have increased more than 265%, where the overdose death rate is 246 per million (population ages 15–64); in parts of Canada the overdose rate is even higher at 285 per million (population ages 15–64) (UNODC, 2017). Recreational, non-medical use of tramadol has been rapidly rising in many African countries (Niger, Sudan, Kenya) and across the Middle East (Iran, Egypt, Jordan, Lebanon, Libya, Mauritius, Saudi Arabia, and the United Arab Emirates). Asia is believed to be the source for much of the illicit tramadol production that reaches Africa and the Middle East (UNODC, 2018). Global seizures of tramadol increased dramatically from about 10 kilograms in 2010 to 125 tons in 2017.

The term "opioids" is a collective term that encompasses natural (raw opium), semi-synthetic and synthetic opiates management medications (e.g. morphine, codeine, oxycontin, oxycodone, oxymorphone, hydrocodone, fentanyl, tramadol) and medication-assisted opioid substitution treatment (buprenorphine, methadone, suboxone). Opioid use is higher than opiate use in most regions of the world. For example, the US has a higher opiate rate than most countries at 1.04% while their opioid use rate is the highest in the world at 5.75%. Serbia has the second highest opioid usage rate in the world at 5.15% but one of the lower rates for opiates at just 0.1%.

During the Soviet–Afghan War, the mujahedeen guerillas increased their production of opium and hashish to fund their fight against the Soviet Union from about 1979 to 1989. The mujahedeen, with encouragement and support from the United States, implemented "Operation Mosquito," which consisted in part of flooding Soviet military bases in Afghanistan with hashish and opium to weaken, addict and demoralize Soviet soldiers. These tactics were similar to those implemented by the Vietnamese during the war between the United States and Vietnam in the 1960s–1970s (Bergen-Cico, 2012). The initiative was as "successful" against the Soviet troops in Afghanistan as it was against American troops in Vietnam, as the proliferation of opium, heroin, and hash in Afghanistan greatly impacted the Soviet troops and their drug use and addiction continued when the Soviet soldiers returned to their homelands. The collapse of the Soviet Union was due in large part to the financial drain and strain of the Soviet–Afghan War. At the same time the Soviet Union collapsed, the former Soviet Union countries which lay in the path from Afghanistan to Russia found themselves without policies, infrastructure and the systems necessary to combat the flow of Afghan opium and hashish across their borders and into Russia. This led to rising rates of alcohol and other drug abuse, which became widespread in the many former countries, notably Azerbaijan, Estonia, Kazakhstan, Republic of Georgia, Romania and the Russian Federation. As the countries re-established policies and the rule of law, drug trafficking and drug use became an organizing focal point as a problem that could be clearly defined as a common societal enemy. Russia and Georgia implemented harsh drug control policies with steep fines and imprisonment for people caught with any drug paraphernalia or even residual amounts of known drugs in their possession. As a result, people developed new synthetic drugs that would not test positive with police testing methods, thereby hoping to skirt the legal system. This has resulted in the development of deadly drugs such as Krokodil, a synthetic opioid-type depressant drug that is produced in small-batch homemade production and administered through injection. Its popularity is primarily limited to Russia and Eurasia. The name Krokodil is in reference to the crocodile-like effect it has on the appearance of the skin of people who use it. The caustic chemicals used in the home brew methods of making it can produce scaly discolored skin that appears eaten away from the inside out. Krokodil served as an opioid-type substitute. Concomitantly, Georgia went through an epidemic of Subutex abuse. Subutex is the brand name for an opioid substitute that is intended to be used to wean people off heroin addiction, but it can also be misused as a recreational drug. The fear of being caught by police with any known drug in one's possession only served as a catalyst for more homemade psychoactive drugs that we will discuss in the section on New Psychoactive Substances (Kirtadze & Otiashvili, 2015; Otiashvili, Kirtadze, & Bergen-Cico, 2017).

New Psychoactive Substances

"New" psychoactive substances (NPS) refer to an ever-changing, diverse, and new emerging category of drugs that lack a "standardization" of terminology (Beselia, Gegenava et al., 2018b). The rapid emergence of NPS, diversity of chemical composition and marketing names, coupled with the lack of users' knowledge regarding the composition of the substances, pose great risk to users and remarkable challenges for researchers worldwide (EMCDDA, 2018).

In many countries the term "bio" is often added as a prefix to the name of a substance to indicate which conventional drug the specific

NPS is mimicking (e.g. bio-amphetamine, bio-MDMA). The NPS markets have emerged in tandem with the use of technology for dealer-driven, internet-based, and mobile app-based drug transactions. New psychoactive substances seemingly are involved in a remarkable share of these new technology-mediated interactions, which may also enable users, dealers and suppliers to skirt law enforcement.

Some of the NPS are synthesized from pharmaceutical formulas such as fenethylline, an amphetamine-type stimulant that goes by the tradename Captagon, and is the leading drug in the Arabian Peninsula and Gulf Region. Captagon is being used to fuel Jihadist fighters, such as ISIS, in the region and its sales are funding conflicts through drug trafficking and illicit economies associated with the instability of wartorn regions like Syria (Kravitz & Nichols, 2016). The violence and trauma stemming from the protracted wars in Syria, Iraq, Afghanistan and the region at large have resulted in pervasive trauma among the societies, thus increasing risks for substance use (Bergen-Cico, 2012; Bergen-Cico, Wolf-Stanton, Filipovic, & Weisberg, 2016). This perpetuating cycle is illustrated in Figure 18.5 below.

Not all NPS are synthetic. There are plant-based psychoactive substances that have been identified and rediscovered. Some are used in their pure plant-based form while others are made through basic extraction methods. Figure 18.1 is an example of betle nut, or areca nut, which is a tropical fruit, or nut, native to warmer regions of Asia and some parts of Africa. Betel nut is a stimulant drug similar to tobacco and caffeine and is used by an estimated 10% of the world population. Kratom is a plant that is also indigenous to Southeast Asia and has become widely marketed throughout Europe and North America. Its legal status varies, and it is not well regulated. Liquid and powder forms of it are sold legally in the US and Europe. Kratom has unusual properties: at low levels it operates as a central nervous system (CNS) stimulant, while at higher doses it is a CNS depressant with opiate-type effects (Bergen-Cico & McClurg, 2016). Figure 18.2 provides a visual reference of retail options for Kratom.

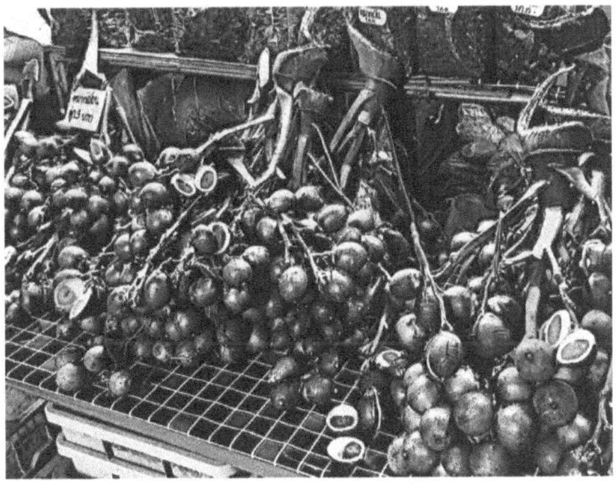

Figure 18.1 Betel nut in a market in Bangkok, Thailand

Datura (aka jimsonweed, moonflower, devil's trumpet) is a plant native to many arid regions of the world. It is a central nervous system depressant and is sought for its psychedelic hallucinatory properties – it is also poisonous. Datura is currently quite popular in the Arabian Peninsula and Middle East. Figure 18.3 provides a visual reference of the datura plant found growing in Tel Aviv, Israel. In Eurasia there is an emerging new homemade psychoactive drug that is synthesized through the conversion of ephedrine to methamphetamine with a reduction of an ephedra-type conifer plant, which is consumed in small batches through injection drug use (Otiashvili, Kirtadz, & Bergen-Cico, 2017). The emergence of this conifer-based ephedra in Georgia is a direct result of strict laws against drug use and is an attempt to develop psychoactive drugs that are not considered illegal. In the following section we discuss the post-Soviet-era drug policies in Georgia, which includes random street-level drug testing for drug possession and the biological presence of psychoactive drugs in one's system (Bergen-Cico, Otiashvili, Kirtadze, Zebransky, & Tsertsvadze, 2017).

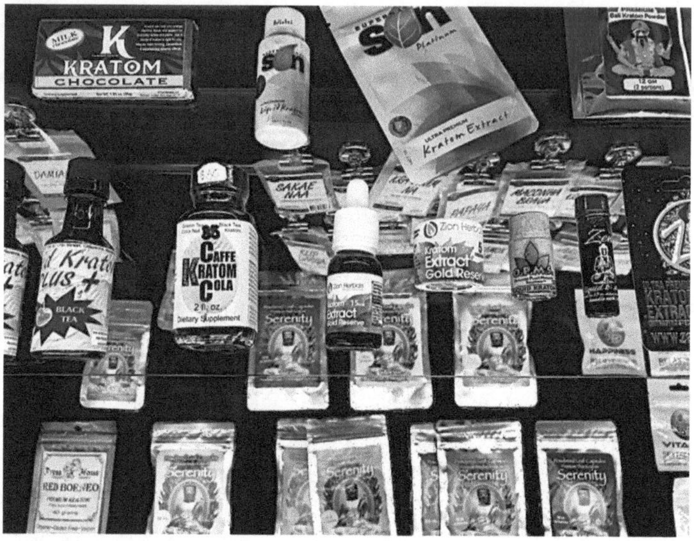

Figure 18.2 Various forms of Kratom as sold legally in the US

POST-COLD WAR CONFLICTS AND DRUG USE: EXAMINING THE EXPERIENCES OF THE UNITED STATES AND THE REPUBLIC OF GEORGIA

We have presented data on drug use trends across the globe, by region and country. Next, we will examine in depth the United States (reflective of North America) and the country of Georgia (reflective of post-Soviet Eastern European and Eurasia). The emerging democracies of the former Soviet Union present a uniquely complex set of socio-cultural, economic, and political factors that have influenced trends and patterns in the use of psychoactive drugs in the region (Kirtadze & Otiashvili, 2015; Otiashvili, Kirtadze, O'Grady, et al., 2014; Otiashvili, Tabatadze, Balanchivadze, & Kirtadze, 2016).

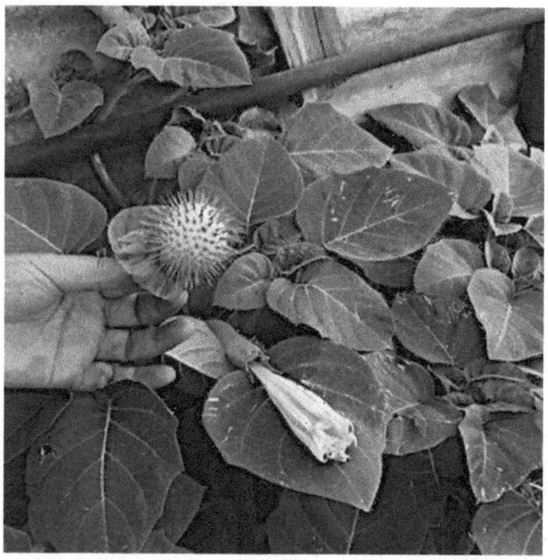

Figure 18.3 Datura growing in the wild in Israel (aka Jimsonweed)

Post-Soviet Regional Conflicts Influence Drug Use and Policy in the Republic of Georgia

The Republic of Georgia presents a clear case in which politics and ideology widely impacted the state's response to drug problems. Many researchers and human rights activists have argued that current Georgian drug policy is deeply rooted in Soviet-style ideology, where drug legislation and treatment approaches often served as mechanisms for social control rather than helping people (Elovich & Drucker, 2008). Advocates for drug policy reform suggest that the focus on enforcement policies rather than public health policies provide clear incentives for the authorities to maintain existing drug policies, whereby they boost the crime-solving rates on paper, they generate revenue (through fines), and they produce a network of informants for other crimes (Bergen-Cico, Otiashvili, Kirtadze et al., 2017; Human Rights Watch, 2018; Otiashvili, Sárosi, & Somogyi, 2008).

The rapid social change and challenges faced by Georgia are representative of the sociological factors that influence trends in drug use and treatment globally and post-Soviet countries in particular. Economic and social transformation following the fall of the Soviet Union in 1991, civil unrest, and relaxation of border control all contributed to the increase in consumption of psychoactive substances (Gamkrelidze et al., 2004; Nizharadze, Stvilia, & Todadze, 2005). As a result of ethnic unrest and separatists-driven military conflicts, 10% of the Georgian population are internally displaced persons (IDPs) (Chikovani et al., 2015). The issue of IDPs and the external forced migration of refugees affects a substantial number of people and countries, with more than 70.8 million people forced to flee their homes. Since 2011 there has been a 2,2490% increase in the number of people from Central America seeking refuge from drug-related gang warfare and violence (UNHCR, 2019). Exposure to armed conflicts and related traumatic events contributed to high levels of trauma, mental disorders and substance use (Bergen-Cico, 2012; Chikovani et al., 2015). The war-related socio-political and psychological factors that increase the risk of substance use among people in Georgia provide us with a framework for understanding and examining problems in many other countries.

Lack of information among the public and healthcare providers, poor referral systems, out-of-pocket costs, and other systemic and structural issues present barriers for access to general health services for the general public, IDPs and particularly people with substance use-related problems (Murphy, Chikovani, Uchaneishvili, Makhashvili, & Roberts, 2018). In addition to wider health system-related issues, there are specific challenges for the provision of substance use-related services in the country of Georgia. The post-Soviet system for addiction medicine is referred to as narcology, and it was completely unprepared to meet the challenges posed by escalations in drug use and associated problems stemming from socio-political changes (Kirtadze & Otiashvili, 2015). The specialized treatment for substance use disorders in post-Soviet countries has historically been fragmented in nature and modeled on detoxification and alleviation of short-term symptoms of withdrawal, with no or very little attention to post-detoxification care and management of lasting psychosocial problems (Latypov, 2011). Knowledge of evidence-based interventions among field professionals as well as demand and utilization from the side of clients has been limited. As a result, relapse rates have been high, specifically in Georgia. In the overall environment of limited resources, state and federal allocations for programs serving individuals with substance use-related problems have been low. As long as ideological, moral and socio-cultural factors dominate over public health perspectives and evidence-informed decision making, it remains politically unpopular to allocate resources to treatment and recovery. As in other places, the availability and accessibility of substance use services was related to the variety of environmental and policy factors, and there was an obvious need for remarkable social and policy changes for progress in this regard to be achieved (Degenhardt et al., 2010; Strathdee et al., 2010).

Injection Drug Use as a Social Activity in Eastern Europe and Russia

Research conducted by Otiashvili, Kirtadze, and Bergen-Cico (2017) documented the communal practice of small-batch homemade drug production and use, whereby people gather in an apartment to cook drugs, such as Krokodil and conifer ephedra described above, often sharing injection equipment. Drug use in Eastern Europe and the former Soviet region has long been a group activity, and injection drug use remains a socializing event. In the 1980s many of the sedative injection drug users in the Soviet Union were well educated, from wealthy families, or individuals who were well-positioned in the power structures. Injection drug use is a socializing event.

Repressive Drug Control Policies Drive Use Underground

Reminiscent of Soviet drug laws, the Georgian law, similarly to the legislation in Russia and some other post-Soviet countries (Levinson, 2008), does not establish a threshold for small quantities for about three-quarters of substances classified as illicit drugs. This means that possession of any detectable quantity of those substances, including the residue of such substances in paraphernalia, qualifies as possession of a large amount, triggering criminal liability and a mandatory minimum five-year prison sentence.

Drug use patterns in Georgia were often shaped by policy response and law enforcement practices implemented at particular periods of time. Advocates for the repressive model have argued that such an approach reduces the demand for drugs. They believe that harsh punitive measures force substance users to stop using and keep youngsters away from trying drugs (United States Department of State, 2015). However, existing evidence suggests that, reactive in its nature, a repressive response that relied heavily on consumer sanctions did not result in any measurable public health benefits in Georgia. With no reduction in the overall scale of illicit substance use, shifts in drug markets and users' behavior in most cases were associated with increased risks and negative consequences for their physical and mental health. The Georgian drug market and its players displayed a remarkable capacity for adapting to the changed legal environment. In many cases, new behavioral patterns were conditioned by users' attempts to substitute the traditional drug of their choice and to make drug use less visible, so that risk of arrest would be reduced. For example, reduction in the availability of conventional substances resulted in drug users rapidly switching to new, mostly domestically manufactured stimulants and opioids (Bergen-Cico et al., 2017; Beselia, Kirtadze & Otiashvili, 2018). This local clandestine production of psychotropic substances did not require involvement with illegal markets – most ingredients for preparation were purchased through pharmacies and convention stores. The shift towards self-manufactured injection preparations has been associated with a number of new risks as the final products often contained highly toxic ingredients (Alves et al., 2015; Gahr et al., 2012; Skowronek, Celiński, & Chowaniec, 2012), complexities with titration posed the risk for overdose (Grund, Latypov, & Harris, 2013), and the vastly group character of home-production and use was linked to increased risks of sharing injection equipment (Abdala, Grund, Tolstov, Kozlov, & Heimer, 2006; Otiashvili et al., 2017).

Georgia presents the case of a small country in which specific policy interventions contributed to prompt and dramatic changes in substance use patterns and user behavior. The end result of these changes did not seem to have led to any improvement in individual or public health. To the contrary, many consumers moved to more toxic preparations and engaged in riskier behavior. The public visibility of drug use has visibly declined at the cost of drug users moving further underground. In such an environment, engaging people with substance use problems with prevention and treatment services can be particularly difficult.

PUBLIC HEALTH IMPACT OF REPRESSIVE DRUG POLICIES

Harms associated with alcohol and other drug use include physical harms and public health risks associated with consumption methods, as well as social harms associated with drug use behaviors deemed illegal. Repressive drug policies, such as those which carry significant punishment for being caught with drug paraphernalia, syringes and illicit drugs, contribute to high-risk drug use behavior. The country of Georgia experienced a hepatitis C (HCV) epidemic that has been fueled by the intersection of risk factors linked to injection drug use (IDU), punitive drug policies, and the country's prison system (Bergen-Cico, Sikharulidze, Ivanashvili, Ivanishvili, & Keshelava, 2017). Transmission of HIV and HCV in former Soviet countries is attributed to the sharing of injection equipment and high rates of imprisonment – Russia has one of the highest rates of imprisonment of any country in the world, second only to the United States (Schwabe & Harrington, 2002).

Since 2010 the annual incidence of human immunodeficiency virus (HIV) has increased in Eastern Europe and Central Asia (EECA) by 60% (UNAIDS, 2017), and the growing epidemic in the region has been driven by people who inject drugs (DeHovitz, Uuskula, & El-Bassel, 2014; Fettig, Swaminathan, Murrill, & Kaplan, 2014). With an estimated 52,000 people who inject drugs (PWID), the prevalence of injection drug use in Georgia (2.24%) ranks third highest in the world (UNODC, 2017). Although HIV prevalence among PWID in Georgia is relatively low (1–4%) (Curatio International Foundation & Public Union Bemoni, 2015), the annual incidence has steadily increased over the last decade by 10–25% (UNAIDS, 2016).

Injection Drug Use

Injection drug use is more common in some parts of the world than others. The estimated global prevalence of injection drug use is 0.27% (Harm Reduction International, 2016; UNODC, 2017). In a sharp contrast, countries in the region of Eastern Europe and Central Asia (EECA) report extremely high rates of injection drug use: 2.24% in Georgia, 1.6% in Kazakhstan, up to 2% in Ukraine, and more than 2% in Russia (Bemoni Public Union & Curatio International Foundation, 2016, 2017; Harm Reduction International, 2016; UNODC, 2017). Globally, IDUs are the group at highest risk for HCV infection; and Georgia is no exception with an estimated 70–92% HCV prevalence rate among people who use drugs, and a 50% HCV prevalence rate among the prison population (Bouscaillou et al., 2014).

There is a long history of home injection of medications and psychoactive drugs in the countries that were part of the Soviet Union. Every home had been issued with a glass and iron syringe that was used for home family medical management, and thus the initiation of injection drug use (IDU) is more normalized in Russia and Eastern Europe than it is in most other regions. As noted, drug use in this region is very much a communal group activity that involves the sharing of drug production and drug injecting equipment. It was also common practice in medicine and among IDUs to reuse the same syringe. These factors contributed greatly to the high rates of HIV, HCV and other blood-borne illnesses in this region. Figure 18.4 shows a home injection drug use kit that was typically disseminated to families throughout the former Soviet Union

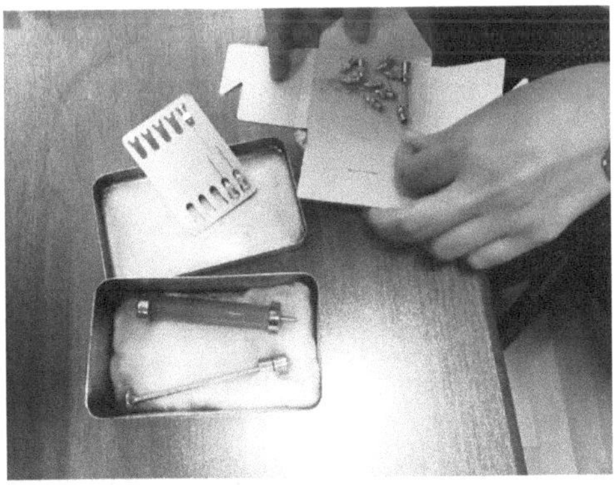

Figure 18.4 Georgian family home medication injection kit. These were typically disseminated to each family in the Soviet Union

and was used for home administration of medications and even vitamin supplements. Individuals, families and healthcare facilities often re-used the same needles on multiple people, and although the needles would likely be cleaned between uses, the risk for transmission of HIV, HCV and other infections was high. It is also notable that because of the home use of injection kits people became very familiar with self-injection or home administration, and this lowered the threshold for likelihood of using injectable drugs.

BEHIND THE DATA: BIO-PSYCHOSOCIAL FACTORS INFLUENCING SUBSTANCE USE TRENDS BY REGION

Geopolitics

Following the collapse of the Soviet Union in 1991, many countries which gained independence from the USSR lacked border and national security systems and structures. Therefore, drug trafficking, particularly with heroin, flooded the region from Afghanistan. Changes in economic security and political transition gave rise to drug trafficking through the opening of borders that allowed heroin to move freely to the Soviet Union through Armenia, Georgia, Azerbaijan, Kazakhstan, and Chechnya from Afghanistan, the world's largest producer of opium (Bird, 2013; Schwabe & Harrington, 2002). Wherever there is drug trafficking, there is also increased drug use, thus the use of opiates in the former Soviet Union, Eastern Europe, and Central Asia escalated following the end of the Cold War (Bergen-Cico, 2012). As referenced previously in this chapter, violence and trauma stemming from wars and political unrest can result in pervasive social trauma, thus increasing the risks for substance use (Bergen-Cico, 2012; Bergen-Cico et al., 2016). This cycle is illustrated in the Figure 18.5. These scenarios illustrate the ways that drugs have been used to achieve the necessary or desired mindset to engage in physically and emotionally stressful

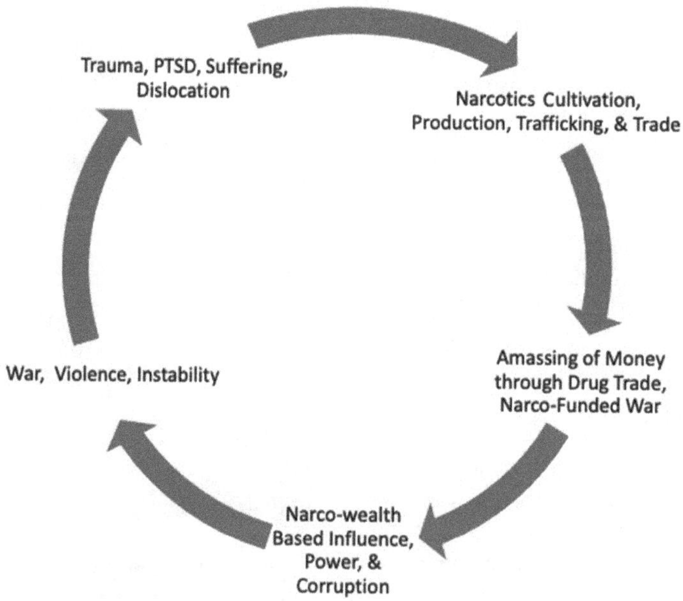

Figure 18.5 Cycle of drug trade, violence, trauma and addiction

fighting. Civilians, as well as warriors, have suffered emotional and physical trauma, and are at increased risk of turning to alcohol and other drugs to numb their pain.

Figure 18.5 depicts the core issues related to war and drugs and their cyclical framework. Cultivation, trafficking, and trade of narcotics *en masse* occur predominantly in countries with unstable governments where power vacuums exist. The drug trade consists of the population demand, production and supply, individual traders, and sometimes government entities. The drug trade generates wealth among groups which can influence and engage law enforcement, governments, and civilians, leading to instability, power struggles, violence, and war or war-like situations. War and conflict produce suffering among soldiers, combatants, and civilians, and this suffering fuels demand for psychoactive substance as a means of coping.

An examination of how large-scale cultivation, trafficking, and trade of narcotics become feasible in some regions illustrates the impact of civil unrest and military conflict. The risk of civil war is greater in low-income economies, and the World Bank recognizes that civil war reflects a failure of economic development (Collier, 2003). Civil war creates territories that are outside the authority of recognized governments and become epicenters of criminal activity, often involving the drug trade. As such, narcotics cultivation and trafficking are most prevalent in countries that characteristically have unstable governments and weak law enforcement. Present-day examples of countries which are affected by civil war and governmental instability and are also leaders in drug production include: Afghanistan, where an estimated 90% of the world's heroin is produced; Myanmar, which is a leading source of amphetamine production; and Syria, which is a major source of captagon production. Instability and conflict in the Middle East contribute to drug trafficking, and the lack of control and monitoring in the region has led to an increase in the manufacture of the stimulant drug captagon, which is a potential source of income for terrorist and insurgency groups throughout the region (UNODC, 2019).

Military incursions and political unrest are in themselves crises that create turmoil, particularly among civilians. The crisis of war creates dangerous opportunities for drug production, sale, distribution and use. Governmental, political, legal, and economic constructs become unstable during a crisis and present the specters of power vacuums, diverted attention of military and law enforcement, and the loss of traditional bases of economic life.

We have become acutely aware of living casualties of war. The human response to the physical and emotional stress of war is better known as post-traumatic stress disorder (PTSD). PTSD is a psychological diagnosis that encompasses a number of symptoms, including depression, anxiety, and heavy alcohol and/or other drug use. There is little dispute that PTSD has affected members of the military, veterans, their families, and civilians for generations. The use of alcohol and other drugs by members of the military to manage the physical and psychological stress of war and subsequent PTSD are accepted but not well-understood facts of war. PTSD among those directly involved in battle has become better understood in recent years (Bergen-Cico, 2012). There is less of an appreciation for the sociological impact of war as reflected in the surge of drug use among civilians during and following wartime. As documented earlier, the spiritual collapse of people, coupled with social and economic dislocation, poverty, and the undermining of traditional authority structures and values, have been the basis for the escalation of alcohol and drug use among regions affected by war and among citizens at home. In this regard, drug use becomes a symbolic gesture against government military actions and a means of expressing political dissent.

At present, there are serious drug problems across the globe. The current escalation of drug use is reflective of geopolitical forces and rapid social change that are out of balance with the social-emotional support needed to counter these risk factors. These problems call for meaningful and significant efforts to reduce the demand for drugs as much as, if not more than, the efforts to reduce supply. The demand for mind-altering substances has risen steadily over the past century and continues to escalate in the context of complex socio-political and psychological factors. When examined through these lenses, it becomes apparent that this is not a problem that can be solved through interdiction, suppression and repressive laws, because these are downstream strategies for addressing a complex problem that needs comprehensive solutions upstream at the roots of the problems that drive demand. As we have seen, even when the supply of an illicit drug is greatly curtailed, people in desperation will develop new homemade drugs like Krokodil (Alves et al., 2015; Georgian Harm Reduction Network, 2015) and plant-based ephedra (Otiashvili et al., 2017) and risk their freedom and their lives because the drive for immediate relief is stronger than the drive for self-preservation and survival for many people. Gabor Maté reframed how we should look at substance use and addiction by suggesting that rather than asking "why the addiction," we should ask what is at the root of why this person is suffering (Maté, 2008). This brings the issue of substance use back to the social and emotional context of the person who is using a psychoactive substance. Which substances they have access to and how much risk is involved in what they may use depends largely on the societal factors and socio-political context of where they are living.

REFERENCES

Abdala, N., Grund, J. P., Tolstov, Y., Kozlov, A. P., & Heimer, R. (2006). Can home-made injectable opiates contribute to the HIV epidemic among injection drug users in the countries of the former Soviet Union? *Addiction*, *101*(5), 731–737.

Alves, E. A., Grund, J.-P. C., Afonso, C. M., Netto, A. D. P., Carvalho, F. I., & Dinis-Oliveira, R. J. (2015). The harmful chemistry behind krokodil (desomorphine) synthesis and mechanisms of toxicity. *Forensic Science International*, *249*, 207–213.

Bemoni Public Union & Curatio International Foundation. (2016). *Population size estimation of people who inject drugs in Georgia*. Retrieved from http://curatiofoundation.org/pse2017/

Bemoni Public Union & Curatio International Foundation. (2017). *HIV Risk and Prevention Behaviors among People Who Inject Drugs in Seven Cities of Georgia*. Retrieved from Tbilisi, Georgia: http://curatiofoundation.org/bss-2017/

Bergen-Cico, D. (2012). *War and Drugs: The Role of Military Conflict in the Development of Substance Abuse*. New York: Routledge.

Bergen-Cico, D., & McClurg, K. (2016). Kratom use, abuse and addiction. p. 903–911. In Victor Preedy (Ed.), *The Neuropathology of Drug Addictions and Substance Misuse*. Volume 3. London, Academic Press.

Bergen-Cico, D., Otiashvili, D., Kirtadze, I., Zebransky, T., & Tsertsvadze V., (2017). Cost analysis of the country of Georgia's street level drug testing policy. *Journal of Drug Policy Analysis*. 10(2), 1–22. https://doi.org/10.1515/jdpa-2017-0003

Bergen-Cico, D., Scholl, S., Invanshvili, N., & Cico, R., (2016). Opioid prescription drug abuse and its relation to heroin trends. In Victor Preedy (Ed.), *The Neuropathology of Drug Addictions and Substance Misuse* (Vol. 1, pp. 878–890). London: Academic Press.

Bergen-Cico, D., Sikharulidze, K., Ivanashvili, N., Ivanishvili, M., & Keshelava, T. (2017). Hepatitis C risk and protective factors associated with drug policies in the Republic of Georgia. *World Medical & Health Policy*, *9*(1), 45–64.

Bergen-Cico, D., Wolf-Stanton, S., Filipovic, R., & Weisberg, J. (2016). Trauma and neurological risks of addiction. In Victor Preedy (Ed.) *The Neuropathology of Drug Addictions and Substance Misuse* (Vol. 1, pp. 61–70). London: Academic Press.

Beselia, A., Gegenava, V., Kirtadze, I., Mghebrishvili,T., Otiashvili, D., Razmadze, M., Stefanishvili, N., Sturua, L., Kutelia, L., &

Javakhishvili, J. (2018). *The Drug Situation in Georgia 2016–2017*. Tbilisi, Georgia. Retreived from www.researchgate.net/publication/330564742_The_Drug_Situation_in_Georgia_2016–17

Bird, M. (2013). Smack in the USSR: how injecting drugs in the Soviet Union was socializing. *The Black Sea: Diving Deep into Stories*. Accessed at: https://theblacksea.eu/stories/smack-in-the-ussr-how-injecting-drugs-in-the-soviet-union-was-socializing/

Bouscaillou, J., Champagnat, J., Luhmann, N., Avril, E., Inaridze, I., Miollany, V., ... & Pataut, D. (2014). Hepatitis C among people who inject drugs in Tbilisi, Georgia: an urgent need for prevention and treatment. *International Journal of Drug Policy*, *25*(5), 871–878.

Chikovani, I., Makhashvili, N., Gotsadze, G., Patel, V., McKee, M., Uchaneishvili, M., ... Roberts, B. (2015). Health service utilization for mental, behavioural and emotional problems among conflict-affected population in Georgia: a cross-sectional study. *PLoS One*, *10*(4), e0122673.

Collier, P. (2003). *Breaking the Conflict Trap: Civil War and Development Policy*. Washington, DC: World Bank Publications.

Curatio International Foundation & Public Union Bemoni. (2015). *HIV Risk and Prevention Behaviours among People Who Inject Drugs in Six Cities of Georgia: Bio-behavioral Surveillance Survey in Tbilisi, Batumi, Zugdidi, Telavi, Gori, Kutaisi in 2014*. Retrieved from Tbilisi, Georgia: http://curatiofoundation.org/wp-content/uploads/2013/06/73.pdf

Degenhardt, L., Mathers, B., Vickerman, P., Rhodes, T., Latkin, C., & Hickman, M. (2010). Prevention of HIV infection for people who inject drugs: why individual, structural, and combination approaches are needed. *Lancet*, *376*(9737), 285–301.

DeHovitz, J., Uuskula, A., & El-Bassel, N. (2014). The HIV epidemic in Eastern Europe and Central Asia. *Current HIV/AIDS Reports*, *11*(2), 168–176. doi:10.1007/s11904-014-0202-3

Elovich, R., & Drucker, E. (2008). On drug treatment and social control: Russian narcology's great leap backwards. *Harm Reduction Journal*, *5*, 23. doi:10.1186/1477-7517-5-23

European Monitoring Centre for Drugs and Drug Addiction (EMCDDA). (2016). *European Drug Report 2016: Trends and Developments*. Luxembourg: Publications Office of the European Union.

European Monitoring Centre for Drugs and Drug Addiction (EMCDDA). (2018). *Monitoring Drug Use in Recreational Settings across Europe: Conceptual Challenges and Methodological Innovations*. Luxembourg: Publications Office of the European Union.

Fettig, J., Swaminathan, M., Murrill, C. S., & Kaplan, J. E. (2014). Global epidemiology of HIV. *Infectious Disease Clinics of North America*, *28*(3), 323–337. doi:10.1016/j.idc.2014.05.001

Gahr, M., Freudenmann, R. W., Hiemke, C., Gunst, I. M., Connemann, B. J., & Schonfeldt-Lecuona, C. (2012). Desomorphine goes "crocodile". *Journal of Addictive Diseases*, *31*.

Gamkrelidze, A., Javakhishvili, J., Kariauli, D., Lejava, G., Stvilia, K., Todadze, K., & Tsintsadze, M. (2004). *Drug Situation in Georgia – 2003*. Tbilisi, Georgia: Southern Caucasus Anti-Drug Programme.

Georgian Harm Reduction Network (GHRN). (2017). *GHRN Program Database*. Tbilisi, Georgia: GHRN.

Grund, J. P. C., Latypov, A. B., & Harris, M. (2013). Breaking worse. the emergence of krokodil and excessive injuries among people who inject drugs in Eurasia. *International Journal of Drug Policy*, *24*(4), 265–274.

Harm Reduction International. (2016). *The Global State of Harm Reduction 2016*. Retrieved from London: www.hri.global/contents/1739

Human Rights Watch. (2018). *Harsh Punishment: The Human Toll of Georgia's Abusive Drug Policies*. New York: Human Rights Watch.

Jones, C. M., Logan, J., Gladden, R. M., & Bohm, M. K. (2015). Vital signs: demographic and substance use trends among heroin users – United States, 2002–2013. *MMWR Morbidity and Mortality Weekly Report*, *64*(26), 719.

Kirtadze, I., & Otiashvili, D. (2015). Changing patterns of drug use in Georgia: a case vignette. In N. el-Guebaly, G. Carrà, & M. Galanter (Eds.), *Textbook of Addiction Treatment: International Perspectives* (pp. 79–86). Milan: Springer.

Kravitz, M., & Nichols, W. (2016). A bitter pill to swallow: connections between captagon, Syria, and the Gulf. *Journal of International Affairs*, *69*(2), 31–44.

Latypov, A. B. (2011). The Soviet doctor and the treatment of drug addiction: a difficult and most ungracious task. *Harm Reduction Journal*, *8*, 32.

Levinson, L. (2008). Half a gram – a thousand lives. *Harm Reduction Journal*, *5*, 22. doi:10.1186/1477-7517-5-22

Maté, G. (2008). *In the realm of hungry ghosts: Close encounters with addiction.* Random House.

Murphy, A., Chikovani, I., Uchaneishvili, M., Makhashvili, N., & Roberts, B. (2018). Barriers to mental health care utilization among internally displaced persons in the republic of Georgia: a rapid appraisal study. *BMC Health Service Research*, *18*(1), 306.

Nizharadze, G., Stvilia, K., & Todadze, K. (2005). *HIV and AIDS in Georgia: A Socio-Cultural Approach.* New York: UNESCO.

Otiashvili, D., Kirtadze, I., & Bergen-Cico, D. (2017). Exploring the new phenomena of home-made extraction and injection of Ephedra plant product in Georgia. *Substance Use and Misuse*, *52*(6), 826–829.

Otiashvili, D., Kirtadze, I., O'Grady, K. E., Zule, W., Krupitsky, E., Wechsberg, W. M., & Jones, H. E. (2013). Access to treatment for substance-using women in the Republic of Georgia: socio-cultural and structural barriers. *International Journal of Drug Policy*, *24*(6), 566–572. https://doi.org/10.1016/j.drugpo.2013.05.004

Otiashvili, D., Kirtadze, I., O'Grady, K. E., Zule, W., Krupitsky, E., Wechsberg, W. M., & Jones, H. E. (2014). Comprehensive women-centered treatment for substance use disorders in Georgia: current status and future directions. *Journal of Substance Use*, *5*(20), 367–374. https://doi.org/10.3109/14659891.2014.923052

Otiashvili, D., Sárosi, P., & Somogyi, G. (2008). Drug control in Georgia: drug testing and the reduction of drug use? *The Beckley Foundation Drug Policy Program, Briefing Paper 15.* https://internationaldrugpolicy.net/

Otiashvili, D., Tabatadze, M., Balanchivadze, N., & Kirtadze, I. (2016). Policing, massive street drug testing and poly-substance use chaos in Georgia – a policy case study. *Substance Abuse Treatment, Prevention, and Policy*, *11*(1), 1–12.

Peacock, A., Leung, J., Larney, S., Colledge, S., Hickman, M., Rehm, J., … & Ali, R. (2018). Global statistics on alcohol, tobacco and illicit drug use: 2017 status report. *Addiction*, *113*(10), 1905–1926.

Schwabe, N. & Harrington, P. (2002). HIV and tuberculosis in the former Soviet Union. *The Lancet*, *360*: S19–S20.

Skowronek, R., Celiński, R., & Chowaniec, C. (2012). "Crocodile" – new dangerous designer drug of abuse from the East. *Clin Toxicol (Phil)*, *50* (4), 269.

Strathdee, S. A., Hallett, T. B., Bobrova, N., Rhodes, T., Booth, R., Abdool, R., & Hankins, C. A. (2010). HIV and risk environment for injecting drug users: the past, present, and future. *Lancet*, *376*(9737), 268–284.

UNAIDS. (2016). *Prevention Gap Report. July 11, 2016* . Retrieved from: www.unaids.org/sites/default/files/media_asset/2016-prevention-gap-report_en.pdf

UNAIDS. (2017). *Ending AIDS: progress towards the 90–90–90 targets*. Retrieved from: www.unaids.org/en/resources/documents/2017/20170720_Global_AIDS_update_2017

United Nations High Commission on Refugees (UNHCR). (2019). *Central American Refugee Crisis*. New York: UNHCR. Accessed on March 6, 2020 at: www.unrefugees.org/emergencies/central-america/

United Nations Office on Drugs and Crime (UNODC). (2009). *Afghanistan Opium Survey Summary Findings, 2010*. New York: United Nations.

United Nations Office on Drugs and Crime (UNODC). (2017). *UNODC World Drug Report 2017*. Vienna, Austria: United Nations.

United Nations Office on Drugs and Crime (UNODC) (2018). *UNODC World Drug Report 2018* (United Nations publication, Sales No. E.18.XI.9).

United Nations Office on Drugs and Crime (UNODC). (2019). *UNODC World Drug Report 2019*. New York: United Nations.

United States Department of State. (2015). *International Narcotics Control Strategy Report*. Washington, DC: United States Department of State.

PART 3

Health Care Systems, Access and Use

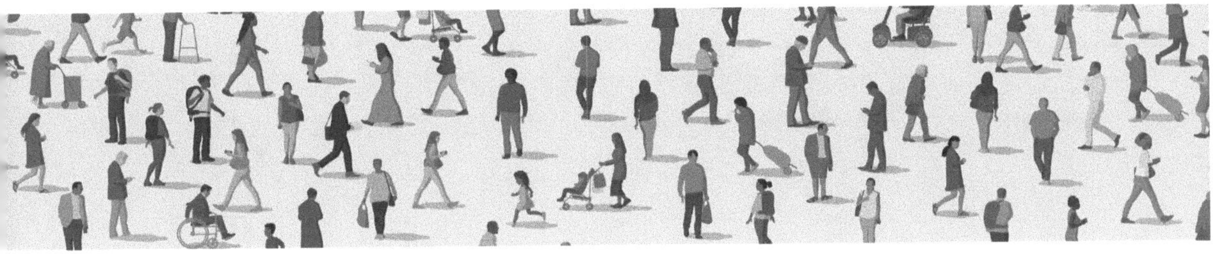

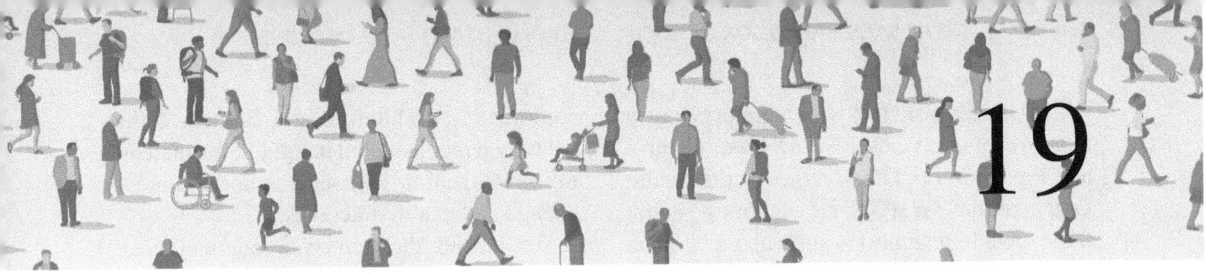

Comparative Health Systems: Paradigm Changes

Cecilia Vindrola-Padros and Linda M. Whiteford

INTRODUCTION

Health care systems and their effectiveness to protect populations has never been more relevant or exciting to observe than it is now. The 2020 deadly arrival and rapid spread of the COVID-19 virus, as it became a global pandemic, put assessments of various government's efforts to confront this 'novel coronavirus' (COVID-19) in front of the public on a moment-by-moment basis. Modern governments are designed to protect the health and well-being of their constituencies through the policies and practices of their health care systems. Previously, understanding and evaluating the efficacy of a government to protect its population was primarily in the purview of social analysists and researchers. However, in 2020, social media made that information available to almost everyone. As a result, people all over the world are comparing health systems, the strategies employed to contain and control the virus, and to protect and prevent the disease from killing people, causing widespread panic, and economic crises.

News agencies, bloggers, Twitter, and other social media outlets provide daily updates on how China, South Korea, Italy, Germany, the UK and the US, for instance, employ their health systems to protect their populations and confront the deadly virus. Around the world, people are reading about and watching in real time how Germany declares a lockdown to control the spread of the virus; how hospitals in Italy are overwhelmed as people are left to die in hospital hallways because there are not enough medical supplies; and how people are being buried in mass graves in cities like Guayaquil, Ecuador (Cabrera and Kurmanaev, 2020; Horowitz and Kirkpatrick, 2020). And they read how early in the pandemic US medical personnel did not have the necessary equipment to protect themselves as they treated patients with the virus. These horrifying outcomes reflect differences in health system paradigms.

In the first nine months of the pandemic, more than 874,717 people died from COVID-19 (Johns Hopkins University, 2020). These deaths are impossible to ignore and people in the US, for instance, who were previously unaware of the Center for Disease Control and Prevention (CDC), or the World Health Organization (WHO), are learning about these health institutions and about contact tracing, contagion, prevention, cures, and herd immunity. They are also learning about health systems quite distinct from their own, and they are comparing them. This interest in comparing health systems is certainly in the public eye in 2020, but scholars and others have been comparing health systems for more than 100 years. This chapter captures the evolution of this type of analysis and describes how it has changed in relation to, and in reflection of, the changes in the world around it.

Health care systems exist in a continuing state of crisis. "Health for all," a 1970s phrase that captured the idealism and hope that health care systems could be designed to provide equal access to good health care for all, no longer dominates comparative health systems (CHS) research. In the 1980s and the 1990s, policy makers turned to scientific metrics to guide health care policies and design practice. By the turn of the millennia, those metrics came under increased scrutiny and challenge. Vaccination programs, the "gold standard" of public health, are resisted in some countries, even as previously managed infectious diseases, such as measles and polio, re-occur.

Responses to the 2020 global COVID-19 pandemic demonstrated this distrust and disdain of science in tragic and excruciating terms as some governments chose to ignore the severity of the threat, while their leaders hawked untested and sometimes dangerously ineffective "cures." But even before the COVID-19 pandemic, hospital-based health care models were being challenged by the popularity of off-site and community-based health care models. Health care systems continue to be in flux as they deal with complex issues, such as global conflict, trade and labor wars, immigration and migration challenges (Mulligan and Castaneda, 2017; Sargent and Larchanche, 2011. Even innovative and successful models such as Cuba's "medicine in community" (Whiteford and Branch, 2008) have been reconsidered in light of the increasing prioritization of concerns about climate change and health outcomes.

We embed the perceived ongoing crisis in health care paradigms in a larger historical and social context and review the origins and history of comparative health system (CHS) research. Two case studies, the first from Chile and the second from the English National Health Service (NHS), provide examples of this type of analysis and show how paradigms that direct health care system change are shaped by global and local histories, perceived needs, and extant technologies.

Research on CHS shows a vast array of models, criteria, concepts, and critiques. The lack of standard definitions and comparability of methods in the field of CHS makes cross-cultural comparisons difficult. Some researchers decry the lack of data available for analysis, while others lament the lack of uniform conceptualizations of the units to be measured, the processes to be investigated, and the outcomes to be compared. The field of CHS analysis, traditionally dominated by social sciences such as sociology, political science, anthropology, economics, and policy and public administration experts, reflects the epistemological and methodological bases of these distinct academic disciplines, as well as the diversity of the subject matter.

The descriptive paradigm of "systems," that formed the basis for CHS analysis from the 1940s through the 1990s is giving way to an emerging paradigm in which the process of health care delivery is being redefined, reformed, and reconceptualized. The new models attempt to include global streams, diversity, allow for structural pluralism, and identify health care methods and evaluations appropriate to their cultural context and articulated goals.

In the early years of CHS research, Eurocentric systems dominated corporate approaches to health care throughout the world. From the 1990s through the early 2000s concepts such "values, vision, and ethics" were viewed as nonessential concerns for corporate managers (Wheatley, 1992). In health care sectors, strict attention to purported and assumed "scientific" objectivity, close data scrutiny, reliable measurement, and prescribed care in the search for absolute answers characterized pre-2000 approaches to health care concerns and practices. Rejection of that paradigm, coupled with global conspiracy theories publicized through social media, created a more fluid and expansive view of health systems.

The formal academic analysis of health care systems began in the 1930s, but did not receive significant attention in the US until the 1970s with the work of medical sociologists such as Milton Roemer, Victor and Ruth Sidel, and other social scientists, economists, and humanists, such as Vincente Navarro, Oscar Gish, Ray Elling, Sander Kelman, Arthur Kleinman, David Mechanic, and Howard Waitzkin. In the late 1970s, medical sociologist Charles Leslie stimulated a parallel interest in comparative medical systems (Leslie, 1978), which culminated in a conference on social science and medicine held in Washington, DC, and the beginning of the journal *Social Science and Medicine*. Researchers at the conference discussed the same shibboleths: lack of shared definitions, methods, concepts, and paradigms. The field of CHS analysis was evolving from an uncritical and unquestioning dominance of the biomedical paradigm as "normal" (using Kuhn's 1970 definition), to an increased understanding of the role played by values in defining the research process. In addition, there was a new focus on the role played by funding agencies and mass media in giving substance and direction to researchers' perceptions and choices of research questions.

HISTORY OF COMPARATIVE HEALTH SYSTEMS RESEARCH

Social scientists have long been interested in the organization of health systems: their economic base, structural compartmentalization, service delivery programs, allocation of resources, decision making, the interactions between physicians, allied health professionals, and the community. Initially motivated by the need to provide outcome data to justify continuing the New Deal social reforms, comparisons of various health care systems were undertaken (Roemer, 1991). In the 1940s and 1950s, health systems reflected the social experimentation of the post-World War II years with, for instance, the Israeli attempts to provide multicultural clinics (Sidney Kark, 1974), the creation of the National Health Service (NHS) (Welch, 2018), and the health system experiments in Cuba and Nicaragua in the 1960s and 1970s. The political left in the United States, Europe, and Latin America gave strength and support to social science analyses of the changing structure of health systems, justifying the social and political restructuring that had occurred. Perhaps in response to the more explicitly polemical writings of the social left, others perceived CHS from a less explicitly articulated political view.

Foremost of those writers was Milton Roemer, whose work shaped CHS analysis for 20 years (Roemer, 1977, 1985, 1991). Roemer's early work focused particularly on the health systems of Europe and the United States, investigating the relationship between national political structure and health system development. Equally powerful in directing the scope of early CHS analysis were Victor and Ruth Sidel (1974), whose work on non-Western health systems, such as those in China, provided powerful counter-examples to the Western models. Anthropologists and sociologists like Ben Paul, Lyle Saunders, Julian Samora, and John Cassel turned their gaze on the role played by the "community" in health programs (Paul, 1955).

In the late 1960s and early 1970s, the CHS paradigm revolved around the issue of *equity*, comprehensive health care availability for entire populations. The writings of the time reflect both an optimistic view of the future and a willingness to challenge past assumptions that economic advantages would "trickle down" to the poor, that overall prosperity would improve health conditions for all, and that established government programs and policies were designed to make "health for all" a realistic goal. The *International Journal for Health Services* epitomized the conceptual changes of the time. It provided a way for the influential social health analysts of that era, such as Vincente Navarro, Oscar Gish, Sander Kelman, Ruth and Victor Sidel, Ray Elling, and Howard Waitzkin, to publish research reports, air opinions, and challenge established ideas by focusing on class relations, non-capitalist health models, and world economic system analyses.

The hopeful optimism of the early 1970s changed to more guarded realism in social analysis following the worldwide oil crisis in the mid-1970s. Social scientists engaged in CHS research turned away from structural analyses of equity, embracing the new paradigm of *cost containment* (Klein, 1991; Sidel, 1980). The Organization for Economic Cooperation and Development (OECD) published a series of comparative health analyses (OECD, 1977, 1985, 1987) as part of their overall research on economic management and public expenditure, which consolidated the shift from equity issues to economic issues. The OECD reports also determined the database that structured the parameters of subsequent research by collecting previously unavailable or inaccessible statistical data on which numerous other studies were based (OECD, 1977, 1985, 1987, 1990, as cited in Klein, 1991). The nature of the data available and the prevailing interests of the OECD in economic indices ensured a continuing focus on cost containment, moving the center of discussion away from issues of equity toward a new paradigm of *efficiency*.

From the late 1970s through the middle 1980s, research demonstrates this clear shift away from equity to new economic indices, such as spending levels, administrative costs, number of beds, and recuperative costs. The shift was, without doubt, influenced by the economic hardships of the times and concomitant emphases on accountability, as well as by the data made available by the OECD. During that decade, economists comparing health inputs in economic terms eclipsed the role of social science analysis from sociologists and anthropologists. Klein (1991), in his discussion of the risks and benefits of comparative studies, suggested that the influence of economists and statisticians reflected both the availability of statistical and economic data, and "…the famine of other data, notably about the impact of different types of health care systems on the *populations* being served" (Klein, 1991: 282, emphasis added).

The impact of differing system paradigms on the actual health of the population was often overlooked as too difficult to measure. However, by the 1980s, as our example of health care reform in Chile shows, negative health outcomes forced significant change. The draconian cuts in Chile's health budgets in the 1980s resulted in increased death and disease for women, children, and other at-risk populations. In some cases, the increase in maternal and child mortality forced decision makers to mediate between the conflicting goals of cost cutting and equity in the provision of services. The decade between the middle 1980s and 1990s shows the beginning of this shift away from cost containment and economic measures to indicators of the *effectiveness* of various health systems. "The assumption of the 1990s was that assuring effectiveness – by eliminating unnecessary, redundant, or low-yield forms of treatment – was a necessary condition for reconciling the demands of economy and equity" (Klein, 1991: 283). Even the 1990 OECD report moved away from the primacy of economic indices to international comparisons of medical practices and health care use. However, unlike some economic indices, health service utilization continued to be problematic to define, difficult to measure, and critical global data were often unavailable.

Since 2010, trends in CHS continued to compare medical practices and use across countries, but showed a greater emphasis on *patient-level outcomes*, health care expenditure, and the state of health care infrastructure (including human resources) (Johnson and Stoskopf, 2010; Levy and Sobolev, 2016). An important component of the comparison of the effectiveness of health services across the globe has become the focus on patient-level treatment outcomes, including patient-reported outcome measures (PROMS) (Levy and Sobolev, 2016). This patient-focused shift was accompanied by a greater emphasis on the improvement of patient experience and reporting of health care quality (Levy and Sobolev, 2016). This trend was exemplified during the 2020 global COVID-19 pandemic that forced the open comparison of different health systems and their abilities to successfully confront the virus, while social media simultaneously exploded with minute-by-minute analyses of their failures.

An increase in health care expenditure at a global scale also led to a more pronounced focus on efficiency (Papanicolas and Smith, 2013). Many health care systems across the world seek to deliver high-quality care at lower costs, but encounter challenges when defining and attempting to measure efficiency in meaningful ways (Papanicolas and Smith, 2013). Furthermore, efficiency is being sought in health care infrastructures characterized by decades of neglect, lack of investment in new technologies, and pressures at the level of human resources (Blank et al., 2017). Therefore, an important component of contemporary CHS research is the concern about the *sustainability* of health care systems, particularly those where medical services are free to the population (Johnson and Stoskopf, 2010).

The early works by Roemer and others (cf. Roemer, 1977; Rostow, 1971) reflected the dominant "modernization" framework common to social policy makers in the 1950s through the 1970s. The modernization framework assumed that all societies desire the same end point – to become "modernized" – and that while they may move at different speeds and through different paths, through time they will become more similar. A related assumption, although not frequently made explicit, was that there was a hierarchy of desirability in health systems, with the US/UK models of affluence setting the standard and the goal for other health systems to emulate. These ideas implicitly deny the validity of alternative directions in health care, denigrate the role of history and culture in shaping national systems, and ignore the value of structured pluralism.

The modernization approach has been thoroughly critiqued by social scientists from a variety of disciplines and fields of concentration. Ray Elling (1981, 1994) pointed out that while Roemer made significant, continual and long-lasting contributions to CHS, his early work in particular reflects an assumption that health systems evolve automatically from diversity and variability, to convergence and conformity, to structures and forms modeled on those from highly industrialized nations. These perspectives of convergence of health systems, along with assumptions of modernization, dominated much of the early writing on CHS in the 1970s (see Field, 1967; Fuchs, 1974; Mechanic, 1975). This view, however, abrogated the role of struggle, particularly class struggle, in the development of systems (Elling, 1981). The case study of health systems development in Chile in this chapter provides an example of how context and culture challenged the modernizationist assumptions of *a priori* models. The UK example highlights the challenges faced by highly industrialized nations in relation to changes in population health and health care systems that have not changed at the same pace. Both examples illustrate the fluidity and complexity of CHS research.

Established views of world order and control were significantly challenged in the 1960s by the global visibility of social movements such as the student-led riots in France, civil rights protests in the US and the war in Vietnam, increasing in the 1970s with the end of the Cold War, the women's movement, the collapse of the Berlin Wall, and intensifying in the 1980s and 1990s with the war in Bosnia, and the genocide in Rwanda. Social media captured live the "Arab Spring" protests across the Middle East in 2010, the capture and death of Osama Bin Laden in 2011, and the 2017 Women's March to protest the election of Donald Trump. The visual immediacy of global events upends the narrow vision of national isolation and exacerbates the engagement and resistance of populations and their push to achieve goals, including the delivery of health care. Systems which may have appeared contained and controlled explode into strange, unrecognizable formations as a result of social media, new technologies, and complex patterns of human migration, dislocation, disasters, and climate change. Old management structures and techniques are increasingly irrelevant as new and novel global linkages and power dynamics emerge, especially when coupled with new distance facilitating technologies.

In the past, health care workers, for example, under the auspices of bureaucratic organizations, were able to organize immunization campaigns and other programs for fairly static populations in countries from the Global South. However, in recent decades those programs and others have been disrupted by large numbers of people migrating from native homelands to resettle in London, Frankfurt, Miami, Marseilles, Caracas, La Paz, Buenos Aires, and other cities in the Global North. Migrations like these overturn traditional assumptions about the health care needs of populations and frustrate established management expectations and norms. Political conflict and complex emergencies create an ever-growing world of refugee populations fleeing places like Syria, Afghanistan, the Democratic Republic of Congo, and with them syndemic health problems that are difficult to treat in traditional health systems. Moreover, because migrations bring diverse populations together and raise compelling new concerns about health care issues, evolving health care paradigms must be prepared to respond quickly and innovatively to global shifts.

By the end of the first quarter of the twenty-first century, CHR has moved from post-industrial, positivistic, post-modern, and relational models to beginning to employ a syndemic model of health. The syndemic model provides a powerful heuristic for health system design and analysis as articulated by medical anthropologist Merrill Singer and others. It focuses on the interactions and co-present and synergistic relationships between multiple diseases and social and environmental factors (Singer et al., 2017).

With the collapse and re-emergence of authoritarian rule, global health conditions change. Some governments have opted to establish new, more participatory governmental forms associated with forecasts for market development and economic vitality. However, advancements in technology, health care, medical knowledge, and global linkages generate corresponding tensions caused by glaring disparities between the affluent and the poor. Internal and cross-border wars in Eastern Europe and Africa, the marginalization of groups of people in Latin America, continued threats to a fragile and seriously damaged environment, and intractable corporate powers are threats to new participatory health models.

While some forces exist that cause health care systems to become more uniform and similar to one another cross-culturally, such as global economic pressures, similar health conditions, and shared health policy goals, there are also important differences that give individuality and identity to the shape and form of health care systems. Cultural systems, while influenced by global interests, still shape how policy makers, practitioners, and populations view their health care needs, and how responses to those needs are structured and evaluated. History, which composes a core portion of a country's identity and shapes its external relations with other countries (Whiteford, 1990, 1992, 1993, 1998a, 1998b), uniquely structures relations between members of the population and their government and defines governmental authority and the role of the central government in the provision of health care. Simultaneously, the very definitions of health and illness, disease and sickness, are culturally constructed, reflecting the cultural interpretations of what it means to become ill, what courses of treatment are possible, and what are the expected roles of the individual and the government alike during illness, disability, and death.

The Cuban "Medicine in Community" model, for instance, builds on the government's control of medical labor and its ability to require physicians and other health professionals to live in local communities for prolonged periods of time (Whiteford and Branch, 2008). The community-based model effectively improves the critical health indicators of infant and child mortality, infectious diseases, and infant birth weights. This innovative and effective model is very much a product of Cuba's history and the US Embargo. Other countries, such as Venezuela, have not achieved the same success with the model as it does not emerge from or fit with the larger, overarching Venezuelan politics and experience in the world market.

CASE STUDY: HEALTH CARE REFORM IN CHILE

While health care systems are strongly influenced by globalizing factors such as sources and conditions of funding and the education and values of policy makers and practitioners, it is local culture, history, and experience that ultimately determine the efficacy and durability of a health care system. The forces of globalization cannot be underestimated, but how they are translated into practice can only be understood through the lens of culture and history. What follows is a brief case study of the Chilean experience.

Several identifiable worldwide trends in health care reform became clear at the end of the millennium. In Latin America in general, and in Chile in particular, four reform strategies were notable: (1) privatization (Chile); (2) decentralization and devolution of central government responsibility (Bolivia, Brazil, and Mexico, among others); (3) deconcentration (Cuba); and (4) delegation of functions to semi-autonomous agencies (Brazil and Mexico) (Frenk and Gonzalez-Block, 1992).

Reichard (1996) pointed out that while market forces and the general health status of a population may be fundamentally linked, it is history and societal values that shape a nation's institutions and through which meaning and conflict are interpreted. In his detailed account of health reforms in Chile from 1873 to 1990s, Reichard (1996) describes how Chile's health care system grew out of early labor movement reforms generated by nitrate miners and, later, railroad workers. Labor strife led to major redistributive laws by the 1920s, and in 1925 social legislation mandated sick pay, disability payments, and free medical coverage for all citizens (Reichard, 1996: 83). Reichard's analysis demonstrates how the establishment of the British National Health Service in 1948 influenced the creation of the Chilean National Health Service in 1952. Clearly, the enduring support for a distributive health system was rooted in Chile's labor history, but the system also found both popular and political support through the political process. The Chilean National Health Service was established to provide comprehensive health care for all citizens, and in so doing established institutions to meet those needs and developed educational and training programs to provide staff for those institutions. A conservative retrenchment of social programs in the 1950s gave rise to the labor alliance that elected President Eduardo Frei (1964–70), and later the Socialist/Communist alliance of President Salvador Allende (1970–73). The 1973 *coup d'état* set the stage for the military dictatorship of General Augusto Pinochet and "dismemberment" of public sector health programs such as health education, sanitation, occupational health service, medical education, and hospital staffing. Between 1974 and 1983 there was an overall reduction of 10% in public health spending (Reichard, 1996: 87) as the Pinochet government brought in economist Milton Friedman and the University of Chicago group of economic theorists to guide Chile's turn toward a market economy.

The Chilean turn toward a market economy at the time was referred to as the "Chilean miracle," a set of economic policies being duplicated throughout Latin America. However, the miracle did not extend to the improvements in Chile's public health system. It is a sad irony that 100 years after the Chilean–Bolivian War of 1873 (when Chile seized lands high in nitrates, initiating nitrate mining and its consequent labor movement, which agitated for health care), President Salvador Allende, physician and former Minister of Health, was assassinated in a bloody *coup d'état* that marked a turn away from comprehensive health coverage for all Chileans. Privatization began in 1982 with the development of private health insurance modeled on the US health maintenance organizations (HMO) and preferred provider organizations (PPO) systems. The government cut subsidies to the public health system, reduced the University of Chile's Medical School budget by 46% and its personnel by 40% in the decade between 1980 and 1990, and ended the previous governments' redistributed tax policies (Reichard, 1996).

The actions reduced the middle class and increased the number of people without access to health insurance. During and following the Pinochet era, health care reform turned toward privatization and decentralization, reducing the influence of grassroots and union organizations. Cost containment became a process as well as an economic goal, which undermined cultural and historical values supporting the state in the delivery of, and access to, health care. Cost containment became a process of social control and marginalization, with far-reaching and long-term health consequences. The turn toward a market economy exacerbated the social, educational, economic, and epidemiological differences within the Chilean population, as exemplified by the disparity of public health services in the rural and urban areas (Montoya-Aguilar and Marchant-Cavieres, 1994: 286).

Previous to 1973, the Chilean National Health Service was financed through the central budget (at about 65%) and by compulsory insurance contributions paid by workers and their employers. The overthrow of the Allende government and the move to neoliberal and structural adjustment policies led to large direct reductions in the central government contributions, leaving a significant gap in funding to be made up by direct user payments and increased compulsory worker insurance premiums, and ever increasingly leaving the poor without health care. In 1980, the increased emphasis on market economy policies resulted in the creation of private, for-profit health organizations that marketed health insurance plans against the compulsory contributions (Montoya-Aguilar and Marchant-Cavieres, 1994). The result was increased epidemiological polarization.

To resolve the "epidemiological polarization" (Frenk and Gonzalez-Block, 1992: 42) that defined health conditions in many parts of Latin America and much of the rest of the world required that health care systems be redesigned to provide for prevention and intervention, maintenance and cure, and programs designed to supplement nutritional needs to children, prevent infectious disease, provide assistance to the elderly, and guarantee access and equity. Instead, what happened in Chile intensively increased the polarization of society, by reducing the prevention and protection of large portions of the population.

The Chilean example continues to reflect the global crisis in health care as in 2000 when Chile enacted another set of reforms (Missoni and Giorgio, 2010). Those reforms focused on enhancing patient rights and increasing equity in the financing system.

However, the solidarity perspective embedded in the post-military health system in Chile was once again challenged by the 2010 government that moved the country and its health priorities to the center-right of the political spectrum, exacerbating differences between social classes (including differences in health outcomes) (Missoni and Giorgio, 2010).

The Chilean example demonstrates the complexity of health system paradigms. Equality and equity are often at odds as health system goals, and both objectives are intrinsically embedded in the larger, overarching national political system, which in itself is a reflection of the tensions emanating from the various global systems. In Chile, as in other countries, proximate variables and indirect causes provided important information for the evolution of health care paradigms. As various authors have pointed out (Montoya-Aguilar and Marchant-Cavieres, 1994; Whiteford, 1992, 1993, 1998a, 1998b), public health systems can withstand radical economic changes for a period of time; health indicators often lag behind practice changes such as the loss of basic sanitation, immunization, prenatal care, health education, and nutritional supplements. In time, however, the health indicators will reflect the changes to show the increase in rates of infectious disease, deterioration of health care infrastructures, reduction of number and quality of health care personnel, and, concomitantly, the loss of faith in the government to provide those basic needs for its population (Whiteford, 1993, 1998a).

CASE STUDY: HEALTH CARE REFORM IN THE UK

In both Chile and the United Kingdom, socialized medicine was introduced in the 1950s. In the UK, the National Health Service (NHS) (organized across the four public health systems of England, Scotland, Wales and Northern Ireland) celebrated its 70th birthday in 2018. The anticipation of that anniversary was shared around the world when the UK hosted the Olympics and the Opening Ceremony was a celebration of the National Health Service (complete with a faux Queen jumping out of an airplane with a faux James Bond). The celebration highlighted the NHS commitment to deliver equitable and high-quality care in the context of patient populations with complex needs, financial austerity, and changing geopolitical landscapes (Stoye, 2018). It was the very description of a highly complex health care paradigm.

As of 2020, the NHS founding principle of delivering care based on need and not the ability to pay continues to be a paramount goal, yet many argue that it will only be possible to maintain if the health care system itself undergoes significant transformations in the ways in which it considers and delivers care. Compared to other health care systems across the world, the NHS health coverage does not depend on patients' financial situation; it is relatively efficient and performs well, managing patients with some long-term conditions (Dayan et al., 2018).

In the UK, the demand for care is increasing due to a growing ageing population with more comorbidities (Oliver et al., 2014). These complex clinical cases of frail elderly patients represent a challenge for a health care paradigm that is often fragmented and unable to deliver adequate care in the community (Oliver et al., 2014). These patients are then required to access care in secondary and tertiary hospitals for prolonged periods of time, contributing to bed shortages and the burden of already overworked staff (Gordon et al., 2014). Their care also requires the combined expertise of different medical professionals in the form of multidisciplinary teams, who might not always be available locally (Gordon et al., 2014).

Despite significant advances, variations in care delivery across the country are still present. Inequalities have been documented in relation to access to screening, timely diagnosis, waiting time for medical procedures and treatments, treatment outcomes, and quality of life (Abel et al., 2015; Cooper et al., 2017; Douglas et al., 2016; Reilly et al., 2015). The most economically deprived areas of the country continue to receive a lower quality of care, experience longer waiting times, have a poorer patient experience and overall lower quality of life (Fowler et al., 2017; Oliphant et al., 2013).

In 2020, developments such as Britain's exit from the European Union (Brexit) could further exacerbate shortages as European health care professionals leave and the UK no longer becomes a popular destination for other professionals seeking jobs in health care (Lintern, 2017; McKenna, 2017; Murray, 2017). The infrastructure of the NHS is also under pressure. In the decade 2010–20, emergency departments from across the country were failing to meet waiting time targets and acute hospitals are encountering issues with bed shortages and the timely delivery of elective care (with long waiting times for outpatient appointments and elective procedures). There are evident crises at the workforce level, with a deficit of nurses, midwives, health visitors and staff working in the social care sector. In 2014, there was an overall staffing shortfall of 5.9%, which equates to 50,000 clinical staff (National Audit Office, 2016). This staff shortage increases the burden on existing staff members and, in extreme cases, could pose a safety concern for patients (The Health Foundation et al., 2018).

In 2014, England published the *Five Year Forward View* (FYFV), outlining a health care model that would bring together different areas of the health and social care sectors to address the challenges outlined above (NHS, 2014). According to the FYFV, the British health care model needed to undergo significant transformations in the following areas:

1 an increase on the focus on prevention and public health,
2 a shift toward giving patients more control over their care and more local management of health service delivery,
3 an emphasis on more care delivered locally (in the community or local hospitals), but certain treatments delivered in specialist centers, requiring a better integration of primary, secondary and tertiary care,
4 a redesign of urgent and emergency care services (with more local options, such as walk-in centers and out-of-hours general practitioner services, to reduce attendance in hospital emergency departments),
5 a reinforcement of primary care as the foundation of NHS care, and
6 promotion of a cost-effective health service with a focus on both efficiency and a high quality of care (NHS, 2014).

Since the FYFV report in 2014, the NHS focused on implementing the changes outlined in the FYFV, testing new models of care in 50 "vanguard" sites, creating 44 geographical "footprints" with sustainability and transformation plans (STPs) and addressing growing financial pressures produced by further funding to health and social care services (Ham et al., 2016). Some "vanguards" focused specifically on developing new models of care in acute hospitals (The Dalton Review; Department of Health, 2014). The acute care collaboration vanguards (ACCs), for instance, sought to test the implementation of hospital group models (i.e., hospital chains) to reduce unwarranted clinical variation and reduce costs through economies of scale (Department of Health, 2014). These hospital group models are currently being evaluated (Vindrola-Padros et al., 2019) to determine if they can be useful models for the NHS to adopt at a national scale in the near future.

Sustainability and transformation plans became the mechanism through which to plan and deliver services locally (Ham et al., 2016). Funding continues to be a problem, however, and most of the increases in funding have been at the tertiary care level and not in prevention and primary care, where the service would see most long-term benefits (Ham et al., 2016). This difficult financial situation is further exacerbated by the uncertainty generated by the UK's initiation of Brexit in

March 2019, where questions will be raised about the government's priorities in relation to health and social care, the sustainability of health care infrastructures and resources, and the improvement of the population's health.

The NHS continues to be viewed internationally as a successful health care paradigm. It provides a considerable amount of coverage for its population; it is relatively cost-effective and has improved in terms of treatment outcomes and patients' quality of life (Dayan et al., 2018). It faces challenges that are similar to those seen in other Western industrialized nations, where the needs of the population are changing, health care infrastructures are requiring additional technological investment to keep abreast of new trends in clinical practice, workforce crises are complicating the delivery of timely and high-quality care and financial resources allocated to health care have been reduced. In light of these pressures, the NHS has opted for a model of care that seeks to prioritize prevention and primary care, integrate all levels of care delivery (from primary to tertiary), involve patients and the public in decision making, and is open to experimenting with new models of care delivery based on different types of partnerships. The increased emphasis on patient involvement reflects the significance of a socio-cultural and syndemic orientation.

CONCLUSION

Globally, health systems are in flux, changing to meet changing population needs, political necessities, rising medical costs, and public distrust. In the US, pop-up, urgent care storefront medical care facilities have become commonplace, and a new breed of physicians who operate only in hospitals ("hospitalists") have become the norm. COVID-19 showed hospitals overwhelmed and practitioners working beyond their limits. Even before the global pandemic challenged perceptions of what a health care paradigm should be able to anticipate and treat, outbreaks of Ebola in Liberia and the Democratic Republic of Congo competed with news stories of outbreaks of diseases long controlled in the US (for instance, an outbreak of measles in Disneyland, CA). Worldwide internet access makes advice available from sources such as WebMD, telemedicine, or home diagnosis laboratories, and symptom-checking websites. Information is more immediate, whether through social media, smart TVs, 24-hour news stations, blogs, and Twitter than ever before. While the web provides an innovative and novel health care delivery system with a wide range of explanatory models and practices, the preventive health practices, previously at the core of Western health care models, are increasingly under attack. In both the Global North and South, groups are actively engaged in rejecting health care services designed to control infectious disease as, for instance, people refuse to be vaccinated against childhood diseases.

As we move toward the middle of the twenty-first century, we see increased responsibility placed on patients to maintain their own health, without concern for the social, cultural and economic factors that shape their capacity to maintain healthy lifestyles and to access the care they need. Globalization, often in conflict with local demands, continues to shape regional, national, and world health paradigms.

CHS research has moved from an unquestioning stance and acceptance of quantitative data collected and categorized by researchers as they struggled to compare what, in essence, were apples and oranges. Early CHS analysts often had to fit their data into pre-constructed categories in order to be able to make comparisons. Current health systems research, on the other hand, while still concerned with measurable outcomes, is more focused on the shapes and forms of health systems as they evolve from the local context. Earlier CHS research used a systems metaphor to compare items (policies, practices, indicators, outcomes, economies) that themselves were not comparable because these comparisons ignored underlying cultural and historical differences.

The most exciting new directions in CHS research build on the ideas of previous CHS analysts but incorporate lessons from contemporary experiences, such as presented by the COVID-19 pandemic. Particularly important in contemporary CHR is the importance of identifying biases in research, including those of the researchers, funders, and participants as well as those who use the data. In a time of rapid social and technological change and newly emerging viruses like COVID-19, as well as re-emerging diseases, health care systems will inevitably struggle to adapt. Our examples of health care reform in Chile and the NHS in the UK attempt to show how critical it is to incorporate social, historical, and political variables in comparative health research. While global health systems may be in crisis, the very diversity and innovative energy that these emerging systems demonstrate provide a hopeful future of energized, innovative, and healthy debates of how best to protect the competing interests embodied in future health system paradigms.

ACKNOWLEDGEMENTS

We would like to thank the editors for encouraging us to develop this chapter on comparative health systems. We would also like to thank Eugenia Brage for her assistance with the development of the chapter draft.

REFERENCES

Abel, G. A., Shelton, J., Johnson, S., et al. (2015) Cancer-specific variation in emergency presentation by sex, age and deprivation across 27 common and rarer cancers. *British Journal of Cancer*, 112(s1), S129–S136.

Blank, R., Burau, V., and Kuhlmann, E. (2017) *Comparative health policy*. New York: Macmillan International Higher Education.

Cabrera, J. M., and Kurmanaev, A. (2020) Ecuador's death tool during outbreak is among the worst in the world. *New York Times*, 23 April.

Cooper, C., et al. (2017) Inequalities in receipt of mental and physical healthcare in people with dementia in the UK. *Age and Ageing*, 46, 393–400.

Dayan, M., Ward, D., Gardner, T., and Kelly, E. (2018) *How good is the NHS?* London: The Health Foundation, Institute for Fiscal Studies, The King's Fund and The Nuffield Trust. www.kingsfund.org.uk/sites/default/files/201806/NHS_at_70_how_good_is_the_NHS.pdf

Department of Health (2014) *Examining new options and opportunities for providers of NHS care: The Dalton Review*. London: HMSO.

Douglas, E., Waller, J., Duffy, S., and Wardle, J. (2016) Socioeconomic inequalities in breast and cervical screening coverage in England: Are we closing the gap? *Journal of Medical Screening*, 23(2), 98–103.

Elling, R. H. (1981) The capitalist world-system and international health. *International Journal of Health Services*, 11, 21–51.

Elling, R. H. (1994) Theory and method for the cross-national study of health systems. *International Journal of Health Services*, 24, 285–309.

Field, M. (1967) *Soviet socialized medicine: An introduction*. New York: Free Press.

Fowler, H., Belot, A., Njagi, E. N., et al. (2017) Persistent inequalities in 90-day colon cancer mortality: an English cohort study. *British Journal of Cancer*, 117(9), 1396–404.

Frenk, J., and Gonzalez-Block, M. A. (1992) Corporatism and health care: A comparison of Sweden and Mexico. *Health Policy*, 21, 167–180.

Fuchs, V. (1974) *Who shall live? Health, economics and social choice*. New York: Basic Books.

Gordon, A., Franklin, M., Bradshaw, L., Logan, P., Elliott, R., and Gladman, J. (2014) Health status of UK care home residents: A cohort study. *Age and Aging*, 43(1), 97–103.

Ham, C., et al. (2016) *Policy changes to implement the NHS five year forward view: A progress report*. London: The King's Fund. www.kingsfund.org.uk/publications/five-year-forward-view-progress-report

Horowitz, J., and Kirkpatrick, D. (2020) Dip in Italy's cases does not come fast enough for swamped hospitals. *New York Times*, March 23.

Johns Hopkins University (2020) *COVID-19 Dashboard by the Center for Systems Science and Engineering (CSSE) at Johns Hopkins University (JHU)*. www.coronavirus.jhu.edu/map (accessed 5 September 2020).

Johnson, J., and Stoskopf, C. (2010) *Comparative health systems: Global Perspectives*. Burlington, MA: Jones and Bartlett Learning.

Kark, S. (1974) *Epidemiology and Community Medicine*. McGraw-Hill Appleton/Lange.

Klein, R. (1991) Risks and benefits of comparative studies: Notes from another shore. *Milbank Quarterly*, 69, 275–291.

Kuhn, T. S. (1970) *The structure of scientific revolutions* (2nd ed.). Chicago, IL: University of Chicago Press.

Leslie, C. (1978) Theoretical foundations for the comparative study of medical systems. *Social Science and Medicine*, April, 12(2B), 65–67.

Levy, A., and Sobolev, B. (2016) *Comparative effectiveness research in health services*. New York: Springer.

Lintern, S. (2017) Exclusive: Leak reveals worst case scenario for nursing after Brexit. *Health Services Journal*, April 6, www.hsj.co.uk/workforce/exclusive-leak-reveals-worst-case-scenario-for-nursing-after-brexit/7019223.article

McKenna, H. (2017) *Brexit: The implications for health and social care*. London: The King's Fund. www.kingsfund.org.uk/publications/articles/brexit-implications-health-social-care

Mechanic, D. (1975) The comparative study of health care delivery systems. *Annual Review of Sociology*, 1, 43–65.

Missoni, Eduardo, and Giorgio Solimano (2010) "Towards universal health coverage: the Chilean experience." *World Health Report* 97, 119–124.

Montoya-Aguilar, C., and Marchant-Cavieres, L. (1994) The effect of economic changes on health care and health in Chile. *International Journal of Health Planning and Management*, 9, 279–294.

Mulligan, Jessica M., and Castañeda, Heidi eds. (2017) *Unequal coverage: The experience of health care reform in the United States*. Vol. 2. NYU Press.

Murray, R. (2017) *Falling number of nurses in the NHS paints a worrying picture*. London: The King's Fund www.kingsfund.org.uk/blog/2017/10/falling-number-nurses-nhs-paints-worrying-picture

National Audit Office (2016) *Managing the supply of NHS clinical staff in England*. London: NAO. www.nao.org.uk/wp-content/uploads/2016/02/Managing-the-supply-of-NHS-clinical-staff-in-England-Summary.pdf

NHS (2014) *Five Year Forward View (FYFV)*, www.england.nhs.uk/wp-content/uploads/2014/10/5yfv-web.pdf

OECD (1977) *Public expenditure on health*. Paris: Organisation for Economic Cooperation and Development.

OECD (1985) *Measuring health care, 1960–1983*. Paris: Organisation for Economic Cooperation and Development.

OECD (1987) *Financing and delivering health care*. Paris: Organisation for Economic Cooperation and Development.

OECD (1990) *Health care systems in transition*. Paris: Organisation for Economic Cooperation and Development.

Oliphant, R., Nicholson, G. A., Horgan, P. G., et al. (2013) Deprivation and colorectal cancer surgery: Longer-term survival inequalities are due to differential postoperative mortality between socioeconomic groups. *Annals of Surgical Oncology*, 20(7), 2132–2139.

Oliver, D., Foot, C., and Humphries, R. (2014) *Making our health and care systems fit for an ageing population*. London: The King's Fund. www.kingsfund.org.uk/publications/making-our-health-and-care-systems-fit-ageing-population

Paul, B. (ed.) (1955) *Health, community, and culture*. New York: Russell Sage Foundation.

Papanicolas, I., and Smith, P. (2013) *Health system performance comparison: An agenda for policy, information and research*. London: Open University Press.

Reichard, S. (1996) Ideology drives health care reforms in Chile. *Journal of Public Health Policy*, 17, 80–98.

Reilly, S., et al. (2015) Inequalities in physical comorbidity: A longitudinal comparative cohort study of people with severe mental illness in the UK. *BMJ Open*, 5(12), e009010. https://bmjopen.bmj.com/content/5/12/e009010

Roemer, M. I. (1977) *Systems of health care*. New York: Springer.

Roemer, M. I. (1985) *National strategies for health care organization: A world overview*. Ann Arbor, MI: Health Administration Press.

Roemer, M. I. (1991) *National health systems of the world* (Vol. 1). New York: Oxford University Press.

Rostow, W. (1971) *The stages of economic growth*. Cambridge, UK: Cambridge University Press.

Sargent, Carolyn, and Larchanché Stephanie (2011) "Transnational migration and global health: the production and management of risk, illness, and access to care." *Annual Review of Anthropology*, 40, 345–361.

Sidel, V. W. (1980) International comparisons of health services: How? who? why? *Policy Studies Journal*, 9, 300–308.

Sidel, V. W., and Sidel, R. (1974) *Serve the people: Observations on medicine in the People's Republic of China*. Boston, MA: Beacon.

Singer, M., Bulled, N., Ostrack, B., and Mendenhall, E. (2017) Syndemics and the biosocial conception of health. *The Lancet*, 389, 941–950.

Stoye, G. (2018) *Does the NHS need more money and how could we pay for it?* London: The Health Foundation, the Institute for Fiscal Studies, The King's Fund and The Nuffield Trust. www.kingsfund.org.uk/sites/default/files/2018-06/NHS_70_does_the_NHS_need_more_money.pdf

The Health Foundation, The King's Fund, and The Nuffield Trust (2018) *The health care workforce in England: make or break?* London: The Health Foundation, The King's Fund, and The Nuffield Trust. www.kingsfund.org.uk/publications/health-care-workforce-england

Vindrola-Padros, C., Capelas-Barbosa, E., Ramsay, A. I. G., Turner, S., Morris, S., Agble, R., Caldwell-Nichols, A., and Fulop, N. J. (2019) Mixed methods evaluation of a hospital group model using an embedded research approach: Study protocol. *BMJ Open* 9(6), June. https://doi.org/10.1136/bmjopen-2018-027086.

Welch, E. (2018) *The NHS at 70: A living history*. London: Pen and Sword.

Wheatley, M. J. (1992) *Leadership and the new science: Learning about organization from an orderly universe*. San Francisco, CA: Berrett-Koehler.

Whiteford, L. M. (1990) A question of adequacy: Primary health care in the Dominican Republic. *Social Science and Medicine*, 30, 221–226.

Whiteford, L. M. (1992) Caribbean colonial history and its contemporary health care consequences: The case of the Dominican Republic. *Social Science and Medicine*, 35, 1215–1222.

Whiteford, L. M. (1993) International economic policies and child health. *Social Science and Medicine*, 37, 1391–1400.

Whiteford, L. M. (1998a) Children's health as accumulated capital: Structural adjustment in the Dominican Republic and Cuba. In N. Scheper-Hughes and C. Sargent (eds), *Small wars: The cultural politics of childhood*. Berkeley, CA: University of California Press.

Whiteford, L. M. (1998b) Sembrando El Futuro: Globalization and the commodification of Health. In M. B. Whiteford and S. Whiteford (eds), *Crossing currents: Continuity and change in Latin America*. Upper Saddle River, NJ: Prentice Hall.

Whiteford, Linda M., and Branch., Laurence G. (2008) *Primary health care in Cuba: the other revolution*. Lanham, MD: Rowman & Littlefield Publishers.

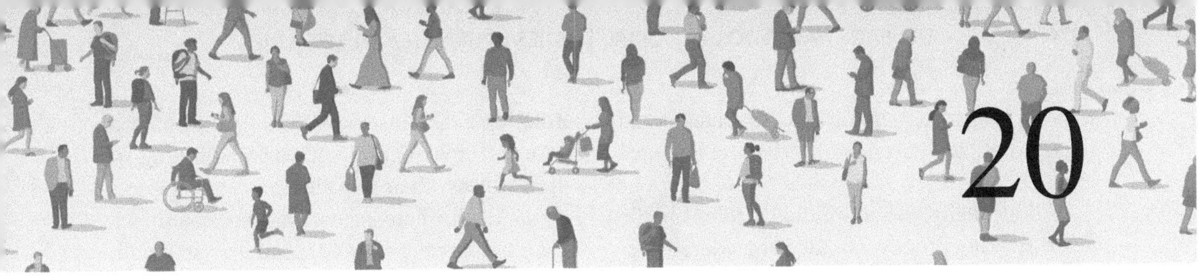

20

Health Service Utilization and Barriers to Health Care

Lutchmie Narine and Ambika Krishnakumar

This chapter explores the landscape of ideas and research that seeks to describe and explain the nature of health service utilization (HSU) and access to services which is informed by a variety of models and frameworks. Some of these models focus on specific constructs that clarify the nature and barriers of health service use, whereas other models incorporate a range of health care constructs and represent hybrid frameworks. Other models focus on the concept of "fit" and propose how a lack of fit between individual health care utilization and availability of health services affects the understanding and assessment of health service access and their use. The various health care utilization models currently available in the literature can be broadly categorized as sociological, social-psychological, institutional, hybrid, and fit frameworks. In this chapter, we describe these frameworks and how they affect health services utilization research. We identify limitations with these models and frameworks and how these, in turn, result in gaps in knowledge about health services utilization. Finally, we highlight more recent work that builds on the concept of health service use as the interaction of the capabilities of individuals and communities with the features of health systems. We also discuss how this perspective is aligned with the growing focus of global health to adopt Amartya Sen's capabilities approach to human development and the related impetus to use human rights-based approaches to improve human health.

SOCIOLOGICAL MODELS

Sociological models postulate that sociological constructs can influence individuals' capacity to pay for health care and thus affect their access to care. These constructs are composed primarily of demographic factors such as age, sex, marital status, and family characteristics (e.g., family size and income), including higher-order constructs such as education, occupation, ethnicity, and family resources.

These constructs are often sub-categorized into what are described as family resource models.

Additionally, the adoption of "roles" in the care-seeking process are also considered predictors of health services use. The adoption of "roles" in the care-seeking process is drawn from the work of Talcott Parsons on the "sick role" and Edward Suchman's model on the stages of illness behavior. Talcott Parsons's (1951) sick role theory conceptualizes illness as an impairment in the body's normal functioning and considers seeking and utilizing health care as a way to return the body to its normal functioning role. Edward Suchman's (1965) five-stage model of illness behavior focuses on the symptom experience, people's behaviors as they access health care, contact with the medical system, and include the person's perception of the "sick role" and their recovery from illness.

The two models highlight the importance of social roles in accounting for people's experience to both seek care and their utilization of health services.

A shortcoming of the Parson's model is that it does not adequately account for variations in sick people's behavior when using health services. It describes the changed role of the sick person but does not account for why some sick people use more and others use fewer services or the types of services they use. The Talcott Parsons "sick role" model and Edward Suchman's stages of illness behavior model do not address the community resources that patients need or take into account the role of aspects of the broader health system that may influence people's access to and use of health care services.

SOCIAL-PSYCHOLOGICAL MODELS

Social-psychological models focus on psychological factors or practices that explain behaviors of individuals when looking for and using health care services. Stoeckle, Zola, and Davidson (1963) suggested that patients' awareness and understanding of their illness; their expectations and opinions about health care providers and health service organizations; and need to get health care, all play influential roles when patients seek and utilize health care services. David Mechanic's model, first described in 1968 and revised in 1978, highlights patients' perceptions of the gravity and responses to their health symptoms as important factors in determining their seeking health care. Like Mechanic's and Stoeckle et al.'s models, the Health Belief Model (Rosenstock, 1966; Rosenstock, Derryberry, & Carriger, 1959) captures important potential psychological determinants of preventive care utilization. The Health Belief Model, put forward in the 1950s and 1960s, suggested that four perceived interrelated factors – vulnerability to illness, acuteness of the illness, advantages of taking action against the illness, along with the perceived impediments to taking action – were central to patients' use of preventative health services. In addition, signals to action are needed for the initiation of health-seeking behaviors.

All three models mentioned above do not take non-psychological factors into account when explaining an individual's behavior in seeking and using health care services. Rosenstock (1974) made further additions to the Health Belief Model, including constructs such as sex, age, race/ethnicity, and social class as exogenous factors that had direct effects on health service use. Subsequent revisions of the Health Belief Model in the 1980s (Rosenstock, Strecher, & Becker, 1988) expanded its focus to the treatment of health problems. However, a major drawback with this and other social-psychological models is the lack of attention that these models pay to the role of the health system and the non-inclusion of health service organizations and health policies on health service access and utilization. Nevertheless, the contribution of the social-psychological models to the literature is to emphasize the relevance of variables such as perceived susceptibility to illness, perceptions about the seriousness of illnesses, the iterative nature of health seeking behavior, the expected benefit from taking action in the face of illness, and the cues that trigger an individual's actions to seek health care.

INSTITUTIONAL MODELS

As described above, the sociological and social-psychological models of health service utilization emphasize the role of individual factors in accessing and using health services. Institutional models, on the other hand, highlight the role of larger social systems that impact access and health service utilization. These include the structure of the health system, such as the availability of a usual source of care, distinctions between universal and other types of health insurance, and the practice styles of health personnel or organizations (Gibson, 1972). Institutional models often encompass "community resource models" that can impact health service utilization, such as the supply of health personnel and health care facilities and the distribution of health care institutions in the community, and the rural-versus-suburban-versus urban character of communities. A newer model, articulated by Derose, Gresenz, and Ringel (2011), underscores the role of the public health system in understanding disparities in health care access and can also be categorized under the umbrella of being an institutional model. Recent models that look at geographical or spatial factors that seek to explain access and barriers to health services can also be typified as institutional. While the focus of geographic models is on the proximity or lack of proximity of patients to health services, the lack of proximity is often due to the availability of community resources such as proper roads and transportation facilities. Also, falling within the construct of institutional models are the various economic models that seek to characterize forces affecting health service access and use along dimensions of supply and demand factors.

In particular, supply factors such as the number of hospital beds, physicians, community workers, and so on are measures of community resources. It is easily acknowledged that the number of community resources available, the nature of health service organizations, and health systems and policies can play important roles in determining individual differences in health care utilization. However, these factors are not seen as completely accounting for individual variations in access and use of health services.

HYBRID MODELS

Andersen Behavioral Model

Coming out of work in the late 1960s and early1970s, Ronald Andersen in collaboration with John F. Newman produced a model of health service use termed the "Behavior Model of Health Services Use" (Andersen & Newman, 1973). Later, with LuAnn Aday (Aday & Andersen, 1974), they developed a behavioral model termed "Framework for the Study of Access to Medical Care." In the first formulation of the model, it was envisioned that an individual's access and use of health services is a function of three factors – predisposing, enabling, and need factors. Predisposing factors include characteristics of individuals that may influence the likelihood of someone using or not using a health service. The predisposing factors include demographic (such as age and gender), social structure (such as education, occupation, and race/ethnicity), and health beliefs (such as the belief that an individual may gain from the health service). This allows for consideration that while individuals may be disposed to accessing health services, their ability to do so may be impacted by their ability to get health insurance and the availability of health care personnel or facilities in their communities.

Need factors are those where the individual recognizes a need to utilize a health service. This need could be subjective, where the individual perceives a threat from illness, or is evaluated, where an individual is clinically diagnosed as having an illness in need of care.

An important feature of the model is the inclusion of the actual use of health services within the framework of the behavioral model. The emphasis on the use of health services was influenced by Donabedian's observation that "The proof of access is the use of service, not simply the presence of a facility" (Donabedian, 1972: 111). Another departure of the model is that while many of the earlier models focused on two major alternative dimensions, i.e., the characteristics of the patient population and their surroundings versus the health delivery system, the Andersen behavioral model sought to incorporate a broader set of factors to transcend this dichotomy of factor choices. Indeed, in response to criticisms and changes in the health care landscape over time, the model was modified several times. First, it was broadened to include factors of the health system. In the subsequent years (Andersen, 1995), factors from the external environment, such as market forces, health policy, and constructs of the physical environment, were incorporated. Also, an individual's "health behaviors" in the form of personal health practices, such as self-care, diet, and exercise, were included in the revised model. In all of these variations of the model, health service use remained the endogenous or dependent variable.

In recognition of the importance of the nature and quality of service received, the model was further revised to include consumer satisfaction and health status as the ultimate endogenous endpoints of the model. Additional revisions to the model focused on how the model was structured and organized. The initial formulation of the model postulated a linear sequence from predisposing to enabling to need factors, and then ultimately ending in impact on health service use. It should be noted that this linear flow to the key factors in the model was not in conformity with Andersen's earlier conception of access, which he saw as operating in a circular causal manner with patients and health systems both gaining from the experience of health service use and thus feeding back onto themselves, resulting in dynamic change. However, this linear flow along the key constructs dominated the early use of the model in the scientific literature. In later versions of the model, Andersen re-emphasized the possibility of feedback loops between constructs. In particular, health behaviors are said to feed back onto the core of the model, i.e., predisposing, enabling, and need factors. Even though the model is in its sixth revision, the linear flow among variables still predominates its conceptualization (Andersen & Davidson, 2007). However, the current version presents a more complex path model in which health service utilization is an intervening variable rather than an outcome variable with the health care system and the larger environmental context being conceptualized as independent variables. The ultimate dependent variables in the current version are health status outcomes.

The Institute of Medicine Access Model

In the early 1990s, the Institute of Medicine (IOM) outlined in its publication (Millman, 1993) a model to understand patients' access to personal health services. The IOM model proposes a unidirectional linear relationship from barriers to mediators, service use, and outcomes. This hybrid model incorporates a variety of constructs having to do with barriers to access to services, use of services, mediators between barriers and service use, and health outcomes. Personal, structural, and financial variables are considered barriers that impede the use of particular health services (rates of patients' utilization of provider visits and procedures delivered). Mediator variables include the appropriateness of the health care received by individuals and encompass such things as the quality of health care providers, whether patients adhere to treatments prescribed (compliance), and the efficacy of treatments and medications prescribed. Health outcomes include the ability of all individuals to receive adequate health care without impediments as well as health status indicators, such as morbidity, mortality, functional ability, and well-being.

Health Care Access Barriers Model

Like the Andersen–Newman behavioral model and the Institute of Medicine model, the Health Care Access Barriers (HCAB) model employs a variety of variables to help understand people's use of health services and the barriers to such services. The model (Carrillo, Carrillo, & Perez et al., 2011) proposes a taxonomy of three categories of variables that serve as barriers to health care use. These include financial, structural, and cognitive barriers. The financial barriers fall broadly into the cost of care and health insurance status factors. Structural variables include variables described for institutional models that have been covered earlier in this chapter. Cognitive barriers cover factors such as patient's beliefs and knowledge of the disease, prevention and treatment, and their capacity to communicate with health care providers. In addition, the HCAB model identifies three intermediary variables between the barriers and health outcomes. These intermediary variables include prevention, timely care, and the nature of the treatment.

The broad intent of the HCAB model is to provide nomenclature and a framework for identifying and categorizing barriers to health service use. However, the focus in identifying barriers is to uncover those that are modifiable and measurable. By targeting modifiable barriers, the HCAB seeks to be a practical tool for root cause and other quality improvement analyses which then allows for the design of effective community-based interventions.

FIT MODELS

5A Model

In the 1980s, Penchansky and Thomas (1981) developed a model of health service use that emphasized the fit between the patient and the health care system. Similar to other health care utilization models, Pechansky and Thomas recognized that individual-level variables such as having health insurance, a source of care, and the patient's income could facilitate or serve as barriers to the use of health services. However, it is the degree of fit between patients and the health care system within which they seek care that ultimately determines the utilization of health services. The degree of "fit" is said to be measured by five aspects – availability, accessibility, accommodation, affordability, and acceptability. Hence, the model is commonly referred to as the 5A model. Availability refers to the volume of physician and other health care services available to the patient whereas accessibility is conceptualized as the geographic proximity between the users of health care services to the providers of those services. Accommodation is conceptualized as the characteristics of the health care organization delivering the services and the ease with which patients can utilize health care in that organization. Affordability refers to the patient's ability to pay for services and their perception of the value of those services, and acceptability refers to the views of the patients toward those who provide care. The outcome posited by the 5A model is patients' satisfaction, which is the fit between patients and each of the five aspects of the health care system.

Patient-centered Model

Levesque, Harris, and Russell (2013) described a model in which they proposed that access to health services was a function of the interaction between five aspects of health services and five aspects of the patient seeking care. Four aspects of health services that include availability, affordability, acceptability, and accommodation are similar to the construct of health services in the 5A model. In the patient-centered model, the fifth aspect of health services is approachability, which replaces the 5A aspect of health service accessibility. Approachability refers to the extent to which health services make themselves known to people who may need care. Features such as information about available treatments and the nature of outreach activities are elements of the concept of approachability.

Although the 5A model suggested the importance of understanding the fit between health services and patients, it did not identify features of patients that fit with its five aspects of health services. Levesque et al.'s patient-centered model addresses that deficiency. The patient-centered model highlights five abilities of people (ability to perceive, the ability to seek, ability to reach, ability to pay, and ability to engage) that match to its five aspects of health services. The ability to perceive the need for health care is affected by people's beliefs about health and illness and their level of health literacy. The ability to seek health services includes patients' knowledge about options for services, their autonomy, and whether they face discrimination in the receipt of services. The ability to reach includes patients' ability to physically reach health service providers and is determined by whether they have restricted physical mobility, the ability to access transportation to services, and have the flexibility from work to easily access health services. The ability to pay for health services includes patients' ability to generate enough financial resources to afford to pay for health services or whether they have insurance or another mechanism that subsidises their ability to pay for such services. Finally, the ability to engage with health services includes patients' ability to participate and be involved in the decision making about the treatment and services they receive.

While not explicitly referred to in the articulation of the patient-centered model, the focus on abilities of people is consistent with Amartya Sen's concept of the capability approach, which argues that people's freedom to achieve better well-being is determined in part by their abilities to convert resources into valuable functionings (Sen, 1999). Thus, models of health service utilization and barriers that only focus on means (characteristics of health services or health systems) without considering what people can do with those means are insufficient to explain the complex phenomena of the use of health services and the barriers that can exist to receive such services.

Use of Utilization Models

At their earlier conceptualizations of the behavioral model, Aday and Andersen (1974) theorized the model more as a political than an operational idea, i.e., as an organizing framework to help understand the variables that affect service utilization and the barriers to such services. Applications of the behavioral model to broad policy work have also been the ways that the IOM and 5A models have been utilized. Some of the concepts from these models have become particularly important in policy discussions such as customary sources of care, continuity of care, delays in obtaining care, and gaps in insurance coverage. There have been empirical tests of these models, often limited to piece-meal tests of the magnitude and strength of associations between the variables and access and health services utilization.

These concepts from these models as well as improved measures of service use outcomes, such as preventive care, patient satisfaction, and general health status, have become routinely incorporated in key population-based health surveys. These surveys have generally been influential in high-income countries, and, principally, in the United States. Eden (1998), Gold (1998) and, more recently, Andersen (2008) detail the major surveys used in the United States that incorporate the constructs of the various general framework HSU-type models, many of which are sponsored by the US federal government. These include the Behavioral Risk Factor Surveillance Survey (BRFSS), the Medical Expenditure Panel Survey (MEPS), and the National Health Interview Survey (NHIS).

Another use of health care utilization model constructs in the United States has been the development of indices to measure the community's access to health care. For example, the System Response Ratio (SRR) and the Use Disability Ratio (UDR) have been used to identify US Federal Health Profession Shortage Areas (HPSA) and Medically Underserved Areas (MUAs) and to evaluate the impact of programs designed to advance access to primary care services (Ricketts & Goldsmith, 2005). Allin, Masseria, Sorenson et al. (2007) describe similar indices developed for use in European countries and the regional surveys in which they are incorporated.

The models derived from the perspective of "fit" approach have more recently been the driving force for studies done to investigate utilization and barriers to service for primary care in Australia (Ward, Humphreys, McGrail et al., 2015). They have been used to conduct cross-national comparisons of primary care between Australia and Commonwealth countries (Corscadden, Levesque, Lewis et al., 2017), outpatient specialist care for chronic illness (Fradgley, Paul, & Bryant, 2015), use of health services for Indigenous people across countries (Davy, Harfield, McArthur et al., 2016) and native peoples in Australia (Bailie, Schierhout, Laycock et al., 2015), and services for people with disabilities in rural areas (Dassah, Aldersey, McColl et al., 2018).

In the study that investigated the use and barriers to primary care in Australia, the researchers used a brief questionnaire to assess four of the 5A dimensions. Community respondents were asked through paired comparisons to rank which of the dimensions were more important given their situation. The studies that looked at determinants of health service use among people living in British Commonwealth countries and among Indigenous Peoples in Australia used the dimensions of the patient-centered model to guide their analysis of secondary data that had been collected by third parties. In the study that examined the use of specialist chronic illness services in high-income countries, the researchers used the concepts from the patient-centered model to conduct a literature synthesis. The literature synthesis revealed the important determinants of chronic illness services. A similar approach was used in Davy, Harfield, McArthur et al.'s (2016) study of primary care service utilization among Indigenous people in seven countries, including two in South America and Papua New Guinea. In their study, Dassah, Aldersey, McColl et al. (2018) assessed the concept of fit but did not focus on one particular HSU model to guide their literature synthesis of factors affecting people with disabilities who live in rural areas. Interestingly, of the 36 studies that were part of the literature synthesis, the majority (26) were conducted in low- and middle-income countries.

Most of the earlier applications of health service utilization models have been limited to studies conducted in high-income countries, but in more recent times the concepts and constructs in these models have been used to investigate service use in low- and

Table 20.1 Framework of interventions to address health service use and barriers in low- and middle-income countries

	Dimensions of Service Utilization and Barriers			
Types of Interventions	Geographical Accessibility	Availability	Affordability	Acceptability
Non-monetary	Outreach services	Counseling and information	Regulation	Counseling and information
	Maternity waiting homes	Peripheral health units		Culturally sensitive care
	Emergency transport	Social marketing		Social marketing
		Deconcentration		Deconcentration
		Accreditation		
	Improved management, including supervision, and feedback mechanisms			
	Community participation, community-based interventions, provision of essential services			
Monetary	Community loan funds		Community loan funds	
			Health insurance subsidies, prepayment schemes	
			Abolishment of fees	
	Needs-based financing			
	Contracting, conditional cash transfers, health equity funds, pay for performance, vouchers			

Adapted from Jacobs, Por, Maryam et al. (2012)

middle-income countries. Similar to the focus in high-income countries, studies conducted in low-income countries have used hybrid-type models to inform surveys on health service utilization. Jacobs, Por, Maryam et al. (2012) have articulated an analytic framework to help researchers and practitioners from low- and middle-income (LMI) countries select monetary and non-monetary interventions to improve access to and use of health services. Jacobs and colleagues used four of the dimensions of the 5A model to further categorize interventions. Table 20.1 is an adaptation of the framework used by Jacobs, Por, Maryam et al. (2012) to identify barriers to access and service use in the districts of Kirivong and Kampon Cham in Cambodia in the context of geographical accessibility, availability, affordability, and acceptability.

Thus, in a general sense, the identification of the usual source of care and continuity of care factors in high-income countries has highlighted the need to create systems that ensure that populations have access to reliable health care in LMI countries. The result has been greater advocacy and funding support by international development organizations toward universal health insurance or in other cases support for microfinancing schemes for health services. In 2005, the World Health Organization member states endorsed a resolution to provide universal coverage defined "as access for all to appropriate promotive, preventive, curative and rehabilitative services at an affordable cost" (Jacobs, Por, Maryam et al., 2012: 288). The World Bank and other development finance organizations have in turn provided technical support and funding to help LMI countries provide universal coverage as their resources allow. The results have been a proliferation of initiatives in LMI countries, with Jacobs, Por, Maryam et al. (2012) using the concepts of HSU models, and particularly those of the 5A model, to develop an analytic framework to help LMI countries select both monetary and non-monetary interventions to improve access to and use of health services.

Box 20.1 The Economic Impact of COVID-19

JEAN-PAUL L'HUILLIER

The emergence of the novel coronavirus SARS-CoV-2 in December 2019 (COVID-19) has drastically affected the normal functioning of human society, generating at the same time a massive disruption of economic activity. To illustrate the scale of the disruption, let us consider a few figures for the United States. By December 2019, the US had seen one of its longest macroeconomic expansions on record. Six months later, by June 2020, GDP had fallen 10%. To put this number in perspective, it is useful to recall that during the Great Recession GDP fell, *in total*, by 4%. Thus, the start of the recession caused by the "Great Lockdown" led to a much larger GDP loss. Moreover, at the time of writing, we have no data on the effects of the second wave of the pandemic. Looking at other macroeconomic variables, such as unemployment, aggregate investment, or trade volume, leads to similar conclusions.

Even though it is to some extent obvious that one should expect a large recession to ensue from any serious pandemic, it is still quite puzzling to observe the scale of the ongoing disruption. Thus, a key question for macroeconomic research is, simply: Why such a large effect? One way to shed light on this question is by comparison to the recession induced by the 1918–1920 Great Influenza Pandemic or "Spanish Flu". According to Barro, Ursua, and Weng (2020), a cross-national study indicates that the typical country suffered a total economic decline of GDP of 6%, with a total death toll of around 2% of world population. It is still early to conclude, but assuming an infection fatality ratio below 2% for COVID-19 (Brazeau et al., 2020), this suggests that either societies have decided to put in place tougher lockdown policies with an eye toward the protection of human lives (and larger economic costs), or that individuals are this time more aware of the dangers of the disease and exercised greater prudence.

Thankfully, and with some variation from county to country, this unprecedented crisis has overall been met by bold economic policies. In this regard, the United States has once again provided an example of unprecedented pragmatism. On the fiscal end, the US Congress enacted the Coronavirus Aid, Relief, and Economic Security (CARES) Act, a multidimensional economic stimulus package targeted at providing emergency assistance to households and business. Allocating $2.2 trillion to this end (or 10% of GDP), it is the largest stimulus package in US history.

On the monetary end, the Federal Reserve, an institution characterized by much restraint in recent years, has been unusually creative by engaging in emergency lending programs in favor of a range of businesses, and by revising its notion of longer-run goals and monetary policy strategy.

An interesting theoretical question that arises in light of the economic shock generated by the pandemic is whether it should be considered an aggregate demand or aggregate supply shortfall? This is a difficult question, because at face value the pandemic has affected both the demand and supply side of the economy. On the demand side, people remaining at home means, for many sectors such as the hospitality industry a loss of revenue. On the supply side, people remaining at home also means that close-contact or physical labor-intensive production is operationally affected, generating a lower supply of goods and services.

This question is important for policy purposes, because a fall in supply is typically associated with another evil, a rise of inflation. This was the case in the two recessions that hit in the 1970s, leading to "stagflation." Instead, a fall in demand leads to a fall in inflation, opening up room for government policy targeted at providing a boost without sacrificing price stability. The evidence thus far strongly speaks in favor of a stronger demand shortfall, mainly due to an observed fall of inflation and a massive rise of unemployment. A recent paper by Guerrieri, Lorenzoni, Straub, and Werning (2020) provides an elegant explanation: supply downfalls in sectors of the economy can propagate as *demand* shortfalls in the rest of the economy, as workers in the affected sectors adjust their overall spending. As explained, the evolution of key indicators after the start of the pandemic give credence to this theory.

I conclude with a very brief discussion of possible long-term effects. By now, it is clear that the pandemic will have marked structural effects as people have adjusted their behavior to a prolonged lockdown. For instance, it is now clear that telework or teleconferencing is not only feasible, but it also has desirable features. A silver lining of the pandemic is that this may accelerate technological change and raise productivity. However, these gains will not be shared equally. Contact-dependent firms and the hospitality industry will continue to suffer from this structural change, and workers who are not able to adjust to these new technologies will be left behind. Thus, we certainly should expect a recovery, but, unfortunately, a recovery toward a different economy, and one featuring higher inequality.

(Continued)

(Continued)

REFERENCES

Barro, Robert J., José F. Ursúa, and Joanna Weng (2020). *The corona virus and the Great Influenza Pandemic: Lessons from the "Spanish Flu" for the corona virus's potential effects on mortality and economic activity*. Working Paper 26866. Cambridge, MA: National Bureau of Economic Research.

Brazeau, Nicholas F., Robert Verity, Sara Jenks, Han Fu, Charles Wittaker, Peter Winskill, Ilaria Dorigatti, Patric Walker, Steven Riley, Ricardo P. Schekenberg, Henrique Hoeltgebaum, Thomas A. Mellan, Swapnil Mishra, H. Juliette T. Unwin, Oliver J. Watson, Zulma M. Cucunubá, Marc Baguelin, Lilith Whittles, Samir Bhatt, Azra C. Ghani, Neil M. Ferguson, and Lucy C. Okell (2020). *Report 34: COVID-19 infection fatality ratio: Estimates from seroprevalence*. London: Imperial College London.

Guerrieri, Veronica, Guido Lorenzoni, Ludwig Straub, and Iván Werning (2020). *Macroeconomic implications of COVID-19: Can negative supply shocks cause demand shortages?* Working paper 26918. Cambridge, MA: National Bureau of Economic Research.

PROBLEMS AND FUTURE WORK

The sociological, psychological, and institutional models of health care utilization had shortcomings because of the limited focus on specific factors without taking into account the broad array of individual and non-individual factors that affect health care access and utilization. Some of these shortcomings were addressed in the Andersen behavioral model, which included a broad range of variables thought to be important to explain access and utilization of health services. Over the years that followed, this model has indeed grown to dominate the field and has helped scholars organize constructs associated with health service access and use. However, much of the empirical research using this model has taken a static linear approach and have not considered the importance of feedback and interaction among variables. In fact, in later versions, the model is envisaged to serve as a learning framework. Most studies using the Anderson behavioral model have tended to use earlier versions of the model. Even with its simplified focus, the application of the Andersen behavior model in health services research has not been without its problems.

Inconsistencies in Study Variables

Babitsch, Gohl, and Lengerke (2012), in a systematic review of 16 studies using the Andersen behavioral model published between 1998 and 2011, found that most studies (13 of 16) were based on secondary data, with inconsistencies in operationalization and the mis-categorization of key variables, e.g., predisposing, enabling or need. For example, neighborhood socioeconomic status was a predisposing factor affecting the demand for services and in other studies it was an enabling factor in association between individual, community income and demand for services. In some studies, age and sex were classified as individual predisposing variables, but then in other studies they served as proxies of need given their association with morbidity.

Identifying Strongest Variables and Effect Sizes

Because of the methodological challenges in extant studies, it is not possible to identify the variables that have the strongest effects on access and utilization of health services. This stems from the fact that complex multivariate statistical methods are not regularly employed, which makes it difficult to control for the effects of confounding factors and to assess the richness of the relationships among variables. Future research would benefit from studies like that of Graham, Hasking, Brooker et al. (2017) that used structural equation modeling techniques to assess the relevance of the Anderson behavioral model to understanding the use of mental health services among Australians who were depressed. In that analysis, it was possible to identify that need factors and social connectedness were the strongest predictors of mental health service utilization. Future work would also benefit from meta-analytic studies that would aggregate the effect sizes across studies on factors associated with health service use. When conducting meta-analysis, researchers should be cognizant that sometimes variables used in studies using the Andersen behavioral model or other HSU models may be specific to the populations being studied (e.g., immigration populations) or specific services such as applications to those seeking mental health or HIV/AIDS services. Indeed, this was part of the reasoning for restricting the systematic review by Babitsch, Gohl, and Lengerke (2012) to studies that dealt with general populations and common services to allow for easier comparison among the associations between factors and health service use.

A Better Study of Macro Variables

Although the Andersen behavior model and other HSU models do posit that health care utilization is determined by societal, contextual, and individual factors, many of the past empirical investigations have tended to focus on individual factors. In cases where macro variables are used, they are often limited to quite broad and unsophisticated measures that do not provide much insight into which variables are most important and consistent in impacting health service utilization. This is partly due to the lack of a clear framework about how macro factors relate to each other and the health system and then in turn impact health services utilization. Derose, Gresenz, and Ringel (2011) highlighted this limitation in their work and have suggested a framework that incorporates macro variables of the social and economic environment along with functions of the public health system to better account for health service access and utilization. The public health functions suggested for study included assurance, assessment, and policy development. Future research would benefit from refinements and elaborations of this initial framework and, most importantly, empirical testing of the framework to validate the nature and degree that such macro variables affect health service utilization.

Variety of HSU Types and Modes

Although recent work on models of health service utilization have included variables relevant for immigrants (Yang & Hwang, 2016), those with mental health concerns (Graham, Hasking, Brooker et al., 2017), adolescents (Ezinwanne, 2016), and the LGBT community (Martos, Fingerhut, Wilson, & Meyer, 2019), more work needs to be done to test how well these models/frameworks explain the unique service use of these specific populations. Nevertheless, this work does show a growing recognition that there is a diversity of users for different types of services. It should be noted that service use is not just about individuals having needs for which they then access services or experience barriers to accessing services. Rather, individuals have a variety of opportunities to react to their needs or perceived risks. In some cases, depending on the level of trust that individuals have in the health system or their experience with health care providers, they may or may not utilize health services. For example, a study by Blanchard and Lurie (2004) indicated that people who felt disrespected by caregivers were more likely to avoid seeking health care in the future. In some instances, having a perceived need or feeling at risk for one's health can lead to overuse of the health system rather than underuse. Ellen, Wilson, Vélez et al. (2018) highlighted studies from high-income countries that report that between 20% and 33% of patients receive treatments and or services that the best evidence suggests are potentially harmful or at the very least unnecessary or ineffective. In addition, seeking and use of health services may not only be driven by overt need or perceived risk. The authors found that some individuals in high-income countries undertake the use of health services to simply maintain their health and not because they see themselves as being susceptible to a specific disease.

It would seem that health service utilization models/frameworks that describe the factors that motivate individuals to seek health care are likely to be different from traditional models based on people believing themselves to be at risk which cue or motivate them to seek care. Additionally, newer models of health service utilization should consider the changing nature and modes by which people connect with health care and use health services. In particular, models are needed that incorporate the use of social media for the seeking of health information and online methods to consult with providers and even access products such as prescriptions. This has taken on added significance given the COVID-19 pandemic and the need for social distancing, which has resulted in the proliferating use of telemedicine for the facilitation of a variety of health services. This enhanced use of telemedicine and other online methods has accelerated forces that were already beginning to take hold and are likely to continue even after the end of the pandemic. Thus, models of health service utilization will need to take into consideration how differing service delivery methods affect patterns of health service use.

HSU as Empowerment

Structural equation modeling studies like that by Graham, Hasking, Brooker et al. (2017) remind us that the relationship among factors affecting health service use is dynamic and likely to involve significant adaptation, learning and feedback. Indeed, this is why the concept of fit and the models derived from the concept of fit present the prospect of better understanding the nature of those relationships. However, the nature of fit and how it is to be measured remains undeveloped in the literature. As previously described, Penchansky and Thomas (1981) proposed fit to be the interaction between the individual's needs and the health care system's ability to meet those needs. Fit was conceptualized as the match between three system-type variables – availability, accessibility and accommodation – and two individual-level variables – affordability and acceptability. Julio Frenk (1992), in his writings, adopted Avedis Donabedian's concept of "fit" (Donabedian, 1972), which referred to the match between the population and the health delivery system, and also highlighted the contrast between the constructs of availability and accessibility to health care systems. Frenk added a third construct, that of resistance, which was conceptualized as the various obstacles that stand in the way of individuals seeking and obtaining health care. He also discussed the utilization power of community members, which was conceptualized as the broadening of the construct of affordability. Levesque, Harris, and Russell (2013), in perhaps the most comprehensive conceptualization of fit to date, described it as the interaction between the five dimensions of the health system (which included the three proposed by Penchansky and Thomas (1981) and the dimensions of approachability and appropriateness) and the five corresponding abilities of individual patients (i.e., the ability to perceive the need for care, the ability to seek care, the ability to reach health services, their ability to pay for health services, and their ability to engage with health service providers). Unfortunately, the operationalization of Levesque et al.'s concept of fit has mainly focused on assessing the five dimensions of the health system.

It should be noted that the concept of fit in the research on health service use has to date shown three significant limitations. First, many studies have focused only on specific components of the health system, e.g., how financing mechanisms affect service use recommendations, policy responses to service delivery, service financing type interventions, etc. This approach has resulted in a lack of recognition of the variations in the levels of use, types of use, underuse, or even overuse of health services. Second, frameworks and models developed to study health service use have neglected to consider the interaction between the health system and the individuals who use the system. Third, by not considering the individuals and their lived experiences as they interact with the health system, researchers have failed to acknowledge the capabilities and capacities of individuals. In so doing, they miss the opportunity to see health service use as involving the capacity to empower individuals and to reinforce their rights and responsibilities as it concerns access to health services.

The abilities of individuals and the dynamic interaction of the fit between these abilities and the health system relate well to Amartya Sen's human capability approach (Sen, 1999). Sen outlines two concerns in this regard. The first concern is that individuals vary in their abilities to convert available resources into useful actions, such as the best ways to utilize available health services. For example, pregnant women have specific nutritional requirements unique to their circumstances to improve their health. With this in mind, it is not sufficient to focus only on expanding the means of acquiring health services, but also consider that different people may need different things from the services available to them. The second concern is that individuals living in harsh and difficult environments may not desire to attain goals that are not realistic. Referred to as "adaptive preferences," Sen suggests that impoverished communities where people are clearly in need of health care may state that they have no need for health services and that their health is fine. On the basis of these and other concerns, Sen highlights the impact of variations in the personal circumstances of individuals and associated capabilities on their "effective freedom." The result is that people often have to choose between available options which may not be the most optimal. When considered from this perspective "freedom" represents the empowerment of an individual to use health services based on the social possibilities (e.g., material, human or social resources) available to them and their agency as represented by their abilities and capacities. Adopting this approach means that it is not sufficient for policy makers to make things available to people, but in addition, they need to actively empower individuals to use those services. This would require a participatory process involving the exchange of information between decision makers at various levels on the one hand and members of the local community on the other. Thus, for example, it would not be sufficient for policy makers to think about health service access and use in terms of location as measured by provider–population ratios. Merely locating providers in a community does not necessarily ensure community members with needs are empowered to receive the services offered by those providers (Wolf & Aron, 2013).

The focus on human capabilities and the five individual abilities proposed in the Levesque et al. (2013) model highlight the potential for health service utilization research to align with the commitment of the global health community and the United Nations (UN) system to taking a human rights-based approach to improving health and empowering marginalized communities to access and use health services (Thomas & Magar, 2018). The United Nations was born out of the Universal Declaration of Human Rights, and over the years the UN and its major agency responsible for health, the World Health Organization, have sought to mainstream a human rights perspective into its operations and how policies and service delivery are implemented. A rights-based approach to health of necessity requires a focus on the abilities and capacities of individuals and communities to make the best use of health services (Marks, 2018). It would seem that the most fruitful advancement of health services utilization research would be to further develop how the interaction of human capabilities and abilities with features of the health system can be better used to improve the delivery of health services to individuals and communities in ways that empower them to take charge of their health and the attendant use of services. Doing this could enhance individuals' and communities' rights to claim services due to them by those who have governance over them and the health systems within which they live.

CONCLUSION

A brief search on almost any research database will reveal a significant number of journal articles and publications on the topic of health services use, access, and barriers to service use. The result is a "zoo" of factors that have been proposed and then in lesser cases empirically assessed. These factors in turn are derived from a multiplicity of health service use models and frameworks. To help the reader gain a more insightful understanding of the field, we described the rationale and features of some of the key HSU models prominent in the literature. We identified contradictions and limitations with the models and outlined how earlier models have contributed to the development of more sophisticated hybrid-type models. In the process, we outlined the key factors espoused by the various models. We then discussed how the various models have been used, and identified that, in the past, they were largely deployed in high-income countries and used as guides to identify variables for use in population surveys. Also, in high-income countries constructs arising from health services utilization have led to the development of measures and indices to help evaluate the outcomes of policies geared to addressing inequalities in health service use. The interest of international organizations such as the World Health Organization and the World Bank in the concept of "health for all" has spurred demonstration projects and research around expanding health insurance to low- and middle-income populations and its attendant enhancement in the use of health services. Interventions to address barriers to health service use have followed. We highlighted a useful example of a framework developed by Jacobs and colleagues (2012), identifying the types of interventions that are possible relative to various dimensions of health service use in developing countries. Finally, we outlined some of the critical issues with how HSU models have been studied and reported in the literature and sought to suggest how the various models might be reconciled and perhaps even unified. We argue that the best prospect for doing so would be the recent patient-centered model articulated by Levesque, Harris, and Russell (2013). Not only does that model seek to synthesize various models into a patient-centered approach, but it has the real potential to foster an approach that sees health services use in the lens of empowerment of individuals and communities. Moreover, this approach would be consistent with recent efforts by Amartya Sen and others to situate human functioning, including health service use, in the context of enhancing individuals' capabilities as entities with a right to health care and health services.

REFERENCES

Aday, L.A., & Andersen, R. (1974). A framework for the study of access to medical care. *Health Services Research*, 9, 208–220.

Allin, S., Masseria, C., Sorenson, C., Papanicolas, I., & Mossialos, E (2007). *Measuring inequalities in access to health care: A review of the indices?* European Commission, Brussels, Belgium. Research Note. London, London School of Economics.

Andersen, R.M. (1995). Revisiting the behavioral model and access to medical care: Does it matter? *Journal of Health and Social Behavior*, *36*, 1–10. doi: 10.2307/2137284.

Andersen, R.M. (2008). National health surveys and the behavioral model of health services use. *Medical Care, 46*, 647–653. doi: 10.1097/MLR.0b013e31817a835d.

Andersen, R.M., & Davidson, P.L. (2007). *Improving access to care in America: Individual and contextual indicators.* In R.M. Andersen, T.H. Rice, & G.F. Kominski (Eds.), *Changing the US health care system: Key issues in health services policy and management* (pp. 3–30). San Francisco, CA: Jossey-Bass.

Andersen, R.M., & Newman, J. (1973). Societal and individual determinants of medical care utilization in the United States. *Milbank Memorial Fund Quarterly Health and Society, 51*, 95–124. doi: 10.2307/3349613.

Babitsch B., Gohl, D., & von Lengerke, T. (2012). Re-revisiting Andersen's behavioral model of health services use: A systematic review of studies from 1998–2011. *Psychosocial Medicine, 9*. Doc. 11. doi:10.3205/psm000089.

Bailie, J., Schierhout, G., Laycock, A., Kelaher, M., Percival, N., O'Donoghue, L., McNeair, T., & Baille, R. (2015). Determinants of access to chronic illness care: A mixed-methods evaluation of a national multifaceted chronic disease package for Indigenous Australians. *The BMJ Open*, 5. http://dx.doi.org/10.1136/bmjopen-2015-008103.

Blanchard, J., & Lurie, N. (2004). R-E-S-P-E-C-T: Patient reports of disrespect in the health care setting and its impact on care. *Journal of Family Practice, 53*, 721–730.

Carrillo, J.E., Carrillo, V.A., Perez, H.R., Salas-Lopez, D., Natale-Pereira, A., & Byron, A.T. (2011). Defining and targeting health care access barriers. *Journal of Health Care for the Poor and Underserved, 22*, 562–575.

Corscadden, L., Levesque, J.F., Lewis, V., Breton, N., Sutherland, K., Weenink, J.W., Haggerty, J., & Russell, G. (2017). Barriers to accessing primary health care: Comparing Australian experiences internationally. *Australian Journal of Primary Health, 23*, 223–228. doi: 10.1071/py16093.

Dassah, E., Aldersey, H., McColl, M.A., & Davison, C. (2018). Factors affecting access to primary health care services for persons with disabilities in rural areas: A 'best-fit' framework synthesis. *Global Health Research and Policy, 3*, 36. doi:10.1186/s41256-018-0091-x.

Davy, C., Harfield, S., McArthur, A., Zachary, M., & Brown, A. (2016). Access to primary health care services for Indigenous peoples: A framework synthesis. *International Journal for Equity in Health, 15*, 1–9. doi:10.1186/s12939-016-0450-5.

Derose, K.P., Gresenz, C., & Ringel, J. (2011). Understanding disparities in health care access – and reducing them – through a focus on public health. *Health Affairs, 30*, 1844–1851.doi:10.1377/hlthaff.2011.0644.

Donabedian, A. (1972). Models for organizing the delivery of personal health services and criteria for evaluating them. *Milbank Memorial Fund Quarterly, 50*, 103–154.

Eden, J. (1998). Measuring access to care through population-based surveys: Where are we now? *Health Services Research, 33*, 685–708.

Ellen, M.E., Wilson, M.G., Vélez, M., Shach, R., Lavis, N.J., Grimshaw, M.J., & Moat, A.K. (2018). Addressing overuse of health services in health systems: A critical interpretive synthesis. *Health Research Policy and Systems, 16*, 48. doi:10.1186/s12961-018-0325-x.

Ezinwanne, C.A. (2016). Using Anderson's model of health service utilization to examine use of services by adolescent girls in south-eastern Nigeria. *International Journal of Adolescence and Youth, 21*(4), 523–529. https://doi.org/10.1080/02673843.2015.1124790.

Fradgley, E.A., Paul, C.L., & Bryant, J. (2015). A systematic review of barriers to optimal outpatient specialist services for individuals with prevalent chronic diseases: What are the unique and common barriers experienced by patients in high income countries? *International Journal of Equity in Health,* 14(52), 9 June. doi:10.1186/s12939-015-0179-6.

Frenk, J. (1992). The concept and measurement of accessibility. In K.L. White (Ed.), *Health services research: An anthology* (pp. 842–855). (Scientific Publication No. 534). Washington, DC: Pan American Health Organization.

Gibson, G. (1972). Explanatory models and strategies for social change in health care behavior. *Social Science and Medicine, 6*, 635–639.

Gold, M. (1998). Beyond coverage and supply: Measuring access to healthcare in today's market. *Health Services Research, 33*, 625–652.

Graham, A., Hasking, P., Brooker, J., Clarke, D., & Meadows, G. (2017). Mental health service use among those with depression: An exploration using Andersen's behavioral model of health service use. *Journal of Affective Disorders, 208*, 170–176. doi:10.1016/j.jad.2016.08.074.

Jacobs, B., Por, I., Maryam, B., Annear, L.P., & Van Damme, W. (2012). Addressing access barriers to health services: An analytical framework for selecting appropriate interventions in low-income Asian countries. *Health Policy and Planning, 27*, 288–300. doi:10.1093/heapol/czr038.

Levesque, J.-F., Harris, M.F., & Russell, G. (2013). Patient-centered access to health care: Conceptualising access at the interface of health systems and populations. *International Journal for Equity in Health, 12*(18). doi:10.1186/1475-9276-12-18.

Marks, S.P. (2018). Integrating a human-rights based approach to development and the right to development into global governance for health. In B.M. Meier & L.O. Gostin (Eds.), *Human rights in global health: Rights based governance for a globalizing world*. New York: Oxford University Press. doi: 10.1093/oso/9780190672676.003.0016.

Martos, A.J., Fingerhut, A., Wilson, P.A., & Meyer, I.H. (2019). Utilization of LGBT-specific clinics and providers across three cohorts of lesbian, gay, and bisexual people in the United States. *SSM-Population Health, 9*, 100505. doi:10.1016/j.ssmph.2019.100505.

Mechanic, D. (1968). *Medical sociology*. New York: Free Press.

Mechanic, D. (1978). *Medical sociology: A comprehensive text* (2nd ed.). New York: Free Press.

Millman, M. (1993). *Access to health care in America*. Washington, DC: National Academies Press, Institute of Medicine.

Parsons, T. (1951). *The social system*. London: Routledge.

Penchansky, R., & Thomas, J.W. (1981). The concept of access: Definition and relationship to consumer satisfaction. *Medical Care, 19*, 127–140.

Ricketts, T.C., & Goldsmith, L.J. (2005). Access in health services research: The battle of the frameworks. *Nursing Outlook, 53*, 274–280.

Rosenstock, I. (1966). Why people use health services. *Milbank Memorial Fund Quarterly, 83*, 1–32.

Rosenstock, I. (1974). Historical origins of the Health Belief Model. *Health Education & Behavior, 2*, 328–335.

Rosenstock, I., Derryberry, M., & Carriger, B. (1959). Why people fail to seek poliomyelitis vaccination. *Public Health Reports, 74*, 98–103.

Rosenstock, I., Strecher, V.J., & Becker, M.H. (1988). Social learning theory and the Health Belief Model. *Health Education Quarterly, 15*, 175–183.

Sen, A. (1999). *Development as freedom*. Oxford: Oxford University Press.

Suchman, E. (1965). Social patterns of illness and medical care. *Journal of Health and Human Behavior, 6*, 114–128.

Stoeckle, J., Zola, I.K., & Davidson, G.E. (1963). Ongoing to see the doctor: The contributions of the patient to the decision to seek medical aid. *Journal of Chronic Diseases, 16*, 975–989.

Thomas, R., & Magar, V. (2018). Mainstreaming human rights across WHO. In B.M. Meier & L.O. Gostin (Eds.), *Human rights in global health: Rights based governance for a globalizing world*. New York: Oxford University Press.

Ward, B.M., Humphreys, J.S., McGrail, M.R., Wakerman, J., & Chisholm, M. (2015). Which dimensions of access are most important when rural residents decide to visit a general practitioner for non-emergency care? *Australian Health Review, 39*, 121–126. doi.org/10.1071/AH14030.

Woolf, S.H., & Aron, L. (Eds.) (2013). *US health in international perspective: Shorter lives, poorer health*. Washington, DC: National Academies Press.

Yang, P.Q., & Hwang, S.H. (2016). Explaining immigrant health service utilization: A theoretical framework. *SAGE Open, 6*, 2. doi.org/10.1177/2158244016648137.

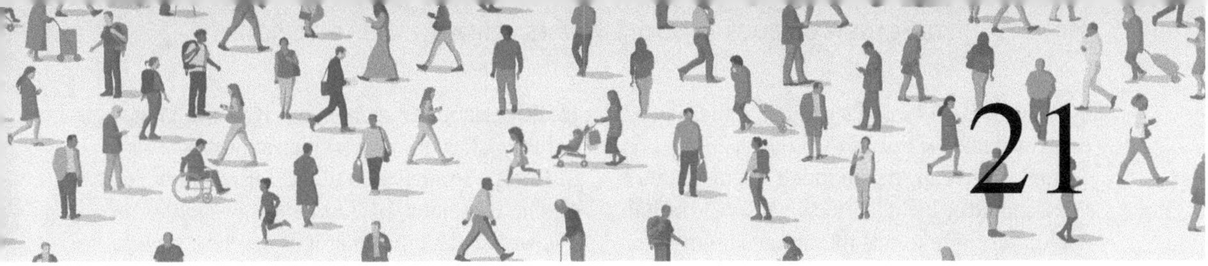

21

Measuring Health and Health Related Quality of Life

Manu Raj Mathur and Deepti Nagrath

EVOLVING DEFINITION OF HEALTH: THE JOURNEY SO FAR

This chapter focuses on definitions of health and methods for the assessment of health since the mid-1940s, after the conclusion of World War II. The chapters in this volume on "The Social Causation of Health and Illness" by Johannes Siegrist, on "The History of the Changing Concepts of Health and Illness" by Bryan Turner, and on "Cultural Variation in the Experience of Health and Illness" by Pamela Erickson and Cynthia Frank provide detailed reviews and analyses of the evolution of health throughout human history as a community responsibility, going beyond individual interests, and thus complement the discussion in this chapter.

The first director-general of the World Health Organization (WHO), Brock Chisholm (1948–1953), contributed to the definition of health included in the WHO Constitution that "we have responsibility for social health, for being able to live in peace and contributing to the welfare of other people. The social responsibility of the individual has never been recognized before on such a wide international basis" (Larson 1996, 181). Chisholm also said that "a new kind of citizen is necessary if the human race is going to survive" (Larson 1996, 181). Hinkle (1961) objected to this definition and argued that an absence of a disease and/or symptoms is not a strong indicator for health. Hinkle argued that "the most healthy people in our society nearly always have dental caries, sometimes have colds, sometimes have accidents, sometimes become anxious or depressed, [and] not infrequently experience an elevated blood pressure or become obese" (Hinkle 1961, 290).

The WHO definition helped shape the thinking around health in the Declaration of Alma-Ata, which led to the focus on Primary Health Care (PHC) as an approach to strengthening health systems. However, Alma-Ata was criticized for being utopian and unrealistic, with Walsh and Warren (1980) highlighting the drawbacks of the declaration of Alma-Ata. Primary health care's expansive but somewhat vague goal, exemplified by its slogan "health for all by the year 2000," made it difficult for researchers to evaluate the results (Marahatta 2010). For example, how can "health for all" be measured? What should be included and what should be left out? In response to this measurement problem, Walsh and Warren put forward the idea of selective primary health, focusing on the elements of primary care that had the strongest association with decreasing infant and child mortality. This shift from global, but somewhat poorly specified, primary care to targeted approaches to decreasing child death attracted strong backing from the academia, donors and agencies. The authors suggested interventions known as GOBI (Growth monitoring, Oral rehydration, Breastfeeding, and Immunization), which led to an inconclusive debate between the supporters of comprehensive primary health care and selective primary health care. These discussions lingered throughout 1980s. In the early 1990s, WHO primary health care proponents acknowledged that health for all would not be achieved by 2000. It was against this background that the World Bank's *World Development Report* of 1993, *Investing in Health*, was published (Klouda 1994). The WHO definition was further examined. They noted that many definitions around health did not allow for the measurement of the social causes of diseases, and the concepts proposed often overlooked the importance of social and cultural concepts of family, beliefs, traditions and customs. In 2014, Frenk and Gómez-Dantés proposed that "given the complex and dynamic nature of health, we cannot aim to generate a once-and-for-all agreement on its precise meaning. Instead, let us work to develop a general framework to guide further explorations to identify and measure the complex components and determinants of that elusive aspiration we call health" (Frenk and Gómez-Danté 2014, 401).

HEALTH MEASUREMENT: THE BEGINNING

> Epidemiology is, therefore, not only a bio-science but is also a social science. (Raj 2016, 6)

Health calamities such as the Bubonic Plague or "Black Death," which killed almost one-third of Europe's population in the 14th century, led to the formation of *Lazarettos* or *houses of quarantine*, and the control of markets, sewage systems, and water supplies. Forming boards of physicians and controlling the activities of beggars and prostitutes were some of the earliest public health measures globally (Rhodes and Bryant 2020). In 1546 Girolamo Fracastoro, published *De contagione et contagiosis morbis* (*On Contagions and the Cure of Contagious Diseases*), more popularly known as *Theory of Contagion* (Fracastoro 1546; Nutton 1990). Fracastoro proposed that many diseases are caused by agents called "*germs*" (seminaria), which propagate themselves in tissues of the infected host and cause disease by setting up chemical processes and are spread by direct or indirect transmission. An outbreak of smallpox in the 16th century was crucial in leading to the three most important contributions in public health, namely: the organization of panels of health, the promulgation of a theory of contagion, and the introduction of health statistics (Rhodes and Bryant 2020).

In 1662, John Graunt was the first to employ quantitative methods, describing in *Nature and Political Observations Made Upon the Bills of Mortality* a population's vital statistics (Britannica 2020). The rural shift to urban settings that accelerated in the 1700s created the conditions for the rapid spread of infectious diseases through communities. Crowded, unhygienic conditions and long hours of work in unsafe industries contributed to outbreaks of cholera, smallpox, typhoid, tuberculosis and yellow fever. However, several key discoveries were made during this period. Significant contributions to the measurement of health were made by Johann Peter Frank, *System of a Complete Medical Policy*, Jeremy Bentham, *Introduction to the Principles of Morals and Legislation, Constitutional Code* (Spector 1963), Edwin Chadwick, *General Report on the Sanitary Condition of the Labouring Population of Great Britain* (Small 2020), and Pierre Charles Louis, a French physician, who was recognised for introducing the use of the numerical method in the field of medicine. In 1884, Robert Koch developed four postulates that further guided the understanding of infectious agents and diseases (Ross and Woodward 2016).

Social science has a long history of measurement. It can be traced back to Pierre Guillaume Frédéric Le Play (1806–82), who is credited for introducing the idea of social surveys (Le Play 1982). The theory of measurements is also often credited to the social and behavioural scientists (Hand 1996). The foundations were laid with the Guttman scales, proposed in the 1950s and 1960s, a precursor to the currently used Item Response Theory (IRT) in behavioural sciences which proposes the development of items that measure various kind of abilities, traits and behavioural characteristics. However, it was Abraham Kaplan's (1964) *The Conduct of Inquiry: Methodology for Behavioral Science* which established foundational work in the field of research methods in 1964. More recently, classifications of measurements such as counts versus measurements, nominal, ordinal, numerical and dichotomous variables were reported by Van den Berg (see Van Manen and Van Manen 2021) in 1991. Nelder described various modes of data, distinguishing continuous counts, continuous ratios, count ratios (Nelder and Wedderburn 1972).

William Farr, an eminent figure in the field of measurement who identified himself as a statistician, laid the foundations for the future analytical models of medicine (Farr 2004). The distinctions between ratio and rates made by Farr continue to provide the basis for today's understanding. The Infant Mortality Rate (IMR) is an indicator of young mortality, which also correlates to socio-economic and environmental improvements. However, calculating rates has a major drawback in comparing subgroups of two or more populations. For example, age standardization allows a better comparison of rates, but it can sometimes be unreasonable to work with a large number of subgroups.

Box 21.1 Rates and measures

Rate

"A measure of the frequency of occurrence of a phenomenon. In epidemiology, demography, and vital statistics, a rate is an expression of the frequency with which an event occurs in a defined population, usually in a specified period of time." (Porta 2014, 239)

$$Rate = \frac{Number\ of\ Events\ in\ a\ Specific\ Period}{Average\ Population\ During\ the\ Period} \times 10^n$$

*For example: Death rate = (number of deaths in one year/mid-year population) *1000*

Ratio

"The value obtained by dividing one quantity by another." (Porta 2014, 240)

Mathematically, it is expressed as :- x: y or x/y

For example, a sex ratio compares proportions of males to females in a population.

Proportion

"A type of ratio in which the numerator is included in the denominator. The ratio of a part to the whole, expressed as a 'decimal fraction' (e.g., 0.2), as a 'common fraction' (1/5), or as a percentage (20%)." (Porta 2014, 229)

*Mathematically, for example, Number of deaths due to diarrhoea in a village/Total number of people in a village *100*

Source: Porta 2014

Epidemiologists seek the support of statisticians for quantitative analysis and other statistical testing. Epidemiologists and biostatisticians use mathematical models to study the measures of disease frequency in order to quantify the measurement of diseases in modern epidemiology. One such concept epidemiologists rely upon is incidence, defined as the number of new cases occurring in a defined population during a specified period of time. Another key measure is prevalence, which is referred specifically to all the current cases (old and new) existing at a given point in time. Doll and Hill estimated ratios from their case-control study, which was advanced by MacMahon et al. in their study "Studies of cases referable to a defined population" (Poole 2015; Schlesselman 2006). In modern epidemiology it is referred to as measures of effects. Odds ratio is used to summarize the link between exposures and outcomes and odds ratios are expressed in relative and absolute terms. The risk ratio is an extension of the concept, and estimates the magnitude of the effect of the exposure on the outcome. It tells us how many times higher or lower the disease risk is among the exposed as compared to the unexposed. It does not have a unit, and ranges from 0 to infinity. It is represented in a standard two by two frequency table similar to odds ratio.

An alternative way to compare occurrence of an outcome in the exposed and unexposed group is the measures of impact. It is based on difference between two measures of frequency and gives information on: the absolute effect of exposure on disease occurrence – the excess disease risk, or disease burden, in the exposed group compared to the unexposed group.

While the WHO definition stressed that health was not just the absence of disease, measurement of health in the early 20th century was predominantly focused on comparing disease occurrence in an exposed group to another group that was not exposed. Measures of occurrence of a disease (morbidity and mortality) were used for health service planning in epidemiology and/or public health.

HEALTH MEASUREMENT: THE 20TH CENTURY

> We have included almost 800 million deaths from 1950 to 2010, and the data came from different sources. The goal was to incorporate "all the available data." (Das and Samarasekera 2012, 628)

Box 21.2 Risk and odds ratios

Risk Ratio

"The ratio of two risks, usually of exposed and not exposed." (Porta 2014, 252)

$$\frac{\textit{Risk of Disease (Incidence Proportion, Attack Rate) in Group of Primary Interest}^{\circ}}{\textit{Risk of Disease (Incidence Proportion, Attack Rate) in Comparison Group}}$$

Odds Ratio

"(Syn: cross-product ratio, relative odds) The ratio of two odds." (Porta 2014, 205)

$$\frac{\textit{Odds of Exposure in Cases}}{\textit{Odds of Exposure in Control}}$$

Source: Porta 2014

The early 20th century saw a rise in public health programs, the development of schools of public health and a rise in philanthropic organizations. Health summary measures were reported at global, national and local levels in a population and formed the core of epidemiological measurements. They provided an overview of the population over a period of time and elaborated on community health, thus helping in identifying affected areas to plan preventive strategies. One such effort was the "The Global Burden of Diseases, Injuries, and Study" (GBD). GBD was an international collaborative effort to organize and publish health-related evidence at the global, regional, sub-regional, national and sub-national levels. It covered 310 diseases and injuries, 2,619 sequelae and 79 risk factors by age and sex globally from 1990 to 2017. The data were extracted by sex (male, female), the age range represented, country and measures (Arthur 2014). Researchers from a variety of disciplinary perspectives created new health metrics that incorporated physical and psychological morbidity and disability (DALYs: Disability Adjusted Life Years) in addition to mortality. DALYs were used in the first Global Burden of Diseases Study in the 1990s and in the World Development Report in 1993, and have evolved from being a rough estimator to an advanced summary measure of the local, regional, and global burden of diseases.

DALYs are used to measure the overall disease burden expressed as the number of years lost due to sickness, disability or early death. DALYs comprises of Years of Lost Life (YLL), which is calculated from the number of deaths at each age multiplied by the expected remaining years of life according to a global standard life expectancy. Years Lost to Disability (YLD) is calculated by the number of incident cases due to injury and illness multiplied by the average duration of the disease and a weighting factor reflecting the severity of the disease on a scale from 0 (perfect health) to 1 (deceased). Another most commonly used measure is HALE (Health Adjusted Life Expectancy), based on expectancy of life at birth with an adjustment for time spent in poor health. It is expressed as the number of years in full health that a new-born can expect to live depending on the current rates of ill-health and mortality. However, getting estimates of the total number of infections in the population due to a specific factor is difficult, so DALYs also fail to capture the subjective outcomes.

Therefore, social scientists often argue the measures of subjective well-being and/or happiness should supplement the usual measures of health. The National Happiness Index of Bhutan is one such measure of well-being.

Box 21.3 Measures of subjective well-being

DALY (Disability Adjusted Life Years) – it is a measure of overall disease burden expressed as the number of years lost due to ill health, disability or early death. DALY comprises of:

Years of Lost Life (YLL) – calculated from the number of deaths at each age multiplied by the expected remaining years of life according to a global standard life expectancy.

Years Lost to Disability (YDL) – calculated by the number of incident cases due to injury and illness multiplied by the average duration of the disease and a weighting factor reflecting the severity of the disease on a scale from 0 (perfect health) to 1 (dead)

$$DALY = YLL + YDL$$

One DALY is a measure of one year of healthy life lost

Source: Porta 2014

It was conceptualized by His Majesty the Fourth King of Bhutan. Described as a multi-dimensional measure, and looking at individual portraits for thousands of Bhutanese people, it provides a snapshot of the quality of life, and how it is changing, for better or worse (Ura and Penjore 2017). The concept thrives on the principle of "creating for others," unlike the western concept where happiness is a personal concept. With a practical application and its linkage to policies, the Gross National Happiness (GNH) survey studies 33 indicators compressed into nine domains that have a direct link to a person's happiness on the scale of zero to one. Implemented with the assistance of the Government of Bhutan's Centre for Bhutan Studies, "The nine domains of GNH are, (1) psychological wellbeing, (2) health, (3) education, (4) time use, (5) cultural diversity and resilience, (6) good governance, (7) community vitality, (8) ecological diversity and resilience, and lastly (9) living standards" (Ura and Penjore 2017, 8).

The index recognizes the limitations of quantitative measures of health and identifies any person as happy who achieves adequacy in six of the nine domains. The index's strength lies in the fact that it recognizes that all people are different and some of the indicators are not relevant, and an individual will perform according to his/her values and/or belief set. The Gross National Happiness measure is also subjective to the achievements of the individual. For example, an illiterate person has a different set of achievements for the pursuit of happiness.

The index uses the Alkire-Foster method with headcount, intensity and an overall GNH index which are decomposable. The scale is categorized into: people who have achieved sufficiency in less than 50% are categorized as "unhappy"; 50–65% of domains are called "narrowly happy"; those who have achieved a sufficiency in 66–76% are categorized as "extensively happy" and those with 77% or more are "deeply happy". Self-reported and personally-answered indicators are given lighter weights in the scale as compared to the objective pointers.

However, the scale has its own advantages and disadvantages. One of the main advantages of the scale is its contribution in the development of the society. It demonstrates the parallelism in materialist and spiritual development. The index also acts as a guiding light in allocating resources to a better sustainable development. A criticism of the index is the definition of happiness, which is subjective and self-reported. The happiness index is suitable for small populations such as that of Bhutan, which is oriented to Bhutanese cultural life. Its translation is not standardized for other cultures.

Taking inspiration from Bhutan, in 2012 the United Nations General Assembly declared March 20th as "World Happiness Day." Subsequently, the first World Happiness Report was released on April 1, 2012. The report highlighted how social inequalities dictate a person's happiness. It describes "the aspiration of society is the flourishing of its members. [The World Happiness Report gives evidence on how to achieve societal well-being. It's not by money alone, but also by fairness, honesty, trust, and good health" (Caspani 2015). The report is published annually, in association with The UN Sustainable Development Solutions Network (SDSN). The latest Happiness report was issued on March 20, 2020 (Helliwell et al. 2020). It ranked 156 countries according to the world poll, and for the first time it ranked cities around the world by their personal well-being.

Another example of subjective measurement is the well-being scale. Well-being provides a vital foundation for human development, and is therefore central to countries realizing their full potential. Greg Anderson describes wellness as "the complete integration of body, mind and spirit. The realization that everything we do, think, feel and believe has an effect on our wellbeing" (Anderson 1995). There is no accepted definition of well-being, and well-being is measured by a variety of indicators, such as the quality of relationships, positive emotions and resilience, realization of self-potential, and/or overall satisfaction with life (Ellison et al. 2014). An example is the WHO well-being scale, a questionnaire that measures current mental well-being (WHO (Five) Well-Being Index {World Health Organization, 1998 #41}.

HEALTH RELATED QUALITY OF LIFE: CONCEPT AND MEASURES

> The quality of life is more important than life itself.
> (Attributed to Alexis Carrel)

To further augment the subjective and quantitative measures of health, the year 2000 saw the introduction of the Millennium Development Goals (MDGs) (World Health Organization 2015). They were proposed with the aim of making the world free from diseases, hunger and poverty. Set up against the backdrop of existing trends and conferences of the 1990s, the MDGs were vital in promoting the collection of standardized measurements of data. Aryeetey and Ackah (2012) highlighted that the MDGs "forced an unrelenting spotlight on the need for better data and that of crisp numerical targets." A set of eight quantifiable goals, 18 targets and 48 indicators were proposed to be achieved by 2015. However, the biggest drawback of the MDGs was their inability to address the inequalities faced by the countries (both nationally and internationally).

Under these premises, in 2012 the Rio +20 conference further asserted a sustainable disease and poverty free world. The summit's final outcome was the call for new Sustainable Development Goals (SDGs) (United Nations Development Programme 2015) to be adopted by the United Nations (UN) post-MDGs. The SDGs were recognized as fundamental to achieving Universal Health Coverage (UHC) by 2030. A set of 17 goals and 169 targets, the SDGs were a "blueprint to achieve a better and more sustainable future for all." The SDGs called for higher investment in health and were proposed with an aim to initiate action, while guiding policy making and accountability for the elimination of poverty, the promotion of prosperity, the furthering of peace and justice, and the conservation of the planet's resources for further generations. While the SDG goals and targets set a global context, they were designed in a way so that they could be adapted locally to meet the specific challenges. Collecting data on sex, socio-economic status, disability, geographic location and various other measurements, they were a hallmark in generating "independent, comparable, valid, and consistent measurements of development indicators."

Another ignored measurement, predominantly in the developing world, is the social determinants of health (SDH). The World Health Organization's Commission on Social Determinants of Health (CSDH) define health inequities as "systematic differences in health" that are "avoidable by reasonable action" and are "quite simply, unfair." Health inequities arise not only from within but also from beyond the domain of health, through other social determinants, including the "unequal distribution of power, income, goods, and services, globally and nationally," the consequent unfairness in the immediate, visible circumstances of people's lives, their access to health care, schools and education, and their conditions of work and leisure.

However, the SDH suffered a major drawback for not having consistent measures globally. For example, experts in a study conducted in 2017 concluded "Without consistent measures across communities, the ability to monitor the influence of SDH on health outcomes, health care utilization, and costs will be limited" (Byholff et al. 2017, 425).

DISEASE- AND POPULATION-SPECIFIC TOOLS FOR MEASURING QUALITY OF LIFE

Health measures, as described previously, are broadly categorized into morbidity and mortality, of which morbidity measures (non-fatal outcomes) are the most difficult to track.

To simplify this, Fryback reviewed some examples of morbidity indicators, and introduced a typology for health measures that focused on the need for standardized "health-related quality of life" (HRQoL) indexes. Fryback argued for less subjective ways of summarization and believed that HRQoL was one of the best ways to represent overall health (Kaplan and Fryback 2010). The concept of health-related quality of life quantifies those aspects of quality of life that affect health, either physically or mentally, as opposed to the GNH index explained earlier in the chapter. It bridges boundaries between various disciplines and between social, medical and mental services. It is related to both self-reported chronic diseases and their risk factors and also helps as an aid to determine the burden of preventable diseases, injuries and disabilities and provide valuable new insights into the relationship between health and risk factors. Health-related quality of life further helps in identifying subgroups with poorly perceived health and acts as a guide in designing interventions to boost their situation, hence forestalling more serious consequences (Nathan and Scobell 2012). It urges health agencies to acknowledge broader areas of public health policy around a common theme in association (Kindig et al. 2010). The most common generic tool for measuring HRQoL is the Centres for Disease Control and Prevention (CDC) tool called the Healthy Days Measures. The tool uses four questions. The first item measures overall self-rated health on a scale from poor through excellent. The second item measures physical health as a global measure of recent physical symptoms. The third item is a global measure of recent mental and emotional distress, and the fourth item is about recent activity limitation, which is a global indicator of perceived disability as well as an indicator of productivity and human capital (Centers for Disease Control and Prevention 2000).

This standard set of questions, which is also known as CDC HRQoL–4, has been used in the State-based Behavioural Risk Factor Surveillance System (BRFSS) of the United States of America since 1993 and in the National Health and Nutrition Examination Survey (NHANES) for persons aged 12 for the period 2000 to 2012. The second most popular tool for measuring HRQoL is the World Health Organization (WHO) instrument. One of the advantages of the tool is that it was drafted on the basis of statements made by patients with a range of diseases, by healthy people and by health professionals in a variety of cultures.

Some of the other tools are Patient Reported Outcome Measures (PROMs), which are for patients undergoing hip replacements, knee replacements, etc. PROMs provide an indication of the outcomes or quality of care delivered to patients and have been collected by all providers of the UK's National Health Service-funded care since April 2009. Another commonly used tool is the mental health measure, the Warwick-Edinburgh Mental Well-being Scales (WEMWS). It was developed to enable the measuring of mental well-being in the general population and the evaluation of projects, programs and policies. The scale has been widely used nationally and internationally for monitoring, evaluating projects and programs, and investigating the determinants of mental well-being (Taggart et al. 2015).

CONCLUSION

The way we measure health has evolved over the years with the evolving definitions and description of health. We have come a long way with respect to the methods of measuring health. From pure numerical to complex epidemiological and econometric concepts transcending now to more social concepts, such as happiness, well-being and quality of life, health now can be defined and described in many forms and dimensions. With the advent of the concept of Universal Health Coverage (UHC), health is now proposed to be measured under the broader lens of access, effectiveness, affordability and equity. While the first three attributes have got set measures in place, equity raises questions in terms of the way the concept is defined and applied with respect to the population served, services rendered and costs covered, especially in the context of "progressive universalization": whether the concept alludes to all population groups being equal beneficiaries of every component of health services or whether greater priority is assigned to more vulnerable and marginalized populations?

There is also a common adage that "what gets measured gets paid for." Some countries have made recent gains with putting in practice advanced health measurements. These are reflected in the way these countries are realigning their health policies and deciding on the annual spending on health. However, global asymmetries exist in the way various indicators of health are recorded, leading to difficulties in global comparisons and effective monitoring of the global goals for health, such as the SDGs. Quality of life and governance systems have also often failed to connect the overlapping indicators and methods from the various fields with each other to achieve a common consensus on measurement.

Efforts have to be made at local, national and regional levels to develop universal comparable measures of health. Along with the standard measures of mortality and morbidity, there is a need to prioritize, develop and fine-tune measures of inequalities, happiness, well-being and quality of life to provide a holistic picture of the health of a country or a region. The current COVID-19 pandemic is a reminder that we need to look beyond the standard measures of case fatality, testing and vaccine rates and develop robust public health measures which truly reflect and capture individual and societal health and well-being.

REFERENCES

Anderson, Greg. 1995. *The 22 Non-Negotiable Laws of Wellness: Feel, Think, and Live Better than you ever Thought Possible*. New York: Harper.

Arthur, Margaret. 2014. "Institute for Health Metrics and Evaluation." *Nursing Standard* 28(42): 32–32.

Aryeetey, Ernest, and Charles Ackah, eds. 2012. *Globalization, Trade, and Poverty in Ghana*. Legon-Accra, Ghana: Sub-Saharan Publishers.

Aryeetey, E., Esty, D., Feulner, E., Geiger, T., Kaufmann, D., Kraemer, A., et Al. Getting to Zero: Finishing the Job the MDGs Started. In *Global Agenda Council, World Economic Forum*. 2012.

Britannica, The Editors. 2020. "John Graunt." *Encyclopedia Britannica* www.britannica.com/biography/John-Graunt: Accessed, 23 February 2021.

Byholff, Elena, Alicia J. Cohen, Mary C. Hamati, Julie Tatko, and Matthew M. Davis. 2017. "Screening for social determinants of health in Michigan health centers." *Journal of the American Board of Family Medicine* 30(4): 418–427.

Caspani, Maria. 2015. "Researchers pinpoint the world's happiest country." *Reuters, US Markets*, www.reuters.com/article/us-global-happiness-report/researchers-pinpoint-the-worlds-happiest-country-report-idUSKBN-0NE2SR20150423: Accessed, 28 February 2021.

Centers for Disease Control and Prevention. 2000. *Measuring Healthy Days: Population Assessment of Health-Related Quality of Life* Atlanta, GA: US Department of Health and Human Services, Centers for Disease Control and Prevention.

Cornfield, Jerome. 1951. "A method of estimating comparative rates from clinical data. Applications to cancer of the lung, breast and cervix." *Journal of the National Cancer Institute* 11(6): 1269–1275.

Das, Pamela, and Udani Samarasekera. 2012. "The story of GBD 2010: a "super-human" effort." *The Lancet* 380(9859): 2067–2270. doi: 10.1016/s0140-6736(12)62174-6. Erratum in: Lancet. 2013 Feb 23;381(9867):628. PMID: 23259158.

Doll, R., Hill, A.B. 1954. The mortality of doctors in relation to their smoking habits; a preliminary report. *Br Med J.* 1954;1(4877):1451–1455. doi:10.1136/bmj.1.4877.1451

Ellison, Crispin, Cate Reynolds, and Charles Alessi. 2014. *Measuring Wellness*. New York: Oliver Wyman.

Farr, William. 2004. "'On Prognosis' (British Medical Almanack 1838; Supplement 199–216)." In *A History of Epidemiologic Methods and Concepts*, edited by Alfredo Morabia, pp. 159–178. Basel, Switzerland: Birkhäuser.

Fracastoro, Girolamo. 1546. *De contagione et contagiosis morbis* (*On Contagion and Contagious Diseases*) Theory of Contagion." *The British and foreign medico-chirurgical review* vol. 45,89 (1870): 128–137. Venice, Italy.

Frenk, Julio, and Octavio Gómez-Danté. 2014. "Designing a framework for the concept of health." *Journal of Public Health Policy* 35(3): 401–406.

Hand, D.J. 1996. "Statistics and the theory of measurement." *Journal of the Royal Statistical Society, Series A* 159(3): 445–492.

Helliwell, John F., Richard Layard, Jeffrey D. Sachs, and Jan-Emanuel De Neve, eds. 2020. *World Happiness Report 2020*. New York: Sustainable Development Solutions Network.

Hinkle, Lawrence. 1961. "Ecological observations of the relation of physical illness, mental illness, and social environment." *Psychosomatic Medicine* 23(4): 289–296.

Kaplan, Abraham. 1964. *The Conduct of Inquiry: Methodology for Behavioral Science*. San Francisco, CA: Chandler.

Kaplan, Robert M., and Dennis G. Fryback. 2010. *Health Related Quality of Life and Health Status* Washington, DC: National Institutes of Health. https://ods.od.nih.gov/pubs/economicanalysis2010/Kaplan.pdf.

Kindig, David A., Bridget C. Booske, and Patrick L. Remington. 2010. "Mobilizing Action Toward Community Health (MATCH): metrics, incentives, and partnerships for population health." *Preventing Chronic Disease: Public Health Research, Practice, and Policy* 7(4): A68.

Klouda, T. 1994. "The World Development Report 1993 and human rights." *Health and Human Rights* 1(1): 101–109.

Larson, James S. 1996. "The World Health Organization's definition of health: social versus spiritual health." *Social Indicators Research* 38(2): 181–192.

Le Play, Frédéric 1982. *Frédéric Le Play: On family, Work, and Social Change*. Edited and translated by Catherine Bodard Silver. Chicago, IL: University of Chicago Press.

Marahatta, S.B. 2010. "Revitalizing primary health care – another utopian goal?" *Kathmandu University Medical Journal* 8(31): 341–344.

Nathan, Andrew J., and Andrew Scobell. 2012. "How China sees America: the sum of Beijing's fears." *Foreign Affairs* 91(5): 32–47.

Nelder, John, and W.M. Wedderburn. 1972. "Generalized linear models." *Journal of the Royal Statistical Society* 135(3): 370–384.

Nutton, Vivian. 1990. "The reception of Fracastoro's theory of contagion: the seed that fell among thorns?" *Osiris*, Second Series, 6: 196–234.

Poole, Charles. 2015. "A history of the population attributable fraction and related measures." *Annals of Epidemiology* 25(3): 147–154.

Porta, Miquel, ed. 2014. *A Dictionary of Epidemiology* (6th edition). London: International Epidemiological Association/Oxford University Press.

Raj, Bhopal S. 2016. *Concepts of Epidemiology: Integrating the Ideas, Theories, Principles, and Methods of Epidemiology* (3rd edition). Oxford: Oxford University Press.

Rhodes, P., and John H. Bryant. 2020. "Public health." *Encyclopedia Britannica*, www.britannica.com/topic/public-health: Accessed, 23 February 2021.

Ross, Lauren N., and James F. Woodward. 2016. "Koch's postulates: an interventionist perspective." *Studies in History and Philosophy of Science Part C: Studies in History and Philosophy of Biological and Biomedical Sciences* 59: 35–46.

Schlesselman, James J. 2006. "The emerging case-control study: lung cancer in relation to tobacco smoking." *Preventive Medicine* 43(4): 251–255.

Small, H. 2020. "Edwin Chadwick: a biographical update." *Journal of Medical Biography* Online first, August 19. https://doi.org/10.1177/0967772020951083

Spector, Benjamin. 1963. "Jeremy Bentham, 1748–1832: his influence upon medical thought and legislation." *Bulletin of the History of Medicine* 37(1): 25–42.

Taggart, Frances, Sarah Stewart-Brown, and Jane Parkinson. 2015. *Warwick–Edinburgh Mental Well-being Scale (WEMWBS): User guide – Version 2*. Edinburgh: NHS Health Scotland.

United Nations Development Program. *Sustainable Development Goal*. 2015. Accessed

September 2, 2020. https://www.undp.org/content/undp/en/home/sustainable-development-goals.

Ura, Dasho Karma, and Dorji Penjore, eds. 2017. *GNH: From Philosophy to Praxis: Proceedings of the Sixth International Conference on Gross National Happiness, 4–6 November 2015, Paro, Bhutan*. Thimphu, BT: Centre for Bhutan Studies and Gross National Happiness.

Van Manen, Michael, and Max Van Manen. 2021. "Jan H. van den Berg." In *Classic Writings for a Phenomenology of Practice*. Edited by Michael Van Manen and Max Van Manen. London: Routledge.

Walsh, Julia A., and Kenneth S. Warren. 1980. "Selective primary care: an interim strategy for disease control in developing countries." *Social Science and Medicine, Part C Medical Economics* 14(2): 145–163.

World Bank. 1993. *Investing in Health*. World Development Report. Washington, DC: World Bank. © World Bank. https://openknowledge.worldbank.org/handle/10986/5976 License: CC BY 3.0 IGO."

World Health Organization. 2015. *The Millennium Development Goals Report 2015*. New York: United Nations.

World Health Organisation (Five) Well-Being Index (WHO-5). SNAP-Ed.1998. Accessed July 19, 2020. https://snaped.fns.usda.gov/library/materials/who-five-well-being-index-who-5.

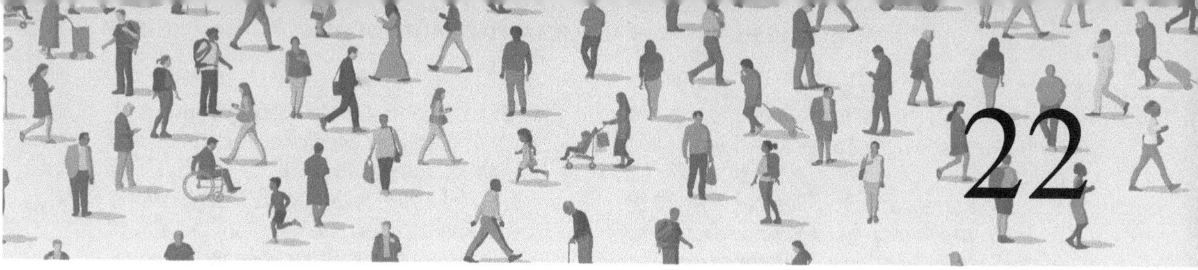

22

Lay Participation in Healthcare Policy, Planning and Practice: To What End?

Deena White

INTRODUCTION

The participation of ordinary people in healthcare policy, planning and practice has continued to rise, since the heady days of popular protest and community action in the 1960s. It takes a multitude of forms: direct citizen participation on decision-making boards and councils, various levels and forms of public consultation, technocratic and deliberative exercises involving "mini-publics", unidirectional strategies such as patient-reported outcome surveys, collaborative partnerships between community-based and public agencies, and, most recently, strategies for promoting the coproduction of healthcare. What these diverse activities share is an invitation to lay or non-professional individuals and groups with a stake in healthcare to contribute experiential knowledge or other resources to improve healthcare systems and practices. Yet countless studies of the implementation of lay participation in healthcare are either equivocal with respect to its influence or effectiveness, or fail to demonstrate any at all.

The reputed value of lay participation for improving health system accountability, service access, responsiveness, quality, equity, and health outcomes, while often reported in the literature, is seldom confirmed by research (Mitton et al., 2011). A large proportion of the massive literature on the subject is normative, based on claims of what lay participation in health could, might, or should accomplish – "more promise than reality", to quote Abelson, Forest and their colleagues (2003). The objectives and justifications put forward by authorities who organize exercises in participation tend to be confusing, and only loosely related to the strategies they adopt (Rowe and Frewer, 2005). Furthermore, participation planning rarely considers how lay input might be translated into action or incorporated into next steps. Given inadequate evidence of effectiveness and efficiency (Crawford et al., 2002; Tempfer and Nowak, 2011; Bolsewicz Alderman et al., 2013; Lever, 2013; Bombard et al., 2018), in a context of shrinking health budgets and calls for evidence-based practice, why do health authorities continue to invest and reinvest in lay participation?

A wealth of recent literature reviews address the forms, dimensions, and outcomes of citizen, community, patient and public participation and engagement in health (Brett et al., 2014; Conklin et al., 2015; Bombard et al., 2018; Harris et al., 2018; Farmer et al., 2018; Haldane et al., 2019). Therefore, this chapter is not itself conceived as a literature review. Instead, it proposes a reading of the literature focused on the question: why do healthcare institutions invest in lay participation? The chapter seeks answers that are nested in the specific and complex healthcare contexts – both local and global – within which all forms of lay participation in healthcare are performed. From an actor-network perspective (Latour, 2005), these contexts can be conceived as "ecologies" of healthcare, a metaphor to describe the somewhat stable, and more or less coordinated assemblage, within and across national spaces, of diverse professional, managerial, administrative, market, non-governmental and political actors, objectives, knowledge and skill sets, platforms, policies, programmes, protocols and practices, budgets, capital, and industries that constitute health systems world wide (Moran, 1999; Hanefeld et al., 2017). Health system ecologies are different in different places, notably in the West and in the Global South, but they are also transnationally interconnected. They are all characterized by complexity, uncertainty, and constant change.

Context includes health spending, which represents almost 9% of GDP in wealthy nations (OECD, 2019), closer to 10% worldwide (World Bank, 2017), and everywhere it is growing more rapidly than GDP, particularly in the richest and poorest countries. To provide perspective, in the USA, healthcare outlays account for almost 18% of GDP, compared to military spending at 3.2%. Most societies want citizens to be able to benefit from the constant gains being made in medical knowledge and technology, spurred by university research and biotechnology industries competing in the global science and technology market. But the definition of quality healthcare is a moving target. Insofar as better and innovative tools, treatments and procedures mean improved diagnoses and prognoses, doctors and hospitals are typically keen to adopt them, and patients are eager to access them. Thus, the cost of healthcare is forever escalating, and moving way beyond the means of low- and middle-income countries. All this contributes to making healthcare and healthcare systems highly complex, international arenas, within which lay participation has a yet-to-be determined place (Peters and Bloom, 2012).

This chapter explores a variety of approaches to address the question: to what end is lay participation in health pursued? A reading of the literature suggests, first, a tension between ideal ends and strategic means. Second, it suggests an evolution of ends over time. In the West, initial concerns for democratic accountability and improved decision-making have moved towards a greater concern for consensus-building to manage change, and capacity-building to manage national deficits. In the Global South, in contrast, consensus-building and capacity-building objectives have always been the impetus behind the promotion of lay participation in health, while more recently, its contribution to democracy-building has become more prominent in the literature. To account for both the tensions between the ends and means of lay participation, and its evolution over time, this chapter will address it within the different contexts that have shaped its meaning and practice.

LAY PARTICIPATION: LAYERS OF CONTEXT AND INTERACTION

The everyday understanding of lay participation has evolved over time, from the autonomous and contentious engagement of citizens in changing healthcare practices and institutions, to administrative mandates and institutional exercises orchestrated by experts, and most recently, to the recruitment of patients and community-based organizations to the co-production of health. Even the question of who lay participants are has changed. We used to think in terms of citizen and community participation, but today, there is a greater emphasis on patient and public participation (Callaghan and Wistow, 2006). Indeed, the word "lay" is seldom used today, though its generic nature suits the needs of the current discussion. A real-world, as opposed to a conceptual, understanding of lay participation will be proposed here, so that the question of its ends, which will be taken up next, can better be explored in context.

A functional definition of participation in health might simply refer to the ways in which different stakeholders engage in the activities of this sector. Stakeholders in the health sector include a vast array of actors, such as doctors, nurses, and numerous other healthcare professionals; politicians, public administrators, managers, and researchers; insurance, health maintenance and non-governmental organizations; the biomedical industries; and finally, patients and potential patients, sometimes referred to as citizens or consumers, or simply the public. Some stakeholders consistently have a significant influence on healthcare and health system decision-making, either directly or remotely, while some have none. When we talk about *lay* participation, we are concerned with system outsiders, those whose considerable stake in the health system very rarely leads to involvement in decision-making, beyond the confines of the interpersonal, dependent, doctor–patient relation. They contrast with health system "insiders", those whose livelihood is assured by that system, who circulate in the arena of healthcare decisions and practices, and who have some access to the human, technological, financial, informational and organizational resources that are concentrated there. Insiders' interests within the health system are normally well-organized through professional orders, business associations, or unions, or by hierarchical status within bureaucracies. Because they are embedded in working relationships, these interests are central to insiders' daily lives (Marmor and Marone, 1980). System outsiders, on the other hand, are peripheral actors, having only limited, intermittent, or tightly circumscribed access to the health system. But exactly who this includes is not fixed in time or space. Some of those who are decidedly insiders today, such as health administrators, were once considered outsiders, or "laymen" [sic], with no right to interfere in decisions that were the preserve of the medical profession (Horrobin, 1977).

Today, the health sector is immensely more populated than it was, and more diversely so. An array of administrators, economists, researchers, global NGOs and biomedical merchants circulate within the core arenas of health system decision-making around the world, and join medical professionals as system insiders at local, national, and international levels of decision-making. In contrast, system outsiders constitute that vague category of "ordinary people" (Martin, 2008) that includes us all – patients, one-time patients and potential patients. Some low-status, though vital, groups of healthcare workers – such as long-term care attendants – are also outsiders. Outsiders' links to the health system are marginal, precarious or sporadic. They are dependant upon it in moments of vulnerability and need. Ideally, lay participation aims to include such powerless stakeholders in healthcare and health system decision-making.

The current conception of "ordinary people" as legitimate lay stakeholders in the health system emerged in the 1960s (Feingold, 1969; Toth, 1996). The radical idea that health professionals should encourage citizens and communities to participate in the planning and delivery of healthcare had already surfaced in the developing world, top down, and was eventually consolidated there in the community health movement (Perry, 2013). Facing autocratic, corrupt or ineffectual governments and public institutions (also present, but less pervasively, in the West), limited allopathic health literacy, constrained resources, and populations sceptical and distrustful of Western medicine, international NGOs sought to improve their effectiveness and legitimacy by promoting the engagement of community members in activities such as identifying needs, planning and managing programmes, or delivering information and services. The World Health Organization's Alma-Ata Declaration (1978) stated that people have the right and duty to participate in the planning and implementation of their healthcare.

In the West, however, the turn to lay participation was rather driven by the growing illegitimacy of a highly developed medical establishment. In emerging post-war welfare states, access to, and the quality of, healthcare had vastly improved. But citizens and patients also witnessed its rampant specialization and bureaucratization, an alienating shift in professional practices and relationships, and the growth and concentration of power in the hands of more and more remote sets of experts. Ordinary citizens were increasingly powerless over medical practices that intimately touched their lives. Citizen engagement was a means to take back some sense of control for ordinary people.

The original call for participation in the West originated in its robust, post-war civil societies, and was born of a critique of the emerging "programmed society" in general (Touraine, 1971), and of the medical establishment in particular. First targeted was psychiatry, accused of being arbitrary, authoritarian, and repressive, and of questionable scientific grounding (Szasz, 1961; Rosenhan, 1973; Conrad and Slodden, 2013). Then followed a vast literature critical of medicine in general as a form of social control (Foucault, 1975; Illich, 1976), particularly from a nascent feminist perspective (Ehrenreich and English, 1973). Finally, the medicalization of more and more conditions and behaviours newly identified as subject to medical intervention, such as attention deficit in children, was seen to have ominous consequences for the society (Conrad, 2005). At first, lay participation in healthcare referred to citizen engagement through social movements, protest, or lobbying, as typified by the anti-psychiatry movement (Crossley, 1998) and the women's health movement (Marieskind, 1975). Such autonomous collective action seeking to impose citizen influence in the health field has had considerable success and has not abated. Note, for example, the disability movement, the HIV-AIDS movement, the anti-vaccination movement and others (Shakespeare, 1993; Haldi, 1999; Blume, 2006; Keefe et al., 2006; Hoffman, 2008). But these civil society movements are not what we mean by lay participation in health today.

Rather, lay participation has come to refer to an institutional practice, organized by health system insiders and the "consultation industry" (Bherer and Lee, 2019; see also Amelung and Grabner, 2017). This construction of a parallel, institutional form of lay participation was born of political and administrative strategies to co-opt, tame and harness autonomous, anti-establishment forms of citizen engagement in health. In the 1960s and 1970s, efforts were already being made to integrate citizens into local or regional health councils and agencies (Lipsky and Lounds, 1976; Checkoway, 1982a, 1982b; Bowl, 1996). Even the earliest evaluations indicated that they rarely presented a challenge to established ways of running health systems (Topliss, 1975; Checkoway et al., 1984; Lupton et al., 1995; Donovan and Coast, 1996). Still, enthusiasm for institutional forms of lay participation in controlled, invited spaces never diminished, despite the mounting and nearly unanimous studies documenting their disappointing performance (Lipsky and Lounds, 1976; Grant, 1989; Milewa 1997; Milewa et al., 1998; Bombard et al., 2018; but see Haldane et al., 2019).

More recently, the discourse of "citizen" and even of health "consumer" participation, both empowering concepts, has given way to that of "patient engagement" (Callaghan and Wistow, 2006). Citizens and consumers can claim power as a right: the right to voice and influence, or the right to choose (whether or not real-life practices of lay participation realize these rights). The legitimacy of "patients" as participants, however, is grounded in the recognition of a need for their collaboration or compliance in healthcare, if it is to become more effective and efficient. Patients as "partners" and their participation in the "coproduction" of healthcare are championed in the literature as essential to achieving the best health outcomes (Karazivan et al., 2015). In addition, their unique experiential expertise can be mobilized to differently evaluate and prioritize healthcare practices and policy decisions, to provide a politically valuable counterweight to the interests of more powerful stakeholders, or to allow decision-makers to share the responsibility for unpopular decisions with "the public" (Abelson, Eyles et al., 2003).

In contrast to citizens' autonomous participation in grassroots and social movement organizations, contemporary lay participation constitutes what we might call "dependent participation", that is, dependent on the goals and strategies of institutions and insiders. In dependent participation, ordinary people are invited into the healthcare arena by organizers of purpose-specific exercises or spaces, to share their experiential knowledge, express their opinions about the issues put to them, and contribute to health system planning and evaluation. These purposes are all vital to health administrators' mandates, but are not necessarily the areas in which citizens themselves might seek to influence policies, programmes, and practices. For the latter, participation in autonomous citizen action remains an option (Crane, 2018). Moreover, since the turn of the twenty-first century, lay participation serving institutional purposes has burgeoned into a multiform industry, as well as a research priority. It is implemented more and more through precise and formal methods, requiring a degree of professional expertise to properly plan, execute and evaluate (Bherer et al., 2017; Bherer and Lee, 2019). Its purposes tend towards confirming or strengthening administrative decisions, and avoiding the risk of public non-cooperation, or of disruptive opposition to institutional and governmental policies (Irvin and Stansbury, 2004).

The gap between the expressed ideal and the actual practice of lay participation in health is universally recognized in the literature, and it has long been noted in passing that understanding this gap requires the consideration of context (Charles and DiMaio, 1993; Hoppe, 2011). Decision-making in different health systems is regulated by specific, complex sets of relations, resources, rules, and imperatives over which local decision-makers may have little control (Moran, 1999). Considering participation in both the West and the South brings context to the forefront. Although formal structures and exercises in participation have evolved principally in the West, they have recently travelled back to the Global South, under the influence of transnational organizations such as the World Health Organization (WHO) and international NGOs, as well as the massive supporting literature based on Western contexts and experiences. While the ecology of health systems in the South is both similar to and different from the West, the burden of disease is different and greater, and the ability to respond, weaker. The same array of local, national, and international stakeholders may be present, but their attributes and capacities, and particularly their power relations, are quite different (Kay and Williams, 2009).

In the Global South, the capacity of public medical institutions is often inadequate compared to that of the private sector, and the administrative apparatus may operate less exclusively on the basis of expertise and more in line with personal interest (García, 2019). Clientelism and patronage may be central to the dynamics of these health systems, generating and consolidating significant inequities in access and quality of healthcare and in population health (Brun and Diamond, 2014). These dynamics dampen any incentive for autonomous organization and popular protest, as disloyalty and dissent can incur heightened insecurity for dependent populations (Wood, 2003). Aiming to expand the reach of modern medicine and improve population health in the Global South, politically and economically powerful "outsiders", such as the WHO, the World Bank, NGOs and their Western funders, have positioned themselves as health system "insiders", and thanks to the resources they bring, their influence on decision-making with respect to policy, programmes and local practices is significant. From this contradictory put powerful position, they promote the establishment of institutional spaces of lay participation (Wallace, 2004). Numerous southern governments now include mandates for lay participation in their health policies, although these typically meet with tacit but effective resistance by those responsible for their implementation (Aiyar, 2010; Bano, 2019). As in the West, then – but for different reasons – dependent lay participation in the South is also known for its ineffectiveness (Golooba-Mutebi, 2005; Bolsewicz Alderman et al., 2013; Kamuzora et al., 2013; but see Bukenya, 2018).

The next sections synthesize a reading of the vast literature on lay participation practices, which focuses almost entirely on the closed spaces within which specific exercises unfold, with little regard for context. Recent systematic reviews regularly catalogue well over 20,000 articles on lay participation in the health sector, overwhelmingly concerned with Western practices. They can be classified according to four ends or orientations. The largest portion is normative, where lay participation is presented as an exercise in democracy with its own intrinsic, taken-for-granted value, and provides guidelines for realizing this end (while recognizing that it is rarely met). A smaller portion of the literature treats it instead as a strategy, or a means to an end, for example, to broaden the knowledge base and protect the legitimacy and prerogatives of medical experts and authorities who are called upon to make consequential decisions for ordinary people. "Technocracy" is the name we apply to these strategic ends, to highlight their contrast with democracy, or "power to the people". More recently, two other ends of lay participation have emerged as salient in the literature: consensus-building and capacity-building. In the first, lay participation appears as a strategy for managing change, and in the second, for mobilizing resources. While resource mobilisation has always been an objective in the Global South, in the context of community health programmes in local villages, it is now increasingly evoked in the West, where fully developed, technocratic health systems have been afflicted by austerity (Reeves et al., 2014). In the following sections, these four "ends" of lay participation in health are taken up in turn.

PARTICIPATION AS DEMOCRACY IN ACTION

In the Western literature, lay participation is understood as an instance of participative democracy, insofar as it gives voice to otherwise powerless stakeholders. Arnstein's (1969) celebrated ladder of participation is the classic framework for those studying lay participation as democratic practice in health and in other arenas. But Arnstein's ladder was founded on the premise that participation is not democratic unless it is able to exert real influence, or even control over decisions directly affecting citizens. It was written as a defence of autonomous citizen participation, in opposition to institutional, dependent lay participation (Stewart, 2013). In some cases, Arnstein argued, participation fulfils purposes that are opposite to democracy. For example, at the "lowest" levels of the ladder, it involves participants in a therapeutic relation, in which their participation is deemed to be "good for them" on a psychosocial level, rather than making it possible for them to contribute to change. It can also be manipulative, when lay input is deployed to achieve ends extraneous to, if not contradictory to, participants' own interests. One-way information-gathering techniques, such as consultations, or claims to transparency by "informing" citizens, often mistakenly pass for participation. Even "partnership" is suspect; citizen control is the summit. Arnstein's ladder is still systematically invoked in the current literature on participation worldwide, representing citizen control as its ideal end (Lauria and Slotterback, 2020). It has inspired adaptation and elaboration for application in the health sector (e.g. Charles and DeMaio, 1993; Thompson, 2007) as well as critical assessment (Tritter and McCallum, 2006). When applied as an analytic framework in the health sector, this approach invariably serves to highlight the fact that, in the real world, lay participation is anything *but* democratic.

Lay participation as a democratizing force for Western health systems is often espoused as the justification for community and public representation in consultations and local, regional or national councils (Crane, 2018). Its failure to influence procedures and outcomes is attributed to implementation problems: who got to participate, and how (Djellouli et al., 2019). Recruitment is difficult, and rarely representative. It tends to be skewed towards more educated, articulate, and interested citizens, while the voices of vulnerable and marginal groups are still not heard (Snow et al., 2018). Procedures tend to ignore the presence and needs of lay participants: the flow of information and the rhythm of meetings, burying participants in documentation, "bulldozing" a committee's way through controversial dossiers, multiplying the number of committees that seem to "do nothing", all serve to obstruct effective democratic lay participation (Aronson, 1993; Bowl, 1996). The question of accountability, or whether and how lay input is actually acted upon, is seldom considered in the literature, except where it notes the absence of any strategy for incorporating the concerns of lay participants in decisions (Aronson, 1993; Fitzpatrick, 1994; Pickard et al., 1995; Milewa, 1997). For all these reasons, lay participation tends to be a parallel process that never meets the decision-making process. It is often perceived by citizens who participate as a "no-destination ship" (Seixas, 2017), an ineffective ritual with no discernable purpose (Stewart, 2016; Komporozos-Athanasiou et al., 2018).

Despite these contradictions, lay participation has in recent years been touted as a democratizing force for the Global South, to promote not only accountability (Cornwall, 2002; Govender and Mooney, 2012), but also "transformative change" (de Freitas, 2017). Decision-making by health authorities in developing countries is often driven by a lack of resources and expertise, leading to improvisation and self-interested behaviour on the part of medical professionals and administrators (Kamuzora et al., 2013). It is also more exposed to external pressures and corrupt practices on the part of governments and officials, international NGOs, and global corporations (Lewis, 2006; Mackey and Liang, 2012). These are all situations conducive to unequal and poor-quality care and seeming indifference to patients. Lay participation is held up as part of the solution to these problems, based on the assumptions that it allows scrutiny over individual and institutional behaviour, provides feedback to decision-makers, and encourages greater responsiveness. However, as in the West, mandated structures and exercises rarely generate the desired processes and outcomes (Morgan, 2001; Piper and Von Lieres, 2008). On the one hand, they are unevenly implemented by the very authorities who are ostensibly targeted by them (Aiyar, 2010). On the other hand, given the deep-rooted, intersectional inequalities, dependencies and social exclusions that characterize many societies in the South, lay participation is often not a very meaningful concept. The opportunity costs of participation – or the time, travel, money, and relational hazards that it would entail – are typically too high for ordinary people living in these societies. This makes recruitment – even if genuine efforts are made – an overwhelming challenge.

The turning of institutional lay participation to democratic ends in the South seems an inversion of its logic. Rather than engendering democracy, it rather emerges under conditions of democracy. For example, Brazil's famously participative health system (Cornwall and Shankland, 2008) was built in the 1980s, in the context of a pervasive, political democratization movement following years of military dictatorship that had interrupted its democratic institutions, and in which health professionals played a leading role. A comparable context has not often existed in the South, where today, democratization movements are either struggling or stillborn, without having reached the point of building democratic institutions. Kerala province in India is another often-cited story of the democratizing power of citizen participation (Franke and Chasin, 1994). However, the preconditions that existed in that province are also rare in the South. Kerala was never under British rule, but existed as an autonomous, matriarchal kingdom until Indian independence, and since the early 1800's, literacy and education for both sexes was promoted (Sen, 1991). These conditions meant that significant barriers to the mobilization and participation of ordinary people prevalent elsewhere in the South were absent in Kerala. The same preconditions led to the eventual election of local governments there that have developed institutions capable of providing a full range of services from schools to banks, and including health centres and hospitals (Franke and Chasin, 1994). In short, two complementary conditions of democracy have exceptionally been present in Kerala and Brazil, as they have in the West: on the one hand, institutions whose functioning and destiny depend on their legitimacy within the population they serve; and on the other hand, capable communities or publics that expect to be able to exert influence on these institutions.

Democratization of healthcare systems may be an ideal goal of lay participation everywhere, but its significance is different in the West and the South. In the West, just giving voice to citizens is deemed sufficient to avoid the potential costs of not doing so. Lay participation is thus a simple transaction cost for institutions: it is worth the investment insofar as it smooths the implementation of potentially unpopular changes and undermines the likelihood of citizens organizing themselves independently to resist, make alternative demands, or hold decision-makers to account. Pointing to a participative process justifies decisions, whether it influenced them or not. Thus, Lehoux and her colleagues (2012) refer to "the unbearable lightness of citizens" in lay participation. For citizens in the West who want real influence, there are effective, autonomous forms of participation in health associations and movements. Such democratic alternatives, however, are not often available in most countries of the Global South, where both institutions and civil society may be weak or fragile.

PARTICIPATION AS CONSENSUS-BUILDING

Much of the more recent literature on democratic participation in the health field recognizes that dependent lay participation is not about empowerment, but rather about legitimacy. Since the 2000s, new forms of governance engaging public authorities, civil society stakeholders as well as experts in collaborative partnerships and networks have been taking root in all sectors of Western democracies (Osborne, 2006; Stoker, 2006). In this light, lay participation has received a boost, and is lately being defined more as a collaborative instrument than an empowering one. In the health sector, this collaborative or consensus-building orientation has largely taken shape under the banner of deliberative democracy. Nabatchi and Leighninger (2015) call this "thick participation". It promotes two-way information-sharing between decision-makers and stakeholders, and thorough, inclusive discussion of the reasons for and against various potential decisions or paths of action (Abelson, Forest et al., 2003).

Ideally, deliberation would make it possible to achieve close to a consensus among diverse publics regarding priority setting, the values and norms that should inform policy decisions, and the relative acceptability of controversial health-related proposals within a society (Niemeyer and Dryzek, 2007; Kornreich et al., 2012). Concretely, it involves increasingly formalized, dedicated, short-term, controlled exercises such as deliberative forums, citizens' juries, citizens' councils and deliberative polling (Davies et al., 2006; Street et al., 2014; Carman et al., 2016; Degeling et al., 2017). Health authorities have turned to deliberative participation, often initiated by researchers, to inform decisions about ethical issues, such as genetic testing (Bennett and Smith, 2007); priority-setting, for example, regarding health technology (Menon and Stafinski, 2008) or health insurance (Goold et al., 2005); and health policy development such as telemedicine (Mort and Finch, 2005) and pandemic communications (Rogers et al., 2009).

Deliberation is said to be the most meaningful form of participation (Mansbridge, 2010), but it is also the most intensive and time-consuming. It calls for the involvement of steering committees, researchers, knowledge brokers, and professional facilitators to promote open discussion and debate among diverse and informed participants, or "mini-publics", under conditions that ensure equal opportunity, equal voice, and equal influence on the outcome (Fishkin, 2003; Deng and Wu, 2010). This requires documenting evidence from a wide range of expert and political perspectives, in order to inform lay participants fully and fairly about all sides of the issue at hand (Safaei, 2015). Thus, although deliberative participation has been enthusiastically prescribed, it has been only occasionally implemented in both the West and the South, often in a research context (Ellen et al., 2017).

"Thick participation" of this type is not only a costly, but also a risky investment, given the potential challenges to established professional interests and political preferences that it ideally presents. But the literature shows that actual processes of deliberative participation are typically "adapted" to the context and instrumental ends of the authorities that sponser them (Kashefi and Mort, 2004; Street et al., 2014). A systematic review of citizens' juries in health policy decision-making found that the process was typically compromised at every step: recruitment did not ensure a representative range of public positions among participants; expert knowledge brokers, who framed the issues and decided what information was relevant for participants, were biased; time allotted for exchanges among participants was limited; the moderation processes were less than open and fair (Street et al., 2014). Clearly, deliberative democracy with lay participants is an even more remote ideal than participative democracy in the context of competing healthcare and health system interests.

Most revealing, however, is the way in which the outcomes of deliberative exercises in lay participation are reported in the literature (and outcomes are more consistently reported for this type of participation than any other). Changes in opinions before and after the exercise are documented, but the changes measured are in the opinions and views of the lay participants themselves, not of decision-makers (Abelson, Eyles et al., 2003; Delli Carpini et al., 2004; Stafinski et al., 2014; Carman et al., 2015). In other words, deliberative lay participation is designed to educate lay participants to better understand and accept the complex, expertly defined factors that must be considered when making decisions in the healthcare field. It helps health authorities understand how to define and publicly disseminate their positions, and to develop strategies to circumscribe and diffuse public debate. The aim is neither to improve accountability to powerless stakeholders, nor to enhance their influence on decisions (Street et al., 2014), but rather, to bolster the public legitimacy of those decisions.

Whether participatory or deliberative, the credibility of lay participation as a democratic practice has perhaps unintentionally taken a beating in the literature. The same authors who report these doubtful politico-administrative objectives and outcomes nevertheless continue to extol the practice's democratic credentials in ritualistic fashion. This invites the question of the extent to which democracy in healthcare decision-making is a pertinent value, and if so, in what contexts and under what conditions? For example, the NIMBY (not in my backyard) phenomenon pits wealthier citizens against programmes for the community integration of people with mental health problems; neo-liberal lobbies have succeeded in legitimating the increasing privatization of health systems, though this serves the interests of only the few (Armstrong, 2001); the anti-vaccine movement thrives against the full weight of scientific evidence and the debunking of a single flawed study (Hobson-West, 2007). Moreover, the COVID-19 pandemic has pitted conflicting health and economic priorities against each other, making public deliberation a risky basis for decision-making. In this context, autonomous lay participation in some societies has opened up a more or less tacit contest between "power to the people" and "power to the scientists". Many consider democracy a poor way to regulate health policy, and would rather put their trust in expertise.

PARTICIPATION AS TECHNOCRATIC PRACTICE

Technocracy as an ideology claims that science and technology hold the promise of a best possible world. Given the advances in hygiene and medicine witnessed over the last century, this is hardly an outlandish idea in the field of health. But the extraordinary pace of scientific and technological developments has driven health practices and systems towards ever-increasing specialization, bureaucratization, and complexification, rendering them impenetrable to all but experts (Sturmberg and Martin, 2013). When decision-makers are selected or otherwise rise to positions of power on the basis of their expertise, rather than their social, economic, or political status, we are talking about a technocracy. In the West, while imperfect, this is a fair description of the health field.

From a technocratic perspective, the democratic management of healthcare has significant downsides, not least because it is seen as inefficient and ineffective compared to traditional, autocratic models of decision-making (Irvin and Stansbury, 2004). Health professionals' and administrators' hostile, resistant, or indulgent attitudes with respect to lay participation have been well documented, as is their limited interest in actually incorporating lay ideas into their decision-making (Frankish et al., 2002; Mitton et al., 2011). Moreover, properly implementing lay participation is problematic for managers, who are expected to arrive at decisions in short timeframes, and in a complex work environment where participation is rarely a priority (Martin, 2012). Lay participation is somewhat mistrusted by authorities because of the unknown quality of citizens' input, their uneven awareness and understanding of health issues, and the risk of disruption to both legitimacy and institutional routines that it represents, for example, if tensions or oppositional positions get out of hand by finding their way into the press (Lipsky and Lounds, 1976; Donovan and Coast, 1996; Milewa, 1997; Rowe and Shepherd, 2002; Crawford et al., 2003; Martin, 2008). It is, however, seen by many as a necessary ritual insofar as the risks involved in not consulting and involving citizens and communities are potentially greater than the costs of doing it

(Aronson, 1993; Bowl, 1996; Komporozos-Athanasiou, 2018). Therefore, it is a process to be tightly circumscribed and controlled. As early as 1979, Steckler and Herzog provided an amusing but accurate compendium of administrative strategies for keeping lay boards "out of your hair and off your back". And administrators will often prefer to solicit lay perspectives using "thin" forms of participation (Nabatchi and Leighninger, 2015), such as surveys and questionnaires, which avoid dynamic interactions altogether.

Yet today, there is an increasing recognition of "lay expertise" in the health sector – a term once considered an oxymoron. Lay expertise is based on experiential knowledge (Castro et al., 2019). As a form of expertise specifically founded on the patient experience, it is less and less contested in the healthcare arena. One exemplary technocratic instrument based on patient expertise is PROMs, or patient-reported outcome measures (Devlin and Appleby, 2010). PROMs are tools, such as questionnaires, used to collect data on patients' perceptions in their areas of expertise, that is, their symptoms, level of functioning, quality of life, or experience of care, typically in relation to a particular disease or condition. These data contribute to the evaluation of old and new methods of providing care, to promoting equity in service delivery, and to ensuring the cost-effectiveness of treatment decisions. In the US, some insurance organizations use PROMs in their reimbursement protocols, as a proxy for accountability (Black, 2013). In both the US and Europe, the use of PROMS is mandated to support drug labelling claims (Weldring and Smith, 2013). In the UK, it is mandatory to use PROMs in cases of elective surgery, with the ultimate objective of providing patient-centred information on the effectiveness of these treatments, thus improving health consumers' ability to make informed choices, but also, reducing the demand for expensive but unproven procedures Controversies abound over what to measure, how to interpret the data, how to disseminate it, and how to use it (Haywood et al., 2016). While such indirect forms of lay participation in health decision-making, under tight expert control, can attain a high degree of acceptance by authorities, they meet with some resistance when used as an instrument to audit healthcare professionals and practices (Browne et al., 2017).

In the South, where adequate expertise is often scarce, and may be undermined by distorted incentive systems and status-based authority, it is the *absence* of efficient health technocracies that is seen to pose the more serious challenge (Bano, 2018; Fanelli et al., 2020). Faced with unyielding obstacles to improvinig population health, transnational-health authorities such as the WHO, NGOs, and international donors generally promote lay participation as a technocratic fix for weak or failed health system governance (Ejaz et al., 2011). But formal structures and exercises in institution-led lay participation, such as citizens' juries, are rarely functional (e.g. Golooba-Mutebi, 2005; Mubyazi et al., 2007; Scott et al., 2017). The misplaced reliance on technocratic lay participation to correct ineffective institutions, entrenched power differentials and counterproductive norms have been accused of rather maintaining and exacerbating them. It is argued that lay participation evades the real political and institutional transformations that would ultimately be required to build reliable, capable and equitable health systems (Cooke and Kothari, 2001). Dependent participation is thus seen to empower Southern health elites, just as it empowers Western ones, insofar as it constitutes little threat to traditional practices and relations, and indeed, supports them.

PARTICIPATION AS CAPACITY-BUILDING

A shortage of medical and public health expertise in the South, and its relatively poor performance in terms of population health, were the impetus for the original promotion of lay participation in developing countries in the 1960s and 1970s. Capacity-building strategies, such as health education and community organization, were adopted to train and enable community leaders to assume health-related responsibilities (Jewkes and Murcott, 1998; Lawn et al., 2008). Unlike in the West, then, the roots of lay participation in the South do not lie in civil society, but in the global healthcare technocracy in which Western NGOs, corporations and transnational authorities have played the leading role (Frenk and Moon, 2013), with the objectives of improving health, but also of transforming community attitudes and practices.

In what appears to be a transfer of ideas from the South, the promotion of lay participation as a capacity-building strategy has recently come to the fore in the West (Butterfoss et al., 1993; Bogue et al., 1997). As with NGO–community partnerships in the South, partnerships with voluntary organizations in the West ideally support communities to identify their own health experiences and concerns, and to gain influence over the conditions that underlie them. But the literature shows that, as in the South, these partnerships typically degenerate into expert-led health promotion and health education interventions, targeting communities and populations profiled as being vulnerable or at risk (Rantala et al., 2014). On Arnstein's ladder, such community health "partnerships" would rather be considered "therapy", and would never realize their promise of shared or delegated citizen control. Despite the "empowerment" rhetoric of this literature (Rifkin and Pridmore, 2001), collaborative partnerships are not deemed valuable as much because of their democratic or deliberative practices *per se* as because of their potential contribution to resourcing healthcare institutions, through the contribution of time, money, materials, and energy to institutional programmes (Rifkin, 2009). As in the South, while the end is surely enhanced population health, collaborative community partnerships constitute in large part a resource mobilization strategy (Zakus, 1998).

The most recent enthusiasm in the literature on lay participation re-conceptualizes health partnerships in terms of "coproduction". This concept elevates lay participants from their outsider status as occasional *consumers* of healthcare, to that of *producers* of healthcare, making clinical, institutional and policy decisions alongside insiders (Nabatchi et al., 2017). A careful reading of the literature reveals the capacity-building objectives of coproduction. Bovaird (2007: 847) defines coproduction as relationships "*where all parties make substantial resource contributions*" (italics added). Boyle and Harris (2009: 14) state that coproduction is about "recognizing people as *assets*". Palumbo (2016: 76) maintains that patients harbour "*untapped resources* which could be exploited for the purpose of service provision". Batalden and her colleagues (2016: 512) suggest that coproduction strategies are "employed to expand access, *decrease utilisation*, improve outcomes, increase patient satisfaction and *grow patient capacity for selfcare*". It would appear that the coproduction discourse is in large part a discourse on resource mobilization, either to augment the capacity of the health system, or to reduce pressure on it by devolving more healthcare responsibilities to patients, potential patients, and outsider organizations.

In developing countries, where access to appropriate healthcare for large swathes of the population remains a serious challenge, coproduction represents the evolution of community health (Cepiku and Giordano, 2014). It is seen by some as imperative in order to supplement the capacity of resource-poor health systems (Zakus, 1998; Joshi and Moore, 2004). In the West, under the political-economic conditions of austerity, a similar resource mobilization logic is taking the place of those democratic ideals that were once the universal impetus for lay participation. According to at least some "evangelical" takes on coproduction (Judge and Bould, 2006), it could virtually put an end to ineffective lay participation as we know it (Boyle and Harris, 2009). It would turn attention instead to self-care and self-management of health and to the complementary role of health-related voluntary organizations, community groups, and cooperatives (Bovaird, 2007). The vast new literature on patient and public engagement in health is largely oriented by this discourse.

Healthcare producers today are generally working under increasingly strained and exploitative conditions, associated with repeated shocks to the world economy, austerity, precarious labour, and reduced welfare protections. They are often not well protected or supported, as past and more recent pandemics, such as SARS and COVID-19, have revealed (Draper et al., 2010; Pappa et al., 2020; Sim, 2020). Indeed, the role of "alternative resources" in helping to manage the COVID-19 pandemic among marginal and excluded populations has everywhere been recognized as indispensable (Miao et al., 2020; Pradana et al., 2020; de Losada and Abdullah, 2020). They are better able to reach otherwise excluded populations (e.g. the homeless or immigrants and refugees), and their practices are more responsive to the particular needs of specific groups (e.g. youth, women, and people with mental health problems). Their strengths highlight public health systems' weaknesses. However, they are largely dependant on precarious grants and donations, and on lay expertise and voluntary participation. Their harnessing to the ends of health systems as coproducers of healthcare is severely under-resourced, compared to those highly technocratic health institutions with which they partner (Pill and Guarneros-Meza, 2018). Some argue that lay participation in the form of coproduction poses a risk of eventual co-*destruction* (Palumbo and Manna, 2018), that is, the erosion of healthcare quality and equity in the name of cost efficiency (Essén et al., 2016; Innes et al., 2019; Blunden and Calder, 2020).

LAY PARTICIPATION IN CONTEXT

Although the literature on lay particiaption in health is hermetic, focusing largely on the microprocesses of implementing lay participation in specific cases, it is nonetheless highly informative about the ends to which lay participation is deployed. The evidence shows that lay participation is ritually championed for its potential democratic influence and its ability to improve health outcomes. But this influence is rarely demonstrated or confirmed. This failure is overtly or tacitly recognized, and blame is typically placed on implementation procedures, such as recruitment biases, asymmetries in the capacity to absorb and analyze the issues, and controlling or manipulative facilitation. But paying attention to implementation strategies (and occasionally, outcome measures) reveals the ends towards which lay participation is oriented. It serves as a device for legitimating complex, technocratic processes and decisions; as a tool for managing public responses to institutional or system change; and as a strategy for resourcing cash-strapped health systems in innovative ways.

These are laudable ends, but both the normative and analytic knowledge base in lay participation may be best advanced by overtly recognizing them, and mobilizing the ample literature that exists on how to effectively analyse and address them. Without the benefit of relevant accumulated knowledge on, for example, policy decision-making, change management, or social innovation, the literature on lay participation in health seems to run in place. We have observed its evolution, with new ideas such as collaborative partnerships and coproduction coming to the fore. But there is not strong evidence of an awareness and questioning of this evolution within the literature, nor of an acknowledgement of relevant knowledge-bases grounded in a realistic and contextualised conceptualisation of participation (but see Bherer et al, 2017; Bherer et al, 2019).

The reading offered here invites us to step out of the dual confines that address lay participation as an ideal or as a practice, to consider it rather within the dynamics of the healthcare ecosystem within which it is mobilized, and to which it is meant to contribute. We have seen how outsiders are invited in by institutions, and how insiders' interests determine the means and the ends of lay participation. But these means and ends emerge within a dynamic health sector ecosystem that operates on a global scale, producing specific local challenges. If the larger environment in which it is nested and the accumulated, relevant political, adminsitrative and sociological knowledge is ignored, exercises in lay participation will likely remain ineffective rituals or experiments, or simply an adminsitrative transaction cost, as much of the literature suggests it is.

What are the sorts of challenges that impinge on the very practicality of lay participation in different contexts? Austerity, or limited resources in relation to healthcare needs or demands, is a reality in both the West and the South, though differently so. Biotechnological advances, such as genetic editing and artificial intelligence applied to medical interventions, are the principal motors behind rising costs and complexity and constitute a significant universe of "unknowns" for decision-makers, driving lay exercises in deliberative priority setting, for example. These developments also bring new ethical dilemmas, an arena in which deliberative lay participation has played an important role, for example, in devising policy for assisted reproductive technologies. Finally, there is the unknown of new health threats, whether generated by the pharmaceutical industry, such as menopause, erectile dysfunction, and childhood attention deficit; by evolving lifestyles, such as obesity, musculoskeletal problems and urban poverty; or by evolving viruses and potential pandemics. All these challenges engage a complex biomedical ecosystem, including the increasing intertwining of university-led and industry-led research, global markets, governments as producers, purchasers and regulators, professionals with ambitions to provide more effective cures, and relatively powerless patients who are increasingly told that their health – and the efficiency of available cures – are substantially within their own hands. This is the case both in the West (with the emphasis on diet, exercise and optimism or hope) and the South (banishing traditional cultural ideas and magical thinking in favour of rational behaviours, for example, to better control AIDS and Ebola). These issues explain why in much lay participation, particularly in the form of community health programmes, the targets of change are not the system, but rather, citizens and communities themselves.

Western health systems are also faced with increasingly knowledgeable, critical, but also susceptible publics – indeed, some prone to conspiracy theories (e.g. regarding the source of COVID-19 and even its very existence, or the effects and even the objectives of vaccines). Patients are less dependent insofar as they have multiple and alternative sources of information, but the question of its credibility and reliability is crucial. In this context, we see lay participation growing less concerned with the democratization of health decision-making, than with increasing health and health system literacy, and health communication in the form of consensus-building. Indeed, effective democratic participation could become a wild card within some health systems, unless subject to even more strategic manipulation than is currently the case.

In the South, addressing the population health deficit remains the priority. However, in a world characterized by massive migration, health threats once confined to developing countries have travelled north and west. Worldwide connections are generated not only by the health ecosystem encompassing governments, transnational authorities, international NGOs and multinational corporations, but increasingly by global networks of contagion. In this context, worldwide, coordinated, functional health governance is imperative, but rare in the South. There is a growing recognition that the barriers to effective health governance lie beyond the local community, where resource and leadership mobilization through lay participation often has some success. Rather, whole healthcare systems need to be transformed, but first, the overall state systems within which they are entrenched need reform. International organizations and donors and many development researchers remain heavily invested in promoting lay participation as a vector of democratic "good governance" in the South (Hickey and Mohan, 2004), but critics see it as a futile sideshow (Cooke and Kothari, 2001).

Lay participation, as a cherished concept and evolving practice, is nonetheless here to stay. The question proposed in this chapter – to what end? – should serve not simply to debunk much of the rhetoric, practice and literature on lay participation, but to suggest ways forward for both knowledge development and practice. It has been argued that significant advancements in understanding the roles that lay participation can and should effectively play depends on context (Charles and DiMaio, 1993; Hoppe, 2011). Context is nested: it includes everything from specific organisational dynamics (Marent et al., 2015) and institutional interests and capacity, to political will, civil society capabilities, and the structures of inequality in any given society, all influenced by global actors and relations. It also includes the extent, validity, and deployment of the knowledge base in all these relevant areas to analyse the realistic potential – and the realistic ends and means – of lay participation in any given context. Even in the West, the definition of realistic ends and how to reach them through lay participation could benefit from openly considering the role of global capitalism in determining health decision-making, and the same sorts of administrative resistance, self-interested behaviour, tacit norms, power games, and disinterest for patients, that are more often pointed to as hampering it in less technocratically developed health systems.

Beyond the local context, the effective ends of lay participation are seriously constrained by the position of the implementing institutions in the larger health ecosystem. For example, a government ministry or national commission will have different leverage to translate particular types of outcomes into action than an NGO, regional council, or single hospital. In each of these contexts, an initial environmental scan is an indispensable tool to explore the full network of actors and their relations within which the exercise is embedded. It should serve to analyze the specific administrative, social, cultural, political, and economic barriers and opportunities that will inevitably shape, and ought to orient, the practice and outcome of lay participation (Higgs, 2019). Results of the scan ultimately inform the following types of questions: what needs to change, what role can lay participation realistically play considering the nested context, who should therefore be included, in what capacity, how can they contribute, and how should the outcomes that emerge be transferred beyond the boundaries of the single exercise, and transformed into action? At this stage, the building of a "logic model" (Chen, 1990) would be another pragmatic tool: it posits a desired end, and then constructs the path by which that end can realistically be achieved, in discreet steps, through the practice of lay participation. These exercises serve to bring achievable ends into focus, to consider whether the necessary conditions are present in the environment, to select the most appropriate methods and the steps required, and, sometimes, to eliminate lay participation as an effective strategy in certain situations, even for reasons of legitimation (Djellouli et al., 2019; Abimbola, 2020).

Finally, the question of who controls the participation process, and therefore, its potential contribution, needs to be addressed. Institutions have defined and often deformed its ends to meet their own interests, by controlling the microprocesses of participation. Since the 1960s, lay participation in the West has passed almost entirely out of the hands of civil society and into institutional hands, which apply increasingly strategic means to ensure institutional legitimacy, while also mobilizing lay resources to support health institutions and practices, and learning to manage the increasingly complex challenges that health systems face. Has the pendulum swung too far? Or was dependent participation designed from the outset to mobilize lay power to strengthen health institutions and support their decision-making tiers?

CONCLUSION

There has been tremendous change over the past fifty years in the relationship between health experts and institutions on the one hand, and ordinary people on the other. These changes, known as "social learning", are only obliquely captured by the literature on individual instances of participation, but become more visible when exploring lay participation as a phenomenon unfolding over time and space within a larger, dynamic health ecosystem. We then can recognize that the ubiquity of lay participation has had significant repercussions, first and foremost for public expectations: the expectation to be consulted and to have one's say – whether it is effective or not – has raised the bar for legitimate institutional functioning and policy decision-making. Lay participation over the long haul has also influenced the health research agenda, and – to a lesser degree so far – medical training. It is also evident that, through years of experience with lay participation, hospital administrators and health system decision-makers are increasingly aware of the nature and potential of lay expertise, as well as the diversity of autonomous health-related organizations in their environment. Together with the dissemination of health and medical information through the internet, lay participation has thus contributed to increasingly symmetrical relations between medical professionals and patients, at least in the West, where the weight of the financial transaction has mostly been eliminated.

Are the huge public investments in lay participation able and likely to take us any further than the long-term, vague and largely undocumented outcomes mentioned above? At this point, the rich knowledge bases on organizational dynamics, intersectoral collaboration, policy networks, and other relevant processes remains to be integrated into future theoretical thinking on lay participation if a more realistic understanding and development of its potential is to be achieved. Still, some literature reliably shows that certain local conditions do have a significant impact on both democratic and strategic ends of lay participation. These include executive commitment, as measured, for example, by the budget, time, and dedicated staff accorded for planning and implementation, but, more importantly, the existence of a feedback strategy, such that participants see how their input is fed into the decision-making process, and its effects (Checkoway et al., 1984; He and Ma, 2020). It has also been established that democratic ends with respect to lay participation in healthcare are met only when lay participants are well organized, delegated by civil society groups, and supported with information and ideas by constituencies to which they feel accountable (Marmor and Marone, 1980; Checkoway et al., 1984). Backed by effective, autonomous organizations with their own interests and sources of knowledge, lay participation becomes less dependent. Indeed, it can in this way become a valuable tool for civil society, infiltrating institutions and effectively disseminated alternative knowledge and ideas (Palumbo, 2017).

As Christens and Speer (2006) have argued, it is perhaps futile to consider that means can be separated from ends. There is a clear tension between lay participation as a democracy-enhancing process versus an effectiveness- or efficiency-enhancing process (Morgan, 2001). Context matters. For example, within the doctor–patient relation patient input and even direction may be desirable, but at other levels it can result in institutional capture, in which one well-organized civil-society group influences decisions in ways that do not necessarily reflect the public interest.

And, as illustrated by the contradictory public responses to the COVID-19 pandemic and the measures proposed to control it, enhancing democratic effects poses the risk of politicizing decisions that, within a well-functioning technocracy, would be based on evidence rather than public pressure.

A healthy ambivalence regarding the democratization of healthcare reminds us of the importance of placing it in context, and of the reasons lay participation was made dependent on institutional ends in the first place. If more power is still to be claimed by the people, research and practice will need to focus more on the legitimacy of public institutions on the one hand, and the culture and dynamic of civil society on the other. In contexts where these interrelated drivers of lay participation are inauspicious, underdeveloped, or absent, there is reason to look elsewhere to effectively improve healthcare practices and systems.

REFERENCES

Abelson, J., Eyles, J., McLeod, C. B., Collins, P., McMullan, C., & Forest, P. G. (2003). Does deliberation make a difference? Results from a citizens' panel study of health goals priority setting. *Health Policy*, 66(1), 95–106.

Abelson, J., Forest, P. G., Eyles, J., Smith, P., Martin, E., & Gauvin, F. P. (2003). Deliberations about deliberative methods: issues in the design and evaluation of public participation processes. *Social Science & Medicine*, 57(2), 239–251.

Abimbola, S. (2020). Beyond positive a priori bias: reframing community engagement in LMICs. *Health Promotion International*, 35(3), 598–609.

Aiyar, Y. (2010). Invited spaces, invited participation: effects of greater participation on accountability in service delivery. *India Review*, 9(2), 204–229.

Amelung, N., & Grabner, L. (2017). Making citizen panels a 'universal bestseller'. In L. Bherer, M. Gauthier, & L. Simard (Eds.), *The Professionalization of Public Participation* (pp. 189–123). London: Routledge.

Armstrong, H. (2001). Social cohesion and privatization in Canadian health care. *Canadian Journal of Law & Society*, 16, 65.

Arnstein, S. R. (1969). A ladder of citizen participation. *Journal of the American Institute of Planners*, 35(4), 216–224.

Aronson, J. (1993). Giving consumers a say in policy development: influencing policy or just being heard? *Canadian Public Policy*, 19(4), 367–378.

Bano, M. (2019). Partnerships and the good-governance agenda: improving service delivery through state–NGO collaborations. *VOLUNTAS: International Journal of Voluntary and Nonprofit Organizations*, 30(6), 1270–1283.

Batalden, M., Batalden, P., Margolis, P., Seid, M., Armstrong, G., Opipari-Arrigan, L., & Hartung, H. (2016). Coproduction of healthcare service. *BMJ Quality & Safety*, 25(7), 509–517.

Bennett, P., & Smith, S. J. (2007). Genetics, insurance and participation: how a citizens' jury reached its verdict. *Social Science & Medicine*, *64*(12), 2487–2498.

Bherer, L., Gauthier, M., & Simard, L. (Eds.). (2017). *The Professionalization of Public Participation*. London: Routledge.

Bherer, L., & Lee, C. W. (2019). Consultants: the emerging participation industry. In S. Elstub & O. Escobar (Eds.), *Handbook of Democratic Innovation and Governance* (pp. 196–208). Cheltenham, UK: Edward Elgar Publishing.

Black, N. (2013). Patient reported outcome measures could help transform health care. *British Medical Journal*, 346, f167.

Blume, S. (2006). Anti-vaccination movements and their interpretations. *Social Science & Medicine*, 62(3), 628–642.

Blunden, N., & Calder, G. (2020). Co-production and person-centred care in neoliberal conditions. *European Journal for Person Centered Healthcare*, 8(1), 75–85.

Bogue, R. J., Antia, M., Harmata, R., & Hall Jr, C. H. (1997). Community experiments in action: developing community-defined models for reconfiguring health care delivery. *Journal of Health Politics, Policy and Law*, 22(4), 1051–1076.

Bolsewicz Alderman, K. B., Hipgrave, D., & Jimenez-Soto, E. (2013). Public engagement in health priority setting in low-and middle-income countries: current trends and considerations for policy. *PLoS Med*, 10(8), e1001495.

Bombard, Y., Baker, G. R., Orlando, E., Fancott, C., Bhatia, P., Casalino, S., … & Pomey, M. P. (2018). Engaging patients to improve quality of care: a systematic review. *Implementation Science*, 13(1), 98.

Bovaird, T. (2007). Beyond engagement and participation: user and community coproduction of public services. *Public Administration Review*, 67(5), 846–860.

Bowl, R. (1996). Legislating for user involvement in the United Kingdom: mental health services and the NHS and Community Care Act 1990. *International Journal of Social Psychiatry*, 42(3), 165–180.

Boyle, D., & Harris, M. (2009). *The Challenge of Co-Production*. London: New Economics Foundation/NESTA.

Brett, J., Staniszewska, S., Mockford, C. et al. (2014). Mapping the impact of patient and public involvement on health and social care research: a systematic review. *Health Expectations*, 17(5), 637–650.

Browne, J. P., Cano, S. J., & Smith, S. (2017). Using patient-reported outcome measures to improve health care: time for a new approach. *Medical Care*, 55(10), 901–904.

Brun, D. A., & Diamond, L. (Eds.). (2014). *Clientelism, Social Policy, and the Quality of Democracy*. Baltimore, MD: Johns Hopkins University Press.

Bukenya, B. (2018). Are service-delivery NGOs building state capacity in the Global South? Experiences from HIV/AIDS programmes in rural Uganda. *Development Policy Review*, 36(51), O378–O399.

Butterfoss, F. D., Goodman, R. M., & Wandersman, A. (1993). Community coalitions for prevention and health promotion. *Health Education Research*, 8(3), 315–330.

Callaghan, G. D., & Wistow, G. (2006). Publics, patients, citizens, consumers? Power and decision making in primary health care. *Public Administration*, 84(3), 583–601.

Carman, K. L., Mallery, C., Maurer, M., Wang, G., Garfinkel, S., Yang, M., … & Gold, M. R. (2015). Effectiveness of public deliberation methods for gathering input on issues in healthcare: results from a randomized trial. *Social Science & Medicine*, 133, 11–20.

Carman, K. L., Maurer, M., Mangrum, R., Yang, M., Ginsburg, M., Sofaer, S., Gold, M. R. et al. (2016). Understanding an informed public's views on the role of evidence in making health care decisions. *Health Affairs*, 35(4), 566–574.

Castro, E. M., Van Regenmortel, T., Sermeus, W., & Vanhaecht, K. (2019). Patients' experiential knowledge and expertise in health care: a hybrid concept analysis. *Social Theory & Health*, 17(3), 307–330.

Cepiku, D., & Giordano, F. (2014). Co-production in developing countries: insights from the community health workers experience. *Public Management Review*, 16(3), 317–340.

Charles, C., & DeMaio, S. (1993). *Lay Participation in Health Care Decision Making: A Conceptual Framework*. CHEPA working paper series No. 92–16, Hamilton, ON: McMaster University.

Checkoway, B. (1982a). Public participation in health planning agencies: promise and practice, *Journal of Health Politics, Policy and Law*, 7(3), 723–733.

Checkoway, B. (1982b). The empire strikes back: more lessons for health care consumers. *Journal of Health Politics, Policy and Law*, 7(1), 111–124.

Checkoway, B., O'Rourke, T. W., & Bull, D. (1984). Correlates of consumer participation in health planning agencies: findings and implications from a national survey. *Policy Studies Review*, 3(2), 296–310.

Chen, H.-T. (1990). *Theory-driven Evaluations*. Newbury Park, CA: Sage.

Christens, B. D., & Speer, P. W. (2006). Tyranny/transformation: power and paradox in participatory development. *Forum: Qualitative Social Research*, 7(2), article 22.

Conklin, A., Morris, Z., & Nolte, E. (2015). What is the evidence base for public involvement in health-care policy? Results of a systematic scoping review. *Health Expectations*, 18(2), 153–165.

Conrad, P. (2005). The shifting engines of medicalization. *Journal of Health and Social Behavior*, 46(1), 3–14.

Conrad, P., & Slodden, C. (2013). The medicalization of mental disorder. In C. S. Aneshensel,

J. C. Phelan, & A. Bierman (Eds.), *Handbook of The Sociology of Mental Health* (pp. 61–73). Dordrecht, NL: Springer.

Cooke, B., & Kothari, U. (Eds.). (2001). *Participation: The New Tyranny?* London: Zed Books.

Cornwall, A. (2002). *Making spaces, changing places: situating participation in development.* IDS Working Paper #170 www.ids.ac.uk/publications/making-spaces-changing-places-situating-participation-in-development/, accessed October 12, 2020.

Cornwall, A., & Shankland, A. (2008). Engaging citizens: lessons from building Brazil's national health system. *Social Science & Medicine*, 66(10), 2173–2184.

Crane, J. (2018). Why the history of public consultation matters for contemporary health policy. *Endeavour*, 42(1), 9–16.

Crawford, M. J., Rutter, D., Manley, C., Weaver, T., Bhui, K., Fulop, N., & Tyrer, P. (2002). Systematic review of involving patients in the planning and development of health care. *British Medical Journal*, 325(7375), 1263.

Crawford, M., Rutter, D., & Thelwall, S. (2003). *User Involvement in Change Management: A Review of the Literature*. Report to the National Co-ordinating Centre for NHS Service Delivery and Organisation R&D (NCCSDO). London: NHS Service Delivery and Organisation Programme.

Crossley, N. (1998). RD Laing and the British anti-psychiatry movement: a socio–historical analysis. *Social Science & Medicine*, 47(7), 877–889.

Davies, C., Wetherell, M., & Barnett, E. (2006). *Citizens at the Centre: Deliberative Participation in Healthcare Decisions*. Bristol, UK: Bristol University Press and Policy Press.

de Freitas, C. (2017). Public and patient participation in health policy, care, and research. *Porto Biomedical Journal*, 2(2), 31–32.

de Losada, A. F., & Abdullah, Hannah. (Eds.). (2020). *Cities on the Frontline: Managing the Coronavirus Crisis*. CIDOB Report #05. Barcelona: Barcelona Centre for International Affairs.

Degeling, C., Rychetnik, L., Street, J., Thomas, R., & Carter, S. M. (2017). Influencing health policy through public deliberation: lessons learned from two decades of Citizens'/community juries. *Social Science & Medicine*, 179, 166–171.

Delli Carpini, M. X., Cook, F. L., & Jacobs, L. R. (2004). Public deliberation, discursive participation, and citizen engagement: a review of the empirical literature. *Annual Review of Political Science*, 7, 315–344.

Deng, C. Y., & Wu, C. L. (2010). An innovative participatory method for newly democratic societies: the 'civic groups forum' on national health insurance reform in Taiwan. *Social Science & Medicine*, 70(6), 896–903.

Devlin, N. J., & Appleby, J. (2010). *Getting the Most Out of PROMS: Putting Health Outcomes at the Heart of NHS Decision-Making.* London: The King's Fund.

Djellouli, N., Jones, L., Barratt, H., Ramsay, A. I., Towndrow, S., & Oliver, S. (2019). Involving the public in decision-making about large-scale changes to health services: a scoping review. *Health Policy*, 123(7), 635–645.

Donovan, J., & Coast, J. (1996). Public participation in priority setting: commitment or illusion? In J. Coast, J. Donovan, & S. Frankel (Eds.), *Priority Setting: The Health Care Debate*. Chichester, UK: John Wiley & Sons.

Draper, H., Sorell, T., Ives, J., Damery, S., Greenfield, S., Parry, J., ... & Wilson, S. (2010). Non-professional healthcare workers and ethical obligations to work during pandemic influenza. *Public Health Ethics*, 3(1), 23–34.

Ehrenreich, B., & English, D. (1973). *Complaints and Disorders: The Sexual Politics of Sickness*. New York: Feminist Press.

Ejaz, I., Shaikh, B. T., & Rizvi, N. (2011). NGOs and government partnership for health systems strengthening: a qualitative study presenting viewpoints of government, NGOs and donors in Pakistan. *BMC Health Services Research*, 11(1), 1–7.

Ellen, M., Shach, R., Kok, M., & Fatta, K. (2017). There is much to learn when you listen: exploring citizen engagement in high- and low-income countries. *World Health Population*, 17, 31–42.

Essén, A., Värlander, S. W., & Liljedal, K. T. (2016). Co-production in chronic care: exploitation and empowerment. *European Journal of Marketing*, 50(5/6), 724–751.

Fanelli, S., Salvatore, F. P., De Pascale, G., & Faccilongo, N. (2020). Insights for the future of health system partnerships in low- and middle-income countries: a systematic literature review. *BMC Health Services Research*, 20(1), 1–13.

Farmer, J., Taylor, J., Stewart, E., & Kenny, A. (2018). Citizen participation in health services co-production: a roadmap for navigating participation types and outcomes. *Australian Journal of Primary Health*, 23(6), 509–515.

Feingold, E. (1969). The changing political character of health planning. *American Journal of Public Health*, 59(5), 803–808.

Fishkin, J. S. (2003). Consulting the public through deliberative polling. *Journal of Policy Analysis and Management*, 22(1), 128–133.

Fitzpatrick, R. (1994). Health needs assessment, chronic illness and the social sciences. In J. Popay & G. Williams (Eds.), *Researching the People's Health* (pp. 183–200). London: Routledge.

Foucault, M. (1975). *The Birth of the Clinic: An Archaeology of Medical Perception*. New York: Vintage Books.

Franke, R. W., & Chasin, B. H. (1994). *Kerala: Radical reform as development in an Indian state*. Oakland, CA: Food First Books, The Institute for food and Development Policy.

Frankish, C. J., Kwan, B., Ratner, P. A., Higgins, J. W., & Larsen, C. (2002). Challenges of citizen participation in regional health authorities. *Social Science & Medicine*, 54(10), 1471–1480.

Frenk, J., & Moon, S. (2013). Governance challenges in global health. *New England Journal of Medicine*, 368(10), 936–942.

García, P. J. (2019). Corruption in global health: the open secret. *The Lancet*, 394(10214), 2119–2124.

Golooba-Mutebi, F. (2005). When popular participation won't improve service provision: primary health care in Uganda. *Development Policy Review*, 23(2), 165–182.

Goold, S. D., Biddle, A. K., Klipp, G., Hall, C. N., & Danis, M. (2005). Choosing health plans all together: a deliberative exercise for allocating limited health care resources. *Journal of Health Politics, Policy and Law*, 30(4), 563–602.

Govender, V., & Mooney, G. (2012). People's policies for the health of the poor globally. *The International Journal of Health Planning and Management*, *27*(2), e92–e103.

Grant, Jane A. (1989). Consumer participation in health planning: policy and political implications. *Nonprofit and Voluntary Sector Quarterly*, 18(2), 147–165.

Haldane, V., Chuah, F. L., Srivastava, A., Singh, S. R., Koh, G. C., Seng, C. K., & Legido-Quigley, H. (2019). Community participation in health services development, implementation, and evaluation: a systematic review of empowerment, health, community, and process outcomes. *PloS One*, 14(5), e0216112.

Haldii, A. (1999). AIDS, anger and activism: ACT UP as a social movement organization. In Jo Freeman & Victoria L. Johnson (Eds.), *Waves of Protest: Social Movements since the Sixties* (pp. 135–150). Lanham, MD: Rowman and Littlefield.

Hanefeld, J., Powell-Jackson, T., & Balabanova, D. (2017). Understanding and measuring quality of care: dealing with complexity. *Bulletin of the World Health Organization*, 95(5), 368.

Harris, J., Cook, T., Gibbs, L., Oetzel, J., Salsberg, J., Shinn, C., Springett, J., Wallerstein, N., & Wright, M. (2018). Searching for the impact of participation in health and health research: challenges and methods. *BioMed Research International*, Art. 9427452. https://doi.org/10.1155/2018/9427452, accessed January 21, 2021.

Haywood, K. L., Wilson, R., Staniszewska, S., & Salek, S. (2016). Using PROMs in healthcare: who should be in driving seat – policy makers, health professionals, methodologists, or patients? *Patient*, 9, 495–498.

He, A. J., & Ma, L. (2020). Citizen participation, perceived public service performance, and trust in government: evidence from health policy reforms in Hong Kong. *Public Performance & Management Review*, 1–23, doi: 10.1080/15309576.2020.1780138.

Hickey, S., & Mohan, G. (2004). *Participation – From Tyranny to Transformation? Exploring New Approaches to Participation in Development*. London Zed Books.

Higgs, J. (2019). Exploring practice in context. In J. Higgs, S. Cork, & D. Horsfall (Eds.), *Challenging Future Practice Possibilities* (pp. 3–16). Leiden, NL: Brill Sense.

Hobson-West, P. (2007). 'Trusting blindly can be the biggest risk of all': organised resistance to childhood vaccination in the UK. *Sociology of Health & Illness*, 29(2), 198–215.

Hoffman, B. (2008). Health care reform and social movements in the United States.

American Journal of Public Health, 98(Suppl 1), S69–S79.

Hoppe, R. (2011). *The Governance of Problems: Puzzling, Powering, Participation*. Bristol, UK: Policy Press.

Horrobin, D. F. (1977). *Medical Hubris: A Reply to Ivan Illich*. Montreal, CA: Eden Press.

Illich, I. (1976). *Limits to Medicine: Medical Nemesis: The Expropriation of Health*. London: Marion Boyars.

Innes, M., Davies, B., & McDermont, M. (2019). How co-production regulates. *Social & Legal Studies*, 28(3), 370–391.

Irvin, R. A., & Stansbury, J. (2004). Citizen participation in decision making: is it worth the effort? *Public Administration Review*, 64(1), 55–65.

Jewkes, R., & Murcott, A. (1998). Community representatives: representing the 'community'. *Social Science & Medicine*, 46(7), 843–858.

Joshi, A., & Moore, M. (2004). Institutionalised co-production: unorthodox public service delivery in challenging environments. *Journal of Development Studies*, 40(4), 31–49.

Judge, K., & Bauld, L. (2006). Learning from policy failure? Health action zones in England. *The European Journal of Public Health*, 16(4), 341–343.

Kamuzora, P., Maluka, S., Ndawi, B., Byskov, J., & Hurtig, A. K. (2013). Promoting community participation in priority setting in district health systems: experiences from Mbarali district, Tanzania. *Global Health Action*, 6(1), 22669.

Karazivan, P., Dumez, V., Flora, L., Pomey, M. P., Del Grande, C., Ghadiri, D. P., Fernandez, N., Jouet, E., Las Vergnas, O., & Lebel, P. (2015). The patient-as-partner approach in health care: a conceptual framework for a necessary transition. *Academic Medicine*, 90(4), 437–441.

Kashefi, E., & Mort, M. (2004). Grounded citizens' juries: a tool for health activism. *Health Expectations*, 7(4), 290–302.

Kay, A., & Williams, O. (2009). Introduction: the international political economy of global health governance. In A. Kay & O. Williams, (Eds.), *Global Health Governance* (pp. 1–23). London: Palgrave Macmillan.

Keefe, R. H., Lane, S. D., & Swars, H. (2006). From the bottom up: tracing the impact of four health-based social movements on health and social policies. *Journal of Health and Social Policy*, 21(3), 5–69.

Komporozos-Athanasiou, A., Fudge, N., Adams, M., & McKevitt, C. (2018). Citizen participation as political ritual: towards a sociological theorizing of 'health citizenship'. *Sociology*, 52(4), 744–761.

Kornreich, Y., Vertinsky, I., & Potter, P. B. (2012). Consultation and deliberation in China: the making of China's health-care reform. *The China Journal*, (68), 176–203.

Krinks, R., Kendall, E., Whitty, J. A., & Scuffham, P. A. (2016). Do consumer voices in health-care citizens' juries matter? *Health Expectations*, 19(5), 1015–1022.

Latour, B. (2005). *Reassembling the Social: An Introduction to Social Life*. Oxford: Oxford University Press.

Lauria, M., & Slotterback, C. S. (Eds.). (2020). *Learning from Arnstein's Ladder: From Citizen Participation to Public Engagement*. London: Routledge.

Lawn, J. E., Rohde, J., Rifkin, S., Were, M., Paul, V. K., & Chopra, M. (2008). Alma-Ata 30 years on: revolutionary, relevant, and time to revitalise. *The Lancet*, *372*(9642), 917–927.

Lehoux, P., Daudelin, G., & Abelson, J. (2012). The unbearable lightness of citizens within public deliberation processes. *Social Science & Medicine*, 74(12), 1843–1850.

Lever, A. (2013). Democracy, deliberation and public service reform: the case of NICE. In? H. Kippin & G. Stoker (Eds.), *Public Services: A New Reform Agenda* (pp. 91–106). London: Bloomsbury Academic Press.

Lewis, M. (2006). *Governance and Corruption in Public Health Care Systems*. Center for Global Development Working Paper #78. doi:10.2139/ssrn.984046

Lipsky, M., & Lounds, M. (1976). Citizen participation and health care: problems of government induced participation. *Journal of Health Politics, Policy and Law*, 1(1), 85–111.

Lupton, C., Buckland, S., & Moon, G. (1995). Consumer involvement in health care purchasing: the role and influence of the community health councils. *Health & Social Care in the Community*, 3(4), 215–226.

Mackey, T. K., & Liang, B. A. (2012). Combating healthcare corruption and fraud with improved global health governance. *BMC*

International Health and Human Rights, *12*(1), 23.

Mansbridge, J. (2010). Deliberative polling as the gold standard. *The Good Society*, 19(1), 55–62.

Marent, B., Forster, R., & Nowak, P. (2015). Conceptualizing lay participation in professional health care organizations. *Administration & Society*, 47(7), 827–850.

Marieskind, H. (1975). The women's health movement. *International Journal of Health Services*, 5(2), 217–223.

Marmor, T. R., & Marone, J. A. (1980). Representing consumer interests: imbalanced markets, health planning, and the HSAs. *Health and Society*, 58(1), 125–165.

Martin, G. P. (2008). 'Ordinary people only': knowledge, representativeness, and the publics of public participation in healthcare. *Sociology of Health & Illness*, 30(1), 35–54.

Martin, G. P. (2012). Public deliberation in action: emotion, inclusion and exclusion in participatory decision making. *Critical Social Policy*, 32(2), 163–183.

Menon, D., & Stafinski, T. (2008). Engaging the public in priority-setting for health technology assessment: findings from a citizens' jury. *Health Expectations*, 11(3), 282–293.

Miao, Q., Schwarz, S., & Schwarz, G. (2020). Responding to COVID-19: community volunteerism and coproduction in China. *World Development*, 137, 105–128.

Milewa, T. (1997). Community participation and health care priorities: reflections on policy, theater, and reality in Britain. *Health Promotions International*, 12(2), 161–167.

Milewa, Timothy, Valentine, Justine & Calnan, Michael (1998). Managerialism and active citizenship in Britain's reformed health service: power and community in an era of decentralization, *Social Science and Medicine*, 47 (4): 507–517.

Mitton, C., Smith, N., Peacock, S., Evoy, B., & Abelson, J. (2011). Integrating public input into healthcare priority-setting decisions. *Evidence & Policy*, 7(3), 327–343.

Moran, M. (1999). *Governing the Health Care State: A Comparative Study of the United Kingdom, the United States, and Germany*. Manchester, UK: Manchester University Press.

Morgan, L. M. (2001). Community participation in health: perpetual allure, persistent challenge. *Health Policy and Planning*, 16(3), 221–230.

Mort, M., & Finch, T. (2005). Principles for telemedicine and telecare: the perspective of a citizens' panel. *Journal of Telemedicine and Telecare*, 11(1 suppl), 66–68.

Mubyazi, G. M., Mushi, A., Kamugisha, M., Massaga, J., Mdira, K. Y., Segeja, M., & Njunwa, K. J. (2007). Community views on health sector reform and their participation in health priority setting: case of Lushoto and Muheza districts, Tanzania. *Journal of Public Health*, 29(2), 147–156.

Nabatchi, T., & Leighninger, M. (2015). *Public Participation for 21st Century Democracy*. New York: John Wiley & Sons.

Nabatchi, T., Sancino, A., & Sicilia, M. (2017). Varieties of participation in public services: the who, when, and what of coproduction. *Public Administration Review*, 77(5), 766–776.

Niemeyer, S., & Dryzek, J. S. (2007). The ends of deliberation: meta-consensus and intersubjective rationality as ideal outcomes. *Swiss Political Science Review*, 13(4), 497–526.

OECD (2019). *Health spending set to outpace GDP growth to 2030*. www.oecd.org/health/health-spending-set-to-outpace-gdp-growth-to-2030.htm, accessed September 26, 2020.

Osborne, S. P. (2006). The new public governance? *Public Management Review*, 8(3), 377–387.

Palumbo, R. (2016). Contextualizing co-production of health care: a systematic literature review. *International Journal of Public Sector Management*, 29(1), pp. 72–90.

Palumbo, R. (2017). *The bright side and the dark side of patient empowerment: Co-creation and co-destruction of value in the healthcare environment*. Springer.

Palumbo, R., & Manna, R. (2018). What if things go wrong in co-producing health services? Exploring the implementation problems of health care co-production. *Policy and Society*, 37(3), 368–385.

Pappa, S., Ntella, V., Giannakas, T., Giannakoulis, V. G., Papoutsi, E., & Katsaounou, P. (2020). Prevalence of depression, anxiety, and insomnia among healthcare workers during the COVID-19 pandemic: a systematic review and meta-analysis. *Brain, Behavior, and Immunity*, 88, 901–907.

Perry, H. (2013). *A Brief History of Community Health Worker Programs*. www.mchip.net/

sites/default/files/mchipfiles/02_CHW_History.pdf, accessed 21 January 2021.

Peters, D. H., & Bloom, G. (2012). Bring order to unregulated health markets. *Nature*, 487(7406), 163–165.

Pickard, S., Williams, G., & Flynn, R. (1995). Local voices in an internal market: the case of community health services. *Social Policy & Administration*, 29(2), 135–149.

Pill, M., & Guarneros-Meza, V. (2018). Local governance under austerity: hybrid organisations and hybrid officers. *Policy & Politics*, 46(3), 409–425.

Piper, L., & Von Lieres, B. (2008). Inviting failure: citizen participation and local governance in South Africa. *Citizenship DRC Special Issue*, 1(1), 1–22.

Pradana, M., Rubiyanti, N., Hasbi, I., & Utami, D. G. (2020). Indonesia's fight against COVID-19: the roles of local government units and community organisations. *Local Environment*, 25(9), 1–3.

Rantala, R., Bortz, M., & Armada, F. (2014). Intersectoral action: local governments promoting health. *Health Promotion International*, 29(suppl. 1), i92–i102.

Reeves, A., McKee, M., Basu, S., & Stuckler, D. (2014). The political economy of austerity and healthcare: cross-national analysis of expenditure changes in 27 European nations 1995–2011. *Health Policy*, 115(1), 1–8.

Rifkin, S. B. (2009). Lessons from community participation in health programmes: a review of the post Alma-Ata experience. *International Health*, 1(1), 31–36.

Rifkin, S. B., & Pridmore, P. (2001). *Partners in Planning: Information, Participation, and Empowerment*. London: Macmillan.

Rogers, W. A., Street, J. M., Braunack-Mayer, A. J., Hiller, J. E., & FluViews Team (2009). Pandemic influenza communication: views from a deliberative forum. *Health Expectations*, 12(3), 331–342.

Rosenhan, D. L. (1973). On being sane in insane places. *Science*, 179(4070), 250–258.

Rowe, G., & Frewer, L. J. (2005). A typology of public engagement mechanisms. *Science, Technology, & Human Values*, 30(2), 251–290.

Rowe, R., & Shepherd, M. (2002). Public participation in the new NHS: no closer to citizen control? *Social Policy & Administration*, 36(3), 275–290.

Safaei, J. (2015). Deliberative democracy in health care: current challenges and future prospects. *Journal of Healthcare Leadership*, 7, 123.

Scott, K., George, A. S., Harvey, S. A., Mondal, S., Patel, G., & Sheikh, K. (2017). Negotiating power relations, gender equality, and collective agency: are village health committees transformative social spaces in northern India? *International Journal for Equity in Health*, 16(84), 1–12.

Seixas, B. V. (2018). The no-destination ship of priority-setting in healthcare: a call for more democracy. *International Journal of Health Policy and Management*, 7(4), 345.

Sen, A. (1991). The Kerala Difference, reply to Barbara H. Chasin and Richard W. Franke. *New York Review of Books*, October 24, 1991. www.nybooks.com/articles/1991/10/24/the-kerala-difference/, accessed October 12, 2020.

Shakespeare, T. (1993). Disabled people's self-organisation: a new social movement? *Disability, Handicap & Society*, 8(3), 249–264.

Sim, M. R. (2020). The COVID-19 pandemic: major risks to healthcare and other workers on the front line. *Occupational and Environmental Medicine*, 77(5), 281–282.

Snow, M. E., Tweedie, K., & Pederson, A. (2018). Heard and valued: the development of a model to meaningfully engage marginalized populations in health services planning, *BMC Health Services Research*, 18, 181.

Stafinski, T., Menon, D., & Yasui, Y. (2014). Assessing the impact of deliberative processes on the views of participants: is it 'in one ear and out the other'? *Health Expectations*, 17(2), 278–290.

Steckler, A. B., & Herzog, W. T. (1979). How to keep your mandated citizen board out of your hair and off your back: a guide for executive directors. *American Journal of Public Health*, 69(8), 809–812.

Stewart, E. (2013). What is the point of citizen participation in health care? *Journal of Health Services Research & Policy*, 18(2), 124–126.

Stewart, E. (2016). *Publics and Their Health Systems: Rethinking Participation*. Dordrecht, NL: Springer.

Stoker, G. (2006). Public value management: a new narrative for networked governance? *The American Review of Public Administration*, 36(1), 41–57.

Street, J., Duszynski, K., Krawczyk, S., & Braunack-Mayer, A. (2014). The use of citizens' juries in health policy decision-making: a systematic review. *Social Science & Medicine*, 109, 1–9.

Sturmberg, J. P., & Martin, C. M. (2013). *Handbook of Systems and Complexity in Health*. Dordrecht, NL: Springer.

Szasz, T. (1961). *The Myth of Mental Illness*. New York: Free Press.

Tempfer, C. B., & Nowak, P. (2011). Consumer participation and organizational development in health care: a systematic review. *Wiener Klinische Wochenschrift*, 123(13–14), 408–414.

Thompson, A. G. (2007). The meaning of patient involvement and participation in health care consultations: a taxonomy. *Social Science & Medicine*, 64(6), 1297–1310.

Topliss, E. (1975). The role of community health councils. *Royal Society of Health Journal*, 95(6), 299–301.

Toth, Ben (1996). Public participation: an historical perspective in Coast, Joanna, Donovan, Jenny, and Frankel, Stephen, eds., *Priority Setting: The Health Care Debate*, Chichester: John Wiley & Sons.

Touraine, A. (1971). *The Post-Industrial Society: Tomorrow's Social History: Classes, Conflicts and Culture in the Programmed Society*. New York: Random House.

Tritter, J. Q., & McCallum, A. (2006). The snakes and ladders of user involvement: moving beyond Arnstein. *Health Policy*, 76(2), 156–168.

Wallace, T. (2004). NGO dilemmas: Trojan horses for global neoliberalism? *Socialist Register*, 40, https://socialistregister.com/index.php/srv/article/view/5818, accessed January 21, 2021.

Weldring, T., & Smith, S. M. (2013). Patient-Reported Outcomes (PROs) and Patient-Reported Outcome Measures (PROMs). *Health Services Insights*, 6, 61–68.

Wood, G. (2003). Staying secure, staying poor: the 'Faustian Bargain'. *World Development*, 31(3), 455–471.

World Bank (2017). *Current Health Expenditure (% of GDP)*. https://data.worldbank.org/indicator/SH.XPD.CHEX.GD.ZS, accessed September 26, 2020.

World Health Organization (1978). *Primary Health Care: Report of the International Conference on Primary Health Care, Alma-Ata, USSR, 6–12 September 1978*. Geneva, Switzerland: World Health Organization.

Zakus, J. D. (1998). Resource dependency and community participation in primary health care. *Social Science & Medicine*, 46 (4–5), 475–494.

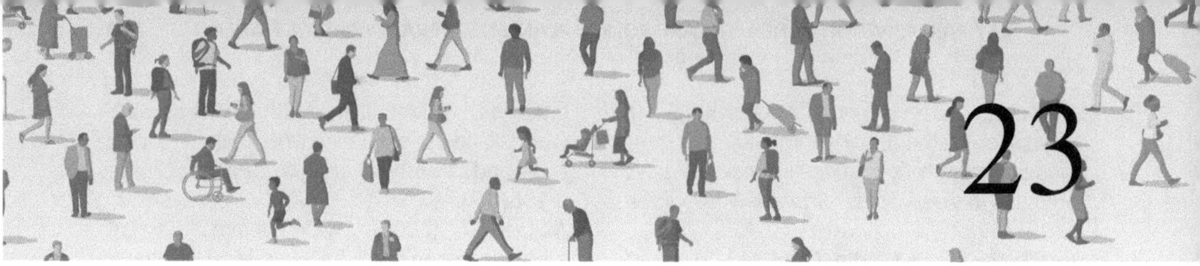

23

Complementary and Integrative Health and Medicine Practices and Systems

Elizabeth A. Goldblatt and Stacy Gomes

INTRODUCTION

There has been tremendous growth in the last twenty years in Complementary and Integrative Health and Medicine (CIHM) in the Western world. What is included in the CIHM (formerly known as complementary and alternative medicine or CAM) disciplines ranges from acupuncture and East Asian medicine, to chiropractic, to naturopathic medicine, to massage therapy to Ayurvedic medicine to mindfulness practices, diet therapies, herbal medicine and more. What makes a system of medicine or a specific healing practice or technique alternative? "Alternative medicine" refers to approaches to health and medicine that are not part of the current dominant Western biomedical system. It is important to keep in mind that medical systems and remedies have roots in historical cultural healing systems, e.g., Chinese medicine, Ayurveda medicine, Tibetan medicine, Humoral medicine, Native American healing traditions. These were in existence long before Western biomedicine, as discussed in Chapter 2 in this volume on *Cultural Variation in the Experience of Health and Illness*.

This chapter presents a global overview of complementary and integrative health and medicine, the implementation of governmental recognition and regulation of CIHM, and World Health Organization policies covering its modalities. CIHM includes a wide variety of herbs, supplements, procedures, and approaches, which we outline, with the understanding that in this chapter we cannot fully describe every strategy or remedy. The chapter also addresses recommendations for testing the efficacy and safety of CIHM with randomized control trials and provides examples of those findings.

GROWTH OF CIHM

The Flexner Report, which established biomedicine as the dominant Western system of medicine, was published in 1910 (Duffy 2011).

It was then that other systems and remedies were labeled as outside mainstream biomedicine and were categorized by the biomedicine community as "alternative medicine."

Many of the CIHM disciplines have existed for centuries, some more prominent in specific areas of the world than others. For example, in East Asia, such as in China, Japan, Vietnam, Thailand and Korea, acupuncture and East Asian medicine (also referred to, at times, as "TCM" or Traditional Chinese Medicine) has existed for over 3,000 years. In China, there is "Western medicine" and "Chinese medicine," and significant collaboration between these two systems (Beinfield and Korngold 1995). China does not use the term "CAM" or "CIHM." There are large TCM and Western medicine universities and hospitals as well. Similar situations exist in Japan, Korea, Thailand and Vietnam where acupuncture and East Asian medicine have existed for centuries and are well integrated into their national health care systems (Kleinman et al. 1975).

While the term Traditional Chinese Medicine (TCM) is used in many countries, as the roots of East Asian medicine came from China, several East Asian countries have each developed unique areas of emphasis that distinguish themselves from the Traditional Chinese Medicine as practiced in China. For example, in Japan, those health professionals who use Chinese herbs are medical doctors (MDs) who extended their formal training in herbal medicine. These MDs are taught separately from those who study and practice acupuncture and moxibustion (an herbal treatment). Whereas in China, TCM practitioners learn all the branches of TCM, which include acupuncture, Chinese herbs, nutrition, moxibustion, cupping, breathing exercise, and body work, after their basic training, they then specialize in one of the TCM branches. Also, in Japan, they generally do not use the term "CAM," but instead refer to integrative medicine in which the health professionals collaborate and work together (Watanabe et al. 2011).

In East Asia, governments regulate both forms of health care systems, include both in their national health care systems, and support university research centers on both systems of medicine. In India, Ayurvedic medicine, a 5,000-year-old approach to health care, is integrated into the Indian health care system. There are many hospitals and out-patient settings in India that use Ayurvedic medicine and government universities that teach Ayurvedic medicine (Lad 1995). In many ways, one could say that Asia and Southeast Asia started integrative medicine. It is important for policy makers, scholars and practitioners to understand how each country or region defines and views the CIHM disciplines. There can be a tendency towards ethnocentricity (the belief that one's own system is the best), and some may believe that conventional medicine is the only viable form of medicine. Yet, it is clear from reviewing many countries' approaches to health care that such a view is limited.

The World Health Organization *Global Report on Traditional and Complementary Medicine* (T&CM), published in 2019, is an excellent resource as 53 out of 194 WHO member states responded to the WHO survey about their use of T&CM by their populations (World Health Organization 2019). This WHO report documents the recent increase in the use of the CIHM disciplines from 2005 to 2018, and offers one of the most comprehensive summaries on the status of CIHM throughout the world.

The 1990s catapulted many of the CIHM health professions into a new level of global recognition, regulation, stature, educational recognition and use, especially in the West. Eisenberg's two seminal studies in the 1990s, which indicated how many persons in the US are accessing the CAM fields and spending out-of-pocket on these health approaches, created significant interest in complementary and alternative medicine (CAM) by the conventional medical world (Eisenberg et al. 1993; Eisenberg et al. 1998). In 1998, the US National Institutes of Health (NIH) created the National Center for Complementary and Alternative Medicine (NCCAM) on research and education about CAM. In 2014, the name of this center changed to the National Center for Complementary and Integrative Health (NCCIH), reflecting the more common, inclusive terminology now in use in several countries (National Center for Complementary and Integrative Health 2019a). Throughout the Western world, a similar growth of the CIHM disciplines as well as research study centers on CIHM have occurred in Canada, the European Union (EU), Australia and New Zealand, South America, Africa, Asia, the USA, Israel and beyond. It is interesting to note that as far back as 1978, the WHO created the Alma-Ata Declaration of Primary Health Care, calling on countries to include traditional medicine into their primary health care approaches (World Health Organization 1978). In addition, the 2009 WHO resolution on traditional medicine urges its members to create national policies, regulations and standards for traditional medicines as part of their comprehensive national health systems (World Health Organization 2013). This resolution has driven the inclusion of traditional medicine into the most recent International Classification of Disease (ICD) codes.

The rapid growth of CIHM/CAM is both consumer-driven and integrative medicine-driven. Integrative health care brings together conventional and complementary approaches in a coordinated way. It emphasizes a holistic, patient-focused approach to health care, and well-being – often including mental, emotional, functional, spiritual, social and community aspects – and treating the whole person rather than, for example, only an organ system. It aims for well-coordinated care between different providers and institutions.

Many of the CIHM professions have established national professional organizations in the last 34 years, created consistent educational standards, accreditation agencies or other government recognition, and recognized testing or certification agencies. It is also important to note that health care regulation varies throughout the world. For example, in the USA, health professional licensure is state by state, in Canada province by province, while in Mexico and China, it is federal. That said, the educational standards tend to be nationally recognized.

There is a growing field of integrative medicine led by physicians, PhDs, nurses and some allied health professionals throughout the US, Canada and the EU, which focuses on being more inclusive of the CIHM/CAM disciplines and has absorbed these health professionals as part of integrative clinics. These may be private or university-based in both in- and out-patient clinics. In their Foreword to the third edition of the *Clinicians' and Educators' Desk Reference on the Integrative Health and Medicine Professions*, Sierpina et al. (2017, xiv) write:

> CIHM providers are well positioned to focus on prevention, lifestyle change, health coaching, and management of certain chronic diseases and painful conditions. The latter problem, chronic pain, has become especially critical to our era as evidenced by an opiate addiction epidemic [which is global] with countless lives affected. In the future, we would like to see more practice and detailed descriptions of interdisciplinary team collaborations between physicians, advanced practice nurses, PAs and CIHM practitioners.

There are a number of resources available which describe the details of regulation of the complementary disciplines internationally, the incidence of utilization of CIHM, as well as research which applies to these fields. These will be discussed throughout this chapter and can be found in the References. In the US and Canada, the five regulated/licensed CIHM professions include acupuncture/Oriental medicine, chiropractic, direct-entry midwifery, massage therapy and naturopathic medicine. Europe regulates homeopathy, reflexology, Anthroposophic medicine, hypnosis and Ayurveda medicine, as well as the five disciplines listed above. In Australia, only chiropractors and TCM practitioners are regulated. In Asia, acupuncture and East Asian medicine are regulated by the government, as is Ayurvedic medicine in India. These are not considered to be CIHM but are integral in their health care system.

The WHO's 2019 *Global Report on Traditional and Complementary Medicine* briefly describes: (1) the national policy on T&CM, (2) the regulatory status of herbal medicines, and (3) the practices, providers, education and health insurance for 149 (of the 194) WHO member states. This report is one of the most comprehensive summaries available on what exists throughout the world and the level of acceptance and the possible regulation of CAM/CIHM. Specific information on which of the CIHM/CAM disciplines are regulated is from surveys circulated to these countries (although, as noted above, only 53 countries responded to this survey) and some list more details than others (World Health Organization 2019). The WHO report covers the following five areas:

1. National framework for traditional and complementary medicine.
2. Regulatory status of herbal medicines.
3. Practice, providers, education and health insurance.
4. Challenges and the need for WHO support.
5. Country summaries.

WHAT DOES CIHM INCLUDE?

What is meant by "complementary and integrative health and medicine"? There are multiple definitions for CIHM. It is important to point out the tendency of societies to be ethnocentric in their definitions of the CIHM disciplines. For example, in the US and most Western countries, acupuncture and East Asian medicine are considered to be in the CIHM category. Whereas throughout East Asia, acupuncture and East Asian medicine are part of their health care systems and recognized by the government as such.

It is important to define and describe each of the relevant CIHM modalities and professional groups in order to establish standards that lend themselves to reproducible research. Moreover, referrals between professional communities and the training of the multidisciplinary teams consisting of both conventional and complementary care practices cannot begin unless and until all participating professional groups learn more about one another (Eisenberg 2017).

The WHO defines traditional medicine as: "The sum total of the knowledge, skills, and practices based on the theories, beliefs, and experiences indigenous to different cultures, whether explicable or not, used in the maintenance of health as well as in the prevention, diagnosis, improvement or treatment of physical and medicine illness" (Che et al. 2017, 15). The terms "complementary medicine" or "alternative medicine" refer to a broad set of health care practices that are not part of that country's own tradition or conventional medicine and are not fully integrated into the dominant health care system. They are used interchangeably with traditional medicine in some countries (World Health Organization 2019).

The US Institute of Medicine (now the National Academy of Medicine) provides one of the most comprehensive definitions of CAM, which defines the many diverse health care systems and modalities that are called CAM. The committee that worked on this project defined CAM thus:

> Complementary and Alternative Medicine (CAM) is a broad domain of resources that encompasses health systems, modalities, and practices and their accompanying theories and beliefs, other than those intrinsic to the dominant health system of a particular society or culture in a given historical period. CAM includes such resources perceived by their uses as associated with positive outcomes. Boundaries within CAM and between the CAM domain and the domain of the dominant system are not always sharp or fixed. (Institute of Medicine 2005, 19)

According to the National Center for Complementary and Integrative Health (NCCIH, formerly NCCAM), CAM therapies can be divided into five different categories:

1. Alternative medical systems (medical treatments that center on specific philosophy, such as Ayurveda, First Nations traditional healing, Traditional Chinese Medicine, homeopathy and naturopathy).

2 Mind–body interventions (treatments that involve fostering the mind–body connection, such as meditation, prayer, relaxation, and art therapy).
3 Biologically based therapies (such as dietary supplements and herbal remedies).
4 Manipulative and body-based methods (such as chiropractic and osteopathic manipulation and massage).
5 Energy therapies (such as bio field therapies – including Qi Gong, therapeutic touch, and reiki – and bio electromagnetic-based therapies, such as magnet therapy or alternating-current or direct-current field therapy).

When describing CIHM approaches, people often use "alternative" and "complementary" interchangeably, but the two terms refer to different concepts. The NIH NCCIH (National Center for Complementary and Integrative Health 2021b) differentiates between the term "complementary" and the term "alternative" in the following way:

- If a non-mainstream practice is used **together with** conventional medicine, it's considered "complementary."
- If a non-mainstream practice is used **in place of** conventional medicine, it's considered "alternative."

As noted earlier, CIHM in the West can mean *all* approaches to health care that are not included in "conventional" or Western biomedicine. There are also mind and body practices included in the promotion of health. This area includes a diverse group of techniques taught by a trained instructor. Such practices include relaxation techniques (such as breathing exercises, guided imagery, and

Box 23.1 CIHM therapies

1 In Complementary and Integrative Health and Medicine systems (medical treatments that center on specific philosophy, such as Ayurveda, First Nations traditional healing, Traditional Chinese Medicine, homeopathy and naturopathy):
   - Acupuncture
   - Anthroposophical medicine*
   - Ayurveda medicine*
   - Direct-entry midwifery (not nurse midwives)
   - Homeopathy*
   - Naturopathy*
   - Tibetan medicine*
   - Traditional Chinese Medicine*
   - Unani medicine*
2 Mind–body interventions (treatments that involve fostering the mind–body connection, such as meditation, prayer, relaxation, and art therapy):
   - Aromatherapy
   - Hypnotherapy
   - Meditation and mindfulness (for stress management and relaxation)
   - Yoga therapy
3 Biologically based therapies (such as dietary supplements and herbal remedies):
   - Herbal therapies (western and China)
   - Homeopathy*
   - Nutritional therapy
   - Supplements
4 Manipulative and body-based methods (such as chiropractic and osteopathic manipulation and massage):
   - Acupressure and shiatsu and Tui Na
   - Chiropractic*
   - Alexander technique
   - Feldenkrais
   - Massage
   - Reflexology
   - Yoga therapy
5 Energy therapies (such as bio field therapies – including qi gong, therapeutic touch, and reiki – and bio electromagnetic-based therapies, such as magnet therapy or alternating-current or direct-current field therapy):
   - Reiki and other healing and energy therapies and therapeutic touch
   - Tai qi and qi gong/breathing exercises (and other movement therapies)

Note: Those entries marked with * are considered whole systems of medicine; the others are considered to be healing remedies and/or healing techniques.

progressive muscle relaxation), tai chi, qi gong, hypnotherapy, meditation, mindfulness-based stress reduction, Feldenkrais method, Alexander technique, Pilates, Rolfing Structural Integration, and Trager psycho-physical integration. Of these, hypnotherapy is regulated in some countries.

Another significant publication is the *Clinicians' and Educators' Desk Reference on the Integrative Health and Medicine Professions* (Goldblatt 2017). This desk reference is published by the Academic Collaborative for Integrative Health. Each chapter on the individual disciplines is authored by scholars, academics and researchers from within their respective fields and approved by their respective councils on education.

BRIEF DESCRIPTION OF CIHM ORIGINS AND HEALING TECHNIQUES

Acupuncture and East Asian Medicine

Acupuncture and East Asian medicine extend back at least 3,000 years with documentation of accumulated knowledge and experience appearing before the Han Dynasty (206 BC to 220 CE), thus providing a long record of traditional use. Since the 1970s Acupuncture and East-Asian Medicine began experiencing increasing popularity in the US when trade began with mainland China. The philosophy of this ancient therapeutic system is based on the concept of *qi*, meaning energy/life force, and its flow through the body along channels or meridians. This traditional medicine, which can interface well with conventional medicine, has its own nomenclature, physiology, pathology and therapeutics, which create a complex system of medicine documented in classical and modern texts (Kleinman et al. 1975).

Acupuncture (needling), cupping, gua sha (scraping), moxibustion (a volatilized Chinese herb with many medicinal uses), nutrition, the modern use of electrical stimulation and cold laser therapy are part of this ancient and modern approach to health care. In addition, there are Asian forms of massage, such as acupressure, shiatsu, tui na and breathing exercises, including qi gong and tai qi, which use many of the same concepts. Chinese herbs play a major role in this form of medicine (Chan, Clancey, and Loy 2002; Goldblatt 2017, 17–42; White and Ernst 2004).

Chiropractic

Chiropractic care seeks to relieve symptoms, restore joint motion, enhance posture and balance, strengthen muscles, improve flexibility and facilitate optimized body function. Also, this approach to health care may also address diet, activities of daily living, lifestyle behaviors and stress reduction.

> A Doctor of Chiropractic practicing in primary health care is qualified to provide independent care to individuals by:
>
> 1. providing direct access to the public,
> 2. establishing a partnership relationship with continuity of care for each individual patient,
> 3. evaluating a patient and independently establishing diagnosis or diagnoses, and
> 4. managing the patient's health care and integrating health care services including specific treatments, recommendations for self-care, referral and/or co-management. (LeFebvre, Peterson, and Haas 2013, 43–44)

Doctors of Chiropractic focus not only on the structural component of a patient's complaint, but also evaluate the overall health of the patient. For example, a lower back complaint may be related locally to a sacroiliac joint dysfunction and general poor posture and obesity, all of which must be taken into consideration in the comprehensive treatment and management plan (Keating, Cleaveland III, and Menke 2004).

Chiropractic was founded by Daniel David Palmer in Davenport, Iowa, in 1895. This led to the formation of a theory relating spinal alignment to states of health and disease, which was similar to that espoused by Andrew Tayler Still, the founder of osteopathy, in 1874 (Palmer 1910). In 1975, the NIH sponsored an interdisciplinary conference called "The Research Status of Spinal Manipulative Therapy" (Goldstein 1975) in Bethesda, Maryland. This meeting brought together the leading practitioners in spinal manipulation from the chiropractic, medical and osteopathic professions.

Chiropractic spread first to Canada, then to the UK, then throughout the world, including in Europe, Africa, Australia, Asia, and North and South America. The educational training is generally at a doctoral level (Goldblatt 2017, 45). Chiropractic was the first of the CIHM disciplines to be accepted into the US Veterans Administration health care system. In 2016, the VA established a formal chiropractic residency program which is accredited by the Council on Chiropractic Education (Lisi and Brandt 2016).

Chiropractors are recognized throughout the world, but not as broadly as practitioners of acupuncture and Traditional Chinese Medicine. The formation of chiropractic can be found on the website of the World Federation of Chiropractors (WFC), which has extensive information on the global status of the chiropractic field including which countries regulate this discipline.

Direct-Entry Midwifery

Direct-entry midwives (DEMs) do not have prior nursing education and may complete a training program to be certified as professional midwives (Certificate of Professional Midwifery). DEMs are distinct from Certified Nurse Midwives. Direct-entry midwives are now legally allowed to practice in 23 US states whereas Certified Nurse Midwives are legally allowed to practice in all 50 states (Cheyney et al. 2014; National Academies of Sciences 2020). The care of DEMs encompasses the normal childbearing cycle of pregnancy, birth and post-partum. Direct-entry midwives are autonomous clinical practitioners who work in partnership with families to provide support, education and care during the pregnancy, labor/birth and post-partum periods. This care includes preventative measures, the promotion of normal physiologic birth, the detection of complications in mother and/or child, the accessing of medical or other appropriate assistance, and the carrying out of limited emergency measures. Midwives have an important task globally in health counseling and education, not only for the individual clients, but also within the family and community. Midwifery is covered in depth in Chapter 24 in this volume on *Childbirth, Midwifery and Obstetrics* by Robbie Davis-Floyd and Ibu Robin Lim.

Massage Therapy

"Massage is the intentional and systematic manipulation of the soft tissue of the body to enhance health and healing" (Benjamin and Tappan, 2009). "Massage therapy uses a variety of touch techniques for intentional and systematic manipulation of the soft tissue of the body to enhance health and healing," according to the American Massage Therapy Association (AMTA). The philosophy encompasses a preference for natural methods of healing, the belief in an innate healing force, and a holistic view of human life (Goldblatt 2017, 101–102).

Massage has been practiced in most cultures throughout the world and human history, from the South Sea Islands to the Mexican peninsula and the indigenous cultures of the Americas to the ancient practice of Ayurveda medicine. In Greece, Hippocrates wrote about the ability of massage to build muscle as well as heal it. The more "modern" practice of massage, known as Western massage or Swedish massage, became prominent in the 19th and early 20th centuries. A Dutch physician named Johann Georg Meager (1838–1909) developed the techniques that are now the basis for Swedish massage. Swedish massage creates relaxation, stress relief through parasympathetic dominance, support of pain and symptom relief and structural/postural balance. Wellness-oriented collaboration with the entire health care team is one goal of this therapy (Goldblatt 2017, 99–122).

Massage training programs vary from 500 hours to over a 1,400 hours. Massage therapists do not diagnose medical conditions. In some countries massage is regulated and has licensure or registration, recognized educational standards and a US Department of Education-recognized accreditation commission. In other countries, massage is not regulated.

Naturopathic Medicine

In 2014, the professional organization, The World Naturopathic Federation, defined naturopathic medicine as "a distinct health care profession, emphasizing prevention, treatment and optimal health through the use of therapeutic methods and substances which encourage the person's inherent self-healing process. The practice of naturopathic medicine includes modern and traditional, scientific, and empirical methods" (Cayleff 2016, 8). According to the *Clinicians' and Educations' Desk Reference on the Integrative and Health Professions*, "Naturopathic medicine is a holistic approach to health care that recognizes and respects the individuality of the Patient" (Goldblatt 2017, 123). The American Association of Naturopathic Medicine (AANP) defines naturopathic medicine as "a distinct primary health care profession, emphasizing prevention, treatment and optimal health through the use of therapeutics methods and substances which encourage the person's inherent self-healing process, the vis medicatrix naturae" (cited in Goldblatt 2017, 124). A recent critique discusses the importance of more rigorous scientific research in order to better evaluate and validate naturopathic therapies and treatments (Logan et al. 2018).

Additionally, an area unique to the educational training of the naturopathic physician is in-depth study on environmental medicine. This area focuses on the various environmental toxins that currently exist and how to cleanse one's body of these toxins. Humans bio-accumulate toxins throughout their lives and many of these toxins create serious illnesses. Common ones would include heavy metals, herbicides and pesticides, and fire retardant and other chemicals known to be neurotoxins and/or carcinogenic. The functional medicine and integrative medicine physicians are also now learning about the importance of environmental medicine (Goldblatt 2017, 123–150).

Reflexology

Reflexology is a subset of massage therapy. It focuses on the feet, hands and ears, which are seen as reflex areas which correspond to the glands, organs and various parts of the human body. It is performed by applying pressure using the thumb and fingers on these reflex areas. It is believed to aid in maintaining homeostasis, by stimulating the reflex areas in order to relieve stress and tension, improve the blood supply to all areas of the body and promote the correct functioning of nerve impulses. In reflexology, the word "stimulate" refers to an action that may produce a response. This response could be sedation, stimulation or no response at all. Reflexology aims to treat the imbalances of each individual and to alleviate and improve symptoms. It does not, however, diagnose a specific medical problem (Blunt 2006). In the US, to be licensed to practice reflexology, one would need to become licensed as a massage therapist. In several countries in Europe, reflexology is regulated separately. Countries that are members of this organization and use reflexology can be found at: www.reflexology-europe.org/members.

For more information on reflexology and its practice in Europe, including a list of national professional associations of practitioners, visit the websites www.efcam.eu and www.reflexology-europe.org, which offer information on specific CAM modalities and national multi-modality CAM associations, such as those for reflexology, as well as definitions of each health profession.

Shiatsu

Shiatsu therapy is a form of manipulation administered by the thumbs, fingers and palms, without the use of any instrument, mechanical or otherwise, to apply pressure to the human skin (Jarmey and Mojay 1999, 8). In addition to pressure, energy transfer is applied to the body's energy channels and points using physical touch to balance the circulation of the body's energy (qi or chi). The website of the European Shiatsu Federation (ESF) (www.europeanshiatsufederation.eu/en/home/), contains more information on shiatsu and its practice in Europe, including a list of national professional associations of practitioners.

Tui Na

Tui na is also part of massage therapy in the US and Canada but is regulated separately in China. According to the World Health Organization, "The practice of Tui na is guided by principles such as yin and yang, five elements, qi, blood and body fluids, and by the identification of syndromes and patterns. Tui na practice involves a range of conventional diagnostic methods, such as imaging, laboratory tests and orthopaedic and neurological assessments. Patient management includes a range of manual techniques, rehabilitative exercises, patient education and other therapeutic advice" (World Health Organization 2010, 4; see also, Prichard 2010).

In ancient China, medical therapy was often classified as either "external" or "internal" treatment. Tui na was one of the external methods, thought to be especially suitable for use on the elderly population and on infants. In modern China, many hospitals include tui na as a standard aspect of treatment, with specialization for infants and adults in orthopedics, traumatology, cosmetology, rehabilitation, and sports medicine.

Anthroposophic Medicine

> Anthroposophic medicine is an integrative medical system. ... It was founded in the early 1920s by Rudolf Steiner and Ita Wegman. It is established in 80 countries worldwide, most significantly in Central Europe. (Kienle et al. 2013, 20)

> Anthroposophic medicine is integrated with conventional medicine in large hospitals and medical practices. It applies medicines derived from plants, minerals, and animals; art therapy, eurythmy therapy, and rhythmical massage; counseling; psychotherapy; and specific nursing techniques such as external embrocation. (Kienle et al. 2013, 20)

> Since 1976, anthroposophic medicine in Germany has been defined, alongside homeopathy and phytotherapy, as a distinct "special therapy system" (*besondere Therapierichtung*) in the Medicines Act and is represented in Germany by its own committee at the Federal Institute for Drugs and Medical Devices. Also, Switzerland and Latvia have recognized anthroposophic medicine as a distinct therapy system. In some countries, legal recognition is restricted to pharmaceutical regulation. (Kienle et al. 2013, 23)

Ayurvedic Medicine

Ayurveda as a system is in its relative infancy in the US and other Western countries, but it has a long and well-established historical tradition in the Indian subcontinent (Tomasko 2017). As mentioned earlier, the WHO created a Benchmark for Training in Ayurvedic medicine. In addition, the WHO 2019 *Global Report on Traditional and Complementary Medicine* indicates which countries include Ayurvedic medical practice within their health system (Lodha and Bagga 2000). Practitioners are considered ayurvedic medicine doctors and traditional training takes seven years. India has universities that offer this level of training. "Ayurveda focuses on an individual's relationship with his/her own body, mind and spirit, and with the natural world" (Tomasko 2017, 161).

Homeopathy

Homeopathy is part of naturopathic medicine training in the US and Canada. Homeopathic medicine is holistic and informed by science. Homeopathy can be used in both acute and chronic disease and can be useful in many emergency situations as well. Homeopathy uses minute doses of natural substances to activate the body's self-regulatory healing mechanisms. It was founded by Dr Samuel Hahnemann in Germany 200 years ago (Bellavite and Signorini 2002).

Homeopathy is used by people from all walks of life, all ages and in countries all over the world. The World Health Organizations has several informative papers on homeopathy, levels of training, and the use and benefits of homeopathy around the world (see Goldblatt 2017, 177–184).

Advanced Nutritionists

> In the late 20th century, as evidence began demonstrating a powerful influence of food and nutrients on health and the pathophysiology of chronic disease, the profession of advanced nutrition emerged. Based on the principles of nutrition science, including biochemistry, cellular and systemic metabolism, and physiology, advanced nutrition has become both a distinct profession and a specialty of other healthcare professionals. (Goldblatt 2017, 155)

"A consortium of professional nutrition organizations is currently helping move nutrition from the periphery to a core component of healthcare practice and policy, by establishing an independent career path for advanced nutrition professionals" (Goldblatt 2017, 155). Advanced nutrition professionals focus on healthy diets to create health, lifestyle changes and they often work in concert with other health care practitioners in patient management.

A master's or doctoral degree is required to become an "Advanced Nutritionist," and in the US, these degrees are regionally accredited, or government recognized. Currently, many advanced nutrition specialists have private practices, while some work in conventional medical settings.

Yoga Therapy

Yoga therapy is the process of empowering individuals to progress towards improved health and well-being through the application of the teachings and practices of yoga. The practices of yoga traditionally include, but are not limited to, asana (postures), pranayama (breath control), meditation, mantra, chanting, mudra, and ritual and a disciplined lifestyle. Yoga therapy is an orientation to the practice of yoga that is focused on healing, as opposed to fitness and wellness (Kepner 2017). Yoga therapy is distinguished from the more general or popular approach to teaching and practicing yoga, is that the yoga therapists are trained to address specific conditions and work with other health professionals. Yoga has been part of Ayurvedic medicine from its inception. It is now generally well recognized for improving health (Kepner 2017). In the US, the field of yoga therapy is self-regulated primarily by the International Association of Yoga Therapists.

Integrative Medicine

Growing numbers of conventional medicine practitioners and CIHM health professionals are engaged together in the integrative medicine and health movement in the US, Canada, the EU, Australia, New Zealand, Israel and elsewhere. These professionals wish to include integrative medicine and health in the national health care systems. Both the conventional medical and CIHM health providers believe that it is time to put a greater focus on health and well-being. The integrative medicine movement has emerged from a collaboration of leaders from conventional medicine academic health centers in association with community-based practitioners from diverse disciplines (Goldblatt 2017, 185–198).

GOVERNMENTAL RECOGNITION AND REGULATION OF CIHM

In most countries, physicians may practice the CIHM disciplines, often under their discipline's medical licensure. In some countries, such as Germany, there are several educational opportunities for physicians to receive education on the CAM fields. In Germany, medical doctors can obtain a variety of qualifications relating to specific CAM therapies (e.g. chiropractic, homeopathy, naturopathy and acupuncture) and are regulated by the regional chamber of physicians. Many general practitioners (GPs) have integrated one or more CAM therapies into their practice and are strong advocates of the CAM disciplines. They believe that the overall costs of the health care system could be reduced by the integration of CAM into the conventional medical settings. In addition, the GPs who practice CAM in Germany believe that the CAM approaches have a lower level of side effects and a more preventive approach to disease, and thus have better health outcomes (Jansen 2017). Medical doctors in the US may now obtain a nationally recognized specialization in integrative medicine and health. Such specialized training for MDs exists now in several countries (World Health Organization 2019).

The European Union tends to use the term "CAM" rather than "CIHM," but some countries refer to "traditional and complementary medicine." There is tremendous diversity of regulation across the EU determining who can practice, what qualifications are required and how services are offered and financed. Some EU member states have government-administered regulations or laws about the practice of CAM in general, some have sections on CAM included in their health laws, some regulate specific CAM therapies, while some national health systems do not recognize or regulate CAM. While CAM professions in some member states are tightly regulated, the same professional categories in other countries are totally unregulated (World Health Organization 2019). This situation makes it almost impossible to establish professional cross-border employment or cross-border health provisions for citizens and patients. The lack of recognized educational standards and regulations of the CIHM disciplines presents concerns with regard to the predictability, quality and safety of health care delivery across Europe for its citizens. In addition, this inconsistency creates challenges for the public to be able to access the CIHM health professionals, even though there are many conventional medicine and independent practitioners of CIHM found throughout Europe (Weidenhammer 2014).

Regulation of acupuncture in the EU demonstrates the variations. In France, only medical doctors can legally diagnose and use acupuncture. However, practitioners of Traditional Chinese Medicine (TCM) who are not medical doctors are tolerated. In Germany, MDs and *Heilpraktikers* (healing practitioners) may do acupuncture. The CIHM disciplines are all in the *Heilpratiker* designation, and for that practitioners need to pass a general state exam to practice.

In the UK, there is no government legislation that covers acupuncture, yet there are professional associations that self-regulate. Health insurance will only cover the cost of treatment by practitioners who also have Western medical qualifications. In Portugal, seven of the CIHM disciplines are regulated, including acupuncture. In Norway, there are presently no restrictions on practicing acupuncture, but the health professionals practicing it need to be authorized. In Romania, the practice of acupuncture is restricted to doctors, although there are practitioners who do not have medical training and, similar to France, they are tolerated. Switzerland does regulate acupuncture.

One of the leading national organizations in integrative medicine in the US and Canada is the Academic Consortium for Integrative Medicine and Health (ACIMH or "The Consortium"). The US/Canadian Consortium is currently composed of over 80 North American academic health centers and health systems which have active programs in at least two of the three areas of education, clinical care and research in integrative medicine and have support at the Dean's level or above. The Consortium holds an International Congress on Integrative Medicine and Health bi-annually. The European "sister" organization – The International Society for Traditional, Complementary and Integrative Medicine Research (www.iscmr.org) – holds its conferences bi-annually, coordinating with the Consortium.

The Consortium defines "integrative medicine and health" as reaffirming "the importance of the relationship between practitioner and patient, focuses on the whole person, is informed by evidence, and makes use of all therapeutic and lifestyle approaches, healthcare professionals and disciplines to achieve optimal health and healing" (www.imconsortium.org/about/introduction).

The Consortium started with eight schools in 1999 and now has over 80 members. The mission of The Consortium is "to advance integrative medicine and health through academic institutions and health systems" (www.imconsortium.org/about/introduction). Now with the voice of over half of the US and Canadian medical schools, The Consortium is poised to continue to advocate within academia for a relevant role for integrative medicine and health, across all institutional missions.

The Academic Collaborative for Integrative Health (ACIH) began in 2004 (www.integrativehealth.org). ACIH educates, collaborates and advocates for the inclusion of the values, practices and disciplines associated with integrative health and medicine (IHM). The ACIH membership includes 18 national organizations, approximately 30 individual colleges, universities and schools, and more than 30 associate members. ACIH thus far has US and Canadian members.

ACIH envisions a health care system that is multidisciplinary and enhances competence, mutual respect and collaboration across all health care disciplines. ACIH fosters collaboration and is engaged in projects with many national organizations. For the past seven years, ACIH has been the only organization (out of over 50 conventional medicine and health organizations) to represent integrative health and medicine as a member of the National Academy of Medicine's Global Forum for Innovations in Health Professional Education.

Some key points for the reader to consider when further exploring the CIHM disciplines and integrative medicine in various countries are as follows:

1. How does a country define CIHM/CAM?
2. Do the CIHM/CAM health professionals have the legal ability to practice?
3. Do these disciplines have well-established and government-recognized educational and regulatory standards?
4. Are the CIHM/CAM health professional services reimbursed either by insurance companies or the government?
5. Does the country support research on the CIHM/CAM disciplines?
6. Does integrative medicine exist in that country? If so, which of the CIHM/CAM disciplines does conventional medicine include?
7. Do conventional medicine practitioners learn about inter-professional education and collaborative practice (IPE/CP)? And, does IPE/CP include any of the CIHM/CAM disciplines?

CIHM: Safety and Risk

The United States NIH office of NCCIH emphasizes randomized controlled trials to study the potential safety, efficacy, and risk of the various CIHM therapeutic strategies.

Their website advises consumers to follow the scientific findings for any alternative modalities, cautioning them that "natural doesn't necessarily mean safer or better" (National Center for Complementary and Integrative Health 2021c). An example of risk identified in a CIHM therapy is with chiropractic neck manipulation. Chiropractic treatment was marginalized in the early 20th century, but has grown in popularity since then (Meeker 2000). Its popularity led to it being officially recognized in all US states prior to World War II and it being funded by both Medicare and Medicaid. Chiropractic therapy has been especially popular for back and neck pain, although recent controlled trials of evidence-based medicine have found its results to be similar to, but not better than, massage (Meeker 2000). Chiropractic neck manipulation presents potential harms that, in some cases, can be life threatening (Biller et al. 2014). In some cases, the neck manipulation can cause ischemic stroke, which involves a dissection (meaning shredding) of arteries that supply the brain with oxygen. This clinical catastrophe is rare, but it has been found in young adults as well as older persons (Meeker 2000). The American Heart Association and the American Stroke Association released a statement in 2014 that reviewed the evidence of chiropractic neck manipulation as a risk factor for ischemic stroke, in which they stated: "Cervical manipulative therapy (CMT) has been demonstrated to be associated with CD [Cervical artery dissections] in several studies" (Biller et al. 2014, 3155). Since this study in 2014, several additional studies on the same subject have been published indicating that such adverse occurrences are rare.

Wiesner, Salamonsen and Fønnebøl (2018) point out these inconsistencies and urge the development of consistent educational and regulatory standards. Their study used as its main source of information the CAMbrella data from 39 European countries (CAMbrella EU FP7). In this study, countries were asked if CAM treatments represented high risk, low risk, very little risk, or no risk. Twelve of the 39 countries considered CAM to represent high risk; 20 countries viewed it as low risk; while the remaining seven countries understood CAM treatments as carrying very little or no risk. The CAMbrella report indicated that the CAM disciplines carrying a high risk warranted professional regulation, and included chiropractic, acupuncture, massage, homeopathy and osteopathy. It is interesting to note that naturopathy is not included in the list of disciplines, whereas it is regulated in three European countries (Wiesner, Salamonsen, and Fønnebøl 2018).

EuroCAM is a foundation uniting European organizations representing complementary and alternative medicine, patients and trained CAM health professionals, including medical doctors, veterinarians, and non-conventional medical practitioners. The aim of EuroCAM is to promote the contribution of complementary and alternative medicine to better health in Europe. This foundation covers a broad spectrum of modalities, including acupuncture, Ayurveda, Anthroposophical medicine, herbal medicine, homeopathic medicine, naturopathic or traditional European medicine, osteopathy, and Traditional Chinese Medicine. The objective of EuroCAM is to promote and facilitate CAM's role in enhancing and maintaining citizens' health and highlighting the health promotional and illness prevention aspects of CAM in order to advance the accessibility, affordability and availability of CAM. EuroCAM calls on member states to create national policies, regulations, education and scope of practice standards as part of comprehensive national health systems to ensure appropriate, safe and effective use of CAM, and equitable access to it by citizens (EUROCAM n.d.).

The CAMbrella report offered a roadmap for European CAM research from 2010 to 2012 (Weidenhammer 2014). CAMbrella is a European research network consisting of 16 partner institutions from 12 European countries. CAMbrella found that acupuncture is the most provided treatment by both doctors (80,000) and non-medical practitioners (16,380), followed by homeopathy (45,000 doctors and 5,250 non-medical practitioners), with both disciplines being dominated by doctors. Herbal medicine is the most reported CAM therapy used by patients, variously categorized as medical herbalism, herbal medicine, Chinese or western herbs, herbal products, herbal therapies, herbal remedies, herbal teas and phytotherapy. Reflexology (24,600) is (by self-declaration) almost exclusively provided by non-medical practitioners. Naturopathy (22,300) is predominately practiced by (15,000 mostly German) doctors. EuroCAM also includes information on Anthroposophic medicine, chiropractors, Ayurvedic medicine and the other recognized CIHM disciplines (EUROCAM n.d.).

The *WHO Traditional Medicine Strategy 2014–2023* (World Health Organization 2013) focuses on the importance of the recognition of professional qualifications and consistencies in educational standards and regulations. The WHO has published several papers on traditional and complementary medicine disciplines as well as some healing techniques, and developed benchmarks for educational training programs on the whole systems of TCM, Chiropractic, Naturopathy, Anthroposophic medicine, Ayurvedic medicine, Unami medicine, as well as tui na and nuad thai, both being bodywork therapies. These reports set the basic educational standards for these specific fields, scopes of practice (tied to levels of training) and safety guidelines for each discipline. In this report, WHO calls for there to be worldwide educational standards, consistent regulation and government recognition.

SUMMARY

This chapter has presented a brief overview of complementary and integrative health and medicine, various definitions of CIHM/CAM, descriptions of several CIHM health professions, levels of government regulation, utilization and recognition, levels of educational and inter-professional training, and some in-depth discussions on the US, Canada and the European Union. It is clear that the lack of consistency of the CIHM/CAM disciplines' educational standards, government recognition and regulation across the world is a barrier to wider use of CIHM and that the barriers are fundamentally based on political and economic decisions. Improved educational standards, scopes of practice and regulation would allow the incorporation of the CIHM disciplines into national healthcare systems, which would contribute to the quality of our healthcare throughout the world.

ACKNOWLEDGEMENTS

The authors wish to recognize Sarita Verma, MD, JD, Margaret Chesney, PhD and Frederica Lofquist, MD for their guidance, recommendations and editorial reviews as well as Jordan Know, a graduate student in Health Science at OSU.

REFERENCES

Beinfield, Harriet, and Efrem Korngold. 1995. Chinese Traditional Medicine: an introductory overview. *Alternative Therapies* 1(1): 44–52.

Bellavite, Paolo, and Andrea Signorini. 2002. *The Emerging Science of Homeopathy: Complexity, Biodynamics, and Nanopharmacology* (2nd edition). Berkeley, CA: North Atlantic Books.

Benjamin, Patricia, and Tappan Frances. 2009. *Tappan's Handbook of Healing Massage Techniques: Classic, Holistic and Emerging Methods* (5th edition, pp. 4) Boston, MA: Pearson Education.

Biller, José, Ralph L. Sacco, Felipe C. Albuquerque, Bart M. Demaerschalk, Pierre Fayad, Preston H. Long, Lori D. Noorollah, Peter D.

Panagos, Wouter I. Schievink, Neil E. Schwartz, Ashfaq Shuaib, David E. Thaler, and David L. Tirschwell. 2014. Cervical arterial dissections and association with cervical manipulative therapy: a statement for healthcare professionals from the American Heart Association/American Stroke Association. *Stroke* 45(10): 3155–3174.

Blunt, Elizabeth. 2006. Foot reflexology. *Holistic Nursing Practice* 20(5): 257–259.

Cayleff, Susan E. 2016. *Nature's Path: A History of Naturopathic Healing in America*. Baltimore, MD: Johns Hopkins University Press.

Chan, Alan K. L., Gregory K. Clancey, and Hui-Chieh Loy, eds. 2002. *Historical Perspectives on East Asian Science, Technology and Medicine*. Singapore: Singapore University Press/ World Scientific Publishing Co.

Che, C.-T, V. George, T.P. Ijinu, P. Pushpangandan, and K. Andrae-Marobela. 2017. Traditional Medicine. In Simone Badal and Rupika Delgoda (eds.), *Pharmacognosy: Fundamentals, Applications and Strategies* (pp. 15–30). New York: Academic Press.

Cheyney, Melissa, Marit Bovbjerg, Courtney Everson, Wendy Gordon, Darcy Hannibal, and Sarawathi Vedam. 2014. Outcomes of care for 16,924 planned home births in the United States: The Midwives Alliance of North America Statistics Project, 2004 to 2009. *Journal of Midwifery and Women's Health* 59(1): 17–27.

Duffy, T.P. 2011. The Flexner Report – 100 years late. *Yale Journal of Biology and Medicine* 4(3): 269–276.

Eisenberg, D. 2017. Preface. In Elizabeth Goldblatt (ed.), *Clinicians' and Educators' Desk Reference on the Integrative Health and Medicine Professions* (3rd edition, pp. ix–xi). Mercer Island, WA: American Collaborative for Integrative Medicine.

Eisenberg, D., R.B. Davis, S.L. Ettner, S. Appel, S. Wilkey, M. Van Rompay, and R.C. Kessler. 1998. Trends in Alternative Medicine use in the United States, 1990–1997. Results of a Follow-up national Survey. *Journal of the American Medical Association* 280(18): 1569–1575.

Eisenberg, D., R.C. Kessler, C. Foster, F.E. Norlock, D.R. Calkins, and T.L. Debance. 1993. Unconventional medicine in the United States: prevalence, cost and patterns of use. *New England Journal of Medicine* 328(4): 246–252.

EUROCAM. n.d. *Complimentary and alternative medicine, CAM for sustainable patient centred heatlhcare*. https://cam-europe.eu/ (accessed, 21 January 2021).

Goldblatt, Elizabeth, ed. 2017. *Clinicians' and Educators' Desk Reference on the Integrative Health & Medicine Professions* (3rd edition). Mercer Island, WA: Academic Collaborative for Integrative Health.

Goldstein, Murray, ed. 1975. *The Research Status of Spinal Manipulative Therapy: A Workshop Held at the National Institutes of Health, February 2–4, 1975*. Washington, DC: US Department of Health, Education and Welfare.

Institute of Medicine. 2005. *Complementary and Alternative Medicine in the United States*. Washington, DC: The National Academies Press.

Jansen, E. 2017. The role of complementary and alternative medicine in the healthcare system: a German paradox. *Complementary Medicine Research* 24(5): 290–294.

Jarmey, Chris, and Gabriel Mojay. 1999. *Shiatsu: The Complete Guide* (Revised edition). New York: Harper Collins.

Keating, Joseph C., Carl S. Cleaveland III, and Michael Menke. 2004. *Chiropractic History: A Primer*. Davenport, IA: Association for the History of Chiropractic.

Kepner, John. 2017. Yoga therapy. In Elizabeth Goldblatt (ed.), *Clinicians' and Educators' Desk Reference on the Integrative Health and Medicine Professions* (3rd edition, pp. 199–204). Mercer Island, WA: Academic Collaborative for Integrative Health.

Kienle, Gunver S., Hans-Ulrich Albonico, Erik Baars, Harald J. Hamre, Peter Zimmermann, and Helmut Kiene. 2013. Anthroposophic Medicine: an integrative medical system originating in Europe. *Global Advances in Health and Medicine* 2(6): 20–31.

Kleinman, Arthur, Peter Kunstadter, E. Russell Alexander, and James L. Gale, eds. 1975. *Medicine in Chinese Cultures: Comparative Studies of Health Care in Chinese and Other Societies*. Washington, DC: John E. Fogarty International Health Center, National Institutes of Health.

Lad, Vasant. 1995. An introduction to Ayurveda. *Alternative Therapies* 1(3): 57–63.

LeFebvre, Ron, David Peterson, and Mitchell Haas. 2013. Evidence-based practice and chiropractic care. *Journal of Evidence-Based Complementary & Alternative Medicine* 18(1): 75–79.

Lisi, Anthony J., and Cynthia A. Brandt. 2016. Trends in the use and characteristics of chiropractic services in the Department of Veterans affairs. *Journal of Manipulative and Physiological Therapeutics* 39(5): 381–386.

Lodha, R., and A. Bagga. 2000. Traditional Indian systems of medicine. *Annals of the Academy of Medicine, Singapore* 29(1): 37–41.

Logan, Alan C., Joshua Z. Goldenberg, Jane Guiltinan, Dugald Seely, and David L. Katz. 2018. North American naturopathic medicine in the 21st century: time for a seventh guiding principle. *Explore* 14(5): 367–372.

Meeker, William C. 2000. Public demand and the integration of complementary and alternative medicine in the US health care system. *Journal of Manipulative and Physiological Therapeutics* 23(2): 123–136.

National Academies of Sciences, Engineering, and Medicine. 2020. *Birth Settings in America: Outcomes, Quality, Access, and Choice*. Washington, DC: The National Academies Press.

National Center for Complementary and Integrative Health. 2019a. *Important Events in NCCIH History*. National Center for Complementary and Integrative Health, www.nih.gov/about-nih/what-we-do/nih-almanac/national-center-complementary-integrative-health-nccih (accessed, 29 January 2021).

National Center for Complementary and Integrative Health. 2021b. *Complementary, Alternative, or Integrative Health: What's in a Name?* National Center for Complementary and Integrative Health, www.nccih.nih.gov/health/complementary-alternative-or-integrative-health-whats-in-a-name (accessed, 8 February 2021).

National Center for Complementary and Integrative Health. 2021c. *Natural Doesn't Necessarily Mean Safer, or Better*. National Center for Complementary and Integrative Health, www.nccih.nih.gov/health/know-science/natural-doesnt-mean-better (accessed, 8 February 2021).

Palmer, Daniel David. 1910. *The Science, Art and Philosophy of Chiropractic*. Portland, OR: Portland Printing House Company.

Prichard, Sarah. 2010. *Tui na: A Manual of Chinese Massage Therapy*. London: Elsevier.

Sierpina, Victor S., Mary Jo Kreitzer, and Adam Perlman. 2017. Foreword. In Elizabeth Goldblatt (ed.), *Clinicians' and Educators' Desk Reference on the Integrative Health & Medicine Professions* (3rd edition, pp. xiii–xv). Mercer Island, WA: Academic Collaborative for Integrative Health.

Tomasko, Felicia Marie. 2017. Ayurvedic Medicine. In Elizabeth Goldblatt (ed.), *Clinicians' and Educators' Desk Reference on the Integrative Health and Medicine Professions* (3rd edition, pp. 161–168). Mercer Island, WA: Academic Collaborative for Integrative Health.

Watanabe, Kenji, Keiko Matsuura, Pengfei Gao, Lydia Hottenbacher, Hideaki Tokunaga, Ko Nishimura, Yoshihiro Imazu, Heidrun Reissenweber, and Claudia M Witt. 2011. Traditional Japanese Kampo Medicine: clinical research between modernity and traditional medicine – the state of research and methodological suggestions for the future. *Evidence-Based Complementary and Alternative Medicine* 2011 (Art. ID 513842): 1–19.

Weidenhammer, Wolfgang. 2014. *The Roadmap for European CAM Research: An Explanation of the CAMbrella Project and its Key Findings*. Munich, DE: CAMbrella.

White, A., and E. Ernst. 2004. A brief history of acupuncture. *Rheumatology* 43: 662–663.

Wiesner, Solveig, Anita Salamonsen, and Vinjar Fønnebø1. 2018. Which risk understandings can be derived from the current disharmonized regulation of complementary and alternative medicine in Europe? *BMC Complementary and Alternative Medicine* 18(11): 1–7.

World Health Organization. 1978. *Primary Health Care: Report of the International Conference on Primary Health Care Alma-Ata, USSR, 6–12 September 1978*. Geneva, Switzerland: World Health Organization.

World Health Organization. 2010. *Benchmarks for Training in Traditional Complementary and Alternative Medicine: Benchmarks for Training in Tuina*. Geneva, Switzerland: World Health Organization.

World Health Organization. 2013. *Traditional Medicine Strategy 2014–2023*. Geneva, Switzerland: World Health Organization.

World Health Organization. 2019. *WHO Global Report on Traditional and Complementary Medicine 2019*. Geneva, Switzerland: World Health Organization.

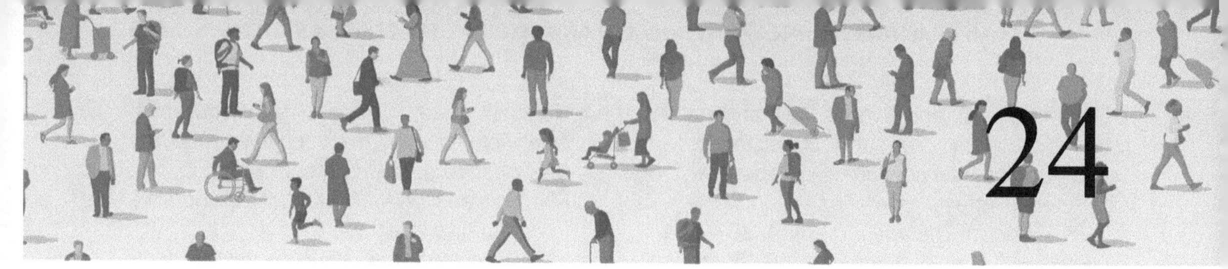

24

Childbirth, Midwifery, and Obstetrics: Global Issues in Maternity Care

Robbie Davis-Floyd with Ibu Robin Lim

CONTEMPORARY BIRTH: A GLOBAL OVERVIEW[1]

From the beginnings of our species, birth was exclusively the work of women as they labored to push their babies from the private inner world of their wombs into the larger worlds of society and culture. Yet today, increasing numbers of women around the world have their babies pulled through the "birth canal" with forceps or vacuum extractors, or cut from their wombs via cesarean section. The medical definition of birth as "the emergence of a fetus from a uterus" ignores all issues of women's involvement and agency.

Cross-cultural comparison is critical to reproductive studies because, globally, the medical management of childbirth has been generally understood to be driven by scientific inquiry and therefore based on "hard fact." Thus, medically managed birth in facilities has been quite commonly seen as the safest, indeed the only, acceptable way to give birth. However, as cross-cultural analyses are adept at revealing, the assumed scientific neutrality of medicalized obstetrics is a fiction. As Jordan (1993 [1978]) pointed out, "Birth is everywhere culturally marked and socially shaped."

This chapter offers cross-cultural comparisons that demonstrate that cultural and social marking and shaping, and provides an overview, with some evolutionary and historical background, of current salient issues in maternity care. The chapter focuses on the current global crisis in maternity care primarily steming from the international development push to move birth into facilities, where poor quality of care and obstetric violence, disrespect, coercion, and abuse of birthing women too often abound. This is particularly true in low- to middle-income countries (LMICs), yet these factors also frequently characterize birth treatment in high-resource nations as well.

Parts of this chapter draw on my (Davis-Floyd's) personal experiences conducting research on childbirth, midwifery, and obstetrics in the US, Latin America, New Zealand, the Netherlands, and various European countries. Midwife Robin Lim and I then offer a case study of effective maternity care in disaster zones that exemplifies many of the points made in the preceding sections. We conclude with a series of lessons learned from successful disaster-zone maternity care. These lessons, if heeded, could erase the problems caused for birthing women by the centralization of care in poor-quality, overly interventive institutions. The lessons conclude with a strong recommendation for the implementation of the *International Childbirth Initiative (ICI): 12 Steps to Safe and Respectful MotherBaby–Family Maternity Care*, launched in 2018, in birthing facilities worldwide (Lalonde et al. 2019). Thus, this chapter constitutes both a scholarly report and a call to action.

INDUSTRIALIZED AND TECHNOCRATIC BIRTH

A technocracy, as I define it, is a post-industrial, late modern, capitalistic, hierarchical, socially stratified, bureaucratic, institution-laden, and (still) patriarchal society organized around the progressive development and use of high technologies and the global flow of information (Davis-Floyd 2001, 2018a). Yet technocratic childbirth arrived only in the later 20th century. Since its inception in the 1700s, hospital birth first went through a long period of industrialization, in which hospitals, mirroring the industrializing process, became baby-producing factories and women's bodies were treated like dysfunctional machines on medical assembly lines – a process still ongoing in many low-resource countries. As one Argentinean obstetrician working in a large public hospital commented to Davis-Floyd:

> Birth is just an assembly line here – we wheel them in, extract their babies, and wheel them out. The doctors are treated like God, but the midwives and nurses do most of the work – we are only there for the last 15 minutes of the birth. But who has time to worry about that? The birthing women just keep coming and we just keep getting those babies out – that's why we like cesareans so much – it's so easy and quick and we don't have to wait around! So our national cesarean rate is around 40%, and we are just fine with that.

In higher-resource countries over the past four decades, "biomedical" (medicine focused on biology) obstetrics has become "technomedical" obstetrics: birth has become heavily technocratized via the insistent application of high-tech machines such as ultrasound and electronic fetal monitors. Such machines are often unavailable in under-resourced nations where the older, industrialized model still prevails. Over the last century, the technocratic facility-based management of childbirth as normative has spread to nearly every corner of the globe. Today we have a transnational/global birth culture of industrialization and technocratization that, along with local cultural variations, shapes the performance of childbirth – often to the point of subsuming or entirely eliminating the traditional birthways that previously predominated everywhere (Selin and Stone 2009; Davis-Floyd and Cheyney 2019; Cheyney and Davis-Floyd 2020a, 2020b). Evidence increasingly indicates that birth is safer in most instances when its normal physiology is understood and supported by laboring women's primary caregivers and when women's emotional states during birth are actively addressed via the care of supportive companions, including doulas (trained labor support companions), family, friends, and practitioners (National Academies of Sciences, Engineering, and Medicine 2020). In this circle of care, midwives emerge as most salient for achieving a brighter future for birth.

MIDWIFERY AND OBSTETRICS: THE CONSEQUENCES OF DEFINITION

"Midwife," an Anglo-Saxon term meaning "with woman," aptly describes the role as birth attendants that women long assumed, traditionally providing direct assistance and support. Attendance at birth has been suggested to be essential in facilitating mother–child survival as the physiology of birth changed during the process of human evolution (Trevathan 2017 [1987]). The upright stance necessary for bipedal locomotion, and other factors (see Cheyney and Davis-Floyd 2020a, 2020b) made human birth more complicated than the births of other higher primates, whose quadrupedal locomotion allows a pelvis aligned for the direct descent of the fetal head, whereas the human infant must rotate as it descends so that its widest parts fit through the mother's pelvis, causing pain to the laboring woman. Immediately after birth, primate babies can climb onto their mothers' backs and cling; human infants, born earlier in their developmental cycle because of their larger brains, are relatively helpless at birth and require immediate nurturance. These factors encouraged the evolution of birth as a highly social process; in few societies do women give birth alone and unaided (for descriptions of some of these societies, see Selin and Stone 2009; Cheyney and Davis-Floyd 2020a). Indeed, it is reasonable to assume that midwifery must have evolved right along with *Homo sapiens* birth. The presence of other females would have enhanced the success of the birth process as they acquired such skills as turning the baby in utero, providing emotional support to the mother through the pain of labor, assisting rotation of the head and shoulders at birth, massaging the mother's uterus, and administering herbs to stop postpartum bleeding. Such skills historically typify the traditional midwifery of thousands of cultures.

Yet birth attendants are not always specialists, and some cultures do not have specifically delineated roles for midwives. In Nepal and Bangladesh, for example, family members often care for the birthing mother (Blanchet 1984; Pigg 1997). But most traditional societies, and almost all industrialized societies, do have a specific category of caregiver that translates into English as *midwife*. Social scientists generally define a "midwife" as a skilled practitioner who learns by apprenticeship or formal training, cares for the mother during pregnancy, birth, and the postpartum period, and is recognized by her government or her community as such. In traditional societies, midwives often serve additional roles as community healers, and in modern societies as specialists in primary health care, gynecologic well-woman care, and sometimes also in complementary therapies such as homeopathy, herbalism, and nutrition. Midwives may practice in hospitals, clinics, health units, freestanding birth centers, homes, or any place their services are needed. Their government, community, insurance companies, or individuals may pay for their services. Traditional midwives often barter for their care, accepting whatever the family might offer. Midwives function best when they can practice autonomously, yet few are allowed by the systems they work in to do so. Thus, the search for autonomy is one of the most important issues contemporary midwives – the vast majority of whom are women – face. (Male midwives constitute only around 1% of the global midwifery workforce. This estimate comes from my repeated inquiries in multiple countries about the percentage of male midwives in that country. The answer is always, "around 1%.")

The social science definition of a midwife as one recognized either by her government *or her community* is rejected by the International Confederation of Midwives (ICM), the World Health Organization (WHO), UNICEF, USAID, and other development agencies, which insist on calling traditional midwives "traditional birth attendants" (TBAs), in order to reserve the appellation "midwife" for professional midwives who graduate from government-recognized programs (ICM 2020). This split has had severe consequences for those "TBAs," which I explore below.

Significantly, the words "obstetrics" and "obstetrician" stem from the Latin term *obstare*, which as a verb means "to oppose," "to hinder," "to stand in the way of" and as a noun means "one who stands opposite to."

Throughout the world, most especially during the 20th century, biomedical obstetrics took over much of the care and "management" of pregnancy and birth, inexorably moving birth from the home to the hospital. Biomedical personnel tend to attribute the dramatic decline in maternal and infant mortality of the 20th century, especially in high-resource nations, to medical and technological advances and hospital birth (Wertz and Wertz 1989). Yet public health experts insist that much of this decline is due to public health measures, such as improvements in sanitation and hygiene, better nutrition, higher education, and better working conditions for women in these high-resource countries. Nevertheless, biomedicalization is regarded as an essential part of modernization, so modern hospitals and clinics continue to be built in modernizing LMICs, with obstetricians normatively in charge – except where they are lacking. (See Pereira and Bergström (2021) for a description of how lower-level Assistant Medical Officers in Tanzania and Mozambique are being trained to perform cesareans due to the "brain drain" of obstetricians.) And governments continue to encourage or insist that women give birth in these facilities, despite their flaws. I have interviewed many obstetricians over the course of my research career (Davis-Floyd 1987, 2018b [2001], 2018c; Davis-Floyd and St John 1998; Davis-Floyd and Georges 2018), and have come to realize the intensity of their socialization into industrial or technocratic models of birth care via years of training in those models. This socialization renders the vast majority of them either unable or unwilling to even read, much less accept and act on, the huge body of scientific evidence against many routine practices, as I will further explain below.

BIRTH, CULTURE, AND WOMEN'S STATUS

Although childbirth is a universal fact of human physiology, the social nature of birth and its importance for survival ensure that this biological and intensely personal process will carry a heavy cultural overlay, resulting in wide variation in childbirth practices: where, how, with whom, and even when a woman gives birth are increasingly culturally determined. In 1908, Arnold van Gennep noted that cultures ritualize important life transitions into what he called *rites of passage* – of which birth is a prime example. Like all rites of passage, including obstetric training, birth practices reflect and reveal the core values and beliefs of the culture, telling the observer a great deal about the way that culture views the world and women's place in it (Davis-Floyd 2003 [1992]).

Where women's status is high, a rich set of nurturant traditions tends to develop around birth; where it is low, the opposite may occur. For example, in the patriarchal Islamic society of Bangladesh, in which the status of women is low, childbirth (like menstruation) has traditionally been regarded as highly polluting (Blanchet 1984; Afsana and Rashid 2009). It was believed that women should give birth on dirty linens, with the baby set aside on a pile of rags until the placenta was delivered, as that was considered the moment of greatest danger; thus, rates of neonatal mortality and puerperal infections have long been high. In contrast, in matrilineal societies such as those of Milne Bay in Papua New Guinea and Micronesia, where the status of women is high, pregnant women are pampered and nurtured (Ward 2004). Skilled traditional midwives administer frequent full-body massages during pregnancy and have a rich repertoire of techniques for assisting women during labor and birth.

Anthropologists such as Roger and Patricia Jeffery and Andrew Lyon (1989) have warned against romanticizing traditional midwives, pointing out that not all their practices are beneficial. Indian *dais* would often put cattle dung on the umbilical stump to dry it; Thai midwives traditionally "roasted" women and their newborns on a mat over a low fire to "purify" them; Mexican *parteras tradicionales* would often encourage a woman to push too early in labor, resulting in a painfully swollen cervix. Yet when compared to contemporary obstetric practices, those of traditional midwives the world over emerge in general as far more efficacious and evidence-based for most births, in the absence of relatively rare complications that traditional midwifery techniques are not equipped to address (Trevathan 2017; Cheyney and Davis-Floyd 2020a, 2020b).

THE EFFECTS OF PLACE OF BIRTH AND OF THE IDEOLOGIES OF BIRTH PRACTITIONERS

> The most scientific birth is also the least technological birth. (Alice Drieger MD)

Brigitte Jordan's (1993 [1978]) comparative study of birthing systems in Holland, Sweden, the United States, and Mexico's Yucatán, was the first to comprehensively document the wide cultural variations in birth. Her "biocultural" approach used *the cultural definition of birth*, the *place of birth*, *birth attendants*, *artifacts* employed to facilitate or control birth, and *differences in knowledge systems about birth* as foci for cross-cultural comparison. Among these, place of birth and the beliefs, ideologies, and knowledge systems of the practitioners who attend births (Hodnett 2002) have emerged as the most salient for how birth happens. Place of birth is so salient that it has recently been the focus of a major report of the US National Academies of Science, Engineering, and Medicine (2020).

In home settings across cultures, from huts to houses, childbirth flows according to the natural rhythms of labor and women's social routines. In early labor, women move about at will, stopping their activities during the 45 seconds or so per contraction, and then continuing to be active (which may include doing chores, cooking, chatting, walking, eating, singing, and dancing). Such activities subside as they begin to concentrate more on the work of birthing, often aided by massage and emotional support from their labor companions – usually midwives and relatives. Many cultures have rich traditions about who should be present (sometimes the father, sometimes only women, sometimes the whole family and/or friends), how labor support should be provided, what rituals should be performed to invoke the help of God(s), Goddesses, and/or ancestor spirits, and what herbs and hand maneuvers may be helpful to assist a birth or stop a postpartum hemorrhage. When birth is imminent, women at home in any culture usually take upright positions, squatting, sitting, standing, or on hands and knees, often pulling on a rope or pole or on the necks or arms of their companions, and work hard to give birth, rewarded by the baby in their arms. These practices are consonant with our evolved biology; they work to facilitate the normal physiology of birth (Cheyney and Davis-Floyd 2020a, 2020b).

Postpartum practices vary widely: some cultures encourage early breastfeeding, whereas some code colostrum as harmful and feed the baby other fluids until the breastmilk comes in (a dangerous practice; many babies die from contaminated water). Most especially in low-resource countries, long-term breastfeeding is essential for infant survival. Steam and herbal baths, and periods of postpartum confinement are often culturally prescribed, varying in length from a few to 40 days (for examples see Selin and Stone 2009; Davis-Floyd and Cheyney 2019).

My research experiences have shown that where freestanding birth centers exist, whether staffed by traditional or professional midwives, the experience of birth is resonant with the experience of birthing at home – a free flow. There are usually no absolute rules for how long birth should take. As long as the mother's vital signs are good and the baby's heartbeat is relatively stable, knowledgeable attendants allow labor to proceed at its own pace, keeping their focus on the needs of the mother for emotional and physical support.

The laboring mother's cervix – the opening to the uterus – must dilate to 10 cm for the infant to pass through. Skilled midwives recognize the difference between the *latent phase of labor* (up to 6 cm of cervical dilation), which can safely take many hours or even days as the uterus tones and prepares for its work of delivery, and the *active phase* (from 6 cm on), which is usually much more rapid.

The movement of birth into hospitals and its concurrent domination by obstetricians resulted in a complete rupture of its normal physiology, as (mostly) viable cultural traditions were replaced by what quickly became biomedical "traditions." Busy technomedically trained practitioners, who either don't recognize the normality of the latent phase of labor (during which, if possible, women should not be admitted to the hospital, as, again, that phase can take hours or days until active labor kicks in at 6 cm) or lack both the time and the patience to nurture the mother through a lengthy latent phase, tend to assume that birth should follow a certain pattern. For example, biomedical practitioners follow a protocol of expecting cervical dilation of one centimeter per hour, although that arbitrary rule remains unsupported by science but consistent with industrial patterns of production (Davis-Floyd 2003; National Academies of Sciences, Engineering, and Medicine 2020).

Obstetric Iatrogenesis and the Obstetric Paradox: The Techno-Medical Ritualization of Labor and Birth

All cultures ritualize birth, and technocratic birthways are no exception. A *ritual* is a patterned, repetitive, and symbolic enactment of a cultural (or group, or individual) belief or value (Davis-Floyd 2003; Davis-Floyd and Laughlin 2016). Many of the "standard procedures for birth" are in fact rituals that enact the core values of the technocracy and that, like rituals everywhere, give humans a sense of control over seemingly uncontrollable natural processes (Davis-Floyd 2003). The following is a description of those standard obstetric procedures/rituals commonly applied to all facility births where the necessary technologies are available.

According to both the industrial and technocratic models of birth, as expressed in *Williams Obstetrics* (Cunningham et al. 2018), the primary textbook in the field, frequent manual checking of cervical dilation is necessary to ensure the mechanical consistency of labor, which, if determined to be proceeding too slowly, will be augmented by breaking the amniotic sac (which introduces the possibility of fetal infection) and intravenous administration of the synthetic hormone Pitocin (syntocinon) to speed labor, thereby interfering with the laboring person's own natural flow of oxytocin. Laboring women are often not allowed to eat – rendering them weak from hunger – or drink, and thus are routinely hydrated through intravenous lines, which also facilitate the administration of Pitocin and other drugs. Use of Pitocin to augment labor can increase the rate of interventions during labor and leads to increased cesareans (Alfirevic, Kelly, and Dowswell 2009). IV lines ritually serve as symbolic "umbilical cords" to the hospital, effectively making the woman dependent on the institution (Davis-Floyd 2003, 2018d). Electronic fetal monitoring (EFM) to record the strength of the mother's contractions and the baby's heartbeat is pervasive in Western-style, technocratic hospitals. Low-risk women subjected to continuous EFM have been shown to have a 20% increase in cesareans and an increase in instrumental vaginal births (with forceps or vacuum extractors) over women who are not – and without reduction in neonatal or maternal mortality (Alfiveric et al. 2017). This high rate of cesarean increase stems from the fact that the EFM records every single fetal heart-rate deceleration, often making it appear that the baby is in distress when it is not (Alfiveric et al. 2017; Devane et al. 2017).

Intermittent auscultation of the fetal heart rate by a human practitioner has been proven to be more effective than EFM at detecting fetal distress (Sholapurkar 2010; Devane et al. 2017; Blix et al. 2019). Yet the EFM is the highest technology applied to birth, and thus is symbolic of the supervaluation (Davis-Floyd 2003) of high technologies in technocratic societies (or those striving to modernize/technocratize) around the world. Its constant use provides an ongoing flow of information, in accordance with the high cultural value the technocracy places on information that comes from high-tech machines such as computers, the EFM, and ultrasound, which is now used by obstetricians to determine fetal size and position, instead of the hands-on uterine palpation midwives are trained in but obstetricians, increasingly, are not. The de-skilling of obstetricians in manual, hands-on techniques is yet another factor in the rising rates of cesarean births around the world. Thus, despite the longstanding and growing body of evidence against its routine use, the EFM continues to be heavily relied on by technocratic practitioners, who become afraid to do without the flow of information and the sense of control that it provides. Another harm posed to the mother by the EFM is her immobilization in bed, which can decrease her own blood supply and hence the oxygen supply to the fetus, leading to heart rate abnormalities and a higher incidence of cesareans; movement is essential for physiologic birth (Morris 2013).

Nevertheless, *for practitioners' convenience and status*, women must lie still in the supine (lithotomy) position, which compresses the pelvic outlet and makes pushing more difficult. This position embodies cultural hierarchies: the woman is "down" and the practitioner is "up," demonstrating the power imbalance between them. Rare are obstetricians who will get down on the floor to attend women laboring and pushing in physiologically efficacious upright positions, which include the hands-and-knees position – called the "Gaskin maneuver" (Meenan, Gaskin et al. 1991; Bruner, Meenan, and Gaskin 1998; Kovavisarash 2006). This position widens the pelvic outlet to its maximum capacity and facilitates the delivery of stuck shoulders (shoulder dystocia) and breech babies, yet remains under-utilized, as it puts practitioners on their knees in front of the woman's rear end – too symbolically demeaning for most. Ironically, world-renowned professional midwife Ina May Gaskin learned this highly efficacious position from Guatemalan traditional midwives, who learned it by watching women about to push instinctively adopt it.

Episiotomies to widen the vaginal outlet at the moment of birth are also common, although scientifically demonstrated to be unnecessary in the vast majority of births (Graham et al. 2005; Friedman et al. 2015). According to *Williams Obstetrics* (Cunningham et al. 2018: 530), because of the preponderance of evidence against routine episiotomy, most US obstetricians have drastically reduced its use – episiotomy rates in the US have dropped by 75% since the 1990s, to 12% in 2012. Yet in many LMICs, including almost all Latin American nations, Romania, Bulgaria, Croatia, and others, as my research experience has shown, the episiotomy rate for vaginal birth is 100%, because obstetricians in these countries are taught that the baby will not come out without the episiotomy and/or that "the perineum will explode" (Davis-Floyd and Georges 2018). Thus, in these sites, literally all birthing women experience either "the cut below" – episiotomy – or "the cut above" – cesarean section – unless they reject obstetrics altogether and choose to give birth in community settings.

None of the routine procedures/rituals described above make *scientific* sense, but, like the lithotomy position, they do make *cultural* sense, both within the culture of obstetrics and within the wider culture, because they consistently enact and display core technocratic cultural values on dominating and controlling nature via technology. Just as rivers are dammed to control flooding, so the flow of labor is dammed to control this equally natural process. Sadly, in imposing technological control over labor and birth, these technocratic rituals in themselves are iatrogenic (see Liese and Davis-Floyd 2021), in what Cheyney and Davis-Floyd (2019) have called the "obstetric paradox" – causing harm to birthing women and babies by interfering with the normal physiology of birth in an effort to make birth safer. Their routine overuse has been given an acronym by Miller and colleagues (2016): TMTS – "too much, too soon."

THE IMPACT OF THE WESTERN TECHNOCRATIC MODEL OF BIRTH IN LOW-RESOURCE COUNTRIES AND THE GLOBAL CESAREAN EPIDEMIC

A growing body of anthropological literature reveals the systematic deconstruction of traditional birthing systems around the world (for example, see Davis-Floyd and Sargent 1997; Ram and Jolly 1998; Luckere and Jolly 2002; Van Hollen 2003; Cosminsky 2016; Davis-Floyd and Cheyney 2019; Ali et al. 2021; Graham and Davis-Floyd 2021). These systems are being replaced by biomedical management, which, as we have seen, often disregards women's individual and physiologic needs in favor of standardized approaches, and which, in low-resource nations, often suffers from such drastic underfunding that basic supplies, clean facilities, and sufficient numbers of trained caregivers are regularly unavailable. The all-too-common result is care that is poor in quality, withheld, or simply unavailable until it is too late. Thus, Miller et al. (2016) contrast TMTS interventions with TLTL ("too little, too late") failures of care. In addition, facility (medical clinics and hospitals) staff members often have little understanding of or respect for local birth traditions and values, with the result that local women often avoid such facilities and their culturally insensitive, TLTL care whenever possible.

From Northern India to Papua New Guinea to Croatia to Mexico, as many anthropologists have recorded, Indigenous and other women echo each other's concerns about biomedical hospitals and clinics in both rural and urban areas: "they expose you," "they shave you," "they cut you," "they leave you alone and ignore you, but won't let your family come in to support you and feed you," "they give you nothing to eat or drink," "they disrespect or ignore you" and "they yell at you and sometimes slap you if you do not do what they say." Such treatment demonstrates why more and more birth activists around the world are using the terms *obstetric violence*, *disrespect*, *abuse*, *coercion*, and *neglect* to characterize such practices, and are insisting that these forms of violence, whether subtle or overt, constitute violations of women's human rights (UNESCO 2006; Sadler et al. 2016; Savage and Castro 2017; Liese et al. 2021). Feminist birth activists have managed to get laws prohibiting obstetric violence passed in several Latin American countries, yet they are rarely, if ever, enforced.

Care providers trained in protocols that emphasize intervention are rarely also trained in the skills and knowledge required to support the normal physiology of labor and birth (Miller et al. 2016). Thus, the trans global imposition of this technocratic model of childbirth, sold to governments as "modern health care" and to women as "managing risk" and "increasing safety in birth," as we have seen, has resulted in an explosion of TMTS interventions in birth – including cesarean births (CBs) – unprecedented in human history (see Reyes 2021). The World Health Organization has shown that, although a national CB rate below 10% means deaths from lack of access to this lifesaving operation, when the rate is higher than 15%, many cesareans are neither necessary nor lifesaving, and can even cost lives due to their iatrogenic side effects, which include infection, blood loss, blood clots, and problems in future pregnancies (World Health Organization 2015). Yet in far too many countries, CB rates are above 40% (Althabe et al. 2006; Belizán et al. 2018).

For example, in most Latin American countries, it is normal for private hospitals to have CB rates of 80% or higher, with rates of 20–40% in public hospitals. Greece has the highest national CB rate in the world, at around 65% (Georges and Daellenbach 2019). CB rates in India and China vary widely, from 100% in some private urban hospitals to dangerously low in rural areas. Giving credit to US obstetricians for choosing to avoid perpetrating the global cesarean epidemic in their country, it should be noted that the US CB rate stopped rising around 2011 and currently stands at (a still-too-high) 32%. Even more evidence-based practices in the UK and New Zealand keep the CB rate in those countries at around 25%, and at around 19% in Japan and the Scandinavian countries.

The WHO standard of 15% is nearly met in the Netherlands, with its cesarean rate of 16%, and is reinforced by the excellence of birth outcomes in that country. This success is entirely cultural: the definition of birth as a normal physiologic process in the Netherlands, in combination with Dutch cultural values on family, midwifery care, and careful attention to scientific evidence, have led to minimal interventions during hospital births and a higher homebirth rate than in any other high-resource nation (13%) (Cheyney et al. 2019). In contrast, in Greece, what Georges (2008) terms the *symbolic domination* of modernity became prevalent after World War II. She shows how Greek women's quest to be viewed as "modern" led them quickly into appreciation for cesarean delivery. They both literally and metaphorically embody modernity as their babies are birthed via this surgical procedure.

Driving Factors behind the Global Cesarean Epidemic

For obstetricians, primary driving forces behind this cesarean epidemic include fear of birth – the deeply ingrained medical belief that birth is a pathological process that could go awry at any moment and must be technologically surveilled and controlled, and in some countries, fear of lawsuits. Other primary drivers include physician convenience (a cesarean takes less than an hour to perform) and economic gain (even where obstetricians are not paid more for cesarean births, the more they perform them, the more time they have to see lucrative private patients), along with the afore-mentioned de-skilling of obstetric residents, who are no longer taught how to use hand maneuvers to deliver babies in breech positions, nor how to turn them in utero before labor begins (see Daviss and Bisits 2021).

For women, the fear of birth, which obstetricians and technocratic culture have instilled in most high-resource countries, is the driving force that sends such women to the hospital for labor and delivery, "just in case." My recent dataset of interviews with 165 US childbearers revealed that the presence and application of high technologies makes many laboring people feel safe (Davis-Floyd 2022). Thus, in most of the developed world, including the US, homebirth rates hover at 1–2% (Cheyney et al. 2019), a rate that saw a large (as-yet unquantified) spike in 2020 as the coronavirus pandemic rendered hospitals – major sites of contagion – far less safe spaces for birth (Davis-Floyd, Gutschow, and Schwartz 2020). Obstetricians, most of whom have never seen a technologically untrammeled birth, are some of the fiercest and most vocal opponents of homebirth in most high-resource countries. They perceive it as a selfish and irresponsible choice to reject "safe" hospital care in favor of a better, more empowering birth experience for the mother, insisting that such mothers are "endangering their babies" (see Wax et al. 2010). During the COVID-19 pandemic, one US obstetrician went so far as to say, "I always thought homebirthers were nuts. Now with this pandemic, I am losing patients to homebirth midwives and birth centers, despite the fact that I tell them that those are completely irresponsible and badly informed choices. Today more than ever, the hospital is the safest place for birth" (cited in Davis-Floyd, Gutschow, and Schwartz 2020).

But the evidence proves otherwise. Large-scale studies (Daviss and Johnson 2005; de Jonge et al. 2009; Stapleton, Osborne, and Illuzi 2013; Cheyney et al. 2014) show that planned, midwife-attended homebirths and births in freestanding birth centers entail few interventions, result in healthier mothers and babies and higher rates of breastfeeding, and carry the exact same risk of perinatal mortality for babies as low-risk hospital births: two baby deaths per 1,000 births (Anderson, Daviss, and Johnson 2021; Daviss, Anderson, and Johnson 2021).[2]

CONTESTING BIOMEDICAL HEGEMONY: OPPOSING MODELS OF CARE

The global hegemony of the technocratic model is heavily contested. For one example, professional midwives around the world are working to develop, articulate, and strive to practice the "midwifery model of care" – a humanistic and physiologic approach to birth based on respect and compassion for the laboring woman and on the large body of scientific evidence that demonstrates the much better outcomes that result when women are encouraged to birth in the place of their choice, to move about freely, eat and drink at will during labor, and adopt upright positions. Application of this midwifery model (fully described in Davis-Floyd 2018a) has been shown in multiple studies to result in far less technological intervention in birth, greater maternal satisfaction, higher rates of breastfeeding after birth, and low rates of cesarean births and perinatal mortality (National Academies of Sciences, Engineering, and Medicine 2020).

In addition to the thousands of local birthing systems still extant, I have long identified three primary paradigms for contemporary childbirth that exist throughout the world: the *technocratic*, *humanistic*, and *holistic* models (Davis-Floyd 2018b [2001]). This chapter began by exploring the effects of the technocratic model. In contrast, the midwifery model of care is a combination of the humanistic and holistic models. The reform effort located in the humanistic model stresses that the birthing body is not a dysfunctional machine but rather an organism influenced by stress and emotion; it calls for relationship-centered care, respect for women's needs and desires, and a physiologic, evidence-based approach to birth. It is essential to distinguish between *superficial humanism*, in which TMTS interventions are applied but with a kinder, gentler approach, and *deep humanism*, in which the *deep physiology* of birth is honored and facilitated (Davis-Floyd 2018b).

A humanistic approach can incorporate epidurals (pain-relieving analgesia that numbs the laboring woman from the chest down and generally prohibits movement), which many women want and are unlikely to cause harm *if* administered after active labor has begun. Epidurals have not been shown to increase cesarean rates in large-scale studies (for example, see Anim-Somuah, Smyth, and Howell 2005); yet a smaller-scale study in one hospital (Klein 2006) found that they did, depending on when they were administered. Giving an epidural too early in labor, as often occurs in the technocratic approach, can slow labor down, thus "necessitating" the administration of Pitocin to speed it back up, in what is known as the TMTS "cascade of interventions" in which one leads to more, often resulting in an "emergency" CB due to the stress to the baby from the more powerful Pitocin-induced contractions, duly registered on the monitors. In many low-resource countries, epidurals are simply not available. In the United States, they are used in around 60% of births, usually upon childbearers' requests (Cunningham et al. 2018), whereas in the equally high-resource country of Japan, the epidural rate is only around 6%, as Japanese midwives and women place value on labor pain, considering it to be an important, "metamorphic" part of the process of transformation into motherhood (Williamson and Matsuoka 2019).

The more radical holistic model defines the body as an energy system, stresses spiritual and intuitive approaches to birth, and places a high value on "the feminine" – without essentializing women as "slaves to their biology." Rather, in both the humanistic and holistic paradigms, as in the midwifery model of care, women are the protagonists and the choices are theirs to make, whereas in the technocratic paradigm, women are passive recipients of whatever kind of care their practitioners choose to provide. In dozens of countries, humanistic and holistic midwives, obstetricians, and consumer members of growing birth activist movements are using scientific evidence and anthropological research to challenge the dominant technocratic model of birth. They seek to combine the best of Indigenous and professional knowledge systems to create healthier, safer, and more cost-effective systems of birth care, using *informed relativism* (Davis-Floyd et al. 2018) – the ability to pick and choose what works in a given birth from a variety of knowledge systems. Some few obstetricians make a complete paradigm shift to humanistic or holistic practice, as Davis-Floyd and Georges (2018) have described in their study of the (self-named) "good guys and girls" of Brazil. Their motivations to make these paradigm shifts include studying and accepting the scientific evidence in favor of supporting normal physiologic birth, personal traumatic birth experiences for themselves or their partners, exposure to midwives and midwifery care, and witnessing untrammeled births. Such witnessing, especially for the first time, can shake obstetricians to their cores. They are trained to *do something*, so doing nothing – besides simply watching the mother push her baby out under her own power – can be a huge, paradigm-challenging shock to them.

For example, obstetrician-interlocutor Ricardo Jones, of Porto Alegre, Rio Grande do Sul, Brazil, was called during residency to attend to a "peasant woman" who had walked into the ER and was squatting in a corner on the floor, already pushing out her baby. He yelled at her to get up on the table, but "she looked right through me, as if I were made of glass." With no time to even put on gloves, Ric caught the baby and immediately handed its wet, sticky body (which grossed him out) to a nurse and then yelled at the woman for dirtying the floor as she pushed out the placenta. The baby was immediately whisked off to the NICU because it was considered "contaminated." Later on, when a nurse said to Ric, "Oh doctor, what a good thing you made it there in time – imagine what might have happened if you had not!" it suddenly hit Ric that without him, she would simply have caught the baby herself and that all he had done was to try to ruin her birth experience, which, in her altered state of consciousness (which many midwives call "laborland," she had simply refused to let him do. And so began his paradigm shift, which led him to 34 years of a highly successful home- and hospital birth practice (described in Jones 2009), during which, despite the 75% CB rate in his city, he and his midwife and doula team achieved a 16.5% cesarean rate – until he was finally driven out of practice by the obstetric establishment in his state. The title of his memoirs, translated from the Portuguese, is *Stories from a Man Made of Glass*.

SOCIO-STRUCTURAL STRATIFICATION VS. A FOCUS ON THE INDIVIDUAL

From a cross-cultural point of view, all three paradigms – technocratic, humanistic, and holistic – are limited by their focus on the care of the individual. For example, mortality resulting from parturition (pregnancy, birth, and the post-partum period) is widely recognized as a massive global problem, costing over 230,000 lives per year. The leading individual causes of maternal mortality include hemorrhage, sepsis, eclampsia, obstructed labor, unsafe abortion, and infectious diseases such as HIV/AIDS and malaria during pregnancy (Nour 2008). All of these are socio-structurally "stratified" (Ginsburg and Rapp 1995) to affect the poor far more than the well-off, as their underlying causes include the structural violences of poverty, malnutrition, the lower status of women – especially women of color and the poor – and lack of education for such women and of access to skilled care. The global infant mortality rate stands at around 29 per 1,000 (World Health Organization 2018a, 2018b). Leading individual causes of neonatal and infant mortality include prematurity, low birthweight, birth asphyxia and injuries, infection, congenital birth defects, sudden infant death, respiratory distress, and gastrointestinal diseases – again also often stemming from the underlying causes listed above (World Health Organization 2018a, 2018b). For example, as pointed out in Gutschow, Davis-Floyd, and Schwartz (2020), in the United States between 2014–2017, the pregnancy-related mortality for Black women (41 deaths/100,000 live births) was three times that of non-Hispanic white women (13.4 deaths/100,000 live births) and quadruple that of Hispanic or Latina women (11.6 deaths/100,000 live births) (CDC 2020). There is ample evidence that these racial disparities in maternal outcomes are caused by the chronic stress of structural racism and providers' implicit racial bias (Bridges 2011; Eichelberger et al. 2016; Davis 2019).

Yet despite their stratified embeddedness in these larger problems, *most maternal and infant deaths are preventable* through a combination of strategies that includes community-based skilled attendance during childbirth from caregivers trained in facilitating the normal physiology of birth and breastfeeding, and access to emergency obstetric care – as will be more explicitly demonstrated in the case study of disaster zone care presented below. Thus far, *the global development push towards facility-based birth in order to "save lives" has often failed to do so precisely because of the poor quality of care provided in such facilities*, particularly in low- to middle-income countries (LMICs).

Recently, there has been increasing focus among international and national organizations on examining the quality of care and highlighting the socially stratified and racialized abuse/neglect of women in biomedical facilities during childbirth and the lack of professional and social accountability among facility-based care providers (UN Office of the High Commissioner for Human Rights 1966a, 1966b; UN General Assembly 1993; UN Entity for Gender Equality and the Empowerment of Women 2009; UN High Commissioner 2010). The *quality of care is directly related to maternal and newborn health outcomes*, including mortality (UN Office of the High Commissioner for Human Rights 1996a, 1966b; UN Entity for Gender Equality and the Empowerment of Women 2009; White Ribbon Alliance 2011). For example, Miller et al. (2003) demonstrated that paradoxically high rates of maternal mortality persisted in the Dominican Republic, despite 98% facility delivery by skilled attendants. The authors showed that lack of quality care and provider accountability was at the root of unnecessary maternal deaths, as did a review series by Bhutta et al. (2014).

BACK TO THE FUTURE: SCIENCE AND MIDWIFERY CARE

Deep in the evolutionary past, our ancestors came to understand the benefits of women helping other women to give birth. Today, the most successful birthing systems combine midwifery – and, increasingly, doula care – with solid scientific research on the physiology of birth, resulting in what Cheyney and Davis-Floyd (2020b) have termed the RARTRW approach – "the right amount at the right time in the right way" – as contrasted with TMTS and TLTL poor quality care. (See

Davis-Floyd et al. 2009 for many examples of highly functional and effective RARTRW birth models, including that developed by "good guy" obstetrician Ricardo Jones.)

In the United States and Canada, obstetricians solidified their control over birth during the first half of the 20th century and had nearly eliminated midwifery by the 1950s. Since then, the demands of many women for the more one-on-one, time-intensive, and humanistic care midwives often provide have generated a small but growing midwifery renaissance in both countries, with US professional midwives currently attending around 10% of births (up from 2% in 1980) (Martin et al. 2019) and Canadian professional midwives attending around 11% of births nationwide – a figure that is much higher in certain Canadian provinces, such as Ontario and British Columbia. A major midwifery renaissance has taken place in New Zealand, where midwives were nearly nonexistent by the 1980s. Yet today, they are present at 100% of births – even at scheduled cesareans performed by obstetricians – and they are chosen as primary caregivers by 94% of pregnant women (Georges and Daellenbach 2019). (Given that midwives must transfer some women to obstetric care, the ratio as achieved in New Zealand and as should be striven for in all countries is midwives: 80% and obstetricians: 20%.) This fact reflects the success New Zealand midwives have achieved at convincing the population that birth is a normal process. (Like the Netherlands, New Zealand was originally a nation of farmers who saw birth as a simple fact of life.) The longstanding midwifery systems of the Netherlands, the Scandinavian countries, Japan, and to some extent, the United Kingdom continue to achieve excellent results. And even in Greece, where cesareans prevail on the Alpha and Beta wards where obstetricians attend to wealthier women, CB rates are low on the Gamma wards for minorities and the poor, where midwives prevail (Georges and Daellenbach 2019).

The WHO, the International Confederation of Midwives (ICM), and other international development organizations have issued a call for 350,000 more professional midwives to be trained by 2035 to meet the global demand for skilled care and evidence-based birth practices and save millions of lives, most especially in LMICs, with a focus on the needs of sub-Saharan Africa. Traditional midwives, formerly the primary care providers for the majority of women in these countries, are being intentionally phased out of practice in most of them because development agencies and Ministries of Health have come to perceive them as generally "untrainable" in best practices and thus unable to lower the still unacceptably high maternal and perinatal mortality rates in those nations. Much research (for example, Buffington et al. 2021; Daviss 2021) addresses the faulty nature of these perceptions and stresses the lamentable fact that traditional midwives are almost never trained in the lifesaving and easy-to-learn proper administration of oxytocin injections, or of Cytotec/misoprostol, to stop post-partum hemorrhages on the ground rather than having to try to transport the bleeding mother to a faraway – and often unreachable – medical facility where TLTL care prevails. Rather, they are taught to transport and then blamed for maternal deaths that occur when transport is impossible. Yet such perceptions of "untrainability" persist to the extent that it seems clear, sadly, that traditional midwives will not accompany us into the future, in spite of their invaluable services in the present and the past. Most Latin American countries, with the exceptions of Bolivia, Guatemala, and the Amazon region, have already succeeded in phasing out traditional midwives. They still predominate in sub-Saharan African nations where maternal and perinatal mortality rates are highest – due not to failures of "TBAs" but to inadequate health infrastructures, TLTL poor quality care, and inadequate training and backup for traditional midwives.

Also sadly, when their training and practice are overly biomedical and their work conditions stressful due to overwork, bullying, and lack of essential supplies, professional midwives and nurses themselves can constitute the sources of the problems of obstetric violence, disrespect, and abuse, sometimes to the same extent as obstetricians (Liese et al. 2021). In contrast, midwives and nurses trained in the midwifery model of care are often the solution. It has repeatedly been demonstrated that practitioners of the RARTRW midwifery model perform fewer interventions, generate less or no iatrogenic damage to mothers and babies, improve outcomes (both psychological and physical), and massively lower costs (de Jonge et al. 2009; Cheyney et al. 2014; Anderson, Daviss, and Johnson 2021). It is to be hoped that eventually the world will pass through the current, modern phase of high-technology interventions in what should and could be normal birth and come full spiral, uniting evolutionary understandings with contemporary science through *postmodern midwives'* (Davis-Floyd et al. 2018) skilled, nurturant, and woman-centered care.

MATERNITY CARE IN A DISASTER ZONE

> When the hospitals are reduced to rubble, electricity is gone, water is not flowing, and people are left homeless, hungry and thirsty, who will receive the babies? Where will the mothers birth? What childbirth protocols will best support life as communities heal in the aftermath? (Ibu Robin Lim)

"Natural" (now often man-made) disasters are powerful revealers of what is truly needed for safe birth. What follows is a case study of effective maternity care in a disaster zone that exemplifies many of the points made above. Most of it is written by midwife Robin Lim, winner of the CNN 2011 Hero of the Year Award. She demonstrates how skilled midwives using low-tech equipment can save lives in the aftermath of a major disaster while following all the Steps of the *International Childbirth Initiative (ICI): 12 Steps to Safe and Respectful MotherBaby–Family Maternity Care*. This initiative, created by the International Federation of Gynecology and Obstetrics (FIGO – its acronym in French) and the International MotherBaby Childbirth Organization (IMBCO), was launched in 2018; it provides a globally relevant template for optimal maternity care (Lalonde et al. 2019).

It would be easy to assume that a great deal of high technology is needed for birth attendance in disaster zones. For example, as Lim and Leggett (2021) describe:

> A team of international relief doctors deployed by the Israeli Defense Forces wrote about their responses to the earthquake disasters in Haiti, 2010 and Japan, 2011 (Pinkert et al. 2013). They reported that they saw 44 pregnant and 24 non-pregnant patients as early responders covering both disasters. They handled 16 births, three of these by cesarean. Half of the births were complicated by preeclampsia and 31% were preterm (30 to 32 weeks gestation), leading them to believe that obstetrical specialists plus technological equipment, including fetal heart monitors, gynecologic chairs (birth tables), and an ample supply of blood for transfusions were necessary in order to effectively attend births in disaster zones.

Yet the account presented below by Lim will demonstrate otherwise.

CASE STUDY: BUMI SEHAT AND ITS DISASTER RELIEF EFFORTS AFTER THE ACEH TSUNAMI – BY IBU ROBIN LIM

Yayasan Bumi Sehat, based in Bali, Indonesia, was founded in 1995. "Yayasan" means "not-for-profit", "bumi" means "earth-mother," and "sehat" translates as "healthy." Thus we are the Healthy Mother Earth Foundation. We operate five Community Health and Education and Childbirth Centers within Indonesia and one in Haiti. At our clinics, we offer a comprehensive range of allopathic and holistic medicine, as well as pre- and post-natal care, breastfeeding support, infant, child and family health services, nutritional education, prenatal yoga, and gentle, loving natural birth services (Lim and Leggett 2021; Lim and Davis-Floyd 2021). And we provide care in the aftermath of major natural disasters, which to date we have done in the Philippines, Haiti, Nepal, and various sites in Indonesia. We distribute food, tools, shelter tarps, solar lanterns, and precious water filters. We treat illnesses and wounds, both physical and psychological. We carry water in buckets. And we receive babies in tents, by the light of solar lanterns and with rudimentary supplies. Our outcomes in all these settings remain far better than the national statistics for these countries.

In Aceh, close to the epicenter of the December 2004, 9.3 earthquake and tsunami that killed 260,000 people (an official estimate – the military in the region claim they bulldozed 400,000 human bodies), during the immediate aftermath of the disaster, we successfully helped over 1,000 mothers give birth. The Bumi Sehat team had very basic traveling birth kits, no whole blood, no fetal monitors or gynecologic chairs. The team consisted of volunteer midwives, one GP (who did not attend births, but treated wounds, as did all the medical volunteers), nurses, plus a support team. We camped close to Ground Zero, where each Acehnese survivor had lost an average of 12 close family members. We found them mostly homeless, with little food and inadequate water. We also found that, even in the worst of circumstances, pregnant women do manage to bravely and safely birth their babies, with just the most basic care (Figure 24.1). It has been our experience that few ob/gyns are needed in disaster zones.

When ob/gyns did join our team, they worked closely with the midwives, providing the most natural, simple model of supportive and respectful care for mothers in labor, birth and post-partum. I suggest that the ob/gyn specialist level of care be focused in the most populated areas of a disaster, where if a birth must be accomplished by cesarean, the midwives have the possibility to transport. Most effective in disasters are sound midwifery skills, select medicines, and simple tools, plus a transport vehicle on standby when possible. Post-birth visits to the dwelling places of the survivors (usually shacks or tents) help support breastfeeding as the only viable way to feed babies, especially when water supplies are undependable and often polluted.

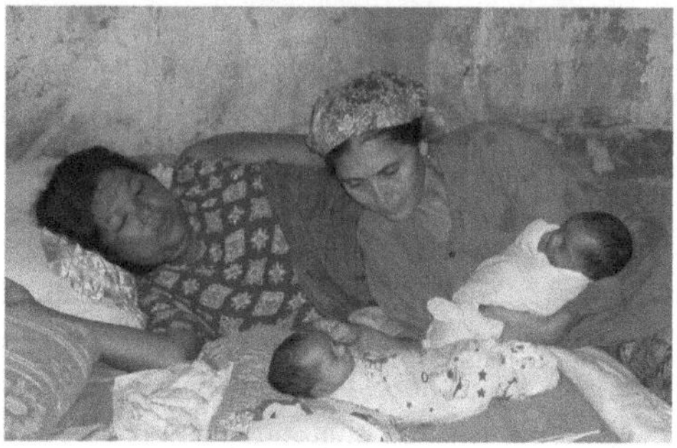

Figure 24.1 Ibu Elly, with midwife Ibu Robin Lim, lost her two daughters in the tsunami waters. Eleven months later, she had twin daughters!

Out of the 1,000 births we attended in the tsunami aftermath where pregnancies were monitored by the Bumi Sehat Aceh midwives, 14 babies died:

- 1 baby was stillborn after intrauterine death during labor at clinic.
- 1 baby died during early labor before our midwives were summoned to help at home.
- 2 stillborn babies were born after transport to hospital (1.5 hours away) for fetal distress.
- 6 premature babies died, ranging from 20–32 weeks gestation; some had birth weights as low as 500g–800g.
- 2 babies died due to congenital abnormalities.
- 1 baby died at term due to shoulder dystocia.
- 1 baby was born healthy but the mother was suffering from what was diagnosed as "smallpox"; one week later the baby died with the same symptoms as the mother. (To our knowledge, smallpox has been eradicated from Indonesia. It is possible that this was measles or some other infectious disease that produced a rash.)

The World Bank reported that in 2013, Indonesia's infant mortality rate was 25 per 1,000 live births – high compared to Bumi Sehat outcomes even in a disaster zone: 14 infant deaths per 1,000 live births. Ikatan Bidan Indonesia (the Indonesian Midwives Association) cites 359/100,000 as the current maternal mortality rate. Bumi Sehat Aceh has had no maternal deaths among the mothers being looked after by our midwives.

The traditional midwives – called *bidan kampong* – of the catchment area of more than 11 villages close to the epicenter of the disaster organized and worked closely with Bumi Sehat. (These women have lifelong skills from mentoring/apprenticeship and their own experiences of supporting mothers in childbirth, but no medical training.) Each *bidan kampong* was given a hand phone along with a paid phone plan from Bumi Sehat. The phones came with hand crank chargers as well as electric chargers, as much of Aceh had no electricity for up to four years following the tsunami, and electricity, where available, is still not dependable. Training these elderly traditional midwives how to use a phone was a long process, but the Bumi Sehat team was determined to give these community leaders a way to communicate. Once they had and could use phones, the traditional midwives could and would call the medically trained midwives of Bumi Sehat to attend births with them in the cases where mothers preferred to birth at home. These *bidan kampong* also come to the Bumi Sehat Aceh clinic to attend their patients in prenatal care and birth, in concert with our midwives, and we continue to conduct monthly training seminars for them. The result: No mothers have died since this partnership between medically skilled and traditionally skilled midwives began (Figure 24.2).

Bumi Sehat does not go into disaster relief with an exit strategy; rather, we attempt to assure continuing care, which is critical for devastated communities and refugees. More than a decade after the earthquake and tsunami, the Bumi Sehat Aceh Community Health and Childbirth Clinic that we constructed there with grant funding is still serving the Aceh community on its long road to healing after the unthinkable happened, as are our clinics in Haiti and on several Indonesian islands that have suffered earthquakes, superstorms, and volcanic eruptions.

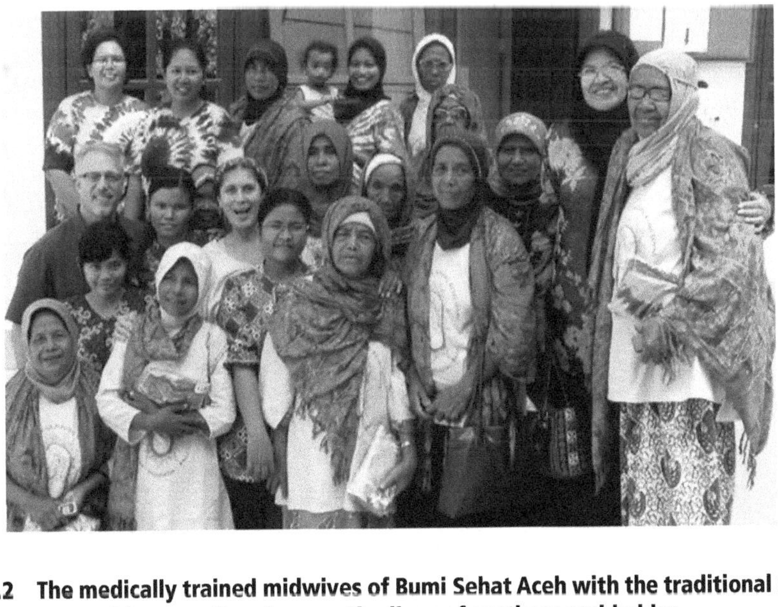

Figure 24.2 The medically trained midwives of Bumi Sehat Aceh with the traditional midwives/ bidan kampong working together to save the lives of mothers and babies

The Bumi Sehat gentle Midwife-to-MotherBaby model of care has proven to be cost-effective, life-saving, and sustainable, even in the context of utter devastation. We suggest widespread embracing of the template behind this model – the *International Childbirth Initiative (ICI): 12 Steps to Safe and Respectful MotherBaby–Family Maternity Care* (IMBCO and FIGO 2018; Lalonde et al. 2019) – as the most viable way to welcome babies and to nurture mothers respectfully, in *all* settings. All Bumi Sehat clinics practice according to the 12 Steps of the ICI (see Lim and Davis-Floyd 2021) and in full compliance with the Baby-Friendly Hospital Initiative (the 10 Steps of which constitute the final Step of the ICI); our sites have achieved 100% breastfeeding before discharge. (The full text of the ICI, along with a list of the many international organizations that have endorsed it to date, can be found at www.ICIchildbirth.org.) We are proud to be able to show that the inherent flexibility of these 12 Steps makes them possible to implement even in the makeshift services provided in disaster zones. Childbirth, even in the Age of the Climate Crisis, can be gentle and must be respectful, holistic, and culturally sensitive and safe. Homeless, hungry, thirsty, traumatized pregnant women need the best of care. When disaster and tragedy strike, and still, mothers must have their babies, the BirthKeepers must be ready (see Figure 24.3).

Lessons Learned from Bumi Sehat's Disaster Care Experiences

> It is a pity that we've lost practicing independent midwives who could deliver babies close to home. We wouldn't have been in such trouble [after the 3/11/11 earthquake and its resultant tsunami and nuclear disaster] if there had been enough midwives in the community. (Japanese midwife, quoted in Matsuoka, 2019)

Ironically, disasters provide valuable opportunities to examine what happens when high technologies cannot be used during labor and birth. In this sense, as was pointed out by Ivry, Takaki-Einy, and Murotsuki (2019) in their article on disaster care in the immediate aftermath of the Great Japanese Earthquake of 3/11/11, disasters emerge as "revealers" (Hoffman 2005; Fortun and Frickel 2012) of the risks embedded in the technological systems on which hyper-modern societies rely – including the risks generated by the technocratic model of birth with its TMTS/TLTL care. RARTRW maternity care in the aftermath of disasters that ends with healthy mothers and babies stands in stark contrast to the insistence of techno-obstetrics that all births are themselves potential disasters-in-the making. *In the face of true disaster, childbirth risk emerges as secondary and the lack of need for high-tech intervention in the majority of births is revealed.*

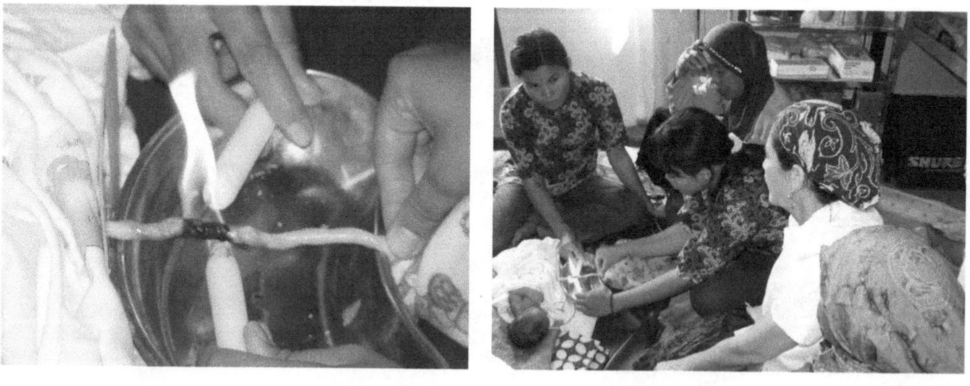

Figure 24.3 Bumi Sehat midwives and Acehenese traditional midwives burning a baby's umbilical cord to prevent tetanus when sterile tools are not available in the disaster zone

Beyond the 2004 Aceh case study reported by Ibu ("Ibu" means "mother") Robin above, in 2018 alone, Bumi Sehat's relief efforts reached 52,121 survivors in the aftermath of disasters that continue to plague Indonesia. The vast majority of the thousands of births attended by Bumi Sehat staff in disaster aftermaths in five countries over the years ended safely, as did the 165 births attended by the staff of the charitable organization Mercy in Action in the immediate aftermath of super-typhoon Haiyan in the Philippines in 2013 (Penwell 2019).

And immediately after the 3/11/11 earthquake in Japan, the women who were in labor in a hospital when the earthquake struck – even very heavy labor or needing to push – were all able to climb down several flights of stairs and walk out into the hospital parking lot on their own (none of them had epidurals) – as did the mothers protectively cradling their just-born babies. Midwives and nurses provided effective birth care in that parking lot, sometimes receiving babies in cars, with only the most minimal of supplies that they were able to grab on their way out of the hospital. The birthing mothers reported that the emotional support provided by the nurses and midwives was far more important to them as they labored and gave birth than any high-tech equipment could ever be. Tellingly, post earthquake, the Japanese Nursing Association (2013) produced a formal recommendation that *all birth professionals learn how to attend "freestyle" childbirth* (Ivry, Takaki-Einy, and Murotsuki 2019) – just as the Bumi Sehat and Mercy in Action midwives do.

Babies born safely in disaster aftermaths teach us many lessons, which include the facts that:

- high technologies are not needed for safe births when complications are absent – only minimal equipment is;
- laboring women are not helpless (unless they have been given epidurals or are otherwise medicated). They can be powerful and the birth process is resilient;
- skilled community midwives in all settings, and skilled traditional midwives in LMICs, constitute invaluable resources in both regular birth care and in disaster care, as do skilled facility-based midwives trained in flexible, low-tech modes of care;
- *traditional and professional midwives must work together*, both for effective disaster response and in normal circumstances. Women want care in their communities, which "TBAs" can provide. Traditional midwives sometimes need the kind of backup that professional midwives can provide. And professional midwives can assist in liaising with obstetricians when needed;
- in general, obstetricians who do not know how to facilitate normal birth should be reserved for truly pathological births, in both disaster zones and otherwise;
- in facilities, breastfeeding and rooming-in after birth are essential both for the overall well-being of mother and baby and for adaptability to disasters, in which mothers themselves must protect and care for their newborns;
- maternity care should be decentralized, everywhere (see below);
- *all birthing facilities should fully implement the 12 Steps of the ICI*, which work under all circumstances to improve quality of care and support normal physiologic birth.

Given the onrushing Climate Crisis, disasters like wildfires, super-storms and tsunamis can be expected to increase. Earthquakes and volcanic eruptions, and disasters like wars and refugee crises, will continue to occur, and may well increase as the Climate Crisis drives millions, or perhaps billions, of people away from lands flooded by rising sea levels and competition for scarce resources arises. There will certainly be more pandemics as ecosystems are disrupted and novel viruses spread. Therefore, we must stress that *de-centralizing birth care* in favor of localized systems of support for normal physiologic birth will better prepare LMICs and high-resource nations alike for effective disaster response. Large tertiary care facilities are: (1) extremely costly and thus often economically unsustainable, especially in LMICs; (2) frequently plagued by both TMTS and TLTL poor quality and iatrogenic care; and (3) especially vulnerable to disaster-caused damage. The push for facility-based birth in LMICs described previously in this chapter should be turned around 180 degrees and transformed into a push for the support and empowerment of local community midwives, homebirths, and births in small, primary or secondary care-level local birth centers, clinics, and hospitals. Instead of being phased out, traditional midwives, wherever they still exist in large numbers, should be phased in – fully incorporated into their country's maternity care system.

It is important to reiterate that, as the models presented in *Birth Models That Work* (Davis-Floyd et al. 2009) clearly demonstrate, *women everywhere want care in their communities*! Community-based care systems are more flexible and adaptable to the upheaval caused by disasters, including pandemics, are more likely to be able to provide high-quality care, are more economically sustainable, and are also more adaptable to women's actual needs, which rarely include technological surveillance and intervention but always include skilled, low-tech care and hands-on physical and emotional support. Midwives should be the primary care providers for the vast majority of births and allowed to practice autonomously. In smaller birth facilities staffed primarily by midwives, or at home, the midwifery model of care can prevail, resulting in vast improvements in the quality of maternity care in general and enormous cost savings. As demonstrated by Daviss, Anderson, and Johnson (2021), in the United States, a whopping $11 billion could be saved per year if only 10% more births there took place at home or in community birth centers (see also Anderson, Daviss, and Johnson 2021).

THE CORONAVIRUS PANDEMIC AND ENSUING CHANGES IN US MATERNITY CARE

During the early stages of the coronavirus pandemic, Andrew Cuomo, governor of New York – then the epicenter of the pandemic in the US – issued Executive Order 202.11 (State of New York Executive Chamber 2020), which allowed midwives licensed in other states to legally practice in New York. This Executive Order was issued in response to the fact that Certified Professional Midwives (CPMs), who practice in the US only outside of hospitals, in homes and freestanding birth centers, are illegal in New York State and so none are licensed there. Yet during the pandemic, there were so many calls made to the few Certified Nurse-Midwives (CNMs) who practice out-of-hospital in New York from pregnant women seeking to transfer to their practices in order to stay out of the hospital that these CNMs rapidly became overwhelmed – hence Governor Cuomo's Executive Order. In addition, the American College of Obstetricians and Gynecologists (ACOG), in an unprecedented step, issued guidelines recommending collaboration with CPMs, whom they had been trying to put out of practice for decades. Said one Florida CPM: "Hilarious to me that now ACOG wants to connect with OOH [out-of-hospital] providers in the community. ... Now [after persecuting midwives like me], you want me during a pandemic!" (quoted in Davis-Floyd, Gutschow, and Schwartz 2020). And yes, CPMs across the US *were* wanted during the pandemic; concomitantly, many independent midwives across Europe were also flooded with calls for transfers to their practices (Kim Frompeyrine, French independent midwife, personal communication, April 2020). Again, we stress that flexible, community-based models of midwifery care are essential during disasters, including pandemics, and during times of normalcy as well, and we repeat our call for the decentralization of maternity care.

The International Childbirth Initiative (ICI)

In conclusion, we repeat our insistence that in *all* birthing models, the Principles and 12 Steps of the *International Childbirth Initiative* should be used as the template for best practice, as they have been shown to work to provide optimal care and their woman-centered, low-tech approach can be fully implemented in any birth setting, even in the aftermath of devastating disasters. Pregnant women should be fully educated about birth and offered the full range of birthing options, which midwives, working collaboratively with obstetricians in cases where they are truly needed, can provide. We must end the global "pandemic" of TMTS/TLTL maternity care and obstetric violence in favor of facilitating the evolved physiology of normal birth by providing RARTRW care in de-centralized settings.

ACKNOWLEDGEMENTS

Robbie Davis-Floyd thanks the editors of this collection for inviting her to contribute this chapter, and midwives Robin Lim and Vicki Penwell for the safe and woman-centered care they have provided, and continue to provide, in the immediate aftermaths of disasters. You are my heroes!

Notes

1 Sections of this chapter are adapted in revised and updated form from an encyclopedia entry, "Birth," written by Davis-Floyd for *The SAGE Encyclopedia of Children and Childhood Studies*, ed. Daniel Thomas Cook et al. (London: Sage, 2020). This chapter also draws on Chapter 1, "Birth as everywhere culturally marked and shaped" – the introduction to *Birth in Eight Cultures* by Melissa Cheyney and Robbie Davis-Floyd (2019), and on "Effective maternity disaster care: Low-tech, skilled touch" by Robbie Davis-Floyd, Robin Lim, Vicki Penwell, and Tsipy Ivry in *Birthing models on the human rights frontier: Speaking truth to power*, eds. Betty-Anne Daviss and Robbie Davis-Floyd (London: Routledge, 2021).

2 The data on perinatal mortality are complicated by different methods for collecting and reporting such data, and the results are not consistent. They are also complicated by different levels of collaboration between providers in different birth settings, and the ability for smooth transfer in the event of need for hospital level care. The data and the variation in outcomes, along with the complexity of assessing outcomes, are discussed in detail in a 2020 National Academy of Sciences Report (National Academies of Sciences, Engineering, and Medicine 2020).

REFERENCES

Afsana, K., & Rashid, S. F. (2009) Constructions of birth in Bangladesh. In H. Selin & P. K. Stone (Eds.), *Childbirth across Cultures: Ideas and practices of Pregnancy, Childbirth, and the Postpartum*. New York: Springer, pp. 123–136.

Alfirevic, Z., Devane, D., Gyte, G. M., & Cuthbert, A. (2017) Continuous cardiotocography (CTG) as a form of electronic fetal monitoring (EFM) for fetal assessment during labour. *Cochrane Database of Systematic Reviews* 2: CD006066.

Alfirevic, Z., Kelly, A. J., & Dowswell, T. (2009) Intravenous oxytocin alone for cervical ripening and induction of labour. *Cochrane Database of Systematic Reviews* 7(4): CD003246.

Ali, I., Sadique, S., Ali, S. & Davis-Floyd, R. (2021) Birthing Between the "Traditional" and the "Modern": Dai Practices and Childbearing Women's Choices During COVID-19 in Pakistan. *Front. Sociol.* 6:622223. doi: 10.3389/fsoc.2021.622223.

Althabe, F. et al. (2006) Cesarean section rates and maternal and neonatal mortality. *Birth: Issues in Perinatal Care* 33: 270.

Anderson, D. A., Daviss, B. A., & Johnson, K. C. (2021) What if another 10% of deliveries in the United States occurred at home or in a birth center? Safety, economics and politics. In B. A. Daviss & R. Davis-Floyd (Eds.), *Birthing models on the Human Rights Frontier: Speaking Truth to Power*. London: Routledge, Chapter 7, in press.

Anim-Somuah, M., Smyth, R., & Howell, C. (2005) Epidural versus non-epidural or no analgesia in labour. *Cochrane Database of Systematic Reviews* 19(4): CD000331.

Belizán, J. M., Minckas, N., McClure, E. M. Saleem, S., Moore, J. L., Goudar, S. S., &

Althabe, F. (2018) An approach to identify a minimum and rational proportion of caesarean sections in resource-poor settings: A global network study. *The Lancet Global Health*, 6(8): e894–e901.

Bhutta, Z. A., Salam, R. A., Lassi, Z. S., Austin, A., & Langer, A. (2014) Approaches to improve Quality of Care (QoC) for women and newborns: Conclusions, evidence gaps and research priorities. *Reproductive Health* 11(Suppl. 2), S5.

Blanchet, T. (1984) *Meanings and rituals of birth in rural Bangladesh*. New York: Routledge.

Blix, E., Maude, R., Hals, E., Kisa, S., Karlsen, E., Nohr, E. A., de Jonge, A., Lindgren, H., Downe, S., Reinar, L. M., Foureur, M., Serine A., Pay, D., & Kaasen, A. (2019) Intermittent auscultation fetal monitoring during labour: A systematic scoping review to identify methods, effects, and accuracy. *PLoS One* 14(7): e0219–573. Online first July 10, 2019. doi: 10.1371/journal.pone.0219573. www.ncbi.nlm.nih.gov/pmc/articles/PMC6619817/

Bridges, K. (2011) *Reproducing Race: An Ethnography of Pregnancy as a Site of Racialization*. Berkeley: University of California Press.

Bruner, J., Drummond, S., Meenan, A. L., & Gaskin, I. M. (1998) All-fours maneuver for reducing shoulder dystocia during labor. *Journal of Reproductive Medicine* 43(5): 439–443.

Buffington, S. T., Sibley, L., Armbruster, D., Beck, D., Lori, J., Dynes, M., & Tadesse, L. (2021) Home based life saving skills: Working with local leaders and families to prevent maternal and perinatal mortality. In B. A. Daviss & R. Davis-Floyd (Eds.), *Birthing models on the Human Rights Frontier: Speaking Truth to Power*. London: Routledge, 110–128.

Centers for Disease Control and Prevention (CDC) (2020) *Pregnancy Mortality Surveillance Program: Pregnancy-Related Deaths by Race/Ethnicity*. https://www.cdc.gov/reproductivehealth/maternal-mortality/pregnancy-mortality-surveillance-system.htm. Accessed Jan 10, 2021.

Cheyney, M., Bovbjerg, M., Everson, C., Gordon, W., Hannibal, D., & Vedam, S. (2014) Outcomes of care for 16,924 planned home births in the United States: The Midwives Alliance of North America statistics project, 2004 to 2009. *Journal of Midwifery and Women's Health* 59(1): 17–27. doi:10.1111/jmwh.12172.

Cheyney, M., & Davis-Floyd, R. (2019) Birth as everywhere culturally marked and shaped. In R. Davis-Floyd & M. Cheyney (Eds.), *Birth in Eight Cultures*. Long Grove, IL: Waveland Press, pp. 1–16.

Cheyney, M., & Davis-Floyd, R. (2020a) Birth and the big bad wolf: A biocultural, co-evolutionary perspective, part 1. *International Journal of Childbirth* 09(4): 177–192.

Cheyney, M., & Davis-Floyd, R. (2020b) Birth and the big bad wolf: A biocultural, co-evolutionary perspective, part 2. *International Journal of Childbirth* 10(2): 66–78. http://dx.doi.org/10.1891/IJCBIRTH-D-19-00029.

Cheyney, M., Goodzari, B., Wiegers, T., Davis-Floyd, R., & Vedam, S. (2019) Giving birth in the United States and the Netherlands: Midwifery as integrated option or contested privilege? In R. Davis-Floyd & M. Cheyney (Eds.), *Birth in Eight Cultures*. Long Grove, IL: Waveland Press, pp. 165–202.

Cosminsky, Sheila (2016) *Midwives and Mothers: The Medicalization of Childbirth on a Guatemalan Plantation*. Austin: University of Texas Press.

Cunningham, F. G., Leveno, K. J., Bloom, S. L., Dashe, J. S., Hoffman, B. L., Casey, B. M., & Spong, C. Y. (2018) *Williams obstetrics* (25th edition). New York: McGraw Hill.

Davis, D. (2019) *Reproductive Injustice: Racism, Pregnancy, and Premature Birth*. New York: New York University Press.

Davis-Floyd, R. (1987) Obstetric training as a rite of passage. *Medical Anthropology Quarterly* 1(3): 288–318.

Davis-Floyd, R. (2001) The technocratic, humanistic, and holistic paradigms of childbirth. *International Journal of Gynecology & Obstetrics* 75(S1): 5–23.

Davis-Floyd, R. (2003 [1992]) *Birth as an American rite of passage* (2nd edition). Berkeley, CA: University of California Press.

Davis-Floyd, R. (2018a) The midwifery model of care: anthropological perspectives. In R. Davis-Floyd, *Ways of Knowing about Birth: Mothers, Midwives, Medicine, and Birth Activism*. Long Grove, IL: Waveland Press, pp. 323–338.

Davis-Floyd, R. (2018b [2001]) The technocratic, humanistic, and holistic models of birth. In R. Davis-Floyd, *Ways of Knowing about Birth: Mothers, Midwives, Medicine, and Birth Activism*. Long Grove, IL: Waveland Press, pp. 3–44.

Davis-Floyd, R. (2018c) Medical training as technocratic initiation. In R. Davis-Floyd, *Ways of Knowing about Birth: Mothers, Midwives, Medicine, and Birth Activism*. Long Grove, IL: Waveland Press, pp. 107–140.

Davis-Floyd, R. (2018d) The rituals of hospital birth: Enacting and transmitting the technocratic model. In R. Davis-Floyd, *Ways of Knowing about Birth: Mothers, Midwives, Medicine, and birth Activism*. Long Grove, IL: Waveland Press, pp. 45–70.

Davis-Floyd, R., & Sargent, C. (1997) *Childbirth and Authoritative Knowledge: Cross-Cultural Perspectives*. Berkeley CA: University of California Press.

Davis-Floyd, R., Barclay, L., Daviss, B. A., & Tritten, J. (Eds.) (2009) *Birth Models That Work*. Berkeley, CA: University of California Press.

Davis-Floyd, R., & Cheyney, M. (Eds.) (2019) *Birth in Eight Cultures*. Long Grove, IL: Waveland Press.

Davis-Floyd, R., & Georges, E. (2018) The paradigm shift of humanistic and holistic obstetricians: The 'good guys and girls' of Brazil. In R. Davis-Floyd, *Ways of Knowing about Birth: Mothers, Midwives, Medicine, and Birth Activism*. Long Grove, IL: Waveland Press, pp. 141–163.

Davis-Floyd, R., Gutschow, K., & Schwartz, D. (2020) Pregnancy, birth, and the COVID-19 pandemic in the United States. *Medical Anthropology* 39(5): 413–427. DOI: 10.1080/01459740.2020.1761804.

Davis-Floyd R., & Laughlin, C. (2016) *The Power of Ritual*. Brisbane, Australia: Daily Grail Publishing.

Davis-Floyd, R., Lim, R., Penwell, V., & Ivry, T. (2021) Effective maternity disaster care: Low-tech, skilled touch. In B. A. Daviss & R. Davis-Floyd (Eds.), *Birthing Models on the Human Rights Frontier: Speaking Truth to Power*. London: Routledge.

Davis-Floyd, R., Matsuoko, E., Horan, H., Ruder, B., & Everson, C. L. (2018) Daughter of time: The postmodern midwife. In R. Davis-Floyd, *Ways of Knowing about Birth: Mothers, Midwives, Medicine, and Birth Activism*. Long Grove, IL: Waveland Press, pp. 221–264.

Davis-Floyd, R., & St John, G. (1998) *From Doctor to Healer: The Transformative Journey*. New Brunswick, NJ: Rutgers University Press.

Daviss, B. A. (2021) Are top down or grassroots solutions better in conflict areas? Two approaches to foreign aid in Afghanistan. In B. A. Daviss & R. Davis-Floyd (Eds.), *Birthing Models on the Human Rights Frontier: Speaking truth to power*. London: Routledge.

Daviss, B. A., & Bisits, A. (2021) Bringing back breech: Dismantling hierarchies and re-skilling practitioners. In B. A. Daviss & R. Davis-Floyd (Eds.), *Birthing Models on the Human Rights Frontier: Speaking truth to power*. London: Routledge, 145–183.

Daviss, B. A., Anderson, D. A., & Johnson, K. C. (2021) Pivoting to Childbirth at Home or in Freestanding Birth Centers in the US during COVID-19: Safety, Economics and Logistics. *Front. Sociol.* 6:618210. doi: 10.3389/fsoc.2021.618210.

de Jonge, A., van der Goes, B. Y., Ravelli, A. C., Amelink-Verburg, M. P., Mol, B. W., Nijhuis, J. G., Bennebroek Gravenhorst, J., & Buitendijk, S. E. (2009) Perinatal mortality and morbidity in a nationwide cohort of 529,688 low-risk planned home and hospital births. *BJOG: An International Journal of Obstetrics & Gynaecology* 116(9): 1177–1184. doi:10.1111/j.1471-0528.2009.02175.x.

Devane, D., Lalor, J. G., Daly, S., McGuire, W., Cuthbert, A., & Smith, V. (2017) Cardiotocography versus intermittent auscultation of fetal heart on admission to labour ward for assessment of fetal wellbeing. *Cochrane Database of Systematic Reviews*, 1. CD005122. doi. 10.1002/14651858.CD005122.pub5.

Eichelberger, K. Y., Doll, K., Ekpo, G. E., et al. (2016) Black Lives Matter: Claiming a Space for Evidence-Based Outrage in Obstetrics and Gynecology. *American Journal of Public Health* 106(10): 1771–72. doi:10.2105/AJPH.2016.303313.

Fortun, K., & Frickel, S. (2012, March) *Making a case for disaster science and technology studies*. An STS Forum on the East Japan Disaster. https://fukushimaforum.wordpress.com/onlineforum-2/online-forum/making-a-case-for-disaster-science-and-technology-studies/

Friedman, A. M., Cande, V., Ananth, V., Prendergast, E., Alton, M. E. D., Wright, J.D., et al. (2015) Variation in and factors associated with use of episiotomy. *JAMA* 313(2): 197–199.

Graham, S., Davis-Floyd R. (2021) Indigenous Midwives and the Biomedical System among the Karamojong of Uganda: Introducing the Partnership Paradigm. *Front. Sociol.* 6:670551. doi: 10.3389/fsoc.2021.670551.

Georges, E. (2008) *Bodies of knowledge: The Medicalization of Reproduction in Greece*. Nashville, TN: Vanderbilt University Press.

Georges, E., & Daellenbach, R. (2019) Divergent meanings and practices of childbirth in Greece and New Zealand. In R. Davis-Floyd & M. Cheyney (Eds.), *Birth in Eight Cultures*. Long Grove, IL: Waveland Press, pp. 129–164.

Ginsburg, F., & Rapp, R. (1995) *Conceiving the new world order: The global politics of reproduction*. Berkeley, CA: University of California Press.

Graham, I. D., Carroli, G., Davies, C., & Medves, J. M. (2005) Episiotomy rates around the world: An update. *Birth: Issues in Perinatal Care* 32(3): 219–223.

Hodnett, E. (2002) Pain and women's satisfaction with the experience of childbirth: A systematic review. In J. Rooks, C. Sakala, & M. Corry (Eds.), *The Nature and Management of Labor Pain: Peer-reviewed papers from an evidence-based symposium*. A special issue of the *American Journal of Obstetrics and Gynecology*, 1086(3), part 2.

Hoffman, S. M. (2005) Katrina and Rita: A disaster anthropologists' thoughts. *Anthropology News* 46: 19.

ICM (International Confederation of Midwives) (2020) *Definitions*. Retrieved from: www.internationalmidwives.org/our-work/policy-and-practice/icm-definitions.html, accessed March 18, 2020.

IMBCO and FIGO (2018) *The International Childbirth Initiative (ICI): 12 steps to safe and respectful MotherBaby–Family maternity care*. International MotherBaby Childbirth Organization and the International Federation of Gynecology and Obstetrics, www.internationalchildbirth.com

Ivry, T., Takaki-Einy, R., & Murotsuki, J. (2019) What disasters can reveal about techno-medical birth: Japanese women's stories of childbirth during the 11 March, 2011 earthquake. *Health, Risk & Society* 21(3–4): 164–184.

Japanese Nursing Association (JNA) (2013) *Bunben shisetsu ni okeru saigai hasseiji no taiou manyuaru sakusei gaido [A guide for the creation of a response manual in maternity facilities at times of disaster]*. Osaka: Medica Shuppan.

Jeffery, R., Jeffery, P., & Lyon, A. (1989) *Labor pains and labor power: Women and childbirth in India*. London: Zed Books.

Johnson, K. C., & Daviss, B. A. (2005) "Outcomes of Planned Home Births with Certified Professional Midwives: Large Prospective Study in North America." *British Medical Journal* 330(7505):1416.

Jones, R. (2009) Teamwork: An obstetrician, a midwife, and a doula. In R. Davis-Floyd, L. Barclay, B. A. Daviss, & J. Tritten (Eds.), *Birth Models that Work*. Berkeley, CA: University of California Press, pp. 271–304.

Jordan, B. (1993 [1978]) *Birth in four cultures: A cross-cultural investigation of childbirth in Yucatan, Holland, Sweden and the United States* (4th edition, revised and updated by R. Davis-Floyd). Long Grove, IL: Waveland Press.

Klein, M. C. (2006) Does epidural analgesia increase rate of cesarean section? *Canadian Family Physician (Medecin de famille canadien)* 52(4): 419–428. www.ncbi.nlm.nih.gov/pmc/articles/PMC1481670/

Kovavisarash, E. (2006) The all-fours maneuver for the management of shoulder dystocia. *International Journal of Gynecology and Obstetrics* 95(2): 153–154.

Lalonde, A., Herschderfer, K., Bonaro, D. P., Hanson, C., Fuchnter, C., & Visser, G. H. A. (2019) The International Childbirth Initiative: 12 steps to safe and respectful MotherBaby–Family maternity care. FIGO Statement. *International Journal of Obstetrics and Gynecology* 146: 65–73.

Liese, K., & Davis-Floyd, R. (2021) Obstetric iatrogenesis in the United States: The spectrum of disrespect, violence, and abuse. Special journal issue on 'Medicine's Shadowside'. Emma Varley and Saiba Varma (Eds.), in press to *Anthropology & Medicine*, 28(2):1–17.

Lim, R., & Davis-Floyd, R. (2021) Implementing the International Childbirth Initiative (ICI) in disaster zones: Bumi Sehat's experiences in Indonesia, Haiti, the Philippines, and Nepal. In B. A. Daviss & R. Davis-Floyd (Eds.),

Birthing models on the human rights frontier: Speaking truth to power. London: Routledge, 253–264.

Lim, R., & Leggett, S. (2021) Bumi Sehat Bali: Birth on the checkered cloth. In B. A. Daviss & R. Davis-Floyd (Eds.), *Birthing Models on the Human Rights Frontier: Speaking truth to power*. London: Routledge, 55–74.

Lukere, V., & Jolly, M. (2002) *Birthing in the Pacific: Beyond Tradition and Modernity?* Honolulu: University of Hawaii Press.

Martin, J. A., Brady, M. H., Osterman, J. K., & Driscoll, A. K. (2018) Births: Final data for 2018. *National Vital Statistics Report* 28(13). www.cdc.gov/nchs/data/nvsr/nvsr68/nvsr68_13-508.pdf

Matsuoka, E. (2019) *Japanese independent midwives and the 3/11/11 Great East Japan Earthquake*. An update on Chapter 8, Maternity homes in Japan: Reservoirs of normal childbirth. Available at: www.understandingbirthbetter.com

Meenan, A., Gaskin, I. M., et al. (1991) A new (old) maneuver for the management of shoulder dystocia. *Journal of Family Practice* 32: 625–629.

Miller, S., Cordero, M., Coleman, A. L., Figueroa, J., Brito-Anderson, S., Dabash, R., et al. (2003) Quality of care in institutionalized deliveries: The paradox of the Dominican Republic *International Journal of Gynecology and Obstetrics* 82(1): 89–103.

Miller, S. et al. (2016) Beyond too little, too late and too much, too soon: a pathway towards evidence-based, respectful maternity care worldwide. *The Lancet* 388(10056): 2176–2192, https://doi.org/10.1016/S0140-6736(16)31472-6

Morris, T. (2013) *Cut it out: The c-section epidemic in America*. New York: New York University Press.

National Academies of Sciences, Engineering, and Medicine (2020) *Birth settings in America: Outcomes, quality, access, and choice*. Washington, DC: The National Academies Press. https://doi.org/10.17226/25636.

Nour, N. M. (2008) An introduction to maternal mortality. *Reviews in Obstetrics and Gynecology* 1(2): 77–81.

Penwell, V. (2019) A birth model for disaster care in the Philippines. An update on Chapter 12, Mercy in action: Bringing mother- and baby-friendly birth centers to the Philippines. In R. Davis-Floyd, L. Barclay, B. A. Daviss & J. Tritten (Eds.), *Birth Models that Work*. Berkeley, CA: University of California Press. Available at: www.understandingbirthbetter.com

Pereira, C., & Bergström, S. (2021) Where there are no doctors: Task shifting of major surgical operations to non-physician clinics for better perinatal outcomes in Tanzania and Mozambique. In B. A. Daviss & R. Davis-Floyd (Eds.), *Birthing Models on the Human Rights Frontier: Speaking truth to power*. London: Routledge, 359–372.

Pigg, S. (1997) Authority in translation: Finding, knowing, naming, and training 'traditional birth attendants' in Nepal. In R. Davis-Floyd & C. Sargent (Eds.), *Childbirth and Authoritative Knowledge: Cross-cultural perspectives*. Berkeley, CA: University of California Press, pp. 233–262.

Pinkert, M., Dar, S., Goldberg, D., Abargel, A., Cohen-Marom, O., Kreiss, Y., & Merin, O. (2013) Lessons learned from an obstetrics and gynecology field hospital response to natural disasters. *Journal of Obstetrics and Gynecology* 122(3): 532–536. www.ncbi.nlm.nih.gov/pubmed/23921856

Ram, Kalpana & Margaret Jolly (Eds.) (1998) *Maternities and Modernities: Colonial and Postcolonial Experiences in Asia and the Pacific*. Cambridge: Cambridge University Press.

Reyes, E. (2021) The global cesarean epidemic: futuristic implications. In R. Davis-Floyd (Ed.), *Birthing Techno-sapiens. Human-technology co-evolution and the future of reproduction*. London: Routledge, 149–162.

Sadler, M., Santos, M. J. D. S., Ruiz-Berdún, D., Rojas, G. L., Skoko, E., Gillen, P., & Clausen, J. A. (2016) Moving beyond disrespect and abuse: Addressing the structural dimensions of obstetric violence. *Reproductive Health Matters* 24(47): 47–55. doi:http://dx.doi.org/10.1016/j.rhm.2016.04.002.

Savage, V., & Castro, A. (2017) Measuring mistreatment of women during childbirth: A review of terminology and methodological approaches. *Reproductive Health*, 14: 1–27. doi:10.1186/s12978-017-0403-5.

Selin, H., & Stone, P. K. (Eds.) (2009) *Childbirth Across Cultures: Ideas and practices of pregnancy, childbirth, and the postpartum*. New York: Springer.

Sholapurkar, S. L. (2010) Intermittent auscultation of fetal heart rate during labour – a widely accepted technique for low-risk pregnancies: But are the current national guidelines robust and practical? *Journal of Obstetrics and Gynaecology* 30(6): 537–540.

Stapleton S. R., Osborne, C., & Illuzzi, J. (2013) Outcomes of care in birth centers: Demonstration of a durable model. *Journal of Nurse Midwifery* 58(1): 3–14.

State of New York Executive Chamber (2020) *Executive Orders No. 202.11 & Executive Order No. 202.12*. www.governor.ny.gov/news/no-20211-continuing-temporary-suspension-and-modification-laws-relating-disaster-emergency

Trevathan, W. (2017 [1987]) *Human birth: An evolutionary perspective* (3rd edition). New York: Routledge.

UNESCO (United Nations Educational Scientific and Cultural Organization) (2006) *Universal declaration on bioethics and human rights*. www.unesco.org/new/en/social-and-human-sciences/themes/bioethics/bioethics-and-human-rights/

UN Entity for Gender Equality and the Empowerment of Women (2009) *Convention on the elimination of all forms of discrimination against women*. www.un.org/womenwatch/daw/cedaw/text/econvention.htm

UN General Assembly (1993) *Declaration on the elimination of violence against women*. New York: United Nations, www.un.org/documents/ga/res/48/a48r104.htm

UN High Commissioner (2010) *Report of the Office of the United Nations High Commissioner for Human Rights on preventable maternal mortality and morbidity and human rights*. www2.ohchr.org/english/bodies/hrcouncil/docs/14session/A.HRC.14.39_AEV-2.pdf

UN Office of the High Commissioner for Human Rights (1996a) *International covenant on civil and political rights*. www.ohchr.org/en/professionalinterest/pages/ccpr.aspx

UN Office of the High Commissioner for Human Rights (1966b) *International covenant on economic, social and cultural rights*. www.ohchr.org/EN/ProfessionalInterest/Pages/CESCR.aspx

Van Hollen, C. (2003) *Birth on the Threshold: Childbirth and Modernity in South India*. Berkeley CA: University of California Press.

Ward, M. (2004) *Nest in the wind: Adventures in anthropology on a tropical island* (2nd edition). Long Grove, IL: Waveland Press.

Wax, J. R., Lucas, F. L., Lamont, M., Pinette, M. G., Cartin, A., & Blackstone, J. (2010) Maternal and newborn outcomes in planned homebirth vs planned hospital births: A meta-analysis. *American Journal of Obstetrics and Gynecology* 203: 243e1–8.

Wertz, R. W., & Wertz, D. C. (1989) *Lying-in: A history of childbirth in America* (2nd edition). New Haven, CT: Yale University Press.

White Ribbon Alliance for Respectful Maternity Care (2011) *The universal rights of childbearing women*. Washington, DC: White Ribbon Alliance for Respectful Maternity Care. www.whiteribbonalliance.org/wp-content/uploads/2017/11/Final_RMC_Charter.pdf

Williamson, K. E., & Matsuoka, E. (2019) Comparing childbirth in Brazil and Japan: Social hierarchies, cultural values, and the meaning of place. In R. Davis-Floyd & M. Cheyney (Eds.), *Birth in Eight Cultures*. Long Grove, IL: Waveland Press, pp. 89–128.

World Health Organization (2015) Statement on caesarean section rates. *Reproductive Health Matters* 23(45): 149–150. doi:10.1016/j.rhm.2015.07.007.

World Health Organization (2018a) *WHO Global Health Observatory Data*. Geneva: WHO. www.who.int/gho/child_health/mortality/neonatal_infant_text/en/

World Health Organization (2018b) *Intrapartum care for a positive childbirth experience*. Geneva: WHO. www.who.int/reproductive-health/publications/intrapartum-care-guidelines/en/

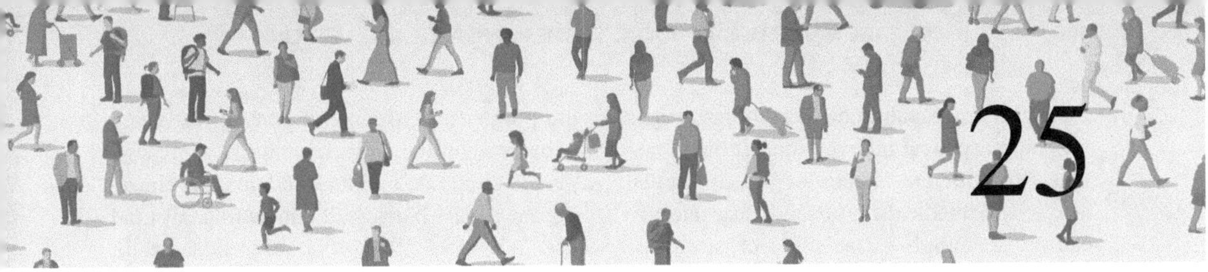

25

Medicalization and Pharmaceuticalization: A Conceptual Analysis

Tom Douglass and Michael Calnan

INTRODUCTION

Medicalization has been one of the major conceptual and empirical interests in medical sociology since the late 1960s (Pitts 1968). A widely accepted definition for medicalization is the process whereby social problems come to be defined and treated as medical conditions (Conrad 2007). During its long history, the concept of medicalization has shifted over time with varying levels of significance given to different actors (Busfield 2017; Conrad 1975, 2005; Williams 2003). In the early scholarship, the medical profession was a central actor in the process of medicalization, but over time other actors, such as the pharmaceutical industry, have gained greater significance in the definition and treatment of disease, even to the extent that the explanatory power of medicalization as a concept has been questioned, with associated arguments made for replacing it with a new concept.

This chapter unpacks the history of medicalization and divides its conceptual development into three phases. The first two phases have broadly been established by other scholars (Lupton 1997; Williams 2003), but this chapter argues that there is now a third phase of scholarship. This section begins by exploring the initial accounts of medicalization, from the late 1960s to early 1980s with a focus on how deviant behaviours came to be socially defined as a medical issue (Conrad and Schneider 1980). It then moves to explore more contemporary arguments beginning in the mid-1980s concerned with how the process of medicalization has shifted increasingly to capture individual lifestyle choices and the risk of disease, and then turns to explore the very latest thought on medicalization in the 2000s and 2010s. The focus here is on the continuing explanatory power of the concept and whether contemporary concepts should replace or can complement medicalization. The section introduces the concept of pharmaceuticalization and its development, defined by Williams, Martin, and Gabe (2011b, 711) as a process concerned with the "transformation of human conditions, capacities or capabilities into opportunities for pharmaceutical intervention." It then illustrates the different strands of the conceptual analysis of medicalization and pharmaceuticalization through a case study of cardiovascular disease (CVD) and the prescription of statins. The chapter concludes by considering how medicalization and pharmaceuticalization can provide one lens to analyse COVID-19 (particularly in terms of risk and vaccination).

INITIAL ACCOUNTS OF MEDICALIZATION

Situating Medicalization

Before exploring the work of the first scholars of medicalization, it is necessary to discuss two key aspects. First, the foundations of the sociological study of deviance and, second, the emancipatory culture of the 1960s and 1970s, which led to critical analysis of powerful actors and institutions, including the medical profession (Gabe, Kelleher, and Williams 2006).

To understand the genesis of the concept of medicalization it is important to appreciate the foundations of the sociological study of deviance, which lie as far back as the work of Emile Durkheim (1895/1933). The ability to define and control deviance was a central issue in the initial work on medicalization. It is important to note that Durkheim did not write in the language of medicalization, and suggested that as societies mature from simple to complex that deviance management transitions from repressive to restitutive, which results not only in a change in how deviance is controlled, but also how it is thought of and defined (Conrad and Schneider 1980). Later, Parsons (1951), in his functionalist account of the sick role, highlighted how the separation of intentional deviance (criminal) and unintentional deviance (sickness) were necessary with regard to appropriate disciplinary or treatment mechanisms. Criminals are punished, with an end goal of reshaping behaviour in line with convention, while sick people are treated with an end goal of removing the illness barriers to convention (Conrad and Schneider 1980). For those that are ill, the existence of a sick role legitimizes the "deviant" behaviour of being sick, suggested Parsons. For society, this sick role helps to manage the potentially damaging and disruptive nature of sickness. The sick role has four parts, comprised of two accepted exemptions and two obligations. The sick individual (1) is exempt from normal responsibilities for the period of illness, and (2) is not held to be personally responsible for their illness. The two obligations, namely that the individual (1) must understand that illness is an undesirable state and (2) that they are obligated to cooperate with relevant medical professionals to aid in their recovering to normal functioning. Parsons focused on how the sick role allowed society to function by restoring individuals to normal social roles.

Later scholars, building on the insights about deviance proposed by Durkheim and Parsons, saw the necessity of going further and critiquing medicine's sphere of social control, which was going beyond what was considered legitimately a medical problem to increasingly encompassing social problems (Conrad and Schneider 1980). In this regard, scholars of medicalization, beginning in the 1960s and 1970s, sought to problematize medical social control and show that disease could also be socially constructed (Williams 2003, 9–28). This was particularly because, as Conrad and Schneider (1980, 8) state, "the greatest social control power comes from having the authority to define certain behaviours, persons, and things."

It is also important to understand that the concept of medicalization developed out of the radical and emancipatory culture of the late 1960s and early 1970s, which, for a short time turned the world, including medicine, upside down (Gabe, Kelleher, and Williams 2006). Indeed, Gerhardt (1989) suggested that (medical) sociologists, inspired and provoked by student revolution and demonstrations of the late 1960s, began to see injustice and inequality as a cornerstone of academic inquiry and applied this to a critique of medicine. In the same period, radical critiques of psychiatry were also emerging that challenged conventional thinking. The anti-psychiatry movement was significant, where it was argued forcefully and critically that a dominant psychiatric lens was increasingly classifying normal behaviours and feelings as illness (Laing 1960, 1961; Szasz 1960; see also, Crossley 1998).

The Birth of Medicalization and the Social Construction of Disease

Social constructionism has been a central tenet in the scholarly development of medicalization. It has been argued that disease is constructed and defined socially and reflects the influence of powerful social forces, not least the professional authority and cultural significance of medicine (Freidson 1970; Pitts 1968; Zola 1972). The first phase of thought about medicalization, which has been described as the "orthodox" position (Lupton 1995; Williams 2003), argued that medicine actually served to reinforce the moral order of society (Conrad and Schneider 1980) despite attempts to portray itself as objective and neutral. In this way, initial medicalization scholarship was concerned with "deviant" behaviours, such as alcoholism, childhood delinquency, child abuse, and hyperactivity, and for a period of time, homosexuality, and the shift in spheres of control of such phenomena from the other institutions of social control (religion and law) to medicine – or from 'badness to sickness' (Conrad and Schneider 1980). This reflected, for example, greater secularization in society, changing social norms and values about what is considered a crime, and the growing social status afforded to the medical profession. Deviant behaviours were becoming increasingly controlled and treated by medicine with the aim of minimizing disruption to society. With these shifts, sociologists developed the concept of medicalization. Early work was primarily concerned with conceptualizing and analyzing how deviant behaviours come to be defined within the sphere of medical control and treatment. They explored whether these behaviours were legitimate medical problems requiring medical treatment or were really social problems requiring social solutions (Conrad 1975; Spector and Kitsuse 1977).

Early Medicalization Thinkers

Zola (1972) and Illich (1975) most famously espouse what we now can think of as the critical and problematizing tendencies of the initial medicalization thesis. Zola suggested that an objective, scientific, supposedly morally neutral medicine was becoming the repository of truth, replacing or incorporating religion and law as the source of judgement. Zola (1972) suggested that the process whereby medicine was displacing other institutions of social control was often a low-key and potentially insidious process. In essence, the attachment of the labels "healthy" and "ill" was argued to be becoming increasingly relevant to ever further elements of human life. Zola saw medicalization not as a reflection of a type of medical imperialism, but rather as our bureaucratic and technological social system having led to a reliance on experts. Illich (1975) also wrote critically about the extension of medicine's sphere of control. He wrote of the threats of the medical establishment to health. Again, writing with a systemic focus, he saw industrial society as expropriating personal responsibility for health and as removing autonomy from the individual.

While some scholars located doctors as seeking out and discovering illness (Freidson 1970), helping to drive medicalization through their professional activity, Conrad and Schneider (1980; see also Conrad 1992) influentially conceptualized medicalization as (potentially) occurring across three distinct levels that may or may not involve professionals. These levels were the conceptual (use of medical vocabulary), the institutional (organizational adoption of a medical approach often with non-medical personnel conducting the routine work), and the interactional (resulting from the doctor–patient relationship where physicians are necessarily involved). This shows importantly that the medicalization critique was not necessarily or solely a critique of the medical profession directly, which is not always involved, or its expansionist tendencies, despite what some have claimed (e.g., Strong 1979).

The period also witnessed an emergent Marxist and feminist scholarship that engaged with the ideas around medicalization. Taussig (1980) and particularly Navarro (1975, 1980) took issue with much of the framing of the social constructionist medicalization critique, suggesting that it had neglected to sufficiently engage with the role that medicine played in reproducing capitalist power relations in society. Feminists (Ehrenreich and English 1973; Martin 1987; Oakley 1986) argued that medicine is a patriarchal institution that has used illness and disease definitions to subjugate and reinforce existing inequality between men and women – by emphasizing female "weakness" and "illness susceptibility" as well as seizing control of areas such as pregnancy/childbirth.

THE MEDICALIZATION OF LIFESTYLE AND RISK

In the late twentieth century the concept of medicalization was expanding to include natural life processes. The medicalization of matters beyond those traditionally considered deviance and the problematizing of the risk of disease arose as a result of health surveillance (Armstrong 1995, 395), where "the dissolution of the distinct clinical categories of healthy and illness … [establish] everyone within its network of visibility." In other words, with an increasing focus on lifestyle as impacting health and preventative medicine, even the idea of "health" was inherently problematized – with bodies both healthy and ill simultaneously (Hughes 1994).

Foucauldian Influence

The work of Michel Foucault went further than the initial scholars of medicalization in terms of asserting the socially constructed nature of disease and, in a sense, challenged biological realities.

Lupton (1997) provides a useful overview of the influence of Foucauldian thought on medicalization. Above all else the scholarship of Foucault influenced a realignment in conceptual understandings of power, which was in itself important for understandings of medicalization. Whereas the institution of medicine had previously been lambasted and castigated by some for wielding a repressive power (Illich 1975), Foucault (1973, 1979) suggested that power is a complex phenomenon that is not reducible to only one entity or set of actors. Rather, it emerges and is propagated by a variety of social actors and institutions, and may be productive and positive, rather than solely repressive. Medicine is part of a wider system of disciplinary techniques in an expanding apparatus of control oriented towards moral regulation rather than more overt forms of violence or coercion – what Foucault terms a panoptic system of surveillance. Power cannot be reduced to dualisms of state versus people, or a powerful medical profession versus patients/lay knowledges (Lupton 1995). Power does not simply constrain or dominate patients/citizens; it works to shape/produce/make-up individuals who have a regulated autonomy/freedom. As such, as Lupton (1995, 99) observes, Foucauldian scholars see medicine as a disciplinary power. This scholarship suggests that medicine provides systems of knowledge/practice whereby we not only understand the body but also shape the way in which we experience it. Power relations "work in and through the human body" (Lupton 1995, 5). In this sense, Foucauldian scholarship suggests that there is no biophysical or authentic body that exists beyond medical discourse – or in other words, that the body is constructed through discourse and the clinical gaze of health professionals and other actors/entities (Lupton 1997). Williams (2001, 147) states, the emergence of this more thorough critique seemed to strip away, or at least critically question, "former acknowledgment or acceptance of an underlying 'natural' or 'biophysical' reality…" which had always existed in the initial analysis of medicalization.

Lifestyle, Risk of Disease and Surveillance

In the final stages of the twentieth century power/control became entrenched at the level of the individual, widening the medical realm into everyday aspects and spaces. Strategies for the individual to affect their own bodies in the name of health, or technologies of the self, became increasingly important (Rose 1996, 1999). As such, this "fundamental remapping of the space of illness" and "the problematization of the normal" (Armstrong 1995, 395), occurring in the latter stages of the second half of the twentieth century, resulted in the distinction between health and illness taking on a new form in terms of a focus on prevention and the relationship between lifestyle and *risk* of disease. In other words, new truths and realities occurring at the site of and through the body have been opened up, and thus influence and shape how we experience health and (potential) illness. In particular there was a growing focus on lifestyle choice as determining disease. This shift might be termed "healthism" (Crawford 1980, 2006) or "lifestylism" (Hansen and Easthope 2007), and central to this focus is a strong moral component/imperative to take responsibility for one's own health, or responsibilization (Crawford 2006; Rose 1999). As Hansen and Easthope (2007, 56) state, "[u]nlike the traditional medical model of disease where understandings are limited to physical aberrations from 'normal', the focus on risk, future disease, individual behaviours mean that under a lifestyle approach almost every aspect of living is seen as health related." It is in this broader context of the medicalization of lifestyle choice and risk that, for example, medical interest in cholesterol and the risk and prevention of future cardiovascular disease (despite lack of disease) emerges (Green 2007; and see case study below). This way of thinking about disease causation emerged out of the broader influences of epidemiological multivariate analysis of chronic disease determinants, public health and government promotional activities, as well as the increasing focus on risk in society.

In the Foucauldian manner discussed above, Nettleton and Bunton (1995, 47) suggested that the methods and techniques of lifestyle-oriented health promotion have fostered "an all-encompassing network of surveillance and observation." Armstrong (1995) similarly discussed the rise of "surveillance medicine" alongside and to an extent as displacing hospital medicine as the hegemonic model of medicine. Surveillance medicine means an expansion of the clinical gaze into an "extra-corporeal space often represented by the notion of lifestyle – to identify the precursors of future illness" (Armstrong 1995, 401). In adopting a lifestyle approach there is a growing penetration of the medical gaze into the everyday lifestyle choices of citizens (Lupton 1997). As discussed above, this surveillance, due to the complex assemblages of power, also occurs at the level of self-surveillance, as well as at the institutional or state levels, as a result of the development of what might be thought of as the health promoting self (Nettleton and Bunton 1995). In other words, the medicalization of everyday lifestyle occurs as citizens became the target of technologies of monitoring, risk assessment and population-level treatment interventions, which in turn make citizens aware in these terms of their own potential contributions to their own health "project" (Nettleton and Bunton 1995).

BEYOND MEDICALIZATION?

Medicalization as a concept has since its inception been subject to critique. For example, the extent to which it is "rampantly" occurring (Fox 1977); of medical sociologists who are no less imperialist than the institution of medicine itself (Strong 1979); through to issues surrounding the regard, reliance, understandings and expectations that lay individuals place on medical technologies (Williams and Calnan 1996), and the particular dismissiveness of constructionist modes of thought surrounding biological realities and the positives and promises of bodies of knowledge such as medicine (Bury 1986; Williams 2001).

Throughout the 2000s the relevance of the explanatory effectiveness of medicalization has been subjected to increasing scrutiny.

Abandon Medicalization?

Medicalization has significant intellectual baggage attached to it, not least due to the initial efforts to frame and explain illness. Rose (2007a; see also Rose 2007b, 2019) argues that medicalization implies medical authority has extended beyond what is legitimate, and that to de-medicalize society is desirable. He suggests that arguing in this manner is of little help to social scientists, calling for a deeper examination starting with an abandonment of the term. He goes on to suggest that medical meaning is entangled with every part of our life and influences how we experience the world.

The Continuing Value of Medicalization: Reconfiguration

Meanwhile, one of the most eminent and influential scholars of medicalization, Conrad (2005, 2007), argues for a reconfiguration and development in understanding of the drivers of medicalization without abandoning the term. Drivers, Conrad argues, include the pharmaceutical industry alongside other biotechnology industries (marketing solutions to new health problems), consumerism (where consumers help shape the scope and demand for medical treatments) and managed care. He argues that these changing drivers of medicalization have served to reduce the influence of medical professionals, but that the broader underpinnings of the medicalization thesis remain valid and important. Broadly, he argues that changes in medicine and society do not invalidate the premise of medicalization, rather that there must be an appreciation of the shifting drivers of medicalization. Davis (2006) offers another argument, suggesting there is a need to reposition the medical profession as a central player in the process of medicalization rather than disconnect from it.

The initial scholarship of medicalization emphasized it as a potentially problematic process, however, this has changed over time. The need for medicalization to be conceptualized neutrally is exemplified in the areas of contested illnesses which are diffuse conditions which fall between labels of physical and mental health, such as chronic fatigue syndrome, repetitive strain injury and fibromyalgia. The patient's experience is problematized so they are required to look for "hard" medical evidence and diagnosis which validates their condition as a clinical disease (Wainwright et al. 2006). In this way, patients themselves fight for appropriate diagnostic recognition – or, in other words, to become medicalized appropriately or at all. As Annandale (2014, 214) states "diagnosis is an arena for struggle where professionals and lay people fight over the roles and functions of illness: diagnostic processes underpin discussions of medicalisation." This quotation highlights how patients have agency and good reasons for both accepting medical labels as well as resisting them

(Wainwright and Calnan 2002; Williams and Calnan 1996), and thus the need for medicalization to be reconfigured and considered a neutral process with both potential positive and negative outcomes.

The Need for a New Concept?

Nevertheless, others have argued for a more radical (re)framing of medicalization (while still utilizing similar terminology) in line with developments in bioscience and technological development. Clarke et al. (2003) have framed such notions as biomedicalization. Biomedicalization has been defined as the "increasingly complex multisited, multidirectional processes of medicalization that are both being extended and reconstituted through the emergent social forms and practices of a highly and increasingly technoscientific biomedicine" (Clarke et al. 2003, 162). They argue that the "bio" in biomedicalization reflects the developments and transitions made possible by various biological and medical sciences and technologies, ranging from genomics to transplant medicine.

Pharmaceuticalization

The explanatory power of both medicalization and biomedicalization has been critiqued by those specifically concerned with the expanding usage of pharmaceuticals and the power, influence and wealth of the pharmaceutical industry in contemporary societies. The concept of pharmaceuticalization has been developed to grapple with a lack of specificity and focus on pharmaceuticals in other concepts (Abraham 2009, 2010; Williams, Gabe, and Davis 2009; Williams, Martin, and Gabe 2011b). Pharmaceuticalization is a sociological process that is defined by Williams et al. (2011b, 711) as the "transformation of human conditions, capacities or capabilities into opportunities for pharmaceutical intervention". Williams, Gabe and Martin (2012) argue that pharmaceuticalization is a more specific term than the "catchall" term of biomedicalization, while they also claim that the extent of the processes of biomedicalization have been overestimated by Clarke et al. (2003), particularly when considering, for example, that the promises attached to genomic development and personalized medicine have as yet not come to fruition.

Pharmaceuticalization is a term that was actually first used in anthropology (see chapter 9, by Mark Nichter "Pharmaceuticals, the commodification of health, and the health care-medicine use transition" in Nichter and Nichter 1989; also Bell and Figert 2012; Gabe et al. 2015), although the term has only really entered widespread academic and particularly sociological usage since the late 2000s and early 2010s (Abraham 2009, 2010; Fox and Ward 2008; Williams, Gabe, and Davis 2009). The sociological study of pharmaceuticals was somewhat limited prior to the twenty-first century. Some scholarships considered pharmaceuticals (e.g., attention deficit hyperactivity disorder drugs) under the auspices of medicalization (Conrad 1975; Conrad and Schneider 1980), but generally not with pharmaceuticals as the primary sociological focus themselves (Gabe et al. 2015). Perhaps the most significant body of medical sociological work on pharmaceuticals prior to the concept of pharmaceuticalization has been within the sociology of prescribing (Gabe 1990; Gabe and Lipshitz-Phillips 1984; Parish 1974). This body of work focused on the social factors shaping prescribing and did empirically engage with pharmaceuticals as analytic entities in and of themselves – although without the sophisticated conceptual apparatus offered by pharmaceuticalization.

The Conceptual Frameworks of Pharmaceuticalization

Two main conceptualizations and frameworks for analysis have been proposed in the literature. First, Abraham (2010) sets up his concept and framework for analysis as concerned with assessing the "real" impacts of pharmaceuticals – arguing that the necessity of expanding pharmaceuticalization can and should be judged against whether or not it meets healthcare need, has efficacy, and is safe for patients. Pharmaceuticalization, according to Abraham (2010, 604), is "the process by which social, behavioural or bodily conditions are treated or deemed to be in need of treatment, with medical drugs by doctors or patients." He argues that in biomedical science, drug development is always seen as the process of meeting objectively defined and established health problems but, in actuality, this is a problematic assumption. For example, it may serve the commercial interests of the pharmaceutical industry rather than public health.

Williams et al. (2011a, 2011b) set out arguably a more theoretically fluid conceptualization and framework for analysis that is not tied to a realist philosophical position – thus arguably possessing greater conceptual dexterity. These authors reject a grand synthesis in favour of an adaptable, eclectic, multilevel and multidimensional conceptual understanding so as to stimulate research with a variety of (interconnected) concerns. Williams, Martin, and Gabe (2011b, 711) conceptualize pharmaceuticalization as a "dynamic and complex heterogeneous socio-technical process that is part of what we might call a pharmaceutical regime." This notion of a "pharmaceutical regime" is vital to their framework, and refers to the networks of actors, institutions, cognitive structures and subprocesses involved in driving and influencing the development and consumption of drugs.

It is not the intention of pharmaceuticalization scholars to argue for the abandonment of the concept of medicalization. The links between medicalization and pharmaceuticalization are "complex and contingent" (Williams, Martin, and Gabe 2011b, 711). Both can occur at the same time through, for example, expansion in pharmaceutical deployment reflecting widening diagnostic criteria (Abraham 2010). Nevertheless, a conceptual assumption apparent in pharmaceuticalization scholarship to date that is that pharmaceuticalization has greater explanatory scope in matters pertaining to drugs (where they are central to the case or disease area under study) than medicalization or biomedicalization (Coveney, Gabe, and Williams 2011, 387; Williams et al. 2017).

CASE STUDY: THE (WIDENING) PRIMARY PREVENTION OF CARDIOVASCULAR DISEASE

In July 2014, the National Institute for Health and Care Excellence (NICE), a regulatory body concerned primarily with cost-effectiveness and standardization, issued an update to its guidance on the assessment and reduction of cardiovascular disease and lipid modification. The most publicly and professionally visible aspect of this guideline was the recommendation to lower the primary prevention risk threshold from ≥20% risk of developing cardiovascular disease (CVD) over ten years to a ≥10% risk over ten years. This was an extremely significant development not least because it vastly expanded the numbers of people eligible to be offered CVD risk assessment and potentially advice on prophylactic measures against CVD, including, saliently, the offer of a pharmaceutical solution. It has been estimated that lowering the risk threshold makes 4.5 million additional people in England eligible for the class of drugs called statins (National Clinical Guideline Centre 2014; National Institute for Health Care Excellence 2021). This is in addition to the millions of individuals already taking a statin at higher thresholds of risk and in the secondary prevention of CVD (to prevent further cardiovascular events). Analysis has suggested that more than 30% of all adults aged 30–84 under this guidance would be deemed at significant enough risk of CVD to be eligible for a statin, with 95% of males and the majority of females aged over 60, and all men and women aged 75–84 being eligible for the drugs (Ueda et al. 2017).

Statins reduce LDL cholesterol (or bad cholesterol), a key risk factor for CVD. A complex picture of risk factors is additionally taken into account within risk calculation by tools such as QRISK2 (a cardiovascular disease prediction algorithm). CVD is strongly associated with age, mostly occurring in people older than 50. QRISK2 risk calculation also takes into account sex, family history, ethnicity, modifiable lifestyle risk factors such as smoking, blood pressure, and geographical factors such as whether an individual lives in the north or south of England (National Clinical Guideline Centre 2014, 5). These risk factors are in part bound up together. For example, modifiable lifestyle risk factors contribute to cholesterol levels in most cases of high cholesterol (or hypercholesterolemia) and broadly statins can be thought of as "risk reducers" that are prescribed as a result of overall risk calculation and strategy.

What drove this changing threshold? First, the widening generic availability of drugs within the statins class at the time of NICE's guideline development process, including the expiry of the patent for atorvastatin, previously marketed by Pfizer as *Lipitor* (in its patented lifetime, the world's most profitable drug). This drug became generic in the UK after its patent expired in 2012. This seems to have influenced NICE's decision to begin in 2012 what was by their standards a relatively early full update of CVD prevention/lipid modification guidance. There was also reanalysis of data that changed understandings of acceptable levels of risk and the associated benefits of statins at lower levels of risk. Rather than the ground-breaking addition of randomized controlled trial (RCT) evidence, this was primarily secondary meta-analyses. This kind of analysis, which suggested benefit at lower levels of risk than codified in clinical practice guidelines, created a widened understanding of unacceptable risk and use of pharmaceuticals to prevent CVD.

Greene (2007) suggests a centrality of pharmaceuticals to fostering the legitimacy of treating risk and gradually widening the numbers of people to treat. Saukko et al. (2012, 562) summarize: "Rather than the risk factor being identified first and treatment second, cholesterol gained traction as a risk factor only after the development of targeted drugs. This co-development of a risk factor and drugs has continued in the last decade, as the category of high cholesterol [and thus risk of CVD] has expanded to encompass increasingly lower levels of cholesterol [and thus lower levels of risk of CVD]." In this regard, there is evidence of both medicalization and pharmaceuticalization occurring (and also arguably evidence of their interconnectedness) in this case.There has been both a widening understanding of unacceptable levels of CVD risk and creation of an opportunity for pharmaceutical intervention to manage or 'treat' this risk. Neither process can be divorced totally from the other in this case.

MEDICALIZATION AND PHARMACEUTICALIZATION IN THE COVID-19 PANDEMIC

How can the concepts of medicalization and pharmaceuticalization be used to understand and provide a framing of the responses to the COVID-19 pandemic? At the time of writing, the world is struggling to contain the COVID-19 pandemic, with several vaccines offering hope. Medicalization is certainly occurring in terms of everyone being labelled as "at risk" of developing and transmitting the virus (Armstrong 1995). Risk of disease has been used to justify increased surveillance of and constraints on the liberty of citizens in many countries around the world.

The development of a COVID-19 vaccine in 2020 has highlighted the explanatory power of pharmaceuticalization. The spread of COVID-19 has led to opportunities for pharmaceutical intervention (with vaccines discussed as an example of pharmaceuticalization in other research (Manca 2018; Mulinari and Vihelmsson 2020)). Vaccines are viewed as the quickest and most effective (in terms of the economy and public health) way to allow a degree of normalcy to return to everyday life. National vaccination programmes need to cover a substantial proportion of the population to control the pandemic. The Williams et al. (2011b) pharmaceuticalization framework, with its focus on the pharmaceutical regime, allows sociologists to analyze all of the moving parts of the COVID-19 pandemic. There are various social forces, actors and interests shaping vaccine development, regulation and if, who and how quickly people can be vaccinated.

Governments and the pharmaceutical industry, motivated by their own aims, are working together in the research and development of a vaccine. As Calnan and Douglass (2020) note, initially some disquiet existed in the scientific community that as a result of the haste required to save lives and protect economies, efficacy and safety might not be given sufficient attention. It was feared, for example, that there would be an emphasis on vaccines that reduce severity of illness rather than protect against infection and provide only short-lived immunity, which might be beneficial for industry profit, and/or political interests (including, for example, election campaigns), but not for global public health (Godlee 2020). Indeed, it normally takes many years to develop a vaccine – although, reflecting the significant impacts on public health and economic interests, vaccine developers have been able to attract unprecedented levels of research funding from governments. The first vaccines have been shown to be safe and effective and have achieved regulatory approval. However, there are still questions about lasting immunity, about the evidence for the use of "mix and match" approaches to vaccination (by the UK government) to the use of different brands for first and second doses (Mahase 2021), and about how inequalities between countries as well as within countries might shape affordability and access to vaccines globally (Calnan and Douglass 2020; Douglass and Calnan 2020).

Traditional print media and web-based media have covered the work of vaccine development and the scientific debate about it, providing widely divergent narratives that seem simultaneously to proffer hope and despair. Also, while people trust that there will be an end to the health and economic threats posed by the pandemic, there is a significant community of people who are hesitant or who hold anti-vaccination views (often due to concern about safety, the unnaturalness of vaccination or because of a lack of trust in governments or commercial actors). Trust in professionals and governments is one highly important factor in public take-up of vaccines (Calnan and Douglass 2020). Whether these complex dynamics, interests and beliefs cohere sufficiently to result in widespread vaccination remains at this point in time unclear.

CONCLUSION

This chapter clearly shows that medicalization is a resilient concept and has been one of the major theoretical and empirical interests in medical sociology since the late 1960s. It has been the focus of considerable debate and the definition of medicalization has shifted over time, with changing conceptual significance given to different actors and drivers. The latest thought and debate about medicalization have focused on the continuing explanatory power of the concept and whether it is necessary for the concept to be abandoned altogether or refined and narrowed in scope or replaced by more sophisticated conceptual apparatus, such as biomedicalization or pharmaceuticalization. As this chapter shows, the diagnostic setting of CVD and the prescription of statins provides an insightful example of the interconnectedness between medicalization and pharmaceuticalization and the utility and importance, as such, of both concepts.

REFERENCES

Abraham, John. 2009. "The pharmaceutical industry, the state and teh NHS." In *The New Sociology of the Health Service*. Edited by Jonathan Gabe and Michael Calnan, pp. 99–121. Abingdon, UK: Routledge.

Abraham, John. 2010. "Pharmaceuticalization of society in context: theoretical, empirical and health dimensions." *Sociology* 44(4): 603–622.

Annadale, Ellen. 2014. *The Sociology of Health and Medicine: A Critical Introduction* (2nd edition). Cambridge, UK: Polity Press.

Armstrong, David. 1995. "The rise of surveillance medicine." *Sociology of Health and Illness* 17(3): 393–404.

Bell, Susan, and Anne E. Figert. 2012. "Medicalization and pharmaceuticalization at the intersections: looking backward, sideways and forward." *Social Science and Medicine* 75(5): 775–783.

Bury, Michael R. 1986. "Social constructionism and the development of medical sociology." *Sociology of Health and Illness* 8(2): 137–169.

Busfield, Joan. 2010. "'A pill for every ill': explaining the expansion in medicine use." *Social Science and Medicine* 70(6): 934–941.

Busfield, Joan. 2017. "The concept of medicalisation reassessed." *Sociology of Health and Illness* 395: 759–774.

Calnan, Michael, and Tom Douglass. 2020. "Hopes, hesitancy and the risky business of vaccine development." *Health, Risk and Society* 22(5–6): 291–304.

Clarke, Adele E., Janet K. Shim, Laura Mamo, Jennifer Ruth Fosket, and Jennifer R. Fishman. 2003. "Biomedicalization: technoscientific transformations of health, illness, and US biomedicine." *American Sociological Review* 68(2): 161–194.

Conrad, Peter. 1975. "The discovery of hyperkinesis: notes on the medicalization of deviant behavior." *Social Problems* 23(1): 12–21.

Conrad, Peter. 1992. "Medicalization and social control." *Annual Review of Sociology* 18(1): 209–232.

Conrad, Peter. 2005. "The shifting engines of medicalization." *Journal of Health and Social Behavior* 46(1): 3–14.

Conrad, Peter. 2007. *The Medicalization of Society: On the Transformation of Human Conditions into Treatable Diseases*. Baltimore, MD: Johns Hopkins University Press.

Conrad, Peter, and Joseph W. Schneider. 1980. *Deviance and Medicalization: From Badness to Sickness*. St. Louis, MO: Mosby.

Coveney, Catherine, Jonathan Gabe, and Simon Williams. 2011. "The sociology of cognitive enhancement: medicalisation and beyond." *Health Sociology Reveiw* 20(4): 381–393.

Crawford, Robert. 1980. "Healthism and the medicalization of everyday life." *International Journal of Health Services* 10(3): 365–388.

Crawford, Robert. 2006. "Health as a meaningful social practice." *Health* 10(4): 401–420.

Crossley, Nick. 1998. "RD Laing and the British anti-psychiatry movement: a socio–historical analysis." *Social Science and Medicine* 47(7): 877–889.

Davis, Joseph E. 2006. "How medicalization lost its way." *Society* 43(6): 51–56.

Douglass, Tom, and Michael Calnan. 2020. "All for vaccination? Vaccination for all?" *Discover Society* https://discoversociety.org/2020/11/23/all-for-vaccination-vaccination-for-all/ (accessed, 2 March 2021).

Durkheim, Emile. 1895/1933. *The Rules of Sociological Method*. New York: The Free Press.

Ehrenreich, Barbara, and Deirdre English. 1973. *Complaints and Disorders: The Sexual Politics of Sickness*. New York: The Feminist Press.

Foucault, Michel. 1973. *The Birth of the Clinic*. London: Tavistock.

Foucault, Michel. 1979. *Discipline and Punishment: The Birth of the Prison*. London: Allen Lane.

Fox, Nick J., and Katie J. Ward. 2008. "Pharma in the bedroom … and the kitchen … the pharmaceuticalisation of daily life." *Sociology of Health and Illness* 30(6): 856–868.

Fox, Renée C. 1977. "The medicalization and demedicalization of American society." *Daedalus* 106(1); 9–22.

Freidson, Eliot. 1970. *Profession of Medicine: A Study of the Sociology of Applied Knowledge*. Chicago, IL: University of Chicago Press.

Gabe, Jonathan. 1990. "Towards a sociology of tranquillizer prescribing." *British Journal of Addiction* 85: 41–48.

Gabe, Jonathan, David Kelleher, and Gareth Williams. 2006. "Understanding medical dominance in the modern world." In *Challenging Medicine* (2nd edition). Edited by David Kelleher, Jonathan Gabe and Gareth Williams, pp. xiii–xxxiv. Abingdon, UK: Routledge.

Gabe, Jonathan, and Susan Lipshitz-Phillips. 1984. "Tranquillisers as social control?" *The Sociological Review* 32(3): 524–546.

Gabe, Jonathan, Simon Williams, Paul Martin, and Catherine Coveney. 2015. "Pharmaceuticals and society: power, promises and prospects." *Social Science and Medicine* 131: 193–198.

Gerhardt, Uta. 1989. *Ideas about Illness: An Intellectual and Political history of Medical Sociology*. New York: New York University Press.

Godlee, Fiona. 2020. "Covid-19 Less haste more safety." *BMJ* 370: m3258.

Green, Jeremy A. 2007. *Prescribing by Numbers: Drugs and the Definition of Disease*. Baltimore, MD: Johns Hopkins University Press.

Hansen, Emily, and Gary Easthope. 2007. *Lifestyle in Medicine*. Abingdon, UK: Routledge.

Hughes, Miranda. 1994. "The risks of lifestyle and the diseases of civilisation." *Annual Review of Health Social Science* 4(1): 57–78.

Illich, Ivan. 1975. *Limits to Medicine. Medical Nemesis: The Expropriation of Health*. London: Marion Boyars.

Laing, R.D. 1960. *The Divided Self*. London: Tavistock.

Laing, R.D. 1961. *Self and Others*. London: Tavistock.

Lupton, Deborah. 1995. *The Imperative of Health: Public Health and the Regulated Body*. London: Sage.

Lupton, Deborah. 1997. "Foucault and the medicalisation critique." In *Foucault, Health and Medicine*. Edited by Alan Petersen and Robin Bunton, pp. 94–110. London: Routledge.

Mahase, Elisabeth. 2021. "Vaccine brands can be mixed in 'extremely rare occasions,' says Public Health England." *BMJ* 372: n12.

Manca, Terra. 2018. "One of the greatest medical success stories:" physicians and nurses' small stories about vaccine knowledge and anxieties." *Social Science and Medicine* 196: 182–189.

Martin, Emily. 1987. *The Woman in the Body: A Cultural Analysis of Reproduction*. Boston, MA: Beacon Press.

Mulinari, Shai, and Andreas Vihelmsson. 2020. "Revisiting the pharmaceuticalisation of pandemic influenza using Lukes' framework of power." *Sociology of Health and Illness* 42(2): 327–341.

National Clinical Guideline Centre. 2014. *Lipid Modification: Cardiovascular Risk Assessment and the Modification of Blood Lipids for the Primary and Secondary Prevention of Cariovascular Disease*. NICE Clinical Guideline CG181. London: National Clinical Guideline Centre, www.nice.org.uk/guidance/cg181/evidence/lipid-modification-update-full-guideline-pdf-243786637.

National Institute for Health Care Excellence. 2021. "NICE recommends wider use of statins for prevention of CVD." *National Institute for Health Care Excellence* www.nice.org.uk/news/article/nice-recommends-wider-use-of-statins-for-prevention-of-cvd (accessed, 2 March 2021).

Navarro, Vicente. 1975. "The industrialization of fetishism or the fetishism of industrialization: a critique of Ivan Illich." *Social Science and Medicine* 9(7): 351–363.

Navarro, Vicente. 1980. "Work, ideology, and science: the case of medicine." *Social Science and Medicine. Part C: Medical Economics* 14(3): 191–205.

Nettleton, Sarah, and Robin Bunton. 1995. "Sociological critiques of health promotion." In *The Sociology of Health Promotion: Critical Analyses of Consumption, Lifestyle and Risk*. Edited by Robin Bunton, Sarah Nettleton and Roger Burrows. London: Routledge.

Nichter, Mark, and Mimi Nichter. 1989. *Anthropology and International Health: Asian Case Studies*. London: Routledge.

Oakley, Ann. 1986. *The Captured Womb: A History of the Medical Care of Pregnant Women*. Oxford: Blackwell.

Parish, Peter A. 1974. "Sociology of prescribing." *British Medical Bulletin* 30(3): 214–217.

Parsons, Talcott. 1951. *The Social System*. London: Routledge.

Pitts, Jesse R. 1968. "Social control: the concept." In *International Encyclopedia of the Social Sciences* (Vol. 14). Edited by David L. Sills, pp. 382–395. New York: Crowell Collier and Macmillan.

Rose, Nikolas. 1996. *Inventing our Selves: Psychology, Power, and Personhood*. Cambridge, UK. Cambridge University Press.

Rose, Nikolas 1999. *Powers of Freedom: Reframing Political Thought*. Cambridge, UK: Cambridge University Press.

Rose, Nikolas. 2007a. "Beyond medicalisation." *The Lancet* 369(9562): 700–702.

Rose, Nikolas. 2007b. *The Politics of Life Itself: Biomedicine, Power, and Subjectivity in the Twenty-First Century*. Princeton, NJ: Princeton University Press.

Rose, Nikolas. 2019. *Our Psychiatric Future*. Cambridge, UK: Polity Press.

Saukko, Paula M., Hannah Farrimond, Philip H. Evans, and Nadeem Qureshi. 2012. "Beyond beliefs: risk assessment technologies shaping patients' experiences of heart disease prevention." *Sociology of Health and Illness* 34(4): 560–575. doi: 10.1111/j.1467-9566.2011.01406.x.

Spector, Malcolm, and John I. Kitsuse. 1977. *Constructing Social Problems*. Menlo Park, CA: Benjamin Cummings.

Strong, P.M. 1979. "Sociological imperialism and the profession of medicine: a critical examination of the thesis of medical imperialism." *Social Science and Medicine. Part A: Medical Psychology and Medical Sociology* 13: 199–215.

Szasz, Thomas. 1960. "The myth of mental illness." *American Psychologist* 15(2): 113–118.

Taussig, Michael T. 1980. "Reification and the consciousness of the patient." *Social Science and Medicine. Part B: Medical Anthropology* 14(1): 3–13.

Ueda, Peter, Thomas Wai-Chun Lung, Philip Clarke, and Goodarz Danaei. 2017. "Application of the 2014 NICE cholesterol guidelines in the English population: a cross-sectional analysis." *British Journal of General Practice* 67(662): e598–e608.

Wainwright, David, and Michael Calnan. 2002. *Work Stress: The Making of a Modern Epidemic*. Buckingham, UK: Open University Press.

Wainwright, David, Michael Calnan, Claire O'Neil, Anna Winterbottom, and Christopher Watkins. 2006. "When pain in the arm is 'all in the head': The management of medically unexplained suffering in primary care." *Health, Risk and Society* 8(1): 71–88.

Williams, Simon J. 2001. "Sociological imperialism and the profession of medicine revisited: where are we now?" *Sociology of Health and Illness* 23(2): 135–158.

Williams, Simon J. 2003. *Medicine and the Body*. London: Sage.

Williams, Simon J., and Michael Calnan. 1996. "The 'limits' of medicalization? Modern medicine and the lay populace in 'late' modernity." *Social Science and Medicine* 42(12): 1609–1620.

Williams, Simon J., Jonathan Gabe, and Peter Davis, eds. 2009. *Pharmaceuticals and Society: Critical Discourses and Debates*. London: John Wiley and Sons.

Williams, Simon J., Jonathan Gabe, and Paul Martin. 2012. "Medicalization and pharmaceuticalization at the intersections: a commentary on Bell and Figert (2012)." *Social Science and Medicine* 75(12): 2129–2130.

Williams, Simon J., Paul Martin, and Jonathan Gabe. 2011a. "Evolving sociological analyses of 'Pharmaceuticalisation': a reply to Abraham." *Sociology of Health and Illness* 33(5): 729–730.

Williams, Simon J., Paul Martin, and Jonathan Gabe. 2011b. "The pharmaceuticalisation of society? A framework for analysis." *Sociology of Health and Illness* 33(5): 710–725.

Williams, Taryn, Coenraad J. Hattingh, Catherine M. Kariuki, Sean A. Tromp, Anton J. van Balkom, Jonathan C. Ipser, and Dan J. Stein. 2017. "Pharmacotherapy for social anxiety disorder (SAnD)." *Chochrane Database of Systematic Reviews* 19(10): CD001206.

Zola, Irving K. 1972. "Medicine as an institution of social control." *The Sociological Review* 20(4): 487–504.

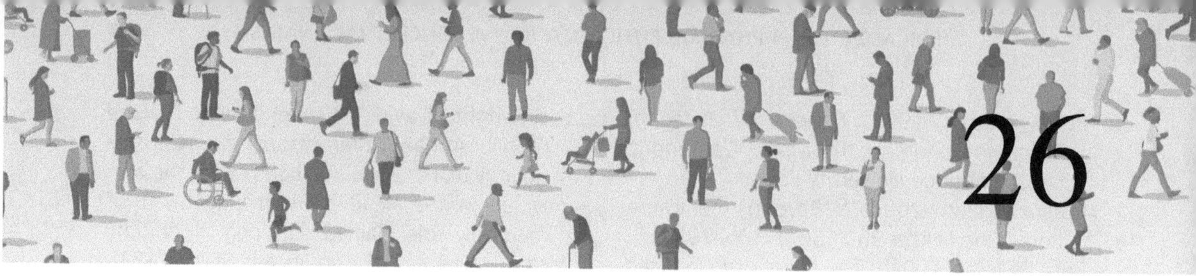

26

Digital Health: An Important Public Health Tool

Lina Williatte-Pellitteri, Nesrine Benyahia, Thierry Moulin and Nicolas Giraudeau

INTRODUCTION

Digital technologies are increasingly prevalent in our personal lives (banking, shopping, social interactions etc.), in our professional lives (videoconferencing, email etc.) and in health care (in our relationships with our physicians and other health care providers). However, the integration of information and communication technologies in health care is not a new phenomenon, and can be traced back to the creation of the first "modern" communication technologies: The arrival of the telephone in the 19th century was quickly followed by the first long-distance medical consultations. In fact, the inventor himself, Alexander Graham Bell, reported that on 10 March 1876 he used the telephone after spilling sulphuric acid on himself during an experiment. Three years later, *The Lancet* reported the first use of the telephone in paediatric medicine, when it was used to communicate the clinical condition of a child suspected of having croup (Anonymous 1879). Nowadays, digital tools are increasingly numerous, increasingly quick and increasingly intrusive. They range from smartphones to wearables such as smartwatches, other wrist devices, buttons and patches. Their increasing use in health care has even led to the creation of the term "digital health", which has essentially become a medical specialty in its own right.

Additionally, digital health is now thought of as a potential response to inequalities in access to health care, and as a factor in meeting sustainable development objectives (World Health Organization 2020). Digital health should therefore be affordable, sustainable, scalable, and accessible to the greatest possible number of people. To this end, it should be thought of as a tool, specifically as a public health tool. For a tool to be used effectively, it must be defined, and its users must know how to wield it. We have therefore decided to structure this chapter on digital health by examining, first, the regulatory aspects of digital health and, second, how it is taught to health professionals.

THE MAJOR REGULATORY PRINCIPLES GOVERNING DIGITAL HEALTH

It is undeniable that new information and communication technologies have become ubiquitous in our hospitals, clinics and medical offices. The "connected" physician is, however, often faced with demanding patients, some of whom expect 24/7 monitoring.

Digitalization of the doctor–patient relationship has progressed at different rates in different countries. Advancements are being spearheaded by countries in the Anglosphere, notably the USA, which is currently on track to become the world leader in the processing of Big Data in health care. Meanwhile, Europe, and France in particular, is weighing up the potential consequences of setting up a (heavily regulated) open health data repository.

Approaches to digital health are undeniably different in different countries. However, the differences are poorly understood by physicians, some of whom would like to develop research projects mirroring those of their Anglosphere counterparts, but feel restricted by incomprehensible standards. The same is true of patients—who embrace the quantified self (i.e. self-monitoring using digital technologies) and remote medical coaching—and start-ups, which are forced to choose where to set up their projects based on the standards imposed by each country.

The parties involved are right to criticize these fundamentally different standards, in that they create unassailable competitive advantages according to how libertarian they are. However, legal experts explain the diversity of the standards by citing the legislative traditions of each country and their policies that protect fundamental rights. These divergent traditions explain the legislative framework of the standards, which applies both to the development of practices that use new technologies, and to the processing and use of the resulting data.

Telehealth: A Different Pattern of Adoption in Different Countries

An in-depth analysis of practices in the health care sector has revealed that the meanings given to telemedicine terminology differ between countries. This means that an identical term may describe different actions in different countries. These actions may fall under a different category of medical act, and may therefore be governed by a different set of standards. The divergence in terminology also leads to differences in the standards that are created and how they are understood. The example of telemedicine and e-health demonstrates this well.

Nowadays, certain terms, expressions and words are used interchangeably to refer to different acts, trends and practices in the field of telehealth. As evidence of this, a recent study (Gallois and Rauly 2015) revealed that the terms "telemedicine", "telehealth" and "e-health" are sometimes used synonymously (Crigger 2006). However, in some cases they describe a remote medical practice and define a medical act (Chandra, Pettry Jr., and Paul III 2013), and in others, they describe the tools and mediation involved in providing the service (Kerleau and Pelletier-Fleury 2002) or e-commerce linked to health (Kirsch 2002). These differences in the meanings ascribed to the terms affect not only the relevant legal framework but also the legislator's perception of the act. As an illustration, let us consider the example of telemedicine.

The Unique Status of Telemedicine in France

There are two opposing understandings of telemedicine: in developed countries, it is essentially clinical, whereas in developing countries it is mostly informative (Simon and Lucas 2013). Clinical telemedicine is defined as "a professional activity that uses digital telecommunication methods, allowing physicians and other health care professionals to perform medical acts remotely to benefit patients" (Croels 2006, Le droit des obligations à l'épreuve de la telemedecine. Presses Universitaires d'Aix-Marseille 2006, p.23), whereas informative telemedicine is defined as "interactive audiovisual communication that enables the dissemination of medical knowledge and protocols for patient care, with the aim of supporting and improving medical activities" (Simon P. Telemedicine is not e-commerce. Communication from ANTEL in partnership with the National Order of Physicians. 22 Nov 2013).

France was one of the first countries to enact a legal basis for the practice of telemedicine: law number 2009-879 of 21 July 2009, known as the Hospital, Patient, Health and Territories law (HPST), and the related decree of 19 October 2010, updated in 2018 (Ministère de la santé et des sports 2010). These two key texts sanction a clinical approach to telemedicine, defining it as a medical act performed by health care professionals by means of information and communication technologies. In other words, in France, telemedicine is a medical act performed by a health care professional. Its effectiveness is recognized and it guarantees the highest level of health care safety in terms of proven medical knowledge. This definition of telemedicine is clearly distinct from that of other countries, which define telemedicine as any health service performed using new technologies. Although this difference may seem small, it reveals a fundamental difference in how telemedicine is understood, as one definition describes a medical act, and the other describes the provision of a medical service more generally. This difference in vocabulary leads to an idiosyncratic regulatory framework: in France, telemedicine is covered by specific legislation, whereas elsewhere in Europe, it falls under the more general category of e-health.

The French understanding of telemedicine is as a medical act performed by health care professionals by means of information and communication technologies. This principle is confirmed by article R.6316-1 of the French Public Health Code, which defines telemedicine as "medical acts performed remotely by means of a device using information and communication technologies". The 2010 decree includes a list of the acts that fall within the category of telemedicine:

1 Teleconsultation, which allows a medical professional to perform a remote consultation for a patient.
2 Tele-expertise, which allows a medical professional to obtain the opinion of one or more other medical professionals remotely, on the basis of medical information related to the patient's care.
3 Medical tele-surveillance, which allows a medical professional to remotely interpret the necessary data for the follow-up of a patient and, if required, to make decisions regarding the patient's treatment.
4 Medical teleassistance, which allows a medical professional to remotely assist a health care professional who is performing a medical act.
5 Medical regulation, which describes medical advice given in the context of medical dispatching (emergency services).

Additionally, in order to meet requirements, telemedicine projects must take into account the deficiencies in the health care services in their regions due to geographical isolation (art. L6316-1 from the French Public Health Code).

In France, legislation classes telemedicine as a "tool" that must meet objectives related to organization, continuity, permanence of care, and safety. Because telemedicine is fundamentally viewed as a medical act, the conditions for practising medicine must be provided for and adhered to. To this end, the 2010 decree requires telemedicine project leaders to respect the fundamental rights of the patient and comply with all legal obligations relating to the practice of medicine, as set out by the French Public Health Code and the medical code of ethics. Because these objectives and obligations have been assessed and verified by the authorities, professionals in contravention of them may be held liable.

Until 2018, telemedicine acts were not covered by health insurance in France, which had a significant impact on the rollout of telemedicine across the country. Since the enactment of the 2018 decrees, two telemedicine acts have been covered. The conditions of reimbursement build upon the condition laid out in the decree of 2010. These conditions draw an even clearer distinction between the practice of telemedicine and practices related to e-health.

WEARABLE TECHNOLOGY AND HEALTH

Telemedicine is increasingly being influenced by devices that people can wear, and which can collect and transmit information to health care providers. We are experiencing a rapid transformation in the availability of devices and applications that people can have on their person and which provide information both to the individual using them, and to health care providers and researchers. A number of these are listed below. It should be noted that access to these devices and applications varies by socio-economic status, and by country or region.

Wearable devices and related applications have been used for the management of diabetes, asthma, obesity, stress, depression, smoking cessation and cardiovascular health, among others (Kumar et al. 2013). Research, including case-control trials, has shown the impact of mobile connective technology in influencing weight loss (Spring et al. 2013). However, in a study of patients with artery disease, there was not sufficient evidence to show that mobile connective technology influenced activity levels. (McDermott et al. 2018).

These technologies can have either push or pull functions, or both. A push function pushes the wearer to engage in a given behavior. For example, tracking steps taken can include notifications to meet specific step goals for a day, a week or a month, or a reminder to take some deep breaths when the device detects stress. A pull function records data and provides it to the wearer, and can also transmit it to a health care provider, a coach, or a researcher (presumably with the permission of the wearer). An example of a pull function is a glucose monitoring device, which provides read-outs of blood glucose levels. This technology-based interaction has been called "engagement" in the literature on health behavior change (Yardley et al. 2016).

- **Wrist devices**: Smartwatches or other devices called trackers, which are designed to be worn on the wrist. All of these track steps and other physical activity. Smartwatches can measure a range of health information, including heart rate, sleep patterns, blood oxygen saturation, ECG, physical activity, skin temperature and more. For example, a combination of ECG and heart rate can be used to detect stress. Watches are also now being used to detect seizures (Thompson, Langer, and Kinte 2019).

  The FDA has cleared an app for the Apple Watch to help people suffering from nightmares or post-traumatic stress disorder (PTSD) get a better night's sleep. Dubbed Nightware, the prescription app monitors the wearer's heart rate and movement while they sleep – and, if they're having a nightmare, gently prods them out of the dream without aiming to wake them up completely, using the smartwatch's vibrations.
- **Wearable monitor strapped to the upper arm**: Uses light sensors to sense blood flow, similarly to many consumer electronics and fitness trackers. Within three to five minutes, it uses an artificial intelligence model to crunch the data on the person's pulse rate and other factors to determine whether their blood could be clotting more easily than normal. Combined with temperature checks, this technology can identify people over the age of 5 who could be carrying COVID-19 without showing any symptoms.
- **"Biobutton"**: An FDA-cleared medical-grade wearable device for continuous vital sign monitoring for up to 90-days (based on configuration). This coin-sized disposable "button" measures temperature, respiratory rate and heart rate.

- **Epidermal electronics**: These are small patches that attach to the skin. They contain electrophysiological, temperature, and strain sensors, as well as transistors, light-emitting diodes, photodetectors, radio frequency inductors, capacitors, oscillators, and rectifying diodes. "The electrodes, electronics, sensors, power supply, and communication components are configured together into ultrathin, low-modulus, lightweight, stretchable 'skin-like' membranes that laminate onto the surface of the skin by soft contact, in a manner that is mechanically invisible to the user, much like a temporary transfer tattoo" (Kim et al. 2011). They can monitor electrophysiological (EP) processes related to activity of the brain [electroencephalograms (EEGs)], the heart [electrocardiograms (ECGs)] and muscle tissue [electromyograms (EMGs)] (Kim et al. 2011). Increasingly, they are used where monitoring equipment can be cumbersome, such as with babies in neonatal intensive care units and people with epilepsy. They are also used to monitor patients who are out of the hospital, but still need close monitoring. Some can also analyze sweat to measure dehydration, electrolytes, calcium, zinc and iron.

  Patches also are being developed using microneedles to measure protein biomarkers. One study measured protein biomarkers in interstitial fluid, and tested anti-cocaine antibody levels in mice that had received a cocaine. The same study also measured cytokines and matricellular proteins in the blood in mice. Cytokine measurement is an established method for evaluating the ability of the immune system to mount an innate inflammatory immune response, and so could be used to study vaccine efficacy. Another potential application is to diagnose myocardial infarction using cardiac troponin. The authors point out multiple uses of this technology, in home, emergency and hospital settings (Wang et al. 2021).
- **Glucose monitoring devices**: These are various forms of "buttons" with internally implanted sensors that can detect blood glucose levels and transmit these to a wearable or handheld device. They can also alert the wearer to abnormally low or high blood glucose levels (Nichols et al. 2013).
- **Multiple devices**: Wearing multiple devices can increase applications, as multiple devices can combine data points. Some things are better measured at different points on the body. As time goes on, it is likely that we will have a constellation of sensors, patches and buttons in places such as shoes and glasses in addition to wrists. For example, tonic-clonic seizures can be detected before they happen if the person wears a device on both wrists. Smartphones are also being used as an additional data point. There are now applications for nutrition research and encouraging healthier eating habits that rely on photos taken with a phone to analyze food intake (Ben Neriah and Geliebter 2019).

HEALTH DATA: 21ST-CENTURY GOLD

Digital health practices have one key element: health data. This digital information is the subject of numerous questions and concerns from both potential patients and political leaders, who fear abuses in the way the data are used. Additionally, the increasingly large streams of data that are available represent a gold mine that is important to regulate.

The development of digital health technologies naturally entails the use of personal health data, either directly or indirectly, notably by providers of digital platforms and solutions, health care professionals and patients themselves.

The large-scale digitalization of health care has revealed shortcomings in the interoperability and security of hospital information systems. These weaknesses were given even more media coverage during the COVID-19 health crisis, at a time when the public was becoming more aware of the idea of privacy protection and IT security.

Personal Health Data: Sensitive Information

Information is categorized as "personal data" when it makes it possible to identify a natural person either directly or indirectly. However, the broadness of this definition makes it difficult to apply the concept of anonymization. Personal health data is any information that makes it possible to know the state of physical or mental health of a natural person. Following the same logic as the previous definition, personal health data can be characterized by the possibility to use it to identify, either directly or indirectly, the state of health of a natural person by inference, correlation or individualization.

In current international legislation, personal health data is often classed as sensitive information, in the same way as genetic information, biometric information or even data related to religious affiliation, political opinions, etc. This idea of sensitivity is interesting, because it is more closely related to the preservation of citizens' fundamental liberties and free-will than to their financial or material assets. Personal health data therefore requires an even higher level of protection and security in order to avoid any confidentiality breaches, and to protect against any attacks on its content or availability.

Personal health data has always been treated distinctly, as evidenced by patients' fundamental right to medical confidentiality. The protection of personal health data is therefore an integral part of the care relationship, and is a keystone of building trust. Because of this, the mediation performed by digital solution platforms between the health care professional and the patient therefore requires careful consideration of shared responsibility, transparency and clarity of the information.

Liabilities in Terms of the Protection of Personal Data

Processing personal health data for telemedicine or artificial intelligence primarily involves three categories of people: the patient, the health care professional and the service provider.

- The health care professional is liable for the protection of the patients' personal health data in the context of a medical or paramedical treatment.
- Health care professionals must be fully aware of their liabilities and contractual relationship with the digital solution provider before any data are processed. The difficulties in this case often stem from the health care professionals' lack of time or lack of knowledge of complex subjects that are not necessarily related to their profession, which creates an imbalance in their contractual relationships with solution providers.
- The solution provider is more broadly liable for any infringement or violation of personal data resulting in particular from negligence, fault, or breach of the applicable laws and regulations.

Patients' Right to be Informed

Health care professionals and digital solution providers have a duty to inform patients regarding the use of their personal data. The information must be clear, honest and transparent. It should include details about the nature of the data processing, the purposes for which the data will be used, and the means of accessing the data in a format readable by a machine, for example. The provision of this information is the consequence of patients exercising their rights concerning their data. All patients have the right to access, rectify, and erase their data. The health care professional is the guarantor of the patient's rights, whereas the solution provider usually intervenes to support the health care professional for the necessary technical operations.

It is essential to obtain patient consent for certain uses of personal data, particularly in the contexts of research or analysis of data for reasons outside the initial scope of the data collection. At the very least, patients must be informed of their right to refuse the future use of their data, and the possibility to refuse must be guaranteed by the health care professional and the digital solution provider.

The Security of Health Data

Personal health data must be protected by appropriate technological and organizational security measures whose robustness is proportional to the sensitivity of the data. The loss of, alteration of, or illegitimate access to the patient's health data can cause physical harm to the patient, or even, in some extreme circumstances, the death of the patient. Data security measures must therefore be integrated into the main pre-existing processing operations: data collection, handling, transmission, storage, archiving, and destruction.

Traceability of the data processing is also a particularly important requirement in digital health, not least because the liability regime is linked to this traceability. The digital service provider must therefore ensure that accurate logs are kept regarding access to the data, as well as functional and technical logs and records of all interventions by all users and administrators of the digital service.

The storage of personal data can be a difficult issue, particularly in terms of the location of the servers that host the data. Because national legislations are different and sometimes impose national data storage rules, the geographical location of data storage facilities is a significant factor in user confidence in the solutions available on the digital health market.

Big Data and Exploitation of Health Data

All digital service providers, alongside the majority of health establishments and health care professionals, are racing to collect large volumes of health data. The potential benefits of exploiting these data are significant, particularly in the field of industrial and academic research.

Huge quantities of high-quality data are contained in digital health solutions. The collection of these data by connected devices, as a result of the Internet of Things (IoT), and the digital interpretation of these data by health care professionals, fuels both research and the development of artificial intelligence. These real-life data, which present a rare opportunity due to their volume and representativeness, are therefore particularly sought-after.

Current regulation by government policies is challenged by the emergence of new uses of existing technologies and new, high-performance technologies, as well as citizens' dissatisfaction with the lack of transparency. As we have seen, the regulation of digital health ensures its proper use. That being said, if a practice is to be performed well, it must be taught well. Teaching in health care and medicine is traditionally based on practical experience, which usually consists of supervised practical exercises before clinical practice. Is this also the case for training in digital health? Until now, very few medical faculties or health care training programmes have included digital health in their basic training. We will now consider in more detail the approach of French universities towards digital health teaching.

CASE STUDY: DIGITAL HEALTH TEACHING IN FRANCE

The advent of digital technologies entails a paradigm shift in medical practices, organizations, and patient management models, from acute pathologies to chronic illnesses and preventive medicine. It is therefore necessary to supplement health care professionals' training and to create new professions and training that are adapted to the digital revolution. Stephen Klasko, President of Thomas Jefferson University, insightfully diagnoses the current state of teaching programmes(https://sklasko.com/2016/07/04/teve-klasko-interview-michael-hoad/):

> We need a longitudinal curriculum … around technology so that the people who get out of medical school really understand how technology can help them communicate with patients, some of which will be telehealth. As an example, when doctors have the ability to understand health care disparities, so many things are possible.

In this period of transition, in which medical practices and organizations are being transformed and new treatment models are becoming available to patients, universities should reflect these changes in the training provided to health professionals. They should also create new training programmes that address connected health solutions and telemedicine.

Klasko affirms that in order to transform communication within care structures, universities must teach students how to behave in society, notably in a society that consumes an ever-increasing amount of health information. He also predicts that the use of science and algorithms in curative medicine will mean that the role of physicians in the future will be increasingly focused on keeping people in good health, i.e. preventative medicine.

It is also worth noting that, as highlighted by Klasko, digitalization goes hand in hand with globalization, and patients will be able to access the physician of their choice from anywhere in the world. This will be supported by applications of artificial intelligence, such as voice recognition systems and machine translation systems, which will break down language barriers. As well as being able to communicate and consult with physicians across the globe, patients will be able to take a more active role in their own health management by using technology such as connected devices and robots in the home. They will be able to monitor their own health using these tools, and send the results to their physician, wherever they may be.

This shift towards digitalization should prioritize the well-being of patients – who are at the centre of the system and are key players in their own health – by adapting to the challenges of a future of connected health care. Finally, we should also consider transhumanism and the effects of merging technomedicine, brought about by NBIC (nanotechnology, biology, information technology and cognitive science), with the integration of the human–machine interface, algorithms, robotics, etc. These scientific and medical developments require careful consideration of the associated ethical questions, which should therefore form a key part of medical students' training.

The Current State of Telemedicine Training

Leaders of the digital technology industry, innovation specialists and transhumanist philosophers are continually proclaiming that medicine is undergoing a significant change, that medical practice in the 21st century will not resemble that of the 20th century, and that digital medicine will be more predictive, preventive, personalized and participative (4Ps), and more complete, chronic, cooperative and connected (4Cs).

Technological innovations are transforming the traditional model of our health care system, strongly influenced by huge investments from Big Tech (Google, Apple, Facebook, Amazon, etc.). Universities should participate in this transformation by providing appropriate training to students who have grown up in the digital revolution. The integration of artificial intelligence and robotics in delivery of care and treatment of patients will be the role of engineers, computer scientists, data scientists, technicians and researchers, who will develop, maintain and secure new systems. Physicians must be prepared to take their place within this framework.

Training throughout students' time at university and their professional careers must anticipate an environment in which artificial intelligences are partners used to improve performance. The shift towards digitalization, which, as stated above, is to the benefit of patients, who are at the centre of the system and are key agents in their own health, must be adapted to the realities of the situation. One way of achieving this is to create 5P and 5C models of medicine by including a "fifth P": proof, or evidence-based medicine, and a "fifth C": collaboration, which includes co-construction. Programmes that teach these developments should include the following key topics: (1) scientific developments in medicine, (2) the various professional organizations and their interactions, (3) interactions between medicine, technology and engineering, and (4) new perspectives on human sciences (economics, law, sociology, psychology, philosophy and ethics).

Actions Already Being Implemented

The very nature of medicine, which is to take care of an ill patient, is not changed by digital innovation, and must be placed at the heart of training for all future physicians and health care workers. The fundamental principles of teaching are to train students to care for patients, basing their practices on data obtained by medical science in an interdisciplinary context.

Digital health has accelerated the dissemination of knowledge and the standardization of practices around the globe, particularly as a result of telemedicine. These changes in practices, which are facilitated by the use of digital tools, should, however, continue to respect both the principles of medical ethics and medical deontology, which is founded in humanism. Initial training must be integrative and cooperative, and should teach delegation, advanced practices, and cooperation between public health stakeholders, between public and private practitioners, and between different specialists. This education should be integrated into the foundations of telemedicine.

Medical faculties in the 21st century should train all health care professionals and move away from traditional approaches that separate different subjects and place a heavy emphasis on individual work. Medical faculties have already entered the digital age by integrating e-learning, the UNESS (Digital University of Health and Sport), the SIDES (Inter-University Digital Assessment System in Healthcare) platform, and Massive Open Online Courses etc.

All these innovations in teaching begin with simulation training (the first time is never on a patient), for all professions, both individually and in group settings, and in synchronous and asynchronous telemedicine. The process of digitalization must be accelerated by the large-scale inclusion of health care simulation centres, which have already seen a great deal of growth in recent years, with more than 100 operational centres in France, spanning all health care disciplines. Simulation training is an effective way to supplement knowledge with role plays and practical skills (e.g. communication, teamwork). It facilitates learning technical skills and makes it possible to reproduce a wide range of clinical situations, particularly high-risk scenarios.

Another trend caused by the development of digital health technologies is the increasing level of automation in practical interventions. Nowadays, we often see situations where a practitioner takes on the role of a "supervisor" during the intervention as part of a team that includes technicians and engineers. These teams perform grafts of living tissues and implantations of artificial organs that are built by 3D printers and equipped with "weak" artificial intelligence (e.g. CARMAT hearts, bionic hands, exoskeletons for people with paraplegia, etc.). These innovations accelerate the development of new uses of technologies.

Teaching the Principles of Telemedicine

Medical faculties are beginning to teach the principles of telemedicine (teleconsultation, tele-expertise, tele-assistance, telemonitoring and medical dispatching) to all health care professionals. Initial and continuing training should develop knowledge and skills in telemedicine and its related fields, such as how to set up a telemedicine project, from the development of a strategy (an understanding of the stakes) to project design (appropriate knowledge for the needs) and implementation of the project (training health care professionals in the required practices). The aim of this is to provide an understanding of the context, the challenges and the different forms of telemedicine, and to ensure high-quality practices, founded on an evidence-based approach. This training encourages cooperative learning between health care professionals, which enables the development of group practices in care homes and medical centres. These structures are prime examples of places where organizational innovation would enable the development of primary care medicine and the use of telemedicine tools in progressive patient care. The emphasis should be on training specialists in the coordination of primary care, which is what general practitioners have become.

Above all, telemedicine is a way to improve access to primary care, to reduce admissions to accident and emergency departments, to avoid unnecessary hospitalizations for patients with chronic illnesses, to consolidate the coordination of care between hospitals and other health care providers, and to develop tele-expertise between primary care physicians and specialists, as is practised during clinical traineeships. In addition to organizational changes, this shift into interdisciplinary working requires effective training.

Embracing Technological Innovations

This requires collaboration with researchers in mathematics, computer science and artificial intelligence, as well as digital manufacturers. Big Data, deep learning, artificial intelligence and blockchain are new concepts that must be integrated into the training of health care professionals in collaboration with other departments in the university. The university itself should be willing to support the physicians that it has trained. It is necessary to blur the lines between initial training and continuing professional development (CPD) as knowledge and skills become obsolete increasingly quickly.

The Challenges

Openness and Multidisciplinarity

Openness and multidisciplinarity are increasingly required in teaching programmes for many reasons. The complexity of treatments for people with chronic illnesses and vulnerable people requires the involvement of teams of professionals from a variety of disciplines. These collaborations could be even more efficient and straightforward if the professionals involved received training together or complementary training. Digital technology could be both the object of this training and a tool to facilitate its implementation. Ideally, this would herald the end of organizational silos from the very beginning of medical training, notably by bringing health care training entirely into universities. The boundaries that currently separate training for certain specialisms will also be broken down, with the use of new equipment and new techniques, such as health care engineering platforms. This will require a redefinition of the boundaries of each specialism, as well as organization of where they overlap.

Physicians should not be content merely to use technology. They should inspire new technologies, design them (either directly or in collaboration with other professionals), test them and evaluate them. This means that physicians need to develop knowledge outside their curriculum, such as in natural sciences and social sciences. At the very least, they should be familiar with the key concepts in these fields.

Universities should also be prepared for the arrival of new careers that bridge the gap between life sciences and engineering, and should facilitate multidisciplinary degree pathways. These should be developed without neglecting training in human sciences (deontology, ethics and human relations), which should in fact be reinforced. The more scientific the training becomes, the more the human aspects should be emphasized.

Using Digital Technology in Teaching

The impact of digital technology in teaching is indisputable. Its benefits include teaching sessions that are more engaging, individualized teaching, lifelong learning and the development of collaborative educational practices. Digital technology also demonstrates the interest of redefining the roles of the teacher and student, as students can take responsibility for their own learning through their access to information online, while teachers can take on the role of a guide, and as such can revitalize the long-standing tradition of mentoring.

Digital technology can also contribute to changes in teaching methods, which could become more varied, perhaps by teachers broadcasting lectures online before in-person classes, which could make the in-person discussions more fruitful and interactive. Digital technology also reinforces collaborative educational practices by encouraging the sharing of experiences and expertise, for example in the context of reverse mentoring, peer-to-peer teaching, etc.

Using digital technology in teaching does, however, present a permanent challenge due to the acceleration of technological innovations and their impact on organizations, teaching, and teachers themselves, who must dedicate time to learning the necessary skills.

Training in Digital Technologies

Training health care professionals in digital technologies is the first step to being able to teach using digital technologies. This training consists of developing an understanding of different tools, thinking critically about the potential applications, and participating in the creation of tools, as part of a team. It should be noted that daily use of a smartphone does not necessarily correspond to a mastery of digital technology. The aim of the training is to develop an understanding of digital culture, and the skills learnt contribute to the development of critical thinking.

Re-igniting Research in Multiple Related Areas

Precision Medicine

Medical research aims to better understand, and ultimately completely control, precision medicine, which would be adapted to each individual at every stage of life, from screening and prevention to treatment and therapy, according to the 5P model. The use of large amounts of data that come from new sources is an opportunity to reduce costs and accelerate the development of new treatments, all while making them safer. Digital technologies aid the progress and optimization of clinical trials, from the recruitment of patients to data collection and quality control.

Big Data and Modelling

The aim is to accelerate clinical research programmes by launching virtual collaboration platforms, which provide an adapted environment that facilitates open and collaborative research. These platforms also enable modelling in addition to biological and chemical simulation, and facilitate a more wide-scale contribution to research programmes focusing on the improvement of patient care pathways.

The use of non-structured data generated by research programmes makes it possible to calibrate and validate scientific models, to develop new practices for virtual clinical trials, and to construct algorithms. This requires large cohorts, all while putting the patient at the centre of the epidemiological research.

We imagine the creation of partnerships within the framework of consortia that bring together the public and private spheres. These would have the aim of launching computer tools for modelling, which could be used for hypothesis testing in clinical research. These kinds of partnership could be set up with a university hospital centre as a hub, and regional hospital groups (GHT) as the spokes, and could be distributed throughout the country according to pathologies, scientific discipline, etc.

Interdisciplinarity

Traditional methods consisting of formulating a hypothesis then testing it on well-defined data sets can now be replaced by analysing of huge amounts of data, even from completely heterogeneous sources (such as social networks), and developing hypotheses on the basis of these analyses. This requires a multidisciplinary approach that creates a field of medicine enriched by theoretical, multidisciplinary and translational research: biologists and clinicians can call upon the expertise of physicists, chemists, mathematicians, bioinformaticians, engineers, and researchers in human and social sciences. The integration of a digital technology department and the creation of professorships in informatics and digital health technologies in medical and biotechnology faculties, as well as in science and technology faculties, are key to creating this future. These approaches are intended to develop strategies for partnerships between public and private enterprises, to fuel translational research and encourage interdisciplinarity.

The link between training and research in digital health and telemedicine is indispensable if we are to share the expertise of French clinical medicine on an international scale.

ACKNOWLEDGEMENT

The authors want to acknowledge Jennifer Dobson for her work in the translation of the document and her participation in the writing process.

REFERENCES

Anonymous. 1879. "Practice by telephone." *The Lancet* 114(2935): 819.

Ben Neriah, Daniela, and Allan Geliebter. 2019. "Weight loss following use of a smartphone food photo feature: retrospective cohort study." *JMIR mHealth and uHealth* 7(6): e11917.

Chandra, Ashish, Charles E. Pettry Jr., and David P. Paul III. 2013. "Telemedecine from a macromarketing viewpoint: a critical evaluation with proposed licensing strategies." In Kimball P. Marshall, William S. Piper and Walter W. Wymer (Eds.), *Government Policy and Program Impacts on Technology Development, Transfer and Comercialization: International Perspectives* (pp. 111–149). New York: Routledge.

Crigger, Bette-Jane. 2006. "e-Medicine: policy to shape the future of health care." *The Hastings Center Report* 36(1): 12–13.

Croels, Jean-Michel. 2006. *Le Droit des obligations à l'épreuve de la télémédecine*. Marseille, FR: Aix Marseille Éditions.

Gallois, Florence, and Amadine Rauly. 2015. "Télémédecine et comparaison des systèmes de santé: questionnements méthodologiques." *Dans Colloque International Recherche & Régulation 2015 LADYSS*, 10–12 June, Paris, 15 pages.

Kerleau, M., and N. Pelletier-Fleury. 2002. "Restructuring of the healthcare system and the diffusion of telemedicine." *The European Journal of Health Economics* 3(3): 207–214.

Kim, Dae-Hyeong, Nanshu Lu, Rui Ma, Yun-Soung Kim, Rak-Hwan Kim, Shuodao Wang, Jian Wu, Sang Min Won, Hu Tao, Ahmad Islam, Ki Jun Yu, Tae-il Kim, Raeed Chowdhury, Ming Ying, Lizhi Xu, Ming Li, Hyun-Joong Chung, Hohyun Keum, Martin McCormick, Ping Liu, Yong-Wei Zhang, Fiorenzo G. Omenetto, Yonggang Huang, Todd Coleman, and John A. Rogers. 2011. "Epidermal electronics." *Science* 333(6044): 838–843.

Kirsch, Gorm. 2002. "The business of eHealth." *The Journal of Medical Marketing* 2(2): 106–110.

Kumar, Santosh, Wendy J. Nilsen, Amy Abernethy, Audie Atienza, Kevin Patrick, Misha

Pavel, William T. Riley, Albert Shar, Bonnie Spring, Donna Spruijt-Metz, Donald Hedeker, Vasant Honavar, Richard Kravitz, R. Craig Lefebvre, David C. Mohr, Susan A. Murphy, Charlene Quinn, Vladimir Shusterman, and Dallas Swendeman. 2013. "Mobile health technology evaluation: the mHealth evidence workshop." *American Journal of Preventive Medicine* 45(2): 228–236.

McDermott, Mary M., Bonnie Spring, Jeffrey S. Berger, Diane Treat-Jacobson, Michael S. Conte, Mark A. Creager, Michael H. Criqui, Luigi Ferrucci, Heather L. Gornik, Jack M. Guralnik, Elizabeth A. Hahn, Peter Henke, Melina R. Kibbe, Debra Kohlman-Trigoboff, Lingyu Li, Donald Lloyd-Jones, Walter McCarthy, Tamar S. Polonsky, Christopher Skelly, Lu Tian, Lihui Zhao, Dongxue Zhang, and W. Jack Rejeski. 2018. "Effect of a home-based exercise intervention of wearable technology and telephone coaching on walking performance in peripheral artery disease: the HONOR randomized clinical trial." *JAMA* 319(16): 1665–1676.

Ministère de la santé et des sports. 2010. *Décret n°2010–1229 du 19 octobre 2010 relatif à la télémédecine. Code de la santé publique, SASH1011044D*. Paris, FR: Ministère de la santé et des sports.

Nichols, Scott P., Ahyeon Koh, Wesley L. Storm, Jae Ho Shin, and Schoenfisch. 2013. "Biocompatible materials for continuous glucose monitoring devices." *Chemical Reviews* 113(4): 2528–2549.

Simon, Pierre, and Jacques Lucas. 2013. *La Télémédecine, ce n'est pas du e-Commerce!* Paris, FR: Association Nationale de Télémédecine and Ordre National Des Medecins.

Spring, Bonnie, Jennifer M. Duncan, E. Amy Janke, Andrea T. Kozak, H. Gene McFadden, Andrew DeMott, Alex Pictor, Leonard H. Epstein, Juned Siddique, Christine A. Pellegrini, Joanna Buscemi, and Donald Hedeker. 2013. "Integrating technology into standard weight loss treatment: a randomized controlled trial." *JAMA Internal Medicine* 173(2): 105–111.

Thompson, Mary E., Jennifer Langer, and Meheret Kinfe. 2019. "Seizure detection watch improves quality of life for adolescents and their families." *Epilepsy & Behavior* 98 (Part A): 188–194.

Wang, Zheyu, Jingyi Luan, Anushree Seth, Lin Liu, Minli You, Prashant Gupta, Pria Rathi, Yixuan Wang, Sisi Cao, Qisheng Jian, Xiao Zhang, Rohit Gupta, Qingjun Zhou, Jeremiah J. Morrissey, Erica L. Scheller, Jai S. Rudra, and Srikanth Singamaneni. 2021. "Microneedle patch for the ultrasensitive quantification of protein biomarkers in interstitial fluid." *Biomedical Engineering* 5: 64–76.

World Health Organization. 2020. *Global Strategy on Digital Health 2020–2025*. Geneva, Switzerland: World Health Organization.

Yardley, Lucy, Bonnie J. Spring, Heleen Riper, Leanne G. Morrison, David H. Crane, Kristina Curtis, Gina C. Merchant, Felix Naughton, and Ann Blandford. 2016. "Understanding and promoting effective engagement with digital behavior change interventions." *American Journal of Preventive Medicine* 51(5): 833–842.

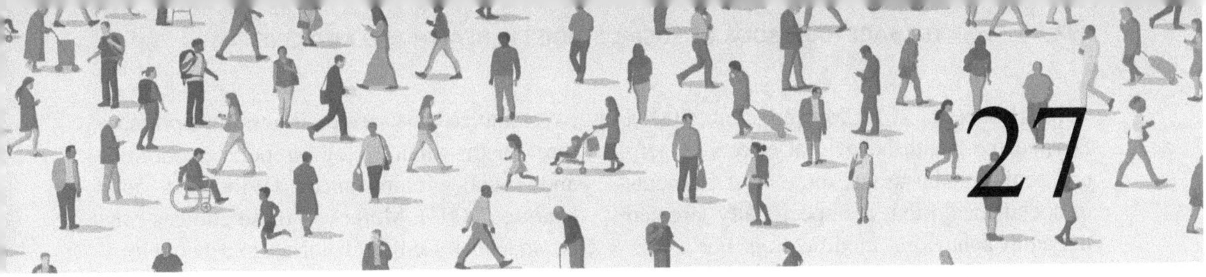

27

Health Behaviors and Social Media

Bhavneet Walia and Christopher Boudreaux

INTRODUCTION

This chapter explores the fundamental ways in which social media influences health behaviors and investigates whether social media's effect on health behaviors differs by participants' demographics, such as age, gender, ethnicity, and country environments. Social media has various and diverse platforms that are constantly evolving with social, economic, and political drivers. Many people, both young and old, view social media as a normal part of daily living (Brown and Bobkowski, 2011; Xenos and Foot, 2008). Social media connects friends and family, governments and citizens, businesses and customers, and even brings together strangers, all of which can positively influence health behavior (Anderson and Jiang, 2018). It also promotes health literacy and the dissemination of important public health information in general. Further, social media applications, such as Strava and Peloton, enable users to share results and data, with the additional benefit of creating virtual communities centered around regular engagement in healthy activities.

On the side of negative impact, however, social media often reinforces gender stereotypes (Rose et al., 2012) and negatively influences health behaviors by providing additional opportunities for bullying and by exacerbating mental health disorders (Anderson and Jiang, 2018). Moreover, users can become addicted to social media (for example, see Blackwell et al., 2017; Hawi and Samaha, 2017; Longstreet and Brooks, 2017), leading to adverse outcomes, such as time distortion (Turel et al., 2018) and withdrawal from in-person social interaction (Al-Menayes, 2015). As a result, heavy social media use among millennials is associated with an increased risk of major depressive disorder (MDD), especially among those who tend to compare themselves to others (Robinson et al., 2019). In turn, the onset of MDD can greatly limit individuals' ability to promote their health through self-care and optimal health decision making (for example, see Cella et al., 2010; Cortena et al.,

2016; Han et al., 2012; Murphy et al., 2001). Beyond the health behavioral effects of general social media usage, there exist elements of social media that are specifically targeted to health behavioral modification. For example, communication campaigns, although often raising awareness of certain issues, are also intended to generate specific outcomes or effects in a large number of individuals within a specified period of time (Institute of Medicine, 2002; Rogers and Storey, 1987). Communication campaigns also use the internet and social media to affect change, educate individuals, and correct information about health behaviors (Porter et al., 2018).

This review and survey study seeks to develop a baseline understanding as to whether the effects of social media use upon health behavior are universal or culturally influenced. In doing so, we survey respondents from a diverse set of countries about their social media usage and health behaviors. We also seek to identify the main positive and negative health behavioral effects of social media use. Hence, it is important to understand the extent to which the observable characteristics of an individual influence their health behavioral response to social media usage. Lastly, we determine how the onset of the COVID-19 pandemic has influenced the usage and health behavioral effects of social media.

Health behaviors are those actions that influence health outcomes, which include tobacco and alcohol use, diet and exercise, the use of social support and safety practices, and efforts to mitigate the onset of disease (Mahalik et al., 2007; Stimson et al., 2003). Studies estimate as much as 50% of morbidity and mortality is due to health behaviors, which are often modifiable (Mokdad et al., 2004). Consequently, understanding why and how people choose their health behaviors is vital to our overall understanding of public health outcomes. In many cases, important health behavioral choices can be influenced by the social environment, and studies have found that individuals face twice the risk of serious illness and premature death when living in poor economic and social circumstances (Wilkinson and Marmot, 2003). Moreover, these choices can be shaped by cultural norms and behaviors in many cases. Through a better understanding of this decision-making process, we can become equipped to offer policy and practice solutions toward improved overall health outcomes.

Despite the important consequences of health behaviors, we still know little about how social media affects health behaviors. In part, this is due to a gap in communication between how experts and the general public understand and interpret messages (Scrimshaw, 2019). This circumstance is concerning because social media has grown considerably in the past decade, from beginnings in internet forums, Facebook, and failed sites such as Myspace and Google's Orkut. In its modern form, social media has proliferated to the point of something close to ubiquity taking many forms. Social media platforms now serve many different functions, including social networking (e.g., Facebook, LinkedIn, Google+), blogging (Twitter, Tumblr), photo sharing (Instagram, Snapchat, Pinterest), video sharing (YouTube, Facebook Live, Periscope, Vimeo), and more. However, social media truly burgeoned with the creation of Facebook and the advent of smartphone technology. In the first quarter of 2020, Facebook topped 2.5 billion monthly active users (Clement, 2020) following two decades of incredible growth. Figure 27.1 illustrates the number of monthly active Facebook users since 2008.

Approximately one in three people now use Facebook on a monthly basis. Despite this incredibly large user base, the company's number of users continues to grow at a steady rate and has not reached the point of diminishing returns to user rates. Figure 27.1 demonstrates that the rate of growth in Facebook's active user base has been much faster than the population growth rate. As such, the percentage of individuals using Facebook has grown substantially over the past decade or more.

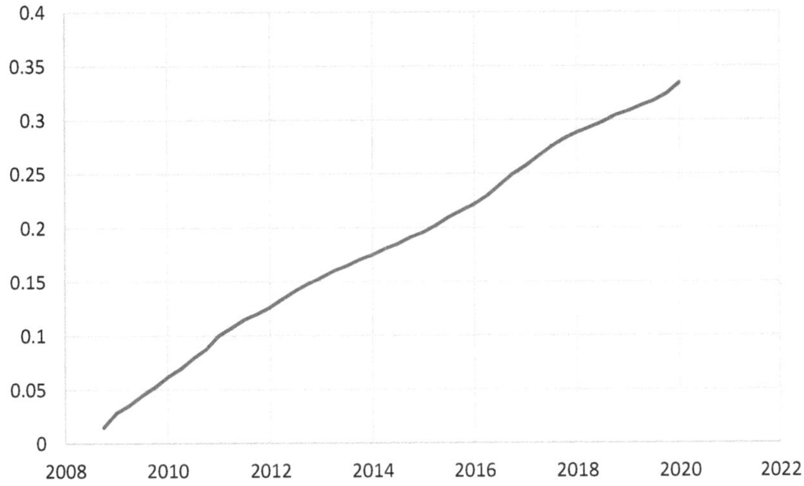

Figure 27.1 Percent monthly active Facebook users

These user rates do not include 0–13-year-olds, who are too young to use Facebook according to the company's terms of service, nor do they include elderly individuals, where both of these groups are expected to have very low user rates. As such, the user rates displayed are actually *downward*-biased. It is clear from the data that Facebook is everywhere in recent years, but is the growth in the Facebook user base confined only to developing countries? The website Internet World Stats (2020), which tracks various global internet use statistics, provides Facebook user penetration data by region. From the data, we render a bar graph of user penetration by region in Figure 27.2.

While rates do vary substantially by region, we find universally substantial Facebook adoption rates across the world, with North America, Latin America/Caribbean, and Oceania/Australia each possessing user penetration rates greater than one-half. In fact, North America's penetration rate is now greater than two-thirds, and that of the Latin America/Caribbean region is not far off this level. While it is clear from Figure 27.2 that Facebook usage rates are positively influenced by level of economic development in a region, it is also clear that Facebook has a hemispheral relationship, with networks proliferating more strongly in the Western hemisphere (the application's region of birth). Even the lowest regional penetration rate – that of Africa – constitutes approximately one-sixth of the continent's population. At this point, social media use is truly a global phenomenon. This is true even beyond Facebook use. For example, YouTube, Twitter, Instagram, Snapchat, and other social media applications now feature user populations of more than a billion. In fact, YouTube topped 2 billion monthly active users in late 2019 (Iqbal, 2020). YouTube, in particular, demonstrates the ability of individuals to engage in herd-like behavior in making content choices (Jiang et al., 2014). Indeed, from this application has come the term "viral video" in reference to a video that is being viewed at high rates explicitly because others have viewed it. As of August 2019, two YouTube videos have received more than 6 billion views, or almost one view per human in the world www.cnn.com/2020/11/02/us/baby-shark-youtube-trnd/index.html). Across several leading applications, social media is a pervasive and powerful tool to transfer information in both well-represented and misrepresented forms.

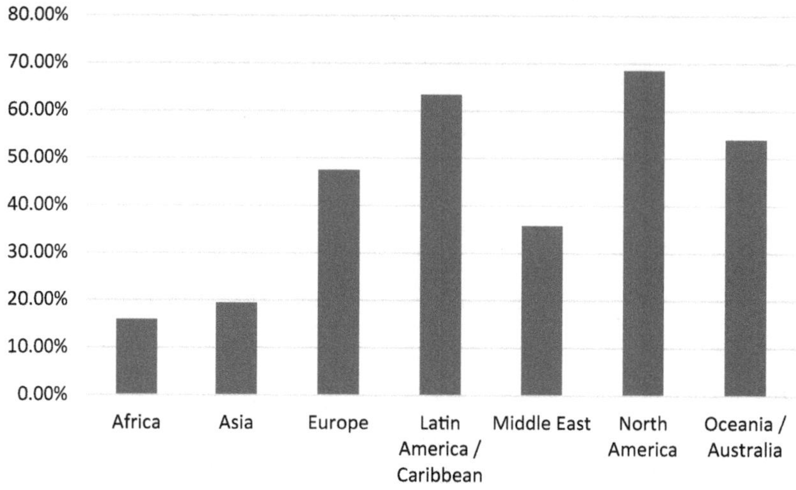

Figure 27.2 Penetration by region (%)

Some studies have found social media to negatively affect health behaviors (Salathé and Khandelwal, 2011). Others have found social media and internet-based interventions to positively affect health behaviors (Murray et al., 2005; Portnoy et al., 2008), and still others have found that the overall effect can go either way (Vaterlaus et al., 2015). These mixed findings suggest that there is further need to examine social media's influence on health behaviors. This is especially true given the recent and sustained COVID-19 pandemic and its effects on social media usage, as well as on mental and physical health levels in populations across the world (Gao et al., 2020; Yao et al., 2020). These mixed findings also pose an interesting question: why does social media usage positively influence health behaviors in some situations and negatively influence them in others?

Mixed findings in the literature are especially problematic because social media usage has shown no signs of slowing down. A 2018 Pew report found that roughly half of teens surveyed used social media "all the time" (Anderson and Jiang, 2018). In other words, it is something like a pervasive part of existence for such teens. Even if they are not directly using social media at all times – a level of use that would appear to be impossible – such teens may remain at least partly in the virtual world of social media essentially during all waking hours. This is one interpretation of the Pew report finding: that half of teens are locked into a sort of digital stream of consciousness.

Social media usage is not simply a trend among teens, however. An IDC Research survey report estimates that 79% of adults between the ages of 18 and 44 "have their phone on or near them for all but up to 2 hours of their waking day" (IDC Research, 2013). Eighty percent of survey respondents report using their phone within 15 minutes of waking up in the morning. The same study also finds social media applications to be the primary driver of smartphone use. In light of this estimate, perhaps the previous Pew finding (of widespread social media use "all the time") should be taken almost literally – the growth in social media usage can be viewed positively if it improves health behaviors and can be viewed negatively if it harms health behaviors. Therefore, it is crucial that we gain a deeper understanding of both the causes and consequences of social media and health behaviors.

POSITIVE IMPACT OF SOCIAL MEDIA ON HEALTH BEHAVIORS: PHYSICAL AND MENTAL

As discussed previously, social media has demonstrated several positive effects upon health behaviors. This section provides a more in-depth review of the literature relating to this result as it pertains to the present survey. For example, social media promotes positive health behaviors, such as proactive health screening and self-protective behaviors toward disease prevention. In addition, activity-based social media, such as Strava and Peloton, allow users to build communities based on health activities, and web-based social support services, such as QuitNet and Free and Clear, allow users to interact through social media to help individuals quit smoking. These peer-to-peer platforms allow users to support each other and provide counseling from members who have already successfully quit smoking (Centola, 2013). Similar peer-to peer programs have been established for support groups related to alcohol abstention, weight control, long-term treatment, and grief and trauma counseling (Kiesler, 1985).

There are other substantial health behavioral benefits from social media, both potential and realized. Perhaps chief among these is the leveraging of social media toward health promotional campaigns. These applications allow users to track, compare, applaud, and even compete with aerobic activity-based accomplishments. Similarly, FitBit users can interact through "Groups" and "Communities" to engage in supportive social media interactions and motivating competitions that track steps per day. Indeed, Zeng et al. (2018) find that online fitness communities increase the expected exercise levels of individuals.

Studies indicate that social media facilitates the emergence of peer-driven health communities. Social media allows individuals to interact with one another and compare detailed records of their health status, treatment programs, and recovery plans (Centola, 2013). Moreover, epidemiology studies find that knowledge about access to medical treatments and technologies can significantly overcome hurdles that might otherwise negatively affect patients' health outcomes (Kawachi and Berkman, 2003).

DESCRIPTION OF THE STUDY'S HEALTH BEHAVIORS AND SOCIAL MEDIA SURVEY INSTRUMENT

For this study, we created an anonymous Health Behaviors and Social Media Survey instrument and uploaded the survey to Qualtrics. The survey included 15 questions, where eight were written to obtain non-identifying information about the respondent's demographic characteristics (i.e., age, gender, country, vacation trips, years of education, smartphone internet access, marital status, race), four were written to obtain general information about the respondent's social media use and physical/mental health behavioral effects therefrom (i.e., social media's influence on physical health, physical appearance, emotional health, lifestyle changes), and three were written to obtain information about how social media use and its health behavioral effects may have changed during the time of the COVID-19 pandemic (i.e., reliance on social media for COVID-19 updates, time spent on social media before COVID-19, time spent on social media after COVID-19). Fittingly, the survey was propagated by accessing broad social media channels via survey link postings. The survey instrument received a strong and swift response, both in terms of overall number of respondents and global reach. Specifically, the survey link was active for one week during July 2020 and obtained 555 complete responses from users who live in 32 countries during that time. In the following two sections, we will summarize the results of the survey through a series of figures and quantitative results.

NEGATIVE PHYSICAL AND MENTAL IMPACT OF SOCIAL MEDIA ON HEALTH BEHAVIORS: REVIEW AND SURVEY RESULTS

As discussed previously, social media has demonstrated some negative effects upon health behaviors. This section provides a more in-depth review of the literature relating to this result as it pertains to the present survey. The literature has found several negative consequences of social media use. Due to social media, people interact in person with non-familial peers much less than before this technology existed (Twenge et al., 2019), which has many implications for physical and mental well-being. Among these, Twenge et al. (2019) and Twenge and Campbell (2019) find that teen social media use in the twenty-first century has, perhaps ironically, been linked to increased feelings of loneliness and lower levels of overall psychological well-being. Twenge et al. (2019: 1892) state, "Adolescents' feelings of loneliness increased sharply after 2011. Adolescents low in in-person social interaction and high in social media use reported the most loneliness."

It appears from these findings that many, or even most, individuals are surrendering substantial REM sleep in exchange for around-the-clock Facebook updates. At the same time, biological needs such as sleep must be reconciled in the physical world. Rather than digital avatars, we are in fact members of a carbon-based life form and therefore cannot simply replace one world with another piece-by-piece. As such, there are potentially substantial consequences from heavy social media use. Given these findings of use proliferation, there is a growing literature on the effects of social media addiction (for example, see Blackwell et al., 2017; Hawi and Samaha, 2017; Longstreet and Brooks, 2017), including time distortion when not directly engaging in social media-related activities (Turel et al., 2018).

In addition to the negative influence of media addictions, social media also has negative consequences on body shaming and cyber-bullying. With bullying no longer confined to a physical time and place, social media can facilitate bullying online. Unfortunately, the consequences of body shaming and cyber-bullying include higher rates of depression and suicide for each demographic group affected, but especially for teenagers (https://afsp.org/suicide-statistics/). Given these findings from the literature, we obtained data on the general emotional health effect of social media through our July 2020 survey (see Figure 27.3), discussed below. We note that all survey responses are reported influences and reported behaviors. Other measures, such as direct observations and measures (e.g., infection rates), would be needed for actual behaviors.

Mirroring the mixed findings of the previous literature, a slight majority of survey respondents report that social media makes them feel happy in some respects and sad in others (i.e., a qualitatively mixed effect on emotional health). This finding suggests that many users may require additional guidance, education, and self-reflection as to the effects of different specific uses of social media and of specific social media behaviors. Nearly one-third of respondents reported that social media use neither makes them feel happy nor sad. These respondents may depend upon social media use for completely non-emotional reasons (e.g., for the gathering of information). Approximately 11% of respondents report that social media has the overriding effect of making them feel happier, while approximately 7% of respondents report that social media has the overriding effect of making them feel sadder. The difference between these percentages is significant in a non-parametric sign test (p-value = 0.044). While the overall emotional effects of social media are largely mixed, we observe significantly more "happy" outcomes than "sad" outcomes in the sample. This sample outcome suggests that processes of positive reinforcement and self-selection may be important in individual decisions to maintain

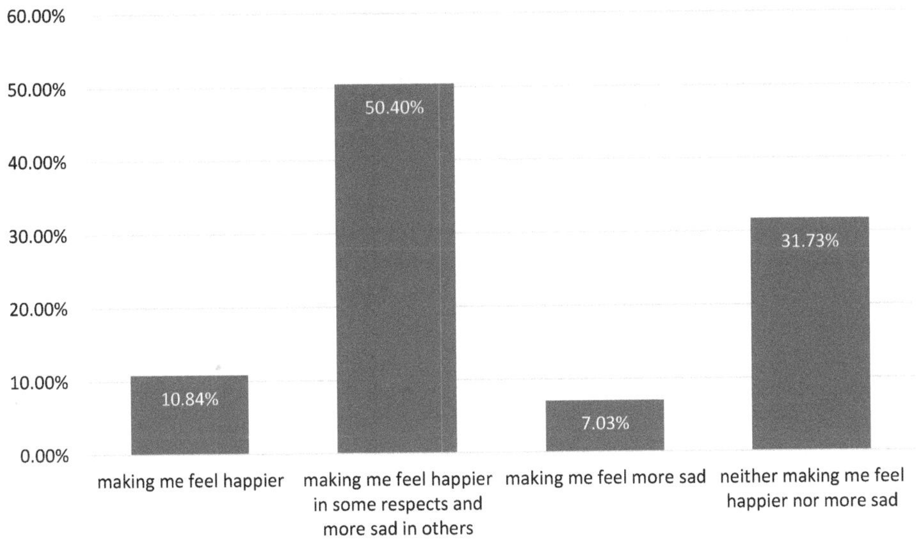

Figure 27.3 General emotional health effect of social media (N = 555; p = 0.044)

social media activity. Figure 27.4 considers the effect of social media on physical exercise choices.

From these data, we conclude that social media use has a neutral effect upon exercise for most users. That is, it has no reported impact on exercise choices for 41.83% of respondents and has a mixed reported impact on exercise level for 23.9% of respondents. Among affected users, however, social media use has the net effect of encouraging exercise. While 32.47% of respondents were encouraged to

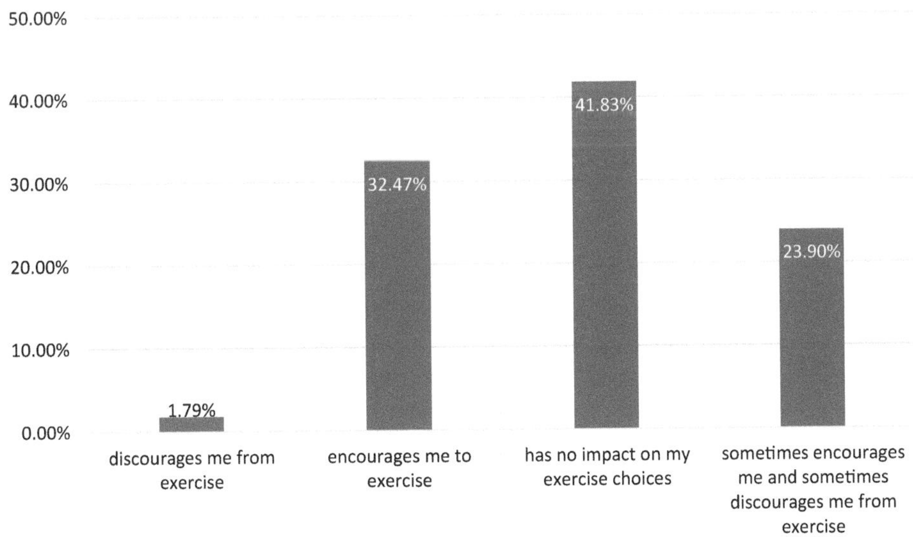

Figure 27.4 Effect of social media on physical exercise choices (N = 555; p = 0.000)

exercise due to social media use, only 1.79% of respondents were discouraged from exercising due to social media use. In a non-parametric sign test, we find that social media encourages exercise significantly more than it discourages exercise (p-value <0.001). From the findings of Figures 27.3 and 27.4, we conclude that (a) social media use has mixed and complex emotional health effects, suggesting that more research on the effects of specific use types and behaviors is needed, and (b) while social media use has no effect or a mixed effect upon exercise behaviors for most respondents, the net effect of social media is to encourage higher levels of exercise.

DOES THE ASSOCIATION BETWEEN SOCIAL MEDIA AND HEALTH BEHAVIORS VARY BY CONTINENT? IS THIS ASSOCIATION STRONGER IN CERTAIN SOCIAL ENVIRONMENTS? REVIEW AND SURVEY RESULTS

Individuals in lower-income countries tend to have fewer health outcomes than those in higher-income countries (Wagstaff, 2002). Furthermore, as discussed previously, social media has the ability to transmit health information to users. Hence, one possibility is that social media can fill a void in health care to help alleviate health inequalities between countries. To assess whether the observed effect of social media on health behaviors varies by region, we report disaggregated survey results in Figure 27.5.

Across all regions, a similarly high proportion of respondents reported that social media use makes them feel happy in some respects and sad in other respects. That is, the mixed emotional health effect of social media is observed in high rates across all world regions within the set of survey responses. To test this result inferentially, we conducted an ANOVA-type logistic regression in which the outcome variable is whether the respondent reports mixed emotions, and the explanatory variables are binary indicator variables for world region. We ran this regression in seven forms, using each possible region as a reference group alternatively, in order to compare each world region with each other world region. At the $\alpha = 0.05$ significance level, we find no significant difference between any world region in terms of propensity to report mixed emotions resulting from social media use. Moreover, the chi-squared test for overall logistic model significance is never significant (p-value = 0.27 in each of the equivalent models run). We conclude that world region does not significantly explain variation in the rate of mixed emotional response from social media use. This mixed emotional health effect of social media appears to be a largely universal outcome. We also observe that the rate of social media use causing sadness as its overriding effect is similarly low throughout the world regions. The roles of positive reinforcement and self-selection in determining who maintains regular social media use may be general across world regions. That is to say, those experiencing negative emotional health effects from social media use may opt out of social media participation in the long run, and this process may be universally observed.

We also consider the effect of social media on physical exercise choices by world region. Figure 27.6 reports these disaggregated survey results.

In each region of the world, the proportion of surveyed individuals reporting encouragement to exercise is higher than the proportion reporting discouragement from exercise. To test the statistical differences, we conducted an ANOVA-type logistic regression in which the outcome variable is whether the respondent reports that social media encourages them to exercise, and the explanatory variables are binary indicator variables for world region. Like before, we ran this regression in seven forms, using each possible region as a reference group alternatively, in order to compare each world region with each other world region. At the $\alpha = 0.05$ significance level, we find no significant difference between any

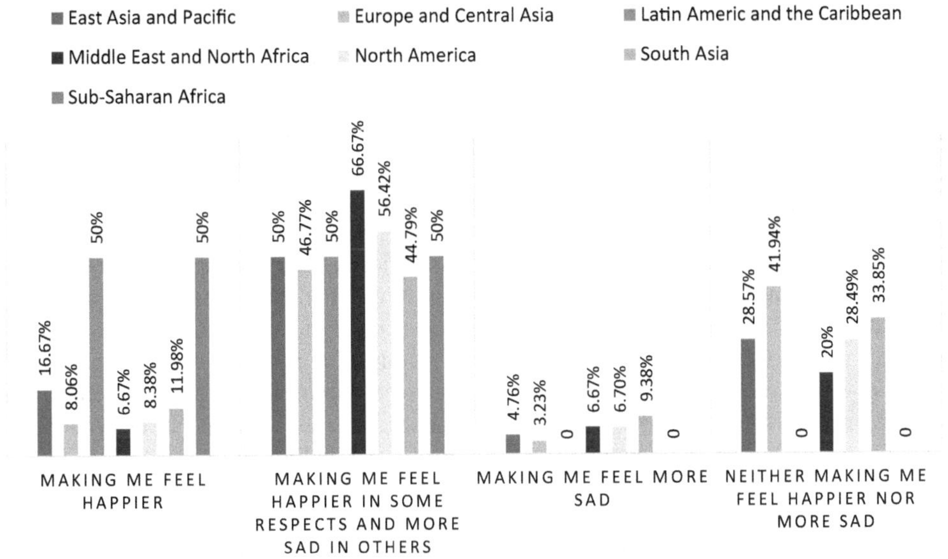

Figure 27.5 General emotional health effect of social media by world region ($N = 555$; $p = .27$)

world region in terms of social media's influence on encouragement to exercise. Moreover, the chi-squared test for overall logistic model significance is never significant (p-value = 0.16 in each of the equivalent models run). Therefore, the net effect of exercise encouragement through social media use is universally observed within the sample of survey

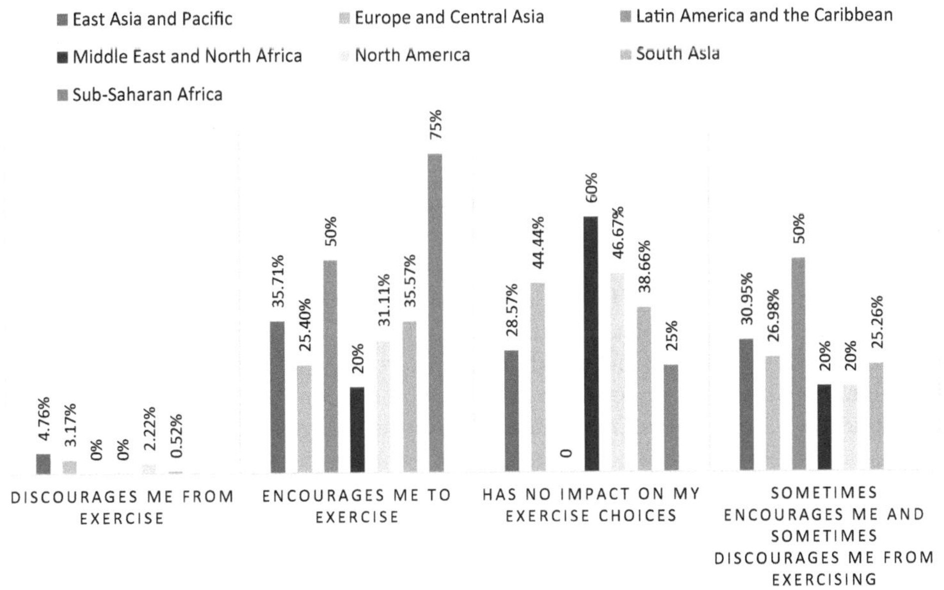

Figure 27.6 Effect of social media on physical exercise choices by world region ($N = 555$; $p = .16$)

respondents. Throughout the world regions, we also observe a fairly high proportion of individuals (20–50%) who report no exercise effects of social media use. It is universally observed within the sample that, for a substantial proportion of individuals, there exists no relationship between social media use and exercise motivation. Across the world regions, it appears that there is a substantial proportion of individuals who use social media for reasons other than exercise choices. This description may also have linkages to the earlier reported findings of Robinson et al. (2019), who find that social media responses can be starkly different for those who tend to compare themselves to others. In the present survey, it may be that individuals have different responses to the observation of those who appear to be physically fit in social media images. Those who tend to compare themselves to others may view some images and consequently be motivated to exercise, whereas those who do not tend to compare themselves to others may have no such response.

ROLE OF SOCIAL MEDIA IN THE TRANSMISSION OF INFORMATION REGARDING COVID-19 AND OTHER IMMINENT PUBLIC HEALTH THREATS: REVIEW AND SURVEY RESULTS

As social media plays a prominent role in transmitting information, recent research has examined how the use of social media affects health behaviors during the COVID-19 pandemic. Does social media spread positive news and increase the accuracy and speed of information about the virus, or does it negatively influence perceptions and information transmission? Recent studies, although early, indicate that social media might potentially negatively influence health behaviors. Depoux et al. (2020) document how news about COVID-19 travels faster than the actual pandemic. This is problematic because information over social media spreads fear-mongering, racism, conspiracy theories, and mass panic. Moreover, other research finds that social media users reported more anxiety compared to non-social media users in China (Gao et al., 2020).

In this study, we examined the association between social media and health behaviors in the wake of the COVID-19 pandemic. Specifically, we asked respondents three questions: (1) How much do you rely on social media for updates regarding COVID-19 compared to other sources, such as TV, radio, or newspaper? (2) On average, how much time did you spend on your social media site before COVID-19? (3) On average, how much time are you spending on your social media site daily during COVID-19? Figure 27.7 reports the results from the first COVID-related question of the survey.

Figure 27.7 demonstrates that people vary widely in their reliance on social media for the purpose of gathering COVID-19 related information. Whereas 30% of the sample exhibits at least 60% reliance, nearly a quarter of the sample does not rely on social media for this purpose whatsoever. In a non-parametric sign test, we find a statistically significant (p = 0.000) difference between those who receive all of their information about COVID-19 (8.98%) from social media and those who receive none of their information about COVID-19 from social media (22.36%). This result again reveals that people use social media for very different reasons. It is therefore no surprise that social media has a wide observed range of effects on health behavior and health outcomes.

Through this time-use comparison, we observe that the percentage using social media 0 hours per week remained essentially unchanged. However, the percentage of respondents using social media up to one hour per week fell by 18.5 percentage points. Almost all of these users shifted to heavier use, which caused the percentage using more than one but less than three hours to rise by 2.7 percentage points and the percentage using social media more than three hours

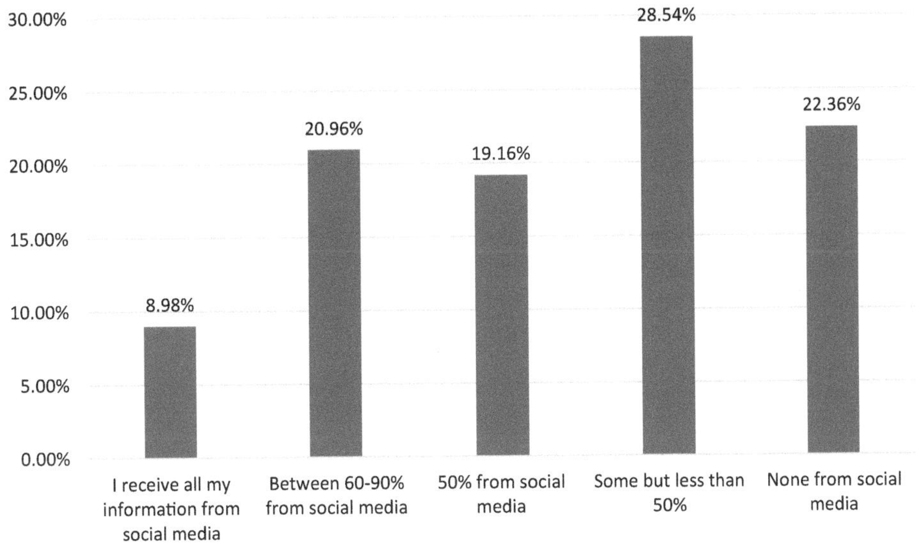

Figure 27.7 Reliance on social media for COVID-19 information/updates (*N* = 555; *p* = 0.000)

per week to rise by 15.6 percentage points. More specifically, we observe from the survey data that most people who changed their social media use during the COVID-19 pandemic shifted from the up to one hour group to the more than three hours group. We conclude that the shift in social media use during the COVID 19 pandemic can be characterized as a substantial increase in time intensity. Before onset of the pandemic, 49.5% of respondents used social media more than one hour per day. Following the pandemic's onset, this percentage rose to 67.8%. In a two-sample t-test where N = 555, this constitutes a significant difference in use intensity across time-period at standard significance levels (p-value < 0.0001; t = 12.97). Specifically, time use significantly increased during the pandemic (e.g., in a one-sided t-test). (See Table 27.1.)

SUMMARY OF OVERALL EFFECTS AND CONCLUSION

This chapter has explored how social media influences health behaviors. Findings in the literature have been mixed, with some documenting a positive influence on health behaviors and others documenting a negative influence on health behaviors. We conducted a survey that asked respondents about their social media use and health behaviors.

Table 27.1 Daily social media time use before and during the COVID-19 outbreak (*N* = 555; *p* = 0.000)

Average daily time use category	*Percentage of respondents before COVID-19*	*Percentage of respondents during COVID-19*
0 hours	3.6	3.8
More than 0 but less than or equal to 1 hour	46.9	28.4
More than 1 but less than or equal to 3 hours	41.3	44
More than 3 hours	8.2	23.8

We also asked whether social media's influence on health behaviors had a different effect before or after the COVID-19 pandemic and whether social media's effect differed by participants' demographics, such as age, gender, ethnicity, and country environments. Mirroring much of the extant literature on the topic, the results from the survey indicated that social media use has mixed and complex emotional health effects, suggesting that more research on the effects of specific use types and behaviors is needed. While social media use has no effect or a mixed effect upon exercise behaviors for most respondents, the survey further shows that the net reported effect of social media is to encourage higher levels of exercise. In the disaggregated analysis by world region, we found these overriding reported effects to be largely universal (i.e., not specific to any particular region).

The reported results from the survey also indicate that people vary widely in their reliance on social media for the purpose of gathering COVID-19 related information. Whereas 30% of the sample exhibits at least 60% reliance, nearly a quarter of the sample does not rely on social media for this purpose whatsoever. This result again reveals that people use social media for very different reasons. It is therefore no surprise that social media has a wide observed range of effects on health behavior and health outcomes. Lastly, we find from the survey the reported result that overall time intensity of social media rose during the COVID-19 pandemic. Most of this reported change is attributable to individuals moving from low to moderate and high social media time allocations.

Overall, this survey and review study identifies and confirms an overriding finding in the literature that the nature of social media use is heterogeneous. As such, the effect of social media upon health behaviors is mixed. We therefore need further investigations on the effects of specific social media uses and use motivation as well as the need to help people distinguish between scientifically based information, misinformation, and bad information.

REFERENCES

Al-Menayes, J. J. (2015). Dimensions of social media addiction among university students in Kuwait. *Psychology and Behavioral Sciences*, *4*(1), 23–28.

Anderson, M., & Jiang, J. (2018). Teens, social media & technology 2018. *Pew Research Center*, *31*.

Blackwell, D., Leaman, C., Tramposch, R., Osborne, C., & Liss, M. (2017). Extraversion, neuroticism, attachment style and fear of missing out as predictors of social media use and addiction. *Personality and Individual Differences*, *116*, 69–72.

Brown, J. D., & Bobkowski, P. S. (2011). Older and newer media: Patterns of use and effects on adolescents' health and well-being. *Journal of Research on Adolescence*, *21*(1), 95–113.

Cella, M., Dymond, S., & Cooper, A. (2010). Impaired flexible decision-making in major depressive disorder. *Journal of Affective Disorders*, *124*(1–2), 207–210.

Centola, D. (2013). Social media and the science of health behavior. *Circulation*, *127*(21), 2135–2144.

Clement, J. (2020). *Number of Facebook users worldwide 2008–2020*. Available online at: www.statista.com/statistics/264810/number-of-monthly-active-facebook-users-worldwide/ Accessed on May 5, 2020.

Cotrena, C., Branco, L. D., Shansis, F. M., & Fonseca, R. P. (2016). Executive function impairments in depression and bipolar disorder: Association with functional impairment and quality of life. *Journal of Affective Disorders*, *190*, 744–753.

Depoux, A., Martin, S., Karafillakis, E., Preet, R., Wilder-Smith, A., & Larson, H. (2020). The pandemic of social media panic travels faster than the COVID-19 outbreak. *Journal of Travel Medicine*, March 3. doi: 10.1093/jtm/taaa031

Gao, J., Zheng, P., Jia, Y., Chen, H., Mao, Y., Chen, S., & Dai, J. (2020). Mental health problems and social media exposure during COVID-19 outbreak. *Plos One*, *15*(4), e0231924.

Han, G., Klimes-Dougan, B., Jepsen, S., Ballard, K., Nelson, M., Houri, A., ... & Cullen, K. (2012). Selective neurocognitive impairments in adolescents with major depressive disorder. *Journal of Adolescence*, *35*(1), 11–20.

Hawi, N. S., & Samaha, M. (2017). The relations among social media addiction, self-esteem, and life satisfaction in university students. *Social Science Computer Review*, *35*(5), 576–586.

IDC Research (2013). *Always connected: How smartphones and social keep us engaged. IDC Research Report*, sponsored by Facebook, April 4. Available online at: www.slideshare.net/ScottValentine1/always-connected-how-smartphone-owners-stay-engaged.

Institute of Medicine (2002). *Speaking of Health: Assessing Health Communication Strategies for Diverse Populations*. Washington, DC: The National Academies Press. https://doi.org/10.17226/10018.

Internet World Stats (2020). *Usage and population statistics*. Available online at: www.internetworldstats.com/facebook.htm Accessed on May 12, 2020.

Iqbal, M. (2020). *YouTube revenue and usage statistics*. Available online at: www.businessofapps.com/data/youtube-statistics/ Accessed on May 14, 2020.

Jiang, L., Miao, Y., Yang, Y., Lan, Z., & Hauptmann, A. G. (2014, April). Viral video style: A closer look at viral videos on youtube. In *Proceedings of International Conference on Multimedia Retrieval* (pp. 193–200). https://doi.org/10.1145/2578726.2578754

Kawachi, I., & Berkman, L. F. (Eds.). (2003). *Neighborhoods and Health*. Oxford: Oxford University Press.

Kiesler, C. A. (1985). Policy implications of research on social support and health. In S. Cohen & S. L. Syme (Eds.), *Social Support and Health* (pp. 347–364). New York: Academic Press.

Longstreet, P., & Brooks, S. (2017). Life satisfaction: A key to managing internet & social media addiction. *Technology in Society*, *50*, 73–77.

Mahalik, J. R., Burns, S. M., & Syzdek, M. (2007). Masculinity and perceived normative health behaviors as predictors of men's health behaviors. *Social Science & Medicine*, *64*(11), 2201–2209.

Mokdad, A. H., Marks, J. S., Stroup, D. F., & Gerberding, J. L. (2004). Actual causes of death in the United States, 2000. *JAMA*, *291*(10), 1238–1245.

Murphy, F. C., Rubinsztein, J. S., Michael, A., Rogers, R. D., Robbins, T. W., Paykel, E. S., & Sahakian, B. J. (2001). Decision-making cognition in mania and depression. *Psychological Medicine*, *31*(4), 679–693.

Murray, E., Burns, J., Tai, S. S., Lai, R., & Nazareth, I. (2005). Interactive Health Communication Applications for people with chronic disease. *Cochrane Database of Systematic Reviews*, *4*.

Porter, E., Wood, T. J., & Kirby, D. (2018). Sex trafficking, Russian infiltration, birth certificates, and pedophilia: A survey experiment correcting fake news. *Journal of Experimental Political Science*, *5*(2), 159–164.

Portnoy, D. B., Scott-Sheldon, L. A., Johnson, B. T., & Carey, M. P. (2008). Computer-delivered interventions for health promotion and behavioral risk reduction: A meta-analysis of 75 randomized controlled trials, 1988–2007. *Preventive Medicine*, *47*(1), 3–16.

Robinson, A., Bonnette, A., Howard, K., Ceballos, N., Dailey, S., Lu, Y., & Grimes, T. (2019). Social comparisons, social media addiction, and social interaction: An examination of specific social media behaviors related to major depressive disorder in a millennial population. *Journal of Applied Biobehavioral Research*, *24*(1), e12158.

Rogers, E. M., & Storey, J. D. 1987. Communication campaigns. In C. R. Berger & S. H. Chaffee (Eds.), *Handbook of Communication Science* (pp. 817–846). Beverly Hills, CA: Sage.

Rose, J., Mackey-Kallis, S., Shyles, L., Barry, K., Biagini, D., Hart, C., & Jack, L. (2012). Face it: The impact of gender on social media images. *Communication Quarterly*, *60*(5), 588–607.

Salathé, M., & Khandelwal, S. (2011). Assessing vaccination sentiments with online social media: Implications for infectious disease dynamics and control. *PLoS Computational Biology*, *7*(10).

Scrimshaw, S. C. (2019). Literacy in a rapidly changing communications landscape. *Proceedings of the National Academy of Sciences*, *116*(16), 7650–7655. doi: 10.1073/pnas.1807218116

Stimson, G. V., Donoghoe, M. C., Fitch, C., & Rhodes, T. J. with Ball, A., & Weiler, G. (2003). *Rapid Assessment and Response*

Technical Guide (Version 1.0). Geneva: World Health Organization, Department of Child and Adolescent Health and Development, and Department of HIV/AIDS.

Turel, O., Brevers, D., & Bechara, A. (2018). Time distortion when users at-risk for social media addiction engage in non-social media tasks. *Journal of Psychiatric Research*, *97*, 84–88.

Twenge, J. M., & Campbell, W. K. (2019). Media use is linked to lower psychological well-being: Evidence from three datasets. *Psychiatric Quarterly*, *90*(2), 311–331.

Twenge, J. M., Spitzberg, B. H., & Campbell, W. K. (2019). Less in-person social interaction with peers among US adolescents in the 21st century and links to loneliness. *Journal of Social and Personal Relationships*, *36*(6), 1892–1913.

Vaterlaus, J. M., Patten, E. V., Roche, C., & Young, J. A. (2015). #Gettinghealthy: The perceived influence of social media on young adult health behaviors. *Computers in Human Behavior*, *45*, 151–157.

Wagstaff, A. (2002). Poverty and health sector inequalities. *Bulletin of the World Health Organization*, *80*, 97–105.

Wilkinson, R. G., & Marmot, M. (Eds.). (2003). *Social Determinants of Health: The Solid Facts*. Geneva: World Health Organization.

Xenos, M., & Foot, K. (2008). Not your father's Internet: The generation gap in online politics. In W. L. Bennett (Ed.), *Civic Life Online: Learning How Digital Media Can Engage Youth* (pp. 51–70). Cambridge, MA: MIT Press.

Yao, H., Chen, J. H., & Xu, Y. F. (2020). Patients with mental health disorders in the COVID-19 epidemic. *The Lancet Psychiatry*, *7*(4), e21.

Zeng, L., Almquist, Z. W., & Spiro, E. S. (2018, July). Stay connected and keep motivated: Modeling activity level of exercise in an online fitness community. In *International Conference on Social Computing and Social Media* (pp. 137–147). Cham, Switzerland: Springer.

PART 4

Health in Environmental and Planetary Context

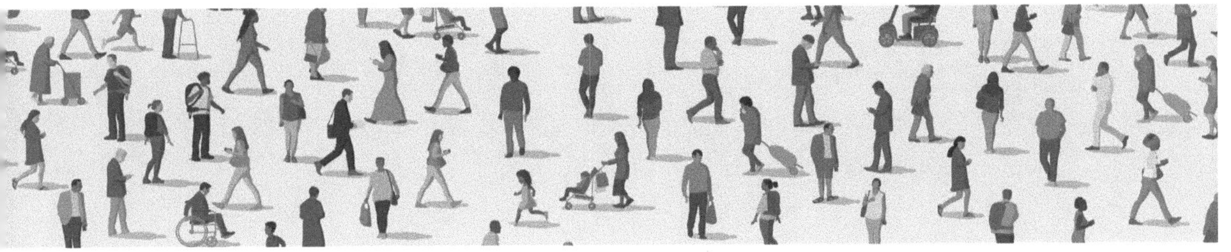

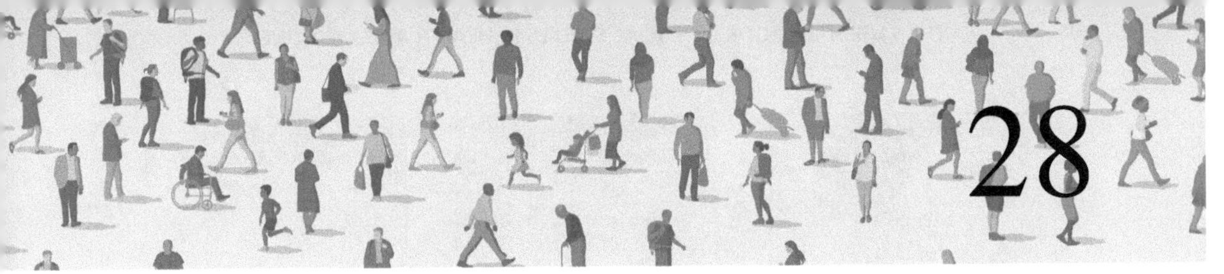

28

The Ecological Paradox: Health and Environment in the 21st Century

Daniel Hryhorczuk and Alex Hryhorczuk

BACKGROUND

In the 21st century we as a species are living longer and enjoying greater well-being than ever before. At the same time, the ecosystem services that sustain us are undergoing dramatic degradation. This divergence between human health and the health of our planet has been called the "ecological paradox" (Raudsepp-Hearne et al., 2010). In the near future, a rapidly growing human population could exceed the carrying capacity of our planet. In 1972, the "Club of Rome," an international group of scientists and policy makers, predicted that without radical changes in our patterns of consumption, we would experience a Malthusian catastrophe by the year 2030 (Malthus [1798] 2004; Meadows et al., 1972). In 1992 the International Union of Concerned Scientists issued their first "Warning to Humanity." They cautioned that "a great change in our stewardship of the Earth and the life on it is required, if vast human misery is to be avoided" (Union of Concerned Scientists, 1992). In 2017, over 15,000 scientists from 184 countries issued a second warning to humanity (Ripple et al., 2017). They presented data showing dramatic declines in key indicators of ecosystem services (Figure 28.1). Since 1992, with the exception of stabilizing the stratospheric ozone layer, humanity has failed to make sufficient progress in generally solving these foreseen environmental challenges, and, alarmingly, most of them are getting far worse.

The concept of sustainability dates back to the ancient writers of China, Greece and Rome, incorporated in the philosophy of living in harmony with nature and neighbors. Plato in the 5th century BC, Strabo and Columella in the 1st century BC and Pliny the Elder in the 1st century AD discussed different types of environmental degradation resulting from human activities such as farming, logging and mining (Du Pisani, 2006). The ancients also recognized that environmental stressors could have negative

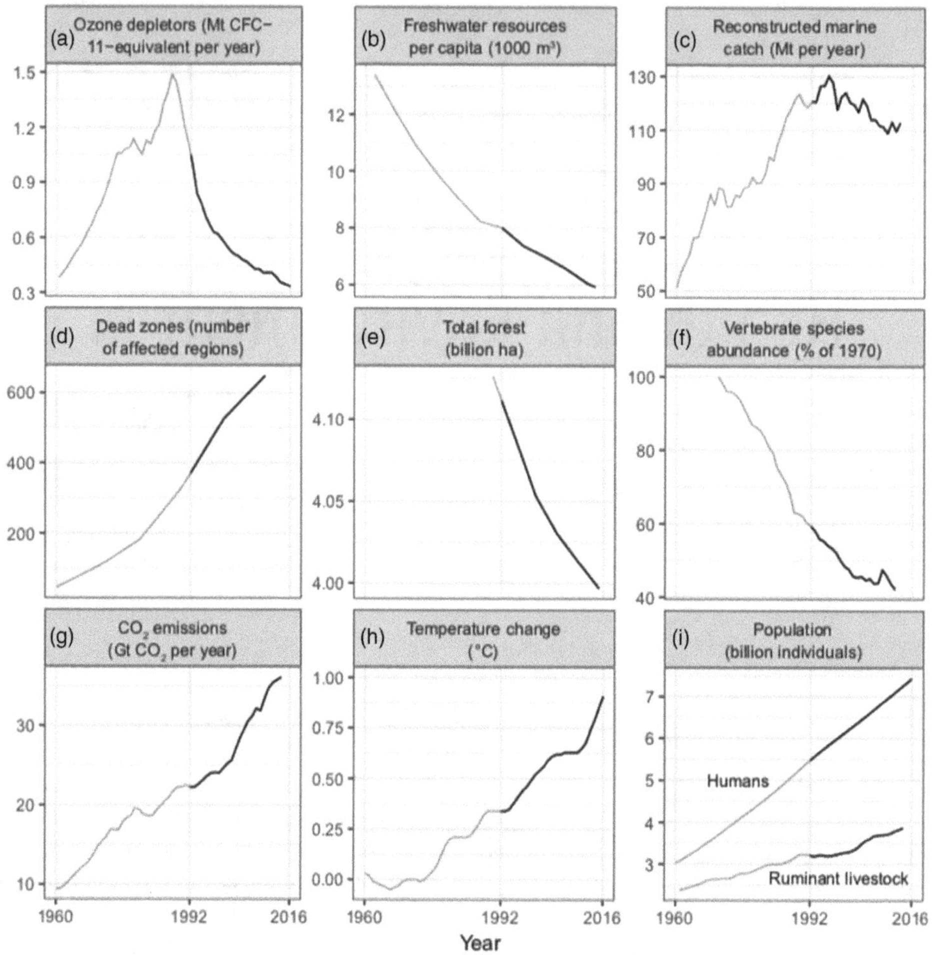

Figure 28.1 Trends over time for environmental issues identified in the 1992 scientists' warning to humanity (see Ripple et al., Bioscience)

impacts on human health. The importance of food safety is written in the Book of Leviticus in the Bible. In "Airs, Waters, and Places," Hippocrates lectured his students that if you want to learn about the health of a population, you need to look at the air they breathe, the water they drink, and the place where they live (Hippocrates, 2020). In 1700, Bernardino Ramazzini in his treatise, "De Morbis Artificum Diatriba," broadened our understanding of the harmful effects of environmental stressors to include occupational hazards (Ramazzini, 1983).

In the 1840s, reformers in England made the connection between income, living conditions, and health. The English Sanitary Report of 1842 paved the way for the Public Health Act in 1848, inaugurating the modern approach to public health (Petrini, 2007). In the 1850s, John Snow traced outbreaks of cholera in London to contamination of water from the Broad Street pump. Sanitary commissions in England and the United States highlighted the responsibility of government to provide essential public health services, most of which, like the supply of clean drinking water, utilization of sewerage, and ensuring the healthiness of dwellings, were environmental in nature.

The outbreak of Minamata disease in Japan in the 1950s and 1960s, which was caused by the discharge of mercury waste into Minamata Bay, and its biomagnification in the aquatic ecosystem, highlighted the devastating human health impacts of the release of toxicants into our environment. The fact that the problem of mercury pollution was not addressed on a global level until 2019 through the Minamata Convention illustrates the shortcomings of our global governance system for the protection of human health and environment. Six years after the index case of Minamata, in her book *Silent Spring*, Rachel Carson described a mythical American town impacted by the pesticide DDT (Carson, 1962). Since her book for the general public was first published, the scientific field of environmental toxicology has made important advances in our understanding of the mechanisms of action, environmental fate, and health impacts of only a small fraction of the tens of thousands of chemicals that are in widespread use today. In 1991, Theo Colburn convened a meeting at the Wingspread Conference Center of the Johnson Foundation in Racine, Wisconsin, where experts compared the impacts of synthetic chemicals on hormone signaling in human and wildlife populations. The conference and her 1997 book, co-authored by Dianne Dumanoski and John Peterson Myers, entitled *Our Stolen Future*, introduced the concept of endocrine disruption and upended our understanding of classic dose–response relationships that were first articulated by Paracelsus in the 16th century (Colburn et al., 1997).

The 1960s and 1970s were a time of great social change in the United States with a confluence of civil rights, women's rights, peace, and environmental movements. Concerns over atom bomb testing, oil spills, and pollution of the Great Lakes became rallying cries for environmentalism in the United States. When debris on the Cuyahoga River caught fire, it inspired the Randy Newman song "Burn On," and brought the issue into the public consciousness. On the first Earth Day, April 22, 1970, millions of people took to the streets to demonstrate against widespread environmental pollution. Eight months later, the United States established the Environmental Protection Agency with a mission of protecting human health and the environment. Landmark legislation, such as the Clean Air Act of 1970 and Clean Water Act of 1972 among others, established a regulatory framework that has resulted in major improvements in the quality of air, water, and places.

The United Nations Conference on Human Health and Environment, held in Stockholm in 1972, moved national environmental concerns into the international political agenda. Globally, these concerns moved beyond environmental quality to a broader emphasis on sustainability and led to the establishment of the United Nations Environment Program (UNEP). In 1987, the Brundtland Commission report on "Our Common Future" addressed the issue of sustainable development and influenced the Earth Summit in Rio de Janeiro in 1992 (Bruntland Commission, 1987; Hanson, 2007). In 2015 the United Nations General Assembly adopted the Sustainable Development Goals (SDGs), which are a set of objectives to end poverty, protect all that makes the planet habitable, and ensure that all people enjoy peace and prosperity, now and in the future (Hanson, 2007). The question remains whether these voluntary agreements, without regulatory enforcement, may be too little, too late.

In the 20th century, environmental health was defined as "the art and science of protecting against environmental factors that may adversely impact human health or the ecological balances essential to long term human health and environmental quality. Such factors include, but are not limited to air, food and water contaminants; radiation; toxic chemicals; wastes; disease vectors;

safety, hazards; and habitat alterations" (Gordon, 1993a, 1993b; Kotchian, 1997). In the beginning of the 21st century, our focus expanded beyond just the protection of our own species to the concept of "One Health," which includes the protection of all living things. We now realize that we have entered the "Anthropocene epoch," a new geological epoch named in recognition of the profound impact that human activity has on the health of the planet that sustains us. Our understanding of the relationship of the harmony between man and nature has evolved from the concept of environmental health, to One Health, to planetary health. The Rockefeller–Lancet Commission on "Safeguarding human health in the Anthropocene epoch" defines planetary health as "the health of human civilization and the state of the natural systems on which it depends" (Whitmee et al., 2015: p.1.

ENVIRONMENTAL RISKS AND THE GLOBAL BURDEN OF DISEASE

The Global Burden of Disease Study attributed 16% of global mortality and 12% of global disability adjusted life years (DALYs) to environmental risks (Forousanfar et al., 2015). Those risks included unsafe water, sanitation and hygiene; air pollution, both ambient and indoor; second-hand smoke; lead; residential radon exposure; and occupational risks. The World Health Organization's assessment of the environmental determinants of the global burden of disease covered a broader range of environmental risks. They considered additional risks from various chemicals, poor housing, the recreational environment, water resource management, land use, the built environment; environmental noise; radiation; and climate change. They also included risks from certain infectious disease that are solely transmitted through pathways, which depend on modifiable environmental conditions. They concluded that in 2012 23% of global deaths and 22% of global DALYs were attributable to environmental risks. These estimates indicate that reducing environmental risks could prevent up to a quarter of the global disease burden (Prüss-Ustün et al., 2017).

The Lancet Commission on Pollution and Health concluded that in 2015 pollution was the world's largest environmental cause of disease and premature death, accounting for 16% of all deaths worldwide as well as for 268 million DALYs (Landrigan et al., 2017). Chemicals that are released into the environment from sources such as industry, agriculture, transportation or household use can pollute the air, soil, and surface and ground water. Their environmental fate and transport depend on their chemical properties. Persistent pollutants can bio-concentrate and biomagnify in trophic levels up the food chain. The major routes of human exposure to chemical pollutants are through ingestion, inhalation, and skin absorption. The toxic effects depend on the dose and the target organs for that specific toxicant. The effects can vary from toxicity to specific organ systems to probabilistic effects, such as increasing the risk of cancer. Environmental regulatory agencies set air, water, and soil quality standards to limit human exposure to doses of pollutants that are unlikely to produce adverse health effects over a lifetime of exposure based on classic dose–response relationships. Theo Colburn's work on endocrine disruption has shown us this approach may be too simplistic for some classes of chemicals (Colburn et al., 1997). Even low doses of chemicals that disrupt endocrine pathways may be sufficient to produce health effects. About 800 chemicals are known or suspected to be endocrine disruptors and many more have not been tested.

Humans differ in their susceptibility to toxicants depending on factors such as genetics, age, gender, and health status. One of the major advances in protecting the public from toxicants was the recognition that children are an especially high-risk population for environmental illness. The 1993 report by the US

National Academy of Sciences, Pesticides in the Diets of Infants and Children, found that children are much more sensitive to the effects of pesticide chemical than adults (National Academy of Sciences, 1993). The report identified four fundamental differences between children and adults that increase their susceptibility. Children breathe more air, drink more water, and eat more food per kilogram body weight than adults, increasing their absorbed dose. Children's metabolic processes are immature, impairing their ability to detoxify and excrete toxicants. Children's blood–brain barrier is less developed than adults and neuro-developmental processes are more easily disrupted. In addition, children have many more future years to develop diseases with long latencies, such as cancer. The National Academy of Sciences publication led to the passage of the Food Quality Protection Act, the only federal statute at the time that contained explicit provisions for the protection of children. In 1997, a presidential executive order required all US federal agencies to consider children's special susceptibilities in all rule making (Landrigan, 2016).

Chemical pollutants have detrimental effects not only on human health, but also on the ecosystems that we depend on for our survival. Ecosystems provide us with food, water, and fuel. They regulate natural systems such as climate and provide cultural, spiritual, and aesthetic value (Raudsepp-Hearne et al., 2010). There are numerous examples of ecosystem disruption from chemical pollutants. Green-house gases emitted from the combustion of fossil fuels lead to global warming, ocean acidification, and destruction of coral reefs. Chloroflourocarbons released into the atmosphere have caused ozone depletion, allowing more ultraviolet radiation to reach the earth's surface. Oil spills have had devastating effects on marine populations. Planetary health scientists have been warning us to abandon our narrow anthropocentric view and focus on the health of the planet as a whole. Global indicators of ecosystem extent and condition have shown a 47% reduction against their estimated baselines (IPBES, 2019). In this age of the Anthropocene, we not only need to protect ourselves from environmental stressors; we need to protect the planet from ourselves.

POPULATION GROWTH

The two major drivers of humanity's ecological footprint are population and consumption (de Sherbinin et al., 2007). The world's population is expected to increase by 2 billion persons in the next 30 years, from 7.7 billion currently to 9.7 billion in 2050. Population growth is a function of fertility rates and mortality rates, which in turn determine the age structure of the population. The factors that affect population projections include age, sex, rural/urban residence, educational attainment, labor force participation, parity status, household status, and health status (Lutz & Samir, 2013).

Globally, mortality and fertility rates are decreasing, resulting in an aging of the world's population. Life expectancy is expected to increase from 72.6 years in 2019 to 77.1 years in 2050. By 2050 one is six people in the world will be over the age of 65. The decreases in mortality and fertility rates are distributed unevenly across countries. Much of the population growth will occur in poorer countries that are less able to sustain the increase. More than half on the projected growth of the global population by 2050 is projected to occur in just nine countries (India, Nigeria, Pakistan, the Democratic Republic of the Congo, Ethiopia, the United Republic of Tanzania, Indonesia, Egypt, and the United States of America). The aging of the population and decline in the proportion of the working age population in other parts of the world strain their social protection systems (United Nations, 2019).

Since 1970, per capita consumption has increased by 45% (IPBES, 2019). Consumption trends per capita depend on global economic conditions, available resources, and efforts to pursue sustainable development (de Sherbinin et al., 2007). These patterns of resource consumption have been highly inequitable, inefficient, and unsustainable (Whitmee et al., 2015). The interactions between human population dynamics and the environment are complex and rely on more than just population numbers. Other factors include technological developments, trade, cultural adaptation and institutional arrangements that have allowed human populations to increase global carrying capacity. Stabilization or even a decline in global population will reduce the strain on ecosystem services. The deceleration of the population growth rate that is occurring in developed countries is primarily due to a drop in fertility rates. The question remains whether this decrease in population growth momentum will be sufficient to prevent collapse of our ecosystem services.

FOOD SECURITY

Malthus's 18th-century prediction that population growth will outstrip food production has not come to pass. This is a result of the massive agricultural land expansion during the past several centuries and the "Green Revolution" of the 20th century. The "Green Revolution" increased crop yields through technological advances in plant biology, the application of fertilizers and pesticides, and the harnessing of energy from fossil fuels to mechanize agriculture. Currently 84% of calories globally come from just 17 crops (Ramankutty et al., 2018). Increased production and increased calories do not necessarily result in adequate nutrition. Reliance on relatively few sources for calories can result in a nutrition gap for micronutrients. Inequalities in food access result in obesity epidemics in some parts of the world and undernourishment in others.

Based on projections of future population growth, estimates of future calorie/protein demand have varied from a 25% increase to a doubling by 2050. Ninety percent of the growth in crop production is expected to come from higher yield, the remainder coming from land expansion. To double global production of the top four crops by 2050 would require an increase in the yield rate of 2.4% per year. A recent study suggests that existing yield rates are insufficient to meet this demand (Ray et al., 2013).

The increase in yield on existing land has been accomplished in large part by the addition of fertilizers containing nitrogen (N) and phosphorus (P). While N and P have natural geochemical cycles, human activity has resulted in a major disruption of these cycles. Large fractions of anthropogenically mobilized N and P in watersheds enter groundwater through leaching and surface runoff and are transported in freshwater toward coastal marine systems. This has resulted in numerous negative impacts on human health and environment, such as groundwater pollution, loss of habitat and biodiversity, an increase in the frequency and severity of harmful algal blooms, eutrophication, hypoxia and coastal dead zones, and fish kills (Bouwman et al., 2013).

In addition to the disruption of natural N and P geochemical cycles, agriculture has been responsible for several other negative environmental impacts. Agriculture has converted 30% of forests worldwide, which decreases biodiversity through habitat replacement. Agriculture accounts for 92% of the human water footprint (Ramankutty et al., 2018). Agricultural pesticides such as DDT persist and biomagnify in the environment, resulting in toxicity to humans and wildlife. Agriculture is an important source of greenhouse gas emissions from deforestation and methane emissions from livestock. Providing adequate nutrition to a growing world population without further degradation of the environment will continue to be a major challenge.

FRESH WATER

Fresh water is a scarce resource. Only 2.5% of the total water on earth is fresh water, of which 69.4% is in the form of ice, snow, or permafrost, and most of the remainder is groundwater. Fresh water in lakes and rivers is only about 1% of fresh water available on earth. Most precipitation is lost through evaporation (Saeijs & van Berkel, 1995. Global water demand has increased by 600% over the past 100 years. At present, 47% of the world's population live in areas that suffer water scarcity at least one month each year. By 2050 that number is expected to increase to 57%. Globally, agriculture accounts for 70% of use and industry for another 20% (Borreti & Rosa, 2019). Demand for fresh water increases with population growth, economic development, and consumption patterns. While water demand is increasing, water availability is decreasing. Water tables in the world's three biggest grain-producing nations are falling in response to unsustainable withdrawals for agriculture (Whitmee et al., 2015). More than 30% of the world's largest groundwater systems are now in distress. In coastal areas, water withdrawal is causing land subsidence and salinization of aquifers.

In addition to shortages of renewable supplies, other major global problems with fresh water include unequal distribution of supplies, problems of water quality, unrestrained construction of dams and reservoirs, and degradation of fresh water ecosystems. Climate change is likely to exacerbate these problems. Increasing temperatures and more variable rainfalls are expected to reduce crop yields in many developing regions where food security is already a problem. By 2030, water scarcity in some arid and semi-arid places will displace between 24 million and 700 million people (United Nations, 2020b).

OCEANS AND FISHERIES

Oceans, seas, and coastal areas form an integrated and essential component of the Earth's ecosystem. They cover more than two-thirds of the earth's surface and contain 97% of the planet's water. The condition or "health" of the coast, oceans and humans are inextricably linked (Sandifer et al., 2013). Nearly 40% of the world's population lives within 100 kilometers of the coast. The global oceans-based economy, which includes employment, ecosystem services provided by the ocean and cultural services, is estimated at between US$3 trillion and $6 trillion per year. Shipping is responsible for more than 90% of the trade between countries. Approximately 50% of all international tourists travel to coast areas. For some developing countries, tourism accounts for over 25% of GDP (United Nations Environment Programme, 2017).

The oceans are crucial for global food security. They provide food for around a third of the global population (Moore et al., 2013). Fish accounted for 15.7% of the global population's intake of animal protein in 2007 (Moore et al., 2013). About 97% of the world's fishermen live in developing countries and fishing is their major source of food and income. Overfishing, however, has a major impact on marine fisheries and their supporting ecosystems. Global catches began to decline in the late 1980s due to overfishing and the resulting broad-based collapse of the underlying ecosystems (Pauly et al., 2005). In 2015, 33% of marine stocks were being harvested at unsustainable levels and 60% at maximally sustainable levels (IPBES, 2019).

The dramatic growth of the human population in the global coastal zone has had significant adverse effects on the quality and sustainability of the coastal marine environment. Oceans, seas, and marine resources are increasingly threatened by human activities (United Nations, 2020a). This degradation of marine ecosystems in turn adversely impacts human health. Human-generated waste from sewage and agricultural runoff results in the influx of pathogenic organisms. The global burden of human disease caused by sewage pollution of coast waters has been estimated at 4 million lost person-years annually

(Moore et al., 2013). Influxes of nutrients can exacerbate naturally-occurring harmful algal blooms that deplete oxygen, block sunlight from reaching the lower depths of the water column, and have the ability to produce potent toxins (Kite-Powell et al., 2008). Fertilizer runoff has produced approximately 400 low-oxygen coastal dead zones, covering more than 245,000 km^2. Each year 300–400 million tons of heavy metals, solvents, toxic sludge and other wastes from industrial facilities are dumped into the world's waters (IPBES, 2019). Some of these, like mercury, can bioconcentrate and biomagnify in aquatic ecosystems, and cause outbreaks of human poisoning from ingestion of contaminated fish. Plastics pollution of the oceans has increased tenfold since 1980. Plastics in marine environments are of increasing concern because of their persistence and effects on the oceans, wildlife and, potentially, humans (Jambeck et al., 2015). Approximately 8 million tons of plastic end up in marine environments every year and make up 80% of all marine debris. Marine species ingest or become entangled in these plastics, resulting in injuries and death (IUPC, 2018).

The oceans have been shielding the earth from the worst effects of rapid climate change by absorbing excess carbon dioxide (CO_2) from the atmosphere (Bijma et al., 2013). This absorption of CO_2 is driving the ocean along the pH gradient toward more acidic conditions. At the same time, ocean warming is having pronounced impacts on the composition, structure, and functions of marine ecosystems, such as bleaching of the coral reefs. Approximately 50% of live coral cover of reefs has already been lost. The ability of the oceans to mitigate climate change through increased carbon sequestration is limited and may decline as the ocean acidifies (Allison & Bassett, 2017). The impacts of climate change on the oceans include rising seas surface temperature; thermal expansion of the oceans and melting sea ice, leading to sea level rise; changes to ocean thermal structure and currents; changes in the periodicity and amplitude of ocean climate cycles; changes in the frequency and severity of hurricanes and typhoons; ocean acidification; and increases in oceanic dead zones (Allison & Bassett, 2017).

LAND COVER CHANGE AND DEFORESTATION

The most visible form of human impact on the environment has been the conversion of natural lands to croplands, pastures, urban areas, reservoirs, and other anthropogenic landscapes. Forty percent of earth's land surface is under agriculture and 75% of the terrestrial environment has been severely altered by human actions (de Sherbinin et al., 2007; IPBES, 2019). Twenty-three percent of land areas have seen a reduction in productivity due to land degradation.

Today, there is 32% less global forest area than in pre-industrial times. Between 1990 and 2015, 290 million hectares of native forest were lost due to clearing and wood harvesting. These losses are partially offset through the planting of 110 million hectares of new forest. Because most developed countries largely deforested their lands in past centuries, much of the current deforestation is occurring in developing countries. From 1980 to 2000, 100 million hectares of tropical forests were lost because of agricultural expansion, mainly due to cattle ranching in Latin America and to conversion to palm oil plantations in Southeast Asia. More than 85% of wetlands present in 1700 had been lost by 2000, which is three times faster in percentage terms than forest loss.

Cities are now the dominant human habitat. Approximately 50% of the world's population is concentrated in urban areas that occupy less than 3% of the earth' surface. While large-scale land cover change is primarily a rural phenomenon, it is driven to a large degree by the consumption demands of urban masses (de Sherbinin et al., 2007).

CLIMATE CHANGE

According to the World Economic Forum's *Global Risks Report* (World Economic Forum, 2016), the failure to mitigate and adapt to climate change will be the most impactful risk facing communities worldwide in the next decade. While the earth has gone through warm and cool cycles long before humans, today's global warming is occurring much faster than ever before and can't be explained by natural causes alone. The vast majority of scientists agree that the greenhouse gases we generate, such as carbon dioxide, methane, and nitrous oxides, play a significant role in global warming. In 2013, the CO_2 concentration in the earth's atmosphere reached 400 ppm (parts per million), a level not seen on earth since the Pliocene Epoch over 2.5 million years ago (McCrink-Goode, 2014). The burning of fossil fuels is the primary source of these emissions. Other important sources include deforestation and agriculture. Fertilizer use is a primary source of nitrous oxide emissions, while livestock are major emitters of methane. The health impacts of climate change will include temperature-related illness due to extreme weather events, the spread of infectious disease vectors; increases in waterborne diseases; and wide-ranging impacts from air pollution. Environmental effects, besides heat and extreme weather events, include rising seas, warmer and more acidic oceans resulting in the loss of coral reefs, drought, and imperiled ecosystems. On land, warmer climates lead to drier conditions, providing ideal kindling for the rapid spread of wildfires. In addition to causing destruction of forest ecosystems and mass property damage, these intense fires impact human health through burns, smoke inhalation, and emotional harm to the fires' victims (Rossiello & Szema, 2019).

In 2018 the Intergovernmental Panel on Climate Change issued a special report on the impacts of global warming of 1.5°C above pre-industrial levels (IPCC, 2018). The report was written and edited by 91 scientists from 40 countries who analyzed more than 6,000 scientific studies. The key findings of the report are that since 1970 the global average temperature has been rising at a rate of 1.7°C per century. The rise in global CO_2 concentration since 2000 is 20 ppm per decade, which is 10 times faster than any sustained rise in CO_2 over the past 800,000 years. Human activities are estimated to have caused approximately 1.0°C of global warming above pre-industrial levels, with a likely range of 0.8°C to 1.2°C. While a rise of 1.5°C will still have substantial impacts, an increase of 2°C will have more severe impacts. With a 2°C rise, sea levels will be 10 centimeters higher than with a 1.5°C rise, a third of the planet will experience extreme heat waves, ice-free summers in the Arctic sea will be ten times more likely, and virtually all of the coral reefs will be lost. Sea level rise threatens the livelihood of 10% of the world's population who live in coastal areas less than 10 meters above sea level.

The pledges under the Paris Agreement are not enough. The current nationally determined contributions (NDCs), extending to 2030, do not limit warming to 1.5°C; they cumulatively track toward a warming of 3–4°C above pre-industrial levels by 2100.

To limit global warming to 1.5°C, net human-caused emissions of carbon dioxide would need to fall by about 45% from 2010 levels by 2030, reaching "net zero" around 2050. Despite these dire predictions, severe global warming is not inevitable. Dramatic reductions in greenhouse gas emissions can limit global warming. The main challenge is the political will and governance capacity of institutions to implement the changes that are needed.

POLLUTION

Environmental pollution is a major cause of disease, disability and death (Landrigan & Fuller, 2016). The leading risk factors include household air pollution, ambient air pollution, and water pollution. While releases of pollutants have caused acute fatalities, such as the Bhopal disaster in 1984, the majority of deaths attributable to pollutants are caused by non-communicable diseases, such as ischemic heart disease, chronic obstructive pulmonary disease, and cancer. The threat of pollution is especially high in low- and middle-income countries, where 70% of chemical manufacture now occurs. Since 1950, an estimated 140,000 new chemicals have been invented. Between 14,000 and 15,000 are in commercial use, and most have not been adequately tested for their toxicity and environmental fate (Landrigan et al., 2018). Pollutants destabilize the earth's support systems and endanger our continuing survival. As an example, honeybees are responsible for nearly one-third of the world's crop pollination. Colony collapse disorder first observed in the United States in 2006 has spread globally, resulting in drastic declines in honeybee populations. While the exact cause is still unknown, potential causes include neonicotinoid pesticides and other environmental stresses (McCrink-Goode, 2014).

Air pollution accounts for 6.5 million premature deaths each year. Particulate matter ($PM_{2.5}$ and PM_{10}) affects more people than any other air pollutant. Inefficient cooking and heating with solid fuels in poorly ventilated homes are a major source of exposure to indoor air pollution in developing countries (Balmes, 2019). Levels of particulate matter from smoke in such homes is often ten times higher than the greatest concentration that occurs in ambient air in developed countries. The greatest burden of household air-pollution premature deaths is in children with pneumonia. The greatest burden in adults is cardiovascular disease, chronic obstructive lung disease, and lung cancer (Balmes, 2019). Nine out of ten people breathe outdoor air polluted beyond acceptable World Health Organization guideline levels (United Nations Environment Program, 2017). The main sources for outdoor air pollution are fossil fuel emissions from coal burning for power and heat, transport, industrial furnaces, brick kilns, agriculture, domestic fuel heating, and unregulated burning of wastes (United Nations Environment Program, 2017). In addition to particulate matter, other major ambient air pollutants include sulfur dioxide, nitrogen oxides, carbon monoxide, ozone, and volatile organic compounds. Air pollutants are also major contributors to climate change.

The primary sources of freshwater body pollution include pathogens from untreated wastewater, agrochemicals, industrial effluents, and metals from mining. Over 80% of the world's wastewater is released into the environment without treatment (United Nations Environment Program, 2017). Globally, 58% of diarrheal diseases are due to a lack of access to clean water and sanitation. Agricultural runoff carries nutrients (nitrates and phosphates) and pesticides into surface waters, contaminating rivers, streams, and lakes. These nutrient overloads cause eutrophication and harmful algal blooms. Toxicants can also leach into groundwater, contaminating aquifers that are used for drinking water and irrigation.

Land and soil can be contaminated through poor agricultural practices, improper waste management, and a range of military and extractive activities. The primary pollutants of concern for soil contamination are toxic metals and persistent organic pollutants. Metals are especially hazardous because they do not degrade in the environment. Numerous examples of outbreaks of childhood lead poisoning have been linked to contamination from lead smelters (Sullivan, 2015). Mercury poisoning from artisanal and small-scale gold mining is a major problem in developing countries (Steckling et al., 2017). In addition to causing elemental mercury poisoning among workers, mercury volatilizes and can be transported large distances, where it deposits in aquatic ecosystems and biomagnifies in the food chain.

Waste generation has more than doubled since 1970. The world generates over 2 billion tons of municipal solid waste annually (World Bank, 2018). At least a third of that is not managed in an environmentally safe manner. At least 2 billion people worldwide lack access to solid waste collection (United Nations Environment Program, 2017). Globally, most waste is dumped or disposed of in some form of landfill. Open dumping accounts for about 33% of waste, the vast majority of which occurs in low-income countries. Dumpsites around the world are sources of complex pollution mixtures. They are home to an estimated 15 million informal waste pickers, who scavenge them for food and recyclables (United Nations Environment Program, 2017). It is estimated that in 2014 the global generation of electrical equipment waste (e-waste) was 41.8 million metric tons. Scavenging e-waste can expose people to toxic metals and pyrolysis products. Mining is the largest source of non-municipal waste. While much of this material is inert, waste streams from mining activities can contain metals and other compounds that can adversely impact ecosystems and human health. Wastes are also dumped into waterways and oceans. An estimated 4.8 to 12.7 million metric tons of land-based plastic waste entered the oceans in 2010. Without waste management the quantity of plastic waste available to enter the ocean from land is expected to increase by an order of magnitude by 2015 (Jambeck et al., 2015). At least 8 million tons of plastic end up in our oceans every year, and make up 80% of all marine debris from surface waters to deep-sea sediments.

LOSS OF BIODIVERSITY

In the age of the Anthropocene, humans are now driving the sixth mass extinction event in earth's history (Isbell et al., 2017). The rate of species extinctions is already tens to hundreds of times higher than the average across the past 10 million years. Up to one million plant and animal species face extinction because of human activities (Tollefson, 2019). The primary drivers of these species extinction rates are habitat loss and fragmentation, over-exploitation of biological resources, pollution, species invasions, and climate change. Because of habitat loss and deterioration, over 500,000 of the world's estimated 5.9 million terrestrial species have insufficient habitat for long-term survival. Among species that have been studied in detail, an average of 25% of species are threatened with extinction across terrestrial, freshwater and marine vertebrate, invertebrate and plant groups. Species at especially high risk include amphibians, reef-forming corals, sharks and shark relatives, and marine animals. Climate change is likely to exacerbate extinction rates. An estimated 5% of all species would be threatened with extinction by 2°C of warming above pre-industrial levels (Tollefson, 2019). Invasive species are taking over ecological niches. Since 1970, there has been a 70% increase of invasive alien species across 21 countries with detailed records.

Biodiversity is essential to ecosystem functioning and stability. Biodiversity is positively correlated with ecosystem productivity by a mechanism known as functional complementarity, which states that the more species there are, the more niches are occupied, and thus the greater productivity of the ecosystem (MIT, 2015). The United Nations Convention on Biological Diversity notes that at least 40% of the world's economy and 80% of the needs of the poor are derived from biological resources (MIT, 2015). Biodiversity contributes to agricultural productivity, moderates climate, and provides sources of new medicines. Biodiversity is critical to cultural ecosystem services that support our spiritual, religious, and aesthetic values. Preserving biodiversity is clearly in our self-interest.

EMERGING INFECTIOUS DISEASES

Infectious diseases can emerge when environmental factors lead to changes in microbial ecological niches and fuel microbial adaptation to human hosts (Nii-Trebi, 2017). These environmental factors include depletion of forests, expansion and modernization of agricultural practices, natural disasters, and climate change. A variety of sociodemographic factors can increase the contact of microbes with human hosts. These include increases in population density, poverty, conflicts and social instability, decline in infrastructure, travel, and killing of wild animals for meat. Many emerging infectious diseases are zoonoses that have reservoir hosts in specific animal species and then adapt to infect humans. These adaptations can be a result of gene mutation, recombination or reassortment. Half of the global emerging infectious disease events of zoonotic origin between 1940 and 2005 are estimated to result from changes in land use, in agricultural practices, and in food production practices (Whitmee et al., 2015). Wet markets that sell live poultry, fish, reptiles and mammals provide optimal conditions for the transfer and evolution of infectious disease agents. In recent years, outbreaks of novel influenza and SARS viruses have been linked to human exposure to reservoir hosts in these types of markets.

Emerging infectious diseases can be new, in that they have been discovered in humans for the first time, or re-emerging, where a disease that had thought to be controlled or eradicated reappears in a new geographic location. Over the past 40 years, over 30 new infectious agents affecting humans have emerged or re-emerged. Most of these have been zoonotic in origin and associated with socioeconomic, environmental and ecological factors (Nii-Trebi, 2017). Pandemics occur when humans have no underlying immunity to these infectious agents and human-to-human transmission is sustained, especially through the respiratory route. Examples include the Spanish influenza epidemic of 1918–19 and the COVID-19 pandemic that began in 2019 and continued through 2021. The COVID-19 pandemic has been the largest global public health crisis in a century, with severe health and socioeconomic impacts.

THE ECOLOGICAL PARADOX

Over the past 50 years, human population growth and unsustainable consumption have negatively impacted the ecosystem services that we depend on for our quality of life (Diaz et al., 2019). Some of these impacts, such as loss of biosphere integrity, disruption of biogeochemical flows of nitrogen and phosphorus, and ocean acidification have exceeded global level boundaries of what we believe to be our planet's "safe operating space" (Whitmee et al., 2015). Yet at the same time, we have seen increases in human life expectancy, decreases in poverty, and increases in the human development index. From 1950 to 2017, the average life expectancy for males increased from 48 years to 71 years and for females from 53 years to 76 years (GBD 2017 Mortality Collaborators, 2018). There has also been marked progress in reducing poverty. Between 1990 and 2015, the percentage of the world's population living in extreme poverty decreased from 1.9 billion people to 734 million (World Bank, 2020). The Human Development Index is a summary measure of human development that incorporates life expectancy and birth, years of schooling, and gross national income per capita. Over the past 100 years, the HDI has been increasing in all regions of the world, including the least developed countries.

This paradox of increasing human well-being while ecosystem services are degrading is referred to as the "ecological paradox." Several alternative hypotheses have been proposed to explain this paradox (Raudsepp-Hearne et al., 2010). The first is that our measures of human well-being are incomplete. The second is that human well-being relies primarily on provision services such as food production, and we have been successful in increasing production to meet demand. The third is that technology and innovation have decoupled us from our dependence on nature's ecosystem services. The fourth and most likely explanation is that there is a time lag after ecosystem degradation before human well-being is affected. For some threats, such as climate change, our time to mitigate the detrimental impacts is measured in a few years to decades rather than centuries and millennia.

CHALLENGES AND SOLUTIONS

The Union of Concerned Scientists has warned us that urgent steps are needed to safeguard our imperiled biosphere. Moreover, they emphasized that time is running out, and soon it will be too late to shift course away from our failing trajectory (Ripple et al., 2017). Why, then, have we failed to act? The Rockefeller-Lancet Commission identifies three major challenges (Whitmee et al., 2015). The first is conceptual and empathy (imagination) failures. Even today, in the face of incontrovertible evidence of global warming, some world leaders continue to cast doubt on climate science and deny the anthropogenic causes. In order to address this conceptual failure, we need a paradigm shift in how we think about human health in the context of planetary health (Al-Delaimy, 2018). The second challenge is knowledge failures and our unwillingness to deal with uncertainty within decision-making frameworks. While more interdisciplinary and transdisciplinary research is needed, we know enough now to develop effective implementation strategies. The third challenge is a failure in governance; we know what changes need to be made, but we fail to implement them.

Human population growth and unsustainable consumption are the greatest drivers of anthropogenic degradation of our ecosystems. The good news is that fertility patterns in the world have been declining over the past few decades. Total fertility is now 2.5 children per woman globally (United Nations Department of Economic and Social Affairs, 2015). The global average masks regional differences. For example, Africa has the highest fertility rate of 4.7 children per woman, while Europe has the lowest of 1.6 children per woman. Historically, fertility has declined in response to increases in well-being associated with economic development (Murdoch et al., 2018). Even though the rate of population growth is slowing, the total population numbers continue to increase. The UN's median projected world population is expected to increase by 4 billion people by 2100. Almost 80% of this increase comes from 37 mid-African countries. The critical question is whether stabilization and reduction in the world's population can occur in time to prevent the catastrophic impacts predicted by the Club of Rome and the Union of Concerned Scientists (Meadows et al., 1972; Ripple et al., 2017).

Reduction in population growth is not sufficient. It needs to be accompanied by policies that reduce our depletion of ecosystem resources and address the imminent threat of climate change (Whitmee et al., 2015). We know how to effectively mitigate many of these threats. For example, in the area of food security, 30–50% of all food produced globally is wasted. Reduction in food waste would enhance food security, as well as substantial additional benefits in terms of reducing use of land, freshwater, fertilizers, energy, and pesticides. The Rockefeller-Lancet Commission identifies disruption of nitrogen and phosphorus geochemical cycles from the application of fertilizers as one of the threats where we have already exceeded the planet's safe operating space. Crops take up between 30% and 50% of applied nitrogen fertilizer and 45% of phosphorus. The remainder leaches into groundwater or is lost by surface runoff and enters aquatic ecosystems where it promotes eutrophication and harmful algal blooms. Strategies to more efficiently apply these fertilizers would help mitigate these negative impacts. As an example of a "win-win" solution for human health and the environment, promotion of plant-based diets would have the dual benefits of improving human health while reducing emissions of the greenhouse gas, methane, from cattle.

Climate change will be the most impactful environmental risk facing communities in the next decade (World Economic Forum, 2016). To limit global warming to 1.5°C, we need to reduce human-caused emissions of carbon dioxide by 45% from 2010 levels and reach a "net zero" emission by 2050. Since fossil fuels account for about 70% of these greenhouse gas emissions, we need to transition to low-carbon energy sources, such as wind power and solar energy. Other strategies include improving energy efficiency, reforestation, and removing carbon dioxide from the earth's atmosphere. We need to make these radical changes now to prevent catastrophic consequences in our own lifetimes.

We also know what actions we need to take to mitigate the other threats to ecosystem integrity. Pollution is preventable and these control technologies can be shared with developing countries and brought to a global scale. We need to protect and restore habitat to maintain biodiversity, curtail illegal poaching and fishing, and establish more land protected areas and marine sanctuaries. We need to invest in the management of freshwater ecosystems and sanitation facilities in developing countries, recycle wastewater, and develop energy efficient desalination plants. We need to invest in pandemic preparedness to prevent the human and economic toll of emerging infectious diseases such as COVID-19. We need to educate on how to reduce consumption and live more environmentally friendly and healthier lifestyles. We need to advocate for policy makers to implement these transformative changes before we exceed the limits of the planet to sustain us. These challenges highlight the critical need to integrate ecosystem governance into national policies and relevant international conventions (Vasseur et al., 2017).

Hanson (2007: n.p.) defined global governance for environment and sustainable development as "organized action on the part of individuals, and organizations such as governments, intergovernmental bodies, private sector, community and non-governmental-organization (NGO) bodies taken to achieve environment and sustainable development objectives concerning problems of global interest, including those affecting the global commons and those of global interest that occur at sub-global or country levels." This definition highlights the fact that global governance is not global government. The authority for global governance is disaggregated across centers of authority in every corner of the world and at every level of community and includes non-state actors, such as NGOs, multinational corporations, and international organizations (Winchester, 2009).

The underpinnings for today's system of governance for environment and sustainable development are derived from more than a 100 years of effort (Hanson, 2007). These began with conservation and natural resource management in the early 1900s; the development of modern public health and sanitation in the 1920s; environmental management in the 1970s; biodiversity management in the 1980s; followed by sustainable development and managing the use of the global commons. The culmination of these international efforts was the adoption of the Sustainable Development Goals (SDGs) by the United Nations General Assembly in 2015 (United Nations Environment Programme, 2020). The SDGs are a set of objectives within a universal agreement to end poverty, protect all that makes the planet habitable, and ensure that all people enjoy peace and prosperity, now and in the future. The 17 SDGs address the five Ps of sustainable development:

people, planet, prosperity, peace, and partnerships. They are to be implemented from 2016 to 2030 (Morton et al., 2017). However, the SDGs are voluntary agreements by governments in contrast to the legally binding Paris Agreement on climate change.

Today there are several hundred Multilateral Environmental Agreements (MEAs) aimed at protecting our global commons. The United Nations Conference on Human Health and Environment, which was held in Stockholm in 1972, moved national environmental concerns into the international political agenda and led to the establishment of the United Nations Environment Programme (UNEP). Declarations from the Stockholm conference, in Principle 21, codify the responsibility to avoid trans-boundary harm to the environment of States and areas beyond the limits of national jurisdiction (United Nations Environment Programme, 1972). Another key component in the Declarations resulting from the Stockholm conference is the principle of intergenerational equity, formalizing the idea that the present generation bears a responsibility to safeguard the environment for future generations (Declarations, Principles 1 and 2). This is the driving force behind sustainable development. Economic arguments based on this principle tend to lose where future costs are severely discounted and difficult to predict compared to present benefits. But, failure of our system to take adequate account of the environment could result in irreparable harm and damage to assets that threatens the financial system itself (Morton et al., 2017). Nevertheless, this idea that we hold the earth in trust as caretakers resonates powerfully with all cultures (Weiss, 1992).

Some other international environmental treaties spanning a wide range of issues include the 1992 Rio Declaration on Environment and Development, the 1973 Convention on International Trade in Endangered Species (CITES), the 1992 Convention on Biodiversity, the 1972 World Heritage Convention, and the 1989 Basel Convention on the Transboundary Movement of Hazardous Wastes.

Arguably, the most successful MEA has been the Montreal Protocol on Substances that Deplete the Ozone Layer (1987) (Winchester, 2009). Negotiated within the framework of the 1985 Vienna Convention for the Protection of the Ozone Layer, these universally ratified treaties are the benchmark for how nations can and ought to cooperate for the benefit of all. Interestingly, controls on CFCs started not with a treaty regime but with a few like-minded nations agreeing to separately ban the use of CFCs in aerosol spray cans (Benedick, 2007). This helped depress the demand for CFCs globally and spearheaded innovation where there was now a recognized market for substitutes. One of the issues with crises around anthropogenic pollutants is that they are initiated more often or in larger share by developed nations. In the case of regulating chlorofluorocarbons (CFCs), developing countries argued that they should not have their own development constrained because they had not created the problem, or else they should be compensated for the cost of switching over to substitutes. The solution was the Multilateral Fund, designed to provide financial and technical assistance to developing nations as an incentive to participate in the treaty. When incentives align with the moral imperative to "do the right thing", success is more likely (McNeill & Otterson, 2015).

The December 2015 Paris Agreement, significant as the first universal agreement on climate change (involving 195 countries and the European Union), was the outgrowth of 21 years of annual conferences of parties to the United Nations Framework for Climate Change (Morton et al., 2017). It embodies many of the procedures and principles that have proven successful in the past, including a bottom-up approach of voluntary "nationally-determined contributions," and a Green Climate Fund pledging assistance to developing countries, calling to mind the Multilateral

Fund from the Montreal Protocol. Instead of installing hard targets, the Paris Agreement includes a commitment at each subsequent meeting only to do more than what was done before, a novel idea which became known as the principle of non-regression (de Chazournes, 2016). The next five years, including the United States' renewed commitment to rejoin the Paris Agreement and its potential to be a leader in setting and achieving its own emissions targets, will be critical to the success or failure of this treaty. In this sense, safeguards not written into the agreement, such as pressure from other nations or pressure from one's own electorate, should be considered when assessing the utility of such a scheme.

As was discussed above, global environmental governance is increasingly characterized by participation of non-state actors, including nongovernmental organizations, scientists and experts, business associations, and even subnational governments (Biermann & Pattberg, 2008). In the United States, states such as California and Hawaii, for example, have set their own climate change targets. This is not to minimize the importance of national and multinational coordination on climate change. It should be encouraging to think that so many are working on this problem, and that the engine or proof of concept to spark worldwide change can originate from almost anywhere. But the overall problem remains at a global and existential scale. Those in positions of power who fail to lead on the issue of climate change will at best be judged as neglectful and ineffectual.

Sustainable development depends on three pillars: economic, social, and environmental. In the vast majority of international agreements, such as trade regimes, foreign investment regimes, and global finance regimes, health and ecosystem integrity play subordinate roles to economics (Morin & Blouin, 2019; Vasseur et al., 2017). The architects of these regimes address human health and environment in terms of avoiding negative externalities. They envision economy, society, and ecosphere as separate, but overlapping, spheres. In this old paradigm that tries to balance positive and negative externalities, economic projects can have the effect of increasing inequities, harming human health, and damaging the ecosphere. We need to envision a new paradigm in which the economic sphere lies with the social sphere, which in turn lies within the ecosphere. This new paradigm, which acknowledges our common dependence on our planet, may lead to more diverse and equitable economic opportunities for all, increasing health and prosperity while concurrently protecting the environment.

The existing system of global governance for environmental and sustainable development has several obvious weaknesses. Many multilateral treaties, like the United Nations Convention on the Law of the Sea (UNCLOS), lack full participation of major stakeholder nations. Enforcement for MEAs is limited and non-compliance results in limited sanctions. MEAs have limited capacity for dispute resolution, limited monitoring, and are poorly funded. But these limitations need not stand in the way of overcoming our environmental challenge. As noted by Richard Benedick, the chief US negotiator of the Montreal Protocol, the ozone science in the 1970s was much more disputed than the climate science of today (Benedick, 2007). Countries lacking capacity to implement change can be incentivized to participate through a scheme of common but differentiated responsibilities. The missing link is not enforcement but leadership. We have the knowledge to act. We have a system, albeit imperfect, for global governance. We need to overcome the imagination challenge. As the world scientists have stated in their second notice: "… time is running out. We must recognize, in our day-to-day lives and in our governing institutions, that Earth with all its life is our only home." (Ripple et al., 2017).

Box 28.1 Case Study: The Chernobyl Nuclear Disaster

The Chernobyl reactor accident is one of the most infamous environmental disasters of the past century. This man-made accident and the events that followed have taught us important lessons about the risks and benefits of nuclear power, disaster response and resilience, and the social, political, and ecological consequences of governments engaging in cover-up and propaganda rather than truth and science.

At 1:26 am on April 26, 1986, a safety experiment at Reactor No. 4 of the Chernobyl Nuclear Power Station in the Ukrainian SSR (Soviet Socialist Republic) went terribly wrong. The plant managers decided to take advantage of a routine maintenance shut-down to determine if, in the event of a loss of station power, the still-spinning turbines could provide enough electrical power to operate emergency equipment and circulate cooling water to the core until the diesel emergency power supply became operative. The operators were not aware that this type of graphite-moderated RBMK reactor becomes unstable at low power. A combination of design failure and human error led to an uncontrolled power surge that destroyed the reactor core and set fire to the graphite moderator. A total of 31 people, including operators and emergency response personnel, died within the first few weeks of accident; 28 of these deaths were from acute radiation syndrome.

The graphite fire was finally extinguished on May 9. By then the initial explosion and plume from the graphite fire emitted more radionuclides than 400 Hiroshima-type nuclear bombs. The predominant radionuclides in the plume included I-131 (Iodine-131) with a half-life of 8 days and Cs-137 (Cesium-137) with a half-life of 30 years. Over the first several days the wind blew the plume north over Belarus and toward the Scandinavian countries, before changing direction and spreading contamination over large swathes of Europe. In addition to direct radiation exposure from the passing plume, a major route of population exposure to radioiodine was through ingestion of contaminated milk from cattle that had grazed on contaminated pastures. Exposure to radioiodine occurred over the first 6–8 weeks. Subsequent population exposure occurred through radiocesium that had been deposited on soil. Areas contaminated with high concentrations of radiocesium would remain uninhabitable for over 100 years. Over 600,000 liquidators were brought in to secure the reactor and remove and bury the contaminated radioactive debris, plants, animals, and soil. Over 350,000 people were eventually evacuated or resettled from contaminated zones in Ukraine, Belarus, and Russia. Among those evacuated were 49,000 people from the city of Pripyat, which was 10 kilometers from the reactor. Pripyat had been built as a model Soviet city to house the workers at the Chernobyl complex.

The long-term health impacts of the Chernobyl accident were subject to considerable debate. Four years after the accident, the rates of thyroid cancer among children in areas with high exposure to radioiodine began to soar. Long-term epidemiological studies have established a clear dose–response relationship between Chernobyl-related radioiodine exposure and risk of thyroid cancer in children. Epidemiological studies have demonstrated increased risks of radiation cataracts and leukemia among liquidators. Models predict that by 2065 about 16,000 cases of thyroid cancer and 25,000 cases of other cancers may be expected in Europe due to radiation from the accident (Cardiss et al., 2006). The accident led to a downward spiral of socioeconomic consequences in the affected communities. In addition to the radiation disease, the psychological impact, and social disruption, the release of radioactive material led to the contamination of the environment and foodstuffs, mandatory resettlement, and economic collapse of the affected communities. Chernobyl produced over 400,000 environmental refugees who had to leave their ancestral homes and resettle in other parts of Ukraine, Russia, and Belarus, often accompanied by the stigma of being a Chernobyl victim.

The Chernobyl accident has taught us several important lessons about radiation safety, radiation health effects, and recovery from nuclear reactor accidents. RBMK reactors, which are still operating in Russia, have been retrofitted to minimize the risk of this type of accident. The risk of accidents, however, is not limited to RBMK reactors. As we have learned from the accidents at Three Mile Island in the US and Fukushima in Japan, western-type reactors, which are moderated by water rather than graphite, and which have an external containment, are still subject to loss of coolant accidents. An interruption of cooling water to the fuel elements caused by operator error, mechanical problems, or natural disasters can lead to the overheating of the core with the potential for substantial releases of radiation. When we calculate the risks and benefits of nuclear power, we need to factor in the low-probability, high-impact scenarios. Additional challenges include the disposal of radioactive waste and reducing the production of isotopes that can be used for nuclear weapons.

From a health standpoint, we have a clearer understanding of the dose–response relationships between exposure to radioiodine and thyroid cancer. The Chernobyl accident has shown us that children are especially susceptible to radiation-induced thyroid cancer. Fortunately, over 98% of the Chernobyl-related thyroid cancers in these children were curable. The studies of radiation-induced cataracts have led to a lowering of permissible exposure limits for workers, including medical personnel that use fluoroscopy. We have learned that the health impacts of nuclear reactor accidents go well beyond direct radiation effects. The psychological stressors among the population included fear

(Continued)

(Continued)

of radiation, distrust of officialdom, the stresses of evacuation and resettlement, and severe economic hardship. In Ukraine and Belarus, large portions of the national budgets went toward compensation for the Chernobyl victims. We learned that following these types of catastrophic accidents, we need to move from a psychology of victimization to a psychology of survivorship. Public health is the health of the community, and recovery efforts should not be restricted to health, but should focus on rebuilding the community.

Chernobyl has shown us what can happen when governments engage in lies and propaganda rather than truth and science. Many of the health impacts could have reduced if the Soviets had evacuated the population sooner and informed them about the risks and how to mitigate them. Mikhail Gorbachev, the Soviet Union's last General Secretary, later admitted that the Chernobyl disaster was a turning point that contributed to the collapse of Soviet communism. The public outrage led to a freedom of expression that could not be contained by the system. It gave rise to an environmental movement that became a potent political force and a rallying point for Ukrainian and Belorusian independence. Chernobyl also taught us that these types of catastrophic accident are not just national events – they are global events. Environmental pollutants do not respect national borders. Remediation of the site required international cooperation and financial investments. The costs of remediation, including the construction of a new sarcophagus over the damaged reactor, totaled billions of dollars, at a time when these newly independent states were going through the hardships of political and economic transition.

The future of the Chernobyl site is still undecided. The new containment is designed to last 100 years. The site will remain radioactive for tens of thousands of years. Paradoxically, wildlife is thriving in the exclusion zone, and the site has become somewhat of an ecological sanctuary. Humans appear to have had a more negative impact on the local ecosystem than radiation. One novel idea is to convert the site into a solar power station given that much of the electrical transmission infrastructure is still intact. Another compelling idea is to designate the site as a UNESCO Dark Heritage site, similar to Hiroshima and Auschwitz (Hryhorczuk, 2018). Chernobyl and the abandoned city of Pripyat are currently a tourist designation. A UNESCO designation would recognize the universal value of the site for future generations and compel the Ukrainian government to preserve it. As a dark heritage site, Chernobyl would continue to teach us that "the lessons learned need to be learned."

REFERENCES

Al-Delaimy, W.K. (2018). Planetary health and population health: the Anthropocene requires different thinking and approaches in serving public health. *Current Environmental Health Reports* 5(4), 397–400. DOI: 10.1007/s40572-018-0222-z

Allison, E.H., & Bassett, H.R. (2017). Climate change in the oceans: human impacts and responses. *Science* 350, 778–782. DOI: 10.1126/science.aac8721

Balmes, J.R. (2019). Household air pollution from domestic combustion of solid fuels and health. *Clinical Reviews in Allergy and Immunology* 143(6), 1979–1987. DOI: 10.1016/j.jaci.2019.04.016

Benedick, R. (2007). Avoiding gridlock on climate change. *Issues in Science and Technology*, 23(2), 37–40. Retrieved December 16, 2020, from www.jstor.org/stable/43314398

Biermann, F., & Pattberg, P. (2008). Global environmental governance: taking stock, moving forward. *Annual Review of Environment and Resources* 33, 277–294. DOI: 10.1146/annurev.environ.33.050707.085733

Bijma, J., Portner, H.-O., Yesson, C., & Rogers, A.D. (2013). Climate change and the oceans – what does the future hold? *Marine Pollution Bulletin* 74(2), 495–505. DOI: 10.1016/j.marpolbul.2013.07.022

Boretti, A., & Rosa, L. (2019). Reassessing the projections of the World Development Report. *Clean Water* 2, 15. DOI: 10.1038/s41545-019-0039-9

Bouwman, L., Goldewijk, K.K., Hoek, K.W., van der Beusen, A.H.W., Vuuren, D.P. van Willems, J., Rufino, M.C., & Stehfest, E. (2013). Exploring global changes in nitrogen and phosphorus cycles in agriculture induced by livestock production over the 1900–2050 period. *Proceedings of the National Academy of Sciences* 110(52), 20882–20887. DOI: https://doi.org/10.1073/pnas.1012878108

Bruntland Commission (1987). *Report of the World Commission on Environment and Development: Our Common Future*. https://

sustainabledevelopment.un.org/content/documents/5987our-common-future.pdf

Cardis, E., Krewski, D., Boniol, M., Drozdovitch, V., Darby, S.C., Gilbert, E.S., Akiba, S., Benichou, J., Ferlay, J., Gandini, S., Hill, C., Howe, G., Kesminiene, A., Moser, M., Sanchez, M., Sorm, H., Voisin, L., & Boyle, P. (2006). Estimates of the cancer burden in Europe from radioactive fallout from the Chernobyl accident. *International Journal of Cancer* 119(6), 1224–1225. https://doi.org/10.1002/ijc.22037

Carson, R. (1962). *Silent Spring*. Cambridge, UK: The Riverside Press.

Colburn, T., Dumanoski, D., & Peterson Myers, J. (1997). *Our Stolen Future: Are We Threatening Our Fertility, Intelligence, and Survival? – A Scientific Detective Story*. London: Penguin Random House.

de Chazournes, L.B. (2016). One swallow does not a summer make, but might the Paris agreement on climate change a better future create. *European Journal of International Law* 27(2), 253–255. DOI: 10.1093/ejil/chw028

de Sherbinin, A., Carr, D., Cassels, S., & Jiang, L. (2007). Population and environment. *Annual Review of Environment and Resources* 32, 345–373. DOI: 10.1146/annurev.energy.32.041306.100243

Diaz, S., Settele, J., Brondizio, E.S., Ngo, H.T., Agard, J., Arneth, A., Balvanera, P., Brauman, K.A., Butchart, S.H.M., Chan, K.M.A., Garibaldi, L.A., Ichii, K., Liu, J., Subramanian, S.M., Midgley, G.F., Miloslavich, P., Molnar, Z., Obura, D., Pfaff, A., Polasky, S., Purivs, A., Razzaque, J., Reyers, B., Chowdhury, R.R., Shin, Y.-J., Visseren-Hamakers, I., Willis, K.J., & Zayas, C.N. (2019). Pervasive human-driven decline of life on earth points to the need for transformative change. *Science* 366(6471). DOI: 10.1126/science.aax3100

Du Pisani, J.A. (2006). Sustainable development – historical roots of the concept. *Environmental Sciences* 3(2), 83–96. DOI: 10.1080/15693430600688831

Forousanfar, H.M., Alexander, I., Anderson, H.R. et al. (2015). Global, regional, and national comparative risk assessment of 79 behavioral, environmental and occupational, and metabolic risks or clusters of risks in 188 countries, 1990–2013: a systematic analysis for the Global Burden of Disease Study (2013). *Lancet* 386(100010), 2287–2323. DOI: 10.1016/S0140-6736(15)00128-2

GBD 2017 Mortality Collaborators (2018). Global, regional, and national age-sex-specific mortality and life expectancy, 1950–2017: a systematic analysis for the Global Burden of Disease Study 2017. *Lancet* 392(10159), 1684–1735. DOI: https://doi.org/10.1016/S0140-6736(18)31891-9

Gordon, L.J. (1993). The future of environmental health, part 1. *Journal of Environmental Health* 55, 28–32.

Gordon, L.J. (1993). The future of environmental health, part 2. *Journal of Environmental Health* 55, 42–45.

Hanson, A.J. (2007). *Global governance for environment and sustainable development*. Unpublished manuscript. Available at: www.iisd.org

Hippocrates (2020). *Airs, Waters, Places*. Available at: https://archive.org/details/b23983139/page/n4/mode/2up (accessed 4/14/2020).

Hryhorczuk, N. (2018). Radioactive heritage: the universal value of Chernobyl as a dark heritage site (2018). *Qualitative Inquiry* 25, 1047–1055. DOI: https://doi.org/10.1177/1077800418787553

International Union for Conservation of Nature (2018). *Marine Plastics*. www.iucn.org/sites/dev/files/marine_plastics_issues_brief_final_0.pdf

IPBES. (2019). *Global assessment report on biodiversity and ecosystem services of the Intergovernmental Science-Policy Platform on Biodiversity and Ecosystem Services (Version 1)*. Zenodo. https://doi.org/10.5281/zenodo.3831674

IPCC (Intergovernmental Panel on Climate Change) (2018). *Global Warming of 1.5°C*. Available at: www.ipcc.ch/sr15/

Isbell, F., Gonzalez, A., Loreau, M., Cowles, J., Diaz, S., Hector, A., Mace, G.M., Wardle, D.A., O'Connor, M.I., Duffy, J.E., Turnbull, L.A., Thompson, P.L., & Lariguaderie, A. (2017). Linking the influence and dependence of people on biodiversity across scales. *Nature* 546(7656), 65–72. DOI: 10.1038/nature22899

Jambeck, J.R., Geyer, R., Wilcox, C., Siegler, T.R., Perryman, M., Andrady, A., Narayan, R., & Law, K.L. (2015). Plastic waste inputs from land into the ocean. *Science* 347, 768–771. DOI: 10.1126/science.1260352

Kite-Powell, H.L., Fleming, L.E., Backer, L.C., Faustman, E.M., Hoagland, P., Tsuchiya, A., Younglove, L.R., Wilcox, B.A., & Gast, R.J. (2008). Linking the oceans to public health: current efforts and future directions. *Environmental Health* 7, S6 https://doi.org/10.1186/1476-069X-7-S2-S

Kotchian, S. (1997). Perspectives on the place of environmental health and protection in public health and public health agencies. *Annual Review of Public Health* 18, 245–259.

Landrigan, P.J. (2016). Children's environmental health: a brief history. *Academic Pediatrics* 16(1), 1–9. DOI: 10.1016/j.acap.2015.10.002.

Landrigan, P.J., & Fuller, R. (2016). Pollution, health and development: the need for a new paradigm. *Review of Environmental Health* 31(1), 121–124. DOI: 10.1515/reveh-2015-0070

Landrigan, P.J., Fuller, R., Acosta, N.J.R., Adeyi, O., Arnold, R., Basu, N., et al. (2017). The Lancet Commission on pollution and health. *Lancet* 391(10119), 462–512. DOI: 10.1016/S0140-6736(17)32345-0

Landrigan, P.J., Fuller, R., Hu, H., Caravanos, J., Cropper, M.L., Hanrahan, D., Sandilya, K., Chiles, T.C., Kumar, P., & Suk, W.A. (2018). Pollution and global health – an agenda for prevention. *Environmental Health Perspectives* 126(8), 084501. DOI: 10.1289/EHP3141

Lutz, W., & Samir, K.C. (2013). *Demography and Human Development*. New York: UNDP. www.hdr.undp.org/sites/default/files/hdro_1304_lutz_kc.pdf

Malthus, T.R. ([1798] 2004). *An Essay on the Principle of Population*. Edited with an introduction and notes by Geoffrey Gilbert. Oxford: Oxford University Press.

McCrink-Goode, M. (2014). Pollution: a global threat. *Environment International* 68, 162–170. DOI: 10.1016/j.envint.2014.03.023

McNeill, D., & Ottersen, O.P. (2015). Global governance for health: how to motivate political change? *Public Health* 129(7), 833–837. DOI: 10.1016/j.puhe.2015.05.001

Meadows, D.H., Meadows, D.L., Randers, J., & Behrens, W.W.W. III. (1972). *The Limits to Growth: A Report for the Club of Rome's Project on the Predicament of Mankind*. Washington, DC: Potomac Associates.

MIT (2015). *Mission 2015: Biodiversity. Benefits of Biodiversity to Humans*. Cambridge, MA: MIT Press. http://web.mit.edu/12.000/www/m2015/2015/benefits_humans.html

Moore, M.N., Depledge, M.H., Fleming, L., Hess, P., Lees, D., Leonard, P., Madsen, L., Owen, R., Pirlet, H., Seys, J., Vasconcelos, V., Viarengo, A., & Marine Board-ESF Working Group on Oceans and Human Health (2013). Oceans and human health (OHH): a European perspective from the Marine Board of the European Science Foundation (Marine Board-ESF). *Microbial Ecology* 65(4), 889–900. DOI: 10.1007/s00248-013-0204-5

Morin, J.F., & Blouin, C. (2019). How environmental treaties contribute to global health governance. *Global Health* 15, 47. https://doi.org/10.1186/s12992-019-0493-7

Morton, S., Pencheon, D., & Squires, N. (2017). Sustainable Development Goals (SDGs), and their implementation: a national global framework for health, development and equity needs a systems approach at every level. *British Medical Bulletin* 124(1), 81–90. DOI: 10.1093/bmb/ldx031

Murdoch, W.W., Chu, F.-I., Stewart-Oaten, A., & Wilber, M.Q. (2018). Improving wellbeing and reducing future world population. *PLoS ONE* 13(9), e0202851. https://doi.org/10.1371/journal.pone.0202851

National Academy of Sciences (1993). *Pesticides in the Diets of Infants and Children*. Washington, DC: NAS. www.nap.edu/catalog/2126/pesticides-in-the-diets-of-infants-and-children

Nii-Trebi, N.I. (2017). Emerging and neglected infectious diseases: insights, advances, and challenges. *Biomedical Research International* 2017: 5245021. DOI: 10.1155/2017/5245021

O'Connell, M.E., Scott, R.F., Roht-Arriaza, N., & Bradlow, D.D. (2015). *The International Legal System: Cases and Materials* (7th ed.). Sunderland, UK: Foundation Press.

Pauly, D., Watson, R., & Alder, J. (2005). Global trends in world fisheries: impacts on marine ecosystems and food security. *Philosophical Transactions of the Royal Society of London B: Biological Sciences* 360(1453), 5–12. DOI:10.1098/rstb.2004.1574

Petrini, C. (2007). Poverty, human development, environmental and health risks: the role of precaution and cautionary policies. *Annali Dell'istituto Superiore di Sanita* 43(4), 320–335. PMID: 18209266.

Prüss-Ustün, A., Wolf, J., Corvalán, C., Neville, T., Bos, R., & Neira, M. (2017). Diseases due to unhealthy environments: an updated estimate of the global burden of disease attributable to environmental determinants of health. *Journal of Public Health* 39(3), 464–475. DOI:10.1093/pubmed/fdw085

Ramankutty, N., Mehrabi, Z., Waha, K., Jarvis, L., Kremen, C., Herrero, M., & Riesenberg, L.H. (2018). Trends in global agricultural land use: implications for environmental health and food security. *Annual Review of Plant Biology* 69, 789–815. DOI: 10.1146/annurev-arplant-042817-040256

Ramazzini, B. ([1700]1983). *Diseases of Workers.* Classics of Medicine Library; Special Edition. ASIN: B0006Y63OC

Raudsepp-Hearne, C., Peterson, G.D., Tengo, M., Bennett, E.M., Holland, T., Benessaiah, K., MacDonald, G.K., & Pfeifer, L. (2010). Untangling the environmentalist's paradox: why is human well-being increasing as ecosystem services degrade? *BioScience* 60(8), 576–589. DOI: 10.1525/bio.2010.60.8.4

Ray, D.K., Mueller, N.D., West, P.C., & Foley, J.A. (2013). Yield trends are insufficient to double global crop production by 2050. *PLoS ONE* 8(6), e66428. https://doi.org/10.1371/journal.pone.0066428

Ripple, W.J., Wolf, C., Newsome, T.M., Galetti, M., Alamgir, M., Crist, E., … 15,364 scientist signatories from 184 countries (2017). World scientists' warning to humanity: a second notice. *BioScience*, *67*(12), 1026–1028. https://doi.org/10.1093/biosci/bix125

Rossiello, M.R., & Szema, A. (2019). Health effects of climate change-induced wildfires and heatwaves. *Cureus* 11(5), e4771. DOI:10.7759/cureus.4771

Saeijs, H.L., & van Berkel, M.J. (1995). Global water crisis: the major issue of the 21st century, a growing and explosive problem. *European Water Pollution Control* 5(4), 26–40. PMID: 12291371

Sandifer, P.A., Trtanj, J.M. & Collier, T.K. (2013). A perspective on the history and evolution of an oceans and human health "metadiscipline" in the USA. *Microbial Ecology* 65, 880–888. https://doi.org/10.1007/s00248-013-0181-8

Steckling, N., Tobollik, M., Plass, D., Hornberg, C., Ericson, B., Fuller, R., & Bose-O'Reilly, S. (2017). Global burden of disease of mercury used in artisanal small-scale gold mining. *Annals of Global Health* 83(2), 234–247. DOI: 10.1016/j.aogh.2016.12.005

Sullivan, M. (2015). Reducing lead in air and preventing childhood exposure near lead smelters: learning from the US experience. *New Solutions* 25(1), 78–101. DOI: 10.1177/1048291115569027

Tollefson, J. (2019). Humans are driving one million species to extinction: one million species face extinction. *Nature* 569, 171. DOI: 10.1038/d41586-019-01448-4

Union of Concerned Scientists (1992). *World Scientists Warning to Humanity*. Cambridge, MA: Union of Concerned Scientists. www.ucsusa.org/resources/1992-world-scientists-warning-humanity

United Nations (2019). *World Population Prospects 2019*. New York: United Nations. www.un.org/development/desa/publications/world-population-prospects-2019-highlights.html

United Nations (2020a). *Sustainable Goals Knowledge Platform, Oceans and Seas*. New York: United Nations. https://sustainabledevelopment.un.org/topics/oceanandseas (accessed 3/31/2020).

United Nations (2020b). *UN Water*. New York: United Nations. https://www.unwater.org/water-facts/scarcity/ (accessed 4/10/2020).

United Nations Department of Economic and Social Affairs, Population Division (2015). *World Fertility Patterns 2015 – Data Booklet* (ST/ESA/SER.A/370). New York: United Nations. www.un.org/en/development/desa/population/publications/pdf/fertility/world-fertility-patterns-2015.pdf

United Nations Environment Programme (2020). *The Sustainable Development Goals in Action. https://www.undp.org/sustainable-development-goals*. Accessed 9-9-2021.

United Nations Environment Programme. *Declaration of the United Nations Conference on the Human Environment. http://docenti.unimc.it/elisa.scotti/teaching/2016/16155/files/file.2017-03-11.7227158899*. Accessed 9-7-2021.

United Nations Environment Programme (2017). *Towards a Pollution-Free Planet*. New

York: UNEP. https://wedocs.unep.org/bitstream/handle/20.500.11822/21800/UNEA_towardspollution_long%20version_Web.pdf?sequence=1&isAllowed=y

Vasseur, L., Horning, D., Thornbush, M., Cohen-Shacham, E., Andrade, A., Barrow, E., Edward, S.R., Wit, P., & Jones, M. (2017). Complex problems and unchallenged solutions: bringing ecosystem governance to the forefront of the UN sustainable development goals. *Ambio* 46(7), 731–742. DOI:10.1007/s13280-017-0918-6

Weiss, E.B. (1992). In fairness to future generations. *American University Journal of International Law and Policy* 8(1), 19–26.

Whitmee, S., Haines, A., Beyrer, C., Boltz, F., Capon, A.G., Dias, B.G., Ezeh, A., Frumkin, H., Gong, P., Head, P., Horton, R., Mace, G.M., Marten, R., Myers, S.S., Nishtar, S., Osofsy, S.A., Pattanayak, S.K., Pongsiri, M.J., Romanelli, C., Soucat, A., Vega, J., & Yach. D. (2015). Safeguarding human health in the Anthropocene epoch: report of the Rockefeller-Lancet Commission on planetary health. *Lancet* 386(10007). www.thelancet.com/commissions/planetary-health

Winchester, N. Brian (2009). Emerging global environmental governance. *Indiana Journal of Global Legal Studies* 16(1), Article 2. Available at: www.repository.law.indiana.edu/ijgls/vol16/iss1/2

World Bank (2018). *What a Waste 2.0*. Washington, DC: The World Bank. https://openknowledge.worldbank.org/handle/10986/30317

World Bank (2020). *Poverty*. Washington, DC: The World Bank. www.worldbank.org/en/topic/poverty/overview

World Economic Forum (2016). *Global Risks Report*. Cologny, Switzerland: WEF. www3.weforum.org/docs/GRR/WEF_GRR16.pdf

World Economic Forum (2020). *A Decade Left: Confronting Runaway Climate Threat*. Cologny, Switzerland: WEF. https://reports.weforum.org/global-risks-report-2020/a-decade-left/

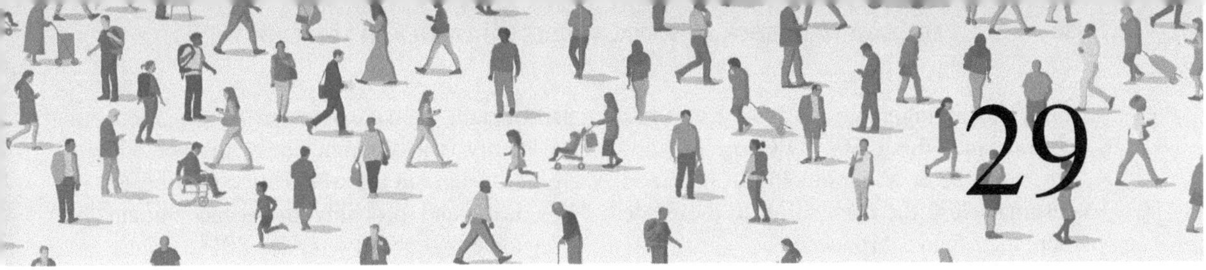

29

Connecting Human Health to Nature Health: The Bridging Potential of Sustainable Food Systems

Theresa Tribaldos and Stephan Rist

MODERN FOOD SYSTEMS AND THEIR IMPACTS

Modern food systems are shaped by an industrial rationale, resulting mechanization, uniformity, reliance on high levels of external inputs and specialization on few food, cash, and flex crops. This rationale applies to all parts within food systems, is interdependent, and creates a diversity of sustainability problems. Intensification of agricultural production at the start of the value chain comes along with high use of agricultural inputs such as pesticides and synthetic and mineral fertilizers to sustain large monocultures of commodity crops. These practices pollute water sources and degrade fertile soils, while biodiversity is shrinking not only among wildlife species but also in agro-biodiversity and soil microorganisms through hybrid and genetically modified crop varieties (Frison & IPES-Food, 2016). The lure of profits for larger businesses from commodity production and trade pushes agricultural frontiers further into forests and other wildlife habitats and increasingly replaces the diversity of small-scale producers (le Polain de Waroux, 2019). Furthermore, land use changes and fossil fuel intense production contribute a large part to global warming (IPCC, 2019).

Related to the intensification of agricultural production are impacts on food processing and trade. Increasing amounts of a uniform production of crops and animals require larger processing facilities to achieve economies of scale (IPES-Food, 2017). To lower prices, these facilities are specialized on few products and leave little room for small amounts of diversified agricultural production. Hence, decreasing diversity in agricultural production goes hand in hand with decreasing numbers of small-scale processors and vice versa. In addition, large amounts of the same crop or animal products cannot be consumed regionally anymore but are meant to be traded to other places of the world. Accordingly, world food trade has doubled since the 1980s (D'Odorico, Carr, Laio, Ridolfi, & Vandoni, 2014) and food consumers lose the connection to the place where their food is produced.

The next step in the value chain is the distribution of food, which is, in modern food systems, based on large supermarket chains. During the last decades, distribution of food has, similar to agricultural production and food processing activities, undergone structural changes from numerous small shops close to where consumers lived to large department stores often located in the outskirts of cities (Gottlieb & Joshi, 2010). These stores sell everything from food products to household goods to clothes. The food offer in such stores is rather standardized and looks alike in most places around the world. Competition among these stores for the best locations and market share is harsh and the constant struggle for cheaper prices has replaced smaller shops not able to compete in this game (Stanton John, 2018). The concentration of a few large stores has also had impacts on consumers and their access to good quality and fresh food depending on the places where they live. As a result, poorer neighbourhoods, who are not among the store chains' preferences, end up as food deserts – a combination of low income and low access to good quality food (Gottlieb & Joshi, 2010).

This concentration of corporate power can be found along the whole food value chain. It is evident with companies that sell agricultural inputs, fewer but increasingly larger agricultural producers, global commodity traders and food companies as well as large department stores and supermarket chains. Left at the end of the chain are consumers who are deluded into thinking that they profit from cheap food. However, this cheap food comes with a price paid for nature and societies. The most striking evidence that modern food systems fail to deliver their core task is human health and nutrition. While food systems are first and foremost meant to feed people with good quality and healthy food, the reality is a different one with over 800 million people in the world affected by food insecurity and probably the same amount of people by obesity (FAO, 2014). These figures are closely related to the seemingly vast variety of supermarket products. Many of these products consists of ultra-processed food items with high proportions of refined sugars, fructose syrups, saturated fatty acids and salt. These products create profits for the agri-food business, but they usually fail to provide healthy nutrition for people (Poti, Braga, & Qin, 2017). The fructose syrups also have especially strong negative environmental impacts as they are made of monoculture corn plantations.

In synthesizing the contexts and components of modern food systems, we find structural determinants sustaining these systems. The first determinant is corporate concentrations of power and small players without big lobbies. A vast number of producers around the world is confronted with enormous financial pressure to produce as cheaply as possible to compete in and serve global market rules. On the other hand, the concentration of power and influence in the agri-food sector increased along the whole value chain over the past decades to the extent that only a few companies worldwide control big chunks of the market (Clapp & Purugganan, 2020). The second determinant is an unequal distribution of capital among food system actors, which is of course closely related to the first point. The bigger a company gets the easier it is to set terms and conditions for other producers and prices, and to acquire new capital on the market. The third structural determinant is the governance and market regulations that often support these structures. For example, agricultural tariffs and subsidies distort market prices and make competition for poorer countries even more difficult (Anderson, Valenzuela, & Martin, 2006). Furthermore, subsidies are often not tied to sustainable production methods and thus, support unsustainable systems (Recanati, Maughan, Pedrotti,

Dembska, & Antonelli, 2019). Lowering or completely eliminating tariffs and subsidies would, however, not change the underlying logic of modern food systems, where food and labour is treated as a commodity that follows international market rules.

The state of modern food systems resembles a deadlock but, fortunately, different actors around the world are increasingly recognizing these problems and are working on alternatives to the dominant system we have today. Agency and resistance to it emerge out of the sense that the system is not in balance with nature or with cultural values and identities. People and even some governments increasingly claim the human right to food, which implies the necessity to also engage in deliberative processes to shape the way they produce and consume food in order to anchor food systems more profoundly within their own perceptions and expectations (Bessa, 2019). This agency manifests in movements of food justice, food democracy or food sovereignty, which are at their core recognizing injustices in food systems and demanding more self-determination to address and correct these problems (Dekeyser, Korsten, & Fioramonti, 2018; Glennie & Alkon, 2018; Patel, 2009). An important step in changing the current system is therefore to acknowledge that the world offers a huge diversity in terms of contexts, cultures, identities and, ultimately, ways of shaping individual relationships between the human and the non-human world. Food systems are at the centre of this relationship because they represent the inevitable link between humans and nature since all of us need to eat.

ASSESSING THE SUSTAINABILITY OF FOOD SYSTEMS

What is a food system? And how can we assess whether a food system is sustainable or not? This chapter will first offer a definition of a food system and its different parts. It will then go on to explain different dimensions of sustainability and justice that have to be considered when assessing sustainability within food systems.

Food systems essentially consist of all the resources, institutions, actors and their activities involved in food production, processing, distribution and consumption (Jacobi et al., 2020). To better distinguish what aspects of the food system are investigated, the definition of subsystems of the food system allows focusing on specific aspects. At the core of every food system definition is the food value chain or the operational subsystem (Jacobi et al., 2019). The first step in this chain is agricultural production, including the necessary inputs. Besides farmers and farm workers, companies that sell seeds, fertilizers and pesticides have to be mentioned here. The context for agricultural production varies strongly between regions. While over 70% of farms worldwide operate on less than one hectare, some extreme cases can reach the size of Austria (FAO, 2014). However, the agricultural input industry has undergone a pronounced concentration process during the last decades, where large international corporations almost completely dominate the market (Clapp & Purugganan, 2020).

The second step in the chain is the processing of agricultural raw products into lightly or ultra-processed food. Depending on the degree of industrialization in the food system, this step contains different sizes of processors from small or medium local and regional companies to large international corporations. The place of processing also varies according to product and the destination for consumption. Local food systems usually process their food close to the place of production and consumption, while products within large international commodity chains often travel around the world before they end up on consumers' plates. The same is valid for the third step in the value chain, the distribution of food, which depending on the character of the food system and the value chain can happen in local farmers markets, large supermarket chains or something in between.

The last step in the value chain is consumption and waste. Although food cultures are as diverse as the world, we can see a global tendency towards increased consumption of ultra-processed food items with high contents of sugar, fat and salt, and added with preservatives and flavour enhancers (Vandevijvere et al., 2019). The health impacts of this diet are well known and range from physical, obesity and related non-communicable diseases, to cognitive (e.g., memory performance) and even psychological effects, such as depression and mental health (Adams, Hofman, Moubarac, & Thow, 2020; Hardman, Kennedy, Macpherson, Scholey, & Pipingas, 2016; Khalid, Williams, & Reynolds, 2016). Furthermore, the alienation of consumers from food production in general and the homogenized international offer of similar food around the world also leads to a devaluation of food in monetary as well as in emotional terms. An outcome of this development is the high amount of food waste, amounting to one third of the food produced globally (Xue et al., 2017), which is, in view of resources used and environmental and social damages inflicted, ethically not acceptable.

Other subsystems, next to the value chain as the operational subsystem, are the natural resource base necessary to produce food, the political context setting the regulatory framework for food system activities, and the information and services subsystem relating to the educational system, infrastructure or logistics (Jacobi et al., 2019). While the resource base sets the context for what plants and animals can be incorporated into food production, the political context is crucial for setting incentives towards more or less sustainability in the food system. This subsystem not only sets the rules for how food production can and should be done, but also targets international standards for trade, and thus favours or impedes the circulation of certain food products. Eventually, the information and services subsystem addresses capabilities and the knowledge base within a food system and determines to what degree the system is able to adapt to global change processes, and which actors can keep up with these processes or are left behind.

All of these subsystems are important when assessing food systems' sustainability or their transformation due to strong interlinkages of food system actors and their activities, which are to a large degree influenced by different societal and cultural contexts. The complexity of food systems requires conceptual approaches that are able to capture the main sustainability dimensions of food systems. One such approach is the food sustainability assessment framework, FoodSAF (Jacobi et al., 2020). It covers five dimensions and is a co-production of a transdisciplinary research project with scientific and societal actors in six Latin American and African countries. The five dimensions are (a) food security defining the degree to which households have access to adequate and nutritious food during the year; (b) the right to food in terms of legal rights and provisions for guaranteeing food security; (c) the reduction of poverty and inequality, which is a crucial point for increasing food security; (d) environmental performance indicating the food system's impacts on the environment; and (e) social-ecological resilience as the ability of a food system to react and cope with shocks (Figure 29.1). A sustainability assessment with FoodSAF includes the definition and mapping of a food system, a discussion of indicators within the five dimensions and the negotiation of values for each of the indicators. Assessing the strong and the weak points within a food system facilitates the finding of entry points for improving the system's sustainability.

Another approach is just transition within food systems, which focuses on different justice dimensions in a transition process towards sustainable, healthy and low carbon food systems (Kaljonen et al., 2021). This approach works with the underlying assumption that the transformation of food systems addressing climate change requires fundamental

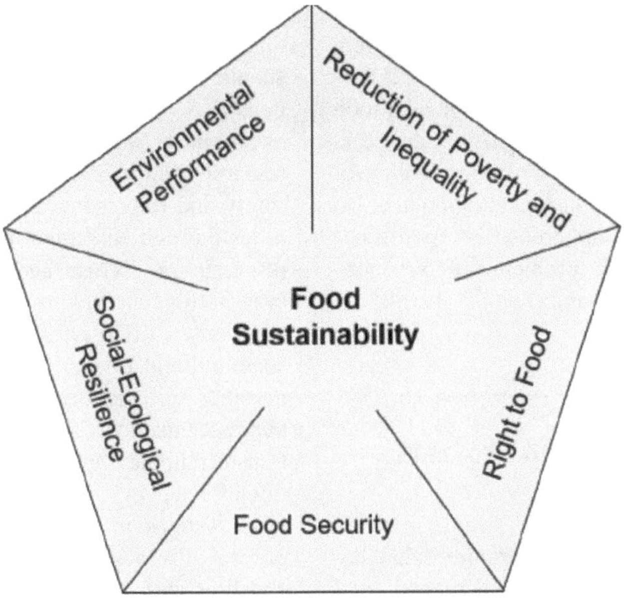

Figure 29.1 The concept of food sustainability with its five dimensions

changes in how food is produced, processed and consumed, and that these changes have to pay special attention to justice and inequality aspects. Current injustices as well as shifts in their distribution during the transitioning process need to be structured in a way that costs are not borne by the most vulnerable parts of society. The main justice dimensions in relation to food systems include distributive justice as the fair distribution of benefits and burdens among the different actors caused by food system activities. and procedural justice as the question of if and how underrepresented and vulnerable groups can participate in food system decisions. Finally, recognitive justice covers the representation of different cultures and world views in food systems as well as the value given to animals and the non-human world in general. Hence the just transition approach focuses on social, economic, structural and cognitive inequalities within food systems.

How food systems are approached conceptually also depends on different world views and the basic features and hierarchies they include. These world views relate to societal and cultural values and are based on fundamental understandings of human–nature relationships that shape our dealings with food systems. Modern food systems are related primarily to technocratic world views emerging from a Western scientific understanding that highlights the instrumental value of nature in serving human needs (Moseley, Schnurr, & Bezner Kerr, 2015). According to this understanding, problems can be solved with and through scientific approaches that build on established disciplines of knowledge. In a food system perspective, this feeds into increasing efficiency and production at all costs in all steps of the value chain (Fouilleux, Bricas, & Alpha, 2017).

A fundamentally different understanding of the existence of human, nature and the related meaning of food can be found in indigenous world views, which do not separate humans from nature but rather see one as an inseparable part of the other (Escobar, 2016). Valuing the non-human world and the environment as such, means valuing one's own existence. This results in tending to nature and animals instead of exploiting them. If nature shows signs of illness, it mirrors the illness of society. Consequently, food systems need to be embedded in nature and society alike. This holistic understanding of human–nature relationships can help us to find entry points to comprehensive approaches addressing both the problems of our modern food systems and health (Lemke & Delormier, 2017).

LINKS BETWEEN FOOD SYSTEMS AND HEALTH

Sustainable food systems require balancing the provision of food and other goods and services to humans and nature. As seen above, this includes considering that sustainable food systems are multidimensional and must simultaneously provide acceptable levels of food security, reduce poverty and inequality, contribute to the enjoyment of the right to food, build resilience without degrading the health of humans, and maintain high levels of environmental performance (Jacobi et al., 2020).

Although there is growing consensus about the need for a broad, multidimensional definition of food sustainability that integrates political, economic and ecological aspects, the specific issue of human health as an important dimension of sustainable food systems is not yet well addressed. It is well known that today over 2 billon people suffer from malnutrition (i.e., all forms from undernourishment to obesity), and that associated diet-related diseases are among the leading causes of death worldwide (Lindgren et al., 2018). However, solutions to diet-related issues of human health are still far from being resolved (Willett et al., 2019).

Linking health issues to the radical transformation of modern, highly unsustainable agro-industrial food systems towards social-ecological and political sustainability poses two challenges that we address in this section. First, sustainable food systems should contribute to optimal public health outcomes. Public health is understood here as an inter- and transdisciplinary field of research and action aiming at protecting safety and improving the health of communities through education, policy making and research for disease and injury prevention (van Teijlingen, Regmi, Adhikary, Aryal, & Simkhada, 2019). It takes account of the socio-cultural diversity of people and communities around the world. It therefore addresses health problems in close inter- and transdisciplinary interaction with communities affected by or interested in co-shaping food systems in such a way that they can prevent diseases and promote healthy food and lifestyles, based on justice, democracy, and freedom from oppression of powerful private or public entities (Williamson, 2019). Such a rather emancipatory and democratic approach to public health in food systems is especially sensible to the biases and power relations emerging from technocratic, top-down, expert-driven (corporate or government) notions of health. An emancipatory and inter-cultural concept of health can overcome materialist and Western culture-based understandings of health and disease and related notions of life, death and its links with meanings of food, eating and nutrition.

Second, due to the manifold entanglements of food provision for human needs with the related eco- and agroecosystems, a public-health orientation of sustainable food systems cannot be reduced to a merely anthropocentric notion of health. Many agroecosystem functions serving human needs are directly involved in the transfer of energy, nutrients, genes, species, and pollutants within or between agroecological habitats. This makes it impossible to understand human health as separated from the health or integrity of eco- and agroecosystems (Augstburger & Rist, 2020; O'Brien, Townsend, Hale, Sharley, & Pettigrove, 2016). In other words, integrating human and ecosystem health means adopting a relational approach to food systems as a dynamic and constantly co-evolving outcome of the unified web of life – an understanding of food systems that does not assume the classical ontological division of human and natural systems. Such an understanding includes all other related entities (i.e., minerals, water, gases and energy). A relational ontology of the food system offers an opening for overcoming the dualist ontological underpinnings of "scientific" food system knowledge (Goodman, 2002).

A "strong One Health" Concept as a New Dimension of Sustainable Food Systems

To address the above-mentioned challenges, we propose to use an enhanced concept of the "One Health" approach that gives systematic attention not only to the biological, but also to the socio-cultural and political sides of health. Hence, the "One Health" approach as a broad system of research and action as well as perspectives from human, animal, and ecosystem health (Rüegg, Häsler, & Zinsstag, 2018) integrates human and ecosystem health into one wider unity of a human–nature relationship.

Van Bruggen et al. (2019) stress the importance of maintaining ecosystem and soil health to keep the complex microbial communities associated with diverse plant communities and plant residues alive. Hence, by including the aspect of soil health, ecosystem health is defined as the result of complex biological networks of relatively healthy individuals and communities. In order to integrate the socio-cultural and political dimension of the concept of human and public health, we draw on the work of Ifejika Speranza et al. (2018), stating that the social sustainability outcomes of the "One Health" approach relate to the positive effects on the basic needs of individuals, such as capabilities and emancipation, environmental justice, solidarity and social cohesion. Making the social sustainability outcomes explicit allows linking the "One Health" concept to biodiversity (in terms of genes, species and habitats of plants, microbes and animals) and the bio-material world to the human side of health. This renders a conceptual framework of "One Health" going beyond the ontological separation of the human from the natural world, which, according to Beever and Morar (2019), would be part of a "strong One Health approach".

Pathways for Operationalizing "strong One Health" in Sustainable Food System Transformation

How can such a "strong One Health" concept become operational for the transformation of modern food systems in view of going beyond the separation of human and natural worlds? We propose to draw on three already existing fields of research and action. The first field is transdisciplinarity, which often relies on the communication between inter-ontological perspectives. The second field is food democracy in the search for integrating and enhancing spaces for deliberation to overcome power relations between key food system actors and to reach an integral democratization of food systems. The third field is agroecology, understood as a science, practice and socio-political movement.

Transdisciplinarity

We understand transdisciplinarity as a collective learning process of key food systems actors on the way to more sustainable food systems. At the centre of this learning process is the co-production of knowledge through dialogue (Rist, Chiddambaranathan, Escobar, Wiesmann, & Zimmermann, 2007), i.e., a process of knowledge co-production in which discursive, political, cultural or economic power is rendered less decisive by a process of deliberation, in which the better argument wins over the exertion of power of the dominant actors. A "strong One Health concept" implies creating equal opportunities for all the key food system actors for participating in the definition of meanings of "health" for humans and nature. This then represents the whole range of socio-cultural orientations. This means that plural notions of health can only be integrated through a transdisciplinary dialogue that is sensible to the manifold intersections of hierarchies between dominant and marginalized actors and their corresponding forms of knowledge (Rist & Dahdouh-Guebas, 2006).

Therefore, a transdisciplinary dialogue could start with spelling out common grounds, differences, tensions, contradictions, or conflicts between different understandings of how health relates to food in particular systems. The inclusive and inter-culturally sensible comparison of different health traditions and their links to human health and death, nature, and food is a first important starting point for transdisciplinary food system transformation.

Food democracy

In general, food democracy is a radical critique of the unilateral imposition of valuing food systems in the operation of large corporations and their varying but often strong alliances with governments. Food democracy proposes that all people should be able to participate in shaping food systems according to their own needs, values and aspirations, instead of those of only a few and powerful actors (Hassanein, 2008). However, food democracy does not automatically take account of the important political question if its principles entail having the right to co-exist along with agro-industrial food systems, or if they rather mean an active engagement across their knowledge systems, as it is proposed by those advocating for "cognitive justice" (Coolsaet, 2016). Assuring the principle of cognitive justice as part of the operationalization of food sustainability means linking the idea of transdisciplinarity to food democracy. This brings us to the second step in promoting food system transformation through dialogue between members of different food traditions. This step concerns co-producing visions, values and norms that should guide the collective action required for transforming modern, mainly technocratic, science and profit-oriented food infrastructures, food products and related institutions. The sustainability potentials of the cultural diversity of communities in concrete food systems build the normative core of this step, around which collective action towards food system transformation can unfold. This core needs to be based on inter-culturally (and hence inter-ontologically) inclusive definitions of visions, values and norms. In this regard, Adelle's (2019) four operational dimensions of food democracy are helpful.

The first dimension concerns the co-production of knowledge with stakeholders. It must include a democratization process of defining what type of knowledge is considered relevant in collective decision making in food systems. If corporate and techno-scientific dominance remains the most relevant cognitive reference in food system transformation, higher levels of political participation and deliberation are not automatically contributing to real transformation. In this case, powerful actors remain the gate keepers for what is regarded as "scientifically valued" food system knowledge ultimately constituting the main reference for food policy making.

Diversifying the definition of relevant knowledge in the context of democracy and the plurality of world views is hence required. This implies defining the relevance of knowledge not only based on an abstract notion of supposedly objective knowledge of sciences, but considering that any form of knowledge is a result of a social construction process. Replacing the notions of "objective" sciences with the more open criteria of socially robust knowledge is an important step forward in overcoming the bias of techno-scientific knowledge as the most prominent reference for carving out food policies (Nowotny, 2000).

The second dimension concerns the need for harnessing non-cognitive knowledge of food system actors in arts and culture. This refers to the insights, wisdom and cultural knowledge expressed in other forms than rationally reasoned texts or discourses. Adelle (2019) considers it essential to mobilize the whole range of the versatility of art genres. The representation of cultural knowledge is often a much more adequate way of harnessing non-cognitive knowledge than the simple participation in often abstract processes of political deliberation. This becomes especially important in non-Western contexts, in which food democracy and deliberation face severe difficulties if people are only allowed to express their own voices in rationalized reasonings, as a characteristic of Western styles of communicative action.

The third dimension is knowledge as a tool of action (Adelle, 2019). Knowledge is perceived as a powerful tool for translating insights gained from sharing food system knowledge to possible common grounds for normative knowledge into collective action. This is often related to taking part in social or political movements, which provide spaces for deepening democracy in the conduct of individual and collective daily life.

The fourth dimension underpins the need for overcoming the "monolithic understanding of knowledge that assumes individual ownership of knowledge enabling exploitative practices that can co-opt and distort indigenous ways of knowing" (Adelle, 2019, p. 219). This can best be done by recognizing that scientific knowledge is just one form of knowledge among many others. Although there are many denominations (e.g. indigenous, endogenous, lay or local knowledge), they show as a common denominator that knowledge can have legitimacy, although – or sometimes even because – it is remaining outside the strict and reductionist forms of knowledge creation of academic institutions.

Agroecology

Agroecology dates back to 1980, beginning in its first phase with the scientific validation of practices used for the biological control of insects in the older social movement of organic agriculture in Europe and Latin America (Altieri & Nicholls, 2017). It has been characterized until now as the historic evolution between and within the scientific community and the practice of engaging farmers and consumers, seeking to establish and develop alternative and more life-friendly forms of food systems in the face of rapid industrialization and later the globally dominating "green" Revolution. Wezel et al. (2009) therefore define agroecology as science, practice and a social movement. Through this, the interdependencies of knowledge creation, politics, resistance and practice are part of the current holistic ecological approach to food systems (Francis et al., 2008).

More concretely, agroecology as a science today offers a huge, differentiated body of disciplinary, inter- and transdisciplinary knowledge about the agronomic, economic, social, political, cultural and ecological challenges, and also many socio-technical and socio-ecological ways of how to address them in the context of the highly diverse array of food systems found around the globe. Research covers scales from local fields, farms, food systems' farming communities, networks and associations at national to global levels. The rich body of research is closely related to the growing number of communities of farmers, processors, retailers and consumers involved in the agroecology movement. It is important to be aware that the social and political movements of agroecology are not the result of agroecology as a science but the other way around. The main legitimacy and trigger of the existence of agroecology and organic agriculture as a science is due to the interactions these movements upheld since their beginnings with representatives of the scientific community. The main legitimacy of scientific agroecology resides in the support of finding concrete and practice-related solutions to agronomic, economic, social, political, and ecological problems that the social movements alone were not able to address.

Hence, agroecology is a field of science that very well meets the criteria of transdisciplinarity and food democracy (Méndez, Bacon, & Cohen, 2013). In contrast to research on transdisciplinarity, agroecology represents a network of different actors that have created considerable social coherence between steering the process of knowledge creation through strong global social and political movements (e.g. Via Campesina), and the needs of their members as practitioners and experts for mobilizing support and facilitation from science and policy in sustainable food system transformations.

Agroecology proposes organizing the process of transforming modern food systems by considering the following five steps. Due to the importance of these aspects for the discussion in this chapter, we cite some of the original text (Gliessman, 2016, p. 187 ff):

Level 1: Increase the efficiency of industrial and conventional practices in order to reduce the use and consumption of costly, scarce, or environmentally damaging inputs. … use industrial inputs more efficiently so that fewer inputs will be needed, and the negative impacts of their use will also be reduced. … considerable modern agricultural technologies, inputs, and practices have been developed. … Although this kind of research has reduced some of the negative impacts of industrial agriculture, they do not help break its dependence on external human inputs and monoculture practices.

Level 2: Substitute alternative practices for industrial/conventional inputs and practices. … replace external input-intensive and environmentally degrading products and practices with those that are more renewable, based on natural products, and more environmentally sound. Organic farming and biodynamic agriculture are examples of this approach. … nitrogen-fixing cover-crops and rotations to replace synthetic nitrogen fertilizers, the use of natural controls of pests and diseases, and the use of organic composts for fertility and soil organic matter management. … many of the same problems that occur in industrial systems also occur in those with input substitution.

Level 3: Redesign the agroecosystem so that it functions on the basis of a new set of ecological processes. … fundamental changes in overall system design eliminate the root causes of many of the problems …. The focus is on prevention of problems before they occur … Agroecosystem structure and function is better understood, and appropriate changes in design can be implemented. Problems are recognized, adjustments made in internal site- and time-specific design and management approaches … reintroduction of diversity in farm structure and management … ecologically-based rotations, multiple cropping, agroforestry, and the integration of animals with crops.

Level 4: Re-establish a more direct connection between those who grow our food and those who consume it. … those who eat must value food that is locally grown and processed, and support with their food dollars the farmers who are attempting to move through Levels 1–3. … Communities of growers and eaters can form alternative food networks around the world … Food once again must be grounded in direct relationships … farmers' markets, community supported agriculture schemes, consumer cooperatives, and other more direct marketing arrangements …

Level 5: On the foundation created … at Level 3 and 4, build a new global food system, based on equity, participation, democracy, and justice, that is not only sustainable but helps restore and protects earth's life support systems. … Level 5 involves change that is global in scope and reaches beyond the food system to the nature of human culture, civilization, progress, and development. … Level 5 thinking and action … provides ways to build upon farm-scale and farmer-driven change processes to a full re-thinking of how we all relate to each other and to the earth that supports us … expanding awareness … extends to other facets of environmental and social relationships beyond food …

CHALLENGES AND SOLUTIONS

We have seen that sustainability problems in modern food systems are multidimensional, multi-scale, dynamic and complex, and that solutions to these problems need approaches that are able to grasp this complexity. Besides the environmental, economic and social aspects, modern food systems are plagued by huge inequalities and the power relations sustaining them. In order to bring food systems onto a more sustainable pathway globally, concerted efforts to address these issues at different levels are deeply needed. However, there is not "one solution fits all". The solutions should be as diverse as our world, with its different ecosystems, societies and cultures, and the solutions must include a rethinking about the relationships between the human and the non-human world and the meaning of health in this relationship. Deliberative theory and practice, combined with food democracy, cognitive justice, agroecology and transdisciplinarity, are paving the ground for the contextualized and participatory bottom-up operationalization of food system transformation that is able to overcome structural core notions of agro-industrial food systems expressed in commodification, specialization and related simplification processes. Their impacts from the individual to the global level are not compatible with just, diverse, resilient and agroecological principles.

In order to better integrate the health dimension into the radical food system transformation, we propose to add a holistic way to rethink the relationships between humans and the non-human, by drawing on the "strong One Health" approach that allows integrating human and ecosystem health into a more comprehensive concept. Transdisciplinarity, food democracy, cognitive justice and agroecology steer us into the right direction. They help to implement deliberative processes that consider optimal outcomes in terms of a strong "One Health" approach. To create enabling environments, local and national governments, as well as the international community, have several instruments they can apply to steer the behaviour of individuals, the public and the private sector. Subsidies and direct payments in agricultural production and processing, for example, can give strong incentives for farmers and companies to produce in a more sustainable way (Piñeiro et al., 2020). Taxation and the labelling of healthy and unhealthy products are, on the other hand, incentives for consumers to consume more or less of these products (Lobstein & Davies, 2009; Niebylski, Redburn, Duhaney, & Campbell, 2015). And trade agreements eventually can support the trade of certain products through preferential treatment of sustainably produced products (Bürgi Bonanomi & Tribaldos, 2020). The question is then how these incentives are set and for what behaviour. Recommendations for healthy and sustainable diets must be brought in line with the sustainability of food systems (Tribaldos, Jacobi, & Rist, 2018), and the aim of any incentives should be to support healthy and sustainable solutions while punishing unhealthy and unsustainable ones.

The type of food system transformation outlined above needs institutional transformation of food systems enacted by governance regimes that unleash the transformative and emancipatory potential of actors and food partnerships (Coulson & Sonnino, 2019). Such an emancipatory-oriented governance of food systems is crucial in this aspect, and it needs connections to other policy fields, such as health, the environment, social security and the economy, and jobs to overcome existing siloes. Hence, policy makers and decision makers should put much emphasis on policy coherence when discussing food system changes and transformations. This is crucial if effective and sustainable changes are to be made.

However, policy coherence also involves more exchange and collaboration between different policy fields. Negotiations and compromises between their perspectives and goals are unavoidable, and therefore much focus must be given to the process of how compromises are reached. To bring the voice of marginalized actors into these processes, more democratic involvement should build the core – at local and national levels. If national governments make their decisions with the inclusion of marginalized voices, they also have a stronger stance and legitimacy when negotiating in international arenas. Vice versa, the international community can put pressure on national decision making towards more sustainability if a common ground exists. Transdisciplinarity and food democracy highlight the practicalities of local processes for realigning humans with the non-human world and research on these fields guides us around the challenges and pitfalls of these processes.

The introduced approaches and their pathways are not equal to a simplified discussion on globalization and de-globalization, which has gained momentum through the COVID-19 pandemic. Although a fundamentally changed, sustainable understanding of food and health will ultimately lead to more local food production and less commodity shipping around the world, its aim is not to support nationalistic tendencies. On the contrary, this holistic understanding of food and health extends to other systems of food and health around the world and acknowledges their interconnections and interdependencies. Receptiveness to other understandings of food and other understandings of culture can facilitate sensitivity for inequalities and ways to address them.

REFERENCES

Adams, J., Hofman, K., Moubarac, J.-C., & Thow, A. M. (2020). Public health response to ultra-processed food and drinks. *BMJ, 369*, m2391. doi:10.1136/bmj.m2391

Adelle, C. (2019). The role of knowledge in food democracy. *Politics and Governance, 7*(4), 214–223.

Altieri, M. A., & Nicholls, C. I. (2017). Agroecology: a brief account of its origins and currents of thought in Latin America. *Agroecology and Sustainable Food Systems, 41*(3–4), 231–237.

Anderson, K., Valenzuela, E., & Martin, W. (2006). *The Relative Importance of Global Agricultural Subsidies and Market Access.* Washington, DC: The World Bank.

Augstburger, H., & Rist, S. (2020). Assessing the capacity of three Bolivian food systems to provide farm-based agroecosystem services. *Journal of Land Use Science, 15*(2–3), 142–171. doi:10.1080/1747423X.2019.1651414

Beever, J., & Morar, N. (2019). The epistemic and ethical onus of "One Health". *Bioethics, 33*(1), 185–194.

Bessa, A. (2019). *The Normative Dimension of Food Sustainability: A Human Rights Based Approach to Food Systems Governance.* Towards Food Sustainability Working Paper 8. Centre for Development and Environment (CDE). Bern, Switzerland: University of Bern, with Bern Open Publishing.

Bürgi Bonanomi, E., & Tribaldos, T. (2020). PPM-based trade measures to promote sustainable farming systems? What the EU/EFTA–Mercosur agreements can learn from the EFTA–Indonesian agreement. *European Yearbook of International Economic Law (EYIEL), 11.*

Clapp, J., & Purugganan, J. (2020). Contextualizing corporate control in the agrifood and extractive sectors. *Globalizations, 17*(7), 1265–1275. doi:10.1080/14747731.2020.1783814

Coolsaet, B. (2016). Towards an agroecology of knowledges: recognition, cognitive justice and farmers' autonomy in France. *Journal of Rural Studies, 47*, 165–171. doi:https://doi.org/10.1016/j.jrurstud.2016.07.012

Coulson, H., & Sonnino, R. (2019). Re-scaling the politics of food: place-based urban food governance in the UK. *Geoforum, 98*, 170–179. doi:https://doi.org/10.1016/j.geoforum.2018.11.010

D'Odorico, P., Carr, J. A., Laio, F., Ridolfi, L., & Vandoni, S. (2014). Feeding humanity through global food trade. *Earth's Future, 2*(9), 458–469. doi:10.1002/2014EF000250

Dekeyser, K., Korsten, L., & Fioramonti, L. (2018). Food sovereignty: shifting debates on democratic food governance. *Food Security, 10*(1), 223–233. doi:10.1007/s12571-017-0763-2

Escobar, A. (2016). Thinking-feeling with the Earth: territorial struggles and the ontological dimension of the epistemologies of the South. *Revista de Antropología Iberoamericana*, *11*(1), 11–32.

FAO. (2014). *The State of Food and Agriculture: Innovation in Family Farming*. Rome: Food and Agriculture Organization. Retrieved from: www.fao.org/3/i4040e/i4040e.pdf (accessed 14 January 2021).

FAO, IFAD, UNICEF, WFP, & WHO. (2020). The *State of Food Security and Nutrition in the World 2020. Transforming food systems for affordable healthy diets*. Retrieved from Rome:

Fouilleux, E., Bricas, N., & Alpha, A. (2017). "Feeding 9 billion people": global food security debates and the productionist trap. *Journal of European Public Policy*, 1–20. doi:10.1080/13501763.2017.1334084

Francis, C. A., Lieblein, G., Breland, T. A., Salomonsson, L., Geber, U., Sriskandarajah, N., & Langer, V. (2008). Transdisciplinary research for a sustainable agriculture and food sector. *Agronomy Journal*, *100*(3), 771–776. doi:10.2134/agronj2007.0073

Frison, E. A., & IPES-Food. (2016). *From Uniformity to Diversity: A Paradigm Shift from Industrial Agriculture to Diversified Agroecological Systems*. Retrieved from: www.ipes-food.org/_img/upload/files/UniformityToDiversity_FULL.pdf (accessed 14 January 2021).

Glennie, C., & Alkon, A. H. (2018). Food justice: cultivating the field. *Environmental Research Letters*, *13*(7), 073003. doi:10.1088/1748-9326/aac4b2

Gliessman, S. (2016). Transforming food systems with agroecology. *Agroecology and Sustainable Food Systems*, *40*(3), 187–189. doi:10.1080/21683565.2015.1130765

Goodman, D. (2002). Rethinking food production–consumption: integrative perspectives. *Sociologia Ruralis*, *42*(4), 271–277.

Gottlieb, R., & Joshi, A. (2010). *Food Justice*. Cambridge, MA: MIT Press.

Hardman, R. J., Kennedy, G., Macpherson, H., Scholey, A. B., & Pipingas, A. (2016). Adherence to a Mediterranean-style diet and effects on cognition in adults: a qualitative evaluation and systematic review of longitudinal and prospective trials. *Frontiers in Nutrition*, *3*(22). doi:10.3389/fnut.2016.00022

Hassanein, N. (2008). Locating food democracy: theoretical and practical ingredients. *Journal of Hunger & Environmental Nutrition*, *3*(2–3), 286–308. doi:10.1080/19320240802244215

Ifejika Speranza, C., Wüthrich, T., Rüegg, S., Zinsstag, J., Keune, H., Boillat, S., & Rist, S. (2018). Evaluating the contributions of One Health initiatives to social sustainability. In S. Rüegg, B. Häsler, & J. Zinsstag (Eds.), *Integrated Approaches to Health: A Handbook for the Evaluation of One Health* (pp. 86–125). Wageningen: Wageningen Academic Publishers.

IPCC. (2019). *Summary for Policymakers*. Retrieved from: www.ipcc.ch/report/sr15/summary-for-policymakers/ (accessed 14 January 2021).

IPES-Food. (2017). *Too big to feed: Exploring the impacts of mega-mergers, concentration, concentration of power in the agri-food sector*. Retrieved from www.ipes-food.org/_img/upload/files/Concentration_FullReport.pdf (accesssed 14 January 2021).

Jacobi, J., Mukhovi, S., Llanque, A., Giger, M., Bessa, A., Golay, C., & Rist, S. (2020). A new understanding and evaluation of food sustainability in six different food systems in Kenya and Bolivia. *Science Reports*, *10*(1), 19145. doi:10.1038/s41598-020-76284-y

Jacobi, J., Wambugu, G., Ngutu, M., Augstburger, H., Mwangi, V. W., Zonta, A. L., & Rist, S. (2019). Mapping Food Systems: a participatory research tool tested in Kenya and Bolivia. *Mountain Research and Development*, *39*(1), R1–R11.

Kaljonen, M., Kortetmäki, T., Tribaldos, T., Huttunen, S., Karttunen, K., Maluf, R., & Valsta, L. (2021). *Just transitions in food systems: widening the research agenda for justice considerations in sustainability transitions*. Environmental Innovation and Societeal Transitions *40*, 474–485.

Khalid, S., Williams, C. M., & Reynolds, S. A. (2016). Is there an association between diet and depression in children and adolescents? A systematic review. *British Journal of Nutrition*, *116*(12), 2097–2108. doi:10.1017/S0007114516004359

le Polain de Waroux, Y. (2019). Capital has no homeland: the formation of transnational producer cohorts in South America's commodity frontiers. *Geoforum*, *105*, 131–144. doi:https://doi.org/10.1016/j.geoforum.2019.05.016

Lemke, S., & Delormier, T. (2017). Indigenous Peoples' food systems, nutrition, and gender: conceptual and methodological considerations. *Maternal & Child Nutrition*, *13*(S3), e12499. doi:https://doi.org/10.1111/mcn.12499

Lindgren, E., Harris, F., Dangour, A. D., Gasparatos, A., Hiramatsu, M., Javadi, F., & Haines, A. (2018). Sustainable food systems: a health perspective. *Sustainability Science*, *13*(6), 1505–1517.

Lobstein, T., & Davies, S. (2009). Defining and labelling "healthy" and "unhealthy" food. *Public Health Nutrition*, *12*(3), 331–340. doi:10.1017/S1368980008002541

Méndez, V. E., Bacon, C. M., & Cohen, R. (2013). Agroecology as a transdisciplinary, participatory, and action-oriented approach. *Agroecology and Sustainable Food Systems*, *37*(1), 3–18.

Moseley, W., Schnurr, M., & Bezner Kerr, R. (2015). Interrogating the technocratic (neoliberal) agenda for agricultural development and hunger alleviation in Africa. *African Geographical Review*, *34*(1), 1–7. doi:10.1080/19376812.2014.1003308

Niebylski, M. L., Redburn, K. A., Duhaney, T., & Campbell, N. R. (2015). Healthy food subsidies and unhealthy food taxation: a systematic review of the evidence. *Nutrition*, *31*(6), 787–795. doi:http://dx.doi.org/10.1016/j.nut.2014.12.010

Nowotny, H. (2000). Re-thinking science: from reliable knowledge to socially robust knowledge. In M. Weiss (Ed.), *Jahrbuch* (pp. 221–244). Zürich: vdf.

O'Brien, A., Townsend, K., Hale, R., Sharley, D., & Pettigrove, V. (2016). How is ecosystem health defined and measured? A critical review of freshwater and estuarine studies. *Ecological Indicators*, *69*, 722–729.

Patel, R. (2009). Food sovereignty: what does food sovereignty look like? *Journal of Peasant Studies*, *36*(3), 663–706.

Piñeiro, V., Arias, J., Dürr, J., Elverdin, P., Ibáñez, A. M., Kinengyere, A., & Torero, M. (2020). A scoping review on incentives for adoption of sustainable agricultural practices and their outcomes. *Nature Sustainability*, *3*(10), 809–820. doi:10.1038/s41893-020-00617-y

Poti, J. M., Braga, B., & Qin, B. (2017). Ultra-processed food intake and obesity: what really matters for health – processing or nutrient content? *Current Obesity Reports*, *6*(4), 420–431. doi:10.1007/s13679-017-0285-4

Recanati, F., Maughan, C., Pedrotti, M., Dembska, K., & Antonelli, M. (2019). Assessing the role of CAP for more sustainable and healthier food systems in Europe: a literature review. *Science of the Total Environment*, *653*, 908–919. doi:https://doi.org/10.1016/j.scitotenv.2018.10.377

Rist, S., Chiddambaranathan, M., Escobar, C., Wiesmann, U., & Zimmermann, A. (2007). Moving from sustainable management to sustainable governance of natural resources: the role of social learning processes in rural India, Bolivia and Mali. *Journal of Rural Studies*, *23*(1), 23–37.

Rist, S., & Dahdouh-Guebas, F. (2006). Ethnosciences: a step towards the integration of scientific and non-scientific forms of knowledge in the management of natural resources for the future. *Environment, Development and Sustainability*, *8*(4), 467–493.

Rüegg, S. R., Häsler, B., & Zinsstag, J. (2018). *Integrated Approaches to Health: A Handbook for the Evaluation of One Health*: Wageningen: Wageningen Academic Publishers.

Stanton John, L. (2018). A brief history of food retail. *British Food Journal*, *120*(1), 172–180. doi:10.1108/BFJ-01-2017-0033

Tribaldos, T., Jacobi, J., & Rist, S. (2018). Linking sustainable diets to the concept of food system sustainability. *Future of Food: Journal on Food, Agriculture and Society*, *6*(1), 71–84.

van Bruggen, A. H., Goss, E. M., Havelaar, A., van Diepeningen, A. D., Finckh, M. R., & Morris Jr, J. G. (2019). One Health-Cycling of diverse microbial communities as a connecting force for soil, plant, animal, human and ecosystem health. *Science of The Total Environment*, *664*, 927–937.

van Teijlingen, E. R., Regmi, P. R., Adhikary, P., Aryal, N., & Simkhada, P. (2019). Interdisciplinary research in public health: not quite straightforward. *Health Prospect: Journal of Public Health*, *18*(1), 4–7.

Vandevijvere, S., Jaacks, L. M., Monteiro, C. A., Moubarac, J.-C., Girling-Butcher, M., Lee, A. C., & Swinburn, B. (2019). Global trends in ultraprocessed food and drink product sales and their association with adult body mass index trajectories. *Obesity Reviews*, *20*(S2), 10–19. doi:https://doi.org/10.1111/obr.12860

Wezel, A., Bellon, S., Doré, T., Francis, C., Vallod, D., & David, C. (2009). Agroecology as a science, a movement and a practice: a review. *Agronomy for Sustainable Development*, *29*(4), 503–515.

Willett, W., Rockström, J., Loken, B., Springmann, M., Lang, T., Vermeulen, S., & Murray, C. J. L. (2019). Food in the Anthropocene: the EAT–Lancet Commission on healthy diets from sustainable food systems. *The Lancet*, *393*(10170), 447–492. doi:10.1016/S0140-6736(18)31788-4

Williamson, C. (2019). The emancipation of patients: a theory whose time has come. *British Journal of General Practice*, *69*(680), 150–151.

Xue, L., Liu, G., Parfitt, J., Liu, X., Van Herpen, E., Stenmarck, Å., & Cheng, S. (2017). Missing food, missing data? A critical review of global food losses and food waste data. *Environmental Science & Technology*, *51*(12), 6618–6633. doi:10.1021/acs.est.7b00401

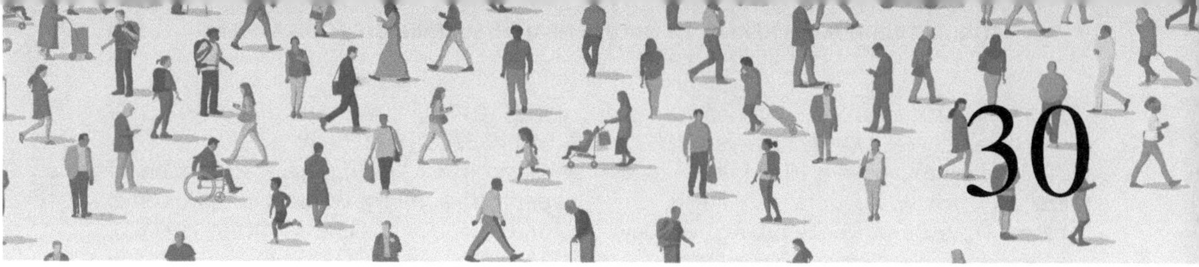

30

Syndemics and Structural Violence

Merrill Singer and Barbara Rylko-Bauer

INTRODUCTION

This chapter focuses on the relationship of two conceptions of social inequality, syndemics and structural violence, that initially emerged or were advanced within medical anthropology but were then broadly applied within the health social sciences as well as in social medicine and public health (Rylko-Bauer & Farmer, 2016; Singer, 2009). Structural violence focuses attention on the ways that structures of inequality, such as poverty, racism, and discrimination, negatively impact the lives and well-being of target populations. The syndemics approach, in turn, deals more specifically with the adverse interactions between two or more diseases or other health conditions, and the broader social and environmental factors – including physical and structural violence – that shape and synergistically exacerbate the negative health effects of any or all of the involved diseases.

One example is the syndemic relationship between tuberculosis and HIV infection, which share a common infectious strategy, interact in various ways to worsen the disease process, and are especially prevalent among the poor and socially disadvantaged (Singer, 2009). Despite several decades of medical awareness of the adverse synergistic consequences of these coexisting infections and despite significant advances in molecular diagnostics, this deadly duo remains a challenge for diagnosis (Méndez-Samperio, 2017; Scott, da Silva, Boehme, Stevens, & Gilpin, 2017). A more recent example is COVID-19, which appears to interact synergistically with other non-communicable diseases or conditions, such as diabetes, obesity, severe asthma, and respiratory and cardiovascular diseases, with serious consequences for morbidity and mortality (Stokes et al., 2020), especially in structurally vulnerable populations (Gravlee, 2020; Williamson et al., 2020).

Syndemics and structural violence both incorporate a biosocial approach to health and disease which stresses the importance of social, structural, and economic contexts that contribute to the vulnerability of disadvantaged populations. A fundamental aspect of these two concepts is the notion of embodiment: "how we literally incorporate biologically – from conception to death – our social experiences and express this embodiment in population patterns of health, disease, and well-being" (Krieger, 2005, p. 104; Csordas, 2009). It is for this reason that both concepts have been especially influential in medical anthropology, a field that considers the biosocial interface as manifest in the health of the bodies that comprise human communities.

Syndemics are found most often under injurious conditions of health inequality, such as poverty, discrimination, marginalization, and environmental injustice – that is, conditions of structural violence (Mendenhall, 2016b; Singer, 2009; Stall, Friedman, & Catania, 2007). In this chapter, we examine syndemics in the context of structural violence, a malignant relationship that has a grave impact on global health, human suffering, and medical practice. We begin with an overview of the latter concept, its emergence, relevant features, and its relationship to other forms of violence. Then we turn to a more in-depth exploration of syndemics, its theoretical development, the complexities of disease interactions, and the wide variety of already-identified syndemics. This is demonstrated with a case study of the cervical cancer/HIV syndemic, followed by a brief discussion of COVID-19. We conclude by examining the utility and multidisciplinary applications of these two concepts and offer some key points for health care professionals.

STRUCTURAL VIOLENCE DRIVES SYNDEMICS

Social disparities (measurable differences between population groups' access to social goods, resources, statuses, and benefits) are a "primary social cause of syndemics," because they create and sustain conditions within which coexisting diseases and health problems concentrate, flourish and interact (Singer, 2009, p. 124). Moreover, the strains they put on bodies makes them vulnerable to disease by weakening internal systems of immunity, recovery, and signaling. The causes of such disparities, when they are unjust, have been described collectively as structural violence. This concept underscores the ways in which social structures (i.e., the stable relations, institutions, laws, and policies that shape how individuals and groups interact and live within a society) can create unfair and unequal social conditions which result in the clustering of diseases and problems that lead to syndemics.

The term structural violence derives from the work of Norwegian sociologist, Johan Galtung, where "violence is built into the [social] structure and shows up as unequal power and consequently as unequal life chances" (1969, p. 171). Various Latin American critical theologians (Gutiérrez, 1983) similarly wrote about the great harm and violence caused by deep poverty, hunger, sexism, class, and racism.

These writings influenced the pioneering work of physician-anthropologist Paul Farmer, who introduced the concept of structural violence to anthropology and social medicine to address social inequities concerning diseases that disproportionately affect the poor, in particular tuberculosis and HIV-AIDS (Farmer, 1997, 2003; Farmer, Nizeye, Stulac, & Keshavjee, 2006). Farmer argues that such diseases – and more recently Ebola in West Africa (Farmer, 2020) – are best understood as biosocial phenomena shaped by history, geography, and political economy, as well as the biosocial context of individuals and their communities – often characterized by poverty, discrimination, social and political marginalization, lack of access to basic resources, and physical violence (Farmer, 2004). These structures of injustice "with their deep histories, become embodied and experienced as violence" (Farmer, 2010, p. 293).

The pervasiveness of structural violence in most societies, including the United States, is partly due to its embeddedness in the day-to-day working of dominant institutions, thus rendering it largely invisible (Gilligan, 1997; Scheper-Hughes & Bourgois, 2004). Structural inequities within housing, the labor market, education, health care, and the justice system – often positively correlated with poverty, racism, or disenfranchisement of select groups – may even seem a natural part of the social order. Such normalization may partly explain why the US is the only wealthy industrialized nation that tolerates lack of access to quality health care for a significant portion of its population, where approximately 27.9 million people have no health insurance, and 34 million of the insured have inadequate coverage (Collins, Bhupal, & Doty, 2019; Tolbert, Orgera, Singer, & Damico, 2019).

Unlike physical violence, which is often criminalized and punished, structural violence occurs with impunity and is often unnoticed by dominant institutions. This normalization is reinforced through social institutions and power structures that promote and sustain discrimination along various axes: ethnicity, race, gender, sexual orientation, religion, class or caste, immigrant status, disability, and age. In this sense, such structures and relations of inequality "can be seen as a form of sanctioned violence" (Singer, 2009, p. 33).

Labeling these social structures of inequality as violent underscores the damage they do by creating conditions that lead to greater human suffering through avoidable deaths, illness, injury, and disability (Gilligan, 1997), and by assaulting people's dignity and limiting their capabilities and agency (Hick & Burchardt, 2016). While these outcomes are "experienced individually, structural violence [like syndemics] targets classes of people and subjects them to common forms of lived oppression. Hence, the experience of structural violence and the pain it produces has been called 'social suffering'" (Singer and Erickson, 2011, p. 1). To put it another way, "social injustice is killing people on a grand scale" (Commission on Social Determinants of Health, 2008, p. 256).

A significant body of literature supports this dire assertion (Angel, 2016; Braveman & Gottlieb, 2014; Hahn, Truman, & Williams, 2018; Krieger, 2014). One example of global consequence is obesity, which is implicated in over 30 diseases, including COVID-19, often via syndemic interactions (Lighter et al., 2020; Singer, 2020; Swinburn et al., 2019). Obesity is disproportionately a problem of the poor and linked to malnutrition, due in part to lack of access to healthy foods (Lane et al., 2008). Instead, the poor buy less expensive and readily-available processed foods high in carbohydrates, fats, and sugar, and low in nutrition (Żukiewicz-Sobczak et al., 2014).

This is certainly the case in the United States, where persistent social disparities are reflected in significantly higher poverty rates for Blacks and Latinx, as compared to non-Hispanic Whites and Asians (Mather & Jarosz, 2014). Moreover, the gap between people at the top and the bottom of income distribution widened by 27% from 1970 to 2016 (Kochhar & Cilluffo, 2018). Such disparities translate into adverse health outcomes, including inequalities in mortality and life expectancy (Levine et al., 2001) for Black as compared to White populations.

The combined effects of racism and low socioeconomic status – often associated with lower quality of education, poorer diets, more stressful social environments, greater incarceration rates, residential instability, exposure to environmental toxins, low-paying jobs, stigmatization, and limited health care access – result in a disproportionately higher burden of disease (Franks, Muennig, Lubetkin, & Jia, 2006; Lane et al., 2004). This includes greater rates of preterm births, infant mortality, stroke and coronary heart disease,

HIV diagnoses, and tuberculosis case rates (Centers for Disease Control and Prevention, 2013). Beyond absolute poverty, studies have shown that relative social and economic inequality is also associated with worse physical and mental health outcomes (Angel, 2016; Commission on Social Determinants of Health, 2008; Pickett & Wilkinson, 2015). These expressions of structural violence can have a cumulative effect: "Inequalities at birth … reiterate biological inequalities in susceptibility to disease throughout the life course. Subsequent structural deprivations only add to the burden of risk" (Singer, 2009, p. 143).

Recent scientific evidence demonstrates that perceptions and experience of discrimination along racial/ethnic lines (Krieger, Jahn, & Waterman, 2017), as well as those of sexual orientation, gender, disability, immigrant status, and age, can have adverse and cumulative effects on physical and mental health through neurobiological stress response and other physiologic, cognitive, or epigenetic pathways (Berger & Sarnvai, 2015; Krieger, 2005, 2014). This is equally true for chronic exposure to social and environmental stressors associated with poverty (Braveman & Gottlieb, 2014; Mendenhall, 2016b), and the impact of such stressors may even begin before birth, threatening fetal development (Collins, David, Handler, Wall, & Andes, 2004; Lane et al., 2008).

Much of this literature has focused on individual experience and interpersonal discrimination, and "coexists with the still-dominant biomedical orientation, also focused on the individual level, which typically ignores social determinants of health and emphasizes genetic causes of disease" (Krieger, 2014, p. 644). However, there is increasing awareness that broader structural factors contribute both independently and synergistically to health inequities and disparities (Commission on Social Determinants of Health, 2008). Successfully addressing these disparities and the unequal differentials in power that sustain structural violence may require an approach that views health and well-being as a human right (Toebes & Stronks, 2016).

Structural violence is often linked to other forms of violence, as McLean and Panter-Brick point out (2018, p. 6372): "toxic social, political, and economic structures breed many forms of violence: it is thus unsurprising that, along the continuum of … forms of violence, we find that interpersonal, structural, and political layers of violence intersect." For example, structural violence can contribute in complex ways to preconditions for political conflicts and war (Singer & Hodge, 2010). The 1994 genocide in Rwanda had its roots in decades of colonial exploitation, facilitated by the construction of ethnic difference and Western development aid that ignored already-existing structural inequities, so that by "the 1990s, the interaction between structural violence and racism created the conditions for genocidal manipulation by the elites" (Uvin, 1999, p. 54). Similarly, the disastrous consequences of political conflict for families and communities are often mediated by pre-existing forms of structural violence, contributing to even greater post-conflict levels of poverty, racism, gendered-violence, and disease (Panter-Brick, 2010; Rylko-Bauer & Singer, 2010; Rylko-Bauer, Whiteford, & Farmer, 2009). Not surprisingly, "war has been a handmaiden of syndemics in many if not all regions of the world" (Singer, 2009, p. 174; Ostrach and Singer, 2012/2013).

Anthropologist Philippe Bourgois (2009) has also shown how structural violence intersects with other forms of less visible violence, most notably normalized everyday violence (Scheper-Hughes, 2007) and symbolic violence, which refers to the ways in which the oppressed naturalize the status quo and blame themselves for their domination. For example, internalized racism – when members of a stigmatized ethnic minority accept negative messages about their abilities and intrinsic worth – has been shown to have negative impacts on mental health (Mouzon & McLean, 2017). Symbolic violence also plays a role in intimate partner violence against women, where the victims question themselves rather than blame the perpetrator (Morgan & Björkert, 2006) and it is often used to justify interpersonal violence. In fact, structural violence and interpersonal violence often go hand in hand, with consequences for physical and mental health and the development of certain syndemics (Singer, 2009; Wies & Haldane, 2018).

What we see as the strengths of structural violence as an analytic construct – its flexibility, inclusiveness, and broad applicability – are viewed by some as limitations. One point of critique is that it is analytically vague, conflating different kinds of violence or serving as a proxy for other forms of injustice (Wacquant, 2004). Within medical anthropology, where structural violence has had the most currency, there are calls for refining this concept by paying attention to the complexities that characterize the lives of the poor (Green, 2004) and to expressions of human agency and resilience (McLean & Panter-Brick, 2018). This suggests a need for specificity with regard to the relationship of structural violence to syndemics: What structural factors are involved in a syndemic? What are the pathways of interaction between structural and biological factors?

SYNDEMICS: A RECONCEPTUALIZATION OF HEALTH AND DISEASE

The syndemics orientation emerged from ethnographic research conducted in the early years of the AIDS pandemic (Singer, 1994) and was shaped by the theoretical orientation of critical medical anthropology, which "emphasizes the importance of political and economic forces, including the exercise of power, in shaping health, disease, illness experience, and health care" (Singer & Baer, 1995, p. 5). The first syndemic to be described in the literature, known as SAVA, involved the interaction of substance abuse, violence, and AIDS (Singer, 1996). This work began in 1988 during the study of injection drug use in Hartford, Connecticut, within the context of the US inner-city health crisis, comprised of a set of closely interrelated epidemic and endemic diseases and social conditions (e.g., HIV, TB, STDs, hepatitis, cirrhosis, drug and alcohol abuse, and street violence). All of these threats to health are strongly influenced and sustained by a set of political-economic and social factors, including high rates of unemployment, poverty, homelessness and residential overcrowding, substandard nutrition, infrastructural deterioration and loss of quality housing stock, forced geographic mobility, family breakup and disruption of social support networks, health care inequality, and violence associated with the illicit drug economy.

Thus, a syndemic is specifically defined as a biosocial grouping of intertwined diseases that work synergistically to significantly affect the overall health status of a population because of noxious social or socially-generated environmental conditions that promote the clustering of such diseases. The term derives from combining the Greek words *synergos* (meaning two or more agents working together to create a greater effect than the sum of each working alone) and *demos* (meaning people). Syndemics involves both biological deleterious interaction (bio-bio) of two or more diseases or other physical or mental health conditions (e.g., malnutrition or depression), and bio-social interaction between these diseases and the social and physical environments of affected populations.

In the SAVA syndemic, for example, AIDS, drug use, and violence (especially domestic or intimate-partner violence as well as childhood sexual abuse) "are so entwined with each other and each is so significantly shaped by the presence of the other two that if one tries to understand them as distinct … it is hard to conceive of them accurately." In addition, "the actual expression of a SAVA syndemic is shaped as well by local social context," which all too often involves the structural violence of poverty, discrimination, and blocked social advancement (Singer, 2009, p. 31). Another example is the VIDDA syndemic that describes how violence, stresses of immigration, depression, type 2 diabetes, and abuse mutually interact to negatively impact the health of Mexican immigrant women in the US (Mendenhall, 2016b).

The existence of comorbidity – the occurrence of two or more diseases or disorders at the same time in a patient – is well recognized in biomedicine (van der Aa, van den Broeke, Stronks, & Plochg, 2017), but not all co-occurring conditions interact and some interactions, such as those between the common cold and influenza, appear to be countersyndemic. In many instances, however, when diseases come together in individuals or in a population, the outcomes are neither neutral nor positive. A syndemic perspective goes beyond awareness of comorbidity to focus on the interactions between these co-existing conditions (Mendenhall, 2016a), including gene mutations, as seen in Knudson's (1971) "two-hit" hypothesis for retinoblastoma and several other cancers. Furthermore, "comorbidity research tends to focus on the nosological issues of boundaries and overlap of diagnoses, whereas syndemic research focuses on communities experiencing cooccurring epidemics that additively increase negative health consequences … [and] on health disparities and the social conditions that perpetrate them" (Mustanski, Garofalo, Herrick, & Donenberg, 2007, p. 38).

Patients with multiple health problems experience burdensome issues in the self-management of their conditions and present significant challenges to health care providers. As reported by Zulman et al. (2014, p. 531), there is a "shortage of clinical trial evidence describing interactions among conditions and treatments in patients with multimorbidity." Moreover, such patients have problems accessing health care because it is not clear to them where they should go and whom they should see. These patients experience a lack of guidance in navigating the medical system, feel unqualified to manage their multiple difficulties alone, and desire a greater degree of assistance (van der Aa et al., 2017).

Problem areas that arise in such cases include medical complexity, the management of polypharmacy, prioritization of treatment of comorbid conditions, reduction of treatment efficacies, lack of time availability to attend to multiple ailments due to payer mandates, and treatment guidelines that are geared to single diseases. Physicians report that treating patients with several serious conditions is "a constant struggle" and "soul destroying" (McNamara et al., 2017; O'Brien, Wyke, Guthrie, Watt, & Mercer, 2011). Moreover, some comorbidities (e.g., restless legs syndrome in psoriasis) are unexpected although they have been shown to occur in statistically significant association (Schell et al., 2015).

Adding to the challenge are cases where multiple diseases are not only co-present but also interact. One example already mentioned is the complex interaction often found between HIV and tuberculosis. Such interacting co-infections, also referred to as cooperative epidemics (Chen, Ghanbarnejad, & Brockmann, 2017), are a frequent aspect of syndemic formation and can lead to explosive contagion.

The term syndemic is sometimes misapplied to cases lacking identified disease interaction (Mendenhall & Singer, 2019; Singer, Bulled, Ostrach, & Mendenhall, 2017), but such interaction is a defining feature of these socially determined global threats to health. Interaction can be unidirectional (one comorbid disease adversely promotes another), bidirectional (two diseases are mutually enhanced by their interaction), and multidirectional (multiple interactions occur in a set of multimorbid conditions). In addition, the interactions are not limited to infectious agents. They can also occur between a disease agent and a health condition (e.g., AIDS and malnutrition or type 2 diabetes and hepatitis C viral infection); or between two non-infectious health conditions (e.g., kidney and cardiovascular diseases or type 1 diabetes and bulimia). The complexity of syndemics cuts across and blurs boundaries between traditional biomedical disease classifications, such as chronic versus acute conditions, behavioral versus physical disorders, infectious versus non-infectious diseases (Singer, 2009).

While the initially described SAVA syndemic continues as an enduring problem of concern (Gilbert et al., 2015; Jones et al., 2019), many other types of behavioral and physical health conditions and diseases have since been identified in syndemic interactions with a wide range of pathways involved in these interactions. These pathways and mechanisms of interaction include the following:

- Access promotion, where one disease facilitates the capacity of another disease – or its agent – to enter and gain access to vulnerable areas of the body, as occurs in the interaction of STIs and HIV.
- Enhanced virulence, where one disease promotes the severity and harmfulness of another, which, in pathogens, can lead to the emergence of a hypervirulent parasite strategy (Alizon & Van Baalen, 2008).
- Alteration of the physical body, where one disease enables another by inducing changes, such as modulation of immune system components, cellular signaling capacity, the integrity of organ systems, and changes in biochemistry, as seen in the role of residual cavities in the upper lobes of the lung caused by tuberculosis and subsequent pulmonary infection by the fungus Aspergillus fumigatus.
- Gene assortment, which promotes disease development through the movement of genes from one strain or subtype of a microorganism to another strain, or the movement of genes across species, as occurred in the triple assortment of viruses involving genes from avian, human and swine influenza viruses in the 2009 H1N1 influenza pandemic.
- Mediation through social behavior, as seen in the diabulimia syndemic, which involves interaction between diabetes and the food disorder, bulimia, where diabetic individuals suffering from bulimia limit their insulin intake to lose weight or minimize weight gain. This occurs within the social context of corporate promotion of a cultural ideal of thinness and of products aimed to achieve this ideal.
- Ecosyndemic interactions triggered by anthropogenic environmental or climatic changes, as seen in the increased likelihood of respiratory disease comorbidity and disease interaction in a time of global warming, or the increased possibility for novel interactions among existing diseases (Bulled, Singer, & Dillingham, 2014).
- Iatrogenic effects, in which clinical intervention for one disease either hampers the treatment of or promotes another disease. This occurred during the clinical trial testing of the efficacy of a prototype HIV vaccine called V520 that possibly resulted in increased risk for HIV infection among participants who were immune to the common cold virus adenovirus type 5 (Hunter, 2010).

Identifying and describing the actual pathways of disease interaction, rather than simply asserting interaction based on multi-disease clustering and enhanced adverse outcomes, is a vital component of syndemic analysis. The following case study demonstrates how the interaction of three different diseases, via several pathways, creates a syndemic that is the cause of significant morbidity and mortality for women worldwide.

CASE STUDY: CERVICAL CANCER/HIV SYNDEMIC

Cancer, a chronic health condition, is the second leading cause of death globally, and was a factor in the deaths of an estimated 9.6 million people in 2018 (World Health Organization, 2018). Receiving a cancer diagnosis commonly provokes intense fear, personal existential crisis, and cancer fatalism, because the disease is bound up in culturally constructed life and death metaphors (Ogle, Swanson, Woods, & Azzouz, 2000). Complicating a cancer diagnosis even further is the presence of comorbid conditions. In a comparison of over 15,000 cancer cases conducted in Detroit, researchers found that comorbidity was present in over 68% (Ogle et al., 2000). Research in Kentucky and in Germany, respectively, found that nearly two-thirds of patients had evidence of at least one comorbidity with survival rates dropping with increased comorbidity burden, and that severe comorbidity is significantly related to the duration of patient survival (Wedding et al., 2007). All cancers are not equal and the effect of comorbidity differs by cancer site and by the type of comorbidities present (Patnaik, Byers, Diguiseppi, Denberg, & Dabelea, 2011).

In the decades preceding the 1960s, diseases were sharply divided into two different sets of human maladies, chronic and infectious. Cancers were firmly established as chronic, noncontagious, nonpathogenic diseases. The American Cancer Society (2019) states on its website that a "healthy person cannot 'catch' cancer from someone who has it," but also allows that "some forms of cancer are found more often in people who are infected with certain viruses." Included on the list of pathogens that are associated with cancers of the cervix, vagina, vulva, penis, anus, and some cancers of the mouth, throat, head, and neck is human papilloma viruses (HPVs). HPVs are the most common sexually transmitted infection and the most common source of viral infection of the reproductive tract.

Cervical cancer, which is almost always associated with HPVs, is the fourth most commonly occurring cancer in women, the fourth most common cause of cancer-related death in women, and the eighth most commonly occurring cancer overall (Bray et al., 2018). Socioeconomic factors are known to negatively influence cervical cancer outcomes. In the US, Black women, for example, have a greater cervical cancer incidence and a higher risk of diagnosis of cervical cancer at advanced stage than White women (Powell et al., 2018). While an HPV vaccine exists, girls in higher poverty states are less likely to be vaccinated (Pruitt & Schoolman, 2010).

Globally, rates of incidence for and mortality from cervical cancer are greater among women living in low-income as compared to high-income countries. Additionally, HPV and HIV are known to interact with adverse outcomes (International Agency for Research on Cancer, 2012). In Brazil, a world leader in the incidence of HPV, co-infection with HIV is highest in non-White women with low education levels (Gaspar, Quintana, Reis, & Gir, 2015). Research in Nigeria indicates that even among health care professionals, awareness concerning HPV, HPV vaccine, and the risks for cervical cancer remains low (Bisi-Onyemaechi, Chikani, & Nduagubam, 2018).

Evidence of a cervical cancer/HIV syndemic has been produced by multiple studies. Research indicates that HIV-positive women face an increased risk of HPV infection, precancerous lesions, cervical cancer, and HPV-associated mortality compared to HIV-negative women with HPV infection (Tartaglia et al., 2017; Whitham et al., 2017). Meta-analyses of the literature on the impact of HIV on HPV natural history have found that HIV-positive women are up to eight times more likely to have cervical cancer than HIV-negative women (Liu, Sharma, Tan, & Barnabas, 2018). This may be in part due to the modifying effect of HIV on HPV pathogenesis. This effect appears to occur because immunosuppression related to HIV infection – particularly the destruction of CD4 cells – plays a role in facilitating HPV acquisition during interpersonal contact, HPV persistence in the body, and progression to low-grade lesions (Massad et al., 2009). Factors that promote HPV persistence are of note because women infected with HPV for longer than six months have a greater chance of developing cellular changes that lead to precancer or cancer (Moscicki, Ellenberg, Farhat, & Xu, 2004). This pattern of syndemic disease interaction exemplifies how one disease changes body biochemistry in ways that facilitate another otherwise unrelated but co-present disease.

SYNDEMICS AND STRUCTURAL VIOLENCE IN COVID-19

COVID-19 is a particularly challenging syndemic (Mendenhall, 2020). While much is still not understood about the novel coronavirus, evidence points toward multi-organ-system involvement and syndemic interactions with a variety of pre-existing non-communicable diseases, such as hypertension, heart disease, obesity, and diabetes (Stokes et al., 2020; Williamson et al., 2020), as well as behavioral factors like vaping (Gaiha, Cheng, & Halpern-Felsher, 2020). This pandemic also demonstrates how structural violence drives syndemics. Social disparities and structural factors are playing an important role in the distribution of serious morbidity and mortality due to COVID-19 infection, both globally and in the United States (Centers for Disease Control and Prevention, 2020; Fisher & Bubola, 2020).

This virus has starkly exposed "the larger pandemic of racial/ethnic disparities in health" (Williams & Cooper, 2020, p. E1) in the US, where both cases and deaths from COVID-19 are disproportionately higher among residents of lower-income neighborhoods and among Black, Latinx, and Native American populations, many of whom live in poverty (American Public Media Research Lab Staff, 2020; Rodriguez-Diaz et al., 2020; Stokes et al., 2020). Such disparities are explained only in part by the fact that these vulnerable populations have higher rates for the diseases associated with severe COVID-19 infection and mortality. Equally important is the role of *pre-existing social-structural* conditions that reflect the structural violence of racism, social class, and poverty (Gravlee, 2020).

These conditions of COVID-19 vulnerability include: lack of health insurance, poor access to quality care, and historical mistrust of biomedicine; Blacks and Latinx are over-represented in many front-line, low-wage, "essential" jobs and do not have the privilege of working from home (Hubler, Fuller, Singhvi, & Love, 2020; Ray, 2020); a larger proportion live in high-density neighborhoods and multi-generational households, making social distancing difficult (Selden & Berdahl, 2020); people living in poverty rely on public transportation; and many poor urban areas are also places of high pollution, food deserts, and unreliable access to clean water – all of which impact immunity and increase risk of disease.

The US is not alone in having disproportionate rates of COVID-19 cases among disenfranchised populations. Ethnic minorities and immigrant groups in various European countries have been unequally impacted by the coronavirus, for reasons similar to those found in the US – poverty, crowded living conditions, use of public transport, and service sector employment (Leicester, 2020; Platt & Warwick, 2020).

This pandemic has also expanded to most parts of the Global South. In Latin America and the Caribbean, for example, where poverty, inequality, and fragmented health systems were long-standing problems, COVID-19 cases are rising sharply (Horton, 2020). In Africa, the pandemic and its economic fallout is decimating the middle class (Dahir, 2020). In fact, income losses in poorer developing nations are projected to exceed US$220 billion, reversing recent gains made in global poverty. This and other pandemic-linked factors may potentially cause twice as many people in low- and middle-income countries to suffer acute hunger by the end of this year, as they did in 2019 (Global Network Against Food Crises, 2020). In addition, many migrant camps housing a significant portion of the world's forcibly displaced people are located in these countries, where resources are limited. The conditions in these camps – overcrowding, lack of sanitation, poor access to clean water, and minimal health care – make social distancing and good hygiene almost impossible, thus increasing the risks of disease outbreaks, including COVID-19 (Kluge, Jakab, Bartovic, D'Anna, & Severoni, 2020). Similar conditions exist in the impoverished slums of major cities in the Global South, such as Dharavi, in Mumbai, India (Sur & Mitra, 2020).

THE ANALYTIC UTILITY OF SYNDEMICS AND STRUCTURAL VIOLENCE

Structural violence and syndemics are both concerned with individual suffering while underscoring the critical importance of broader societal factors and forces – also referred to as the social determinants of health and health equity – that interact in complex and often harmful ways to shape the social milieu within which individuals and families live. The structural violence framework challenges traditional explanatory models, including those in biomedicine and public health, that focus on individual-level proximate causes (biology, behavior, attitudes, culture) or on assumptions of power, agency, or choice for vulnerable populations. At the same time, it expands the analytic gaze to the historic, root causes of inequalities and the processes and relations that create and sustain them (Peña, 2011; Singer, 2008). It redefines the notion of risk by shifting attention to "the factors that put people at risk of risks" (Link & Phelan, 1995, p. 85).

Similarly, "addressing syndemics requires public health, biomedical, and health development models that move beyond individual risk, individual diseases, and individual behavior change" (Singer, 2009, pp. 199–200). And it encourages a focus not only on disease interactions, but on the social and physical conditions within communities that foster disease clustering and interface, especially in cases where structural violence plays a critical role in the generation of syndemics (Lerman, Ostrach, & Singer, 2017; Ostrach, Lerman, & Singer, 2017).

As noted earlier, both concepts originated or were advanced within critical medical anthropology, but their analytic utility and multidisciplinary applicability has since been recognized by scholars and practitioners of other disciplines (Rylko-Bauer & Farmer, 2016; Singer, Bulled, & Ostrach, 2020). For example, a project conducted in Ecuador during the cholera epidemic in the 1990s integrated ethnography, epidemiology, non-formal education, community participation, and a structural violence framework into a synergistic model of social change, with significant health benefits for the involved communities (Whiteford & Vindrola-Padros, 2015). Another case study, concerning environmental degradation, labor safety, and health risks associated with a chemical plant in Mexico, integrated structural violence, historical analysis, and environmental justice (Morales, Grineski, & Collins, 2012).

Structural violence has been especially relevant in examining how poverty, racism, or gender inequity became embodied or expressed as disease and illness. A number of studies have focused on how these factors increased risk for HIV infection or decreased access to prevention and treatment among vulnerable populations (e.g., Abadía-Barrero & Castro, 2006; Lane et al., 2004; Mukherjee, 2007; Shannon et al., 2008). A recent survey of the health and medical care literature also found significant use of this concept across a wide range of other topics and disciplines (Rylko-Bauer & Farmer, 2016).

The embrace of a syndemics approach, beyond medical anthropology, has been especially impressive (Singer, Bulled, & Ostrach, 2020). The concept can be found in the literatures of medicine (Clearfield, Davis, Weis, Gayer, & Shubrook, 2018), nursing (Dobbs & Fogger, 2018), and dentistry (Ryan, 2016), where syndemics research has shown how interaction among oral pathogens and malnutrition in a context of poverty and limited access to dental care diminishes oral health (Kline, 2012). Syndemics has also informed public health (Maju, Sharma, Beeram, & Ostrach, 2019), psychology (Parsons et al., 2017), epidemiology (Diderichsena & Andersena, 2019), and environmental health (Singer, 2016; Talman, Bolton, & Walson, 2013), among others. The concept has also promoted multidisciplinary collaboration in research and practice (Rock, Buntain, Harfield, & Hallgrimsson, 2009), including the examination of the role of social stigmatization in driving syndemic interactions (Lerman, Ostrach, & Singer, 2017; Ostrach, Lerman, & Singer 2017).

CONCLUSION AND KEY POINTS FOR HEALTH PROFESSIONALS

In this chapter, we have examined the relationship of two conceptions of social inequality, syndemics and structural violence, that emerged or advanced within medical anthropology and have had notable impact more broadly within the social sciences of health and beyond. Both syndemics and structural violence challenge the dominant biomedical conceptualization of diseases as distinct entities in nature, separate from other diseases, and independent of the social contexts in which they are found. Rather than individual diseases being the primary drivers of poor health in global populations that are subjected to structural violence, often it is syndemically interacting diseases that produce the greatest health disparities. A unified syndemics/structural violence approach examines the clustering of diseases within a population; the biological, behavioral, and other pathways through which diseases interact; and the ways in which social environments – with structurally maintained conditions of social inequality and injustice – contribute to vulnerability and disease clustering that escalates a population's overall disease burden.

Ten key points emerge concerning the relevance of the syndemics/structural violence approach for health care professionals.

1 **Syndemic awareness**: Recognize the deleterious synergistic interactions of two or more diseases or health conditions and the importance of social, environmental, or economic contexts that promote such interactions and worsen disease. For example, in discussing the standard clinical approach to non-occupational HIV post-exposure prophylaxis (nPEP), Morrison et al. (2018, para. 1) observe that clinical care tends to focus on biomedical aspects of intervention, "but may overlook co-occurring or 'syndemic' psychosocial problems that reinforce future vulnerability to HIV." Similar understanding of adverse disease interactions will improve global health responses.
2 **Structural violence awareness**: Gain awareness of structural barriers to treatment adherence and structural factors in disease promotion within the community. Be particularly aware of how these barriers and factors create conditions for disease clustering, vulnerability, and synergistic disease interaction in patient populations that are vulnerable because of poverty, discrimination, stigmatization, and injustice.
3 **Identify best practices for the simultaneous treatment of co-morbid conditions**: Entwined diseases tend to reduce treatment efficacies and increase treatment costs. Moreover, doctors do not have the luxury of practicing in one-disease silos in a world of co-morbid and syndemic disease contexts. As the number of patients with multiple threats to health increases, it is critical to assemble, teach, and utilize multiple disease treatment guidelines.
4 **Address patient issues in managing multimorbidity and syndemicity**: Anticipate patient uncertainty and the potential of multimorbidity and syndemicity to overwhelm patient self-management.
5 **Avoid iatrogenic syndemics** by considering suspected or identified co-present diseases in a population and possible adverse interactions of specific treatment regimes.
6 **Develop multifactorial models** that recognize the role of social and environmental factors in disease interactions and disease clustering.
7 **Remember that structural and physical violence often go hand-in-hand**: These oppressive

conditions create both positive and negative coping responses in affected populations.

8 **Focus on interrupting pathways and mechanisms of disease interaction to diminish** the potential for **negative disease interactions**.
9 **Develop comprehensive and multidimensional health care and disease prevention responses** designed to identify and address disease clusters in a population.
10 **Expand and refine syndemic/structural research** to enhance understanding of how social-structural conditions and diseases interact and the pathways of such biosocial interaction.

Finally, a syndemic approach "provides a very different orientation to clinical medicine and public health by showing how an integrated approach to understanding and treating diseases can be far more successful than simply controlling epidemic disease or treating individual patients" (Singer, Bulled, Ostrach, & Mendenhall, 2017, p. 947). It encourages a broader awareness of disease clustering and interactions within biological, environmental and social contexts, which can lead to correspondingly broad-based public health and policy initiatives.

REFERENCES

Abadía-Barrero, C. E., & Castro, A. (2006). Experiences of stigma and access to HAART in children and adolescents living with HIV/AIDS in Brazil. *Social Science & Medicine* 62(5), 1219–1228.

Alizon, S., & Van Baalen, M. (2008). Multiple infections, immune dynamics, and the evolution of virulence. *American Naturalist* 172(4), E150–E168.

American Cancer Society (2019). *Is cancer contagious?* Retrieved from www.cancer.org/cancer/cancer-basics/is-cancer-contagious.html

American Public Media Research Lab Staff. (2020, July 22). *The color of coronavirus: COVID-19 deaths by race and ethnicity in the US*. American Public Media (APM) Research. Retrieved from www.apmresearchlab.org/covid/deaths-by-race

Angel, R. J. (2016). Social class, poverty and the unequal burden of illness and death. In D. Brady & L. M. Burton (Eds.), *The Oxford handbook of the social science of poverty* (pp. 660–683). New York: Oxford University Press.

Berger, M., & Sarnyai, Z. (2015). "More than skin deep": Stress neurobiology and mental health consequences of racial discrimination. *Stress* 18(1), 1–10.

Bisi-Onyemaechi, A. I., Chikani, U. N., & Nduagubam, O. (2018). Reducing incidence of cervical cancer: Knowledge and attitudes of caregivers in Nigerian city to human papilloma virus vaccination. *Infectious Agents and Cancer* 13(29). https://doi.org/10.1186/s13027-018-0202-9

Bourgois, P. (2009). Recognizing invisible violence: A thirty-year ethnographic retrospective. In B. Rylko-Bauer, L. Whiteford, & P. Farmer (Eds.), *Global health in times of violence* (pp. 17–40). Santa Fe, NM: School for Advanced Research Press.

Braveman, P., & Gottlieb, L. (2014). The social determinants of health: It's time to consider the causes of the causes. *Public Health Reports* 129(Suppl 2), 19–31.

Bray, F., Ferlay, J., Soerjomataram, I., Siegel, R. L., Torre, L. A., & Jemal, A. (2018). Global cancer statistics 2018: GLOBOCAN estimates of incidence and mortality worldwide for 36 cancers in 185 countries. *CA Cancer Journal for Clinicians* 68(6), 394–424.

Bulled, N., Singer, M., & Dillingham, R. (2014). The syndemics of childhood diarrhea: A biosocial perspective on efforts to combat global inequities in diarrhea-related morbidity and mortality. *Global Public Health* 9(7), 841–853.

Centers for Disease Control and Prevention. (2013). CDC health disparities and inequalities report – United States, 2013. *Morbidity and Mortality Weekly Report* 62(3), 1–186.

Centers for Disease Control and Prevention. (2020, June 25). *COVID-19 in racial and ethnic minority groups*. Retrieved from https://stacks.cdc.gov/view/cdc/89820

Chen, L., Ghanbarnejad, F., & Brockmann, D. (2017). Fundamental properties of cooperative contagion processes. *New Journal of Physics* 19(10), 103041.

Clearfield, M., Davis, G., Weiss, J., Gayer, G., & Shubrook, J. H. (2018). Cardiovascular disease as a result of the interactions between obesity, climate change, and inflammation: The COCCI syndemic. *Journal of the American Osteopathic Association* 118(11), 719–729.

Collins, J. W., Jr., David, R. J., Handler, A., Wall, S., & Andes, S. (2004). Very low birthweight in African American infants: The role of maternal exposure to interpersonal racial discrimination. *American Journal of Public Health* 94(12), 2132–2138.

Collins, S. R., Bhupal, H. K., & Doty, M. M. (2019). *Health insurance coverage eight years after the ACA*. Commonwealth Fund. Retrieved from https://doi.org/10.26099/penv-q932

Commission on Social Determinants of Health. (2008). *Closing the gap in a generation: Health equity through action on the social determinants of health*. Final Report. Geneva: World Health Organization. Retrieved from https://apps.who.int/iris/bitstream/handle/10665/43943/9789241563703_eng.pdf;jsessionid=B860C85DDD8C42ABDC0979F3B9B0BAB4?sequence=1

Csordas, T. (2009). Embodiment as a paradigm for anthropology. *Ethos* 18(1), 5–47.

Dahir, A. L. (2020, June 29). Coronavirus is battering Africa's growing middle class. *New York Times*. Retrieved from www.nytimes.com/2020/06/29/world/africa/Africa-middle-class-coronavirus.html

Diderichsen, F., & Andersen, I. (2019). The syndemics of diabetes and depression in Brazil: An epidemiological analysis. *Population Health* 7, 100318. https://doi.org/10.1016/j.ssmph.2018.11.002

Dobbs, G., & Fogger, S. A. (2018). Caught in the crossfire of the syndemic. *Journal of Addictions Nursing* 29(3), 205–210.

Farmer, P. (1997). On suffering and structural violence: A view from below. In A. Kleinman, V. Das, & M. Lock (Eds.), *Social suffering* (pp. 261–283). Berkeley, CA: University of California Press.

Farmer, P. (2003). *Pathologies of power: Health, human rights, and the new war on the poor*. Berkeley, CA: University of California Press.

Farmer, P. (2004). An anthropology of structural violence. *Current Anthropology* 45(3), 305–325.

Farmer, P. (2010). [Introduction to part 3]. In H. Saussy (Ed.), *Partner to the poor: A Paul Farmer reader* (pp. 293–297). Berkeley, CA: University of California Press.

Farmer, P. (2020). *Fevers, feuds, and diamonds: Ebola and the ravages of history*. New York: Farrar, Straus and Giroux.

Farmer, P. E., Nizeye, B., Stulac, S., & Keshavjee, S. (2006). Structural violence and clinical medicine. *PLoS Medicine* 3(10), e449. https://doi.org/10.1371/journal.pmed.0030449

Fisher, M., & Bubola, E. (2020, March 15). As coronavirus deepens inequality, inequality worsens its spread. *New York Times*. Retrieved from www.nytimes.com/2020/03/15/world/europe/coronavirus-inequality.html

Franks, P., Muennig, P., Lubetkin, E., & Jia, J. (2006). The burden of disease associated with being African-American in the United States and the contribution of socio-economic status. *Social Science & Medicine* 62(10), 2469–2478.

Gaiha, S. M., Cheng, J., & Halpern-Felsher, B. (2020). Association between youth smoking, electronic cigarette use, and coronavirus disease 2019. *Journal of Adolescent Health*. https://doi.org/10.1016/j.jadohealth.2020.07.002

Galtung, J. (1969). Violence, peace, and peace research. *Journal of Peace Research* 6(3), 167–191.

Gaspar, J., Quintana, S. M., Reis, R. K., & Gir, E. (2015). Sociodemographic and clinical factors of women with HPV and their association with HIV. *Revista Latino-Americano de Enfermagem* 23(1), 74–81.

Gilbert, L., Raj, A., Hien, D., Stockman, J., Terlikbayeva, A., & Wyatt, G. (2015). Targeting the SAVA (substance abuse, violence, and AIDS) syndemic among women and girls: A global review of epidemiology and integrated interventions. *Journal of Acquired Immune Deficiency Syndromes* 69, S118–S127.

Gilligan, J. (1997). *Violence: Reflections on a national epidemic*. New York: Vintage Books.

Global Network Against Food Crises. (2020). 2020 *global report on food crises. World Food Programme*. Retrieved from www.wfp.org/publications/2020-global-report-food-crises

Gravlee, C. C. (2020). Systemic racism, chronic health inequities, and COVID-19: A syndemic in the making? *American Journal of Human Biology*. https://doi.org/10.1002/ajhb.23482

Green, L. (2004). Commentary on an anthropology of structural violence. *Current Anthropology* 45(3), 319–320.

Gutiérrez, G. (1983). *The power of the poor in history*. R. R. Barr, Trans. Maryknoll, NY: Orbis Books.

Hahn, R., Truman, B. I., & Williams, D. R. (2018). Civil rights as determinants of public health and racial and ethnic health equity: Health care, education, employment, and housing in the United States. *SSM – Population Health* 4, 17–24.

Hick, R., & Burchardt, R. (2016). Capability deprivation. In D. Brady & L. M. Burton (Eds.), *The Oxford handbook of the social science of poverty* (pp. 660–683). New York: Oxford University Press.

Horton, J. (2020, July 31). Coronavirus: What are the numbers out of Latin America? *BBC News*. Retrieved from www.bbc.com/news/world-latin-america-52711458

Hubler, S., Fuller, T., Singhvi, A., & Love, J. (2020, June 26). Many Latinos couldn't stay home. Now virus cases are soaring in their communities. *New York Times*. Retrieved fromwww.nytimes.com/2020/06/26/us/coronavirus-latinos.html

Hunter, P. (2010). Vaccine outlooks. *EMBO Reports* 11(10), 738–741.

International Agency for Research on Cancer. (2012). *Cervical cancer: Estimated incidence, mortality and prevalence worldwide in 2012*. Retrieved from http://globocan.iarc.tr/old/FactSheets/cancers/cervix-new.asp

Jones, A. A., Gerke, T., Striley, C. W., Osborne, V., Whitehead, N., & Cottler, L. B. (2019). A longitudinal analysis of the substance abuse, violence, and HIV/AIDS (SAVA) syndemic among women in the criminal justice system. *Journal of Psychoactive Drugs* 51(1), 58–67.

Kline, N. (2012). "There's nowhere I can go to get help, and I have tooth pain right now": The oral health syndemic among migrant farmworkers in Florida. *Annals of Anthropological Practice* 36(2), 387–401.

Kluge, H. H. P., Jakab, Z., Bartovic, J., D'Anna, V., & Severoni, S. (2020). Refugee and migrant health in the COVID-19 response. *The Lancet* 395(10232), 1237–1239, March 31. doi: 10.1016/S0140-6736(20)30791-1

Knudson, A. G. (1971). Mutation and cancer: Statistical study of retinoblastoma. *Proceedings of the National Academy of Sciences* 68, 820–823.

Kochhar, R., & Cilluffo, A. (2018). Income inequality in the US is rising most rapidly among Asians. *Pew Research Center. Social & Demographic Trends*. Retrieved from www.pewsocialtrends.org/2018/07/12/income-inequality-in-the-u-s-is-rising-most-rapidly-among-asians/

Kreiger, N. (2005). Embodying inequality: A review of concepts, measures, and methods for studying health consequences of discrimination. In N. Kreiger (Ed.), *Embodying inequality: Epidemiologic perspectives* (pp. 101–158). Amityville, NY: Baywood.

Krieger, N. (2014). Discrimination and health inequities. *International Journal of Health Services* 4, 643–710.

Kreiger, N., Jahn, J. L., & Waterman, P. D. (2017). Jim Crow and estrogen-receptor-negative breast cancer: US-born Black and White non-Hispanic women, 1992–2012. *Cancer Causes Control* 28(1), 49–59.

Lane, S. D., Keefe, R. H., Rubinstein, R., Levandowski, B. A., Webster, N., Cibula, D. A., & Brill, J. (2008). Structural violence, urban retail food markets, and low birth weight. *Health & Place* 14, 415–423.

Lane, S. D., Rubinstein, R. A., Keefe, R. H., Webster, N., Cibula, D. A., Rosenthal, A., & Dowdell, J. (2004). Structural violence and racial disparity in HIV transmission. *Journal of Health Care for the Poor and Underserved* 15(3), 319–335.

Leicester, J. (2020, July 7). In France, study shows virus hits African immigrants hardest. *AP News*. Retrieved from https://apnews.com/e926cfab68103a92d2c07152e8842853

Lerman, S., Ostrach, B., & Singer, M. (Eds.). (2017). *Foundations of biosocial health: Stigma and illness interactions*. Lanham, MD: Lexington Books.

Levine, R. S., Foster, J. E., Fullilove, R. E., Fullilove, M. T., Briggs, N. C., Hull, P. C., & Hennekens, C. H. (2001). Black–White inequalities in mortality and life expectancy, 1933–1999: Implications for Healthy People 2010. *Public Health Reports* 116(5), 474–483.

Lighter, J., Phillips, M., Hochman, S., Sterling, S., Johnson, D., Francois, F., & Stachel, A. (2020). Obesity in patients younger than 60 years is a risk factor for Covid-19 hospital admission. *Clinical Infectious Diseases* 71(15), 896–897.

Link, B. G., & Phelan, J. (1995). Social conditions as fundamental causes of disease. *Journal of Health and Social Behavior* 35(Extra Issue), 80–94.

Liu, G., Sharma, M., Tan, N., & Barnabas, R. V. (2018). HIV-positive women have higher risk of human papilloma virus infection, precancerous lesions, and cervical cancer: A systematic review and meta-analysis. *AIDS* 32(6), 795–808.

Maju, M., Sharma, A., Beeram, A., & Ostrach, B. (2019). A colonial legacy of HIV/AIDS, NTD, and STI super-syndemics: Eugenicist foreign aid and intertwined health burdens in Nigeria. *Global Public Health* 14(9), 1221–1240.

Massad, L. S., Seaberg, E. C., Watts, D. H., Minkoff, H., Levine, A. M., Henry, D., & Hessol, N. (2009). A Long-term incidence of cervical cancer in women with human immunodeficiency virus. *Cancer* 115(3), 524–530.

Mather, M., & Jarosz, B. (2014). The demography of inequality in the United States. *Population Bulletin* 69(2), 1–16. Retrieved from www.prb.org/united-states-inequality/

McLean, K. E., & Panter-Brick, C. (2018). Violence, structural and interpersonal. In H. Callan (Ed-in-chief), *The International Encyclopedia of Anthropology* (Vol. 7, pp. 6368–6375). Wiley Online Library. https://doi.org/10.1002/9781118924396.wbiea2028

McNamara, K. P., Breken, B. D., Alzubaidi, H. T., Bell, J. S., Dunbar, J. A., Walker, C., & Hernan, A. (2017). Health professional perspectives on the management of multimorbidity and polypharmacy for older patients in Australia. *Age and Aging* 46(2), 291–299.

Mendenhall, E. (2016a). Beyond comorbidity: A critical perspective of syndemic depression and diabetes in cross-cultural contexts. *Medical Anthropology Quarterly* 30(4), 462–478.

Mendenhall, E. (2016b). *Syndemic suffering: Social distress, depression, and diabetes among Mexican immigrant women*. New York: Routledge.

Mendenhall, E. (2020). Why social policies make coronavirus worse. *Think Global Health*. Retrieved from: www.thinkglobalhealth.org/article/why-social-policies-make-coronavirus-worse

Mendenhall, E., & Singer, M. (2019). The global syndemic of obesity, undernutrition, and climate change. (letter). *The Lancet*. https://doi.org/10.1016/S0140-6736(19)30310-1

Méndez-Samperio, P. (2017). Diagnosis of tuberculosis in HIV co-infected individuals: Current status, challenges and opportunities for the future. *Scandinavian Journal of Immunology* 86(2), 76–82.

Morales, O., Jr., Grineski, S. E., & Collins, T. W. (2012). Structural violence and environmental injustice: The case of a US–Mexico border chemical plant. *Local Environment* 17(1), 1–21.

Morgan, K., & Björkert, S. T. (2006). "I'd rather you'd lay me on the floor and start kicking me": Understanding symbolic violence in everyday life. *Women's Studies International Forum* 29(5), 441–452.

Morrison, S., Yoong, D., Hart, T., MacPherson, P., Bogoch, I., Sivarajah, V., & Tan, D. H. S. (2018). High prevalence of syndemic health problems in patients seeking post-exposure prophylaxis for sexual exposures to HIV. *PLoS One* 13(5). https://doi.org/10.1371/journal.pone.0197998

Moscicki, A. B., Ellenberg, J. H., Farhat, S., & Xu, J. (2004). Persistence of human papillomavirus infection in HIV-infected and -uninfected adolescent girls: risk factors and differences, by phylogenetic type. *Journal of Infectious Diseases* 190, 37–45.

Mouzon, D. M., & McLean, J. S. (2017). Internalized racism and mental health among African-Americans, US-born Caribbean Blacks, and foreign-born Caribbean Blacks. *Ethnicity & Health* 22(1), 36–48.

Mukherjee, J. (2007). Structural violence, poverty and the AIDS pandemic. *Development* 50(2), 115–121.

Mustanski, B., Garofalo, R., Herrick, A., & Donenberg, G. (2007). Psychosocial health problems increase risk for HIV among urban young men who have sex with men: Preliminary evidence of a syndemic in need of attention. *Annals of Behavioral Medicine* 34(1), 37–45.

O'Brien, R., Wyke, S., Guthrie, B., Watt, G., & Mercer, S. (2011). An "endless struggle": A qualitative study of general practitioners' and practice nurses' experiences of managing multimorbidity in socio-economically deprived areas of Scotland. *Chronic Illnesses* 7, 45–59.

Ogle, K., Swanson, G., Woods, N., & Azzouz, F. (2000). Cancer and comorbidity: Redefining chronic diseases. *Cancer* 88(3), 653–663.

Ostrach, B., Lerman, S., & Singer, M. (Eds.). (2017). *Stigma syndemics: New directions in biosocial health.* Lanham, MD: Lexington Books.

Ostrach, B., & Singer, M. (2012/2013). Syndemics of war: Malnutrition-infectious disease interactions and the unintended health consequences of intentional war policies. *Annals of Anthropological Practice* 36(2), 256–272.

Panter-Brick, C. (2010). Conflict, violence, and health: Setting a new interdisciplinary agenda. *Social Science and Medicine* 70(1), 1–6.

Parsons, J. T., Millar, B. M., Moody, R. L., Starks, T. J., Rendina, H., J., & Grov, C. (2017). Syndemic conditions and HIV transmission risk behavior among HIV-negative gay and bisexual men in a U.S. national sample. *Health Psychology* 36(7), 695–703.

Patnaik, J. L., Byers, T., Diguiseppi, C., Denberg, T. D., & Dabelea, D. (2011). The influence of comorbidities on overall survival among older women diagnosed with breast cancer. *Journal of the National Cancer Institute* 103(14), 1101–1111.

Peña, D. G. (2011). Structural violence, historical trauma, and public health: The environmental justice critique of contemporary risk science and practice. In L. M. Burton, S. P. Kemp, M. C. Leung, S. A. Matthews, & D. T. Takeuchi (Eds.), *Communities, neighborhoods, and health: Expanding the boundaries of place* (pp. 203–218). New York: Springer.

Pickett, K. E., & Wilkinson, R. G. (2015). Income inequality and health: A causal review. *Social Science & Medicine* 128(March), 316–326.

Platt, L., & Warwick, R. (2020). *Are some ethnic groups more vulnerable to COVID-19 than others?* London: Institute for Fiscal Studies. Retrieved from www.ifs.org.uk/inequality/chapter/are-some-ethnic-groups-more-vulnerable-to-covid-19-than-others/

Powell, T. C., Dilley, S. E., Bae, S., Straughn, J. M., Kim, K. H., & Leath, C. A. (2018). The impact of racial, geographic, and socioeconomic risk factors on the development of advanced-stage cervical cancer. *Journal of Lower Genital Tract Disease* 22(4), 269–273.

Pruitt, S., & Schoolman, M. (2010). Geographic disparity, area poverty and human papillomavirus (HPV) vaccination. *American Journal of Preventive Medicine* 38(5), 525–533.

Ray, R. (2020, April 9). Why are Blacks dying at higher rates from COVID-19? *Brookings.* Retrieved from www.brookings.edu/blog/fixgov/2020/04/09/why-are-blacks-dying-at-higher-rates-from-covid-19/

Rock, M., Buntain, B. J., Hatfield, J. M., & Hallgrímsson, B. (2009). Animal–human connections, "one health," and the syndemic approach to prevention. *Social Science & Medicine* 68, 991–995.

Rodriguez-Diaz, C. E., Guilamo-Ramos, V., Mena, L., Hall, E., Honermann, B., Crowley, J. S., & Millett, G. A. (2020). Risk for COVID-19 infection and death among Latinos in the United States: Examining heterogeneity in transmission dynamics. *Annals of Epidemiology.* https://doi.org/10.1016/j.annepidem.2020.07.007

Ryan, M. (2016). Diet, obesity, diabetes, and periodontitis: A syndemic approach to management. *Current Oral Health Reports* 3(1), 14–27.

Rylko-Bauer, B., & Farmer, P. (2016). Structural violence, poverty, and social suffering. In D. Brady & L. M. Burton (Eds.), *The Oxford handbook of the social science of poverty* (pp. 47–74). New York: Oxford University Press.

Rylko-Bauer, B., & Singer, M. (2010). Political violence, war, and medical anthropology. In M. Singer & P. I. Erickson (Eds.), *A companion to medical anthropology* (pp. 219–249). Malden, MA: Wiley-Blackwell.

Rylko-Bauer, B., Whiteford, L., & Farmer, P. (2009). *Global health in times of violence.* Santa Fe, NM: School for Advanced Research Press.

Schell, C., Schleich, R., Walker, F., Yazdi, A. S., Lerche, H., Röcken, M., & Eberle, F. C.

(2015). Restless legs syndrome in psoriasis: An unexpected comorbidity. *European Journal of Dermatology* 25(3), 255–260.

Scheper-Hughes, N. (2007). The gray zone: Small wars, peacetime crimes, and invisible genocides. In A. McLean & A. Leibing (Eds.), *The shadow side of fieldwork: Exploring the blurred borders between ethnography and life* (pp. 159–184). Malden, MA: Blackwell.

Scheper-Hughes, N., & Bourgois, P. (2004). Introduction: Making sense of violence. In N. Scheper-Hughes & P. Bourgois (Eds.), *Violence in war and peace: An anthology* (pp. 1–31). Malden, MA: Blackwell.

Scott, L., da Silva, P., Boehme, C., Stevens, W., & Gilpin, C. M. (2017). Diagnosis of opportunistic infections: HIV co-infections-tuberculosis. *Current Opinion in HIV and AIDS* 12(2), 129–138.

Selden, T., & Berdahl, T. (2020). COVID-19 and racial/ethnic disparities in health risk, employment, and household composition. *Health Affairs* 39(9), 1624–1632.

Shannon, K., Kerr, T., Allinott, S., Chettiar, J., Shoveller, J., & Tyndall, M. W. (2008). Social and structural violence and power relations in mitigating HIV risk of drug-using women in survival sex work. *Social Science & Medicine* 66(4), 911–921.

Singer, M. (1994). AIDS and the health crisis of the US urban poor: The perspective of critical medical anthropology. *Social Science and Medicine* 39(7), 931–948.

Singer, M. (1996). A dose of drugs, a touch of violence, a case of AIDS: Conceptualizing the SAVA syndemic. *Free Inquiry in Creative Sociology* 24(2), 99–110.

Singer, M. (2008). *Drugging the poor: Legal and illegal drug industries and the structuring of social inequality*. Prospect Heights, IL: Waveland Press.

Singer, M. (2009). *Introduction to syndemics: A critical systems approach to public and community health*. San Francisco, CA: Jossey-Bass.

Singer, M. (Ed.). (2016). *A companion to the anthropology of environmental health*. San Francisco, CA: Wiley-Blackwell.

Singer, M. (2020). Deadly companions: Diabetes and COVID-19 in Mexico. *Medical Anthropology* 39(8), 660–665.

Singer, M., & Baer, H. (1995). *Critical medical anthropology*. Amityville, NY: Baywood.

Singer, M., Bulled, N., & Ostrach, B. (2020). Whither syndemics? Trends in syndemics research, a review 2015–2019. *Global Public Health*, 15(7), 943–955.

Singer, M., Bulled, N., Ostrach, B., & Mendenhall, E. (2017). Syndemics and the biosocial conception of health. *The Lancet* 389, 941–950.

Singer, M., & Erickson, P. I. (2011). [Introduction]. In M. Singer & P. I. Erickson (Eds.), *A companion to medical anthropology* (pp. 1–5). Malden, MA: Wiley-Blackwell.

Singer, M., & Hodge, G. D. (Eds.). (2010). *The war machine and global health*. Lanham, MD: AltaMira.

Stall, R., Friedman, M. S., & Catania, J. (2007). Interacting epidemics and gay men's health: A theory of syndemic production among urban gay men. In J. Wolitski, R. Stall, & R. Valdiserri (Eds.), *Unequal opportunity: Health disparities affecting gay and bisexual men in the United States*. Oxford: Oxford University Press.

Stokes, E. K., Zambrano, L. D., Anderson, K. N., Marder, E. P., Raz, K. M., Felix, S. E. B., & Fullerton, K. E. (2020). Coronavirus disease 2019 case surveillance – United States, January 22–May 30, 2020. *Morbidity and Mortality Weekly Report* 698(24), 759–765.

Sur, P., & Mitra, E. (2020). Social distancing is a privilege of the middle class. For India's slum dwellers, it will be impossible. *CNN*. Retrieved from www.cnn.com/2020/03/30/india/india-coronavirus-social-distancing-intl-hnk/index.html

Swinburn, B. A., Kraak, V. I., Allender, S., Atkins, V. J., Baker, P. I., Bogard, J. R., & Dietz, W. H. (2019). The global syndemic of obesity, undernutrition, and climate change: The Lancet Commission report. *The Lancet* 393, 791–846.

Talman, A., Bolton, S., & Walson, J. (2013). Interactions between HIV/AIDS and the environment: Toward a syndemic framework. *American Journal of Public Health* 103(2), 253–261.

Tartaglia, E., Falasca, K., Vecchiet, J., Sabusco, G. P., Picciano, G., Di Marco, R., & Ucciferri., C. (2017). Prevalence of HPV infection among HIV-positive and HIV-negative women in Central/Eastern Italy: Strategies of prevention. *Oncology Letters* 14(6), 7629–7635.

Toebes, B., & Stronks, K. (2016). Closing the gap: A human rights approach towards social determinants of health. *European Journal of Health Law* 23(5), 510–524.

Tolbert, J., Orgera, K., Singer, N., & Damico, A. (2019). Key facts about the uninsured population. *Kaiser Family Foundation Issue Brief*. Retrieved from www.kff.org/uninsured/issue-brief/key-facts-about-the-uninsured-population/

Uvin, P. (1999). Development aid and structural violence: The case of Rwanda. *Development* 42(3), 49–56.

van der Aa, M., van den Broeke, J., Stronks, K., & Plochg, T. (2017). Patients with multimorbidity and their experiences with the healthcare process: A scoping review. *Journal of Comorbidity* 7(1), 11–21.

Wacquant, L. (2004). Commentary on an anthropology of structural violence. *Current Anthropology* 45(3), 322.

Wedding, U., Roehrig, B., Klippstein A., Steiner, P., Schaeffer., T., Pientka, L., & Höffken, K. (2007). Comorbidity in patients with cancer: Prevalence and severity measured by cumulative illness rating scale. *Critical Reviews in Oncology/Hematology* 61(3), 269–276.

Whiteford, L. M., & Vindrola-Padros, C. (2015). *Community participatory involvement: A sustainable model for global public health*. Walnut Creek, CA: Left Coast Press.

Whitham, H. K., Hawes, S. E., Chu, H., Oakes, J. M., Lifson, A. R., Kiviat, N. B., & Kulasingam, S. L. (2017). A comparison of the natural history of HPV infection and cervical abnormalities among HIV-positive and HIV-negative women in Senegal, Africa. *Cancer Epidemiology, Biomarkers & Prevention* 26(6), 1–9.

Wies, J. R., & Haldane, H. J. (2018). Structures of violence throughout the life course: Cross-cultural perspectives of gender-based violence. In N. E. Riley & J. Brunson (Eds.), *International handbook on gender and demographic processes* (pp. 329–340). Dordrecht, NL: Springer.

Williams, D. R., & Cooper, L. A. (2020). COVID-19 and health equity: A new kind of "herd immunity." *Journal of the American Medical Association*, 323(24), 2478–2480.

Williamson, E. J., Walker, A. J., Bhaskaran, K., Bacon, S., Bates, C., Morton, C. E., & Goldacre, B. (2020). OpenSAFELY: Factors associated with COVID-19 death in 17 million patients. *Nature*. https://doi.org/10.1038/s41586-020-2521-4

World Health Organization. (2018). *Cancer: Key facts*. Retrieved from www.who.int/news-room/fact-sheets/detail/cancer

Żukiewicz-Sobczak, W., Wróblewska, P., Zwoliński, J., Chmielewska-Badora, J., Adamczuk, P., Krasowska, E., & Silhy, W. (2014). Obesity and poverty paradox in developed countries. *Annals of Agricultural and Environmental Medicine* 21(3), 590–594.

Zulman, D. M., Asch, S. M., Martins, S. B., Kerr, E. A., Hoffman, B. B., & Goldstein, M. K. (2014). Quality of care for patients with multiple chronic conditions: The role of comorbidity interrelatedness. *Journal of General Internal Medicine* 29(3), 529–537.

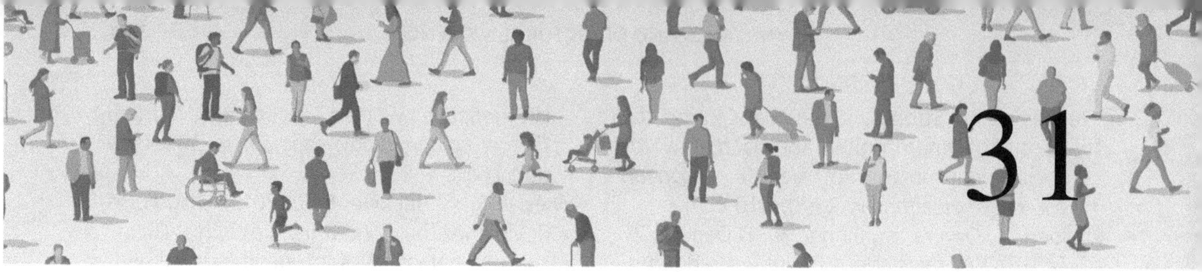

31

Disaster and Health

Robert A. Rubinstein

The United Nations Office for the Coordination of Humanitarian Affairs estimates that 167.6 million people will have been affected by disasters in 2020, and that responding to the needs of the majority of those people will require investments of US$28.8 billion (OCHA, 2020, p. 28).

During the decade between 2009 and 2018, the United Nations High Commissioner for Refugees (UNHCR) estimates that the population of forcibly displaced people nearly doubled, reaching about 71 million. Among these were roughly 26 million refugees, 41 million internally displaced persons, and 4 million asylum seekers. Nearly 14 million people were displaced in 2018 alone (UNHCR, 2018).

This chapter discusses the health consequences of disasters, the ways in which social and cultural factors influence those consequences for better or worse, and the approaches to dealing with disasters, with special focus on health implications. Disaster includes a variety of situations and events that have distinct causes but which have overlapping consequences and responses. Among these calamities are ecological events (such as drought, earthquake, and hurricane, for example), complex emergencies resulting from civil conflict, and epidemics and pandemics resulting from emerging or resurgent infectious disease.

Despite the considerable differences among the ways in which ecological events, complex emergencies, and epidemics and pandemics come about, their effects on morbidity and mortality, and in the production of human suffering, share similarities, discussed in this chapter. As well, local, national, multilateral, and private responses are all subject to political and economic pressures that shape the effectiveness of those responses.

This chapter is structured as follows. The following section describes the situation of Haiti in the early 21st century. The Haiti case includes many of the different kinds of disasters discussed in this chapter, including those resulting from violent conflicts, ecological events, and resurgent disease. The material in this case is illustrative of considerations discussed later in the chapter.

The next section of this chapter is devoted to distinguishing among different types of disaster. It considers first the humanitarian disasters created by complex emergencies resulting from civil-military conflicts. It next considers the nature of disasters resulting from ecological processes, and stresses the important contribution of social and cultural activities to the health consequences of those disasters. This second section concludes with a discussion of epidemic, resurgent, and emerging disease. The third section of the chapter adds a discussion of climate change, its anthropogenic, nature, and some of its health consequences.

The fourth section of this chapter is devoted to describing some of the major health challenges created by disasters. It includes four subsections which discuss: first, the ways in which disasters affect public health infrastructure; second health challenges of population displacement; third, challenges to sanitation, food, and water created by disasters; and, fourth, communicable and non-communicable diseases in the context of disaster.

The chapter concludes with a discussion of health and disaster. Also incorporated into the chapter are four informational boxes and two figures. The informational boxes describe international efforts to address disaster and a typology of diseases after disaster. The figures provide graphic illustrations of the interconnected health challenges of disaster, and the relationships among sanitation, water, nutrition, and health.

HAITI IN THE EARLY 21ST CENTURY

Many of the themes discussed in this chapter are reflected in the experience of Haiti during the first decades of the 2000s. Haiti has long been known as the poorest country in Latin America, and has experienced decades of dictatorships where little attention was paid to the health and welfare of the population. In 2004, Haitian President Jean-Bertrand Aristide left Haiti under duress following an armed insurrection supported by political factions opposing his 2001 election (Farmer, 2004). During the years between 2001 and 2004 international aid to Haiti was restricted, mainly for ideological reasons. The Haitian economy stagnated, political violence and human rights abuses were widespread, and food insecurity and lack of potable (drinking) water were common, all leading to a humanitarian crisis. In response, the United Nations deployed missions to Haiti to support the stabilization of the country. Initially, in the aftermath of President Aristide's departure, the UN presence was a short-term Multinational Interim Force led by the United States. This force was soon replaced by the United Nations Stabilization Mission in Haiti (MINUSTAH). MINUSTAH was active from 2004 until 2017, being replaced at that time by a smaller mission focused on supporting Haitian rule-of-law institutions.

MINUSTAH's early tenure was often contentious within Haitian civil society. The mission carried out attacks in Cite Soleil in 2006. Although the peacekeepers reported that they were responding to being fired upon from that area, because Cite Soleil was an especially impoverished area associated with opposition to the government, this account was disputed. This, and other actions, crystalized for many Haitians the view that MINUSTAH was an occupying force rather than a humanitarian action (Diceanu, 2006; Frerichs, 2017, p. 41; Pingeot, 2020).

Grinding poverty, food shortages, and human rights violations continued after MINUSTAH's deployment. Then, at the beginning of 2010, Haiti was struck by a 7.0 magnitude earthquake, which further devastated the country. At least 200,000 people died when the earthquake struck and more than a million and a half people were internally displaced by the collapse of their homes (Katz, 2013; Schuller, 2012). The earthquake also decimated the Haitian government, destroying buildings – including the Presidential Palace, the seat of government – vital records, and killing a substantial percentage of government workers (Fisher et al., 2018). Following the earthquake Haiti experienced a rise in some infectious diseases, such as tuberculosis (Koenig et al., 2015). The earthquake also exacerbated the already tenuous food security situation facing many Haitians. Thousands of Haitians took refuge in Internally Displaced Persons (IDP) camps. The world responded. The international community quickly pledged billions of dollars in aid. Much of the pledged funding never made it to Haiti. By 2018, only about 40% of funds pledged in response to United Nations Coordinated Appeals had reached Haiti (Fisher et al., 2018, p. 114).

Haiti had long been the focus of humanitarian and development efforts run by nongovernmental organizations (NGOs), often with involvement from high-profile US political and government foundations, including the Clinton Foundation, and supporters (McIntire, 2016). The number of NGOs working in Haiti had risen dramatically in the two decades prior to the earthquake (Schuller, 2012). Following the 2010 earthquake the number of NGOs ballooned even further as NGOs rushed to provide assistance (Kristoff & Panarelli, 2010). Heavy reliance on NGOs brings with it a number of challenges. In Haiti's case, the provision of basic services by NGOs and the funneling of funds through them rather than through the government created challenges to political stability and governance (Kristoff & Panarelli, 2010; Schuller, 2012), as it does in other countries where NGO expertise replaces local knowledge and institutional capacity and growth (Autesserre, 2014).

The complex political and humanitarian situation became even more difficult in October 2010 when an outbreak of cholera was confirmed. In only two months, by early December, cholera had spread throughout the country. The Haitian Ministry of Public Health and Population reported 91,770 cases from all over the country. Of those 43,243 (47.1%) of patients had been hospitalized, and 2,071 (2.3%) had died (Morbidity and Mortality Weekly Report, 2010, p. 1586). These numbers were most likely an undercount due to difficulties in case detection, surveillance, and reporting. All of these were complicated by the politics surrounding the identification of the source of the cholera outbreak. Epidemiological work, later confirmed by genetic sequencing, traced the origins of the cholera outbreak back to the Nepalese military contingent of MINUSTAH (Frerichs, 2017), in which the "camp contaminated the Meille [River] tributary with fecal matter by their unsanitary practice of sewage drainage" (Orata, Keim, & Boucher, 2014, p. 1).

Haiti had not experienced cholera for more than a century; the infection spread rapidly through the population (Centers for Disease Control and Prevention, 2014; Morbidity and Mortality Weekly Report, 2010). The spread was facilitated by a lack of safe water and an inadequate sanitation infrastructure in the country. In the face of this daunting public health crisis, the response was mixed. Case identification was inconsistent. Real-time reporting of the incidence and prevalence of cholera was flawed for a variety of reasons. Among these were lack of public health infrastructure, local politicians with interests in minimizing the numbers, competition among NGOs, and political posturing and denialism locally and at the international level (Frerichs, 2017). Nonetheless, efforts to address the cholera outbreak met with some success (Ivers, Farmer, Almazor, & Léandre, 2010; Periago et al., 2012).

Progress on controlling cholera was interrupted, as were other public health initiatives, when Haiti was struck in 2016 by Hurricane Matthew, a category 4 storm. Hurricane Matthew destroyed much of south Haiti – one account estimated 90% destroyed, with effects for other regions of the island nation, dispossessing about 350,00 people (Elvey, 2016), and once again elicited a complex of international response from governments, specialized agencies, and NGOs.

The Haitian case involves many of the features that are reflected in disasters around the world. Moreover, despite disparate initiating circumstances, ecological events, complex emergencies, and epidemic and pandemics share in the shaping of morbidity and mortality, and in the production of human suffering. Nonetheless, it is important to distinguish among types of disasters so that the differences among them are not lost in the discussion. Accordingly, the next section distinguishes among disasters as background for later addressing the health implications of each.

DISTINGUISHING DISASTERS

This chapter considers in a single framework the common consequences and diversity of responses to many different kinds of disasters. Yet, each disaster, and each type of disaster, can only be understood contextually. Thus, this section describes the different origins and kinds of disaster as a way of contextualizing the specific health effects that result. There are four general types of disaster distinguished.

Complex Emergencies

Especially since the dissolution of the Soviet Union in 1991, which was accompanied by a rise in poverty, general homelessness, and child homelessness, neglect, orphanhood, street children, child prostitution and human trafficking (Fujimura, Stoeck, & Sudakova, 2005), there has been a noted decrease in the number of violent interstate conflicts along with an increase of intra-state conflicts, some becoming long civil wars. The emergence of these intra-state conflicts of various types (civil wars, internal rebellions, border disputes, transnational armed actors) caught many analysts unprepared to account for them. Explanations offered ranged widely. For example, analysts saw the war in the former Yugoslavia variously as an expression of Balkan "ancient hatreds," to the failure of free market pluralism, to the local conditions at the end of the Cold War which made the confederation unsustainable (Schwartz, 1999; Udovicki & Ridgeway, 2000). Similarly, other conflicts, like those in Rwanda, Somalia, the Democratic Republic of Congo, and Sierra Leone, were attributed, for example, to conflicts over resources, resurgent tribalism, corruption, and loss of political patronage from the Soviet Union and the United States that had allowed states to "keep a lid" on these and other tensions. Elsewhere, such as in Somalia, the conflict was viewed variously as expressing tribalism, colonial legacies, resource competition, disease, and corruption (Autesserre, 2010; Kaplan, 1994; Prunier, 1995; Rubinstein, 2008). Intra-state conflicts such as these led to a variety of humanitarian crises, including genocides, famines, displaced persons, and resurgent disease. International responses framed these as resulting from troubled or "failed states," countries where government institutions are unable to provide for the safety and security of their citizens (Gros, 1996). Individual humanitarian organizations, specialized multilateral agencies, or bilateral aid were overwhelmed and had difficulty responding.

When humanitarian crises are such that they can only be addressed by multiple organizations, they are named Complex Emergencies. The term was first used in the 1980s to describe situations that showed "unprecedented levels of abject poverty, political insecurity, conflict, state disintegration and population displacement" (Duffield, 1994, p. 3), and came to more common use in the 1990s in response to situations like those described above. The United Nations Inter-Agency Standing Committee defines a complex emergency as "a humanitarian crisis in a country, region, or society where there is a total or considerable breakdown of authority resulting from internal or external conflict and which requires an international response that goes beyond the mandate or capacity of any single agency and/or the ongoing UN country programme" (IASC, 2008, p. 8).

Sometimes these are also referred to as "complex humanitarian emergencies" because they characteristically involve humanitarian crises that grip the attention of the international community. Yet, including the term "humanitarian" in the designator is inappropriate. Doing so suggests inappropriately that the "solution lies with humanitarian relief (rather than with tackling the underlying human rights abuses for example)" (Keen, 2008, p. 1). And, as Albala-Bertrand points out, the inclusion of the term "humanitarian" suggests the "connotation of philanthropic, altruist, selfless[ness], which … would be highly misleading. Even if there are unselfish elements in all emergency responses … all emergency [sic] can be easily put within a mostly utilitarian framework, especially the response coming bilaterally from abroad" (Albala-Bertrand, 2000b, p. 18; see also, Rubinstein & Kudesia, 2012).

In mortality and morbidity and the social organization of responses to them, the effects of complex emergencies share many features with those of ecological calamities and epidemic and resurgent disease. In the context of complex emergencies, these include, especially, displacement, human rights abuses, sexual violence, scarcity of food and water, damaged infrastructure, diminished or no access to health services, and resurgent infectious disease (Aggarwal, 2018; Keen, 2008; Onyango & Uwase, 2017; Toole, Waldman, & Zwi, 2006).

Ecological Calamities

There is a wide range of environmental exposures that become ecological calamities affecting human populations. These include, for example, drought, earthquakes, hurricanes, typhoons, floods, tornados, tsunamis, landslides, fires, volcanic eruptions, and intensified weather linked to climate change, like extreme heatwaves and coastal storms. Recognizing that disasters were causing increasing suffering, in December 1989 the United Nations passed Resolution 44/236 designating the 1990s as the International Decade for Natural Disaster Reduction. The Annex to the resolution describes the objectives and goals of the decade, which are described in Box 31.1.

Box 31.1 Objectives and Goals of the International Decade for Natural Disaster Reduction

1. The objective of the International Decade for Natural Disaster Reduction is to reduce through concerted international action, especially in developing countries, the loss of life, property damage and social and economic disruption caused by natural disasters such as earthquakes, windstorms, tsunamis, floods, landslides, volcanic eruptions, wildfires, grasshopper and locust infestations, drought and desertification and other calamities of natural origin.
2. The goals of the Decade are:

   (a) To improve the capacity of each country to mitigate the effects of natural disasters expeditiously and effectively, paying special attention to assisting developing countries in the assessment of disaster damage potential and in the establishment of early-warning systems and disaster resistant structures when and where needed;
   (b) To devise appropriate guidelines and strategies for applying existing scientific and technical knowledge, taking into account the cultural and economic diversity among nations;
   (c) To foster scientific and engineering endeavours aimed at closing critical gaps in knowledge in order to reduce loss of life and property;
   (d) To disseminate existing and new technical information related to measure for the assessment, prediction and mitigation of natural disasters;
   (e) To develop measures for the assessment, prediction, prevention and mitigation of natural disasters through programmes of technical assistance and technology transfer, demonstration projects, and education and training, tailored to specific disasters and locations, and to evaluate the effectiveness of those programmes.

Source: Annex to United Nations Resolution 44/236

These objectives and goals are reflected in the work of the 1994 World Conference on Natural Disaster Reduction. Held in Yokohama, Japan, the final report of the conference set out a variety of actions for achieving the goals of the Decade (United Nations, 1994).

The second UN World Conference on Disaster Risk Reduction took place in Hyogo, Japan, in 2005. The report of that conference, the Hyogo Framework for Action 2005–2015: Building the Resilience of Nations and Communities to Disasters, focused on actions that would help communities at all socio-political levels – from nations to local communities – better cope with and be more resilient to disasters (United Nations, 2005). That decade-long plan focused on five action areas:

1 Ensure that disaster risk reduction is a national and a local priority with a strong institutional basis for implementation.
2 Identify, assess and monitor disaster risks and enhance early warning.
3 Use knowledge, innovation and education to build a culture of safety and resilience at all levels.
4 Reduce the underlying risk factors.
5 Strengthen disaster preparedness for effective response at all levels. (United Nations, 2005)

A decade later, in March 2015, a third conference took place in Sendai, Japan, to update the Hyogo Framework. The Sendai Framework for Disaster Risk Reduction 2015–2030, the final report of the conference, set out a 15-year plan, the goal of which is "The substantial reduction of disaster risk and losses in lives, livelihoods and health and in the economic, physical, social, cultural and environmental assets of persons, businesses, communities and countries" (UNDRR, 2015, p. 12). The outcome of the report is summarized in Box 31.2.

During these decades, international activity in framing conceptions of what needed to be done to address disaster shifted. The changing focuses of the Yokohama, Hyogo, and Sendai frameworks suggest a shift in emphasis from disaster risk management to disaster risk reduction. Shifting disaster priorities are also reflected in the changes introduced with each updated edition to the United Nations Office of Disaster Risk Reduction compilation of terminology related to that work (United Nations, 2016). These changes shift the focus from responding to disasters, to specifying ways to better prepare for and recover from disaster, to the addition of a concern about understanding and addressing sources of risk. Even the "core concepts from disaster risk science-hazard, vulnerability, risk focusing on disaster and disaster risk management (DRM)," are reinterpreted in each update (Kelman, 2018, p. 289), reflecting the shift "away from probabilistic notions of risk and their management rationales" (Staupe-Delgado, 2019, pp. 4–5).

The scholarly and research communities that focus on disaster also shifted their focus during the last three decades. Those literatures contain spirited debates about how to best think about disaster (Perry & Quarantelli, 2005; Quarantelli, 1998). For some, these definitional discussions detract from efforts to address disaster and its consequences, while for others the definitional debates are key to finding better ways to understand and coordinate responses to disaster.

The general trend in this literature is a recognition that the term "natural disaster" is often something of a misnomer. The basic idea is that the risks resulting from and exposure to ecological calamities are influenced by human activities in the social and cultural organization of societies (e.g., Bobrowsky, 2013; Button, 2010; Cutter et al., 2012; Oliver-Smith & Hoffman, 2020). As Anthony Oliver-Smith (2017, p. 469) notes:

> It is also now well established that disaster risk and eventual disaster are social constructs based on the presence of potentially damaging physical events but seriously and dominantly conditioned by society's perceptions, needs, demands, decisions and practices. However, the understanding of risk and disaster is still severely impeded by visions of "natural" disaster, the dominance of the physical

Box 31.2 Chart of the Sendai Framework for Disaster Risk Reduction, 2015–2030

Chart of the Sendai Framework for Disaster Risk Reduction
2015-2030

Scope and purpose

The present framework will apply to the risk of small-scale and large-scale, frequent and infrequent, sudden and slow-onset disasters, caused by natural or manmade hazards as well as related environmental, technological and biological hazards and risks.
It aims to guide the multi-hazard management of disaster risk in development at all levels as well as within and across all sectors

Expected outcome

The substantial reduction of disaster risk and losses in lives, livelihoods and health and in the economic, physical, social, cultural and environmental assets of persons, businesses, communities and countries

Goal

Prevent new and reduce existing disaster risk through the implementation of integrated and inclusive economic, structural, legal, social, health, cultural, educational, environmental, technological, political and institutional measures that prevent and reduce hazard exposure and vulnerability to disaster, increase preparedness for response and recovery, and thus strengthen resilience

Targets

Substantially reduce global disaster mortality by 2030, aiming to lower average per 100,000 global mortality between 2020-2030 compared to 2005-2015	Substantially reduce the number of affected people globally by 2030, aiming to lower the average global figure per 100,000 between 2020-2030 compared to 2005-2015	Reduce direct disaster economic loss in relation to global gross domestic product (GDP) by 2030	Substantially reduce disaster damage to critical infrastructure and disruption of basic services, among them health and educational facilities, including through developing their resilience by 2030	Substantially increase the number of countries with national and local disaster risk reduction strategies by 2020	Substantially enhance international cooperation to developing countries through adequate and sustainable support to complement their national actions for implementation of this framework by 2030	Substantially increase the availability of and access to multi-hazard early warning systems and disaster risk information and assessments to people by 2030

Priorities for Action

There is a need for focused action within and across sectors by States at local, national, regional and global levels in the following four priority areas.

Priority 1 Understanding disaster risk	Priority 2 Strengthening disaster risk governance to manage disaster risk	Priority 3 Investing in disaster risk reduction for resilience	Priority 4 Enhancing disaster preparedness for effective response, and to «Build Back Better» in recovery, rehabilitation and reconstruction
Disaster risk management needs to be based on an understanding of disaster risk in all its dimensions of vulnerability, capacity, exposure of persons and assets, hazard characteristics and the environment	Disaster risk governance at the national, regional and global levels is vital to the management of disaster risk reduction in all sectors and ensuring the coherence of national and local frameworks of laws, regulations and public policies that, by defining roles and responsibilities, guide, encourage and incentivize the public and private sectors to take action and address disaster risk	Public and private investment in disaster risk prevention and reduction through structural and non-structural measures are essential to enhance the economic, social, health and cultural resilience of persons, communities, countries and their assets, as well as the environment. These can be drivers of innovation, growth and job creation. Such measures are cost-effective and instrumental to save lives, prevent and reduce losses and ensure effective recovery and rehabilitation	Experience indicates that disaster preparedness needs to be strengthened for more effective response and ensure capacities are in place for effective recovery. Disasters have also demonstrated that the recovery, rehabilitation and reconstruction phase, which needs to be prepared ahead of the disaster, is an opportunity to «Build Back Better» through integrating disaster risk reduction measures. Women and persons with disabilities should publicly lead and promote gender-equitable and universally accessible approaches during the response and reconstruction phases

Guiding Principles

Primary responsibility of States to prevent and reduce disaster risk, including through cooperation	Shared responsibility between central Government and national authorities, sectors and stakeholders as appropriate to national circumstances	Protection of persons and their assets while promoting and protecting all human rights including the right to development	Engagement from all of society	Full engagement of all State institutions of an executive and legislative nature at national and local levels	Empowerment of local authorities and communities through resources, incentives and decision-making responsibilities as appropriate	Decision-making to be inclusive and risk-informed while using a multi-hazard approach

Coherence of disaster risk reduction and sustainable development policies, plans, practices and mechanisms, across different sectors	Accounting of local and specific characteristics of disaster risks when determining measures to reduce risk	Addressing underlying risk factors cost-effectively through investment versus relying primarily on post-disaster response and recovery	«Build Back Better» for preventing the creation of, and reducing existing, disaster risk	The quality of global partnership and international cooperation to be effective, meaningful and strong	Support from developed countries and partners to developing countries to be tailored according to needs and priorities as identified by them

www.preventionweb.net/go/sfdrr
www.unisdr.org
isdr@un.org

UNISDR
The United Nations Office for Disaster Risk Reduction

factors affecting risk and the marginalization of more fundamental social processes. This means that disaster risk management practice is still very much dominated by reaction and response, to the detriment of development-based risk reduction and avoidance interventions.

The recognition that the effects of disaster are exacerbated or limited by human social and cultural activities does not diminish the reality of the suffering experienced by people as a result of the disaster. Rather, this recognition reframes the discussion so that better public policies can be developed to guard against the (worst) effects of disasters (Cutter et al., 2012).

A developing parallel area of research focuses on understanding the cultural construction of risk and how that affects the creation of and exposure to response preparedness (Douglas & Wildavsky, 1983; Lupton, 2013; Samimian-Darash & Rabinow, 2015). Whether the causes of ecological calamities can be traced variously to natural phenomena or to human activity that alters the geophysics leading to them, such as sea levels rising as a result of global warming, or to a combination of both, the sequela of such events lead to increases in morbidity and mortality. Some of those result from the resurgence of disease resulting in epidemics.

Epidemic, Resurgent, and Emerging Disease

Human history, and many of our cultural and social organizational practices have been shaped by infectious disease. Indeed, much of the way that human societies have organized themselves and created systems of meaning through which they deal with the world is in response to the maladies and morbidities caused by disease (Evans-Prichard, 1937; McElroy & Townsend, 2015; McNeill, 1976). This section briefly reviews epidemics, resurgent diseases, and emerging infectious diseases.

Epidemics, incidences of illness in an area that are clearly in excess of its normal rates (for a more technical definition, see Porter, 2014, pp. 93–94), have throughout history shaped societies. When an epidemic extends over a wide area, crosses international borders, and affects a large number of people, it is characterized as a pandemic (for a more technical definition, see Porter, 2014, p. 209).

Developments in the Control of Disease

Epidemics and pandemics have significant effects on the course of history. Hays (2005), for example, describes the effects of epidemics on societies from half a millennium BCE to the 20th century. Among the epidemics he considers are malaria in ancient Rome, syphilis in Europe in the 16th century, and cholera in the 19th century. Responses to infectious diseases, like polio and tuberculosis, also shaped many aspects of social life, from architecture, to patterns of personal interaction, to where people went for holidays (Dubos, 1952; Oshinsky, 2005; Zinsser, 2008). Infectious diseases, especially in contexts of epidemics and pandemics, may lead to those with them being stigmatized, as moral valuations are placed on the diseases (Herring & Swedlund, 2010). For example, as far back as biblical times there are examples of infectious diseases leading people to be ostracized from their communities, in part because their conditions were thought to reflect moral failings. Regarding leprosy, "Although leprosy is not very contagious, since Biblical times the public has tended to drive lepers from their communities and to exile them to remote islands and villages" (Battin, Francis, Jacobson, & Smith, 2009, p. 32).

Public health developments in the late 19th and early 20th centuries relating to better sanitation made major strides in reducing mortality and morbidity even in the absence of belief in germ theory (Prizzi, 2002; Rosen, 2015). Despite the prevailing belief that disease was caused by vapors and bad air (miasma) and immorality, the 1842 sanitary movement was strengthened when Edwin Chadwick published *The Report from the Poor Law Commissioners on an Inquiry into the Sanitary Conditions of the Laboring Population of Great Britain* (Morley, 2007). Control of cholera was an early success of the sanitarian movement.

The beginnings of modern epidemiology are traced back to the work of John Snow, who identified contaminated water supplies as the cause of the 1848 cholera outbreak in London. Once making this finding, he was able to contain the outbreak by controlling access to the contaminated water (Fine, Goldacre, & Haines, 2013; Snow, 2008 [1854]). Yet, "Despite staggering progress in the fight against infectious diseases during the latter half of the 19th century, there were still few advances in treatment" (Gaynes, 2011, p. 235).

Successful management and treatment of infectious diseases accelerated with the wider acceptance of germ theory in the early 20th century (Gaynes, 2011). Among the important health innovations flowing from that development were the identification of viruses as causes of disease, the development of antibiotics to control infection, advances in vaccine development, and the creation of more effective public health systems and techniques.

Box 31.3 Water: quality, availability and access

SANDRA D. LANE, SUSAN C. SCRIMSHAW, AND ROBERT A. RUBINSTEIN

Water is essential for human survival in multiple ways. We need it to drink, for personal cleanliness, for food preparation and for cleaning everything from clothing to food utensils. Safe drinking water prevents the spread of disease and the effects of contamination like the lead poisoning which occurred in Flint, MI (Hanna-Attisha et al., 2016).

Contaminated water can also contaminate crops and lead to disease or exposure to dangerous substances such as pesticides. Water is required for hygiene, and disease spreads in its absence, as demonstrated by work on trachoma in Egypt (Rubinstein et al., 2006). Water cleans our homes, factories and workplaces and helps dispose of human waste. Water is involved in food preparation and food safety. Not only does it irrigate our crops, but to do so safely it must be free of parasites, bacteria and other infectious agents and toxic substances. We use water to farm fish and to sustain the animals raised for food.

Waterways are important as well to the health of many societies. They connect communities for commerce. Travel on them helps people stay in contact with one another, and facilitates the spread of ideas and innovations, but also, pathogens (Anderson et al., 2019; Frerichs, 2017).

In 2010 the United Nations General Assembly approved Resolution 64/292 recognizing the right to adequate and safe water, and sanitation, for all (United Nations General Assembly, 2010). Perhaps the most important historic intervention promoting human health was the 19th century sanitation movement that cleaned up stagnant wastewater in New York, Boston, and London (Fair, 1952). A similar sanitation intervention in the mid-20th century in Japan demonstrated that water purification led not only to decreases in water-borne disease deaths from typhoid, but also to decreased mortality from tuberculosis and pneumonia (Inoue & Ogasawara, 2020). Cleaning up the water supply, in that case, probably led to fewer diarrheal diseases, which in turn led to stronger immune systems.

International agencies have calculated the minimum and optimal amounts of water to assure each individual's health (Tarrass & Benjelloun, 2012). Not surprisingly, vulnerable and impoverished populations in many countries, including in the United States, have less access to clean water, which is a major social determinant of poorer health and survival. Despite the importance of clean water for maintaining health, many people live without access to improved water sources (UNICEF, 2021). In 2019 Oxfam estimated that 2.1 billion people were without access to clean water, and estimated that "On average, women and children in developing countries walk 3.7 miles and carry five gallons every day to bring clean water to their families" (Sakakeeny, 2019, 1). In common with other crises, lack of access to clean water places a disproportionate burden on women and children. This burden increases when lack of access to improved sanitation is added, which the Centers for Disease Control and Prevention estimates to be the case for 2.5 billion people (CDC, 2016). Women and children are at increased risk as they seek water, exposing them

(Continued)

(Continued)

to abduction, rape, and other forms of violence. Their lack of access to clean water sources leads to social practices that expose them to toxins, bacteria, and parasites (Drechsel et al., 2009; El Katsha & Watts, 2002).

Water use varies widely by geographical area and by socio-economic status. In affluent countries, water is often used as though it were an infinite resource, even as agricultural areas and communities experience shortages. In low-income communities in many regions of the world, running water may not be available, and sometimes, any water at all is scarce. For example, using satellite imagery, Hasan and colleagues estimate that 37% of the African population will experience fresh water scarcity by 2025, and that figure will be 57% by 2050 (Hasan et al., 2019). In Bolivia, the municipal government of the city of Cochabamba awarded a contract for water and sanitation services to a private for-profit company. The company immediately increased charges for these services. When people in low-income areas of the city were charged when it rained on the assumption that they would collect rainwater, they revolted, and ultimately, the contract was cancelled (Nickson & Vargas, 2002).

Water access is a factor in civil conflict (Zemmali, 1998). Water supplies can be destroyed in war, accidently or intentionally, in which case it may be labeled as a war crime (International Law Association, 2004). Destruction of safe, adequate water supplies inevitably increases sickness and death in the most vulnerable, including children's mortality due to dehydration from diarrhea.

The tragedy of Flint, MI, for example, was created when the safe water from Lake Huron was switched to the contaminated Flint River without adding anti-corrosives that would have reduced the harm. This led to a doubling of lead poisoning in the largely low-income and minority children who were forced to drink the water (Hanna-Attisha et al., 2016).

Water conflict happens when countries engage in armed interaction, or threaten such militant responses, over access to water, as documented by the Pacific Institute in their extensive five millennia chronology of wars over water (Water Conflict – World's Water, worldwater.org). Among the water-based conflicts they describe since 2010, are the Palestinian West Bank water needs and Israeli governmental responses that limit that access, the destruction of water supplies in South Sudan by Sudan during the civil war that led to South Sudan's independence, and the dispute among Ethiopia, Sudan, and Egypt over the potential damming of the Blue Nile.

REFERENCES

Anderson, Elizabeth P., Sue Jackson, Rebecca E. Tharme, Michael Douglas, Joseph E. Flotemersch, Margreet Zwarteveen, Chicu Lokgariwar, Mariana Montoya, Alika Wali, Gail T. Tipa, Timothy D. Jardine, Julian D. Olden, John Conallin, Barbara Cosen, Chris Dickens, Dustin Garrik, David Groenfeldt, Jane Kabogo, Dirk J. Roux, Albert Ruhi, & Angela H. Arthington. (2019). Understanding rivers and their social relations: a critical step to advance environmental water management. *WIREs Water*, *6*(e1381), 1–21.

CDC. (2016). *Global water, sanitation & hygiene (WASH)*. Washington, DC: Centers for Disease Control and Prevention, www.cdc.gov/healthywater/global/wash_statistics.html (accessed March 29, 2021).

Drechsel, Pay, Christopher A. Scott, Liqa Raschid-Sally, Mark Redwood, & Akiça Bahri, eds. (2009). *Wastewater Irrigation and Health: Assessing and Mitigating Risk in Low-income Countries*. London: Earthscan.

El Katsha, Samiha, & Susan Watts. (2002). *Gender, Behavior, and Health: Schstosomiasis Transmission and Control in Rural Egypt*. Cairo, Egypt: The American University in Cairo Press.

Fair, Gordon M. (1952). Shattuck, Chadwick, and the engineer in public health. *Public Health Reports*, *67*(5), 443–449.

Frerichs, Ralph S. (2017). *Deadly River: Cholera and Cover-Up in Post-Earthquake Haiti*. Ithaca, NY: Cornell University Press.

Hanna-Attisha, Mona, Jenny LaChance, Richard Casey Sadler, & Allison Champney Schnepp. (2016). Elevated blood lead levels in children associated with the Flint drinking water crisis: a spatial analysis of risk and public health response. *American Journal of Public Health*, *106*(2), 283–290.

Hasan, Emad, Aondover Tarhule, Yang Hong, & Berrien Moore III. (2019). Assessment of physical water scarcity in Africa using GRACE and TRMM satellite data. *Remote Sensing*, *11*(8), 904–924.

Inoue, Tatsuki, & Kota Ogasawara. (2020). Chain effects of clean water: the Mills-Reincke phenomenon in early 20th-century Japan. *Economics and Human Biology*, *36*, 100822.

International Law Association. (2004). *Berlin Rules on Water Resources*. London: International Law Association.

(Continued)

(Continued)

Nickson, Andrew, & Claudia Vargas. (2002). The limitations of water regulation: the failure of the Cochabamba Concession in Bolivia. *Bulletin of Latin American Research*, *21*(1), 99–120.

Rubinstein, Robert A., Sandra D. Lane, Sunny A. Sallam, Ahmed S. Sheta, Zahira M. Gad, Aida R. Sherif, Mohammed Selim, Ashry Gad, Ahmed Sharma, Julius Schachter, & Chandler R. Dawson. (2006). Controlling blinding trachoma in the Egyptian Delta: integrating clinical, epidemiological and anthropological understandings. *Anthropology and Medicine*, *13*(2), 99–118.

Sakakeeny, Kria. (2019). *World water day: how far would you walk for water?* London: Oxfam, www.oxfamamerica.org/explore/stories/world-water-day-how-far-would-you-walk-water/ (accessed March 29, 2021).

Tarrass, Faissai, & Meryem Benjelloun. (2012). The effects of water shortages on health and human development. *Perspectives on Public Health*, *132*(5), 240–244.

UNICEF. (2021). Water. *UNICEF for Every Child*, www.unicef.org/wash/water (accessed March 29, 2021).

United Nations General Assembly. (2010). *Resolution Adopted by the General Assembly on 28 July, 64/292. The Human Right to Water and Sanitation*. New York: United Nations.

Zemmali, Ameur. (1998). Dying for water. In Sarah Fleming (ed.), *Forum: War and Water* (pp. 31–35). Geneva, CH: International Committee of the Red Cross.

The mass production of penicillin in the mid-1940s marked the start of the modern antibiotic era. Infections from cuts, wounds, and burns that had once routinely killed people or left them disfigured became easily treatable.

Many infectious diseases that had scourged human society for millennia became treatable and were brought under control with antibiotics. Tuberculosis, once so feared that it affected the organization of human societies, shaping the way people interacted with one another and the design of the built environment, also influenced popular culture. Hays (2005, p. 202) points out regarding tuberculosis, "the pale, wan, frail look of the consumptive became in the early and middle nineteenth century an ideal of beauty that the florid, the heavy, and the entirely healthy envied," and was referred to as "The White Plague" as a consequence (see, for further discussion of the effects of tuberculosis on society, Dubos, 1952). Tuberculosis first became amenable to antibiotic treatment with the discovery of streptomycin in the mid-1940s, though it did not receive widespread clinical use because of the quick development of resistance (Murray, Schraufnagel, & Hopewell, 2015, pp. 1753, antibiotic resistance is discussed further below; Ramachandran & Swaminathan, 2015). Shortly after, in 1954, isoniazid was introduced to clinical use for the treatment of tuberculosis, and remains an important component of tuberculosis antibiotic treatment regimens (Acquisto, 2014, p. 1135).

Sexually transmitted infections that caused tremendous human suffering, such as gonorrhea, chlamydia, and syphilis could be successfully treated with antibiotics. The success of modern antibiotics contributed to a consolidation of medical authority, which helped spur the development of public health infrastructure, and propelled the further professionalization of the public health profession.

The acceptance of germ theory, the development of modern vaccines, and the professionalization of public health also led to support for efforts to control viral diseases, even though they were not susceptible to antibiotic treatment. Smallpox, caused by the variola virus, had long devastated human societies (for descriptions of the effects of smallpox epidemics dating from as far back at 735 CE, see Hays, 2005). Despite developments in smallpox vaccination, it remained a terrifying disease into the 20th century (Riedel, 2005). In 1959 the decision of the 12th World Health Assembly initiated the global smallpox eradication programme. Leveraging public health strategies (like education, surveillance, case identification, contact tracing, and isolation), and advances in vaccine and treatment, these efforts led to the eradication of smallpox, with the last naturally occurring case of smallpox in 1977 (Fenner, Henderson, Arita, Zdeněk, & Ladnyi, 1988).

Although the eradication of smallpox stands out as a singular success, the strategies and tactics used in the campaign against that disease informed other public health efforts. As a result, many formerly epidemic diseases – tuberculosis, leprosy, plague, malaria, typhus fever, and cholera, among them – have been controlled and all but eliminated.

Setbacks and New Challenges

At the start of the last quarter of the 20th century infectious diseases were so diminished as threats to human health that these scourges, which had once loomed large in people's daily lives receded far from many people's awareness. Yet, even at the advent of the modern antibiotic era, there were already clear indications that this situation would change.

Antibiotic Resistance

As early as 1945, Sir Alexander Fleming, the discoverer of penicillin, warned about the rise of penicillin-resistant organisms. He said, speaking in the idiom of his day, "the thoughtless person playing with penicillin treatment is morally responsible for the death of the man who finally succumbs to infection with the penicillin-resistant organism. I hope this evil can be averted" (*New York Times*, 1945, p. 21). Fleming was reflecting on what he saw as the inevitable shifts in how penicillin was administered from injection in a hospital setting to oral administration. He suggested that such developments would lead to easier access, self-administration of the drug, and its use on infections for which it was not effective. Fleming's hope that antibiotic resistance and its consequences might be avoided were in vain.

In the half century following the introduction of antibiotics into clinical care, antibiotics saved uncounted numbers of lives. At the same time, Fleming's fears were realized in the growing number of antibiotic-resistant bacteria. A full discussion of the sources of antibiotic resistance is beyond the scope of this chapter (for a full discussion of antibiotic resistance, see Levy, 2002). However, since the disaster that antibiotic resistance represents is caused in large part by human actions, four such actions are noted here.

First, since antibiotics act quickly to end the pain, discomfort, and general symptoms of an infection, people sometimes do not complete the entire course of antibiotic treatment, creating a biome in which resistant bacteria are able to survive and flourish.

Second, the dosing schedule for antibiotics, needing to be taken multiple times per day, or requiring refrigeration for storage, can also lead to patients not completing the full course of treatment. This creates conditions for the development of organisms resistant to the antibiotic.

Third, in many parts of the world, antibiotics are available for over-the-counter purchase. Where this is possible people often purchase antibiotics to treat self-diagnosed conditions. Different bacteria are sensitive to different antibiotics; indiscriminant and inappropriate use creates the conditions for resistant bacteria to flourish. People also will sometimes take antibiotics for viral infections, again creating conditions for resistant bacteria to grow. The inappropriate application of antibiotic therapy is also a problem where healthcare providers – pharmacists, physicians, nurses, traditional healers – may recommend an antibiotic in response to patient expectations or requests without knowing what organisms are causing the infection.

Fourth, the observation that putting antibiotics into animal food supplies resulted in healthier animals, higher yields, and longer times before spoilage led to the wide use of antibiotics in food production. This includes the widespread use of antibiotics in animal feed to promote growth, especially for cows, pigs, and poultry. Antibiotics are incorporated into animal feed in low doses, 10 to 100 times below their therapeutic level, and for longer periods of time than when administered to treat specific infections. This practice creates contexts in which antibiotic-resistant organisms survive while those susceptible to the antibiotics die off, resulting in the emergence of antibiotic resistance (see Levy, 2002).

Vaccinations (immunization)

The development and use of vaccinations contributed greatly to the control of a variety of infectious diseases. Indeed, "Perhaps the single most dramatic and controversial public health measure of the age [the Age of Enlightenment] was smallpox inoculation, followed by Edward Jenner's revolutionary discovery of vaccination" (Fee, 2015, p. xxiii; see also Riedel, 2005). Vaccine use was especially effective in controlling childhood infectious diseases, for which vaccination conferred life-long immunity. Despite the contribution that vaccination made to the control of infectious diseases, some challenges threaten that progress.

Under vaccination: Vaccination protects the individual. In addition, there will always be people in society who cannot be vaccinated – because of their age or underlying health conditions. For these people, living among those who have high vaccination rates (approaching 95% coverage) gives protection by creating community immunity (Levin, Kershner, Lytton, Salmon, & Omer, 2020). If high enough coverage rates in the population at large are not achieved, these under vaccination rates pose a threat to those who cannot be vaccinated.

Vaccine refusal: Despite the great effect that vaccination had on the control of disease, people opposed using vaccinations almost as soon as they were developed. Early objections to vaccination and widespread vaccination use were based on a variety of views, resonant with those expressed today. These ranged from questions about the efficacy of vaccinations and their basis, fears that vaccination would cause harm, to religiously grounded objections, to concerns about maintaining individual liberty (see Rosen, 2015, p. 104).

Refusal to take vaccines was reflected in the media of the day. For example, the US National Library of Medicine collection contains an etching by James Gillray, entitled "The cow-pock, or, The wonderful effects of the new inoculation!", published in *Vide-the Publications of ye Anti-Vaccine Society* [permanent link: http://resource.nlm.nih.gov/101395166], which depicts the various ills attributed to smallpox vaccination. The etching depicts a chaotic scene in which cows sprout from various parts of those vaccinated.

Despite the resonances and continuities seen in vaccine refusal, as Dubé and her colleagues note:

> there are distinct differences between anti-vaccine promoters then and now. Whereas in the past anti-vaccination activists were mostly proletarians who were opposed to the state intervention in their bodies and their children's bodies, anti-vaccination groups in today's world, at least in HIC [high-income countries], are mostly well-educated middle- and upper-income parents who claim the right to make an "informed decision" about vaccination. Many contemporary anti-vaccination groups were also formed by parents who believed that their child has been seriously harmed by vaccine in order to seek compensation from the industry or the government. Other anti-vaccination groups are lead [sic] by alternative practitioners who are opposed to biomedicine and who sell "natural solutions" to replace vaccination. (Dubé, Vivion, & MacDonald, 2015, p. 106)

In contemporary settings, the spread of the anti-vaccine movement is facilitated by the increased interconnectivity that comes with social media, which give a platform for the spread of misinformation, conspiracy theories, anti-science tropes, and the promotion of alternatives to vaccines that are at best harmless and at worst harmful (Dubé et al., 2015; Fee, 2015; Kata, 2012; Larson, 2020; Lilienfeld, Marshall, Todd, & Shane, 2014). One point of historical continuity, however, likely remains distrust in state and public institutions, an ongoing problem for public health and public health practitioners.

Climate Change

The reality of climate change – that the earth's climate is warming – is a settled consensus within the scientific community (Costello et al., 2009). Within this consensus there are disagreements about how to best model the effects of climate change, where the problems are most acute, and, hence, what interventions are most helpful, and, as a result, what the best estimates of those effects may be (Palmer & Stevens, 2019). Not understanding the nature of scientific consensus, or the contingent nature of knowledge that leads to revisions of models and iterative forecasts as greater understanding develops (Beatty, 2006; Lefsrud & Meyer, 2012), some seize upon the variations among models and in policy prescriptions to support the wholesale rejection of climate science (Boykoff, 2007; Lewandowsky, Oberauer, & Gignac, 2013). As with vaccine refusal, such views are advanced through social media, the politics of anti-elitism attached to anti-science, and by media coverage that misstates scientific understandings of climate science and climate change (Bast & Spencer, 2014; Oreskes & Conway, 2010; Steffen, 2013).

Increasingly, the effects of climate change are observable around the globe, with implications for public health (e.g., see Chapter 28 by Hryhorczuk and Hryhorczuk in this volume; and Goodell, 2020). The debate over whether climate change is driven by human activities (i.e., is anthropogenic or not) is not relevant to the health effects of environmental changes, which are observable. In general, the effects of warming or volatile climate fall into three or four categories. We observe (1) wetter, (2) hotter, (3) more extreme weather, and (4) these developments interact in synergistic ways.

Maslin (2004, pp. 83–101) further describes the effects of global warming by noting that it affects (1) coastlines, (2) storms and flooding, (3) general weather patterns, such as the El Nino-Southern Oscillation, (4) agriculture, (5) and biodiversity, all of which, in turn, affect (6) health. Various reports from the Intergovernment Panel on Climate Change (IPCC) set out in greater detail how climate change is setting off observable perturbations in the ecosystem that affect life on the planet (see, for example, IPCC, 2014, 2019). Some of the health challenges due to climate change follow from the resulting change in the physical environment.

The rising temperature of oceans, for example, leads to ice melts which contribute to rising water levels. Over recent decades we have seen as a result increased risks of coastal flooding, and sea level rise threatening the lifeways of island dwelling peoples (IPCC, 2019; Letman, 2018). Changing water temperature can result in environments more conducive to the growth of pathogens. Studies examining increases in Korean coastal water temperatures linked to global warming showed increases in Vibro vunificus bacterial populations (Chu et al., 2011). This leads to increases in infected fish, which in turn leads to human infection with this zoonotic disease. In people, Vibrum vunificus can infect wounds. The infection may be mild, but it can result in necrotizing fasciitis that can require surgical intervention, amputations of limbs, or death (Harper, 2016, p. 4). Global warming also affects vector-borne diseases, like malaria, dengue, and leishmaniasis, by extending the range of the physical environments that are congenial for pathogen-bearing hosts, like mosquitos and ticks (Barclay, 2008; Bouchard et al., 2019; Ng et al., 2019; Ostfeld & Brunner, 2015; Reiter, 2001).

HEALTH CHALLENGES OF DISASTERS

Although there are important differences among the health challenges posed by disasters of different origin, there are commonalities and overlapping patterns of suffering, morbidity, and mortality in the health that affect people in all of the disasters. All disasters involve health effects that are short term, acute, and requiring immediate action, as well as other health effects which are long term, and requiring continuing attention and care. Complicating this picture is that some of the acute short-term effects have long-term sequelae. This is true too for those effects that may be thought of as direct and indirect effects of disaster. Further, in all of the various kinds of disaster, women and children are disproportionately affected, as are other vulnerable populations, such as those with physical and cognitive disabilities (Eisenman et al., 2009). Thus, although the health effects of disasters may be characterized in ways that make them appear distinct, they may well interact with one another in synergistic ways that intensify the consequences of each. Taken individually, many of the health consequences of disasters are described in detail in other chapters in this *Handbook.* With these considerations in mind, this section highlights a few of the health effects of disasters shown in Figure 31.1, many of which are seen in the Haitian experiences described at the outset of this chapter.

Infrastructure, Social, and Public Health System Destruction

Civil conflict and ecological disasters like those experienced in Haiti hinder the development of physical and social infrastructure. A consistent research finding shows that investments in materiel to prepare for or prosecute civil conflicts uses funds that could otherwise be put towards infrastructure for water and sanitation systems. In situations where the necessary physical infrastructure has been developed, fighting during civil conflict and the acute phases of other disasters can destroy or severely limit the capacity of these systems to effectively support population health (Comes et al., 2016; Pinxten, 1986; Urlainis, Shohet, Levy, Ornai, & Vilnay, 2014). Disasters may make communication difficult when the cell phone networks are overloaded or destroyed or the disruption of the power grid may cause widespread power outages, as also happened, for example, during the 1999 earthquake in Izmit, Turkey (Barka, 1999). In the Haitian case, fighting in Cite Soleil caused considerable infrastructure damage, and the 2010 earthquake damaged or destroyed buildings, including those essential to government functioning (Fisher et al., 2018).

In addition to the destruction of physical infrastructure, disasters affect the ability of societies to provide for the health of their citizens. Not only are the actual facilities used to ensure safe water and food damaged, but so too are health clinics and hospitals. As in the Haiti case, vital statistics and health records can also be damaged or destroyed. The public health workforce is not immune from the travails affecting the population generally. Healthcare workers die and are injured as a result of disaster, making it difficult or impossible to carry out important public health activities like disease surveillance and vaccination programmes. In the context of complex emergencies, health workers can also be targets for opposing groups who see an attack on them as advancing their political ends (Barry & Jefferys, 2002; Rubinstein & Zoli, 2019; Slim, 1997). During disasters resulting from epidemics, resurgent, and emerging diseases, frontline healthcare workers are also at risk. For example, a joint study conducted by Kaiser Health News and *The Guardian* newspaper identified 1,423 healthcare workers in the United States who died as of December 2020 fighting the COVID-19 epidemic (The Guardian and Kaiser Health News, 2020). During the fight against the 2014 Ebola epidemic in Sierra Leone an estimated 221 healthcare workers died, comprising about 21% of the country's healthcare workforce (Raven, Wurie, & Witter, 2018, p. 252). Beyond deaths, during disasters the efficacy of public health efforts is compromised by misinformation spread among populations, fatigue and trauma, increased sickness and physical injury, and loss of social connections (Morren, Dirkzwager, Kessels, & Yzermans, 2007). Additionally, conflicts can occur between intervenors and local populations who work from different ideas about the right way to deal with a wide

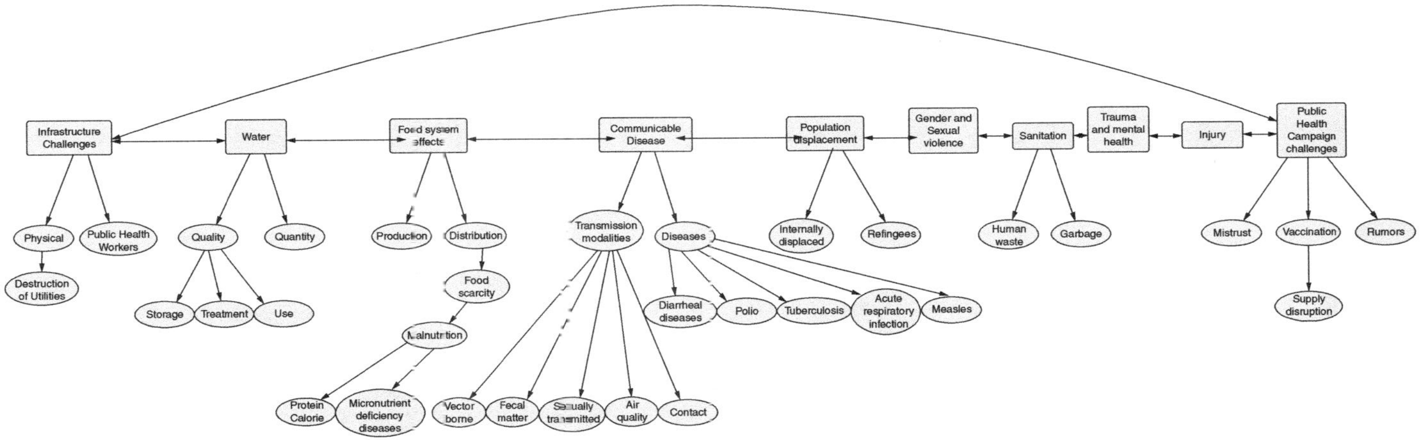

Figure 31.1 Some interconnected health challenges due to disasters

range of activities that are important for ameliorating the effects of disaster. For instance, Omidian, Tehoungue and Monger (2014) describe socio-cultural factors that influenced ways in which communities in Liberia addressed Ebola, including tensions between medical and local understandings of the disease, healthcare providers, and messaging, and the ways in which local practices, like burial customs, contributed to the spread of disease (see also Pailey, 2017).

Population Displacement

Among the most devastating effects of disaster is population displacement. People move within their states, becoming internally displaced persons, or seek safety by fleeing across national borders, becoming asylum seekers and refugees. (These population movements are treated in depth in this *Handbook* in Chapter 13 by McDaniel, Shaw, and Jok.)

Ecological calamities can lead to massive relocations of people within a state as lack of access to resources and economic opportunities lead to people seeking to improve their life chances, such as people whose homes have been destroyed by earthquake, or those who can no longer make a living. Following the 2016 earthquake in Haiti, as described earlier, many people fled from their destroyed homes seeking shelter elsewhere, including as refugees and immigrants to the Dominican Republic (DR). Egyptian farmers in the Nile Delta area face declining agricultural prospects because of the increasing salinization of ground water due to rising water tables contaminated with salt water from rising coastal waters due to global warming (Frihy, Deabes, Shereet, & Abdalla, 2010). This has had the consequence of disrupting the agricultural communities in the Delta, one of the world's most intensively farmed regions, because crops that have traditionally thrived in the Delta's three growing seasons are becoming less viable. This has led to social and economic disruption and the movement of rural people within Egypt, often to cities.

Often these movements are from rural areas to urban settings, where people face additional challenges, including living in informal housing which lacks basic sanitation, access to water, and utilities in areas of high population density and poverty. These circumstances increase the risk of violence, sexual exploitation, and communicable diseases like tuberculosis, HIV/AIDs, and diarrheal disease (Dos Santos, Ouédraogo, & Soura, 2015; Farmer, 1996; Nix et al., 2020; Shortt & Hammett, 2013).

During complex emergencies, where attacks on the civilian population may be part of the strategies of warring parties, people flee their homes in search of safety. Those who escape to neighboring countries may find shelter in refugee camps. Health challenges in such camps abound due to poor infrastructure, crowding, and the overwhelming of health and other services. Too frequently mental health services to help people deal with continuing trauma are limited or unavailable (Catani et al., 2009). Overcrowding increases the risk of communicable diseases. For instance, the Syrian civil war has increased the number of cases of tuberculosis, both inside Syria and, especially, in neighboring refugee camps. For example, the Turkish Ministry of Health reported that one refugee camp saw "an increase in pulmonary TB cases from 25.1% to 34.6% within a 4-year period (2010–2013)" (Ismail, Rafei, Dabboussi, & Hamze, 2018, p. 3). Additionally, women and children in refugee camps are at increased risk for gender-based and sexual violence (Buckley-Zistel & Krause, 2017).

Food, Water, and Sanitation

The complex and important role of food and water in health are discussed in chapters on food and water of this *Handbook*. Safe and adequate food and water are necessary for sustaining human life and for allowing it to flourish. By their ecological character some disasters create problems for access to food and water. Some of these challenges follow from the sudden destruction of the physical infrastructure or disruption of the social institutions related to these necessities. Others result from the disruptions resulting from longer-term trends, including those linked to climate change. Droughts, floods, and rising water tables can all affect access to food and water, though the effects vary regionally and locally (Adedeji, Gieck-Bricco, & Kehayova, 2016; Paris, Reboredo, Ramalho, Pessoa, & Lidon, 2020). Violence related to the context of complex humanitarian emergencies can affect the availability of food and water. These resources are sometimes targeted strategically to force opponents to capitulate, or to disrupt supplies being distributed by humanitarian agencies (Rubinstein & Zoli, 2019; Sahnoun, 1994). For example, in South Sudan the World Food Program reported numerous attacks on food aid, including the killing of humanitarian workers. Similarly, food is weaponized in Syria and Yemen (Human Appeal, n.d.) and the World Food Program reports that as a result "an estimated 17 million are food insecure (including 6.8 million severely food insecure); 14.5 million lack adequate access to clean water or sanitation; 14.8 million people lack sufficient access to healthcare; an estimated 2 million children under the age of five are acutely malnourished" (Alamnew, 2017, p. 4).

During disasters, access to food is disrupted at multiple points. With the food system, the ability to produce, distribute, and have food available can all be disrupted. The resulting food insecurity can lead to protein-calorie malnutrition, micronutrient deficiencies, and starvation, as in Yemen, Somalia, or South Sudan. Access to potable water can also be disrupted by disaster. Infrastructure destruction, loss of technically proficient personnel, and the purposeful targeting of water supplies can also lead to water scarcity. Due to the effects of disaster on a community's ability to safely store and treat water to ensure it is potable, the quality of what water is available may provide a vector for infection (Burkle Jr., Martone, & Greenough, 2014; Wisner, Blaikie, Cannon, & Davis, 2003).

The ways that societies organize themselves in relation to the food and water are complex, as are the roles and meaning which are ascribed to these resources (Ballestero, 2019; Klein & Watson, 2016; Scrimshaw & Lane, 2020). Among the challenges facing those responding to disasters of all types are providing the kinds of food acceptable to the population in need, understanding local patterns of distribution and consumption, and overcoming the complications presented by the politics of international response (Edkins, 2000; Pouligny, 2006; Rubinstein, 2008), as reflected in the Haiti example.

Not only does inadequate, inappropriate food and non-potable water damage health directly, the lack of these resources has indirect effects as well. Interrelationships among water, food, sanitation, and health care are shown in Figure 31.2. People produce waste. In circumstances where the regular mechanisms of dealing with waste are damaged or have not been adequately established – as happens with refugee camps – garbage and human excreta create health hazards. Lack of easily available water affects hygiene practices. Fecal contamination of drinking water can lead to diarrheal disease. Poor management of waste creates conditions in which animal vectors of infectious disease may flourish (Cronin et al., 2008). Lack of appropriate ways to dispose of water may in some climates lead to conditions favorable to mosquito breeding and the spread of malaria. For instance, Bayoh and associates report that in Kakuma refugee camp in Kenya, malaria became hyperendemic "in an area with otherwise low risk of malaria given prevailing climate" (Bayoh et al., 2011, p. 1).

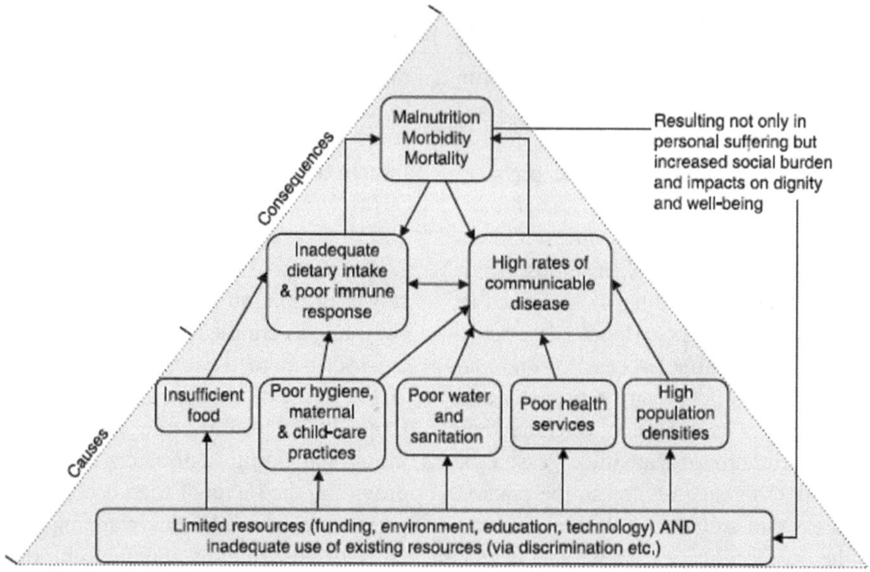

Figure 31.2 Relationships among sanitation, water, nutrition and health sectors. Reproduced from A. A. Cronin et al. 2008. *Journal of Water & Health* 6(1), 1–13, with permission from the copyright holders, IWA Publishing.

Non-communicable and Communicable Disease

Disasters of all types affect the prevalence of non-communicable disease. The suddenness of ecological calamities, or the violence of complex emergencies result in varying degrees of trauma. Women and children are at higher risk due to their particular vulnerability to gender-based violence and sexual assault. Although circumstances differ depending upon the disaster context, the World Health Organization has documented: (1) increases in child abuse and neglect, not infrequently including the infliction of traumatic brain injury; (2) risk for intimate partner and sexual violence; (3) and sexual exploitation (Krug, Dahlberg, Mercy, Zwi, & Lozano, 2002). These, and the trauma that the acute phases of disaster and the longer-term conditions they create, lead to a variety of psychological consequences that require long-term care (Krug et al., 2002).

The sudden, catastrophic nature of earthquake, flooding, fires, tornados and other ecological calamities or of organized violence in civil conflicts results in increased levels of physical injuries. Persons managing chronic diseases may as a result of disaster also be cut off from the sources of help that sustained them prior to the disaster.

Exposure to communicable diseases is increased in many types of disaster, for instance, overcrowding in refugee camps or in shelters made available to people after ecological calamities. Ligon (2006; see also Burnham, 2013) presents a useful typology for infectious disease following disasters. These are: (1) resulting from compromised personal hygiene; (2) respiratory infection; (3) infections linked to contaminated food and water; (4) vector- and insect-borne disease; (5) infections resulting from contact with dead bodies. Box 31.4 expands on this typology and gives a more detailed view of common infectious disease after disaster.

Box 31.4 Infectious diseases after disaster: a typology*

- Infections from Compromised Personal Hygiene
- Respiratory and Airborne Infection
  - Measles
  - Meningitis
  - Severe Acute Respiratory Syndrome
  - Tuberculosis
- Infections due to Accident, Violence, and Sexual Assault
  - Chlamydia
  - Gonorrhea
  - HIV
  - Syphillis
  - Tetanus
- Infections from Contaminated Food and Water
  - Cholera
  - Diarrheal disease
  - Hepatitis A
  - Hepatitis E
  - Leptospirosis
  - Parasitic diseases
    - Amebiasis
    - Cryptosporidiosis
    - Cyclosporiasis
    - Giardiasis
    - Rotavirus
    - Shigellosis
    - Typhoid fever
- Vector- and Insect-borne Disease
  - Dengue
  - Malaria
  - Rabies
  - St. Louis Encephalitis
  - West Nile Virus
  - Infections from Contamination Associated with Dead Bodies

*Some infectious diseases fit into more than one of the categories. After: Ligon, 2006; Perrin, 1996; Toole & Waldman, 1997; Waldman, 1999.

The case of Haiti, described at the beginning of the chapter, illustrates the complex relationships among the variety of health consequences of disaster. For example, in the aftermath of the 2010 earthquake, Doocy and her colleagues found an increase in the injury rate per 1,000, and a reported 300,000 injuries during the period of their study (Doocy, Jacquet, Cherewick, & Kirsh, 2013). Similarly, following the 2010 earthquake, tuberculosis in Haiti rose from already being among the highest incidence in the hemisphere. For example, research carried out in a tent camp to house those who had lost their homes showed The estimated tuberculosis incidence in the camp was 693 cases per 100,000 person-years, about three times the 2010 World Health Organization estimate for Haiti (Koenig et al., 2015, p. 499). And, of course, the destruction of physical infrastructure and social institutions meant that the country was less prepared to deal with the cholera outbreak that swept the country and for the subsequent hurricane.

CONCLUSIONS

Disaster is a broad category, encompassing events brought on by diverse causes. At a broad scale, disasters can be grouped together into groups with similar causes. Nonetheless, disasters are in many ways unique in their origin and in the social and physical circumstances in which they occur. As described in this chapter, the health consequences of disasters are complex, overlapping, dynamic, and specific. This means that preparing for and responding to disasters is especially challenging.

Multilateral organizations, national agencies, nongovernmental organizations, militaries, and consortia of elements of all of these communities, work to develop best practices for disaster preparation and response. These efforts are reflected in efforts like those flowing from the Sendai Framework and in other work (Albala-Bertrand, 2000a; Cutter et al., 2012; Debarre, 2019; Onyango & Uwase, 2017). Preparation and response are complicated also by differing epistemological commitments, perhaps reflected in the value and role accorded to local knowledge (Autesserre, 2014; Omidian et al., 2014), in tensions between the organizations involved, as, for example, between military and humanitarian interveners (Barry & Jefferys, 2002; Rubinstein & Zoli, 2019), or geopolitical considerations that shape decisions to acknowledge and act upon noxious events.

Within this dynamic system of relationships among different kinds of disaster and socio-political and economic processes, the public health system is always stressed. Efforts to deal effectively with disasters often have to confront inaccurate or degraded information (e.g., rumors, gossip, and conspiracy theories). Loss of facilities and personnel often interrupts vaccination programmes. As happened in Haiti, the loss of vital records that were needed to fully address population health needs created data gaps. The disease surveillance effort can be disrupted by making it difficult to fully track the emergence of infectious diseases, which was among the reasons that the cholera in the Haitian case spread so quickly and effective intervention was made more difficult. Local practices and cultural understandings have to be acknowledged and addressed, and members of the affected communities need to be engaged and involved for an effective response, as shown regarding the response to Ebola in Liberia discussed earlier.

Understanding disasters and their health effects is a complex undertaking. The organization and delivery of effective aid to those suffering from the disasters too is a complex undertaking. With estimates that disasters of all types will increase, this is a challenging, rewarding, and essential area of professional work.

REFERENCES

Acquisto, N. M. (2014). Isoniazid. In P. Wexler (Ed.), *Encyclopedia of Toxicology* (3rd edition, Vol. 2, pp. 1135–1137). London, UK Academic Press/Elsevier.

Adedeji, O. S., Gieck-Bricco, J., & Kehayova, V. (2016). *Natural Disasters and Food Crises in Low Income Countries: Macroeconomic Dimensions*. Washington, DC: International Monetary Fund.

Aggarwal, V. (2018). The role of oral health in complex emergencies and disaster rehabilitation medicine. *Disaster Medicine and Public Health Preparedness*, *12*(6), 772–777.

Alamnew, E. (2017). *Yemen: Emergency Food Security and Nutrition Assessment*. Rome: World Food Program.

Albala-Bertrand, J. M. (2000a). Responses to complex humanitarian emergencies and natural disasters: An analytical comparison. *Third World Quarterly*, *21*(2), 215–227.

Albala-Bertrand, J. M. (2000b). *What is a 'Complex Humanitarian Emergency'? An Analytical Essay*. Working Papers 420. London: Queen Mary University of London, School of Economics and Finance.

Autesserre, S. (2010). *The Trouble with the Congo: Local Violence and the Failure of*

International Peacebuilding. Cambridge, UK: Cambridge University Press.

Autesserre, S. (2014). *Peaceland: Conflict Resolution and the Everyday Politics of International Intervention*. New York: Cambridge University Press.

Ballestero, A. (2019). The anthropology of water. *Annual Review of Anthropology, 48*, 405–421.

Barclay, E. (2008). Is climate change affecting dengue in the Americas? *The Lancet, 371*(973–974).

Barka, A. (1999). The 17 August 1999 Izmit earthquake. *Science, 285*(5435), 1858–1859.

Barry, J., & Jefferys, A. (2002). *A Bridge Too Far: AID Agencies and the Military in Humanitarian Response*. Humanitarian Practice Network Paper 37. London: Humanitarian Practice Network.

Bast, J., & Spencer, R. (2014). The myth of the climate change '97%'. *Wall Street Journal, [Eastern edition]*, May 27 (A13).

Battin, M. P., Francis, L. P., Jacobson, J. A., & Smith, C. B. (2009). *The Patient as Victim and Vector*. Oxford: Oxford University Press.

Bayoh, M. N., Akhwale, W., Ombok, M., Sang, D., Engoki, S. C., Koros, D., & Hamel, M. J. (2011). Malaria in Kakuma refugee camp, Turkana, Kenya: facilitation of Anopheles arabiensis vector populations by installed water distribution and catchment systems. *Malaria Journal, 10*, 149–160.

Beatty, J. H. (2006). Masking disagreement among experts. *Episteme: A Journal of Social Epistemology*, 3, 1–2.

Bobrowsky, P. T. (Ed.) (2013). *Encyclopedia of Natural Hazards*. Dordrecht, NL: Springer Reference.

Bouchard, C., Dibernardo, A., Koffi, J., Wood, H., Leighton, P., & Lindsay, L. R. (2019). Increased risk of tick-borne diseases with climate and environmental changes. *Canadian Communicable Disease Report, 45*(4), 81–89.

Boykoff, M. T. (2007). From convergence to contention: United States mass media representions of anthropogenic climate change science. *Transactions of the Institute of British Geographers, NS 32*, 477–489.

Buckley-Zistel, S., & Krause, U. (Eds.). (2017). *Gender, Violence, Refugees*. Oxford and New York: Berghahn Books.

Burkle, Jr., F. M., Martone, G., & Greenough, P. G. (2014). The changing face of humanitarian crises. *Brown Journal of World Affairs, 20*(2), 19–36.

Burnham, G. (2013). Epidemiology of disease in natural disasters. In P. T. Bobrowsky (Ed.), *Encyclopedia of Natural Hazards* (pp. 285–288). Dordrecht, NL: Springer Reference.

Button, G. (2010). *Disaster Culture: Knowledge and Uncertainty in the Wake of Human and Environmental Catastrophe*. Walnut Creek, CA: Left Coast Press.

Catani, C., Kohiladevy, M., Ruf, M., Schauer, E., Elbert, T., & Neuner. (2009). Treating children traumatized by war and tsunami: a comparison between exposure therapy and meditation-relaxation in North-East Sri Lanka. *BMC Psychiatry, 9*, 22–33.

Centers for Disease Control and Prevention. (2014). *Cholera in Haiti*. Retrieved from www.cdc.gov/cholera/haiti/index.htm

Chu, C., Do, Y., Kim, Y., Sito, Y., Lee, S.-D., Park, H., & Lee, J.-K. (2011). Mathematical modeling of *vibrio vulnificus* infection in Korea and the influence of global warming. *Osong Public Health and Research Perspectives, 2*(1), 51–58.

Comes, M., Cubbert, M., Garschagen, M., Hagenlocher, M., Sabelfeld, R., Lee, Y. J., & Birkmann, J. (2016). *World Disaster Report 2016: Logistics and Infrastructure*. Berlin: Bündnis Entwicklung Hilft.

Costello, A., Abbas, M., Allen, A., Ball, S., Bell, S., Bellamy, R., & Paterson, C. (2009). Managing the health effects of climate change. *The Lancet, 373*, 1692–1733.

Cronin, A. A., Shrestha, D., Cornier, N., Abdalla, F., Ezard, N., & Aramburu, C. (2008). A review of water and sanitation provision in refugee camps in association with selected health and nutrition indicators – the need for integrated service provision. *Journal of Water and Health*, 6(1), 1–13.

Cutter, S. L., Ahern, J. A., Amadei, B., Crawford, P., Eide, E. A., Galloway Jr., G. E., & Zoback, M. L. (2012). *Disaster Resilience: A National Imperative*. Washington, DC: National Academy Press.

Debarre, A. (2019). *Delivering Healthcare amid Crisis: The Humanitarian Response in Myanmar*. New York: International Peace Institute.

Diceanu, A. (2006). Haiti deserves better from the United Nations: for many Haitians, MINUSTAH has been closer to a foreign occupation force than a UN peacekeeping mission. *Peace Magazine, 22*(2), 16–19.

Doocy, S., Jacquet, G., Cherewick, M., & Kirsh, T. D. (2013). The injury burden of the 2010 Haiti earthquake: a stratified cluster survey. *Injury, 44*, 842–847.

Dos Santos, S., Ouédraogo, F. d. C., & Soura, A. B. (2015). Water-related factors and childhood diarrhoea in African informal settlements: a cross-sectional study in Ouagadougou (Burkina Faso). *Journal of Water and Health, 13*(2), 562–574.

Douglas, M., & Wildavsky, A. (1983). *Risk and Culture: An Essay on the Selection of Technological and Environmental Dangers*. Berkeley, CA: University of California Press.

Dubé, E., Vivion, M., & MacDonald, N. E. (2015). Vaccine hesitancy, vaccine refusal and the anti-vaccine movement: influence, impact and implications. *Expert Reveiw of Vaccine, 14*(1), 99–117.

Dubos, R. (1952). *The White Plague: Tuberculosis, Man, and Society*. Boston, MA: Little, Brown and Company.

Duffield, M. (1994). Complex emergencies and the crisis of developmentalism. *IDS Bulletin, 25*(4), 1–15.

Edkins, J. (2000). *Whose Hunger? Concepts of Famine, Practices of Aid*. Minneapolis, MN: University of Minnesota Press.

Eisenman, D. P., Zhou, Q., Ong, M., Asch, S., Glik, D., & Long, A. (2009). Variations in disaster preparedness by mental health, perceived general health, and disability status. *Disaster Medicine and Public Health Preparedness, 3*(1), 33–41.

Elvey, S. (2016). Hurricane Matthew continues to wreak havoc after destroying 90 per cent of south Haiti. *Express [Online]*, October 8, 1–3, www.express.co.uk/news/weather/719047/Hurricane-Matthew-Haiti-havoc-destroying-719090-per-cent-south-Carolinas, accessed January 7, 2020.

Evans-Prichard, E. E. (1937). *Witchcraft, Oracles and Magic among the Azande*. Oxford: Oxford University Press.

Farmer, P. (1996). On suffering and structural violence: a view from below. *Daedalus, 125*(1), 261–283.

Farmer, P. (2004). What happened in Haiti? Where past is present. In N. Chomsky, P. Farmer, & A. Goodman (Eds.), *Getting Haiti Right this Time: The U.S. and the Coup* (pp. 11–36). Monroe, ME: Common Courage Press.

Fee, E. (2015). Introduction: a shared social vision. In G. Rosen (Ed.), *A History of Public Heatlh* (revised expanded edition, pp. xiii–lii). Baltimore, MD: Johns Hopkins University Press.

Fenner, F., Henderson, D. A., Arita, I., Zdeněk, J., & Ladnyi, I. D. (1988). *Smallpox and its Eradication*. Geneva: World Health Organization.

Fine, P. E. M., Goldacre, B. M., & Haines, A. (2013). Epidemiology – a science for the people. *The Lancet, 381*(13 April), 1249–1252.

Fisher, D., Hagon, K., Lattimer, C., O'Callaghan, S., Swithern, S., & Walmsley, L. (2018). *Leaving No One Behind: World Disaster Report 2018*. Geneva: International Federation of Red Cross and Red Crescent Societies.

Frerichs, R. S. (2017). *Deadly River: Cholera and Cover-Up in Post-Earthquake Haiti*. Ithaca, NY: Cornell University Press.

Frihy, O. E. S., Deabes, E. A., Shereet, S. M., & Abdalla, F. A. (2010). Alexandria–Nile Delta coast, Egypt: update and future projection of relative sea-level rise. *Environmental Earth Sciences, 61*, 253–273.

Fujimura, C. K., Stoeck, S., & Sudakova, T. (2005). *Russia's Abandoned Children: An Intimate Understanding*. Westport, CT: Praeger.

Gaynes, R. P. (2011). *Germ Theory: Medical Pioneers in Infectious Disease*. Washington, DC: ASM Press.

Goodell, J. (2020). How climate change is ushering in a new pandemic era. *Rolling Stone*, www.rollingstone.com/culture/culture-features/climate-change-risks-infectious-diseases-covid-19-ebola-dengue-1098923/amp/?fbclid=IwAR0AwW2bRanIzJZ8xcgPST7ok-r5D8I-a5OZwnpfhALvHxtoWYObF3NOzlo (accessed December 10, 2020).

Gros, J.-G. (1996). Towards a taxonomy of failed states in the New World Order: decaying Somalia, Liberia, Rwanda and Haiti. *Third World Quarterly, 17*(3), 455–471.

Harper, K. J. (2016). *Marine Zoonotic Disease and You*. Atlanta, GA: Marine Aquarium Societies of North America Educational Series.

Hays, J. N. (2005). *Epidemics and Pandemics: Their Impacts on Human History*. Santa Barbara, CA: ABC-CLIO, Inc.

Herring, D. A., & Swedlund, A. C. (Eds.). (2010). *Plagues and Epidemics: Infected Spaces Past and Present*. Oxford: Berg.

Human Appeal. (n.d.). *Hunger as a Weapon of War*. Cheadle, UK: Human Appeal.

IASC (Inter-Agency Standing Committee). (2008). *Civil-Military Guidelines & Reference for Complex Emergencies*. New York: United Nations.

IPCC. (2014). *Climate Change 2014 Impacts, Adaptation, and Vulnerability. Part A Global and Sectoral Aspects*. Contribution of Working Group II to the Fifth Assessment Report of the Intergovernmental Panel on Climate Change [Edited by C. B. Field, V. R. Barros, D. J. Dokken, K. J. Mach, M. D. Mastrandrea, T. E. Bilir, M. Chatterjee, K. L. Ebi, Y. O. Estrada, R. C. Genova, B. Girma, E. S. Kissel, A. N. Levy, S. MacCracken, P. R. Mastrandrea, & L. L. White]. Cambridge, UK: Cambridge University Press.

IPCC. (2019). *Global Warming of 1.5° C. An IPCC Special Report on the Impacts of Global Warming of 1.5°C above Pre-industrial Levels and Related Global Greenhouse Gas Emission Pathways, in the Context of Strengthening the Global Response to the Threat of Climate Change, Sustainable Development, and Efforts to Eradicate Poverty* [Edited by V. Masson-Delmotte, P. Zhai, H.-O. Pörtner, D. Roberts, J. Skea, P. R. Shukla, A. Pirani, W. Moufouma-Okia, C. Péan, R. Pidcock, S. Connors, J. B. R. Matthews, Y. Chen, X. Zhou, M. I. Gomis, E. Lonnoy, T. Maycock, M. Tignor, & T. Waterfield]. New York: The Intergovernmental Panel on Climate Change/ United Nations.

Ismail, M. B., Rafei, R., Dabboussi, F., & Hamze, M. (2018). Tuberculosis, war, and refugees: spotlight on the Syrian humanitarian crisis. *PLOS Pathogens*, *14*(6), e1007014; 1007011–1007016.

Ivers, L. C., Farmer, P., Almazor, C. P., & Léandre, F. (2010). Five complementary interventions to slow cholera: Haiti. *The Lancet*, *376*(9758), 2048–2051. doi:10.1016/S0140-6736(10) 62243-X

Kaplan, R. (1994). The coming anarchy. *The Atlantic Monthly*, *273*(2), 44–76.

Kata, A. (2012). Anti-vaccine activists, Web 2.0, and the postmodern paradigm: an overview of tactics and tropes used online by the anti-vaccination movement. *Vaccine*, *30*, 3778–3789.

Katz, J. M. (2013). *The Big Truck that Went By: How the World Came to Save Haiti and Left Behind a Disaster*. New York: St Martin's Press.

Keen, D. (2008). *Complex Emergencies*. Cambridge, UK: Polity Press.

Kelman, I. (2018). Lost for words amongst Disaster Risk Science vocabulary? *International Journal of Disaster Risk Science*, *9*, 281–291.

Klein, J. A., & Watson, J. L. (Eds.). (2016). *The Handbook of Food and Anthropology*. London: Bloomsbury.

Koenig, S. P., Rouzier, V., Vilbrun, S. C., Morose, W., Collins, S. E., Joseph, P., & Pape, J. W. (2015). Tuberculosis in the aftermath of the 2010 earthquake in Haiti. *Bulletin of the World Health Organization*, *93*, 495–502.

Kristoff, M., & Panarelli, L. (2010). *Haiti: A Republic of NGOs?* Washington, DC: United States Institute of Peace.

Krug, E. G., Dahlberg, L. L., Mercy, J. A., Zwi, A. B., & Lozano, R. (Eds.). (2002). *World Report on Violence and Health*. Geneva: World Health Organization.

Larson, H. J. (2020). *Stuck: How Vaccine Rumors Start – and Why They Don't Go Away*. Oxford: Oxford University Press.

Lefsrud, L. M., & Meyer, R. E. (2012). Science or science fiction? Professionals' discursive construction of climate change. *Organization Studies*, *33*(11), 1477–1506.

Letman, J. (2018). Rising seas give island nation a stark choice: relocate or elevate. *National Geographic [Online]*, November, www.nationalgeographic.com/environment/2018/11/rising-seas-force-marshall-islands-relocate-elevate-artificial-islands/#close

Levin, H. Y., Kershner, S. P., Lytton, T. D., Salmon, D., & Omer, S. B. (2020). Stopping the resurgence of vaccine-preventable childhood diseases: policy, politics, and law. *University of Illinois Law Review*, *2020*(1).

Levy, S. B. (2002). *The Antibiotic Paradox: How the Misuse of Antibiotics Destroys Their Curative Powers* (2nd edition). Cambridge, MA: Perseus Pubishing.

Lewandowsky, S., Oberauer, K., & Gignac, G. (2013). NASA faked the Moon Landing – therefore, (climate) science is a hoax: an anatomy of the motivated rejection of science. *Psychological Science, 24*(5), 622–633.

Ligon, B. L. (2006). Infectious diseases that pose specific challenges after natural disasters: a review. *Seminars in Pediatric Infectious Disease, 17*, 36–45.

Lilienfeld, S. O., Marshall, J., Todd, J. T., & Shane, H. C. (2014). The persistence of fad interventions in the face of negative scientific evidence: facilitated communication for autism as a case example. *Evidence-Based Communication Assessment and Intervention, 8*(2), 62–101.

Lupton, D. (2013). *Risk* (2nd edition). New York: Routledge.

Maslin, M. (2004). *Global Warming: A Very Short Introduction*. Oxford: Oxford University Press.

McElroy, A., & Townsend, P. K. (2015). *Medical Anthropology in Ecological Perspective* (6th edition). Boulder, CO: Westview Press.

McIntire, M. (2016). Line between public and private blurs for inner circle of Clinton. *The New York Times,* October 17, A1, A14.

McNeill, W. H. (1976). *Plagues and Peoples*. New York: Anchor/Doubleday.

Morbidity and Mortality Weekly Report (MMWR). (2010). Update: outbreak of cholera – Haiti, 2010. *Morbidity and Mortality Weekly Report, 59*(48), 1586–1590.

Morley, I. (2007). City chaos, contagion, Chadwick, and social justice. *Yale Journal of Biology and Medicine, 80*(2007), 61–72.

Morren, M., Dirkzwager, A. J. E., Kessels, F. J. M., & Yzermans, C. J. (2007). The influence of a disaster on the health of rescue workers: a longitudinal study. *Canadian Medical Association Journal, 176*(9), 1279–1283.

Murray, J. F., Schraufnagel, D. E., & Hopewell, P. C. (2015). Treatment of tuberculosis: a historical perspective. *Annals of the American Thoracic Society, 12*(12), 1749–1759.

New York Times. (1945). Penicillin's finder assays its future. *New York Times*, June 26, 21.

Ng, V., Rees, E. E., Lindsay, L. R., Drebot, M. A., Brownstoen, T., Sadeghieh, T., & Khan, S. U. (2019). Could exotic mosquito-borne diseases emerge in Canada with climate change? *Canadian Communicable Disease Report, 4*(45), 98–107.

Nix, E., Paulose, J., Shrubsole, C., Altamirano-Medina, H., Davies, M., Khosla, R., & Wilkinson, P. (2020). Evaluating housing health hazards: prevalence, practices and priorities in Delhi's informal settlements. *Journal of Urban Health, 97*(4), 502–518.

OCHA (Office for the Coordination of Humanitarian Affairs). (2020). *Global Humanitarian Overview 2020: United Nations Coordinated Support for People Affected by Disaster and Conflict*. Geneva: United Nations Office for the Coordination of Humanitarian Affairs.

Oliver-Smith, A. (2017). The social construction for disaster risk: seeking root causes. *International Journal of Disaster Risk Reduction, 22*, 469–474.

Oliver-Smith, A., & Hoffman, S. M. (Eds.). (2020). *The Angry Earth: Disaster in Anthropological Perspective* (2nd edition). Abingdon, UK: Routledge.

Omidian, P., Tehoungue, K., & Monger, J. (2014). *Medical Anthropology Study of the Ebola Virus Disease (EVD) Outbreak in Liberia/West Africa*. Geneva: World Health Organization.

Onyango, M. A., & Uwase, M. (2017). Humanitarian response to complex emergencies and natural disasters. In S. R. Quah (Ed.), *International Encyclopedia of Public Health* (2nd edition, (Vol. 4, pp. 106–116). New York: Elsevier.

Orata, F. D., Keim, P. S., & Boucher, Y. (2014). The 2010 cholera outbreak in Haiti: how science solved a controversy. *PLoS Pathogens, 10*(4), e1003967, 1–5. doi:10.1371/journal.ppat.1003967

Oreskes, N., & Conway, E. M. (2010). *Merchants of Doubt: How a Handful of Scientists Obscured the Truth on Issues from Tobacco Smoke to Climate Change*. New York and London: Bloomsbury.

Oshinsky, D. M. (2005). *Polio: An American Story*. Oxford: Oxford University Press.

Ostfeld, R. S., & Brunner, J. L. (2015). Climate change and *Ixodes* tick-borne diseases of humans. *Philosophical Transactions of the Royal Society B, 370*(20140051), 1–11. http://dx.doi.org/10.1098/rstb.2014.0051

Pailey, R. N. (2017). Liberia, Ebola and the pitfalls of state-building: reimagining domestic and diasporic public authority. *African Affairs, 116/465*, 648–670.

Palmer, T., & Stevens, B. (2019). The scientific challenge of understanding and estimating climate change. *Proceedings of the National Academy of Sciences, 116*(49), 24390–24395.

Paris, I. P., Reboredo, F. H., Ramalho, J. C., Pessoa, M. F., & Lidon, F. C. (2020). Potential impact of climate change on agriculture: a review. *Emirates Journal of Food and Agriculture, 32*(6), 397–407.

Periago, M. R., Frieden, T. R., Tappero, J. W., DeCock, K. M., Aasen, B., & Andrus, J. K. (2012). Elimination of cholera transmission in Haiti and the Dominican Republic. *The Lancet, 379*(9812), e12–e13. doi:10.1016/S0140-6736(12)60031-2

Perrin, P. (1996). *War and Public Health*. Geneva: International Committee of the Red Cross.

Perry, R. W., & Quarantelli, E. L. (Eds.). (2005). *What is a Disaster? New Answers to Old Questions*. Philadelphia, PA: Xlibris.

Pingeot, L. (2020). International peacebuilding as a case of structural injustice. *International Peacekeeping, 27*(2), 263–288.

Pinxten, R. (1986). The developmental dynamics of peace. In M. L. Foster & R. A. Rubinstein (Eds.), *Peace and War: Cross-Cultural Perspectives* (pp. 269–280). New Brunswick, NJ: Transaction.

Porter, M. (2014). *A Dictionary of Epidemiology* (6th edition). Oxford: International Epidemiological Association and Oxford University Press.

Pouligny, B. (2006). *Peace Operations Seen from Below: Un Missions and Local People*. Bloomfield, CT: Kumarian Press.

Prizzi, R. A. (2002). Apostles of cleanliness: the 19th-century Sanitary Movement denied the germ theory of disease, yet created our public health infrastructure. *Modern Drug Discovery, 5*(5), 51–55.

Prunier, G. (1995). *The Rwanda Crisis: History of a Genocide*. New York: Columbia University Press.

Quarantelli, E. L. (Ed.) (1998). *What is a Disaster? Perspectives on the Question*. New York: Routledge.

Ramachandran, G., & Swaminathan, S. (2015). Tuberculosis. In S. Padmanabhan (Ed.), *Handbook of Pharmacogenomics and Stratified Medicine* (pp. 835–857). London: Academic Press/Elsevier.

Raven, J., Wurie, H., & Witter, S. (2018). Health workers' experiences of coping with the Ebola epidemic in Sierra Leone's health system: a qualitative study. *BMC Health Services Research, 18*, 251–259.

Reiter, P. (2001). Climate change and mosquito-borne disease. *Environmental Health Perspectives,* 109(Supplement 1), 141–161.

Riedel, S. (2005). Edward Jenner and the history of smallpox and vaccination. *Baylor University Medical Center Proceedings, 18*, 21–24.

Rosen, G. (2015). *A History of Public Health* (revised expanded edition). Baltimore, MD: Johns Hopkins University Press.

Rubinstein, R. A. (2008). *Peacekeeping under Fire: Culture and Intervention*. Boulder, CO: Paradigm.

Rubinstein, R. A., & Kudesia, S. (2012). Transnational transfers and peace operations: the empirically elusive quality of the analytic categories. In S. Brown (Ed.), *Transnational Transfers and Global Development* (pp. 182–201). London: Palgrave Macmillan.

Rubinstein, R. A., & Zoli, C. (2019). Military culture and humanitarian actions: short-term gains and long-term losses. In H. C. Breede (Ed.), *Culture and the Soldier: Identities, Values and Norms in Military Engagements* (pp. 125–143). Vancouver, BC: University of British Columbia Press.

Sahnoun, M. (1994). *Somalia: The Missed Opportunities*. Washington, DC: United States Institute of Peace.

Samimian-Darash, L., & Rabinow, P. (Eds.). (2015). *Modes of Uncertainty: Anthropological Cases*. Chicago, IL: University of Chicago Press.

Schuller, M. (2012). *Killing with Kindness: Haiti, International Aid, and NGOs*. New Brunswick, NJ: Rutgers University Press.

Schwartz, S. (1999). Beyond 'ancient hatreds': what really happened to Yugoslavia. *Policy Review, 97*, 39–51.

Scrimshaw, S. C., & Lane, S. D. (2020). Culture, behavior, and health. In M. H. Merson, R. E. Black, & A. J. Mills (Eds.), *Global Health: Diseases, Programs, Systems, and Policies* (pp. 43–74). Burlington, MA: Jones and Bartlett Learning.

Shortt, N., & Hammett, D. (2013). Housing and health in an informal settlement upgrade in Cape Town, South Africa. *Journal of Housing and the Built Environment, 28*(4), 615–627.

Slim, H. (1997). Relief agencies and moral standing in war: principles of humanity, neutrality, impartiality, and solidarity. *Development in Practice, 7*(4), 342–352.

Snow, J. (2008 [1854]). On the mode of communication of cholera (revisited classics). *Hygeia: Revista Brasileira de Geografia Médica e da Saúde, 4*(6), 1–11.

Staupe-Delgado, R. (2019). Analysing changes in disaster terminology over the last decade. *International Journal of Disaster Risk Reduction, 40*(2019), 1–5.

Steffen, W. (2013). The myths of climate change-science. *Proceedings of the Royal Society of Victoria, 125*(1/2), 4.

The Guardian and Kaiser Health News. (2020). Lost on the frontline: hundreds of US healthcare workers have died fighting Covid-19. We count them and investigate why. *The Guardian*, August 11, www.theguardian.com/us-news/ng-interactive/2020/aug/11/lost-on-the-frontline-covid-19-coronavirus-us-healthcare-workers-deaths-database, accessed December 7, 2020.

Toole, M. J., & Waldman, R. J. (1997). The public health aspects of complex emergencies and refugee situations. *Annual Review of Public Health, 18*, 283–312.

Toole, M. J., Waldman, R. J., & Zwi, A. (2006). Complex emergencies. In M. H. Merson, R. E. Black, & A. J. Mills (Eds.), *International Public Health: Diseases, Programs, Systems, and Policies* (2nd edition, pp. 445–511). Sudbury, MA: Jones and Bartlett Publishers.

Udovicki, J., & Ridgeway, J. (Eds.). (2000). *Burn This House: The Making and Unmaking of Yugoslavia*. Durham, NC: Duke University Press.

UNDRR. (2015). *Sendai Framework for Disaster Risk Reduction 2015–2030*. New York: United Nations (United Nations Office for Disaster Risk Reduction).

UNHCR. (2018). *Global Trends: Forced Displacement in 2018*. Geneva: UNHCR (United Nations High Commissioner for Refugees).

United Nations. (1994). *Report of the World Conference on Natural Disaster Reduction, Yokohama, Japan 23–27 May 1994 (A/CONF.172/9)*. New York: United Nations.

United Nations. (2005). *Hyogo Framework for Action 2005–2015: Building the Resilience of Nations and Communities to Disasters, 22 January 2005 (A/CONF.206/6)*. New York: United Nations.

United Nations. (2016). *Terminology Related to Disaster Risk Reduction – Updated Technical Non-paper*. New York: United Nations Office of Disaster Risk Reduction.

Urlainis, A., Shohet, I. M., Levy, R., Ornai, D., & Vilnay, O. (2014). Damage in critical infrastructures due to natural and man-made extreme events – a critical review. *Procedia Engineering, 85*, 529–535.

Waldman, R. (1999). Public health and complex emergencies: new issues, new conditions. *American Journal of Public Health, 89*(10), 1483–1485.

Wisner, B., Blaikie, P., Cannon, T., & Davis, I. (2003). *At Risk: Natural Hazards, People's Vulnerability and Disasters* (2nd edition). London: Routledge.

Zinsser, H. (2008 [1935]). *Rats, Lice and History*. New Brunswick, NJ: Transaction.

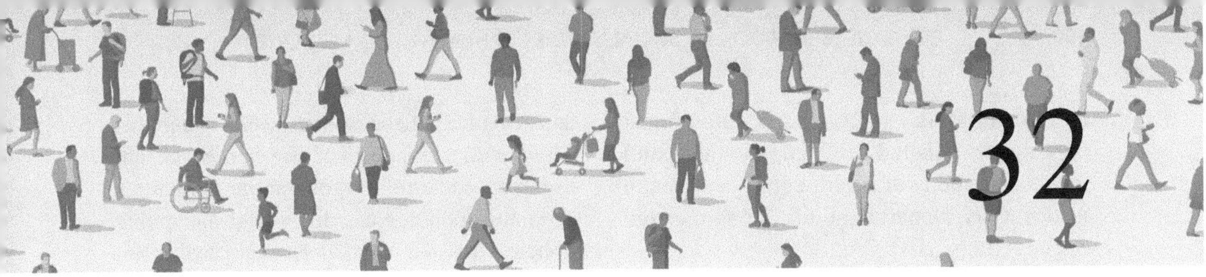

32

Occupational Health in the 21st Century

Lorraine M. Conroy and Linda Forst

INTRODUCTION

Occupational Health from antiquity through the 21st century has been formed by the evolution of social, economic, and demographic forces that determine job tasks, hazardous exposures, illnesses and injuries, preventive strategies, compensation, social benefits, and social position. A 1600 BCE papyrus scroll has illustrations of finger and wrist guards used by Bronze Age archers (Breasted, 1991 [1930]). Pliny described facial protection for miners in the 1st century (Pliny the Elder, 2012) and Paracelsus wrote about the toxicity of chemical agents based on dose (de Vries, 1977; Gochfeld, 2005). The seminal work of Ramazzini (1633–1714) laid the foundation of our modern understanding of health hazards caused by dusts, metals, chemical agents, and work postures, and the importance of collecting information on work in the medical history; he also established the idea that primary prevention is the optimal approach to controlling disease (Franco, 2020).

The public health movement in 19th-century Europe focused on the terrible conditions in factories and workhouses and the consequent impacts on housing, nutrition, stress, poverty and general ill health of individuals and communities (Morley, 2007). The cyclical relationship between opportunities for work, working conditions and societal status is implicit in writings around the globe and throughout history.

In its most fundamental form, Occupational Health covers the recognition, diagnosis, and prevention of illnesses, injuries and fatalities that occur at work. A more recent, holistic approach understands Occupational Health as a social determinant, influenced by structural drivers that determine the potential for individuals and communities to live healthy lives. In the US, occupational illnesses and injuries are not equitably distributed across the entire workforce, with people of color holding a disproportionate number of jobs in the most hazardous sectors of the economy. The United Nations 2030 Agenda for Sustainable Development – Strategic Development Goal

8, Decent Work – recognizes the critical importance of including Occupational Health in considerations of health equity and health justice (UN Department of Economic and Social Affairs, 2015).

WORK AS A DETERMINANT OF HEALTH

The World Health Organization's Commission on Social Determinants of Health has established the following framework to describe the relationship between occupation and health (Solar & Irwin, 2010: 3) and is intended to "guide empirical work to enhance our understanding of determinants and mechanisms and guide policy-making to illuminate entry points for interventions and policies" (Figure 32.1).

This model provides a useful illustration of the social production of health and disease and the role of work and work-related policies in determining equity in health and well-being. The model differs from some other models and frameworks in that it places emphasis on the unequal distribution of power, prestige, and resources that result in health inequities. Those with a high level of power, prestige, and resources determine governance structures, economic policies and the social and public policies that, in turn, determine health and health inequities. Dominant cultural and societal values reflect the values of individuals and groups with high levels of power, prestige and resources. Social and public policies, along with dominant cultural values, result in a hierarchy of socioeconomic positions and those individuals and groups with high socioeconomic positions influence social and public policies that continue to maintain this hierarchy, as illustrated by the two-way arrows between the left-most columns in the model (Figure 32.1). In the US, as in much of the world, these positions are determined by social class, gender, race and ethnicity, education level, occupation, and income. Occupation, in turn, is determined by education, which is determined by parents' social class, education, and income. Public policies, such as those that maintain racial and ethnic segregation, determine where people live, and education funding policies that rely on local property taxes reinforce inequities in educational investment and opportunities, thereby limiting occupational opportunities

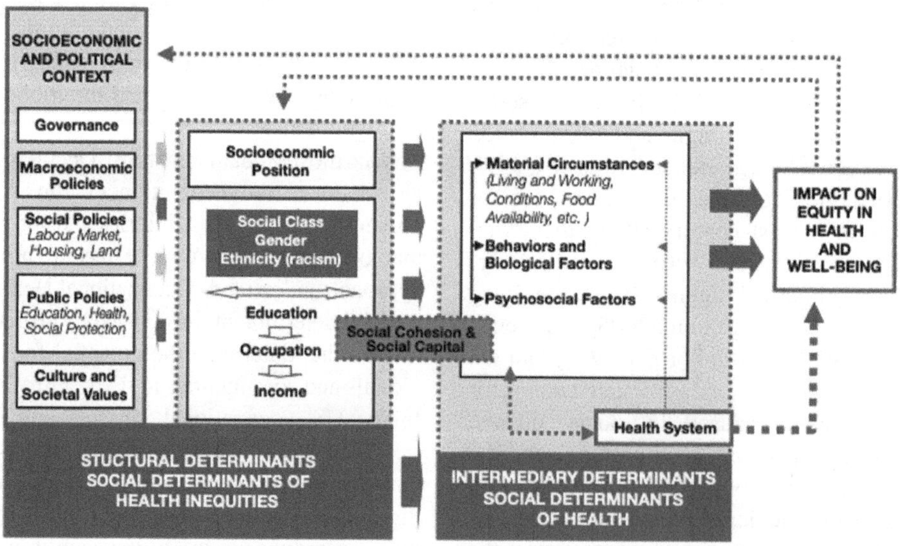

Figure 32.1 Social Determinants of Health Framework (Solar & Irwin, 2010)

for people in low-income communities. Since occupation, in most cases, determines income, occupation determines individuals' and families' material circumstances, which are proximate causes of health and health inequities. Another important role of occupation, unique to the US among high-income countries, is access to healthcare. In the US, inequities in access to and quality of healthcare are determined by employer-provided health insurance and this healthcare benefit is determined by occupational status.

Occupational hazards in the workplace are not randomly or equally shared and public action is often taken only after a tragedy. There are numerous examples of those who know about hazards withholding that information to prevent action – on the part of government in the form of additional regulation and from workers who may act toward organizing into unions, engaging in strikes, or filing lawsuits. Power dynamics in the workplace influence working conditions, resulting in disproportionate impact on workers with limited power. Organized workers can more easily take action or bargain for safer work (Boal, 2009; Frick & Walters, 1998; Yi et al., 2011). Worker advocates play a critical role in improving worker health and working conditions. Throughout US history, African Americans and immigrants have been exposed to the most dangerous jobs. Race, immigration status, class, and gender influence who has access to which jobs, what kinds of exposures they have at work, and their ability to speak up without consequences of losing their job (Friedman & Forst, 2008; Friedman et al., 2012; Loomis & Richardson, 1998; Michaels, 1983; Seabury et al., 2017).

FUTURE OF WORK

Demographics

The United Nations estimates that the world's population will continue to grow, but at a slowing rate (Vollset et al., 2020). Some countries and regions, however, will experience rapid population growth driven by high fertility. The global population is expected to reach 8.5 billion by 2030 and 9.7 billion by 2050. Two-thirds of this population growth will be the result of current age structures in countries expected to have the largest population growth, those countries where the large population of children will reach childbearing age in the next few decades. Life expectancy at birth for the world's population reached 72.6 years in 2019, although wide gaps persist between the least developed and more developed countries. The population will also become older, but the impact of an aging population and workforce is, and will continue to be, greater in more developed countries. Worldwide, the population aged 65 years or older outnumbered children under age 5 for the first time starting in 2018 (UN Department of Economic and Social Affairs, Population Division, 2019). In the US, 16.5% of the population is over 65 years old, with 6.5% less than 5 years of age (US Census Bureau, 2019). The US population is also becoming increasingly diverse, with the highest percentages of people of color in the age groups less than 44 years old.

With an aging population, we are seeing an aging workforce in the US. Of particular note, the percentage of workers over the age of 75 has doubled in the past 20 years, although the numbers are relatively small compared to the total workforce (US Bureau of Labor Statistics, n.d.a.). With fertility decline and a large increase in the proportion of older people in the population, the workforce may continue to see an increase of older workers in coming decades (Vollset et al., 2020). Educational level plays an important role in workforce participation. Not surprising, higher education levels have higher labor force participation and lower unemployment, but the increase in labor force participation over the past two decades is among those with the lowest education level. These jobs are more likely to be low-wage, low-skill jobs (US Bureau of Labor Statistics, n.d.b.). Urbanization is expected to continue with more than half of the world's population now living in urban areas (International Monetary Fund, 2006). The rate of migration is projected to level off some, but net migration will continue to be from less developed to more developed countries, driven by two social phenomena: labor migration where people seek employment, and insecurity and conflict where people migrate for safety.

The global working age population (15 years and older) is estimated to be 5.7 billion people (United Nations, Department of Economic and Social Affairs, Population Division, 2019). Approximately 57% are employed, 39% are not in the labor force, and about 188 million were unemployed. Another 165 million people are employed but want to work more paid hours (International Labour Organization, 2020).

More than 2 billion people work informally, representing more than 60% of global employment: 90%, 67%, and 18% of employment in low-income, middle-income, and high-income countries, respectively (International Labour Organization, 2018). Informal work is associated with income insecurity and lack of social protections. More than 600 million workers live in extreme (daily per capita income below US$1.90 in purchasing power parity (PPP) terms or moderate (daily per capita income between US$1.90 and US$3.20 in PPP terms) poverty (International Labour Organization, 2020).

Technological Advances

In addition to the changing demographics of the workforce, the nature of work is also rapidly evolving, with increased automation, use of artificial intelligence, and use of robotics. Forty-seven percent of US workers have jobs at risk of being replaced by automation (Frey & Osborne, 2015). Sixty-seven percent of jobs in developing countries are susceptible to automation (World Bank, 2016). In the Association of Southeast Asian Nations (ASEAN), 56% of jobs are at risk of automation in the next 20 years (Chang & Phu, 2016). Worldwide, 50% of companies expect that automation will lead to fewer full-time workers by 2022 (World Economic Forum, 2018).

We often picture robotics as replacing tedious, lower skill jobs, but use of robots is happening in all fields, including very highly skilled jobs such as surgery. In many cases, automation has allowed for increases in occupational safety by reducing worker exposures to hazardous chemicals and dangerous lifting tasks. However, the increased use of robots and collaborative robots may also introduce new hazards into the workplace (Catanzarite et al., 2018;; US Department of Health and Human Services (DHHS), 1984; US Department of Labor, n.d.a.).

An area of concern with increasing reliance on technology is its possible impact on income inequality. Globally, only 54% of households have internet access and that number drops to 15% in least developed countries (International Telecommunication Union, 2017). In the US, 62% of households had "high connectivity," meaning they had three key computer and internet items: a desktop or laptop, a handheld computer or smartphone, and a broadband internet subscription, with connectivity increasing to close to 80% for one of these devices. However, disparities in access exist and are dependent on age, income, and location (urban vs. rural) (US Census Bureau, 2017).

Alternative Work Arrangements

Simultaneously with, and often aided by, technology advances, there has been a significant shift in work arrangements. In the US, beginning in the 1930s and through the 1960s, a number of labor and social protection laws and regulations related to civil rights and occupational health and safety were enacted (e.g., Social Security Act,

National Labor Relations Act, Fair Labor Standards Act, Civil Rights Act, Occupational Safety and Health Act) (Howard, 2017). These laws coincided with and promoted what is now referred to as Standard Employment, characterized by jobs that are full-time with the same employer, work that is exclusive to one employer with a predictable work schedule at the employers' places of business with mutual expectations of long-term career development, with workplace and social protections, and in which there is an unambiguous employer–employee relationship (Benach et al., 2014; Broschak & Davis-Blake, 2005). Nearly all US policies and regulations are developed with the assumption of this type of work arrangement – where there is a clear employer–employee relationship – and the policies and regulations set rules for employers and employees and define the rights of employees.

Beginning in the late 1970s and continuing through the present day, the nature of work has been changing. Macro-level political and economic forces, including adoption of neoliberal policies, privatization of state-owned industries and services, global economic deregulation and weakening of labor unions, drove societal transformation, resulting in a reduction in social safety nets, job losses in the public sector, growth of precarious employment and a weakening of regulatory protections (Ahonen et al., 2018; Quinlan et al., 2010). These macro-level forces are coupled with micro-level power differentials related to social position (race/ethnicity, class, gender, and immigration status) that explain the unequal distribution of precarious employment and subsequent adverse health outcomes (Benach et al., 2010; Muntaner, Solar et al., 2010). Beginning in about 1980, economic forces emerged that placed more emphasis on companies' core competencies (Prahalad & Hamel, 1990) and short-term shareholder value, which resulted in: (1) a reduction or outsourcing of cost centers, such as human resources, information technology, and occupational health and safety; (2) the elimination or outsourcing of the peripheral workforce, including landscaping, janitorial, maintenance, and security jobs; and (3) the outsourcing of distribution operations, leading to what David Weil refers to as a "Fissured Workplace" where the lead business no longer hires employees, and instead they buy services from other firms (Weil, 2014).

The fissuring of workplaces, however, is not without consequences. We have seen a decline in attachment to employers, increases in long-term unemployment, and increased job insecurity. We have also seen increases in non-standard and contingent work with the subsidiary firms more likely to hire contingent or temporary workers to increase their flexibility to respond to the needs of lead industries (Kalleberg, 2009; Weil, 2014). In the US, estimates of workers engaged in non-standard work ranges from 5% to 33% (US Bureau of Labor Statistics, 2005; see also Alterman et al., 2013; Jeszeck, 2015; Katz & Krueger, 2018) with about 19% of workers reporting that their primary job was in a non-standard work arrangement and 40% of all workers having a non-standard job (Alterman et al., 2013; Pofeldt, 2015). A 2018 employer survey by Deloitte found that 50% of respondents employed a significant number of contractors, 23% had significant numbers of freelancers, and a smaller percentage, 13%, reported a significant number of gig or app-based workers (Agarwal et al., 2018). At the same time, only 16% reported that they have established policies and practices to manage a variety of worker types, pointing to an enormous gap in capabilities.

We have always seen high levels of non-standard work arrangements in some economic sectors – construction, professional business (such as lawyers and accountants), and other services – but in the past two decades, we have seen large increases in alternative work arrangements across the economic spectrum (Katz & Krueger,

2016). In 2020, a California lawsuit to re-classify ride-share drivers (Uber, Lyft and others) as employees, rather than independent contractors, was based on a three-prong test to determine whether a worker is independent: the worker (1) is free from the control and direction of the hiring entity, (2) does work outside the usual course of the hiring entity's business, and (3) is customarily engaged in an independently established trade, occupation, or business of the same nature as that involved in the work performed. This lawsuit failed.

The combined result of workplace fissuring and increases in non-standard work arrangements has been to shift risks from employers to employees. These risks include traditional occupational health and safety risks (Koranyi et al., 2018), but also risks associated with unemployment or underemployment (Brydsten et al., 2018; Córdoba-Doña et al., 2016; Vancea & Utzet, 2017). These conditions have also led to lower unionization rates, increased income inequality as corporate profits and gross domestic product continued to increase as before, but with wages held constant or decreasing (Federal Research Economic Data, 2017), and a decrease in the share of adults living in middle-income households from 61% in 1971 to 50% in 2015; and the share of overall income held by the middle class decreasing from 62% in 1970 to 43% in 2014 (Pew Research Center, 2015). All of this is important because there is a gradient of health where people who have fewer resources are less healthy than those with more money and social status. This gradient is apparent almost universally across racial and ethnic groups and for many different diseases and conditions. Individuals with jobs that do not pay a living wage have higher rates of stress and anxiety, obesity and diabetes, asthma, adverse birth outcomes, hypertension and heart disease, preventable injuries, and premature death (Benach et al., 2014; National Collaborating Centre for Determinants of Health, 2013).

WORKING CONDITIONS

Leading Causes of Occupational Illness and Injury

A number of factors are important to guide our understanding and ability to prevent workplace illness, injury, and mortality:

- The work environment poses definable and preventable risks.
- The health of workers is generally legislated by departments of labor, rather than departments of health.
- Worker protection standards allow workers to be exposed to higher levels of hazardous agents (e.g., chemicals) than is allowable for the general population.
- Costs to businesses are usually considered in legislating workers' exposure limits.
- The cost of worker mortality (death benefits) is built into bids for construction projects.
- Individual workplaces are rarely inspected, and this often depends on workers filing a complaint.

Small businesses and self-employment provide most jobs in the US and globally; health and safety oversight in these employment conditions is limited. Three in 10 US jobs are held by self-employed individuals (14.6 million) and the workers they hire (44 million) (US Bureau of Labor Statistics, 2018). There were 25.5 million nonfarm sole proprietorships in 2016 (Dungan, 2016).

Work-related injuries are much easier to identify than diseases because of the short time lag between hazardous exposure and adverse health event.

There are many factors that limit case capture in occupational settings: willingness to report on the part of the worker; willingness to report on the part of the employer; recognition of the relationship between a hazardous exposure and an adverse health effect (Azaroff et al., 2002).

Occupational fatalities

Worldwide, hazardous conditions in the workplace are responsible for approximately

2.3 million deaths, annually (International Labour Organization, 2015). In the US, there were 5,333 work-related deaths among the approximately 156 million people working in 2019. Values shown in Table 32.1 are similar in numbers and proportions for each of the preceding four years.

Causes of death are highest for transportation incidents (39.8%), falls, slips, trips (16.5%), violence (15.8%), contact with objects and equipment (13.7%), exposure to harmful substances or environments (12.0%), and homicides, fires and explosions (1.9%). Notably, about 10% of employed individuals are self-employed, implying they have control over their tasks and working conditions, yet they experience 20% of the fatalities (US Bureau of Labor Statistics, 2016). Mortality in male workers is 10 times higher than in women, but a more granular view shows that 22% of occupational fatalities in women are due to homicide, compared to 8% in men. Fatal work injuries rise with age, with 55- to 64-year-old workers dying at 1.5 to 2 times the rate of younger workers and those workers over 65 at 2.5 to 5 times the rate of younger age groups. These facts need to be considered in context: the safest workplaces are indoors and the safest occupations require education beyond high school. The most hazardous occupations are outdoors and entail operating equipment. Gender-based violence against women is more prevalent in the general population; violence spreads from home to work and women also work in customer service jobs that put them at risk for violence.

A look at economic sectors shows the industries with the highest number and rate of fatalities (Tables 32.2 and 32.3). Construction has the highest number, while Agriculture, Forestry, Fishing and Hunting, with significantly smaller workforces, have the highest rate.

Non-fatal occupational illnesses and injuries

The US Bureau of Labor Statistics Survey of Occupational Illnesses and Injuries captures data on non-fatal injuries and illnesses as well (see Table 32.4). Like the occupational fatalities data, agriculture, with its relatively low number of workers, has the highest rate, while healthcare assistance has the highest number of illnesses and injuries, followed by manufacturing and retail.

Though employment in private industry is much more common in the US than work in the public sector, public sector jobs (e.g., firefighting, law enforcement, trash collection, maintenance of public buildings, roads and green spaces) have much higher incidence rates of non-fatal occupational illness and injury (Table 32.5).

Injuries are much more prevalent in occupational surveillance data because they are easier to identify: the proximate relationship between an acute event and an injury outcome is much more easily connected, whereas hazardous exposures to chemicals and physical agents (e.g., noise, radiation) can have a long latency, where the adverse health effect, such as cancer or lung disease, can take decades to develop. In terms of non-fatal injury and illness, there were 2.8 million non-fatal workplace injuries and illnesses reported by industry, occurring at a rate of 2.8 cases to 100 FTE (Full Time Equivalents) workers.

The US Occupational Safety and Health Administration (OSHA) requires employers to maintain a log of workplace injuries and illnesses (US Department of Labor, n.d.b.). Recordable cases include those that require more than first aid, loss of consciousness, days away from work, restricted work, or transfer to another job. The incidence of total recordable cases has shown a gradual downward trend from 2003 to 2018 (Figure 32.2). Notably, 67% of cases with days away from work were in manufacturing and material moving (transportation and warehousing) workers. Workplace hazards are easier to link to injury than illness (disease) because of obvious mechanisms of injury, the brief time from exposure/event to health effect (latency), and the fact that these events are often witnessed.

Table 32.1 Work-related fatalities in the US by event or exposure type, 2019 (US Bureau of Labor Statistics, 2019b)

		Event or exposure[1]					
Worker Characteristics	*Total fatal injuries (%)*	*Transportation incidents*[2]	*Falls, slips, trips*	*Violence and other injuries by persons or animals*[3]	*Contact with objects and equipment*	*Exposure to harmful substances or environments*	*Fires and explosions*
Total	5333 (100%)	2122 (39.8%)*	880 (16.5%)*	841 (15.8%)*	732 (13.7%)*	642 (12.0%)*	99(1.9%)*
Employee status wage and salary[4]	4240 (79.5%)+	1735	683	632	545	548	83
Self-employed[3] Genderf*)	1093 (20.5%)+	387	197	209	185	94	16
Women	437 (8.2%)+	170	65	120	18	59	3
Men	4896 (91.8%)+	1952	815	721	714	583	96
Age(t-) Under 16 years	17(0.3%)+	8	–	–	5	2	–
16 to 17 years	17 (0.3%)	9	–	–	3	–	–
18 to 19 years	50 (0.9%)	19	5	8	7	11	–
20 to 24 years	325 (6.1%)	127	–	79	39	43	–
25 to 34 years	866 (16.2%)	328	92	149	110	164	–
35 to 44 years	967 (18.1%)	360	112	173	134	165	22
45 to 54 years	1082 (20.3%)	428	180	179	153	125	14
55 to 64 years	1212 (22.7%)	484	255	163	169	109	23
65 years and over Race or ethnic origin[6]	793 (14.9%)	355	203	88	112	20	10
White, non-Hispanic	3297(61.8%)	1377	505	487	467	388	60
Black or African-American, non-Hispanic	634(11.9%)	257	58	160	67	79	10
Hispanic or Latino	1088 (20.4%	368	267	111	174	149	–
American Indian or Alaska Native, non-Hispanic	30 (0.6%)	14	6	–	–	5	–
Asian, non-Hispanic	181 (3.4%)	57	30	63	16	10	5
Native Hawaiian or Pacific Islander, non-Hispanic	14 (0.3%)	–	5	–	–	4	–

[1]*Based* on the BLS Occupational Injury and Illness Classification System (OIICS) 2.01 implemented for 2011 data forward.

[2]*Includes* roadway, nonroadway, air, water, rail fatal occupational injuries, and fatal occupational injuries resulting from being struck by a vehicle.

[3]*Includes* violence by persons, self-inflicted injury, and attacks by animals.

[4]*May* include volunteers and workers receiving other types of compensation. Cases where employment status is unknown are included in the counts of wage and salary workers.

[5]*Includes* self-employed workers, owners of unincorporated businesses and farms, paid and unpaid family workers, and may include some owners of incorporated businesses or members of partnerships.

[6]*Persons* identified as Hispanic or Latino may be of any race. The race categories shown exclude data for Hispanics and Latinos. Cases where ethnicity is unknown are included in counts of non-Hispanic workers.

(*) Listed event/cause as a % of total injuries; row percent

(+) Characteristic as % in that category; column percent

Table 32.2 Number and rate of fatal work injuries, by industry sector, 2019 (US Bureau of Labor Statistics, 2019b)

Industry	*Number of fatal work injuries*	*Fatal work injury rate (per 100,000 full-time equivalent workers)*
Construction	1,061	9.7
Transportation and warehousing	913	13.9
Agriculture, forestry, fishing, and hunting	573	23.1
Government	426	1.8
Retail trade	291	2
Leisure and hospitality	271	2.2
Other services (exc. Public admin.)	210	3
Educational and health services	197	0.8
Wholesale trade	178	4.9
Mining, quarrying, and oil and gas extraction	127	14.6

Table 32.3 Safest and most dangerous occupations (US Bureau of Labor Statistics, 2019b)

Top 20 Safest Occupations/ Industries	*Deaths*	*Rate/ 100,000 FTE*	*Top 20 Most Dangerous Occupations/Industries*	*Deaths*	*Rate/ 100,000 FTE*
Computer and mathematical occupations	11	0.2	Fishers and related fishing workers	41	99.8
Hospitals	21	0.3	Logging workers	55	84.3
Business and financial operations occupations	29	0.4	Aircraft pilots and flight engineers	59	48.6
Education, training, and library occupations	30	0.4	Roofers	91	45.2
Registered nurses	14	0.5	Refuse and recyclable material collectors	30	35.0
Finance and Insurance	32	0.5	Structural iron and steel workers	14	33.4
Legal occupations	11	0.6	Coal mining	17	30.3
Healthcare practitioners and technical occupations	57	0.6	Truck transportation	599	28.0
Office and administrative support occupations	101	0.6	Farmers, ranchers, and other agricultural managers	258	24.0
Professional, scientific, and technical services	69	0.6	First-line supervisors of landscaping, etc. workers	53	21.0
Architecture and engineering occupations	23	0.7	Electrical power-line installers and repairers	26	18.7
Health care and social assistance	146	0.8	First-line construction & extraction supervisors	121	17.4
Life, physical, and social science occupations	13	0.9	Water transportation	13	16.9
Healthcare support occupations	28	0.9	Landscaping services	214	16.9
Ambulatory health care services	65	0.9	Maintenance and repair workers, general	87	16.6
Construction managers	12	1.0	Miscellaneous agricultural workers	154	16.4
Chemical manufacturing	13	1.0	Animal production and aquaculture	152	16.4

(Continued)

Table 32.3 (Continued)

Top 20 Safest Occupations/ Industries	*Deaths*	*Rate/ 100,000 FTE*	*Top 20 Most Dangerous Occupations/Industries*	*Deaths*	*Rate/ 100,000 FTE*
Transportation equipment manufacturing	24	1.0	Helpers, construction trades	11	15.7
Educational services	43	1.0	Grounds maintenance workers	191	15.5
Social assistance	28	1.0	Mining (except oil and gas)	31	15.5

Other Notable Occupational Fatality Rates	Deaths	Rate per 100K FTE	**Notes**
Police and sheriff's patrol officers	95	12.9	Ranked as the 25th-most-deadly job or industry in 2017
Drinking places (alcoholic beverages)	26	12.0	Ranked as the 27th-most-deadly job or industry in 2017
Oil and gas extraction	8	7.9	Ranked as the 43rd-most-deadly job or industry in 2017
Firefighters	34	3.6	The occupation with the fatality rate closest to the national average in 2017

Note: These are pre-COVID-19 pandemic data. Risks associated with SARS-CoV-2 exposure are not reflected here. The pandemic has resulted in increased risk for workers in many essential services: healthcare, healthcare support, manufacturing, transportation and warehousing, retail trade (grocery).

Table 32.4 Non-fatal injuries, illnesses and incidence rates, US, 2018 (US Bureau of Labor Statistics, 2019c)

Industry Sector	*Injuries*	*Illnesses*	*Total Injuries + Illnesses*	*Incidence rate per 100 FTE workers*
Agriculture, forestry, fishing and hunting	51.8	2.6	54.4	5.3
Transportation and warehousing	213.1	8.3	221.4	4.5
Arts, entertainment, and recreation	54.4	3.5	57.9	4.1
Health care and social assistance	544.8	32.7	577.4	3.9
Retail trade	401.1	8.8	409.9	3.5
Manufacturing	395.3	35	430.3	3.4
Accommodation and food services	271	7.6	278.5	3.1
Construction	195.6	3.6	199.1	3
Wholesale trade	157.1	3.7	160.8	2.9
Administrative and waste services	112.8	5.8	118.6	2.3
Real estate and rental and leasing	45.2	0.9	46.1	2.3
Other services (except public administration)	70.8	1.9	72.8	2.2
Educational services	35.1	1.8	36.9	1.9
Utilities	9.6	1	10.6	1.9
Mining, quarrying, and oil and gas extraction	9.4	0.4	9.8	1.4
Information	31.7	1.6	33.3	1.3
Management of companies and enterprises	16.8	0.8	17.5	0.8
Professional and technical services	66.1	4.4	70.5	0.8
Finance and insurance	26.1	2.5	2	0.5

In the last decade, work has been done to better understand the global burden of occupational disease. A project of the World Health Organization (WHO), the Global Burden of Disease, includes occupational diseases. Presentation of this program and its findings are beyond the scope of this chapter but can be explored further by going to: www.healthdata.org/gbd/2019.

Beyond the human toll of workplace injuries and illnesses, the economic burden on employers and governments (as representative of the public) is also substantial. The most recent, comprehensive assessment of costs in the US is from 2007 (Leigh, 2011). That study found that, in the United States alone, the cost of workplace injuries and illnesses was approximately $250 billion per year in medical and indirect costs (future lost earnings, fringe benefits, and home production) (Leigh, 2011). US$67 billion alone was for direct medical costs associated with injury and illness. Additionally, Leigh (2011) estimated that less than 25% of the costs were covered by workers' compensation, the insurance system intended to pay the costs for workplace injuries and illnesses. The author describes three factors to explain the discrepancy: compensation pays considerably less than the legal average of about 66% of wages, there is widespread underreporting of work-related injuries, and workers' compensation does not provide benefits for more than 95% of fatal diseases (Leigh, 2011).

Table 32.5 Non-fatal occupational injury and illness incidence rates and number of cases with days away from work, by ownership, 2018 (US Bureau of Labor Statistics, n.d.d.)

Ownership	*Incidence rate per 10,000 full-time workers*	*Number of days away from work cases*[1]
All ownerships	98.4	1,133,670
Private industry	89.7	900,380
State government	142.6	56,170
Local government	163.9	177,120

[1]*Days-away-from-work* cases include those that resulted in days away from work, some of which also included job transfer or restriction.

Inequities in Occupational Illness and Injury

The United Nations Sustainable Development goals, founded on the principle of equity in all aspects of human existence, include

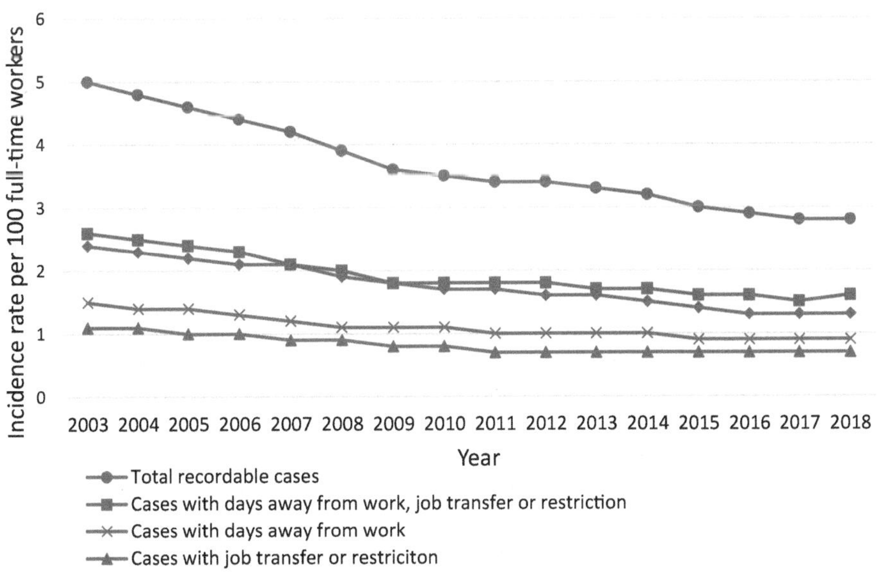

Figure 32.2 Non-fatal occupational injury and illness incidence rates by case type, private industry, US 2003–2018 (US Bureau of Labor Statistics, 2019a)

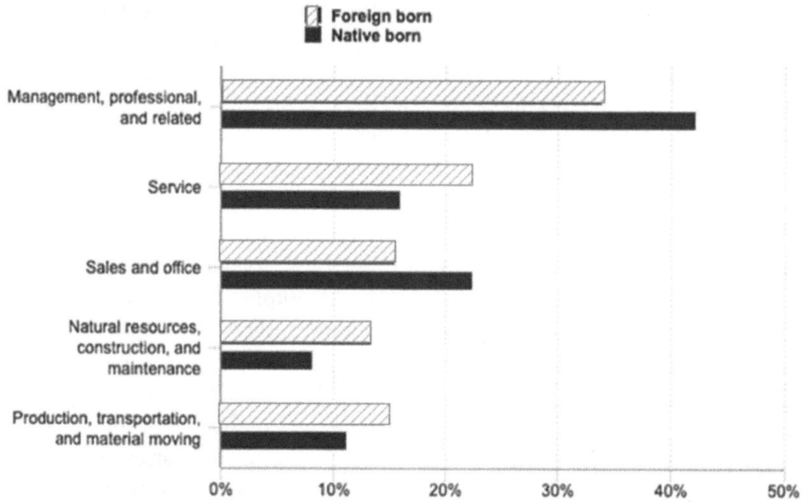

Figure 32.3 Foreign-born and native-born workers by occupation, 2019 (US Bureau of Labor Statistics, 2019e)

several that are related to Occupational Health (UN Department of Economic and Social Affairs, 2015). Goal 8, Decent Work and Economic Growth, is the most obvious. According to the International Labour Organization (ILO) (n.d.), decent work entails: opportunities for work that are productive and deliver a fair income; security in the workplace; social protection for families; better prospects for personal development and social integration (where newcomers or minorities are incorporated into the social structure of the host society); freedom for people to express their concerns, organize and participate in the decisions that affect their lives; and equal opportunity and treatment for all women and men. Less explicit are Sustainable Goal 3, Good Health and Well-being, and Goal 11, Sustainable Cities and Communities.

Apropos to the sections in the first part of this chapter, occupational illnesses and injuries are not equitably distributed across the entire workforce, even within sectors and occupations. First, the composition of the labor force varies by race and ethnicity. The definition of the labor force is those who are employed or seeking employment. In the US, Whites make up the majority of the labor force (77%), while Blacks and Asians comprise 13% and 6%, respectively. Hispanics, who may be of any race, constitute 18% of the labor force, overall. Labor force participation is just above 63%, each, for Blacks and Whites. For Hispanics, labor participation is above 67%. In 2019, the ratio of employment to population was 64% for Hispanics, 61% for Whites and 59% for Blacks (US Bureau of Labor Statistics, 2019d).

Variations in the jobs workers hold – and thus, the wages, benefits and workplace hazards they face – are associated with a number of factors, many of which are hidden. Educational attainment, occupations and industries, geographic areas of the US where various groups are concentrated, rural versus urban residences, and proportion that are foreign born versus native US born are measurable demographic factors that are likely to influence employment sectors and employment arrangements (US Bureau of Labor Statistics, 2019d). More difficult to measure are discrimination based on race and ethnicity, work authorization, prior incarceration,

Table 32.6 Non-fatal occupational illnesses by major industry, 2018 (US Bureau of Labor Statistics, 2019c)

	Total cases		*Skin diseases/ disorders*		*Respiratory Conditions*		*Poisonings*		*Hearing Loss*		*All other illnesses*	
Industry Sector	*# cases[1]*	*IR[2]*	*# cases[1]*	*IR[2]*	*# cases[1]*	*IR[2]*	*# cases[1]*	*IR[2]*	*# cases[1]*	*IR[2]*	*# cases[1]*	*IR[2]*
All industries including private, state and local government[3]	170.9	14.6	24.9	2.1	15.1	1.3	2.4	0.2	16.9	1.4	111.6	9.5
Private industry[3]	127.2	12.4	18.2	1.8	10.8	1.1	1.7	0.2	14.5	1.4	82.0	8.0
Goods-producing[3]	41.2	19.0	5.6	2.6	2.2	1.0	0.6	0.3	11.6	5.4	21.2	9.8
Natural resources and mining[3,4]	3.0	17.1	0.9	4.9	0.3	1.4	0.1	0.4	0.2	1.1	1.6	9.3
Construction	5.2	7.3	1.3	1.8	0.6	0.9	0.4	0.6	0.4	0.5	2.5	3.5
Manufacturing	33.0	25.8	3.5	2.7	1.3	1.0	0.1	0.1	11.0	8.6	17.1	13.4
Service-providing	86.0	10.7	12.6	1.6	8.6	1.1	1.2	0.1	2.9	0.4	60.7	7.5
Trade, transportation, and utilities[4]	23.0	10.0	3.0	1.3	2.0	0.9	0.3	0.1	2.2	1.0	15.5	6.7
Information	1.5	5.6	0.2	0.8	(- 5 -)	0.1	0.1	0.3	0.1	0.4	1.1	4.1
Finance, insurance, and real estate	–	–	0.4	0.5	0.9	1.2	(- 5 -)	0.1	–	–	2.2	2.8
Professional and business services	9.1	5.5	1.6	1.0	0.9	0.6	0.2	0.1	0.3	0.2	6.0	3.6
Educational and health services	34.8	20.6	4.4	2.6	3.6	2.1	0.2	0.1	0.1	0.1	26.6	15.7
Leisure, entertainment, and hospitality	12.0	11.5	2.5	2.4	0.7	0.7	0.4	0.4	0.1	0.1	8.3	8.0
Other services (except public administration)	2.1	6.4	0.6	1.7	0.4	1.1	–	–	0.1	0.3	1.1	3.3
State and local government[3]	43.7	29.7	6.7	4.6	4.3	2.9	0.6	0.4	2.4	1.6	29.7	20.2
State government[3]	10.3	26.3	1.0	2.5	1.0	2.6	0.1	0.2	0.5	1.3	7.7	19.6
Local government[3]	33.3	30.9	5.8	5.3	3.2	3.0	0.5	0.5	1.9	1.7	21.9	20.4

[1]*Number* of cases in thousands.

[2]*The* incidence rates represent the number of illnesses per 10,000 full-time equivalent workers and were calculated as: (N/EH) x 20,000,000, where N = number of illnesses; EH = total hours worked by all employees during the calendar year; 20,000,000 = base for 10,000 equivalent full-time workers (working 40 hours per week, 50 weeks per year).

[2]*Excludes* farms with fewer than 11 employees.

[3]*Data* for Mining (Sector 21 in the North American Industry Classification System – United States, 2017) include establishments not governed by the Mine Safety and Health Administration rules and reporting, such as those in Oil and Gas Extraction and related support activities. Data for mining operators in coal, metal, and nonmetal mining are provided to BLS by the Mine Safety and Health Administration, U.S. Department of Labor. Independent mining contractors are excluded from the coal, metal, and nonmetal mining industries. These data do not reflect the changes the Occupational Safety and Health Administration made to its recordkeeping requirements effective January 1, 2002; therefore, estimates for these industries are not comparable to estimates in other industries.

[4]*Data* for employers in railroad transportation are provided to BLS by the Federal Railroad Administration, U.S. Department of Transportation.

[5]*Data* too small to be displayed.

NOTE: Because of rounding, components may not add to totals. Dash indicates data do not meet publication guidelines.

Source: U.S. Bureau of Labor Statistics, U.S. Department of Labor.

substance use recovery, mental illness, and disability.

Educational attainment. Approximately 25% of Hispanics have less than a high school education and only 21% have a bachelor's degree or higher. This is contrasted with Blacks – 6% less than high school, 31% bachelor's or above; and with Whites – 7% below high school and 41% at or above bachelors.

Nativity. Foreign born workers are more likely to work in service sector, natural resources, construction and maintenance, and production, transportation and material moving (US Bureau of Labor Statistics, 2019e). As shown in Tables 32.2–32.5, these industries are more highly associated with work-related illnesses and injuries. They are also paid generally lower wages than the management, sales, and office jobs held by their native-born counterparts.

Rural/Urban Divide. In 32 states, the median household income was higher for rural households than urban households. However, in 14 states the opposite was true. Non-Hispanic Whites and American Indian and Alaska Natives living in rural areas had higher poverty rates compared to their urban counterparts. For African Americans and Hispanics, there was, overall, no difference. However, there is considerable geographic variation (Bishaw & Posey, 2016).

The impact of these disparities is felt in the form of higher risk of occupational illness and injury, as well as lower wages, lack of social protections, and irregular work arrangements, described above. Contextualized in the WHO Social Determinants model, these factors live within a political, social and economic context and contribute to inequities in health and well-being.

Evaluating Occupational Hazards

Work-related injuries and illnesses are a major public health concern because the majority of people work, occupational illness and injury are prevalent, and these illnesses and injuries are preventable. In order to prevent workplace injuries, it is useful to categorize them by hazard, exposure, risk, and adverse health outcome.

All workplace hazards may be put into the following categories: Chemical, Physical, Biological, Biomechanical, Psychosocial, and Economic-Social-Political (Table 32.7). Chemical, Physical, Biological, Biomechanical, and Psychosocial hazards are associated with Proximate Causes of harm while Structural Influences include Economic and Social Policies.

This framework makes it easy to consider hazardous working conditions whether dealing with individuals in a workplace or in a clinical encounter; groups of workers with the same job title, same workplace; or populations of workers across workplaces. The proximate causes are the focus of workers, employers, insurance companies, and enforcement agencies, such as the Occupational Safety and Health Administration in the US. Structural

Table 32.7 Hazard categories related to work

Proximate Causes					*Structural Influences*
Chemical	Physical	Biological	Biomechanical	Psychosocial	Economic-social-political
Pesticides	Radiation	Bacteria	Overexertion	Bullying	Low wages
Solvents	Cold	Viruses	Awkward posture	Harassment	Lack of health insurance
Metals	Heat	Fungi	Repetition	Violence	Unstable employment
	Noise		Work at heights	Shift work	No opportunity for advancement
			Moving machinery		No sick leave
					Limited legislation/oversight of health and safety

influences, certainly experienced by individual workers, are more in the purview of legislators and other policymakers, unions, community-based organizations like workers' centers, and communities, rather than Public Health. Low-wage work and unstable employment concentrates these workers in impoverished communities and is part of a feedback loop that sustains inequities in employment and health (Forst et al., 2015; Forst et al., 2020; Velonis et al., 2020).

Considering primary prevention of proximate causes, alone, occupational illnesses and injuries can be categorized in a number of ways, particularly if public health practitioners are framing data to guide preventive efforts. Consider the following scenarios:

Case 1. A worker in an automobile body shop spray-paints cars daily and has developed signs of asthma.
Case 2. A roofer applies shingles on a slanted roof and falls off the roof, becoming quadriplegic and subsequently dying of this injury.
Case 3. A nurses' aid sprains her back lifting a heavy patient.
Case 4. A factory worker with long-term exposure to solvents develops leukemia.
Case 5. A healthcare worker develops COVID-19.

Each scenario has a job title, an industry (not made explicit), a hazardous exposure associated with the job task, a mechanism of injury, and an adverse health effect. Table 32.8 illustrates how these are organized for each case.

If the Occupational Safety and Health Administration, the US's enforcement agency located in the US Department of Labor, wanted to decide where to put its scarce resources to prevent these injuries, it might focus on one of these categories: a job title or industry, a particular hazardous agent or condition, a disease or injury type or affected organ system (that may have a variety of causes). In thinking about cost-effective approaches, Occupational Safety and Health Administration (OSHA) might want to consider the number, rate or trends of specific illnesses or injuries and it may put injury severity into its calculation. OSHA may also want to know how often a certain industry experiences injuries or illnesses – how widespread is the hazard? Or who are the "bad actors"? Finally, emerging hazards – new processes or products, or known products used in new processes – are best detected in a real-time surveillance system that allows detection of single or a few unusual events.

How can public health practitioners – industrial hygienists, safety professionals, occupational health nurses, occupational medicine physicians, and public health agencies – prevent workplace illness and injury? It helps to use a stepwise approach.

The first step in the analysis is awareness that there may be a hazard. Awareness may

Table 32.8 Organizing framework for considering prevention of occupational illness and injury

Case	*Job title*	*Industry*	*Hazard*	*Mechanism of injury*	*Adverse health effect*	*Organ system*
1	Spray-painter	Auto repair	Solvent-based paint	Inhalation	Asthma	Respiratory system
2	Roofer	Construction	Work at height	Fall	Quadriplegia, death	Multiple
3	Nurses' aide	Healthcare	Lifting	Sprain	Back injury	Musculoskeletal
4	Factory worker	Manufacturing	Chemicals, unspecified	Inhalation? Skin absorption? Ingestion?	Leukemia, cancer	Hematopoietic
5	Healthcare worker	Healthcare	Coronavirus	Inhalation	COVID-19	Multiple

be the result of a worker who becomes ill, because workers or managers recognize a hazardous situation, because a change in process or product is planned, or because a major event, such as chemical release, has occurred.

The next step is to examine the situation/hazard qualitatively. The overall goal of this step is to characterize the workplace, workers, tasks, agents, potential exposures and potential health effects. This step involves understanding the process(es) leading to potential exposures, developing an inventory of chemical, physical, biological, psychosocial agents and cumulative or acute traumatic hazards. Most health and safety programs are resource strapped and it is desirable to maximize the resources available for controls and prevention. The goal is to make a decision about the need for interventions or controls through an understanding of the process and observation of the workplace. Resources about common industrial processes, occupational exposures, chemical and physical agents, and exposure–disease relationships are available to aid a qualitative hazard or exposure judgement. And this might involve walking through the facility and judging the risk level (e.g., is it very loud so that you can't communicate easily, is it very dusty, are there slipping and tripping hazards that could be corrected without any additional investigation or assessment?).

The qualitative assessment might involve looking at historical data to determine if exposures are increasing, staying the same, or decreasing. It might involve looking at injury rates to determine if there has been change in injury rates and examining where those injuries occurred, what workers were doing when they got injured. Review of new toxicological information might indicate that exposure levels that were considered acceptable might now be considered unacceptable.

The next step is to make a judgement using the information evaluated in the qualitative exposure assessment. The goal of this step is to determine: (1) is the exposure acceptable, (2) is the exposure unacceptable, or (3) is the exposure uncertain? For exposure deemed acceptable, no additional interventions or exposure reductions are needed, and exposures should be periodically re-evaluated. For exposures deemed unacceptable, exposure controls are warranted; examples of exposure controls are described below. In many cases, however, the qualitative exposure assessment does not result in a definitive judgement but instead the acceptability of the exposure is uncertain. In these cases, quantitative exposure assessment is needed. In many cases this involves doing a quantitative exposure assessment, measuring exposures in the workplace and trying to quantify the magnitude of those exposures or conducting a health assessment of workers and trying to quantify the workplace risks. The results of the quantitative exposure or health assessment is again used to make a judgement about the acceptability of the workplace exposures.

Population-level Occupational Surveillance

Occupational surveillance at the population level is the systematic monitoring of hazardous exposures or adverse health effects in the workplace for the purpose of prevention. The components of a surveillance system include: gathering information on exposure and disease (considering, what is the best way to collect this information?); analyzing the data (what are the number, rates, and trends for a given injury or illness?); disseminating results in an organized format (based on who needs to know this information); using these results to target areas for intervention (where is this occurring, what are the circumstances, and, thus, what is the best way to intervene?); and following the data over time (did the intervention help?). Why might you start an occupational surveillance program? For many reasons: you might want to (a) detect a problem and estimate its magnitude; (b) identify groups at risk – as described above, occupational health inequities exist, and this is a way to detect differences in the burden of disease or injury among groups at risk due to structural racism; (c) identify cases, workplaces, and industries for attention – are amputations more common in certain workplaces? Can you direct your scarce resources to those workplaces, rather than casting a wider net? New/emerging illnesses can come from newly used hazardous agents, but also from a new use of an existing agent. For example, toluene diisocyanate, which can cause severe asthma, is used in plastic manufacturing and spray-painting automobile bodies and is controlled through ventilation systems; a worker died when he used this chemical to spray-paint the inside of a tanker vehicle (Chester et al., 2005). This last scenario is an example of a Sentinel Health Event (Rutstein et al., 1983) – that is, an untoward event that signals a failure of prevention and indicates that others are at risk.

The Occupational Safety and Health Administration (OSHA), in the US Department of Labor, is the US's enforcement agency for worker health and safety. The Bureau of Labor Statistics (BLS), the data arm of the US Department of Labor, is responsible for collecting data related to employment and is the national source of occupational illness and injury surveillance in the US. In 1992, the BLS began the Survey of Occupational Illnesses and Injuries, sampling records from companies across the 50 states. Prior to data collection, BLS sends a notice to select employers asking them to maintain a careful OSHA-required injury log (OSHA 301) and provide an annual summary (300A) to BLS at the end of a calendar year (US Bureau of Labor Statistics, n.d.c.). The cases in this sample are weighted to establish numbers and rates of various injuries and can be stratified by demographics, state, industrial sectors and illness/injury type. Workplace deaths, amputations, and acute hospitalizations must be reported to the OSHA within 24 hours. The BLS collects mortality data and corroborates workplace deaths with two other pieces of data (e.g., death records), publishing results in the Census of Fatal Occupational Injury (CFOI).

There are other sources of occupational illness and injury surveillance that cover smaller geographic areas. The National Institute for Occupational Safety and Health funds State-based surveillance in 27 states for some 28 occupational health indicators (Council of State and Territorial Epidemiologists, n.d.).

Hazard surveillance starts with the knowledge that an agent or a mechanism might be hazardous, is present in the environment, and an individual may be exposed through skin absorption, inhalation, or ingestion. Exposure surveillance relates to contact by the host such that the agent reaches target tissue and produces an adverse health effect. Adverse health effects can be detected through clinical signs and symptoms or through clinical testing (e.g., hearing test for noise exposure).

An active Occupational Health surveillance system should provide data to "inform the development of policy, guide educational and regulatory activities, develop safer technologies, and focus research and preventive strategies that protect workers" (National Academies, 2018). Globally, data on work-related illness and injury are patchy. The Global Burden of Disease project includes data on occupational illnesses but are beyond the scope of this chapter (GBD, 2013; Rushton, 2017).

Worker Screening

Occupational surveillance can be done at an individual level, as well. Also called "screening," the goal is detection of a disease or body dysfunction before a worker would normally seek medical care. To achieve primary prevention, workers with potential for exposure who do not have disease are targeted with the goal of changing exposure conditions to reduce risk to zero. In the workplace, an example is lubricating moving machinery so that noise levels are reduced; or covering a chemical container to prevent inhalation. Secondary prevention targets workers with early stage of disease but no symptoms, with the goal of reversing the disease process. Testing iron-workers or building demolition workers for blood lead levels can detect high levels and allow for the removal of the worker before there are systemic effects. Tertiary prevention addresses clinical disease and seeks to cure or control the disease.

In the US, OSHA mandates screening of workers exposed to specific hazardous agents and conditions, including:

1 Acrylonitrile
2 Arsenic (Inorganic
3 Asbestos (General Industry)
4 Asbestos (Construction and Shipyards)
5 8 Benzene
6 Bloodborne Pathogens
7 1,3 Butadiene
8 Cadmium
9 Carcinogens (Suspect)
10 Chromium (VI), Hexavalent Chromium
11 Coke Oven Emissions
12 Compressed Air Environments
13 Cotton Dust
14 1,2dibromo3chloropropane
15 Ethylene Oxide
16 Formaldehyde
17 HAZWOPER
18 Hazardous Chemicals in Laboratories
19 Lead
20 Methylene Chloride
21 Methylenedianiline
22 Noise
23 Respiratory Protection
24 Crystalline Silica
25 Vinyl Chloride

The items that are considered for each of these exposures include a pre-placement medical exam, periodic exam, emergency/exposure examination and tests, termination exam. An exam includes emphasis on respiratory, gastrointestinal (GI), thyroid, skin, and nervous system; work and medical history, chest x-ray, pulmonary function test, other tests, evaluation of respirator use, additional tests if deemed necessary, a written medical opinion, employee counseling regarding exam results, conditions of increased risk; and a medical removal plan.

The International Labor Organization's *Technical and Ethical Guidelines for Workers' Health Surveillance* provides guidance for worker screening as an international standard (International Labor Organization, 1998).

Prevention

As described above, control of hazardous exposures is the basic method for protecting workers. Figure 32.4 provides a graphic, developed by the National Institute for Occupational Safety and Health, which describes this approach.

Following this hierarchy, it is important to try first to eliminate or control the hazard through changes to the process or engineering approaches to reduce exposure. Use of personal protective equipment is considered only while more permanent engineering controls are implemented or for situations where engineering controls are not technically or economically feasible, for example, during non-routine operations that are not at a fixed location, or during emergency situations.

Another way to prioritize exposure reduction controls is thinking about where the controls are implemented. Controls can be applied to Source, in the Pathway between the source and worker, or at the Worker.

Source controls are most effective because the hazardous exposure is eliminated or reduced before it is introduced into the workplace. Whenever possible, the best solution to a hazardous chemical exposure is to remove it entirely from the workplace to prevent all exposure. This is often possible, as demonstrated by the use of water-based paint instead of oil-based paints and the use of insulation fluids other than those that contain PCBs. Care must be taken to ensure that the substituted chemical is significantly safer than the original and that one hazardous condition is not being replace by another

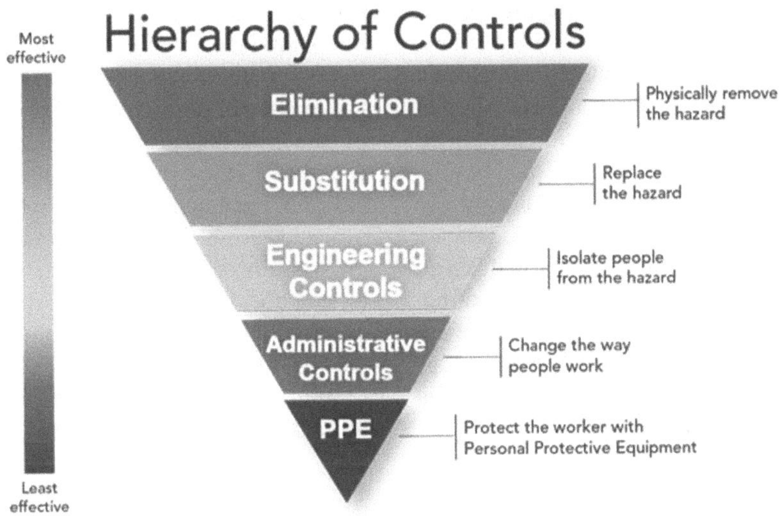

Figure 32.4 Hygiene Hierarchy of Controls (NIOSH, n.d.)

hazardous condition. In many cases the danger or exposure hazards associated with a job are inherent in the set-up of the job or the organization of the work process itself. The process design can often be changed, resulting in potentially dramatic improvements in health and safety, without using personal protection equipment or installing ventilation. Process redesigns are common to improve efficiency and/or to accommodate new technologies and should also be considered to minimize worker exposure to hazards. Automating an operation, or phases of an operation, may be the best approach, especially for extremely dangerous operations. This type of control is used widely in the chemical and nuclear industries. However, it is important that new hazards (e.g., machine hazards) are not introduced. Toxic substances can be controlled through use of local exhaust ventilation applied at a point as close to the source of emission as possible and enclosing as much of the source of emission as possible. An example of this type of control is a laboratory fume hood. If removal of the hazard is not possible, then the process should be enclosed. Process enclosure keeps the contaminant out of the workplace air and effectively away from the worker. Work areas that require only occasional attention can be very effectively controlled without interfering with operations. Additional controls (e.g., ventilation and/or personal protective equipment) may be needed when entry into the isolation area is necessary. Wet methods can be used to reduce dust exposures when dust-generating material is handled if water will not interfere with the process. By keeping the material damp or by using fogging sprays at transfer points, very little material is released to the general air. Also, high-pressure water washing of the inside surfaces of vessels and tanks can be an effective control measure because it can reduce the amount of manual cleaning which potentially exposes workers to chemical hazards.

Pathway controls are used to either dilute the concentration of chemical agents in the workplace or to interrupt the transmission of physical agents through the workplace. Dilution ventilation is not applicable to the control of toxic materials because it does not prevent them from being generated and introduced into the workplace, but only reduces the concentration of the agent. The main use for general ventilation is in office environments or in areas where toxic materials are not used. In these areas, general ventilation is used to circulate fresh air and control temperature for comfort. Another isolation technique is to provide controlled rooms for the workers. This is possible when the process is very large and mostly automated. Workers may be able to operate the process from control rooms with clean and conditioned air and/or sound proofing. Barriers and diking are used where there are process or storage units which contain significant amounts of highly toxic materials and where a spill or leak could be potentially catastrophic. However, this type of control will not reduce exposure for those workers in close proximity to the leak or spill. A routine and preventive maintenance program for process and exposure reduction equipment and machinery is necessary to ensure proper operation of equipment and machinery and effective control of hazardous exposures. Shielding can be effective for physical agents such as radiation or excessive heat. Distance can also be effective for physical agents such as radiation or noise – the further you are from the source, the lower the exposure intensity will be.

When source and pathway controls are being implemented or are not completely protective, use of personal protective equipment may be necessary. Consideration needs to be given to matching the particular piece of equipment to the hazard; fit; training; maintenance; replacement and repair; storage; and record-keeping.

Personal protective equipment (PPE) includes respirators, hearing protection, and traditional safety equipment like safety glasses and hardhats. There are different types of respirators for different types of contaminants and it is crucial that the respirator matches the hazard. PPE is the least protective approach to exposure reduction. In order for PPE to be effective, every worker must comply with the program. They have to have the appropriate PPE available to them in the right size and at the time it is needed. It has to fit correctly and be maintained in good working order. The more people whose exposure you are trying to control through PPE, the more complicated the PPE program will be. With the use of PPE, the exposures in the workplace have not been controlled, the worker is just protected from those exposures. If the respirator fails or if it leaks or the hearing protection doesn't fit correctly or doesn't work exactly right, workers will be exposed to the hazard.

With all of these controls there is a need for administrative controls to ensure that the controls are effective. Examples of administrative controls include training and education to ensure workers understand the risks and understand how to protect themselves; the use of continuous monitors with alarms for chemicals that are highly toxic; the use of personal monitoring devices to alert workers to hazardous exposure situations; and good housekeeping assists in keeping the work environment cleaner and prevents materials left on walking and working surfaces from getting into the air. Housekeeping depends on three basic things: having adequate work time to allow for work area clean up, being provided with proper cleaning equipment, and using proper equipment and procedures. Housekeeping can reduce the risks for things like slips, trips and falls, which may seem minor but are one of the leading causes of injury in the workplace. Medical surveillance, described above, complements exposure reduction strategies described here. The goal is not only to reduce exposures through the use of the hierarchy of controls, but also to monitor for early signs of disease so that early treatment can be implemented.

Policy interventions can be very helpful in both garnering the resources for reducing exposure and for legally requiring a reduction exposure. For example, if OSHA passes a new exposure limit, more resources directed toward reducing exposure will be required.

CASE STUDY: COVID-19 PANDEMIC OF 2019–2021

The recognition of Occupational Health as a critical component of Public Health has been no more evident than during SARS CoV-2 pandemic of 2019–2021. Outbreaks and deaths have occurred among workers in healthcare, first response, correctional facilities, nursing homes, animal slaughter, processing and meatpacking facilities, warehouses, public transportation systems, retail, and migrant/seasonal farm work. These are places where frontline workers directly care for infected individuals or work in congregate living facilities, in workplaces where employees stand shoulder to shoulder, and in jobs that serve the public. All businesses that have remained open during public health shutdowns have put workers at risk.

Mitigating occupational risk of contracting and spreading COVID-19 fits within the long-accepted industrial hygiene hierarchy of controls (Figure 32.4). This framework is used to determine how to implement feasible and effective control solutions, starting at the top of the inverted pyramid – the most effective approaches – and moving toward the bottom when feasibility of optimal approaches is limited. With chemical and physical hazards, this approach to control and prevention is intuitive. In the face of an infectious disease pandemic like SARS-CoV-2, elimination of the hazard (while keeping the economy open) can only be achieved by telecommuting; this is an approach adopted by many companies and is recommended in some jurisdictions. Engineering controls would entail improving ventilation (why outdoor work is preferred) or putting panes of plastic between workers and others. Administrative controls could involve altering shifts such that only part of the workforce is present at one time, spacing workers farther apart, rationing customer access/entry into the space, providing and recommending the use of hand sanitizer, and scheduling frequent cleaning. Online teaching from elementary through graduate school became the norm.

Personal protective equipment (PPE) – masks and face shields – are used where processes are difficult to control. As witnessed in the SARS-CoV-2 pandemic, adequate supply is essential; workers need to be fit-tested and trained on appropriate use, and changing behaviors can be challenging. PPE, an acronym previously known by occupational health experts, alone, is now in the lexicon of the general public. More importantly, the public is now aware of the challenges of prolonged use of respiratory protection, particularly in warm and indoor environments, problems which would be magnified by more protective respirators. Behavioral approaches to prevention – in the case of the SARS-CoV-2 pandemic, mask use and handwashing – are shown to have much lower rates of effectiveness given personal choice, hence their position on the bottom of the pyramid. OSHA provides a guidance document on how to prepare workplaces for COVID-19 (/www.osha.gov/Publications/OSHA3990.pdf).

Figure 32.5 contextualizes specific issues to consider, contextualized by the hygiene hierarchy model. Consideration of the listed items can guide the planning and modification of workplaces, working conditions, and additional factors.

In a broader sense, infectious disease outbreaks in workplaces, and our failure to anticipate and prevent these, highlight a limited understanding of occupational health, a lack of will to control business interests, and ignoring the impact of work on communities and vice versa. The intersection of work, community, home, and personal factors has been made obvious during the pandemic. A combination of personal, home, community, and work factors are displayed in Table 32.9.

The WHO Social Determinants of Health model (Figure 32.1) frames the profound impact of occupational health inequities and injustice made obvious during the SARS-CoV-2 pandemic. Those who are able to telecommute, who have internet connectivity,

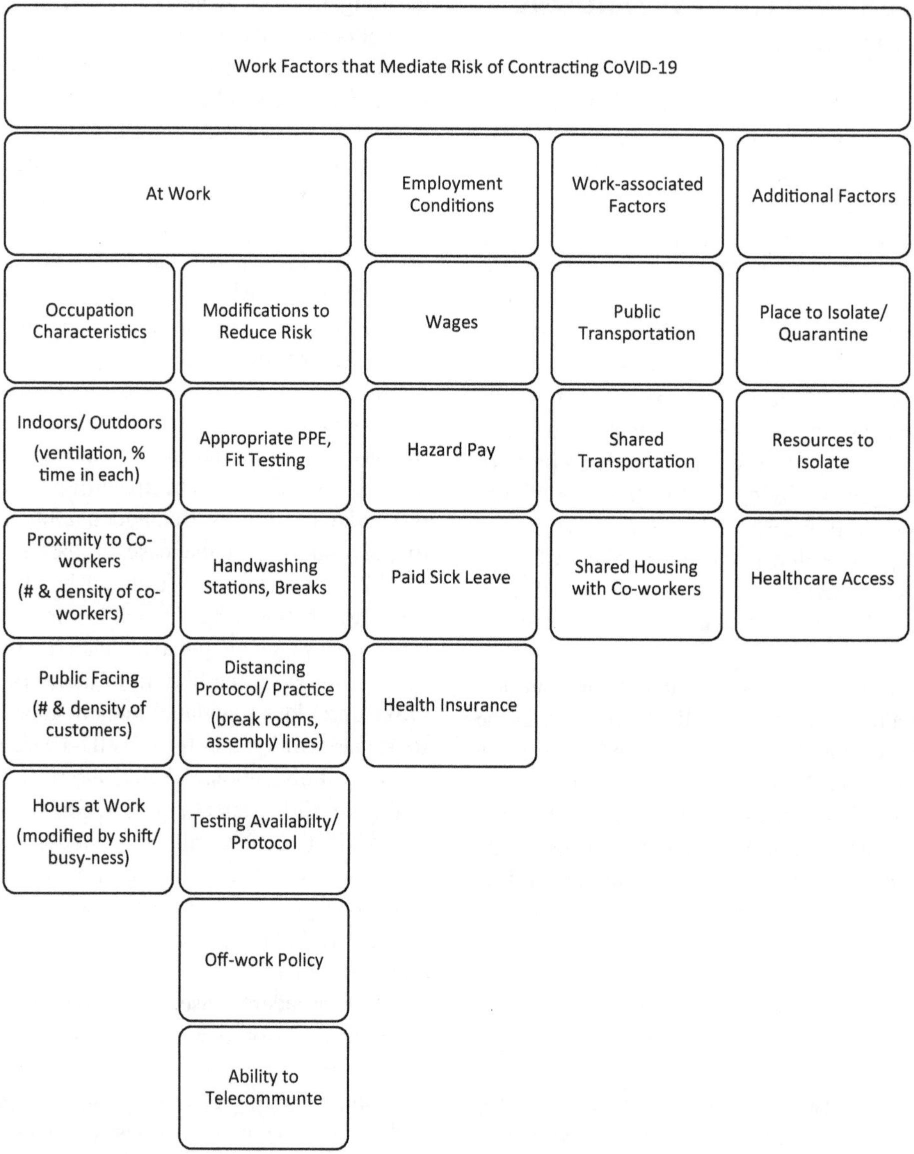

Figure 32.5 Work factors that mediate risk for contracting COVID-19

who have full-time jobs with social protections (health insurance, paid sick leave), who own their own cars and homes, and live in places with well-supported schools, are faring better than their counterparts, both in their ability to withstand the economic challenges and to keep themselves safe. Healthcare workers at obvious risk are the nurses and physicians who care for infected patients. However, there are many supportive, low-wage jobs that are populated by individuals with low educational attainment, and often people of color. Outside of healthcare, which is obviously risky, the occupational COVID-19 outbreaks are occurring in manual labor and low-paying jobs, where workers cannot

Table 32.9 Factors contributing to exposure, contagion and health outcomes related to COVID-19

Personal Health Factors	*Home Factors*	*Community Factors*	*Work Factors*
Age	Roommates/family health	Prevalence of COVID-19	see Figure 6
Chronic diseases	Roommates/family behavior	Resources for isolating, quarantining	
Immune system	How shopping is accomplished	Testing availability	
Genetics	How home services are acquired	Healthcare availability	
Behavior	Place to isolate, quarantine, convalesce		

afford to stay home and rarely have paid sick leave, who live in high economic hardship communities with challenged school systems, and who take public transportation or carpool to work. The lack of available testing for the first 4–6 months of the pandemic fell more heavily on those with fewer resources – in the beginning of the pandemic, one needed a regular provider to find testing, had to pay for testing, and were required to display negative tests to their employers. The intersection of work, high economic hardship and race/ethnicity are no better displayed than in the statistics associated with the pandemic.

The essential/frontline jobs, aside from high acuity, hospital healthcare and first response, are done by a higher proportion of African Americans and Hispanics than their overall representation in the workforce. Table 32.10 represents a sample of high-risk occupations – those prevalent in the news and on various state health department websites – and the racial, ethnic, and gender makeup of those occupations. While Blacks/African Americans make up only 12.3% of the US workforce, they are significantly over-represented in urban transit occupations, home healthcare services, and nursing

Table 32.10 Employed persons by detailed industry, sex, race, and Hispanic or Latino ethnicity (USBLS Current Population Survey, 2019)

	2019					
		Percent of total employed				
Industry	*Total employed*	*Women*	*White*	*Black or African American*	*Asian*	*Hispanic or Latino*
Total, 16 years and over	157,538	47.0	77.7	12.3	6.5	17.6
Agriculture, forestry, fishing, and hunting	2,425	26.2	93.0	2.2	1.7	27.5
Crop production	1,261	26.7	93.8	2.2	1.7	34.0
Construction	11,373	10.3	88.1	6.4	1.9	30.4
Manufacturing	15,741	29.4	79.5	10.4	6.8	16.8
Food manufacturing	1,834	41.5	76.0	14.3	5.7	29.7
Sugar and confectionery products	86	34.0	75.5	18.6	4.6	22.2
Fruit and vegetable preserving and specialty food manufacturing	153	46.7	78.2	10.8	6.2	38.9

(Continued)

Table 32.10 (Continued)

Industry	*2019*					
		Percent of total employed				
	Total employed	*Women*	*White*	*Black or African American*	*Asian*	*Hispanic or Latino*
Dairy product manufacturing	145	23.2	93.2	3.9	1.6	23.8
Animal slaughtering and processing	585	38.7	66.4	21.9	5.6	35.3
Retail bakeries	230	66.6	82.2	7.4	5.6	25.7
Bakeries and tortilla manufacturing, except retail bakeries	232	44.8	73.2	14.5	8.6	36.1
Wholesale and retail trade	19,742	44.2	78.6	11.7	5.7	18.1
Retail trade	16,217	47.6	77.6	12.3	5.7	18.3
Grocery stores	2,670	47.5	76.1	12.6	6.2	20.5
Specialty food stores	225	45.5	81.4	5.3	8.6	20.8
Transportation and warehousing	7,614	24.8	68.7	22.0	5.8	20.1
Bus service and urban transit	492	37.1	59.1	31.4	7.2	18.7
Taxi and limousine service	703	18.2	52.5	29.9	15.6	23.5
Postal Service	669	41.7	62.1	27.2	7.8	11.3
Couriers and messengers	938	22.7	66.6	25.1	4.1	19.5
Warehousing and storage	788	33.0	65.3	23.8	5.2	32.2
Hospitals	7,425	74.9	71.9	16.0	8.9	10.8
Home health care services	1,412	88.5	59.7	30.5	6.1	18.4
Nursing care facilities (skilled nursing facilities)	1,663	83.7	64.4	27.6	4.3	12.6
Residential care facilities, except skilled nursing facilities	995	76.0	67.5	23.9	4.8	12.6
Social assistance	3,430	83.8	71.0	20.1	4.6	19.4
Individual and family services	1,753	78.3	69.6	20.7	5.0	18.1
Community food and housing, and emergency services	125	63.8	72.2	21.5	3.0	15.3
Vocational rehabilitation services	99	56.7	69.2	26.6	0.4	15.2
Child day care services	1,452	94.0	72.7	18.9	4.5	21.5

n.e.c. = not elsewhere classified.

NOTE: Estimates for the above race groups (White, Black or African American, and Asian) do not sum to totals because data are not shown for all races. Persons whose ethnicity is identified as Hispanic or Latino may be of any race. Updated population controls are introduced annually with the release of January data. Dash indicates no data or data that do not meet publication criteria (values not shown where base is less than 50,000).

home care, occupations that have been hard hit by COVID-19. Latinx/Hispanics make up 17.6% of the US population and are more highly over-represented in food/bakery manufacturing, animal slaughter, crop production, and warehousing.

Health inequities have been well described in the public health and healthcare literature, rarely taking into account "work" as an indicator of risk for adverse health effects. The approach described in this chapter can be used to examine differential risk of exposure to SARS-CoV-2, by occupation. Notably, the highest risk of contracting COVID-19 falls on the same groups who have been compelled to work during the pandemic, who are considered "essential critical infrastructure workers"

(Cybersecurity & Infrastructure Security Agency (CISA), 2020). These groups are at highest risk for chronic diseases, limited healthcare access, poorer health outcomes and community-level challenges like poor access to transportation and walkable areas, food deserts, and others.

An economic analysis of the listed occupations – wages, hours, availability of paid sick leave, health insurance and workers' compensation – are salient to understanding the contribution of "work" to risk of contracting and dying from COVID-19. However, such an analysis is beyond the scope of this chapter.

DEDICATION

This chapter is dedicated to Leslie Nickels. As a fierce champion of workers' health and human rights, she would have been a co-author.

REFERENCES

Agarwal, D., Bersin, J., Lahiri, G., Schwartz, J., & Volini E. (2018). The workforce ecosystem: managing beyond the enterprise, 2018 Global Human Capital Trends. *Deloitte Insights*, March 28.

Ahonen, E.Q., Baron, S.L. Brosseau, L.M., Vives, A. (2018). *Health and Safety Issues for Workers in Nonstandard Employment*. Oxford Research Encyclopedias. Oxford: Oxford University Press.

Alterman, T., Luckhaupt, S.E., Dahlhamer, J.M., Ward, B.W., & Calvert, G.M. (2013). Prevalence rates of work organization characteristics among workers in the US: data from the 2010 National Health Interview Survey. *American Journal of Industrial Medicine* 56: 647–659.

Azaroff, L.S., Levenstein, C., & Wegman, D.H. (2002). Occupational injury and illness surveillance: conceptual filters explain underreporting. *American Journal of Public Health* 92(9): 1421–1429. doi: 10.2105/ajph.92.9.1421.

Benach, J., Castedo, A., Solar, O., et al. (2010). Methods for the study of employment relations and health inequalities in a global context. *International Journal of Health Services* 40(2): 209–213.

Benach, J., Vives, A., Amable, M., Vanroelen, C., Tarafa, G., & Muntaner, C. (2014). Precarious employment: understanding an emergin social determinant of health. *Annual Review of Public Health* 35: 229–253.

Bishaw, A., & Posey, K.G. (2016). *A Comparison of Rural and Urban America: Household Income and Poverty*. Available at: www.census.gov/newsroom/blogs/random-samplings/2016/12/a_comparison_of_rura.html

Boal, W.M. (2009). The effect of unionism on accidents in US coal mining, 1897–1929. *Industrial Relations Journal* 48: 97–120.

Breasted, James Henry (1991 [1930]). *The Edwin Smith Surgical Papyrus. Published in facsimile and hieroglyphic transliteration with translation and commentary in two volumes*. University of Chicago Oriental Institute Publications, v. 3–4. Chicago, IL: University of Chicago Press.

Broschak, J.P., & Davis-Blake, A. (2006). Mixing standard work and nonstandard deals: the consequences of heterogeneity in employment arrangements. *Academy of Management Journal* 49(2). https://doi.org/10.5465/amj.2006.20786085

Brydsten, A., Hammarström, A., & San Sebastián, M. (2018). Health inequalities between employed and unemployed in northern Sweden: a decomposition analysis of social determinants for mental health. *International Journal of Equity Health* 17(1): 59. doi: 10.1186/s12939-018-0773-5.

Catanzarite, T., Tan-Kim, J., Whitcomb, E.L., & Menefee, S. (2018). Ergonomics in surgery: a review. *Female Pelvic Medine and Reconstructive Surgery* 24(1): 1–12. doi: 10.1097/SPV.9781473939523456.

Chang, J.-H., & Phu, H. (2016). *ASEAN in Transformation: The Future of Jobs at Risk of Automation*. Bureau for Employers' Activities Working Paper No. 9. Geneva: International Labour Office.

Chester, D.A., Hanna, E.A., Pickelman, B.G., & Rosenman, K.D. (2005). Asthma death after spraying polyurethane truck bedliner. *American Journal of Industrial Medicine* 48: 78–84. https://doi.org/10.1002/ajim.20183

Córdoba-Doña, J.A., Escolar-Pujolar, A., San Sebastián, M., & Gustafsson, P.E. (2016). How are the employed and unemployed affected by the economic crisis in Spain? Educational inequalities, life conditions and mental health in a context of high unemployment. *BMC Public Health* 16: 267. doi: 10.1186/s12889-016-2934-z.

Council of State and Territorial Epidemiologists. (n.d.). *Occupational Health Indicators*. Atlanta, GA: Council of State and Territorial Epidemiologists (https://www.cste.org/page/OHIndicators). Atlanta GA

Cybersecurity & Infrastructure Security Agency (CISA). (2020). *Critical Infrastructure Sectors*. Available at: www.cisa.gov/critical-infrastructure-sectors

Damiano, J., & Mulhausen, J.R. (1998). *A Strategy for Assessing and Managing Occupational Exposures* (2nd edition). Fairfax, VA: AIHA Press.

de Vries, A. (1977). Paracelsus: sixteenth-century physician-scientist-philosopher. *New York State Journal of Medicine* 77(5): 790–798.

Dungan, A. (2016). *Sole Proprietorship Returns, Tax Year 2016*. Washington, DC. Internal Revenue Service, Statistics of Income Division (www.irs.gov/pub/irs-soi/soi-a-inpr-id1905.pdf).

Federal Research Economic Data. (2017). *Federal Reserve Bank of St. Louis, 1984–2016*. St. Louis, MO: Federal Research Economic Data (https://fred.stlouisfed.org/graph/?g=caWq).

Forst, L., Friedman, L., Chin, B., & Madigan, D. (2015). Spatial clustering of occupational injuries in communities. *American Journal of Public Health* 105(Suppl 3): S526–S533. doi: 10.2105/AJPH.2015.302595.

Forst, L., Grant, A., & Hebert-Beirne, J. (2020). Work as a social determinant of health: a landscape assessment of employers in two historically disinvested urban communities. *American Journal of Industrial Medicine* 63(11): 1038–1046. doi: 10.1002/ajim.23174.

Forst, L., Nickels, L., & Conroy, L. (2009). The WHO modules in occupational safety and health: training for prevention. *Public Health Reports* 124(1): 169–176. doi: 10.1177/003335490912400122.

Franco, G. (2020). Revisiting the past strengthens the present: Bernardino Ramazzini and the new occupational health. *Public Health* 181(April): 180–181. doi: 10.1016/j.puhe.2019.12.016.

Frey, C.B., & Osborne, M. (2015). *Technology at Work: The Future of Innovation and Employment*. Citi Global Perspectives and Solutions (Citi GPS). Oxford and New York: University of Oxford and CitiGroup.

Frick, K., & Walters, D.R. (1998). Workers representation on health and safety in small enterprises: lessons from a Swedish approach. *International Labour Review* 137: 367–389.

Friedman, L.S., & Forst, L. (2008). Ethnic disparities in traumatic occupational injury. *Journal of Occupational and Environmental Medicine* 50(3): 350–358. doi: 10.1097/JOM.0b013e3181617324.

Friedman, L.S., Ruestow, P., & Forst, L. (2012). Analysis of ethnic disparities in workers' compensation claims using data linkage. *Journal of Occupational and Environmental Medicine* 54(10): 1246–1252. doi: 10.1097/JOM.0b013e31825a34d1.

GBD 2013 Risk Factors Collaborators, Forouzanfar, M.H., Alexander, L., Anderson, H.R. et al. (2015). Global, regional, and national comparative risk assessment of 79 behavioural, environmental and occupational, and metabolic risks or clusters of risks in 188 countries, 1990–2013: a systematic analysis for the Global Burden of Disease Study 2013. *Lancet* 386(10010): 2287–2323. doi: 10.1016/S0140-6736(15)00128-2. Epub 2015 Sep 11. PMID: 26364544; PMCID: PMC4685753.

Gochfeld, M. (2005). Chronologic history of occupational medicine. *Journal of Occupational and Environmental Medicine* 47(2): 96–114. doi: 10.1097/01.jom.0000152917.03649.0e.

Howard, J. (2017). Nonstandard work arrangements and worker health and safety. *American Journal of Industrial Medicine* 60: 1–10. http://dx.doi.org/10.1002/ajim.22669

International Labor Organization. (1998). *Technical and Ethical Guidelines for Workers' Health Surveillance*. Occupational Safety and Health Series No. 72. Geneva: International Labour Office (www.ilo.org/wcmsp5/groups/public/-ed_protect/-protrav/-safework/documents/normativeinstrument/wcms_177384.pdf).

International Labor Organization. (2015). *Global Trends on Occupational Accidents and Diseases*. Geneva: International Labour Office (www.ilo.org/legacy/english/osh/en/story_content/external_files/fs_st_1-ILO_5_en.pdf).

International Labour Organization. (2018). *Women and Men in the Informal Economy: A Statistical Picture* (3rd edition). Geneva: International Labour Organization.

International Labour Organization. (2020). *World Employment and Social Outlook: Trends 2020*. Geneva: International Labour Organization.

International Labour Organisation. (n.d.). *Decent Work*. Geneva: International Labour Organisation (www.ilo.org/global/topics/decent-work/lang–en/index.htm).

International Monetary Fund, External Relations Department. (2006, August 23). Finance and Development, September 2006. *Finance & Development* 43(3).

International Telecommunication Union. (2017). *ICT Facts and Figures 2017*. Geneva: International Telecommunication Union (https://about.fb.com/wp-content/uploads/2018/08/ICTFactsFigures2017.pdf).

Jeszeck, C.A. (2015). Contingent workforce: Size, characteristics, earnings, and benefits. GAO-15-168R. *GAO@100*, April 20. US Government Accountability Office.

Kalleberg, A. (2009). Precarious work, insecure workers: employment relations in transition. *American Sociological Review* 74(February): 1–22.

Katz, L.F., & Krueger, A.B. (2016). The rise and nature of alternative work arrangements in the United States, 1995–2015. *Journal Title* 72(2), March 29: 382–416.

Koranyi, I., Jonsson, J., Rönnblad, T., Stockfelt, L., & Bodin, T. (2018). Precarious employment and occupational accidents and injuries: a systematic review. *Scandinavian Journal of Work and Environmental Health* 44(4): 341–350. doi: 10.5271/sjweh.3720.

Leigh, J.P. (2011). Economic burden of occupational injury and illness in the United States. *Millbank Quarterly* 89(4): 728–772. doi: 10.1111/j.1468-0009.2011.00648.x

Loomis, D., & Richardson, D. (1998). Race and the risk of fatal injury at work. *American Journal of Public Health* 88(1): 40–44. doi: 10.2105/ajph.88.1.40.

Michaels, D. (1983). Occupational cancer in the black population: the health effects of job discrimination. *Journal of the National Medical Association* 75(10): 1014–1018.

Morley, I. (2007). City chaos, contagion, Chadwick, and social justice. *The Yale Journal of Biology and Medicine* 80(2): 61–72.

Muntaner, C., Chung, H., Solar, O., et al. (2010). A macro-level model of employment relations and health inequalities. *International Journal of Health Services* 40(2): 215–221.

Muntaner, C., Solar, O., Vanroelen, C., et al. (2010). Unemployment, informal work, precarious employment, child labor, slavery, and health inequalities: pathways and mechanisms. *International Journal of Health Services* 40(2): 281–295.

National Academies. (2018). *A Smarter National Surveillance System for Occupational Safety and Health in the 21st Century*. Washington, DC: National Academies (www.nap.edu/read/24835/chapter/1#vi).

National Collaborating Centre for Determinants of Health. (2013). *Let's Talk: Health Equity*. Antigonish, NS: National Collaborating Centre for Determinants of Health, St. Francis Xavier University.

National Institute for Occupational Safety and Health, Centers for Disease Control and Prevention (n.d.), https://www.cdc.gov/niosh/topics/hierarchy/default.html.

NIOSH. *Preventing the Injury of Workers by Robots*. DHHS (NIOSH) Publication Number 85-103. December 1984.

OSHA. Robotics. Standards. https://www.osha.gov/robotics/standards Accessed 7/12/2021

Pew Research Center (2015). *Social and Demographic Trends, December 9, 2015. The American Middle Class is Losing Ground*. Washington, DC: Pew Research Center (www.pewsocialtrends.org/2015/12/09/the-american-middle-class-is-losing-ground/)

Pliny the Elder. (2012). *The Natural History*. Trans. by John Bostock & H.T. Riley. London:

Taylor and Francis. Available at the Perseus Digital Library: www.perseus.tufts.edu/hopper/text?doc=Perseus:text:1999.02.0137:book=33:chapter=40&highlight=face%2C masks

Pofeldt, E. (2015). Shocker: 40% of workers now have 'contingent' jobs, says U.S. government. *Forbes*, May 25.

Prahalad, C.K., & Hamel, G. (1990). The core competence of the corporation. *Harvard Business Review* 68(3): 79–91.

Quinlan, M., Muntaner, C., Solar, O., et al. Policies and Interventions on Employment Relations and Health Inequalities. *International Journal of Health Services*. 2010;40(2):297–307. doi:10.2190/HS.40.2.i

Rushton, L. (2017). The global burden of occupational disease. *Current Environmental Health Reports* 4(3): 340–348. doi: 10.1007/s40572-017-0151-2.

Rutstein, D.D., Mullan, R.J., Frazier, T.M., Halperin, W.E., Melius, J.M., & Sestito, J.P. (1983). Sentinel Health Events (occupational): a basis for physician recognition and public health surveillance. *American Journal of Public Health* 73(9): 1054–1062. doi: 10.2105/ajph.73.9.1054.

Seabury, S.A., Terp, S., & Boden, L.I. (2017). The work/health relationship: racial and ethnic differences in the frequency of workplace injuries and prevalence of work-related disability. *Health Affairs* 36(2).

Solar, O., & Irwin, A. (2010). *A Conceptual Framework for Action on the Social Determinants of Health*. Social Determinants of Health Discussion Paper 2 (Policy and Practice). Geneva: World Health Organization.

UN Department of Economic and Social Affairs. (2015). *Transforming Our World: The 2030 Agenda for Sustainable Development*. A/RES/70/1. New York: United Nations (https://sdgs.un.org/2030agenda)

UN Department of Economic and Social Affairs, Population Division (2019). *World Population Prospects 2019: Highlights*. (ST/ESA/SER.A/423). New York: Department of Economic and Social Affairs Departments (https://population.un.org/wpp/DataQuery/).

US Bureau of Labor Statistics. (n.d.d.) *Labor Force Statistics from the Current Population Survey*. https://www.bls.gov/cps/tables.htm

US Bureau of Labor Statistics. (2019e) *Labor Force Statistics from the Current Population Survey*. https://www.bls.gov/cps/tables.htm

US Bureau of Labor Statistics. (n.d.a). *Current Population Survey: Demographics – Age*. Washington, DC: US Bureau of Labor (https://data.bls.gov/PDQWeb/ln) (https://www.bls.gov/cps/tables.htm#annual)

US Bureau of Labor Statistics. (n.d.b). *Current Population Survey: Demographics – Educational Attainment*. Washington, DC: US Bureau of Labor (https://population.un.org/wpp/Publications/Files/WPP2019_10KeyFindings.pdf) (https://www.bls.gov/cps/tables.htm#annual) (https://www.bls.gov/cps/tables.htm#charemp_m)

US Bureau of Labor Statistics. (n.d.c). *Survey of Occupational injuries and Illnesses*. Washington, DC: US Bureau of Labor (bls.gov/iif).. https://www.bls.gov/iif/soii-overview.htm

US Bureau of Labor Statistics. (2005, February). *Contingent and Alternative Employment Arrangements*. Washington, DC: US Bureau of Labor (www.bls.gov/news.release/history/conemp.txt)

US Bureau of Labor Statistics. 2019c *Survey of Occupational Illnesses and Injuries*. https://www.bls.gov/iif/soii-data.htm

US Bureau of Labor Statistics. (2016). *Self employment in the US*. Washington, DC: US Bureau of Labor (www.bls.gov/spotlight/2016/self-employment-in-the-united-states/home.htm).

US BLS. National Census of Fatal Occupational Injuries. *News Release*. 12/16/2020. https://www.bls.gov/news.release/pdf/cfoi.pdf

US Bureau of Labor Statistics. (2018). *Current Population Survey, 2018*. Washington, DC: US Bureau of Labor.

US Bureau of Labor Statistics. (2019a). *Survey of Occupational Injuries and Illnesses Data*. Washington, DC: US Bureau of Labor (www.bls.gov/iif/soii-data.htm).

US Bureau of Labor Statistics. (2019b). *Census of Fatal Occupational Injuries, 2019*. Washington, DC: US Bureau of Labor (www.bls.gov/iif/oshcfoi1.htm, accessed 01/15/21).

US Bureau of Labor Statistics. (2019c). *The Economics Daily*. https://www.bls.gov/opub/ted/2020/foreign-born-workers-made-up-17-point-4-percent-of-labor-force-in-2019.htm

US Bureau of Labor Statistics. (2019d, November 7). *Survey of Occupational Injuries and Illnesses*. Washington, DC: US Bureau of Labor (https://www.bls.gov/iif/soii-data.htm

US Bureau of Labor Statistics. (2019e) *Labor Force Statistics from the Current Population Survey*. https://www.bls.gov/cps/tables.htm

US Bureau of Labor Statistics. (2020, December). Labor Force Statistics from the Current Population Survey. https://www.bls.gov/cps/tables.htm US Census. (2017). *American Community Survey*. Washington, DC: US Census Bureau.

US Census. (2019). *American Community Survey*. Washington, DC: US Census Bureau.

US Department of Health and Human Services (DHHS). (1984). *Preventing the Injury of Workers by Robots*. National Institute for Occupational Safety and Health (NIOSH) Publication No. 85–103, December.

US Department of Labor. (n.d.a). *Occupational Safety and Health Administration. Robotics*. Washington, DC: US Department of Labor (www.osha.gov/robotics, accessed 01/27/21).

US Department of Labor. (n.d.b). *Occupational Safety and Health Administration. Recordkeeping Requirements*. Washington, DC: US Department of Labor (www.osha.gov/recordkeeping, accessed 01/27/21).

Vancea, M., & Utzet, M. (2017). How unemployment and precarious employment affect the health of young people: a scoping study on social determinants. *Scandinavian Journal of Public Health* 45(1): 73–84. doi: 10.1177/1403494816679555.

Velonis, A.J., Hebert-Beirne, J., Conroy, L.M., Hernandez, M., Castaneda, D., & Forst, L. (2020). Impact of precarious work on neighborhood health: concept mapping by community/academic partnership. *American Journal of Industrial Medicine* 63: 23–35. doi: 10.1002/ajim.23055

Vollset, S.E., Goren, E., Yuan, C.W., Cao, J., Smith, A.E., Hsiao, T., Bisignano, C., Azhar, G.S., Castro, E., Chalek, J., Dolgert, A.J., Frank, T., Fukutaki, K., Hay, S.I., Lozano, R., Mokdad, A.H., Nandakumar, V., Pierce, M., Pletcher, M., Robalik, T., Steuben, K.M., Wunrow, H.Y., Zlavog, B.S., & Murray, C.J.L. (2020). Fertility, mortality, migration, and population scenarios for 195 countries and territories from 2017 to 2100: a forecasting analysis for the Global Burden of Disease Study. *Lancet* 396(10258), October 17: 1285–1306. doi: 10.1016/S0140-6736(20)30677-2.

Weil, D. (2014). *The Fissured Workplace: How Work Became So Bad for So Many and What Can be Done to Improve It*. Cambridge, MA: Harvard University Press.

World Bank. (2016). *World Development Report 2016: Digital Dividends*. Washington, DC: World Bank.

World Economic Forum. (2018). *The Future of Jobs Report 2018*. Geneva: World Economic Forum.

Yi, K.H., Cho, H.H., Kim, J. (2011). An empirical analysis on labor unions and occupational safety and health committees' activity, and their relation to the changes in occupational injury and illness rate. *Safety and Health at Work* 2(4), December: 321–327. doi: 10.5491/SHAW.2011.2.4.321.

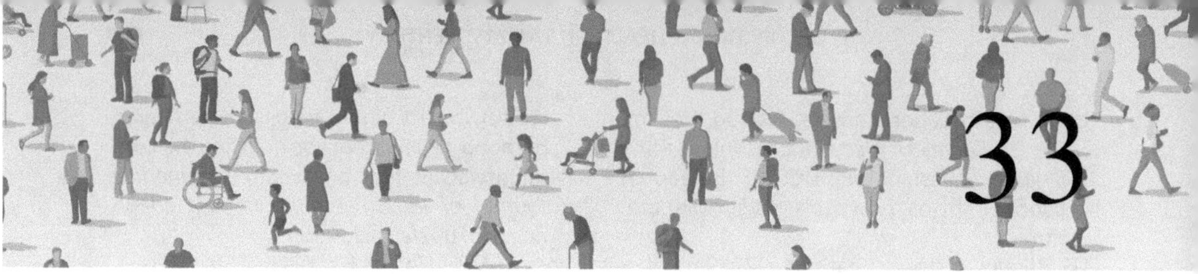

Economic and Health Policy in the Context of the Sustainable Development Goals 2030 Agenda

Jesús Gómez Rossi and Falk Schwendicke

AN INTRODUCTION TO ECONOMIC THEORY AND ITS ROLE IN THE DEVELOPMENT OF SOCIAL AND HEALTH POLICIES WITHIN THE SDG AGENDA

Welfare in Economics and Market Intervention in Social Policy

One of the fathers of neoclassical economics, Alfred Marshall (1890), helped to establish in this discipline that human welfare is inherently material and frequently associated with the cumulative "societal perspective" expressed through markets by individuals. Well-being under this economic perspective is derived from the relationship between the prices of a certain good or service and a buyer's willingness-to-pay (WTP) in a market. The "consumer surplus" that an individual obtains for paying less for a good or service than the maximum WTP they had pre-established is the welfare that he or she derives from a transaction in a certain market. As a certain good or service becomes more abundant, the price of that good is reduced, allowing more units to be purchased at a lower price, increasing overall societal welfare (Figure 33.1).

This definition of economic welfare builds on the assumption that individuals have a number of wants and needs that can be met through consumption of material goods, and that higher consumption directly correlates with higher societal well-being a person or society enjoys. This also assumes that consumption increases well-being regardless of who is consuming a good or service. According to classical economists such as Pareto (1906), if a market follows some criteria (all actors know all details of the goods produced, there are no interventions regarding prices, etc.) the societal outcomes generated by a certain market will result in an efficient allocation of resources for society. Economic efficiency, in this case, known as "Pareto efficiency," is achieved when it is

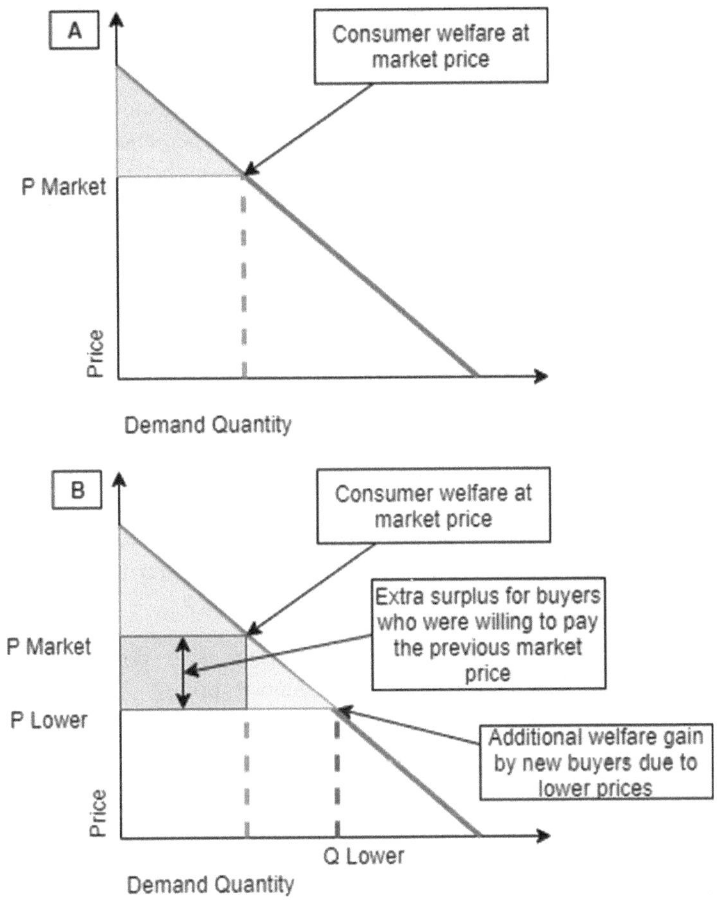

Figure 33.1 Buyer's willingness to pay

not possible to make an individual better off, without making another individual worse-off.

In social policy, though, the discussed definition of an "efficient economy" does not necessarily link to the best results for a society. For example, an "efficient" housing market where most of the houses at a given high price are occupied by those that can pay it, is compatible with the parallel existence of empty houses and homelessness, something which is not desirable from a societal perspective (Lux, 2003). Moreover, the overall well-being of a society could be affected by reducing the consumption of a certain good (e.g., sugar, alcohol or tobacco) or increasing it (e.g., fruits, vegetables or sports) above what the market would provide, generating conflicts between market efficiency and societal health outcomes. Some other goods impose costs not directly on the person consuming them, but on the environment or those around them, such as with smokers and passive smokers. These costs are known as "externalities", and when they are present, efficiency in the markets may not be possible without intervention.

Social policy often aims to address these externalities, for example via taxation or subsidies. A specific form of taxation, the so-called "Pigouvian tax" (1932), aims to improve overall societal well-being by decreasing or increasing the consumption of certain goods via making them more expensive (using taxes) or less expensive (via subsidies) (Pigou, 1932) (Figure 33.2). A Pigouvian tax therefore considers the inclusion of the cost of the externalities and adds them (or discounts them) to the private cost to achieve a societal equilibrium.

Importantly, differences in the access or quality of the goods or services produced can be informed by evidence but remain to a great extent a consequence of political preferences that are defined by the subjective judgement of a decision-maker. The potential interventions to tackle a certain problematic are then instrumentalized in the form of regulation or laws that are not purely scientific, but rather a reflection of political preferences that despite not being objective, could in some cases be informed by scientific evidence. Importantly, the political component in policy-making is frequently framed according to the political scientist Harold Lasswell (1936), who referred to politics as "Who gets what, when, how?" (Foreign Affairs, 1937), or in other words, what political groups should be favoured or prioritized with receiving a certain benefit (good or service), and how should these interventions be funded? These political questions (who should get healthcare, what should they get, and who should pay for it?) should be weighed carefully, considering that all societies have limited resources, as there may be trade-offs between the government intervention in a market and the efficiency in the production of a certain good (e.g., excessively low prices due to price control could generate a reduced incentive to produce that good and service).

Do Economic Growth and Economic Efficiency Lead by Themselves to the Best Societal Outcomes?

The normative political preferences that influence policy-making are always constrained by the finite nature of economic resources. The allocation of a budget in favour of healthcare will be at the expenses

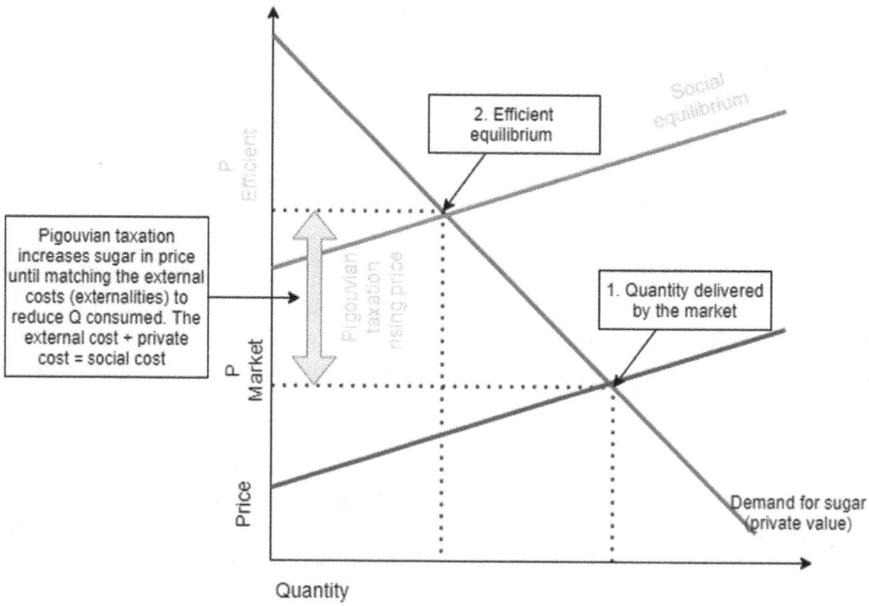

Figure 33.2 Pigouvian Tax

of the alternative allocation of the same resources for education or infrastructure. Health, as discussed in the chapters in this volume on *Comparative Health Systems: Paradigm Changes* (Chapter 19) and on *The Intersectional Impact of Race, Class, Ethnicity, and Place on Social Determinants of Health across the Life Course* (Chapter 3), as well as in the "Introduction" is strongly correlated with income and several social determinants that fuel systematic differences in health outcomes within a given society (WHO, 2018a). Because of that, some policy-makers decide to postpone the investment in healthcare in favour of prioritizing economic growth, under the assumption that in the process of becoming wealthier, a society would re-distribute wealth and improve health outcomes thanks to the free market. But does economic growth reduce health inequality and improve health outcomes on its own?

The concept that economic growth would reduce inequality was first developed by Nobel prize economist Simon Kuznets. He helped to develop the theory that inequality and income per capita would follow the shape of an "inverted-U" as societies develop (Kuznets, 1955) (Figure 33.3).

According to this theory, as societies develop economically, they would first experience an increase in economic inequality that would progressively decrease as they continue to grow wealthier. Kuznets developed this theory based on the empirical observation of Western economies in the period after the Second World War. In a conclusion, policies that aimed to reduce the intervention of markets seemed justified at the time, and to a certain degree successful. Policies that reduced governmental interference in markets coupled with global trade have helped China to lift over 850 million individuals out of poverty (World Bank, 2020). The resulting increased influence and power of multinational corporations at the expenses of governments, with countries competing for lower labour and environmental standards, as well as reducing taxation to attract investment, however, is increasingly faced with scrutiny (Rudra, 2008).

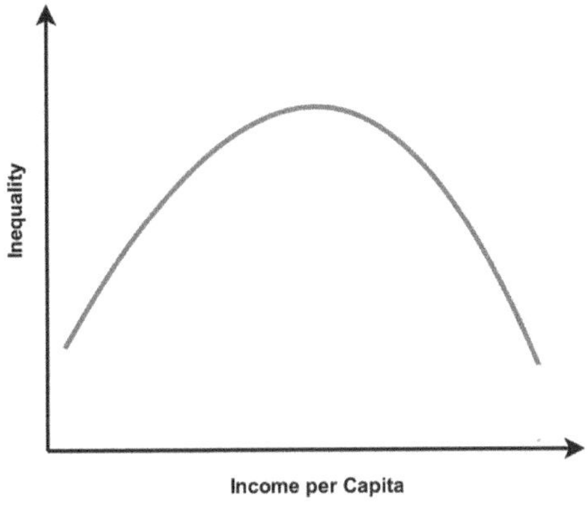

Figure 33.3 Inverted-U theory

Moreover, and especially in high-income countries with limited economic growth (1–3% of the GDP per year), the returns on investment of wealth increasingly exceed the returns generated by labour (Piketty, 2014), driving inequality despite economic growth: owning wealth oftentimes comes with the means of furthering that wealth, while not owning wealth will often not allow fostering an individual's economic growth beyond what is possible by labour. Disparities in the ownership of capital, as in the US, where the top 10% wealth owners in 2012 owned 75% of all wealth, are both a result of and reason for further inequality (World Inequality Report, 2018), and contribute to partially invalidating the "U-shaped theory" of Kuznets, who had predicted a reduction in inequality as societies would grow wealthier. Nowadays, institutions such as the World Bank, the United Nations or even the International Monetary Fund (IMF) differentiate between economic growth and the reduction of inequality as different policy objectives. The implications for social and health policy are significant; economic growth on its own does not suffice to improve health outcomes of those least well-off by reducing health inequalities, but rather economic policies are to be integrated within health policy interventions that aim to secure better societal outcomes than those purely delivered by the free market.

The Limits to Growth

The consideration for social and human development put forward by Marshall, Pareto and Kuznets rely upon a set of common assumptions. They hinge on the continuous economic growth of a globalized system that disregards aspects such as the finite nature of many materials and environmental resources. In other words, even if the "inverted-U" theory of Kuznets were to reduce global inequality, continuing the growth in income per capita of all societies would at this point demand an ever-increasing consumption of natural resources that is neither compatible with the regenerative capacity of our planet, nor with the productive practices deemed as "economic" by our current economic system.

Because all decisions are taken in a context of limited resources, the Club of Rome, as early as the 1970s, commissioned a report that analyzed the so-called "limits to growth". Using computer simulations, the commissioned team warned about the risks of exponential economic and population growth within a finite supply of resources and proceeded to update the model at the 30- and 40-year marks. The authors increasingly attempted to call attention to the fact that policy action should be focused on reducing the risks that overshooting our planet's regenerative capacities could have not only in economic terms, but also in aspects important for the social determinants of health, such as global food and services per capita (Meadows et al., 1972).

Economic activities can have consequences that may be destructive and can negatively affect future life on our planet without fully being reflected in market prices. An example of such "externalities" is carbon dioxide emission to the atmosphere when driving a car. Although the driver may pay for the cost of extraction and transport of the oil at market prices, the environmental damage of the accumulated carbon dioxide is not fully considered when filling the tank at a gas station. Because of the invisible nature of air pollution, carbon-tax markets could appear as a pragmatic way of tackling these externalities via market prices – another example of "Pigouvian taxation".

Currently, the accumulation of negative externalities is regularly quantified by the Intergovernmental Panel on Climate Change (IPCC) across different environmental problems, such as ocean acidification, chemical pollution, loss of biological diversity and land conversion. Scientists currently agree on the risks of trespassing several "tipping points" of no return in the collective damage to fundamental ecosystems of the planet (Lenton et al., 2019). Although modern climate modelling is not fully conclusive as to where precisely the line for these tipping points should be drawn, scientific evidence is informing a civil society increasingly organized to address environmental impacts of human activity (WHO, 2017). Nowadays, there is increasing evidence suggesting that environmental depletion could be followed by a societal collapse (Cumming & Peterson, 2017). Despite that, some voices continue to relativize the importance of rapid policy action against the environmental disruption that human activity can generate on the planet, on the grounds that technological advancement will compensate for shortages of resources in the long term (Bendell, 2020).

Rising temperatures, climate change and environmental depletion are trends whose consequences can affect important dimensions of social determinants of health and generate global tensions. The impact by externalities such as carbon emission is felt the most in regions that contributed the least to cause it. As a result, these trends can further strengthen pre-existing health, social and economic inequalities. Because of the political nature of the policies required to address these environmental processes, countries most affected are poorly equipped to solve these globalized problems. This constitutes an example of a market failure: the externalities generated by consuming in rich countries are felt in a different part of the world without jurisdiction to impose any form of regulatory or Pigouvian taxation capable of correcting these inefficiencies.

The Doughnut Economics and the SDG Economic Agenda

The Sustainable Development Goals (SDGs) set by United Nations include 17 goals that range from economic aspects related to consumption and production, food security, and clean energy over social development, such as improving health and education, and reducing inequality to environmental goals that seek to protect different ecosystems from climate change. This last goal is especially remarkable. In neoclassical economics, ecological resources were mainly seen as raw materials for the production of goods to be sold in the market. Their preservation was not a goal by itself but, at best, a means to an economic end.

The need to take into account environmental impact on individual and societal well-being in policy decision-making motivated policy analysts and economists from Oxfam (Raworth, 2012) to generate frameworks that relate the impact of economic and social policies with the most pressing environmental challenges: the "Doughnut" of social and planetary boundaries (Figure 33.4).

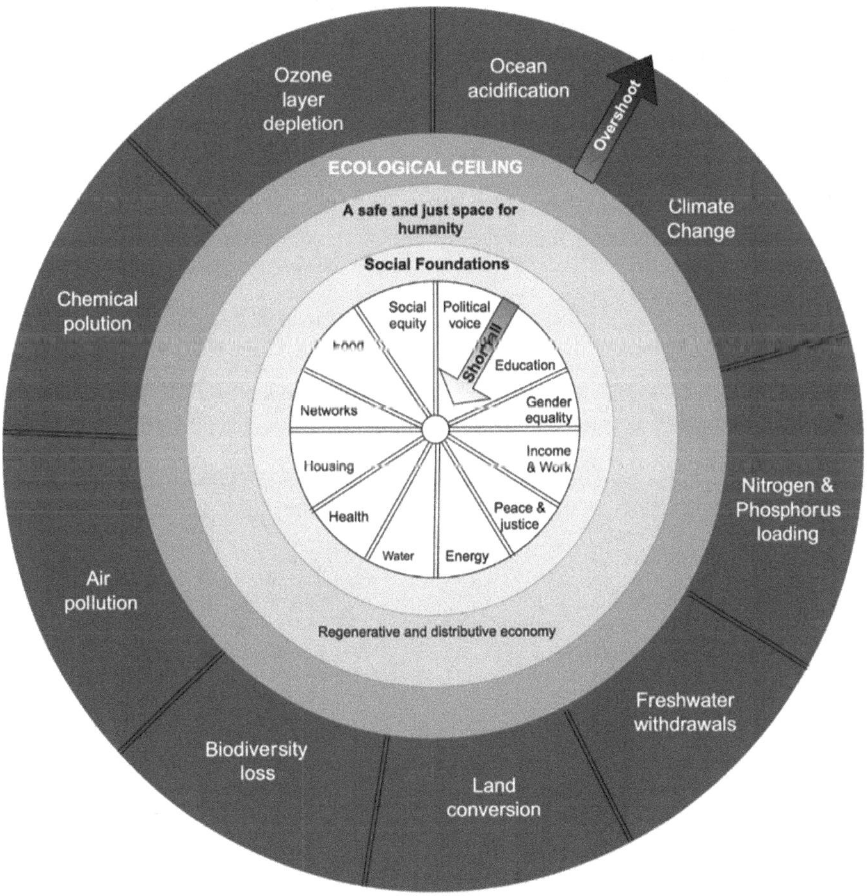

Figure 33.4 "Doughnut" of social and planetary boundaries

The internal ring of the framework establishes the societal goals necessary for obtaining acceptable living standards, derived from the SDGs. The external part of the ring represents the ecological ceiling determined by climate scientists. The middle section highlights the boundaries for human development while avoiding damaging critical environmental dimensions.

This framework has been well received by economists, governments and institutions alike, who use it for analyzing policy alternatives that seek to organize society beyond standard neoclassical economics (Figure 33.5). For example, it can be used to assess how far different countries come to achieving various SDGs at their current use of resources. Policy action according to this framework should focus on bringing countries to the quadrant "D", combining high levels of social development and respecting biophysical boundaries. Currently, the Netherlands announced their desire to work with this framework to redesign its economy (The Guardian, 2020).

The outlined framework forces an expansion of human welfare beyond the standard economic definition suggested by Marshall at the beginning of this chapter to include the normative considerations of well-being agreed by the broad majority of countries in the SDG agenda.

AN INTRODUCTION TO SOCIAL AND HEALTH POLICY FROM AN ECONOMICS PERSPECTIVE

Definition of Health from a Healthcare Perspective and its Relationship with Economic Policy

Different definitions can have implications in the way in which a policy is measured and generate tensions between competing interests

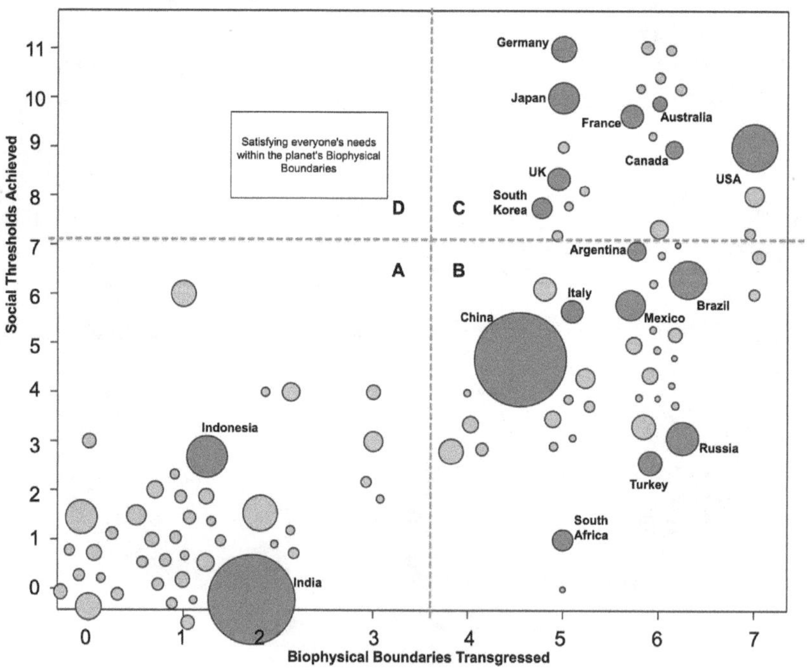

Figure 33.5 "Doughnut model" and policy alternatives

in health, social or economic policies. The Constitution of the World Health Organization (1946) asserts that health is "a state of complete physical, mental and social well-being and not merely the absence of disease or infirmity" and that "Governments have a responsibility for the health of their peoples which can be fulfilled only by the provision of adequate health and social measures". This is in fundamental tension with the economic definition of welfare. In economics, the individual perspective is preferred, while in health policy a societal perspective with a multidimensional assessment of individual and collective indicators, some of which are not material, is usually needed.

Furthermore, these tensions in the policy-design are also present between different areas of policy. As discussed in previous chapters of this volume, seeking to improve health-related indicators by building hospitals while disregarding access to infrastructure providing clean water can be considered not only ineffective but also wasteful. When discussing how to allocate a certain budget, epidemiological and setting-specific aspects and the wider social determinants of health should be weighted.

Moreover, it should be considered that improving the well-being of a society is not a goal attained linearly; the first dollar invested in health has a greater effect than the one millionth. As financial resources available on health policy are limited, the next section of this chapter will aim to provide a summary of the principles guiding the financing of healthcare and how aspects of budget allocation are currently analyzed to secure sustainability.

Financing Healthcare: What are Insurances and How are They Structured?

In healthcare, individuals suffer from significant uncertainty around their future need for services and the resulting costs. Financial protection is important as the top 5% of healthcare users accumulate 50% of the costs of healthcare (WHO, 2019), justifying the creation of health insurances to cover not only the costs of falling ill, but to help to reduce the associated individual uncertainty (Jack, 2002). The goal of generating a sustainable and better future for humanity has positioned not only universal health coverage (UHC) but also financial risk protection as targets 3.8 within the Sustainable Development Goal (SDG) agenda.

Because the likelihood of falling ill is not entirely random and can to a certain degree be predicted by social determinants of health, including income, there are two main pricing options around health insurance: prices can be determined on an individual or a societal basis. Individual determination of prices based on one's risk profiles comes with limitations. First, individuals know more than insurances about the expected true risk of falling ill (Ehrlich & Becker, 1972), meaning that those who are elderly and sick derive inherently more utility from being insured than those who are young and healthy (Einav & Finkelstein, 2018), generating information asymmetry that challenge market outcomes and trigger a debate on moral preferences (Rawls, 1971; see also Follesdal, 2014). Second, it means that smaller, more segmented insurance pools will have less contracting capacity to negotiate with providers for services and supplies, and this will have an impact on quality and efficiency (Layton, 2017; WHO, 2004). Third, because contracting insurance is sensitive to price (US Congressional Budget Office, 2005), those who are more likely to need insurance are at greater risk of not being able to afford it, generating issues of coverage and access due to high prices inhibiting access.

Societal determination of prices (Mossialos, 2002), a practice frequently found for publicly or governmentally regulated insurances, on the other hand, means that the prices are determined according to the overall healthcare need of a much larger risk pool with a more diverse risk profile.

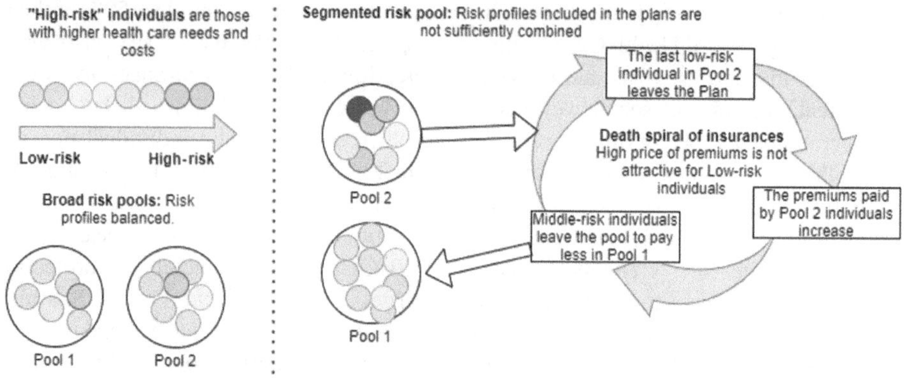

Figure 33.6 Risk pools: broad and segmented

This can prevent the "death spiral of insurances" (Cutler & Zeckhauser, 1998), often found in private insurance markets, where too many high-risk individuals are retained in an insurance company with constant price increases, which force those with less risk to opt-out (Figure 33.6).

Most of the public insurance programs in the European Union hence enforce mandatory contributions to health insurance by all citizens. This form of determining prices decouples the individual need for healthcare from premium prices (Busse et al., 2017), and can also act as a wealth transfer that tackles inequality by generating redistribution from healthy to sick, from young to old or from employed to unemployed (Mossialos, 2002). Moreover, insurance programs become actors in the provision of healthcare services with negotiating power to contain costs on pharmaceutical and medical products (Mossialos et al., 2004).

When deciding on the coverage of insurances, three dimensions need to be considered: who is covered (breadth), what is covered (depth), or to what extent are services covered and/or individual co-payments necessary (height) (Figure 33.7). This framework, known as the "Cube of coverage" helps to make explicit coverage decisions that depend to a large degree on political priorities. Low-income countries may struggle with issues of breadth of coverage while in high- or middle-income countries the height of services may be actively reduced to guide healthy behaviour (via increasing an individual's participation in paying for its consequences) and contain costs.

Limitations to Health Coverage: The Competing Interests for Resources

Given the dimensions of coverage and the assumptions that resources are limited, any services given to an individual covered by his/her health insurance means that alternative services to another individual may not be covered. As a result, any decision of coverage raises questions between competing interests among the beneficiaries of interventions. Coverage decisions – i.e., how to alter breadth, width and height of coverage – should therefore be systematically taken, considering the cost and benefits of different interventions for different groups and interventions (WHO, 2018b), allowing the weighing up of decisions objectively, transparently and explicitly.

Health Technology Assessment (HTA) agencies are governmental institutions that assess the available evidence on potential costs and benefits for specific interventions

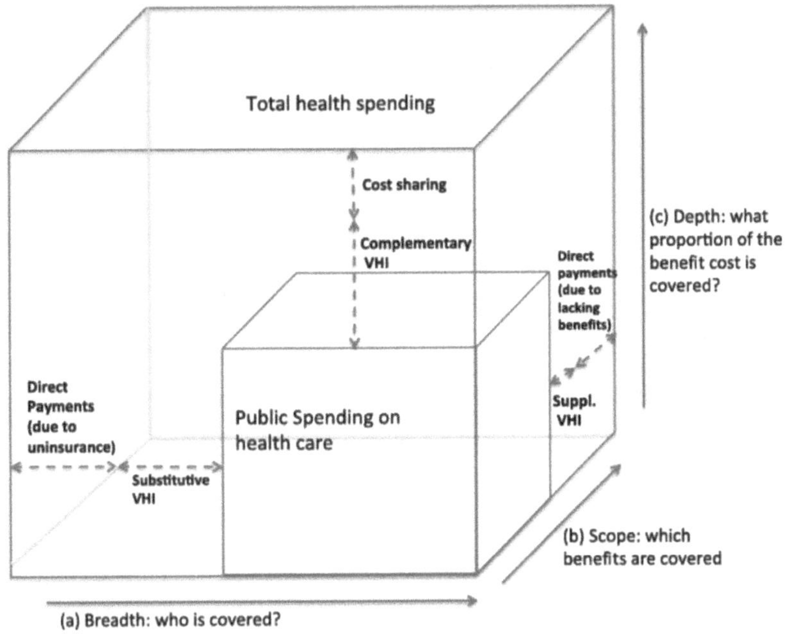

Figure 33.7 Three dimensions of universal coverage

Source Rice, T., Quentin, W., Anell, A. *et al.* Revisiting out-of-pocket requirements: trends in spending, financial access barriers, and policy in ten high-income countries. *BMC Health Serv Res* 18, 371 (2018). https://doi.org/10.1186/s12913-018-3185-8

https://bmchealthservres.biomedcentral.com/articles/10.1186/s12913-018-3185-8

to inform coverage decisions by insurances. First, available evidence has to be collected or commissioned via randomized trials to generate real-world data on the effectiveness and safety of a certain intervention. Then, available information has to be synthesized, for example in the form of meta-analysis or network meta-analysis in the case that more than two comparing interventions exist for treating the same condition (Roever & Biondi-Zoccai, 2016). The impact of these interventions can then be translated into monetary terms by studying the different levels of cost an actor is willing to pay provided the effects (effectiveness, benefit, utility, etc.) of a certain therapy has obtained (Drummond et al., 2002). Finally, these analyses should consider the long-term effects on patients over a longer horizon of time, which usually involve extrapolation models.

The involved analyses, and especially extrapolation via modelling, force many assumptions that increase the uncertainty around decisions. Hence, the robustness of any models should be appraised, for example via sensitivity analyses that assess how changes in a certain parameter would influence the whole model. Despite these known limitations, health technology assessments allow improving transparency in the decisions of coverage by explicitly informing on the variables that justify the coverage of a certain therapy.

Trends in Health Policy: Where Financing Healthcare Meets Epidemiology and Demographics

A Global Burden of Diseases study by Chang and colleagues (2019) modelled future expenditures on healthcare in 195 different countries, including governmental spending, out-of-pocket patient expenditure and development assistance for health (DAH). Based on this study, it can be expected that by 2050 DAH will constitute the main source of funding of healthcare for lower-income settings.

Importantly, in many high-income settings, high healthcare expenditures are not translated into proportionally longer life expectancy (Nixon & Ulmann, 2006), requiring further study and policy design around the role of expenditure and social determinants of health (WHO, 2011b).

One main conclusion of the GBD analysis was that to ensure or achieve universal health coverage (UHC), the most relevant factor is to increase government health expenditure globally, thus expanding the breadth of insurance coverage (Carapinha et al., 2011). The analysis further concluded that reducing the out-of-pocket expenditure in favour of governmental expenditure, especially in low- and middle-income settings, is necessary to sustainably improve health. Particularly, healthcare interventions that tackle Noncommunicable diseases (NCDs) are required in this setting. NCDs cause 70% of global deaths, 85% of which occur in low- and middle-income countries, remaining the most common cause of death worldwide (WHO, 2018c). In low- and middle-income countries, even a moderate increase in investment in healthcare could yield significant results to reduce NCD. Other authors have additionally highlighted the importance of providing not only financial means for health, but the required infrastructure for healthcare (Falchetta et al., 2020).

CONCLUSION

The tension between the concepts of well-being and economic welfare forced by economic and health policy agendas is likely to worsen as ecological resources dwindle. Understanding the trade-offs in policy design and improving the assessment of progress using new economic frameworks is fundamental in maintaining health policy aspects aligned with the purposes of sustainability laid out by the SDG.

REFERENCES

Bendell, J., 2020. *The Collapse of Ideology and the End of Escape*. https://jembendell.com/2020/06/28/the-collapse-of-ideology-and-the-end-of-escape/ (accessed 3.3.21).

Busse, R., Blümel, M., Knieps, F., & Bärnighausen, T., 2017. Statutory health insurance in Germany: a health system shaped by 135 years of solidarity, self-governance, and competition. *The Lancet* 390, 882–897. https://doi.org/10.1016/S0140-6736(17)31280-1

Carapinha, J.L., Ross-Degnan, D., Desta, A.T., & Wagner, A.K., 2011. Health insurance systems in five sub-Saharan African countries: medicine benefits and data for decision making. *Health Policy* 99, 193–202. https://doi.org/10.1016/j.healthpol.2010.11.009

Chang, A.L, Cowling, K., Micah, A.E., & the Global Burden of Disease Health Financing Collaborator Network, 2019. Past, present, and future of global health financing: a review of development assistance, government, out-of-pocket, and other private spending on health for 195 countries, 1995–2050. *The Lancet* 393, 2233–2260. https://doi.org/10.1016/S0140-6736(19)30841-4

Cumming, G.S., & Peterson, G.D., 2017. Unifying research on social–ecological resilience and collapse. *Trends in Ecology & Evolution* 32, 695–713. https://doi.org/10.1016/j.tree.2017.06.014

Cutler, D.M., & Zeckhauser, R.J., 1998. *Adverse Selection in Health Insurance (No. c9822)*. Cambridge, MA: National Bureau of Economic Research.

Drummond, M., Sculpher, M., Torrance, G., O'Brien, B., & Stoddart, G., 2002. *Methods for the Economic Evaluation of Health Care Programmes*. Oxford: Oxford Medical Publications.

Ehrlich, I., & Becker, G.S., 1972. Market Insurance, self-insurance, and self-protection. *Journal of Political Economy* 80, 623–648. https://doi.org/10.1086/259916

Einav, L., & Finkelstein, A., 2018. Moral hazard in health insurance: what we know and how we know it. *Journal of the European Economic Association* 16, 957–982. https://doi.org/10.1093/jeea/jvy017

Falchetta, G., Hammad, A.T., & Shayegh, S., 2020. Planning universal accessibility to public health care in sub-Saharan Africa. *Proceedings of the National Academy of Science* 117, 31760–31769. https://doi.org/10.1073/pnas.2009172117

Foreign Affairs, 1937. Review: *Politics: Who Gets What, When, How*, by H.D. Lasswell (1936). *Foreign Affairs* January. [WWW document], www.foreignaffairs.com/reviews/capsule-review/1937-01-01/politics-who-gets-what-when-how (accessed 2.3.21).

GBD, 2019. *Lancet* https://www.thelancet.com/journals/lancet/article/PIIS0140-6736(19)30841-4/fulltext

Jack, W., 2002. Public intervention in health insurance markets: theory and four examples from Latin America. *World Bank Research Observer* 17, 67–88.

Kuznets, S., 1955. Economic growth and income inequality. *American Economic Review* 45, 1–28.

Lasswell, H.D., 1936. *Politics: Who Gets What, When, How*. New York: Whittlesey House.

Layton, T., Ellis, R.P., McGuire, T.G., & van Kleef, R. 2017. Measuring efficiency of health plan payment systems in managed competition health insurance markets. *Journal of Health Economics* 56, 237–255. https://10.1016/j.jhealeco.2017.05.004. [WWW document], www.ncbi.nlm.nih.gov/pmc/articles/PMC5737816/ (accessed 3.7.21).

Lenton, T.M., Rockström, J., Gaffney, O., Rahmstorf, S., Richardson, K., Steffen, W., & Schellnhuber, H.J., 2019. Climate tipping points – too risky to bet against. *Nature* 575, 592–595. https://doi.org/10.1038/d41586-019-03595-0

Lux, M., 2003. Efficiency and effectiveness of housing policies in the Central and Eastern Europe countries. *European Journal of Housing Policy* 3, 243–265. https://doi.org/10.1080/14616710310001603712

Marshall, A. (1890) *Principles of Economics* – great mind series. Prometheus books.

Meadows, D.H., Meadows, D.L., Randers, J., & Behrens, W.W.W. III. (1972). *The Limits to Growth: A Report for the Club of Rome's Project on the Predicament of Mankind*. Washington, DC: Potomac Associates. [WWW document], https://link.springer.com/article/10.2307/2060819 (accessed 3.3.21).

Mossialos, E. (Ed.), 2002. *Funding Health Care: Options for Europe*. European Observatory on Health Care Systems series. Buckingham, UK & Philadelphia, PA: Open University Press.

Mossialos, E., Mrazek, M., & Walley, T., 2004. *Regulating Pharmaceuticals in Europe: Striving for Efficiency, Equity and Quality*. European Observatory on Health Care Systems series. Buckingham, UK & Philadelphia, PA: Open University Press. [WWW document], www.euro.who.int/en/publications/abstracts/regulating-pharmaceuticals-in-europe-striving-for-efficiency,-equity-and-quality-2004 (accessed 3.7.21).

Nixon, J., & Ulmann, P., 2006. The relationship between health care expenditure and health outcomes. *European Journal of Health Economics* 7, 7–18. https://doi.org/10.1007/s10198-005-0336-8

Pareto, 1906. *Manual of political economy*. The economic equilibrium, 326–345. Oxford: Oxford university press.

Pigou A., 1932. *The Economics of Welfare* (4th edition). London: Macmillan. Available at the Online Library of Liberty [WWW document], https://oll.libertyfund.org/title/pigou-the-economics-of-welfare (accessed 2.3.21).

Piketty, T., 2014. *Capital in the Twenty-First Century*. Cambridge, MA: Harvard University Press.

Rawls, J., 1971. *A Theory of Justice*. Cambridge, 83. Oxford: Oxford university press.

Raworth, K., 2012. *A Safe and Just Space for Humanity: Can We Live within the Doughnut?* [pdf]. https://doi.org/10.1163/2210-7975_hrd-9824-0069

Roever, L., & Biondi-Zoccai, G., 2016. Network meta-analysis to synthesize evidence for decision making in cardiovascular research. *Arquivos Brasileiros de Cardiologia* 106(4), 333–337. https://doi.org/10.5935/abc.20160052

Rudra, N., 2008. *Globalization and the Race to the Bottom in Developing Countries: Who Really Gets Hurt?* Cambridge, UK: Cambridge University Press. https://doi.org/10.1017/CBO9780511491870

The Guardian, 2020. Amsterdam to embrace "doughnut" model to mend post-coronavirus economy. *The Guardian*, April 8. [WWW document]. www.theguardian.com/world/2020/apr/08/amsterdam-doughnut-model-mend-post-coronavirus-economy (accessed 3.3.21).

US Congressional Budget Office, 2005. *Background Paper: The Price Sensitivity of Demand for Nongroup Health Insurance*. [WWW document], www.cbo.gov/publication/17110 (accessed 3.7.21).

WHO, n.d.a. *Health Technology Assessment*. Geneva: World Health Organization. [WWW document], /www.who.int/medical_devices/assessment/en/ (accessed 2.7.21).

WHO, n.d.b. *The Determinants of Health Expenditure*. Geneva: World Health Organization. [WWW document], www.who.int/health_financing/documents/cov-report_e_11-deter-he/en/ (accessed 3.4.21).

WHO, 1946. *Constitution*. Geneva: World Health Organization. [WWW document], www.who.int/about/who-we-are/constitution (accessed 2.7.21).

WHO, 2004. *What are the equity, efficiency, cost containment and choice implications of private health-care funding in western Europe? July*. Copenhagen: WHO Regional Office for Europe. [WWW document], www.euro.who.int/__data/assets/pdf_file/0003/74694/E83334.pdf (accessed 2.7.21).

WHO, 2017. *Global Climate and Health Alliance*. Geneva: World Health Organization. https://climateandhealthalliance.org/workinggroup/

WHO, 2018a. *Health Inequities and Their Causes*. Geneva: World Health Organization. [WWW document], www.who.int/news-room/facts-in-pictures/detail/health-inequities-and-their-causes (accessed 3.2.21).

WHO, 2018b. *Universal Coverage – Three Dimensions*. Geneva: World Health Organization. [WWW document], www.who.int/health_financing/strategy/dimensions/en/ (accessed 2.7.21).

World Health Organization, 2018c. *Noncommunicable Diseases*. [WWW document], www.who.int/news-room/fact-sheets/detail/noncommunicable-diseases (accessed 3.4.21).

WHO, 2019. *Global Spending on Health: Weathering the Storm*. Geneva: World Health Organization. [WWW document], www.who.int/publications/i/item/9789240017788 (accessed 3.3.21).

World Bank, 2020. *The World Bank in China*. Washington, DC: The World Bank. [WWW document], www.worldbank.org/en/country/china/overview (accessed 3.15.21).

World Inequality Report, 2018. [WWW document], https://wir2018.wid.world/part-4.html (accessed 3.17.21).

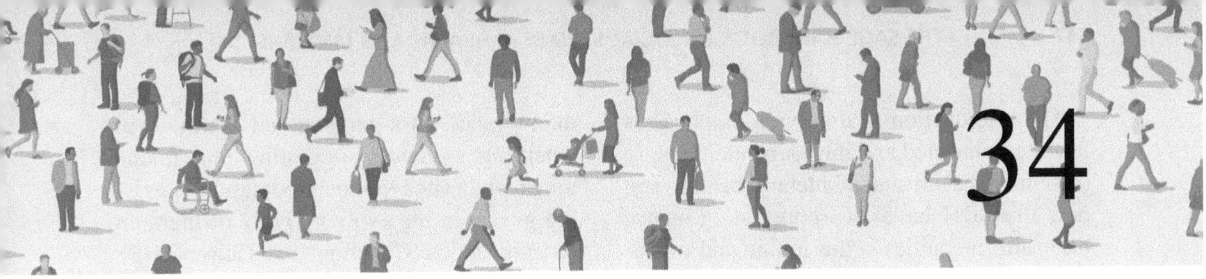

The Social Determinants of Lifelong Learning

Julian Fisher, Patricia Cuff, Ian Couper, Klaus von Pressentin, Roger Strasser, Lionel Green-Thompson and Aparna Roy

> There is no end to education. It is not that you read a book, pass an examination, and finish with education. The whole of life, from the moment you are born to the moment you die, is a process of learning. (Jiddu Krishnamurti)

INTRODUCTION: LOOKING BACK TO MOVE FORWARD

This chapter was written in the midst of the COVID-19 pandemic, which began in early 2020. The pandemic is likely to have profound and far-reaching social, cultural, economic and political consequences, particularly for children and young adults whose education and learning opportunities have been disproportionately impacted by the social measures to control the spread of the virus. It has yet again exposed well-documented and long-standing inequalities in and among countries (The Lancet Public Health 2021).

Countries and their health systems are facing an ever-increasing number of highly complex challenges ranging from protracted system stressors, such as the crippling social and economic burden of non-communicable diseases, and the impact of environmental pollution, climate change, and unsustainable lifestyles. The authors draw attention to a key theme running through many chapters of this *Handbook* which revolves around the social determinants of health. The World Health Organization (WHO) describes the social determinants of health (SDH) as "the non-medical factors that influence health outcomes." They are the conditions in which "people are born, grow, work, live, and age, and the wider set of forces and systems shaping the conditions of daily life. These forces and systems include economic policies and systems, development agendas, social norms, social policies and political systems" (World Health Organization n.d.).

Substitute education for health in the paragraph above, and the same could equally apply to education outcomes and lifelong learning opportunities.

The introduction to this book emphasizes the interconnected and interdependent nature of human health and planetary health, and how the SDH have an important influence on health inequities – the unfair and avoidable differences in health status seen within and between countries. For example, a robust and sustainable water supply is intimately linked with food security, productive capacity, and livelihood stability. Water beyond the household is essential for ecological system sustainability, which in turn provides input for the production system that ultimately maintains livelihoods (United Nations Environment Programme 2021; World Health Organization n.d.). It reinforces how measuring and understanding the social determinants of health, one of the three overarching recommendations of the Commission on Social Determinants of Health, will require a multisectoral approach, one that takes into account ideas such as planetary health and its emerging evidence base (Whitmee et al. 2015). Other chapters in this volume support this broader framing of health, including the growing understanding of genetic risk, gene expression, and epigenetic changes (see Chapter 11 in this volume by Zhang et al. *Historical Trauma and Epigenetics*) and historical trauma as a continuum of multi-, inter-, and intra-generational harm, with emerging evidence suggesting that trauma may be inherited via the modulation of existing genes, in the evolving body of literature on epigenetics (Conching and Thayer 2019).

The idea of looking back to look forward seeks to recognize the multi-generational aspect of historical trauma and the legacy of discrimination inequities, as well as the damage to the integrity of natural systems during the Anthropocene Epoch and resulting ecological stress memory. These form part of the lives and living experiences of people and communities, which are in turn influenced by the prevailing social determinants of health and lifelong learning. These historical and actual determinants are accumulative with health, social and economic consequences over an individuals lifecourse.

Lifelong learning is based on integrating learning and life. It is a continually evolving concept with new thinking around lifelong learning moving beyond school- or college-university-based education, and is catalyzing policies and strategies that are advocating and advancing lifelong learning as the conceptual framework and organizing principle for education reforms in the 21st century. This is particularly relevant in addressing complex challenges such as climate change,

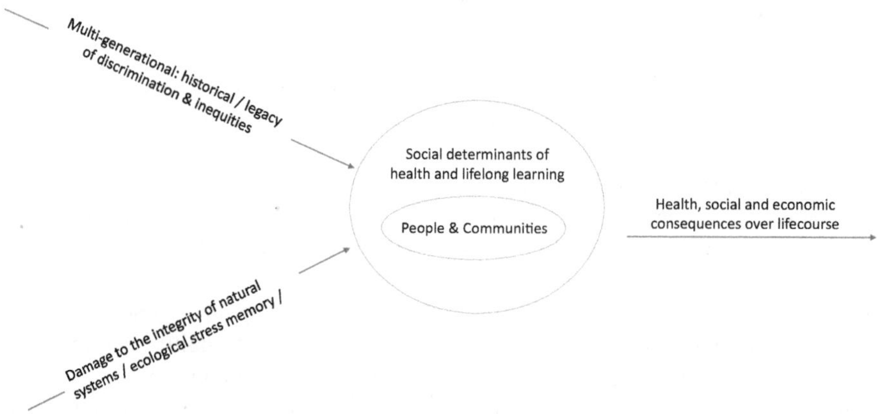

Figure 34.1 The social determinants of health and lifelong learning; the multi-generational aspects of historical trauma and ecological stress memory

which will require all learners to 'learn to transform'.

Lifelong learning with respect to health workforce education is often referred to as the learning that takes place after graduation from pre-service health workforce education, and is synonymous with continuing education (CE), continuing professional development (CPD) and in-service education in the health sector. This chapter explores how health workforce educators have grappled with how to express the key concept that all health professionals, students, and trainees are "learners" when it comes to the social determinants of health. The notion that even veteran educators could be learners was difficult to externalize.

New thinking across the health and education sectors around lifelong learning can help pivot health workforce education and training towards promoting health equity through action on the social determinants of health. Similarly, the WHO conceptual framework on the social determinants of health can help inform education curricula and lifelong learning opportunites in schools and adult learning.

This collaborative approach can support wider application and implementation of social accountability across the health and education sectors to achieve greater health and education equity for the population that these sectors have a mandate to serve.

THE EDUCATION AND HEALTH NEXUS

Nexus, a connection or series of connections linking two or more things.

Historically there has always been a strong link between health and education sectors, particularly at the community level where health workers and teachers often move between education and health facilities as they carry out their daily work. While there is close cooperation and collaboration between individuals at a grass-roots level, adoption of these ways of working across systems is very often constrained by entrenched institutional and sectoral boundaries. These boundaries have fostered the rise in sector-specific terminology, which can lead to gaps in understanding within and between government ministries. These barriers hamper successful analysis and negotiation for intersectoral policy and programming at the national level, which in turn can lead to poor implementation and reinforce siloed interventions at local administrative levels, as well as limiting closer working relationships between health workers and teachers in schools and communities.

A series of major global reports examining health professionals and health workforce education have consistently stressed the need to orient the health workforce "towards the social determinants of health, health promotion, disease prevention, primary care and people-centred, community services" (World Health Organization 2016b, 31). While education is noted as a social determinant of health in the conceptual framework of the WHO Commission on Social Determinants of Health, this framing constrains opportunities for synergistic action to address inequities more broadly as set out in the UN 2030 Agenda for Sustainable Development and the 17 Sustainable Development Goals (SDGs). The report of the WHO Commission, *Closing the Gap in a Generation*, provided the WHO definition of SDH and support for the WHO conceptual framework for action on SDH (World Health Organization 2008). It rightly poses the question: is it sufficient to treat people's illnesses, without changing the conditions that made them sick in the first place?, However, the question raises a more fundamental question: is it sufficient to educate and train health workers to treat people's illnesses, without educating and training them to change the conditions that make people sick in the first place? These questions challenge us to consider complex global issues such as climate change as falling within the social determinants of health i.e., the conditions in people are born, grow, work, live, and age.

Beyond health workforce education and training, these questions also have implications for: health financing and the recruitment, development, training and retention of the health workforce, and how health workers acquire knowledge and skills needed to promote sustainable development, including among others through education for sustainable development and sustainable lifestyles, human rights, gender equality, promotion of a culture of peace and non-violence, global citizenship, and appreciation of cultural diversity and of culture's contribution to sustainable development (UNESCO 2020).

Understanding the nexus of health and education could provide an opportunity to adopt common guiding and organizational principles for health and education that can be applied in a consistent and reinforcing manner in all settings. As noted above, the principles and rationale underpinning the WHO conceptual framework for action on the social determinants of health could equally be applied to social determinants of lifelong learning. The structural determinants of education and lifelong learning opportunities are the same as those for structural determinants of health. The ideas of differential exposure and vulnerability, as well as outcomes and consequences – intermediary determinants – have parallels in education and lifelong learning. Other ideas around the social gradient and social cohesion are well documented in education literature, but are published in education sector journals and use sector-specific terminology.

Education and lifelong learning opportunities are critical to enabling people to be and keep healthy, and actively participate in changing the conditions and circumstances that impact their daily lives, including "learning by doing" (Leicht, Heiss, and Byun 2018). This is central to the thinking underpinning the development and articulation of sustainable development goal (SDG) 4 on Education, namely "Ensure inclusive and equitable quality education and promote lifelong learning opportunities for all." The UN political declaration underpinning the 2030 Agenda and its five overarching themes emphasizes the need for "learning to transform" at all levels, sites and settings, and across all of government and all of society. Translating the idea of "learning to transform" into curricula will be key to addressing complex global challenges. The political will, and commitment to do so, is emerging. SDG target 4.7 calls for all learners to acquire the knowledge and skills needed to promote sustainable development, including among others through education for sustainable development (ESD) and a global citizenship education (GCE). ESD and GCE are viewed as key to addressing complex global challenges such as climate change. They are lifelong learning processes that require opportunities to gain knowledge and skills, as learners move from informative to formative through to transformative learning (Bhutta et al. 2010).

The Berlin Declaration on Education for Sustainable Development (2021) was signed by participants from governments, international, intergovernmental and nongovernmental organizations, civil society, youth, the academic community, the business sector and all spheres of teaching and learning. It notes that "urgent action is needed to address the dramatic interrelated challenges the world is facing, in particular, the climate crisis, mass loss of biodiversity, pollution, pandemic diseases, extreme poverty and inequalities, violent conflicts, and other environmental, social and economic crises that endanger life on our planet". Education systems and national education policies and curricula that are sensitive to mainstreaming an understanding and knowledge of ESD and GCE, and nurture the ability to think and act multi-sectorally, could make a fundamental contribution to transformative education across schooling, tertiary and university education, and technical and vocational training levels. Strengthening collaboration and coordination between education and health systems will be critical in tackling climate change over the long term.

CASE STUDY CLIMATE CHANGE AND WATER

> The risks and impacts of climate change, as well as the capacity to respond to it, vary considerably among countries. The baseline health status of a country, or a community, is the single largest determinant of the likely impact of climate change and the cost of adapting to it. (World Bank 2010)

The exacerbating effects of climate change manifest in multifold ways and affect various systems. Water is no exception to this, with water supply ecosystems being the primary medium which serve as an indicator of climate change. With the impact of climate change on water supply, protracting, irreversible, and highly unstable effects have emerged. The availability of water is becoming less predictable with the frequent occurrences of floods, which destroy sanitation facilities, contaminate water sources and destroy useful water points. Extreme and increasingly unpredictable weather conditions and high temperatures affect the distribution of groundwater, river flows, rainfall, and snowmelt, with the further deterioration of water quality. Increasing droughts as a result of climate change will also necessitate increased demand for water for agriculture, and other purposes, while rising sea levels will demand appropriate infrastructure to ensure resilience of coastal communities.

The Indian subcontinent is on the brink of an extreme water crisis as the country supports 17% of the world's populations and only 4% of its freshwater (Arcanjo 2019). Demand has continued to increase, accompanied by a steady decrease in supply due to temperature fluctuations and dryness. Therefore, the per capita availability has fallen by 70% (presently below 1,500 cubic meters) since 1950, officially making India a water-stressed country, by definition (GIZ 2021). Within the Indian context the implication of climate change has led to several direct and indirect effects on water supply. According to the Global Climate Index, India occupies the sixth position, indicating how vastly it is affected by climate change (Eckstein, Künzel, and Schäfer 2017). Also, according to India's Composite Water Management Index (GIZ 2021), around 600 million people are suffering from an acute water shortage in the country. This has resulted in severe social and economic issues, with vast populations unable to survive with low adaptive capacities, quickly disappearing water resources, unsustainable water management, and large-scale wetland degradation. The changing rainfall patterns has led to surface water deterioration, thereby increasing dependency on groundwater. Furthermore, the Sabarmati and Luni basins, which comprise a vital part of water supply to a large part of the country, have been experiencing water withdrawal of over 60% of potentially utilizable resources. This will make extraction of water more difficult, thus rendering these basins as economically scarce, with implications in the food, livelihoods, income, social and political spheres.

As the challenges of climate change and water scarcity illustrate, the conditions in which people are born, grow, work, live, and age will impact health and learning. The wider set of forces and systems shaping the conditions of daily life will shape people's education and learning opportunities, and health throughout the life course.

THE SOCIAL DETERMINANTS OF LEARNING

> Inclusion and education: All Means All. (UNESCO 2020)

Lifelong learning is based on integrating learning and life. It includes learning activities for people of every age, in all contexts (family, school, community, workplace, etc.)

and using different modalities (formal, non-formal and informal education), which together respond to a wide range of learning-related needs and demands. This new thinking around lifelong learning moves beyond school- or college-based education, and is catalyzing policies and strategies that are advocating and advancing lifelong learning as the conceptual framework and organizing principle for education reforms in the 21st century. Equity in education and learning is the extent to which access and opportunities for children and adults are just and fair. This implies a reduction of disparities based on gender, poverty, residence, ethnicity, language, and other characteristics (UNESCO 2008).

The conventional pipeline model presents health workforce education as a linear and stepwise sequence (i.e., from primary to tertiary education). A more integrated and networked lifelong learning system model frames health workforce development as a progressive and inclusive effort. It extends and expands the pool of people able to enter the health workforce, by supporting inclusive and equitable education and learning opportunities to children, youth and adults (Figure 34.2). This new model could help challenge conventional thinking around health workers and community relationships and working spaces, and shape social dialogue for lifelong learning.

What do we mean by lifelong learning in health workforce education and training? In moving forward, it is important to consider the origin of words and how the meaning of words gives form and function to practice.

Lifelong learning with respect to health workforce education is often referred to as the learning that takes place after graduation from pre-service health workforce education,

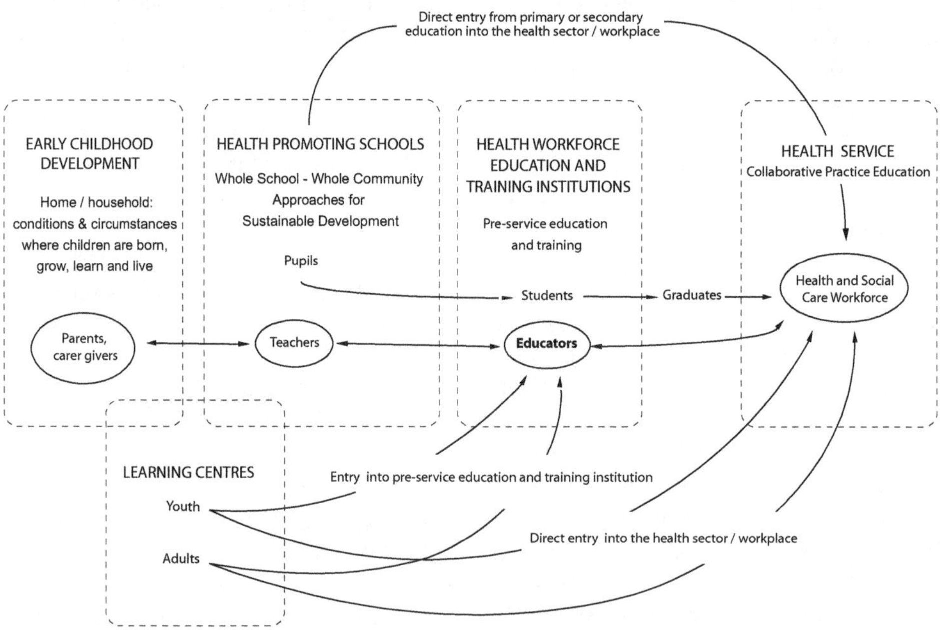

Figure 34.2 Integrated and networked lifelong learning systems model for the production and development of a health workforce (WHO 2021)

Adapted from Chapter 3. The production and development of a health workforce in support of Universal Health Coverage. J Fisher et al. in the Handbook for strengthening the collection, analysis and use of health workforce data and evidence: guidance for countries (forthcoming Nov 2021) World Health Organization, Geneva, Switzerland.

and is synonymous with continuing education (CE), continuing professional development (CPD) and in-service education in the health sector. This compartmentalization has significant implications for the quality and relevance of health workforce education throughout a health worker's professional working life.

Mandatory CE and CPD are developed and delivered by a wide variety of providers, and are to a large extent driven by regulatory bodies that almost exclusively focus on the number of hours spent doing an educational activity. Increasingly, there are moves to align mandatory CE and CPD with core clinical competencies within occupation groups, but at a national level there is little alignment with the evolving health needs of the populations or consideration given to interprofessional education for collaborative practice. The regulatory system itself is not comprehensive or inclusive, with many cadres of health worker, for example community health workers, not covered. This leads to siloed approaches, fragmentation of CE and CPD activities across occupations, and a learning environment that restricts interprofessional learning opportunities. This in turn leads to a situation where agencies have focused attention on subjects considered relevant to health service delivery and provision of care provided by a specific occupation, and with a focus on provision of care to patients, rather than mutual collaboration and learning with, in and from communities. This situation is frequently compounded by inequities in respect of the degree of out-of-pocket expenses borne by participants and time allowed away from the workplace to participate in learning.

In order for the system to change, national education plans for the health and social care workforce, including pre-service education and training curricula, continuing professional development (CPD), continuing education (CE) and in-service training should be aligned with national health plans. For example, recent work on lifelong learning systems could support health services to become providers of health workforce education (Fisher, Holmes, and Chakroun 2017). Generally, health service providers have access to a broader range of data on health needs and concerns of communities, including the social determinants of health, than pre-service health workforce education institutions. Interprofessional education for collaborative practice is well established in pre-service education but is less well applied in health services and the workplace. Health service providers are potentially able to develop education and training through real-world and data-driven processes, which could better respond to evolving community health needs and concerns. The learning could be tailored to health workforce teams at specific sites and settings based on information from health workforce information systems. Its delivery could benefit from existing health information systems to provide a variety of formal, informal and non-formal learning across a range of platforms and channels. Collaborative Practice (CPE) recognizes the goal of inclusive and equitable quality education and promoting lifelong learning opportunities for all (SDG4) and supports learning with and from communities and other sectors to address the social determinants of health.

The current framing of lifelong learning in health workforce education limits its role, utility, and relevance in helping health systems to evolve and address the complex health and development challenges of the 21st century. This includes the knowledge and skills needed to promote sustainable development, including through education for sustainable development and sustainable lifestyles, human rights, gender equality, promotion of a culture of peace and nonviolence, global citizenship and appreciation of cultural diversity and of culture's contribution to sustainable development.

Action on the social determinants of lifelong learning seeks to engage the education sector in health workforce education, and vice versa health workers in education systems.

At the same time, it helps guide and inform joint SDG 3–SDG 4 decision-making to create an enabling environment for action on the social determinants of health and lifelong learning in communities and schools. An example of the co-benefits of such an approach would be addressing the commercial determinants of health and of lifelong learning in a consistent manner. While the authorship of health journal articles and books may be inclusive, cost to the reader/learner in accessing journals and technical books are often prohibitive, particularly for health workforce education institutions in many low- and middle-income countries which may not be party to university libraries agreements. These barriers impact not only lifelong learning opportunities, but also potentially the quality of care. The social determinants of learning are perpetuated and reinforced, in the same way as structural inequities of health, as highlighted in other chapters in this volume.

The next section explores how lifelong learning can help pivot health workforce education and training towards promoting health equity through action on the social determinants of health. The final section examines how lifelong learning systems can enable social accountability to achieve greater health equity for the population that the schools have a mandate to serve.

LEARNING WITH AND FROM OTHERS

> We now accept the fact that learning is a lifelong process of keeping abreast of change. And the most pressing task is to teach people how to learn. (Peter Drucker)

Society's interaction with, and understanding of, the social determinants is constantly evolving. It is the responsibility of educators in the health professions to stay abreast of the newest research and thinking on the topic so they can help guide learners and seasoned health professionals on their roles in addressing underlying causes of disease (i.e., the social determinants of health). The purpose of this section of the chapter is to reflect on new thinking around lifelong learning, and how this could enable institutional and instructional reforms as called for by global health workforce strategies and action plans (World Health Organization 2016a, 2018).

In 2015, the then Institute of Medicine (NASEM) in the US convened a diverse committee of experts to develop a framework for educating health professionals to address the social determinants of health (National Academies of Sciences 2016). While all of the issues written into the committee's framework are still relevant today (see Figure 34.3), reflections on the framework in 2020 revealed gaps, some of which were realized due to the coronavirus pandemic and its spotlight on racial disparities and inequities in the US and around the world.

Background

In developing the framework, NASEM committee members grappled extensively with how to express the key concept that all health professionals, students, and trainees are "learners" when it comes to the social determinants. The notion that even veteran educators could be learners was difficult to externalize. That is, until lifelong learning (LLL) was proposed. LLL was quickly adopted as a central theme to their work and a focal point of the framework. With this concept, health professionals would gain a deeper understanding of the SDH as they progress through education and careers in alignment with those in and out of the health sector, and in respectful partnership with communities. Figure 34.3 shows how all these various aspects interact in the committee's framework.

The framework, comprised of three fluid domains (education, community, and organization) and nine components, is underpinned by not only dynamic partnerships and lifelong

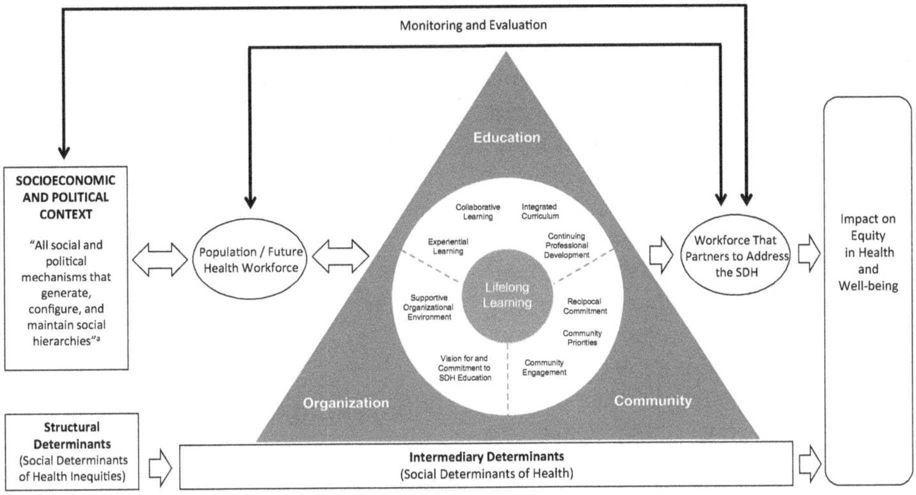

Figure 34.3 Conceptual model for strengthening health professional education in the social determinants of health. (National Academies of Sciences, Engineering, and Medicine. 2016. A framework for educating health professionals to address the social determinants of health. Washington, DC: The National Academies Press. doi: 10.17226/21923.)

learning, but also transformative learning. A goal of transformative learning is the creation of innovative and adaptive change agents who internalize the need to be responsive to the needs of communities. In the end, SDH education is about connecting with community members in a sort of role reversal where the community educates providers and health professions educators on what they need to better serve the community. It is through a trusted relationship that community members educate and providers gain a greater understanding of the social determinants of health.

Applying the Framework – Active Learning

The first recommendation by the NASEM committee was to "use the framework presented in this report as a guide for creating lifelong learners who appreciate the value of relationships and collaborations for understanding and addressing community-identified needs and for strengthening community assets." As the report acknowledges, such education comes with challenges.

Implementing the framework can be time-consuming and labor-intensive for faculty, and given the lack of financial resources, community-engaged learning can also be difficult to initiate and sustain. Even after great efforts are made to offer transformative, community-engaged learning opportunities, some learners will continue to push for a traditional, lecture-only format. This was also a finding from Lane et al. (2018), who described their experiences at Syracuse University in applying the NASEM framework to a course on reproductive health and a course on global health. Considerable time was spent by the main instructor working with learners outside of the classroom, in some instances, more than 10 hours for one student. But despite the intense faculty effort, there were still a small number of learners who desired a more passive education.

Resistance to active learning is not an uncommon phenomenon. In studying active versus passive learning Deslaurier et al. (2019) found a negative correlation between learners' perceptions of learning through active techniques and their actual learning, meaning students learned more with active learning techniques but felt like they learned less. The authors described how being forced to struggle through a difficult educational task can be frustrating for learners as they become aware of their lack of understanding of an issue. This intensified effort is what leads to deeper cognitive processing and understanding compared to lectures that risk confirming an inflated self-perception of one's abilities. This concept supports other study findings where learners overwhelmingly felt the active learning in courses provoked thought and stimulated critical thinking (Lane et al. 2018; Lane et al. 2019).

Applying the Framework – Community Engagement

Possibly the most critical aspect of the framework to the NASEM committee was engagement of the community in a respectful manner. Several chapters in this volume emphasize the critical importance of community-engaged and community-based education, which is examined in detail in the final section of this chapter on social accountability. When community members are the teachers, learners gain a much deeper appreciation for the multi-generational struggles of those impacted by the social determinants. Malotky et al. (2020) further commented that community-centered projects offer learners an opportunity to reflect upon broader economic, social, and political influences that affect daily life – both negatively and positively (Malotky et al. 2020). The NASEM report emphasized how working with communities must be "reciprocal" to avoid even the appearance of volunteer tourism. With that as a foundation, community engagement goes beyond student understanding and appreciation, to actually benefitting the community. During times of "community distrust and turmoil," the report notes, "creating strong partnerships that demonstrate support over time could help ease tensions within communities." It can also create pathways for community members to enter the health professions, facilitate a more aware health workforce attuned to the needs of the community they serve, and create a keener recognition of the importance of cooperation and coordination within the health professions and across sectors.

Addressing Gaps

After releasing the framework in 2016, it became clear that while the report is comprehensive, there were areas that could have been more deliberately emphasized. One glaring gap is mental health. The report does mention mental and physical impacts of racism and inadequate or unsafe living conditions, but fails to explore the psychological ramifications of these exposures in any depth. This is what Shim and Compton (2018) called the social determinants of mental health (SDMH). Just as with SDH, SDMH prioritizes a focus on the underlying causes of psychological distress in affected individuals and communities. Shim and Compton listed multiple factors – income inequality, adverse early life experiences, food insecurity, and racism – that when taken together, create the perfect conditions for major depression and post-traumatic stress. Exposure to such conditions can also lead to other forms of depression, anxiety, and substance use as a coping mechanism.

Care providers and learners working with individuals and communities affected by the social determinants are not immune to the mental health challenges associated with their work, particularly if a provider over-identifies with the people they are serving. While this was not mentioned in the report, it is an important point to highlight. The condition has been referred to by Katsantoni et al. (2019) as compassion fatigue, secondary trauma, or vicarious traumatization, all basically describing the "cost of caring." A result of compassion fatigue for educators or any health care worker is a disassociation from the people they are trying to help, and diminished joy in their work that can be outwardly exhibited as a lack of empathy, emotional distancing, defensiveness or even displays of anger. Burnout is another risk that deserves mentioning. Unlike compassion fatigue that results from the stress of working with traumatized individuals and communities, burnout is more about the long-term effects of being exposed to emotionally draining situations. Educators working with learners on community-engaged initiatives addressing social determinants will need to be acutely aware of their own personal and environmental circumstances or risk experiencing the adverse effects of compassion fatigue and burnout.

Future Exploration

Another important component of LLL is reflection. The NASEM report talks about using "guided reflection" to help learners connect their community experience with academic goals and objectives. It also opens a dialogue for faculty and other educators to consider using reflection to self-examine their own biases as the face of learners change over time to reflect an older, more ethnically and racially diverse population. Creating a safe space for learners and educators to explore personal feelings and challenge assumptions, as described (Carter et al. 2020), can possibly be a conduit to lifelong learning. If the safe space is extended to community members, it might open opportunities to healing deep divisions between universities and communities, and to creating community-engaged pathways into the health professions.

Building a more diverse health workforce could potentially counter some of the health system weaknesses exposed during the COVID-19 pandemic that disproportionately impacted people of color and other at-risk populations. However, a more diverse health workforce is not enough. The pandemic also exposed digital inequalities that placed certain communities at greater risk of coronavirus exposure. Consideration is needed on how education can enlighten health professionals and learners on this and other newly emerging topics, such as biases contained in artificial intelligence algorithms, and how to leverage health professions education to reach underserved communities during a public health crisis.

LIFELONG LEARNING SYSTEMS ENABLE SOCIAL ACCOUNTABILITY TO ACHIEVE GREATER HEALTH EQUITY FOR THE POPULATION

Social and health disparities across the world, and the many global calls for a well-trained, skilled health workforce to close health service access gaps, particularly in rural and underserved areas, highlight the need for social accountability in education and the training of that workforce (Boelen and Woollard 2009; Larkins et al. 2018). The number and distribution of medical schools around the world are not well matched with existing physician numbers and distribution (Duvivier et al. 2014), and the same applies across other health worker groupings. The current international standard is that health workforce graduates have the capability to be appointed as interns or first-year graduates in the teaching hospitals of North America and Europe. For many low- and middle-income countries (LMICs), this means that a medical or nursing degree is a "passport out of the country." It also means that new graduates in any country often lack the experience, skills, and preparation to provide health care in rural and underserved community settings (Strasser, Kam, and Regalado 2016).

An alternative standard is needed, premised on social accountability of health workforce education, to achieve greater health equity for the population that the schools have a mandate to serve. The equitable representation of rural and underserved urban populations in the health workforce and their impact on future practice intentions cannot be overstated. Recruiting students from and training them in underserved areas fosters a desire to practice and provide long-term, sustainable services in these communities.

Accreditation as a Catalyst for Change

To promote lifelong learning, many countries have developed a national qualifications framework as an enabler of effective education, training and employment policies. Qualifications frameworks have been adopted to address various policy issues, including coordinating and improving education and training quality and assisting citizens who have been historically excluded from national education. Lifelong learning is facilitated by systems for the recognition, validation and accreditation of learning and competencies. National quality assurance and accreditation agencies, and other bodies can contribute to regulation through accreditation, licensing and registration processes. For example, the relicensing of health workers could be linked to in-service training, continuing education and professional development to ensure that competencies relevant to the evolving health needs of populations are maintained and updated (World Health Organization 2011).

Accreditation processes should thus value the relevant distribution of graduates as well as their retention in the country of origin (Academy of Science of South Africa (ASSAf) 2018). Community perspectives within and outside the student body can help health professional schools to ensure that the WHO's health care principles of quality, equity, relevance and effectiveness are met, and that health determinants are central to the strategic development of health professional schools and curricula (Boelen and Heck 1995).

The purpose of accreditation is to assure the quality and effectiveness of education and training programs. Increasingly, accreditation procedures have moved beyond quality assurance to an emphasis on quality improvement. Over the last decade, there has been growing encouragement for social accountability to be included among the accreditation standards (Boelen and Woollard 2009, 2010) and Canada implemented this in 2015 (Committee on Accreditation of Canadian Medical Schools (CACMS) 2020).

The starting point is defining standards, which can be applied both globally and locally, without becoming an end in itself (Galukande et al. 2013). WHO's global accreditation standards and standards for health workforce education (HWFE) and training provide an organizing framework for countries shifting towards Universal Health Coverage, but it is not clear to what extent these have been incorporated into accreditation systems, and there is little evidence of monitoring either their implementation or their impact. The challenge is to collect data that will demonstrate this. In South Africa, the Collaboration for Health Equity through Education and Research (CHEER) (Reid 2004) proposed that funding for medical education should, in part, be determined by the extent to which a school's graduates work at all levels of the health care system (community, primary, secondary, tertiary, quaternary), are employed in the public health service, and are serving in rural areas (Couper et al. 2013).

Accreditation has been proposed as a mechanism for achieving quality and relevance of HWFE (Ventres, Boelen, and Haq 2018). In other words, accreditation is thereby intended to drive the issues of social accountability and equity, while not ignoring the role health workforce training schools and students themselves can play in leading transformation (Murray et al. 2012). The extent to which this is incorporated in national data collection processes, by both education and health ministries, however, is not reported. In addition, it is recognized that the gap between well-informed intention and sustained commitment to change remains wide (Ventres, Boelen, and Haq 2018), but the task of evaluating and assessing the extent to which medical schools are socially accountable is recognized to be a complex one (Leinster 2011).

Over half of all countries with medical schools indicate that they have a national process for accrediting medical education programs, but the nature of the various authorities and levels of enforcement vary considerably (Van Zanten et al. 2008), and less is known about many other health professions training programmes. In general, little is known about accreditation processes and systems in Africa (Galukande, Nakasujja, and Sewankambo 2012). Training of mid-level workers in Africa, by way of example, was found to be lacking because of the absence of formal accreditation or agreed-upon standards (Couper et al. 2018), and serious challenges with nursing education in South Africa have been raised using a social accountability lens (Armstrong and Rispel 2015).

There is growing interest in social accountability and understanding how it can support integrating the social determinants into health workforce education. WHO National Health Workforce Accounts have accreditation standards for both social accountability and social determinants of health, which provides an enabling environment for coordinated data collection and analysis, which in turn can help to inform curriculum development with the active participation of local communities. Research on social accountability at the global and national level has been well documented. The Training for Health Equity network (THEnet) is an international community of practice led by health workforce education institutions with social accountability mandates to address health inequities and local health priorities. The THEnet Framework for Socially Accountable Health Professional Education (Larkins et al. 2013; Pálsdóttir et al. 2017) provides assistance with implementing socially accountable health workforce education and is based on 10 core educational and social principles. The THEnet Framework has been promoted and adapted to measure and implement socially accountable education in different countries, including Canada (Association of Faculties of Medicine of Canada (AFMC) 2010), Australia (Worley and Murray 2011), South Africa through the Collaboration for Health Equity through Education and Research (CHEER) (Michaels, Reid, and Naidu 2014) and internationally through the Association for Medical Education in Europe (AMEE) ASPIRE program (see www.aspire-to-excellence.org). In addition, the International Federation of Medical Students Associations (IFMSA) has adapted the THEnet Framework into a toolkit for students to assess the social accountability of their schools (Dijk and Glasner 2017). In Canada, two medical schools have demonstrated success in implementing socially accountable education (Rourke et al. 2018; Strasser et al. 2018).

Community Engagement

An important aspect of social accountability is the process of the democratization of knowledge, ensuring that health workers at all levels have access to the information they need. This is a central tenet of the University of New Mexico's Project Extension for Community Healthcare Outcomes, ECHO. The ECHO model aims to increase access to specialty treatment in rural and underserved areas by providing frontline clinicians with the knowledge and support they need to manage patients with complex conditions. It does this by engaging clinicians in a continuous learning system and partnering them with specialist mentors at an academic medical centre. It aims to help address inadequate access to care, systemic inefficiencies, and unequal or slow diffusion of best practices. This model has expanded its global reach, with hubs all over the world, including at the University of Cape Town and Stellenbosch University's Africa Cancer Institute in South Africa, where the presentation and management of viral hepatitis and cancer, respectively, are the focus.

Understanding how best primary care can be supported by academic health systems requires a shared perspective of the health system as an interconnected whole, based on the notion of support and partnership rather than hierarchical processes. The resources of academic health centres can be offered to assist with the analysis and interpretation of data that are collected at primary care, with joint planning, based on a just culture (no blame) approach, to design appropriate, context-based solutions, which might include developmental support and education. Increasingly, health-related digital data from electronic health records have the potential to benefit communities using informatics and big data tools to create and share digital information (Gamache, Kharrazi, and Weiner 2018).

However, some LMICs may need support from international partners, such as the World Health Organization, to help them realize the true potential of digital health (Knight et al. 2019). Ensuring that LMICs remain current with technological advances may slow down further deterioration of global health inequalities (Cory and Stevens 2020). Conversely, collaboration at international level needs to be balanced with an appreciation for the resources available at the local level. For example, the University of New Mexico Health Sciences Center developed Health Extension Rural Offices (HEROs) as a vehicle for its model of health extension. Health extension agents are in rural communities across the state and are supported by regional coordinators at the Health Sciences Center (Kaufman et al. 2010). These agents are tasked with working with different sectors of the community in identifying high-priority health needs and linking those needs with university resources in education, clinical service, and research. Developing local capacity to address local needs includes ensuring that guideline development is an inclusive process that incorporates more evidence from primary care and contextual adaptation as well as the development of practical and integrated tools (Pather and Mash 2019). Such clinical governance initiatives should be focused on the major disease burdens in the situation to address population health needs.

Active community participation or community engagement places student learning at the centre of partnerships between the academic institutions and the communities in which they learn (Strasser et al. 2015). Community engagement involves true interdependent partnerships between academic institutions and communities in the development and delivery of the education programs, helping students to appreciate the social determinants of health at the local level, and contributing to the "service learning" aspects of the program. In addition, the community plays a critical role in hosting the students.

Members of the community have the capacity to identify their own health needs. A review of strategic and tactical approaches to the empowering of citizens through social accountability showed that collective action needs to be encouraged so that the voices of communities influence the positive responses of policy makers (Fox 2015), including those who educate health professionals. Communities have the capacity to articulate the social determinants of their health, but are unable to give voice to holding doctors to account. Their construct of social accountability emerges through an expectation that good doctoring is manifest through the empowerment of communities (Green-Thompson, McInerney, and Woollard 2017). Community members in South Africa describe the need to teach the spirit of *ubuntu* (African humanism) to medical graduates in order that they understand communities when they graduate. Graduating students, on the other hand, deepen their understanding of the community through relationships only when they are immersed in such communities through their learning. This linking with the community also ensures the retention of their compassion (Green-Thompson, Mcinerney, and Woollard 2018). The extent to which communities are engaged with the education process may have significant implications for improved health outcomes. In Malawi, the *bwalo* (a traditional method of dialogue) was used to evaluate the impact of social accountability strategies. It became an important forum for inter-level engagement between the state and the citizens, enabling resolutions for maternal and perinatal health issues (Butler et al. 2020). In Alberta, a series of curricular modules across indigenous health, addiction medicine and organ donation were transformed, and by including community stakeholders in their development and regular review resulted in graduates feeling better prepared for work among diverse communities (Goez et al. 2020).

IN CONCLUSION

Lifelong learning has been a feature of health system thinking for over 50 years and is referenced in health systems literature, mostly in relation to health workforce education and training. However, conventional understanding has led lifelong learning to be compartmentalized, as the learning that takes place after graduation from pre-service health workforce education, and synonymous with CE, CPD and in-service education. Health sector policy reflects this perspective.

At an individual level, new thinking around lifelong learning can help health workers imagine new ways of working and promote understanding and commitment to address the social determinants of health as a part of everyday clinical practice. At a national level, adopting appropriate SDH-informed lifelong learning approaches could help create an enabling multisectoral policy environment to support the implementation of the UN High-level Commission five-year action plan for health employment and inclusive economic growth. Similarly, lifelong learning approaches could help improve and support governance, regulation, accreditation and quality-improvement mechanisms to ensure safe, ethical, effective and people-centred practice that protects the public's interests and rights.

A model for educating the health workforce oriented towards promoting human health and planetary health through sustainable livelihood approaches would ensure a deeper understanding of the synergies of health in all policy approaches and lifelong learning approaches, and closer working relationships between health workers and teachers in schools and communities.

REFERENCES

Academy of Science of South Africa (ASSAf). 2018. *Reconceptualising Health Professions Education in South Africa*. Pretoria, ZA: Academy of Science of South Africa (ASSAf), https://doi.org/10.17159/assaf.2018/0021.

Arcanjo, Marcus. 2019. *The Future of Water in India*. Washington, DC: Climate Institute. Available at: http://climate.org/wp-content/uploads/2019/10/The-Future-of-Water-in-India.pdf.

Armstrong, Susan J., and Laetitia C. Rispel. 2015. Social accountability and nursing education in South Africa. *Global Health Action* 8(27879): 1–9.

Association of Faculties of Medicine of Canada (AFMC). 2010. *The Future of Medical Education in Canada (FMEC): A Collective Vision for MD Education*. Ottawa, ON: Association of Faculties of Medicine of Canada. Available at: https://cou.ca/wp-content/uploads/2010/01/COU-Future-of-Medical-Education-in-Canada-A-Collective-Vision.pdf.

Bhutta, Zulfiqar A., Lincoln Chen, Jordan Cohen, Nigel Crisp, Timothy Evans, Harvey Fineberg, Julio Frenk, Patricia Garcia, Richard

Horton, Yang Ke, Patrick Kelley, Barry Kistnasamy, Afaf Meleis, David Naylor, Ariel Pablos-Mendez, Srinath Reddy, Susan Scrimshaw, Jaime Sepulveda, David Serwadda, and Huda Zurayk. 2010. Education of health professionals for the 21st century: a global independent Commission. *The Lancet* 375(9721): 1137–1138.

Boelen, Charles, and Jeffery E. Heck. 1995. *Defining and Measuring the Social Accountability of Medical Schools*. Geneva: World Health Organization.

Boelen, Charles, and Bob Woollard. 2009. Social accountability and accreditation: a new frontier for educational institutions. *Medical Education* 43(9): 887–894.

Boelen, Charles, and Bob Woollard. 2010. *Global Consensus for Social Accountability of Medical Schools*. Vancouver, BC: Global Consensus for Social Accountability of Medical Schools. Available at: http://healthsocialaccountability.sites.olt.ubc.ca/files/2011/06/11-06-07-GCSA-English-pdf-style.pdf

Butler, Nadia, Giner Johnson, Asiyati Chiweza, Kyaw Myint Aung, John Quinely, Katherine Rogers, and Jeliet Bedford. 2020. A strategic approach to social accountability: Bwalo forums within the reproductive maternal and child health accountability ecosystem in Malawi. *BMC Health Services Research* 20(568): 1–16.

Carter, Kennita R., Sandra Crewe, Mildred C. Joyner, Angelo McClain, and Carl J. Sheperis. 2020. Educating health professions educators to address the "isms". *NAM Perspectives* https://nam.edu/educating-health-professions-educators-to-address-the-isms/.

Committee on Accreditation of Canadian Medical Schools (CACMS). 2020. *Standards for Accreditation of Medical Education Programs Leading to the M.D. Degree*. Ottawa, ON: Committee on Accreditation of Canadian Medical Schools (CACMS). Available at: https://cacms-cafmc.ca/sites/default/files/documents/CACMS_Standards_and_Elements_AY_2021-2022.pdf.

Conching, Andie Kealohi Sato, and Zaneta Thayer. 2019. Biological pathways for historical trauma to affect health: a conceptual model focusing on epigenetic modifications. *Social Science and Medicine* 230: 74–82.

Cory, Nigel, and Philips Stevens. 2020. *Building a Global Framework for Digital Health Services in the Era of COVID-19*. Washington, DC: Information and Technology and Innovation Foundation. Available at: https://itif.org/publications/2020/05/26/building-global-framework-digital-health-services-era-covid-19.

Couper, Ian, Sunanda Ray, Duane Blaauw, Gideon Ng'wena, Lucy Muchiri, Eren Oyungu, Akinyinka Omigbodun, Imran Morhason-Bello, Charles Ibringira, James Tumwine, Daphney Conco, and Sharon Fonn. 2018. Curriculum and training needs of mid-level health workers in Africa: a situational review from Kenya, Nigeria, South Africa and Uganda. *BMC Health Services Research* 18(1): 553–565.

Couper, Ian, S. Reid, J. Hugo, and CHEER Collaboration. 2013. *Orientating doctors towards primary care and rural medicine: Proposals for transforming the training of medical students in South Africa*. Unpublished Report to the National Health Council.

Deslauriers, Louis, Logan S. McCarty, Kelly Miller, Kristina Callaghan, and Greg Kestin. 2019. Measuring actual learning versus feeling of learning in response to being actively engaged in the classroom. *PNAS: Proceedings of the National Academy of Sciences of the United States of America* 116(39): 19251–19257.

Dijk, Stijntje, and Jeremy Glasner (eds.). 2017. *Students' Toolkit: Social Accountability in Medical Schools*. Amsterdam, NL: International Federation of Medical Students' Associations (IFMSA).

Duvivier, Robbert J., John R. Boulet, Amy Opalek, Marta Van Zanten, and John J. Norcini. 2014. Overview of the world's medical schools: an update. *Medical Education* 48(9): 860–869.

Eckstein, David, Vera Künzel, and Laura Schäfer. 2017. *Global Climate Risk Index 2018*. Berlin: GermanWatch. Available at: https://germanwatch.org/en/node/14987.

Fisher, Julian, Keith Holmes, and Borhene Chakroun. 2017. Transforming the health workforce: unleashing the potential of technical and vocational education and training. In James Buchan, Ibadat S. Dhillon, and James Campbell (eds.), *Health Employment and Economic Growth: An Evidence Base* (pp. 281–306). Geneva: World Health Organization.

Fox, Jonathan A. 2015. Social accountability: what does the evidence really say? *World Development* 72: 346–361.

Galukande, Moses, Noeline Nakasujja, and Nelson Sewankambo. 2012. Social accountability: a survey of perceptions and evidence of its expression at a sub-Saharan African university. *BMC Medical Education* 12(96): 1–6.

Galukande, Moses, Kenneth Opio, Noeline Nakasujja, William Buwembo, Stephen C. Kijjambu, Shafik Dharamsi, Sam Luboga, Nelson K. Seswankambo, and Robert Woollard. 2013. Accreditation in a sub-Saharan medical school: a case study at Makerere University. *BMC Medical Education* 13: 73–79.

Gamache, Roland, Hadi Kharrazi, and Jonathan P. Weiner. 2018. Public and population health informatics: the bridging of big data to benefit communities. *Yearbook of Medical Informatics* 27(1): 199–206.

GIZ. 2021. Water security and climate adaptation in rural India (WASCA). *Deutsche Gesellschaft für Internationale Zusammenarbeit (GIZ) GmbH*, www.giz.de/en/worldwide/75372.html: Accessed 19 April 2021.

Goez, Helly, Hollis Lai, Joanne Rodger, Pamela Brett-MacLean, and Tracey Hillier. 2020. The DISCuSS model: creating connections between community and curriculum – a new lens for curricular development in support of social accountability. *Medical Teacher* 42(9): 1058–1064.

Green-Thompson, Lionel, Patricia McInerney, and Robert Woollard. 2017. The social accountability of doctors: a relationship-based framework for understanding emergent community concepts of caring. *BMC Health Services Research* 17(1): 269–276.

Green-Thompson, Lionel, Patricia McInerney, and Robert Woollard. 2018. Envisioning a socially accountable doctor: a three-axis curriculum emerging from final-year medical student reflections. *Scholarship of Teaching and Learning in the South* 27(1): 76–94.

Katsantoni, Kalliopi, Afroditi Zartaloudi, Dimitrios Papageorgiou, Marianna Drakopoulou, and Evdokia Misouridou. 2019. Prevalence of compassion fatigue, burn-out and compassion satisfaction among maternity and gynecology care providers in Greece. *Materia Socio Medica* 31(3): 172–176.

Kaufman, Arthur, Wayne Powel, Charles Alfero, Mario Pacheco, Helene Silverblatt, Juliana Anastasoff, Francisco Ronquillo, Ken Lucero, Erin Corriveau, Betsy Vanleit, Dale Alverson, and Amy Scott. 2010. Health extension in New Mexico: an academic health center and the social determinants of disease. *Annals of Family Medicine* 8(1): 73–81.

Knight, S.R., R. Ots, M. Maimbo, T.M. Drake, C.J. Firfield, and E.M. Harrison. 2019. Systematic review of the use of big data to improve surgery in low-and middle-income countries. *British Journal of Surgery* 106(2): e62–e72.

Lane, Sandra D., Robert H. Keefe, Robert A. Rubinstein, Meghan Hall, Kathleen A. Kelly, Lynn Beth Satterly, Andrea Shaw, and Julian Fisher. 2018. Integrating the social determinants of health into two interprofessional courses. *Journal of Interprofessional Care* 32(4): 505–508.

Lane, Sandra D., Robert A. Rubinstein, Tracey Reichert Schimpff, Robert H. Keefe, Timothy Jennings-Bey, Sydney Russell Leed, Brady Iles, Patricia A. Cuff, and Lynn Beth Satterly. 2019. Bringing in the community: a university-community endeavor to teach marital and family therapy students about community-based violence and trauma. *Contemporary Family Therapy* 41: 147–156.

Larkins, Sarah, Karen Johnston, John Hogenbirk, Sara Willems, Salwa Elsanousi, Marykutty Mammen, Kaatje Van Roy, Jehu Iputo, Fortunato Cristobal, Jennene Greenhill, Charlie Labarda, and Andre-Jaques Neusy. 2018. Practice intentions at entry to and exit from medical schools aspiring to social accountability: findings from the Training for Health Equity Network Graduate Outcome Study. *BMC Medical Education* 18(261): 1–12.

Larkins, Sarah, Robyn Preston, Marie C. Matte, Iris C. Lindemann, Rex Samson, Filedito D. Tandinco, David Buso, Simone J. Ross, Björg Pálsdóttir, Andre-Jaques Neusy, and THEnet. 2013. Measuring social accountability in health professional education: development and international pilot testing of an evaluation framework. *Medical Teacher* 35(1): 32–45.

Leicht, A., J. Heiss, and W.J. Byun (eds.). 2018. *Issues and Trends in Education for Sustainable Development*. Paris: United Nations Educational, Scientific and Cultural Organization.

Leinster, Sam. 2011. Evaluation and assessment of social accountability in medical schools. *Medical Teacher* 33(8): 673–676.

Malotky, Michele K.H., Kayla M. Mayes, Kailyn M. Price, Gustavo Smith, Sherese N. Mann, Mesha W. Guinyard, Sarina Veale, Vung Ksor, Lek Siu, H'Lois Mlo, Andrew J. Young, Maura B. Nsonwu, Sharon D. Morrison, S. Sudha, and Kelsie M. Bernot. 2020. Fostering inclusion through an interinstitutional, community-engaged, course-based undergraduate research experience. *Journal of Microbiology and Biology Education* 21(1): 1–13.

Michaels, Desireé, Stephen John Reid, and Claudia Susan Naidu. 2014. Peer review for social accountability of health sciences education: a model from South Africa. *Education for Health* 27(2): 127–131.

Murray, Richard B., Sarah Larkins, Heather Russell, Shaun Ewen, and David Prideaux. 2012. Medical schools as agents of change: socially accountable medical education. *The Medical Journal of Australia* 96(10): 653.

National Academies of Sciences, Engineering, and Medicine. 2016. *A Framework for Educating Health Professionals to Address the Social Determinants of Health*. Washington, DC: The National Academies Press.

Pálsdóttir, Björg, Nadia Cobb, Julian Fisher, John H.V. Gilbert, Lyn Middleton, Carole Reeve, Mariela Licha Salomon, and Roger Strasser. 2017. Enabling universal coverage and empowering communities through socially accountable health workforce education. In James Buchan, Ibadat S. Dhillon and James Campbell (eds.), *Health Employment and Economic Growth: An Evidence Base* (pp. 307–338). Geneva: World Health Organization.

Pather, Michael K., and Robert Mash. 2019. Family physicians' experience and understanding of evidence-based practice and guideline implementation in primary care practice, Cape Town, South Africa. *African Journal of Primary Health Care and Family Medicine* 11(1): e1–e10.

Reid, S. 2004. A cheerful group: the Collaboration for Health Equity through Education and Research. *South African Family Practice* 46: 3.

Rourke, James, Shabnam Asghari, Oliver Hurley, Mohamed Ravalia, Michael Jong, Wendy Graham, Wanda Parsons, Norah Duggan, Danielle O'Keefe, Scott Moffatt, Katherine Stringer, Carolyn Sturge Sparkes, Janelle Hippe, Kristin Harriss Walsh, Donald McKay, and Asoka Samarasena. 2018. Does rural generalist focused medical school and family medicine training make a difference? Memorial University of Newfoundland outcomes. *Rural and Remote Health* 18(1): 4426–4445.

Shim, Ruth S., and Michael T. Compton. 2018. Addressing the social determinants of mental health: if not now, when? If not us, who? *Psychiatric Services* 69(8): 844–846.

Strasser, Roger, John Hogenbirk, Kristen Jacklin, Marion Maar, Geoffrey Hudson, Wayne Warry, Hoi Cheu, Tim Dubé, and Dean Carson. 2018. Community engagement: a central feature of NOSM's socially accountable distributed medical education. *Canadian Medical Education Journal* 9(1): e33–e43.

Strasser, Roger, Sophia M. Kam, and Sophie M. Regalado. 2016. Rural health care access and policy in developing countries. *Annual Review of Public Health* 37: 395–412.

Strasser, Roger, Paul Worley, Fortunato Cristobal, David C. Marsh, Sue Berry, Sarah Strasser, and Rachel Ellaway. 2015. Putting communities in the driver's seat: the realities of community engaged medical education. *Academic Medicine* 90(11): 1466–1470.

The Lancet Public Health. 2021. Editorial: COVID-19 – breaking the cycle of inequality. *The Lancet Public Health* 6(2): e82.

UNEP (United Nations Environment Programme). 2021. *Making Peace with Nature: A Scientific Blueprint to Tackle the Climate, Biodiversity and Pollution Emergencies*. Nairobi, KE: United Nations Environment Programme. Available at: https://www.unep.org/resources/making-peace-nature.

UNESCO (United Nations Educational, Scientific and Cultural Organization). 2008. *Education for All by 2015: Will We Make it?* Paris: UNESCO. Available at: https://unesdoc.unesco.org/ark:/48223/pf0000154743.

UNESCO (United Nations Educational, Scientific and Cultural Organization). 2020. *Global Education Monitoring Report. Inclusion and Education: All Means All.* Paris: UNESCO. Available at: https://unesdoc.unesco.org/ark:/48223/pf0000373718/PDF/373718eng.pdf.multi.page=289.

Van Zanten, Marta, John J. Norcini, John R. Boulet, and Frank Simon. 2008. Overview of accreditation of undergraduate medical education programmes worldwide. *Medical Education* 42: 930–937.

Ventres, William, Charles Boelen, and Cynthia Haq. 2018. Time for action: key considerations for implementing social accountability in the education of health professionals. *Advances in Health Science Education Theory and Practice* 23(4): 853–862.

Whitmee, Sarah, Andy Haines, Chris Beyrer, Frederick Boltz, Anthony G. Capon, Braulio Ferreira de Souza Dias, Alex Ezeh, Howard Frumkin, Peng Gong, Peter Head, Richard Horton, Georgina M. Mace, Robert Marten, Samuel S. Myers, Sahia Nishtar, Steven A. Osofsky, Subhrendu K. Pattanayak, Montira J. Pongsiri, Cristina Romanelli, Agnes Soucat, Jeanette Vega, and Derek Yach. 2015. Safeguarding human health in the Anthropocene epoch: report of The Rockefeller Foundation – *Lancet* Commission on planetary health. *The Lancet* 386(10007): P1976–2028.

World Bank. 2010. *World Development Report 2010: Development and Climate Change*. Washington, DC: The International Bank for Reconstruction and Development/The World Bank. Available at: https://reliefweb.int/sites/reliefweb.int/files/resources/A6C69B344D-0E2C1D492576330019775B-WB_Sep2009.pdf.

World Health Organization. 2008. *Closing the Gap in a Generation: Health Equity through Action on the Social Determinants of Health*. Geneva: World Health Organization. Available at: https://apps.who.int/iris/bitstream/handle/10665/70573/WHO_HSS_HRH_HEP2011.01_eng.pdf?sequence=1.

World Health Organization. 2011. *Transformative Scale up of Health Professional Education and Training*. Geneva: World Health Organization. Available at: https://apps.who.int/iris/bitstream/handle/10665/70573/WHO_HSS_HRH_HEP2011.01_eng.pdf?sequence=1.

World Health Organization. 2016a. *Global Strategy on Human Resources for Health: Workforce 2030*. Geneva: World Health Organization. Available at: https://apps.who.int/iris/bitstream/handle/10665/250368/9789241511131-eng.pdf?sequence=1.

World Health Organization. 2016b. *Working for Health and Growth: Investing in the Health Workforce. Report of The High-Level Commission on Health Employment and Economic Growth. Geneva: World Health Organization.* Available at: https://apps.who.int/iris/bitstream/handle/10665/250047/9789241511308-eng.pdf;jsessionid=0FBE066AF585A10B77F7BDF7FD1C011C?sequence=1.

World Health Organization. 2018. *Five-Year Action Plan for Health Employment and Inclusive Economic Growth (2017–2021)*. Geneva: World Health Organization. Available at: https://apps.who.int/iris/bitstream/handle/10665/272941/9789241514149-eng.pdf?ua=1.

World Health Organization. n.d. *Social Determinants of Health*. Geneva: World Health Organization. Available at: www.who.int/health-topics/social-determinants-of-health#tab=tab_1 (accessed: 19 April 2021).

Worley, Paul, and Richard Murray. 2011. Social accountability in medical education – an Australian rural and remote perspective. *Medical Teacher* 33(8): 654–658.

Index

Page numbers in *italic* indicate figures and in **bold** indicate tables.

Kolibri 360 GmbH
Ferdinand-Jühlke-Straße 7
99095 Erfurt, Deutschland
produktsicherheit@kolibri360.de